Managing the Canine Cancer Patient

A Practical Guide to Compassionate Care

Veterinary Learning Systems

Managing the Canine Cancer Patient
A Practical Guide to Compassionate Care

Gregory K. Ogilvie, DVM

Diplomate ACVIM
(Internal Medicine and Oncology)

Director, Angel Care Cancer Center
California Veterinary Specialists
Carlsbad, California

President, Special Care Foundation
for Companion Animals
San Marcos, California

Antony S. Moore, BVSc, MVSc

Diplomate ACVIM (Oncology)

Co-Director, Veterinary Oncology Consultants Pty Ltd
Wauchope, New South Wales, Australia

Adjunct Professor, Faculty of Veterinary Science,
University of Sydney

Consulting Oncologist, Animal Referral Hospital
Sydney, Australia

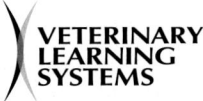

Editor: Robin A. Henry
Designer: Kimberly van Mourik
Production Artist: Stephaney Weber
Bioillustrators: Felecia Paras and Tom Vojt, Biomedical Visuals, Columbus, Ohio

All rights reserved. No part of this publication may be reproduced, stored in a retrieval system, or transmitted, in any form or by any means, electronic, mechanical, photocopying, recording, or otherwise, without prior written permission from Veterinary Learning Systems.

The authors would like to thank the following individuals for sharing their photographs, slides, illustrations, or personal experience:

John Berg, Tufts University; Philip J. Bergman, Donaldson-Atwood Cancer Clinic, New York, NY; Randy Boudrieau, Tufts University; Kimberly J. Caruso, California Veterinary Specialists, Carlsbad, CA; John Chretin, VCA West Los Angeles Animal Hospital; Susan M. Cotter, Tufts University; Gregory B. Daniel, University of Tennessee; Anne G. Evans, Veterinary Information Network; Angela E. Frimberger, Veterinary Oncology Consultants, Wauchope, New South Wales, Australia; Sarah Goldsmid, Animal Referral Hospital, South Strathfield, New South Wales, Australia; Mark Hitt, Atlantic Veterinary Internal Medicine, Annapolis, MD; Marc Kent, University of Georgia; Kim E. Knowles, Veterinary Neurological Center, Phoenix, AZ; Susan L. Kraft, Colorado State University; Karl Kraus, Tufts University; Christopher R. Lamb, Royal Veterinary College, London, England; Julius M. Liptak, Ontario Veterinary College; Bruce R. Madewell, University of California, Davis; Lenore Anderson Mohammadian, California Veterinary Specialists; Nicole Northrup, University of Georgia; Dominique G. Penninck, Tufts University; Kenneth M. Rassnick, Cornell University; Scott H. Schelling, Wyeth Research, Andover, MA; Gordon H. Theilen, University of California, Davis; Donald E. Thrall, North Carolina State University; Amy S. Tidwell, Tufts University; David C. Twedt, Colorado State University

NOTICE: Every effort has been made to ensure that the drug dosage schedules and current therapy contained herein are accurate and in accord with the standards accepted at the time of publication. However, as new research and experience broaden our knowledge, changes in treatment and drug therapy occur. Therefore, the reader is advised to check the product information sheet included in the package of each drug he/she plans to administer to be certain that changes have not been made in the recommended dose or in the contraindications. This is of particular importance in regard to new or infrequently used drugs.

Veterinary Learning Systems
A Division of MediMedia USA
780 Township Line Road
Yardley, PA 19067

Copyright © 2006 Veterinary Learning Systems, a division of MediMedia USA

Library of Congress Control Number: 2005938962

ISBN 1-884254-56-X

Dedication

To my precious Karla—
Love of my life, mother of our Torrie:
Our adventures have just begun!

Gregory K. Ogilvie

To Dodger, the most patient of dogs,
and to Arthur and Harvey,
the gentlest of souls.

Antony S. Moore

Acknowledgments

This book reflects the direct and indirect input of a number of researchers, educators, veterinary students, graduate students, colleagues, and, of course, the remarkable people at Veterinary Learning Systems. In short, this is an acknowledgment of friends who helped directly and indirectly in the creation of a truly unique book that was designed to be an easy-to-read, practical, up-to-date resource for compassionate, progressive veterinarians.

The first friend is coauthor Antony S. Moore, who cannot be thanked adequately in words. Dr. Moore has profoundly influenced the current state of global, modern veterinary oncology with his vision, humor, research, clinical acumen, and skill as an educator. His authority and knowledge have shaped this book and a generation of students, interns, residents, and advanced caregivers who owe all they are to Tony. I am grateful for our friendship over the past 18 years and for his contribution to our profession and to the heart of this book. Tony is not only a superb clinician scientist, he is also an accomplished hunter of exotic butterflies, gardener, apiarist, connoisseur of fine foods and wine, lover and collector of old books, and a kind and sensitive human being. Above all, Tony is a special friend to many, including his wife Angela, son Alexander, and daughter Ivy. This book has also been profoundly influenced by Angela Frimberger, who selflessly gave of her time, wisdom, intelligence, and skill as a veterinary oncologist and scientist to contribute to many aspects of this text.

Associate dean, clinical pathologist, first veterinarian in space, and friend Dr. Martin J. Fettman has contributed indirectly to many aspects of this book through his insightful understanding of nutrition, cancer, and metabolism. Marty's collaborative efforts fused with his undying friendship yielded many discoveries on how cancer impacts animals and how nutrients can enhance quality of life and response to therapy. Marty's work and that of special friends and research colleagues Dr. Rod Hansen and Kristi Richardson spanned almost 15 years, changed my life, and is outlined in many pages of this book. A note of appreciation and acknowledgment also goes to special friends, colleagues, and coinvestigators Drs. Philippe Bougnoux, Jean Yves Le Guennec, and the rest of the INSERM team at the Laboratoire Nutrition, Croisance et Cancer at the Université François Rabelais in Tours, France. The important work done by this team to explore the benefits of fatty acids such as docosahexaenoic acid is outlined in many chapters of this book.

The first half of this book would not have been possible without the impact of many people who define compassionate care on a daily basis via their work. First: Ken Crump, an extraordinary individual who is not only my friend but also a gifted veterinary caregiver, teacher, leader, artist, fisherman, and sensitive human being. Ken has profoundly touched my life and thousands of others' lives as he defines compassionate care through meeting the medical needs of his patients and the nonmedical needs of the families that bring their pets to Colorado State University. Second: The foundation of the cancer care team at CVS Angel Care Cancer Center—friends and team leaders Wendy Minor, Jen Mosca, and Tammy Herald. They and the rest of the veterinary health care team at Angel Care define excellence in compassionate care. Third: The nucleus of California Veterinary Specialists, Drs. Don Krawiec, Amy Carr, and Tim Concannon, and finally, the gentle being Sarit Dhupa. These leaders, along with Drs. Proulx, Mohammadian, Pollard, Mallery, Maher, Herndon, Jaeger, and our own James Herriot Glen Grady, define "Special Care from the Heart."

The pages of this book directly or indirectly reflect the knowledge, experience, and wisdom of a number of people who have impacted my life tremendously. Dr. Susan Cotter, my residency mentor and heroine, gently guided me to understand the magic and mysteries of medicine and oncology. Drs. S.J. Withrow, Edward L. Gillette, Rod Straw, Dennis Macy, Sue LaRue, Barbara Powers, and Sue Lana all have contributed significantly to this book during my 15 years at the Animal Cancer Center at Colorado State University. The pages of this book also reflect the input, enthusiasm, and knowledge of the medical residents, graduate students, thousands of veterinary students, and tens of thousands of veterinarians I have met worldwide during my lectures. Each of these veterinarians kept me running to keep up while I attempted to provide them with some mentorship and knowledge. Special recognition goes to former medical oncology residents and friends Drs. Donna Vicini, M.K. Klein, David Vail, Robyn Elmslie, Steve Atwater, Joyce Obradovich, Phyllis Ciekot, Philip Bergman, Elizabeth McNiel, Karina Valerius, Christine Anderson, Victoria Bregazzi, Nicole Liebman, Mary Kay Blake, Kim Selting, Kathy Kazmerski, and Monika Jankowski. Finally, thank you to the greatest professors I have ever had: four-legged Terry, Amber, and Cocoa.

Last, but not least, a special acknowledgment must go to my parents, Bev and Stan, who gave me the gift of independence to achieve my heart's desires, and to my wife Karla and daughter Torrie, who have graced my life and granted me the time and opportunity to complete this book.

Gregory K. Ogilvie

Over the 10 years since Greg and I wrote our first book, there has been a huge increase in the amount of available information about veterinary oncology. As the veterinary profession has embraced the concept of evidence-based medicine, I believe that oncology has led the way in providing a reevaluation of previously accepted dogma and executing prospective studies of exceptional worth. That information is summarized in this book, but as the explosion of new knowledge continues, interested veterinarians will find that they need to rely on the support of specialists to keep themselves updated. In my experience both speaking at scientific meetings and through our consultation service, I am thrilled to find veterinarians embracing new knowledge.

In 2003, I left academia to return to a gentler life in Australia. With my wife and colleague, Angela Frimberger, and our spectacular children, Alexander and Ivy, we have made the "sea change." A consequence of living far from an urban area is that we needed to find a way to use our knowledge that did not rely on patients walking into our office. One of the problems we had found with academic and private clinical oncology practice is that there is little time to answer the questions posed by other veterinarians about what to tell a client or how best to stage or treat a patient. By setting up a service that is primarily consultation based (rather than clinic based), we hope to fill that gap. Nothing can replace referral to a veterinary oncologist, but so much can be done by talented and interested practitioners, often far from such a specialist, and with a dedicated owner who will not accept palliative treatment. With that in mind, Veterinary Oncology Consultants' mission is to assist other veterinarians in providing the highest possible quality of life for pets with cancer and their human families by making evidence- and compassion-based recommendations for their care and by providing educational materials.

It is without a doubt one of the most rewarding experiences to treat an animal with cancer. I have always enjoyed the practice of oncology, and since moving from academia, I have also returned to private clinical practice and have rediscovered the simple joy of sitting on the ground with a patient, giving chemotherapy, and chatting with caring pet owners. The cures are still few, but we are getting better and better at preserving and extending quality of life for our patients. Attention to the needs of the patient and caregiver is paramount to a successful oncology practice. Forming bonds with the patient and caregiver means gaining the trust of both parties; it takes dedication and compassionate listening. However, without up-to-date knowledge about the way a cancer behaves, the prognostic factors for the individual patient, and the backing of experienced specialists, it is difficult to provide the very best in care. As a companion volume to *Feline Oncology*, this book aims to provide that necessary and practical information in a readable, easy-to-understand format.

As always, this book would not have been possible without the support of many people, not just recently, but throughout my career to date. As with the previous books, Trena Haroutunian was an enthusiastic supporter in the initial stages of manuscript preparation and in teaching me to use a reference managing program. Suzanne Duncan gave me support and access to the resources of the library at Tufts University and made finding the literature painless. Of particular note, I would like to thank the residents I worked with at Tufts over the past years for their enthusiasm, hard work, and critical minds that have made them all into oncologists that make me proud to have been part of their careers. Dave Ruslander, Carrie Wood, Laurel Williams, Orna Kristal, Nicole Northrup, Johnny Chretin, Sarah Payne, and Tony Calo have all had a part in this book. Their own careers speak to the quality of these individuals and their talents. Angela Frimberger deserves special mention as my partner both in our oncology consulting business and in the joy of raising our children.

I wish to specially thank Sue Cotter, whose enthusiasm and knowledge are unrivalled, and Ken Rassnick, an extremely talented oncologist who taught me the meaning of organization. Both have shaped the way I think and the way I practice oncology. As always, I am indebted to Bruce Madewell and Gordon Theilen for taking a chance on me and offering me a residency when I still couldn't even spell "onclogoist."

Finally, I thank Greg Ogilvie, who understands not only veterinary oncology but also people, and who is a leader in all aspects of patient care and meeting the needs of clients. As someone who sometimes found Greg's ideas challenging, I admit that I now embrace many of them as self-evident truths. I have been proud to call Greg a friend for the past 18 years and hope to do so for many more years to come.

Antony S. Moore

About the Authors

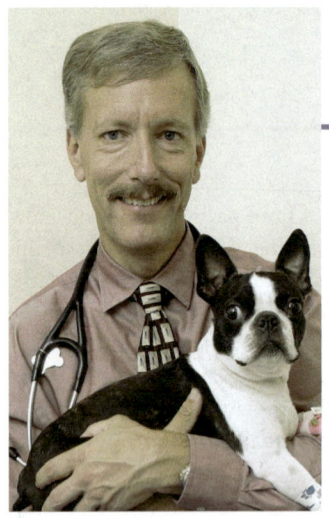

Gregory K. Ogilvie, DVM, Diplomate ACVIM (Internal Medicine, Oncology)

Dr. Ogilvie was a full tenured professor, internist, head of medical oncology, and director of the medical oncology research laboratory Animal Cancer Center at Colorado State University (CSU) from 1987 until he followed his dream to join the team at California Veterinary Specialists (CVS) in 2003 as director of the CVS Angel Care Cancer Center and president of the Special Care Foundation for Companion Animals. Dr. Ogilvie continues to teach interns, residents, and veterinary students and has an active cancer research program. Dr. Ogilvie is also on the advisory board of the College of Veterinary Medicine at Western University in California and has been a full member of the University of Colorado Cancer Center under the directorship of Dr. Paul Bunn. During this 16-year period at CSU, Dr. Ogilvie spent 1 year on sabbatical teaching and developing new, innovative cancer therapies at the medical school and the Laboratoire Nutrition, Croisance et Cancer at the Université François Rabelais in Tours, France.

Dr. Ogilvie received his DVM from CSU and was in private practice in Connecticut before completing a residency at Tufts University/Angell Memorial Animal Hospital. From there, he joined the faculty as a professor at the University of Illinois before moving back to Colorado. Dr. Ogilvie is board certified in the specialties of internal medicine and oncology by the American College of Veterinary Internal Medicine.

He is coauthor with his friend, Dr. Antony Moore, of two other books, *Managing the Veterinary Cancer Patient: A Practice Manual* (Veterinary Learning Systems, 1995, in English, French, and Japanese) and *Feline Oncology: A Comprehensive Guide to Compassionate Care* (Veterinary Learning Systems, 2001); more than 200 scientific articles and chapters; and more than 120 scientific abstracts and posters. He has been awarded two international patents and $9.5 million in research as a principal investigator or coinvestigator. Dr. Ogilvie is the recipient of many awards, including the Arnold O. Beckman Research Award, the Beecham Research Award, the Purina Small Animal Research Award, the Samuel F. Scheidy Memorial Research Award, and the American Veterinary Medical Association/American Kennel Club Award.

Dr. Ogilvie has lectured to many thousands of students, veterinarians, physicians, and scientists in Africa, Australia, Asia, Europe, the Middle East, South America, and North America, where he shares his love for the practice of veterinary medicine and oncology. Dr. Ogilvie's teaching skills have also been frequently recognized. He is the recipient of the Outstanding Teachers Award, two Norden Distinguished Teacher Awards, the MSD Agvet Award for Creativity in Teaching, and the SCAVMA Award for "Dedication to Students and the Profession," and he was named Outstanding Companion Animal Speaker for 1999 at the North American Veterinary Conference.

Dr. Ogilvie has also been recognized with the AVMA Veterinarian of the Year (1995), the American Animal Hospital Association's Veterinarian of the Year (1996), the Colorado Veterinary Medical Association Outstanding Faculty Award (1996), and the 1999 SHARE Human Animal Bond Companion Animal Award. Dr. Ogilvie was also awarded the World Small Animal Veterinary Association Hills Award for Excellence in Veterinary Healthcare for 2001.

When not caring for pets and their people, Dr. Ogilvie is a certified ski instructor and enjoys camping, scuba diving, and long-distance cycling. He has volunteered for 15 years as a counselor at the Sky High Hope Camp for children who have cancer. His greatest joys are his daughter, Torrie; his wife, Karla; and, of course, Cocoa the wonderdog.

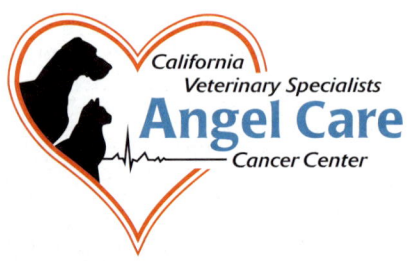

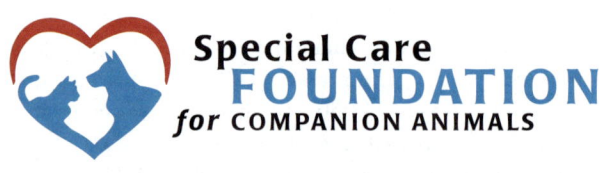

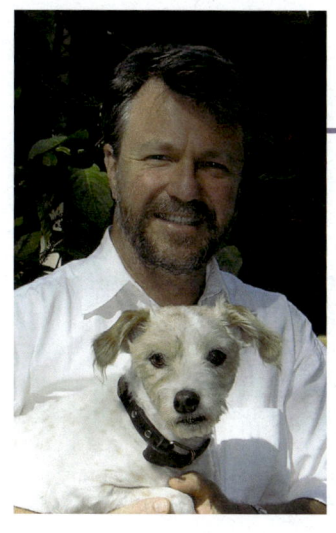

Antony S. Moore, BVSc, MVSC, Diplomate ACVIM (Oncology)

Dr. Moore received his veterinary degree in 1981 and his master's degree in feline hematology in 1986, both from the University of Sydney. After completing a residency in veterinary oncology at the University of California, Davis, in 1988, he joined the faculty at Tufts University. During his 15 years at Tufts, he achieved the rank of full professor and trained seven residents to careers in veterinary oncology. After leaving Tufts in 2003, he partnered with Angela Frimberger in establishing Veterinary Oncology Consultants (www.vetoncologyconsults.com), a Web-based consulting company that assists other veterinarians in providing the highest possible quality of life for pets with cancer and their human families by making evidence- and compassion-based recommendations for their care and providing educational materials.

Dr. Moore has spoken at meetings in the United States, Australia, Japan, Europe, and South and Central America. He is the author of more than 75 articles in the veterinary literature and has coauthored two other books with Dr. Gregory Ogilvie, *Managing the Veterinary Cancer Patient: A Practice Manual* (in English, Japanese, and French) and *Feline Oncology: A Comprehensive Guide to Compassionate Care* (in English and Japanese). Dr. Moore has received awards for creativity in teaching and clinical research and is particularly interested in the epidemiology of cancer in companion animals. His other interests include entomology and collecting antiquarian veterinary and butterfly books; he still likes the *idea* of running.

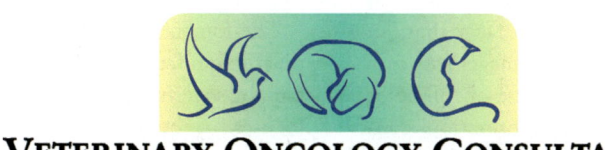

Foreword

Managing the Canine Cancer Patient: A Practical Guide to Compassionate Care is designed to provide veterinary practitioners with clinically relevant details about the diagnosis and management of the canine cancer patient in an easy-to-read format. While this book unlocks the secrets to meet the needs of the cancer patient, it also explores ways to support the client through the emotionally challenging process of dealing with cancer. The book is a companion to *Feline Oncology: A Comprehensive Guide to Compassionate Care*. While that book amassed a huge amount of data regarding cats with cancer, it was often hard to provide a "bottom line," purely due to the paucity of information. In contrast, the available literature regarding canine cancer is impressive in its detail. We have endeavored to summarize up-to-date information about canine oncology by organizing each chapter into major subdivisions, which facilitates easy access to practical information and the most common problems encountered in clinical canine oncology. As with *Feline Oncology,* clinical briefings are used throughout the sections to give the reader information about the most commonly asked clinical questions. Key points are also included throughout the text to reinforce facts that, in many cases, are critical to the successful management of a dog with cancer. New to this book is the use of full-color illustrations that enhance the critical information contained in the text; additionally, color tabs on the side of the pages speed access to needed information.

The first section, **Fundamentals of Cancer Care: Cancer Prevention, Philosophy, Staging, and Compassionate Care**, reviews current information regarding the epidemiology of canine cancer and sets out our philosophy of the approach to caring for both the patient and the client. The goal is to direct the reader to meet the medical needs of patients while meeting the nonmedical needs of caregivers and the cancer treatment team.

The second section, **Cancer Diagnostics**, is highly illustrated and provides the busy practitioner with an easy reference guide for executing diagnostic methods essential for the management of the canine cancer patient. The updated chapter on clinical cytology contains a series of color plates and accompanying keys that will assist the practitioner in general cytologic interpretation. In addition to the practical techniques, this chapter also discusses how best to build a partnership with the surgical pathologist and how to get the most out of advanced imaging and blood work to completely evaluate the canine patient. The reader will also find guidance about newer pathology testing, such as immunohistochemistry, flow cytometry, and molecular medicine.

The third section, **Common Therapeutic and Supportive Procedures**, details practical and important information needed to treat and support dogs with cancer. Topics include newer methods of safe handling and administration of chemotherapeutic agents as well as the use of biologic response modifiers, radiation therapy, and hyperthermia. With most clients opting for complementary and alternative medicine in addition to more traditional medicine, the chapter on such treatments will assist practitioners in understanding the basis for many of these treatment strategies. Sections on bone marrow transplantation and emerging new therapies will keep the reader up-to-date in these fast-growing areas of cancer treatment. Management of complications of cancer in dogs, such as pain, vomiting, and side effects of treatment, is key to providing compassionate care. Information about the nutritional needs of dogs with cancer is provided. Also helpful is a list of toxicities associated with anticancer drugs and hormones used to treat dogs with cancer.

The fourth section, **Diagnosis and Therapy: Paraneoplastic Syndromes and Oncologic Emergencies**, is essential for veterinarians who deal with cancer. This section focuses on the diagnosis and treatment of life-threatening problems that can arise during the course of cancer and its treatment. Tables provide easy access to information on drugs and dosages that may be needed in an emergency situation. The successful diagnosis and management of these conditions affect the patient's quality of life and survival as much as the management of the malignant condition itself.

The fifth section is **Management of Specific Diseases**. In the past 10 years, there has been an exponential increase in clients' use of the Internet to obtain information about their pet's condition, often before they consult a veterinarian. Being able to find summarized information about different cancer types and the best treatments is invaluable to the busy practitioner in helping clients sort through the often conflicting information they have available. Extraordinary efforts have been made to provide only the most important, up-to-date, and clinically relevant data to assist the practitioner in understanding how to determine the extent of cancer and how best to treat affected dogs.

The sixth section contains an updated and complete **formulary** to assist busy practitioners in meeting the needs of the canine cancer patient and a guide to the **abbreviations** used in this book.

Finally, the seventh section, **Client Information Series**, provides material that can be photocopied and distributed to clients and caregivers to empower them with information and knowledge about cancer.

This manual is an up-to-date, comprehensive reference guide to the management of the most common natural cause of death in dogs: cancer. We have also worked to include information on how to support the client through the difficult, often emotional process of dealing with a dog with cancer. Our belief is that it will prove to be an easy-to-use, practical resource for the progressive practitioner who seeks the very best for his or her patients. We are confident that this book has captured the torrent of new information about dogs and their cancers and will provide a basis for general practitioners in understanding these perplexing conditions, guiding their clients, and helping their patients maintain an excellent quality of life.

The authors, editors, and publisher of this manual have made every effort to ensure that all therapeutic modalities are recommended in accordance with accepted standards at the time of publication and that all drug dosages and regimens are correct. Nevertheless, anyone not familiar with cancer treatment should consult a veterinary oncologist before administering or prescribing any form of cancer treatment.

G. K. Ogilvie
A. S. Moore

Quick Reference: Hematology

General Rule: Amount of Blood to Transfuse

Note: 2.2 ml of whole blood/kg or 1 ml/kg of packed red blood cells raises the packed cell volume (PCV) 1% (transfused whole blood has a PCV of 40%).

$$\text{ml donor} = [(2.2 \times \text{wt}_{kg}) \times (40)] \times \frac{PCV_{desired} - PCV_{recipient}}{PCV_{donor}}$$

General Rule: Rate of Blood Transfusion

0.5 ml/kg/h or faster (22 ml/kg/day) with close patient monitoring.

Blood Products for Red Cell Replacement

Product	Storage Conditions	Shelf Life	Dosage Guidelines
Fresh whole blood	Room temperature	<8 hr	12–20 ml/kg
Whole blood	Refrigeration	20–35 days	12–20 ml/kg
Packed RBCs	Refrigeration	20–35 days	5–10 ml/kg

IV Potassium Supplementation to Correct Hypokalemia

Serum Potassium (mEq/L)	KCl Added to Each Liter of Fluid (mEq)	Maximum Rate of Infusion (ml/kg/hr)[a]
<2	80	6
2.1–2.5	60	8
2.6–3.0	40	12
3.1–3.5	28	16

[a]Above this rate, the risk of life-threatening complications increases.

Treatment of Hypercalcemia[a-d]

Treatment	Dosage	Suggested Use
Volume expander IV saline (0.9%)	>66 ml/kg/day to achieve urinary output of 2 ml/kg/hr	Moderate to severe hypercalcemia Monitor serum potassium
Diuretic Furosemide	2–4 mg/kg PO, SC, IV bid to tid	Moderate to severe hypercalcemia
Bone resorption inhibitor Calcitonin	4–6 IU/kg SC bid to tid	Hypervitaminosis D toxicity
Glucocorticoids Prednisone Dexamethasone	1–2 mg/kg PO, SC, IV bid 0.1–0.22 mg/kg IV, SC bid	Moderate to severe hypercalcemia Moderate to severe hypercalcemia
Bisphosphonate Pamidronate	1–2 mg/kg in 150 ml 0.9% NaCl as a 2-hr IV infusion; can repeat in 1–3 wk. Package insert suggests giving during diuresis to reduce nephrotoxicity.	Moderate to severe hypercalcemia
Mithramycin	25 μg/kg IV in 5% glucose in water over 2–4 hr q2–4wk	Severe hypercalcemia

[a]Ogilvie GK: Metabolic emergencies and the cancer patient, in Wingfield WE (ed): *Veterinary Emergency Medicine Secrets*. Philadelphia, Hanley and Belfus, 2001, pp 247–251.
[b]Hostutler RA, Chew DJ, Jaeger JQ, et al: Uses and effectiveness of pamidronate disodium for treatment of dogs and cats with hypercalcemia. *J Vet Intern Med* 19(1):29–33, 2005.
[c]Milner RJ, Farese J, Henry CJ, et al: Bisphosphonates and cancer. *J Vet Intern Med* 18(5):597–604, 2004.
[d]Feldman EC, Nelson RW: Hypercalcemia and primary hyperparathyroidism in dogs, in Bonagura JD (ed): *Kirk's Current Veterinary Therapy XIII*. Philadelphia, WB Saunders, 2000, pp 345–348.

Quick Reference: Chemotherapy

General Concepts in Calculating and Administering Chemotherapy Doses

1. Convert weight in pounds to weight in kilograms by dividing by 2.2. A 22-lb dog weighs 10 kg (22 ÷ 2.2 = 10).
2. Look up weight in kilograms on the weight–to–body surface area (BSA) table at right.
3. Determine the dose of the drug by multiplying the dosage (e.g., 0.5–0.7 mg/m^2) by the patient's body surface area (m^2).
4. Before drawing up or obtaining the quantity of chemotherapeutic drug, check the concentration (mg/ml, mg/pill, or mg/capsule).
5. Before administering the drug, double-check the dose and results of the complete blood count.

For more details, see Chapter 20.

General Treatment Guidelines for Extravasated Chemotherapeutic Drugs

Minimize amount of drug at site:

- Do not remove the catheter or needle.
- With a syringe, immediately withdraw as much drug as possible from the tissue, tubing, and catheter.
- Administer antidote or sterile saline to neutralize or dilute the drug.

For treatment of extravasation of specific drugs, see page 296.

Level of Myelosuppression of Chemotherapeutic Drugs

High	Moderate	Mild
Doxorubicin	Melphalan	L-Asparaginase
Vinblastine	Chlorambucil	Vincristine
Cyclophosphamide	5-Fluorouracil	Bleomycin
Lomustine	Methotrexate	Corticosteroids

Conversion of Body Weight to BSA for Dogs[a]

Weight (kg)	BSA (m^2)	Weight (kg)	BSA (m^2)
0.5	0.06	26	0.88
1	0.10	27	0.90
2	0.15	28	0.92
3	0.20	29	0.94
4	0.25	30	0.96
5	0.29	31	0.99
6	0.33	32	1.01
7	0.36	33	1.03
8	0.40	34	1.05
9	0.43	35	1.07
10	0.46	36	1.09
11	0.49	37	1.11
12	0.52	38	1.13
13	0.55	39	1.15
14	0.58	40	1.17
15	0.60	41	1.19
16	0.63	42	1.21
17	0.66	43	1.23
18	0.69	44	1.25
19	0.71	45	1.26
20	0.74	46	1.28
21	0.76	47	1.30
22	0.78	48	1.32
23	0.81	49	1.34
24	0.83	50	1.36
25	0.85	51	1.38

[a]Most chemotherapeutic agents are dosed on a BSA basis.

Quick Reference: Drugs

Selected Analgesics

Drug	Dosing Regimen
Opioid Agonists	
Fentanyl	2–5 µg/kg IV bolus before CRI
Postoperative	2–5 µg/kg/hr CRI for the duration of infusion
Operative	10–45 µg/kg/hr CRI for the duration of infusion
Patch	2–3 mg/kg/hr topical application; replace q3–5d
Hydromorphone	0.05–0.2 mg/kg IV, SC, or IM q2–6h
Meperidine	3–5 mg/kg SC or IM q1–2h
Methadone	1–1.5 mg/kg IV, SC, or IM once
Morphine	0.5–2 mg/kg PO, IM, or SC q2–4h
Morphine, sustained-release	2–5 mg/kg PO q1–4h
Oxymorphone	0.05–0.4 mg/kg IV, SC, or IM q2–4h
Remifentanil	4–10 µg/kg IV bolus before CRI q2–6h
Postoperative	4–10 µg/kg/hr CRI for the duration of infusion
Operative	20–60 µg/kg/hr CRI for the duration of infusion
Sufentanyl	5 µg/kg IV bolus before CRI q2–6h
Postoperative	0.1 µg/kg/hr CRI for the duration of infusion
Opioid Agonist–Antagonists	
Buprenorphine	0.005–0.02 mg/kg IV, IM, or SC q8–12h
Butorphanol	0.1–0.4 mg/kg IV, IM, or SC q1–4h or 0.5–2 mg/kg PO q6–8h
Nalbuphine	0.5–1 mg/kg IV, IM, or SC q4h
Pentazocine	1–3 mg/kg IV, IM, or SC q2–4h
NSAIDs	
Carprofen	2.2 mg/kg PO q12h
Deracoxib	1–2 mg/kg PO q24h
Etodolac	10–15 mg/kg PO q12h
Ketoprofen	1–2 mg/kg IV, IM, or SC q24h or 1 mg/kg PO q24h
Meloxicam	0.1–0.2 mg/kg IV, IM, or SC q24h; 0.1 mg/kg PO q24h
Piroxicam	0.3 mg/kg PO q24–48h
Tolfenamic acid	4 mg/kg PO or SC q24h for 3 days on, 4 days off

Drug	Dosing Regimen
α_2-Agonists	
Medetomidine	5–10 µg/kg IM or SC once or 1–4 µg/kg IV once
Romifidine	10–20 µg/kg IM or SC once
Xylazine	0.2–0.5 mg/kg PO q12h
Other Drugs	
Acetaminophen (paracetamol)	5–10 mg/kg PO q12h
Amantidine	3–5 mg/kg PO q24h
Amitriptyline	1–4 mg/kg PO q24h
Glucosamine, chondroitin	13–15 mg/kg PO q24h
Ketamine	0.5–1 µg/kg IM q30min or 1 µg/kg/min CRI for the duration of infusion and postinfusion
Pamidronate	1 mg/kg slow IV as needed q3–6wk with diuresis
Tramadol	2–4 mg/kg PO q6–8h

Selected Antiemetics

Recommended
- Butorphanol: 0.4 mg/kg IM q8h
- Dolasetron: 0.1–0.3 mg/kg IV, PO 15 min before chemotherapy then daily to bid
- Metoclopramide: 1–2 mg/kg CRI IV over 24 hr
- Ondansetron: 0.1–0.5 mg/kg IV, PO 15 min before chemotherapy then daily to bid

Less Effective
- Chlorpromazine: 0.5 mg/kg IM, SC, rectal suppository q6–8h
- Dimenhydrinate: 8 mg/kg PO q8h
- Diphenhydramine: 2.0–4.0 mg/kg PO q8h
- Domperidone: 0.1–0.3 mg/kg IM, IV bid
- Prochlorperazine: 0.1–0.5 mg/kg IM, SC q6–8h or 1.0 mg/kg rectally q8h
- Prochlorperazine–isopropamide: 0.5–0.8 mg/kg IM, SC q12h
- Trimethobenzamide: 3 mg/kg IM q8h
- Yohimbine: 0.25–0.5 mg/kg SC, IM bid

Antibiotics Used to Treat Sepsis[a-d]

Antibiotic	Potential Toxicoses
Gram-negative bacteria	
Gentamicin (2.2–4.4 mg/kg IV tid)	• Nephrotoxicity, especially when renal damage is present; ototoxicity; ensure adequate hydration and check frequently for renal damage during use
Cefazolin (22 mg/kg [10 mg/lb] IV q8h)	• Phlebitis, muscle pain after IV or IM administration; rare prevalence of nephrotoxicity
Cefoxitin (22 mg/kg IV tid)	• Phlebitis; discomfort with rapid IV injection; rare prevalence of nephrotoxicity
Gram-positive bacteria	
Sodium or potassium penicillin (22,000 U/kg IV qid)	• Allergy to penicillin can cause anaphylaxis, hives, fever, and pain; neurologic signs may occur with rapid infusion
Cefoxitin (22 mg/kg IV tid)	• Same as above
Enrofloxacin (10 mg/kg IV bid)	• Hives, fever, and pain
Anaerobic bacteria	
Metronidazole (15 mg/kg IV or IM tid)	• Anorexia, vomiting, and neurologic signs
Cefoxitin (22 mg/kg IV tid)	• Same as above

[a]Couto CG: Management of complications of cancer chemotherapy. *Vet Clin North Am Small Anim Pract* 4:1037–1053, 1990.
[b]Woodlock TJ: Oncologic emergencies, in Rosenthal S, Carignan JR, Smith BD (eds): *Medical Care of the Cancer Patient,* ed 2. Philadelphia, WB Saunders, 1993, pp 236–246.
[c]Hughes WT, Armstrong D, Bodey GP: Infectious Diseases Society of America: Guidelines for the use of antimicrobial agents in neutropenic patients with unexplained fever. *J Infect Dis* 161(3):381–390, 1990.
[d]Quadri TL, Brown AE: Infectious complications in the critically ill patient with cancer. *Semin Oncology* 27(3):335–346, 2000.

Anticonvulsants Used in an Acute Situation to Treat Seizures[a-c]

Anticonvulsant	Recommended Dosage	Half-Life	General Indications	Precautions
Phenobarbital	5–16 mg/kg/day, divided bid or tid	40 hr	Long-term seizure control; grand mal and partial seizures; effective in delaying progressive activity (kindling)	Monitor for sedation, ataxia, polydipsia, and polyuria (usually abate over time)
Primidone	15–80 mg/kg/day, divided bid	Metabolized to phenobarbital, then 40 hr	Not as effective as phenobarbital for emergency therapy Grand mal and partial seizures, status epilepticus; effective in delaying progressive activity (kindling)	Expensive Monitor for sedation, ataxia, polydipsia, polyuria, and personality trait changes (usually abate over time); hepatotoxicity
Diazepam	5–15 mg tid	2–4 hr	Grand mal seizures and status epilepticus	Monitor for sedation

[a]Fenner WR: Diseases of the brain, in Birchard SJ, Sherding RG (eds): *Saunders Manual of Small Animal Practice.* Philadelphia, WB Saunders, 1993, pp 1126–1146.
[b]Woodlock TJ: Oncologic emergencies, in Rosenthal S, Carignan JR, Smith BD (eds): *Medical Care of the Cancer Patient,* ed 2. Philadelphia, WB Saunders, 1993, pp 236–246.
[c]Bunch SE: Anticonvulsant drug therapy in companion animals, in Kirk RW (ed): *Current Veterinary Therapy IX, Small Animal Practice.* Philadelphia, WB Saunders, 1986, pp 836–844.

Contents

Acknowledgments vi
About the Authors viii
Foreword x
Quick Reference Sheets xii

SECTION 1 FUNDAMENTALS OF CANCER CARE: CANCER PREVENTION, PHILOSOPHY, STAGING, AND COMPASSIONATE CARE

1. Introduction to Managing the Canine Cancer Patient: A Practical Guide to Compassionate Care 3
2. The Role of Cancer Prevention in Health and Wellness Programs 6
3. Philosophy of Cancer Care 11
4. Approach to the Cancer Patient: Staging 15
5. Commandments of Cancer Care to Improve Quality of Life 18
6. Setting Goals for Compassionate Care 23
7. Pet Loss and Bereavement 25
8. Compassion Fatigue 29

SECTION 2 CANCER DIAGNOSTICS

9. The Veterinary Oncologic Pathologist 35
10. Clinical Chemistries and Tumor Markers 40
11. Veterinary Cancer Imaging 44
12. Biopsy, Biopsy, Biopsy! Theory and Practice ... 56
13. Skin Biopsy 61
14. Lymph Node Biopsy 66
15. Respiratory Tract Biopsy 70
16. Bone Marrow Aspiration and Biopsy 78
17. Lower Urogenital Tract Biopsy 82
18. Digestive System Biopsy 87
19. Clinical Cytology and Neoplasia 96

SECTION 3 COMMON THERAPEUTIC AND SUPPORTIVE PROCEDURES

20. Drug Handling and Administration 111
21. Chemotherapy: Properties, Uses, and Patient Management 126
22. Radiation Therapy: Properties, Uses, and Patient Management 148
23. Biologic Response Modifiers: Properties, Uses, and Patient Management 167
24. Surgical Oncology: Properties, Uses, and Patient Management 174
25. Complementary and Alternative Veterinary Medicine: Properties, Uses, and Patient Management 179
26. Bone Marrow Transplantation 190
27. Hyperthermia, Cryotherapy, and Photodynamic Therapy: Properties, Uses, and Patient Management 197
28. Emerging Cancer Therapies: Gene Therapy, Cancer Vaccines, and Molecularly Targeted Therapies 204
29. Prevention and Treatment of Pain 213
30. Prevention and Treatment of Nausea and Vomiting 225
31. Nutritional Support 230
32. Transfusion Support 246
33. Hematopoietic Growth Factor Support 251

SECTION 4 DIAGNOSIS AND THERAPY: PARANEOPLASTIC SYNDROMES AND ONCOLOGIC EMERGENCIES

34. Paraneoplastic Syndromes and Oncologic Emergencies: Overview 259
35. Chemotherapy- or Radiation-Induced Congestive Heart Failure 261

#	Title	Page
36	Metabolic Manifestations of Malignancy: Hypercalcemia, Hypocalcemia, Hypoglycemia, and Hyponatremia (SIADH)	266
37	Hematologic Manifestations of Malignancy	277
38	Hypergammaglobulinemia	292
39	Extravasation of Chemotherapeutic Agents	295
40	Chemotherapy-Induced Anaphylaxis and Hypersensitivity	298
41	Cancer Therapy–Induced Renal Failure	301
42	Acute Tumor Lysis Syndrome	306
43	Disseminated Intravascular Coagulation	309
44	Cancer-Related Disorders of the Central Nervous System	314
45	Cancer Cachexia as a Manifestation of Malignancy	320
46	Fever, Hypertrophic Osteopathy, and Hypercortisolism	323

SECTION 5 MANAGEMENT OF SPECIFIC DISEASES

#	Title	Page
47	Lymphoma	329
48	Bone Marrow Neoplasia	359
49	Tumors of the Nervous System	379
50	Tumors of the Eye and Ear	396
51	Tumors of the Respiratory Tract	405
52	Cardiac Tumors	420
53	Tumors of the Gastrointestinal Tract	425
54	Melanoma	457
55	Tumors Affecting the Liver, Pancreas, and Spleen	470
56	Tumors of Blood and Lymph Vessels	479
57	Tumors of the Endocrine System	495
58	Tumors of the Reproductive System	522
59	Mammary Neoplasia	537
60	Tumors of the Urinary Tract	549
61	Tumors of Bone	565
62	Soft Tissue Sarcomas	590
63	Tumors of the Body Cavities	603
64	Tumors of the Skin and Surrounding Structures	620
65	Mast Cell Tumors	643

SECTION 6 ABRIDGED FORMULARY AND GUIDE TO ABBREVIATIONS

Abridged Formulary	659
Abbreviations	669

SECTION 7 CLIENT INFORMATION SERIES

Client Handouts	675
Glossary for Caregivers	701

SECTION 8 INDEX

Index	707

SECTION 1

FUNDAMENTALS OF CANCER CARE: CANCER PREVENTION, PHILOSOPHY, STAGING, AND COMPASSIONATE CARE

Chapter 1	Introduction to Managing the Canine Cancer Patient: A Practical Guide to Compassionate Care	3
Chapter 2	The Role of Cancer Prevention in Health and Wellness Programs	6
Chapter 3	Philosophy of Cancer Care	11
Chapter 4	Approach to the Cancer Patient: Staging	15
Chapter 5	Commandments of Cancer Care to Improve Quality of Life	18
Chapter 6	Setting Goals for Compassionate Care	23
Chapter 7	Pet Loss and Bereavement	25
Chapter 8	Compassion Fatigue	29

INTRODUCTION TO MANAGING THE CANINE CANCER PATIENT: A PRACTICAL GUIDE TO COMPASSIONATE CARE

Gregory K. Ogilvie and Antony S. Moore

CLINICAL BRIEFING

Prevalence	• Cancer causes more deaths in dogs than any other disease, yet it is the most curable of all chronic diseases. Cancer is the number one health concern of families that have dogs.
Goals	• Establishment of a cancer prevention program enhances health and wellness and meets the concerns of most clients. • Dispelling the myths about cancer and cancer care is the first and possibly the most important step to providing quality, compassionate cancer care.
Evidence-based medicine	• A discipline that formalizes the long-practiced principle of managing cancer and other patients based on current scientific evidence as well as expert and personal experience.
Planning for the future	• Continuing education and links to resources such as the Internet can enhance and improve knowledge base and patient care.

Overview

Cancer is one of the most common causes of death in geriatric dogs in Australia, Europe, Japan, and the United States.[1] Cancer has been reclassified as a chronic disease much like hypertension, chronic renal failure, and valvular heart disease, all of which have one thing in common: They can be successfully controlled without being cured. This reclassification is of profound importance in this day and age of molecular therapeutics, such as inhibitors of matrix metalloproteinases, epidermal growth factor, and angiogenesis, which induce their effects primarily by arresting the growth and metastasis of cancer.

The importance of cancer in any practice is highlighted by the knowledge that cancer is the number one health care concern of pet owners.[2-7] This fact alone should be taken seriously to (1) develop health and wellness programs that begin with pet selection, including identification of breeds and lines that have a lower risk of cancer; (2) initiate cancer prevention programs; and (3) initiate screening programs for early detection and diagnosis. These are not only logical steps to protect the health of animals in our care but also the right things to do for the people who entrust their pets to our care.

The popularity of oncology is increasing dramatically in veterinary medicine, partly because of the many advances in veterinary cancer diagnostics and therapeutics.[2-7] These advances have been made readily available by the dramatic increases in access to advanced veterinary care centers. Advanced cancer care used to be available exclusively at veterinary schools. Today, however, private practice specialty centers are often more highly equipped and staffed than many university veterinary hospitals, which has resulted in an increased ability to help a larger number of animals with a wide variety of malignancies. This in turn has increased the awareness of veterinarians and clients alike regarding the availability of sophisticated veterinary cancer care. Despite the proliferation of centers that can provide advanced cancer care, veterinary oncology and advanced medicine and surgery exist primarily because of the importance of companion animals in our society. Veterinarians and the rest of the veterinary health care team who recognize and act on this pivotal fact will succeed personally, professionally, and financially.

Cancer care will succeed if the profession is active in developing health and wellness programs that incorporate cancer prevention and screening.[3,4] Cancer prevention and early detection and diagnosis are the keys to reducing cancer-related deaths in veterinary medicine.

The question before each veterinarian faced with a patient that has cancer is when and how to treat the patient. The answer begins with the understanding that each and every patient can and should be helped regardless of the financial, time, or philosophical capabilities of the client. Each client should be given all the appropriate options, including supportive care, curative treatment, palliative therapy, hospice care, and euthanasia.[1-5] Furthermore, each client or caregiver can be helped through this difficult process with the support, education, and empowerment

> **KEY POINT**
>
> *Every patient can be helped regardless of finances, time, and the underlying diagnosis through supportive care, curative treatment, palliative therapy, hospice care, or euthanasia. Furthermore, each client or caregiver can be helped through education and empowerment with realistic, honest information.*

that realistic, honest information brings (see Section 7).[3] Therefore, by meeting the medical needs of the patient and the nonmedical needs of the client, the veterinary health care team can enhance, celebrate, and enrich the relationship between animals and humans. This relationship—the human–animal bond—is the very reason why veterinary medicine and advanced veterinary cancer care exist and flourish. Some may consider this verbiage "evangelical." Others consider the concept of caring from the heart and the science so obvious that it is unnecessary to even mention. Regardless, the human–animal bond is the foundation of the veterinary profession and worthy of note, especially in a book about caring for cancer patients.

Perhaps the greatest barrier to enhanced cure and control of cancer is that the caregiver and the veterinary health care team often have preconceived notions about cancer and its treatment.[2-9] This is true regardless of whether you are talking about cancer prevention or treatment. There are few words as frightening as *cancer*, unless perhaps the word is *chemotherapy*, yet this fear is often unfounded. The first and possibly most difficult task facing the veterinary health care team is the dissolution of the negative myths and misperceptions regarding cancer and the efficacy and toxicity of cancer therapy. Within the past 10 years, dramatic advances in cancer treatment have resulted in improved response rates, disease-free intervals, and survival times. Despite these strides, many caregivers and veterinarians are not aware that a huge percentage of dogs with cancer can be cured or at least rendered free of their disease for significant periods. With appropriate care, dogs undergoing cancer treatment often experience limited to no toxicity and an improvement in their quality of life due to the control of their cancer. Finally, when cure or control is not possible, then the lives of our patients and their families can be enhanced by embracing palliative, supportive, and hospice care.

Every practitioner wants to provide the very best care for their patients with cancer. The caring professional often asks how to find the essence of truth in all the data. This is especially true in veterinary medicine, where the studies are often small, uncontrolled, and underpowered. In human medicine, conclusions are often not made unless studies have been conducted on much larger data sets and then confirmed by other individuals and subsequently published in peer-reviewed, refereed journals of high integrity.

The question becomes how to assess the information at hand to make clinical judgments for patients coming into our clinics and hospitals today. Evidence-based medicine is a clinical discipline that has emerged in the 1990s as one very important way for health care professionals to make conclusions about patient care.[10,11] Evidence-based medicine is often defined as a conscientious, explicit, and judicious discipline that formalizes the long-practiced principle of managing patients based on current scientific evidence as well as expert and personal experience.[10,11] The practice of evidence-based medicine requires the integration of individual clinical expertise with the best available external clinical evidence from systematic research and our patient's unique values and circumstances. Because this type of decision making is based on the most up-to-date information available, its success is only as good as the practitioner's access to the latest information and a dedication to lifelong learning skills. In essence, the management of each patient evolves over time as the knowledge about the disease, patients, diagnostics, and therapeutics evolves.

When evaluating the available information, there is a general hierarchy of information based on the probability of its accuracy and applicability to the population as a whole. The hierarchy is as follows:

Personal experience	Least reliable
Case reports	
Case series	
Retrospective studies (cross-sectional, case–control)	
Uncontrolled clinical trials	
Nonrandomized controlled clinical trials	
Randomized controlled clinical trials	Most reliable

The authors of this book have taken great steps to provide readers with practical, up-to-date information and personal experience in the management of malignant disorders in dogs. That said, information is continually expanding and new evidence-based medicine conclusions are continually being made. Keeping up with the literature and with our

Internet Resources for Cancer Treatment and Care[a]	
Angel Care Cancer Center at California Veterinary Specialists www.cvsangelcare.com	Memorial Sloan-Kettering Cancer Center www.mskcc.org
Veterinary Oncology Consultants www.vetoncologyconsults.com	University of Colorado Cancer Center www.uccc.info
Veterinary Information Network www.vin.com	Association of Cancer Online Resources www.acor.org
Veterinary Cancer Society www.vetcancersociety.org	The Susan G. Komen Breast Cancer Foundation www.komen.org
Guide to Internet Resources for Cancer www.cancerindex.org/clinks1.htm	Brain Tumor Society www.tbts.org
American College of Veterinary Internal Medicine www.acvim.org	CancerCare www.cancercare.org
American College of Veterinary Surgeons www.acvs.org	Ronald McDonald House Charities www.rmhc.com
Sprecher Institute for Comparative Cancer Research www.vet.cornell.edu/cancer/index.html	Animal Cancer Care www.animalcancercare.com.au
National Cancer Institute and the National Institutes of Health www.nci.nih.gov	Animal Cancer Institute www.animalci.com
American Cancer Society www.cancer.org	

[a]The most useful resources are presented first.

clients is a continuous effort. Active participation in conferences and online resources is key. The box on this page lists a few of the many Internet resources available to seek information on caring for animals with cancer and other disorders.

The objectives of this section are to:

- Discuss the integration of cancer prevention into health and wellness programs to increase cancer cure rates.
- Examine how clients and the veterinary health care team perceive cancer, dispel the myths associated with cancer treatment, and replace these myths with accurate concepts about how dogs with cancer and their caregivers should be approached, supported, and treated.
- Discuss how cancer cure and control rates can be enhanced through the processes of staging and of understanding the type, extent, and consequences of the malignancy.
- Establish the goals of cancer care, including prevention, cure, palliation, hospice care, and euthanasia.
- Briefly review "compassion fatigue," a condition that may be a debilitating consequence of caring for a pet with cancer.

REFERENCES

1. Animal health survey, in: *Companion Animal News*, Englewood, CO, Morris Animal Foundation, March 1998, pp 1–2.
2. Ogilvie GK, Moore AS: Compassionate care of the cancer patient, in Ogilvie GK, Moore AS (eds): *Feline Oncology: A Comprehensive Guide for Compassionate Care*. Yardley, PA, Veterinary Learning Systems, 2002, pp 1–6.
3. Ogilvie GK: Préservation de la santé des animaux âgés, in *Gériatrie vétérinaire*. Les Editions du point vétérinaire. Nantes, Intervet, 2004, pp 51–56.
4. Ogilvie GK: Pris en charge du cancer chez l'animal âgé, in *Gériatrie vétérinaire*. Les Editions du point vétérinaire. Nantes, Intervet, 2004, pp 61–66.
5. Ogilvie GK: The care of animals with cancer, in Dobson JM, Lascelles BD (eds): *BSAVA Manual of Canine and Feline Oncology*, ed 2. Gloucester, UK, British Small Animal Veterinary Association, 2003, pp 68–72.
6. Mitchener KL, Ogilvie GK: Rekindling the bond. *Vet Econ* 40:30–36, 1999.
7. Mitchener KL, Ogilvie GK: Giving cancer patients hope. *Vet Econ* 40:84–88, 1999.
8. Downing R: *Pets Living with Cancer: A Pet Owner's Resource*. Denver, American Animal Hospital Association, 2000, pp 1–8.
9. Ogilvie GK: Meeting the needs of patient and client through compassionate care, in Ettinger SJ, Feldman EC (eds): *Textbook of Veterinary Internal Medicine*, ed 6. Philadelphia, WB Saunders, 2005, pp 535–537.
10. Rosenberg W, Donald A: Evidence based medicine: An approach to clinical problem-solving. *BMJ* 310:1122–1126, 1995.
11. Sacket DL, Richardson WS, Rosenberg W, Haynes RB: *Evidence-Based Medicine. How to Practice and Teach EBM*. New York, Churchill Livingstone, 1997, pp 21–34.

THE ROLE OF CANCER PREVENTION IN HEALTH AND WELLNESS PROGRAMS

Gregory K. Ogilvie and Antony S. Moore

CLINICAL BRIEFING

Key to increased cure rates	• Early detection and diagnosis, especially via cancer screening programs for all stages of life.
Nutrition and prevention	• Restrict daily intake to maintain a thin body weight throughout life. • Feed a balanced diet specifically for dogs; consider the use of n-3 polyunsaturated fatty acids.
Reproduction and prevention	• Early ovariohysterectomy or orchiectomy is recommended.
Pet selection	• Encourage adoption of dogs that have a low risk of cancer (especially mixed breeds) and fit the family environment.
Reducing carcinogens	• Eliminate exposure to environmental carcinogens such as pesticides, coal or kerosene heaters, herbicides such as 2,4-dichlorophenoxyacetic acid, environmental (passive) tobacco smoke, asbestos, radiation, and strong electromagnetic fields.

Health and wellness programs for pets, especially those that focus on cancer prevention, are gaining momentum worldwide. This is in part because veterinarians are being reminded by their clients that their pet is generally considered a member of the family.[1-8] Early detection and diagnosis of many diseases, including cancer, often result in enhanced cure rates. This chapter outlines why health care and cancer screening is so vital in all stages of the life of an animal. Included is a reminder of the reason it is important to meet not only the medical needs of the patient but also the nonmedical needs of the client. In addition, a brief summary is provided of a few select, essential points about the importance of epidemiology in guiding health and wellness programs. Finally, one example of a health and wellness program is presented to be freely adapted to the needs of the individual hospital or clinic.

The Pet and the Bond

The veterinary profession is in the middle of a renaissance: an era in which the profession is reconnecting itself with that which is the single most important unifying force that defines it and gives it purpose.[5,6] This force is known by many names, including the *human–animal bond*. This bond is often the most palpable in aging pets and their families and is the key to every veterinarian's aspirations of personal, professional, and financial success. The bond is almost indefinable, yet it is often described as the unique relationship between people and animals and is described using such terms as companionship, unconditional love and affection, protection, and nurturance. The bond is present in some form between each and every caregiver and his or her pet and is at the heart of why we need to provide the best veterinary care possible. Because cancer is the biggest health care concern in the hearts and minds of our clients, it is vital to include cancer screening and prevention programs in veterinary practice.

The question remains: How does one best incorporate health care, including cancer screening, into veterinary practice? The first step in incorporating heath and wellness programs is to educate veterinary students and graduate veterinarians about the unique needs of the aging pet.[2,3] The second step is to enhance understanding of the tools, drugs, and procedures, including cancer screening, that can be used successfully to enhance the health and wellness of the aging animal.[4-6] Throughout this process, it is important that the entire team understand that age is a number and not a disease, but along with age comes a complex of disorders and diseases that increase the risk associated with the management of other diseases or the way drugs are metabolized.

It is beyond the scope of this chapter to review a summary of age-associated health changes in dogs. It can be said, however, that age is associated with some definable changes in body function, susceptibility, and response to diseases such as cancer. What this means is that age itself is not a disease, but that conditions such as cancer, which are associated with increasing age, need to be accounted for when dealing with geriatric patients. Following are some examples of how to initiate the prevention of cancer and other diseases:[8]

- Initiate a health and wellness program for all stages of life, and always include cancer screening as a vital aspect of that program.
- Recognize that aging patients have unique changes in organ function, susceptibility to complications for routine procedures, and altered metabolism of drugs and other agents.
- Identify clinically silent diseases, such as early evidence of cancer, and initiate measures to sustain health and wellness.
- Identify clinically evident diseases and initiate therapy to treat these conditions.
- Counsel clients about how to prevent cancer and other diseases associated with aging.

Epidemiology and Cancer

One of the most common questions clients ask their veterinarian is, "What caused my dog's cancer?" That question is difficult to answer, but as in humans, the etiopathogenesis of cancer in dogs often involves genetics and environmental risk factors. Indeed, golden retrievers have recently been pointed out as having a high death rate from cancer when compared with other breeds. Similarly, exposure to cigarette smoke, asbestos, and other environmental contaminants has been associated with an increased risk of developing cancer in dogs.[9] Therefore, cancer prevention is based on the identification of at-risk animals with certain familial/genetic and environmental influences and elimination of those influences. Epidemiology is the science that begins to identify these genetic and environmental influences that can then be used for cancer prevention. Before venturing into the world of cancer epidemiology, a few key definitions are in order:

- **Cancer incidence:** The number of new cases of cancer occurring in an animal population at risk for this disease over a set period of time.
- **Incidence rate:** Measure of the absolute risk for a disease (in this case, cancer).
- **Annual cancer mortality rate:** The number of animals dying from cancer in 1 year per the population of animals at risk during that time period.
- **Odds ratio:** Statistical odds that animals with a specific cancer were exposed to a parameter in question compared with the odds that animals without the cancer were exposed to the same parameter. This measurement of association is determined in a case–control study.
- **Relative risk:** Ratio of the incidence or mortality rate in an exposed group to the incidence or mortality rate in an unexposed group. Relative risk is determined in prospective studies.

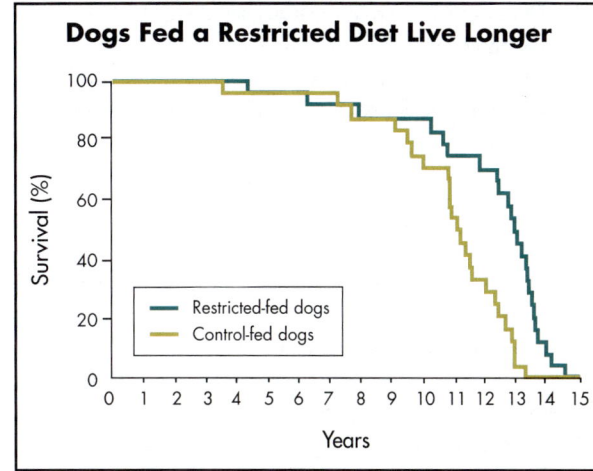

Figure 2-1. Survival curves from a lifetime study of restricted daily food intake in a total of 48 control-fed versus paired restricted-fed (25% less intake) dogs. The median life span of the restricted-fed group was significantly longer than that of the control-fed dogs. The mean age of death due to cancer-related illness was 2 years older in the dogs that received the restricted diet.

> **KEY POINT**
> *Lifelong weight control enhances the overall survival time of dogs, and the prevalence of cancer has been shown to be less in dogs that tend not to be overweight.*

The identification of factors associated with an increased risk of developing cancer is in its infancy in veterinary epidemiology and oncology. Despite this early state of development, several important observations can be made.[9–26] Clients should be educated that increased risk may or may not be equated with causality; in other words, exposure to a risk factor may not have *caused* their pet's cancer. These factors should be included during counseling sessions. Following are a few of the many factors, including guidelines on the best ways to decrease the potential for cancer:

- **Nutrition:** A lifetime study of restricted daily intake of the same food was done with a total of 48 control-fed versus paired restricted-fed (25% less intake) Labrador retrievers that came from seven litters.[10,11] The median life span of the restricted-fed group was significantly longer (Figure 2-1). While the prevalence of cancer between groups was similar, the mean age due to cancer-related deaths was 2 years older in the dogs that received the restricted diet. The long-chain eicosapentaenoic and docosahexaenoic acids have been shown consistently to inhibit the proliferation of breast and prostate cancer cell lines in vitro and to reduce the risk and progression of these tumors in many species.[12,13]

— Restrict daily intake to maintain a thin body weight throughout life.

— Feed a balanced diet made specifically for dogs with possible consideration of the use of polyunsaturated fatty acids of the n-3 series.

- **Ovariohysterectomy/orchiectomy:** Ovariohysterectomy has long been demonstrated to be a markedly effective method of preventing mammary tumors if it is performed before the first estrus.[13,14] Spaying is moderately effective if performed before the dog is 2.5 years of age. Spaying may also be therapeutic when treating dogs with mammary tumors.[16] Orchiectomy will reduce the risk of testicular tumors. Gonadectomy may not uniformly protect against all cancers. A study of rottweilers was conducted to examine the effect of elective gonadectomy and the spontaneous development of appendicular bone sarcomas.[15] In that study, male and female rottweilers that underwent gonadectomy before 1 year of age had an approximate 25% lifetime risk for bone sarcoma and were significantly more likely to develop bone sarcoma than dogs that were sexually intact.

— Early ovariohysterectomy and orchiectomy is recommended.

- **Genetics:** There is little doubt that cancer occurs more often in certain breeds than in others and that environmental factors may have an influence.[9] German shepherds have been shown to have bilateral cystadenocarcinomas. Flat-coated retrievers and Bernese mountain dogs have been shown to have a high incidence of cancer, including malignant histiocytosis.[17] Scottish terriers, especially those with exposure to herbicides, have an increased risk of developing transitional cell carcinomas of the bladder.[18]

— Encourage adoption of dogs that have a low risk of cancer and fit the family environment.

> **KEY POINT**
> *Limiting or eliminating environmental carcinogens such as pesticides, tobacco smoke, and asbestos may decrease the risk of developing cancer in many species, including dogs.*

- **Environmental carcinogens:** Dogs have been shown to have an increased risk of developing cancer of the respiratory tract, especially of the lung and nasal cavity, when exposed to coal and kerosene heaters and passive tobacco smoke.[19–21] Mesothelioma is more common in dogs owned by people who worked in the asbestos industry.[22] The use of chemicals by owners, specifically 2,4-dichlorophenoxyacetic acid, paints, asbestos, or solvents, and radiation and electromagnetic field exposure were associated with an increased risk for several types of cancer in pet dogs.[24–26] In another study, application of insecticides (but not in a spot-on formulation) increased the risk for bladder cancer in Scottish terriers.[23]

— Eliminate exposure to environmental carcinogens such as pesticides, coal or kerosene heaters, herbicides such as 2,4-dichlorophenoxyacetic acid, passive tobacco smoke, asbestos, radiation, and strong electromagnetic fields. These steps may be particularly important for clients with susceptible breeds (e.g., a Scottish terrier and herbicide exposure).

> **KEY POINT**
> *Incorporating principles of cancer prevention into health and wellness programs brings a good chance of enhancing early detection and diagnosis of cancer, thereby increasing cure rates.*

Setting up a Health and Wellness Program

Cancer is one of the biggest health care concerns in the hearts and minds of most people, regardless of the age of their dog.[5,6] Despite this fact, few veterinarians include cancer education and screening for all age groups. If cancer prevention and early detection and diagnosis were incorporated in health and wellness programs for all patient age groups, it would not only meet the needs and concerns of the client but also be the right thing for the pet.

Setting up a health and wellness program for all stages of life, including senior patients, is an important endeavor and one that takes a great deal of thought and effort. Once the team has made a decision to provide a health and wellness program for their older patients, the following steps should be considered:

- Select a name for the program, ensuring that the name does not have a negative connotation. Golden Years, Evergreen, and Best Friends are some examples.
- Identify someone who can initiate this program and will see it through to the end.
- Determine a fee for this service.
- Ensure that this is a team approach, with nurses, receptionists, and veterinarians all on board.
- Clearly identify the job descriptions and tasks for everyone involved.
- Initiate a training session, and repeat it regularly.

Table 2-1 **Components of Health and Wellness Programs by Age**

<1 Year of Age	1–7 Years of Age	>7 Years of Age
Preadoption counseling to select breeds and lines with a reduced risk of cancer and to meet the needs of the adopting family Behavioral counseling and suggestions regarding obedience classes		
A complete history	A complete history every 12 mo	A complete history at least every 6 mo
A complete physical examination	A complete physical examination every 12 mo	A complete physical examination at least every 6 mo
Body weight evaluation and body condition scoring	Body weight evaluation and body condition scoring	Body weight evaluation and body condition scoring
Nutritional counseling to include discussion of optimum diet, weight, and exercise	Nutritional counseling to include discussion of optimum diet, weight, and exercise	Nutritional counseling to include discussion of optimum diet, weight, and exercise
Select diagnostics, including complete blood count and biochemical profile	Select diagnostics, including a *minimum* of: • Complete blood count • Biochemical profile, including creatinine, potassium, serum alanine aminotransferase, and serum alkaline phosphatase • Complete urinalysis by cystocentesis • Blood pressure • Fine-needle aspiration and mapping of any masses or swelling • Counseling to reduce exposure to carcinogens such as passive tobacco smoke, industrial chemicals, direct constant sunlight, etc.	Select diagnostics, including a *minimum* of: • Complete blood count • Full biochemical profile, including electrolytes • Thyroid panel (optional) • Complete urinalysis by cystocentesis • Blood pressure • Miscellaneous diagnostic testing such as chest radiographs, as needed • Fine-needle aspiration and mapping of any masses or swelling • Counseling to reduce exposure to carcinogens such as passive tobacco smoke, industrial chemicals, direct constant sunlight, etc.
Education on critical issues such as vaccination scheduling, ovariohysterectomy, orchiectomy, cancer screening, nutrition, dental screening, and obesity prevention.	Education on critical issues such as vaccination scheduling, cancer screening, nutrition, dental screening, and obesity prevention.	Education on critical issues such as vaccination scheduling, cancer screening, nutrition, dental screening, and obesity prevention.

- Contact industry representatives to obtain handout materials, samples, and posters to enhance effectiveness of the program.
- Decide where and when this program will be held each week.

After the team has been identified and educated, and *after* several months of practice, a concerted promotion effort should be initiated.

Model Health Care Programs[2,3]

Most veterinary health care centers that are providing health and wellness programs divide their programs into those for dogs younger than 1 year of age, dogs 1 to 7 years of age, and dogs 7 years of age and older (Table 2-1).

Conclusion

Cancer prevention is a mainstay of human health care, and it should be the cornerstone of veterinary health care. This is not only the correct type of care for our patients but also the right thing to do for our patients' human family members who are rightfully concerned about cancer in their pets and themselves. More information will become available as the years roll by, and more specific recommendations will become part of the standard screening process.

REFERENCES

1. Ogilvie GK, Moore AS: Compassionate care of the cancer patient, in Ogilvie GK, Moore AS: *Feline Oncology: A Comprehensive Guide for Compassionate Care.* Yardley, PA, Veterinary Learning Systems, 2002, pp 1–6.
2. Ogilvie GK: Préservation de la santé des animaux âgés, in *Gériatrie vétérinaire. Les Editions du point vétérinaire.* Nantes, Intervet, 2004, pp 51–56.
3. Ogilvie GK: Pris en charge du cancer chez l'animal âgé, in *Gériatrie vétérinaire. Les Editions du point vétérinaire.* Nantes, Intervet, 2004, 61–66.
4. Ogilvie GK: The care of animals with cancer, in Dobson JM, Lascelles BD (eds): *BSAVA Manual of Canine and Feline Oncology,* ed 2. Gloucester, UK, British Small Animal Veterinary Association. 2003, 68–72.
5. Mitchener KL, Ogilvie GK: Rekindling the bond. *Vet Econ* 40:30–36, 1999.
6. Mitchener KL, Ogilvie GK: Giving cancer patients hope. *Vet Econ* 40:84–88, 1999.
7. Epstein M, Kuehn NF, Landsberg G, et al: AAHA senior care guidelines for dogs and cats. *JAAHA* 41(2):81–91, 2005.
8. Ogilvie GK: Meeting the needs of patient and client through compassionate care, in Ettinger SJ, Feldman EC (eds): *Textbook of Veterinary Internal Medicine,* ed 6. Philadelphia, WB Saunders, 2005, pp 535–537.
9. Craig LE: Cause of death in dogs according to breed: A necropsy survey of five breeds. *JAAHA* 37(5): 438–443, 2001.
10. Kealy RD, Lawler DF, Ballam JM, et al: Influence of diet restriction on life span and age-related changes in Labrador retrievers. *JAVMA* 220:1315–1320, 2002.
11. Lawler DF, Evans RH, Larson BT, et al: Influence of lifetime food restriction on causes, time and predictors of mortality of dogs. *JAVMA* 226:225–231, 2005.
12. Terry PD, Rohan TE, Wolk A: Intakes of fish and marine fatty acids and the risks of cancers of the breast and prostate and of other hormone-related cancers: A review of the epidemiologic evidence. *Am J Epidemiol* 141(4):352–359, 1995.
13. Sonnenschein EG, Glickman LT, Goldschmidt MH, McKee LJ: Body conformation, diet, and risk of breast cancer in pet dogs: A case–control study. *Am J Epidemiol* 133(7):694–703, 1991.
14. Ferguson HR: Canine mammary gland tumors. *Vet Clin North Am Small Anim Pract* 15(3):501–511, 1985.
15. Cooley DM, Beranek BC, Schlittler DL, et al: Endogenous gonadal hormone exposure and bone sarcoma risk. *Cancer Epidemiol Biomarkers Prev* 11(11):1434–1440, 2002.
16. Sorenmo KU, Shofer FS, Goldschmidt MH: Effect of spaying and timing of spaying on survival of dogs with mammary carcinoma. *J Vet Intern Med* 14(3):266–270, 2000.
17. Morris JS, Bostock DE, McInnes EF, et al: Histopathological survey of neoplasms in flat-coated retrievers, 1990 to 1998. *Vet Rec* 147(11):291–295, 2000.
18. Glickman LT, Raghavan M, Knapp DW, et al: Herbicide exposure and the risk of transitional cell carcinoma of the urinary bladder in Scottish terriers. *JAVMA* 224(8):1290–1297, 2004.
19. Bukowski JA, Wartenberg D, Goldschmidt M: Environmental causes for sinonasal cancers in pet dogs, and their usefulness as sentinels of indoor cancer risk. *J Toxicol Environ Health A* 54(7):579–591, 1998.
20. Reif JS, Bruns C, Lower KS: Cancer of the nasal cavity and paranasal sinuses and exposure to environmental tobacco smoke in pet dogs. *Am J Epidemiol* 147(5):488–492, 1998.
21. Reif JS, Dunn K, Ogilvie GK, Harris CK: Passive smoking and canine lung cancer risk. *Am J Epidemiol* 135(3):234–239, 1992.
22. Glickman LT, Domanski LM, Maguire TG, et al: Mesothelioma in pet dogs associated with exposure of their owners to asbestos. *Environ Res* 32(2):305–313, 1983.
23. Raghavan M, Knapp DW, Dawson MH, et al: Topical flea and tick pesticides and the risk of transitional cell carcinoma of the urinary bladder in Scottish terriers. *JAVMA* 225:389–394, 2004.
24. Gavazza A, Presciuttini S, Barale R, et al: Association between canine malignant lymphoma, living in industrial areas, and use of chemicals by dog owners. *J Vet Intern Med* 15(3):190–195, 2001.
25. Hayes HM, Tarone RE, Cantor KP: On the association between canine malignant lymphoma and opportunity for exposure to 2,4-dichlorophenoxyacetic acid. *Environ Res* 70(2):119–125, 1995.
26. Reif JS, Lower KS, Ogilvie GK: Residential exposure to magnetic fields and risk of canine lymphoma. *Am J Epidemiol* 141(4):352–359, 1995.

PHILOSOPHY OF CANCER CARE

Gregory K. Ogilvie and Antony S. Moore

3

FUNDAMENTALS OF CANCER CARE

CLINICAL BRIEFING

Three steps of cancer care

Step 1: Dispel the myths: the client's, the team's, and yours.
Step 2: Establish the team, including the client.
Step 3: Deliver compassionate care to patient and client.

Clients arrive at our clinics and hospitals frightened about the possible loss of their pet's life to the disease called cancer. In their minds, cancer is, in effect, a one-word death sentence. Sadly, many members of the veterinary health care team, including some clinicians and nurses, also believe that cancer is a one-way trip to death. In reality, that is just not true. In fact, compared with heart disease and renal disease, cancer is the most curable of all chronic diseases, and cancer care can be provided while enhancing quality of life for the vast majority of patients. In short, each and every patient can and should be helped.

> **KEY POINT**
>
> *Most of the fears and misconceptions about cancer and cancer care are wrong or out of proportion. The devastating consequence of these myths is that they serve as a barrier that often precludes early, decisive therapy from the veterinary health care team and client.*

Each member of the veterinary health care team plays a critical role in providing compassionate care for cancer patients. Before compassionate care with specific therapeutics can be initiated, three steps of cancer care need to be undertaken.[1-8] The first is to dispel the myths that blind us to the possibilities of providing exceptional care for the cancer patient. The second is to build a team to care for the owner and the patient with equal focus. After these two steps have been accomplished, the third step—true compassionate care—can begin.

Step One: Dispel the Myths

Regardless of our culture, nationality, or religion, most of us are indoctrinated from an early age that cancer and cancer therapy are horrible. Therefore, clients, nursing staff, and even veterinarians often perceive cancer and its therapy as something dark and hopeless. The truth is that most of the fears and misconceptions about cancer and cancer care are wrong or out of proportion. These myths serve as barriers that often preclude early, decisive therapy. They envelop the disease in a cloud that obscures true understanding and vision and blocks out all hope. Such surgical procedures as amputation, chest wall resection, hemipelvectomy, and maxillectomy are perceived as traumatic to patient, client, and health care providers. We imagine chemotherapy protocols as being inevitably linked with horrible side effects. We fear that therapy will be financially devastating and physically debilitating, with little benefit for client or patient. In essence, we are often frozen in indecision as we, our team, and our clients wonder, "Is it all worth it?"

The initial steps in providing compassionate cancer care are to first identify the myths and misconceptions in the heart of each member of the veterinary health care team, including receptionists, nurses, veterinarians, and other allied team members, and then erase them. We all drag in our own misconceptions, prejudgments, and preconceived notions that can stifle the hope in cancer care. The consequence of not dispelling these myths is that the patient and caregiver are hurt by shortsighted or ineffective care.

> **KEY POINT**
>
> *The consequence of not dispelling the myths associated with cancer care is that the patient and caregiver are hurt by shortsighted or ineffective care.*

Few would debate that the goal of most veterinary health care teams is to enhance, maintain, or improve quality of life for their patients. While it is true that small sacrifices in quality sometimes have to be made, these sacrifices must be temporary and made only to gain significant, additional length of life. We must assure our staff members, the client, and ourselves that quality time during cancer therapy is a reality, and we must always work to maintain that quality throughout treatment. It is then that hope begins to supplant the myths and misconceptions.

> **Ways to Dispel Preconceived Notions of Clients That Have Animals with Cancer**[8]
>
> - Provide an audio transcript of actual discussions regarding the disease and its treatment. Many hospitals lend pocket dictation recorders to their clients to record discussions with the veterinary health care team.
> - Give clients written "bullet points" of discussions.
> - Provide information about the most common disorders and treatments.
> - Keep an updated list of clients whose pets have undergone cancer treatment and who are willing to discuss the realities of care and disease with others. It is best to match clients based on common diseases in their pets.
> - Carefully prescreen and review Web site information on diseases to ensure that your clients can obtain truthful, accurate facts about cancer and cancer care.
> - Take new clients on a tour of the hospital and introduce them to the staff.
> - Include the client in as much patient care as law and ethics allow.
> - Encourage clients to summarize critical information.

Step Two: Establish the Team

The second step of compassionate cancer care, establishing the team, is a crucial move toward providing care from the heart as well as from science. A dedicated, trained, cohesive, caring veterinary health care team is essential to adequately care for cancer patients and their owners and to fight the disease. All members of the staff, including office personnel, nurses, and other staff, must understand that they play a vital role in caring for cancer patients and the people who bring them to us. Everyone must be united in focus, philosophy, and the ultimate goal of enhancing and improving the quality of life for the cancer patient while supporting each other. Each veterinarian, nurse, and receptionist within a facility must be prepared to accept a role as part of the team. This team must then reach out beyond the walls of the practice to specialists and consultants such as pathologists, pharmacists, and veterinary oncologists when appropriate. Finally, the most vital members of the team are the clients themselves. They must be incorporated through education, support, and empowerment to provide ongoing day-to-day care and assessment (see the box on this page). Without their input, attention, care, and ongoing assessment, care of the cancer patient cannot be optimal.

In our society, cancer, no matter who it affects, is associated with many negative feelings. The presence of these feelings in staff and colleagues often results in a mental roadblock to hope, care, and cure. It is imperative that these feelings are acknowledged by everyone on the veterinary health care team. Cancer treatment is not easy. It requires total dedication of all staff involved and often can be emotionally taxing. Preconceived notions about cancer and the toxicity and efficacy of cancer therapy must be acknowledged. It is vital for the team members to openly discuss these matters and to provide realistic information about cancer and its therapy. Once the health care team overcomes these misconceptions, comprehensive, team-based client education is possible. As mentioned, all involved must overcome their biases and ingrained feelings about cancer before rationally approaching cancer and cancer care. Ongoing support, information, and care must be provided to all members of the veterinary health care team to prevent burnout and "compassion fatigue" and to retain individuals who will provide quality, compassionate care on a continuous basis (see Chapter 8). After the misconceptions have been replaced with realities and options for cancer care, the health care team and caregiver can begin to make decisions and provide the necessary care of the cancer patient.

> **KEY POINT**
>
> *A dedicated, trained, cohesive, caring veterinary health care team is essential to adequately care for the cancer patient and client and to fight the disease.*

Care of the cancer patient requires unique skills, knowledge, drugs, procedures, and philosophies. The health care team must dedicate itself to an aggressive continuing education program to maximize care of their canine patients. Canine cancer patients usually have a dynamic course to their disease; thus, ongoing communication is essential to maximize care for both the patient and the caregivers. Communication during hospitalization should be a daily procedure, but ongoing communication by multiple members of the veterinary health care team can greatly improve the patient's quality of care by providing the veterinarian with ongoing reassessments and progress reports. These and other policies and procedures regarding patient care should be established long in advance and applied in a team approach to maximize seamless care for each patient and build the team.

Clients are perhaps the most vital—and often most overlooked—members of the health care team. Once their misconceptions have been dispelled and they are able to make rational, educated decisions regarding cancer care, clients must know that they are empowered and necessary members of the team. Quality of life assessments, administration of medication, and daily or even hourly patient monitoring can be appropriately accomplished only by the clients and are most effective when clients are empowered and educated and know that they are a vital extension of the health care team at home. Emergency preparedness as well as prevention is only possible with an informed, alerted client. Cancer care takes a tremendous leap forward when 24-hour outpatient care is provided by the client. In addition, including clients as members of the health care team gives them an active responsibility and restores the bond between them and their beloved pet.

Following are a few examples of ways to form, empower, and enhance the veterinary health care team[8]:

- Identify, reward, and promote only the best, most compassionate people.
- Openly celebrate, review, and revise the mission statement and goals written by the team.
- Ensure that the team participates in all interviews and assists in decisions to hire new applicants.
- Share and celebrate when a team member is recognized by clients or others.
- Meet at least weekly to listen to team members; value their input, feelings, and thoughts.
- Introduce clients to the team, including nurses and receptionists, during the first visit.

Step Three: Delivering the Care[1-8]

Once the caring team is forged to include at least the veterinarian, veterinary health care staff, and client and the misconceptions of cancer are shed, the emotional component of the disease is defeated. Stripped of its emotional cloud, cancer is attackable, diagnosable, treatable, manageable, and, in many cases, curable. In fact, as stated earlier, it is the most curable of all chronic diseases. At this point, the team is prepared for the third step: delivering the care (see the box on this page).

> **KEY POINT**
> *Compassionate care is the single most important term in veterinary medicine. It is achieved by meeting the medical needs of the patient and the nonmedical needs of the client.*

Compassionate care is the single most important term in veterinary medicine and is imperative in cancer care. The first phase of compassionate care is defining and describing the disease and the health status of the patient through diagnostics and staging (i.e., determining the extent of the cancer in the body; see Chapter 4). The second phase is providing caring support by responding to the pet's needs and client's concerns through the commandments of cancer care (see Chapter 5). The final phase is providing direct therapy for the underlying disease using the appropriate tools, such as surgery, chemotherapy, or radiation therapy. Each step of the process of compassionate care is dependent on the others.

> **Steps for Delivering Cancer Care[8]**
>
> - Do not prejudge client desires and capabilities; give all options regardless of cost or outcome.
> - Review team philosophy for patient care with the client, nurses, and others if indicated.
> - Define the importance of preventing toxicity or illness and the steps to do so.
> - Outline contingency plans for when problems occur. Include plans for weekends, nights, and holidays.
> - Empower clients with information about cancer and its treatment; the goal should be to have them know as much as the rest of the team.
> - Listen and respond to the client's needs, goals, concerns, desires, fears, time commitments, financial limitations, and philosophy regarding quality and quantity of life.
> - Call clients days to weeks after euthanasia to ensure they are coping reasonably well.

The average client caring for a patient with cancer will visit the clinic frequently over the next year; therefore, a bond of trust must be developed between the veterinary health care team and the client. This bond must begin with communication, which requires time and an open, honest discussion with all parties involved. Ideally, sufficient time should be set aside during the first visit to discuss the dog's condition, prognosis, and options for therapy. It is helpful for the client to see the facility and meet any involved staff. During this initial office visit, information should be provided in oral and written form. Preprinted information sheets in plain language are essential and should describe the practice, the patient's disease, and the treatments that may be used. The client may be encouraged to take notes and ask questions, or the veterinarian can take notes during the discussion and give them to the client. A summary of all major discussions with the caregiver should be either typed or written so that a copy is available for the patient record and the client.

The members of the health care team should realize that most clients are overwhelmed by emotion and are not able to make a rational decision or even completely absorb or comprehend the information provided to them during the first visit. Therefore, the written or recorded information and a follow-up telephone call or personal conference is of tremendous value. Clients should not be forced to make quick or immediate decisions but should be allowed to think about the options available for their dog. By providing the client with an accurate prognosis, information regarding quality of life and duration of therapy, and treatment choices, you restore a sense of control and power to the client. When discussing the option of euthanasia, information about the philosophy, procedures, and aftercare of the animal's body should be provided in both oral and written forms. Cancer by itself can engender many feelings of loss and bereavement, even though treatment is a viable option and the patient's prognosis may not be guarded. However, the emotional and physical impact of pet loss and bereavement should be discussed at some point during the care of the canine cancer patient.

REFERENCES

1. Ogilvie GK, Moore AS: Compassionate care of the cancer patient, in Ogilvie GK, Moore AS: *Feline Oncology: A Comprehensive Guide for Compassionate Care*. Yardley, PA, Veterinary Learning Systems, 2002, pp 1–6.
2. Ogilvie G: Préservation de la santé des animaux âgés, in *Gériatrie vétérinaire. Les Editions du Point Vétérinaire*, Nantes, France, Intervet, 2004, pp 51–56.
3. Ogilvie GK: Pris en charge du cancer chez l'animal âgé, in *Gériatrie vétérinaire. Les Editions du Point Vétérinaire*. Nantes, France, Intervet, 2004, pp 61–66.
4. Ogilvie GK: The care of animals with cancer, in Dobson JM, Lascelles BD (eds): *BSAVA Manual of Canine and Feline Oncology*, ed 2. Gloucester, UK, British Small Animal Veterinary Association, 2003, pp 68–72.
5. Mitchener KL, Ogilvie GK: Rekindling the bond. *Vet Econ* 40:30–36, 1999.
6. Mitchener KL, Ogilvie GK: Giving cancer patients hope. *Vet Econ* 40:84–88, 1999.
7. Downing R: *Pets Living with Cancer: A Pet Owner's Resource*. Denver, American Animal Hospital Association, 2000, pp 1–8.
8. Ogilvie GK: Meeting the needs of patient and client through compassionate care, in Ettinger SJ, Feldman EC (eds): *Textbook of Veterinary Internal Medicine*, ed 6. Philadelphia, WB Saunders, 2005, pp 535–537.

APPROACH TO THE CANCER PATIENT: STAGING

Gregory K. Ogilvie and Antony S. Moore

CLINICAL BRIEFING

Cancer staging
- Obtain a tissue and/or cytologic diagnosis.
- Determine the location and extent of the cancer.
- Determine the patient's condition and general health.
- Empower the client and the veterinary health care team with staging information.

Staging describes the process of diagnosing and assessing an individual patient's cancer and its consequences to the body.[1-4] The process of staging introduces the veterinary health care team to the "enemy" (cancer) and is an essential prelude to effectively designing a treatment strategy. The three components of the staging process are to identify the following:

1. **Tissue diagnosis:** Each tumor is unique and thus must be identified with a biopsy.
2. **Location and extent of the tumor:** This component of staging is the process of assessing the extent of the malignancy locally and at distant sites through the metastatic process. Although this assessment will vary among tumor types, the staging process always begins with a thorough physical examination to identify any enlarged lymph nodes or other obvious areas of cancer spread. The exam is often combined with a complete blood count (CBC), biochemical profile, urinalysis, thoracic radiographs (right and left lateral and ventrodorsal views), and abdominal radiographs. In addition, ancillary diagnostics such as ultrasonography, computed tomography (CT), magnetic resonance imaging (MRI), or other, more specialized tests may be required.
3. **Condition of the patient:** Any neoplastic process may result in a number of paraneoplastic conditions that affect the well-being of the cancer patient. In addition, these dogs are generally geriatric patients with the potential for a number of underlying conditions and problems, including renal disease, cognitive dysfunction disorders, and degenerative myelopathy, which may adversely affect their health or the potential success or course of therapy. It is all too easy to claim that "the patient has cancer; that's why it's sick." In many instances, correcting underlying problems such as renal failure, urinary tract infections, heart disease, and metabolic disturbances may significantly improve the overall health of the patient and thus improve the potential for successful cancer care.

> **KEY POINT**
>
> *Staging the patient by determining the histologic diagnosis of the tumor by biopsy or cytology, defining the extent of the primary tumor and any metastasis, and assessing the patient's condition is essential to treating dogs with cancer.*

The World Health Organization and other groups traditionally describe the process of staging using the TNM system:

- Size of the primary tumor (T)
- Lymph node metastasis (N)
- Distant metastasis (M)

These components are further modified by the use of subscript numbers to indicate increase in tumor size (T_0, T_1, T_2, and T_3), progressive involvement of regional lymph nodes (N_0, N_1, and N_2), and presence or absence of distant metastasis (M_0 and M_1). To obtain this information, ancillary diagnostic tests are very important and sophisticated imaging techniques are often used.

Physical Examination

A complete physical examination is essential to the staging process. All lymph nodes, especially those that provide lymphatic drainage from the site of the primary tumor (referred to as regional lymph nodes), should be palpated. The primary tumor and involved lymph nodes should be measured, and those measurements should be recorded to assist the veterinarian in assessing response to therapy or in planning surgery and adjunctive therapy.

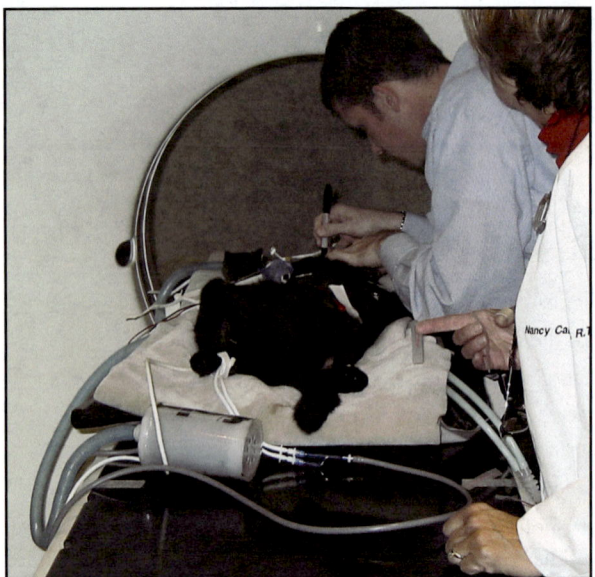

Figure 4-1. *The availability of advanced diagnostics such as CT has enhanced the ability to stage cancer patients and direct therapy while reducing morbidity and mortality.*

Clinical Pathology

The results of a CBC, biochemical profile, or urinalysis rarely provide definitive information regarding the type of cancer or whether it has metastasized. In this book, such information is discussed in the Staging and Diagnosis section for each tumor type only if specific prognostic information can be obtained. Routine blood work and a urinalysis should be conducted as part of a general health screen for every animal with cancer.

Anemia in animals with cancer is common, but it is usually low grade and characterized as normocytic–normochromic, which is compatible with anemia of chronic disease. Moderate to severe anemia may be present in animals experiencing blood loss from gastrointestinal involvement with the tumor, coagulopathies, or, occasionally, paraneoplastic immune-mediated destruction. White cell counts and differentials rarely assist the clinician in staging a dog with cancer. Neutrophilia may result from inflammation, tumor necrosis, or stress and does not automatically imply infection, but it should prompt further investigation for an underlying cause. Similarly, abnormalities in other cell lines may not be specific for the animal's tumor but should be investigated by thoracic radiography, ultrasonography, or possibly bone marrow aspiration. Some tumors cause changes in the hemogram or biochemical profile as a paraneoplastic syndrome, and these changes are noted in the relevant chapters.

Biochemical profiles are essential to establish the health of an animal with cancer. When complicated surgical procedures or multiple radiation therapies that require repeated or prolonged anesthesia are planned, acceptable renal and hepatic functions are vital. In addition, some chemotherapeutic agents that are metabolized or excreted by the liver or kidneys may require reduction in dosage if these organs are functionally compromised (see Chapters 20 and 21). Paraneoplastic conditions, such as hypercalcemia or hypoglycemia, may be observed and may direct the clinician to search for an otherwise unsuspected neoplasm (see Section 4).

Urinalysis may disclose evidence of infection that can occur as a consequence of tumor-related immunosuppression or general debility. Initiation of appropriate antibiotic therapy is recommended, particularly when myelosuppressive chemotherapy is anticipated as a treatment modality.

Radiography and Ultrasonography

Radiographs of the thorax and abdomen are valuable in determining the clinical stage of disease. Thoracic radiographs may permit identification of lymphadenopathy of sternal or tracheobronchial nodes. In addition, they may reveal a mediastinal mass, pulmonary metastasis, or pleural effusion. Proper radiographic assessment of the lungs requires right and left lateral views as well as a dorsoventral view. Radiographs of the abdomen are used to identify a mass, organomegaly, or lymphadenopathy, particularly of the sublumbar nodes. Some tumors are calcified and are easily visualized on radiographs.

If biopsy of a mass located in one of the body cavities is considered (particularly if effusion is present), ultrasonography provides an accurate and relatively safe guide for obtaining a tissue or fluid sample. In addition, when involvement of abdominal viscera is suspected, ultrasonography allows evaluation of organ homogeneity and architecture and can be used to detect the presence of enlarged lymph nodes as well as gastrointestinal involvement. Ultrasonography has the advantage of providing no risk of exposure to radiation and does not require an anesthetized patient.

Computed Tomography and Magnetic Resonance Imaging

CT and MRI are becoming more widely available for veterinary use, particularly at teaching institutions and large specialty practices (Figure 4-1). The major advantage of CT and MRI over conventional radiography is their ability to discriminate between tissues that have only minor differences in radiodensity that would not be appreciated on plain radiographs. For example, CT and MRI can discriminate hepatic metastases from normal liver tissue. Objects that are close together, however, may be difficult to depict separately. CT and MRI have advantages over ultrasonography in imaging lesions that are shielded by bone or gas (e.g., lung or intracranial tumors); however, unlike ultrasonography, CT and MRI require general anesthesia.

Imaging Tumors of Specific Sites

For diagnostic purposes, conventional radiography, preferably with high-detail film, is effective in imaging nasal and oral tumors, whereas ultrasonography is often useful for retrobulbar lesions. CT is probably the modality of choice for imaging tumors of the brain as well as nasal, oral, and retrobulbar tumors. CT is particularly useful when the veterinarian is trying to determine tumor margins in these sites before surgery or radiation therapy. In fact, CT is very useful in assessing margins of large soft tissue tumors anywhere in the body. However, lesions of the brain stem may be difficult to image accurately with CT.

Ultrasonography is the imaging modality of choice for tumors of the heart. For most other thoracic lesions, conventional radiography provides a more global view. CT is best for assessing tumor margins and the tissue of origin (e.g., mediastinum versus lung). CT may also detect pulmonary metastases that are too small to be seen or are equivocal lesions on conventional radiographs.

Ultrasonography is considered by some to be the first choice for imaging the abdomen, although conventional radiography will provide a global aspect. CT may be useful if organs are obscured by gas. An even newer modality to the veterinary field, MRI is often available to veterinarians through regional veterinary referral centers. MRI provides excellent resolution and is particularly useful for imaging tumors of the brain or spine.

Conclusion

Once the cancer has been staged, appropriate options for therapy and prognosis can be determined. The client or caregiver is given information and education regarding the name of the disease, its extent, the options for care, and the prognosis. The veterinary health care team is given the information it needs to formulate an appropriate plan of care, including the prevention and/or treatment of potential problems.

REFERENCES

1. Mitchener KL, Ogilvie GK: Rekindling the bond. *Vet Econ* 40:30–36, 1999.
2. Mitchener KL, Ogilvie GK: Giving cancer patients hope. *Vet Econ* 40:84–88, 1999.
3. Ogilvie GK, Moore AS: Compassionate care of the cancer patient, in Ogilvie GK, Moore AS (eds). *Feline Oncology: A Comprehensive Guide for Compassionate Care.* Yardley, PA, Veterinary Learning Systems, 2001, pp 1–6.
4. Ogilvie GK: The care of animals with cancer, in Lascelles BD, Dobson J (eds). *BSAVA Manual of Canine & Feline Oncology,* ed 2. Gloucester, UK, British Small Animal Veterinary Association, 2003, pp 68–72.

COMMANDMENTS OF CANCER CARE TO IMPROVE QUALITY OF LIFE

Gregory K. Ogilvie and Antony S. Moore

CLINICAL BRIEFING

Prevent misperceptions	• Meet the medical needs of the patient and the nonmedical needs of the client. Educate each client. Recognize client fears, and take action to enhance quality of life for the pet.
Prevent and treat pain	• Prevention of discomfort is essential whenever possible. NSAIDs, opiates, nerve blocks, and comfort care are important options.
Prevent and treat nausea and diarrhea	• Prevent nausea with drugs such as metoclopramide and serotonin antagonists.
Prevent anorexia	• Appetite stimulants and specific nutritional support for the cancer patient are essential to enhance quality of life.

Cancer is a word that frightens us all. It evokes images of pain, discomfort, baldness, nausea, vomiting, cachexia, and anorexia. These fears and feelings fill the minds of clients and the veterinary health care teams of hospitals worldwide, yet few animal patients that are responsibly treated ever suffer from these adverse effects. In fact, experienced health care teams work hard to ensure that their cancer patients endure few, if any, side effects of cancer therapies. They accomplish this by instituting proactive programs to prevent problems before they ever happen. Similarly, if these unfortunate adverse effects do happen, clients should be informed that their pet will be aggressively and efficiently treated to limit these problems and thus enhance and improve their pet's quality of life. In addition, future treatments will be altered to prevent recurrences of the same side effect. Developing proactive strategies to prevent and treat pain, discomfort, nausea, vomiting, anorexia, weight loss, and starvation is not only the right thing to do for the patient but also vital for meeting the fears and concerns of the people who bring these animals to us.

This discussion reviews the three commandments of cancer care.[1-4] In addition, it is normal for many fears to fill the hearts and minds of caregivers. One of the most frequently mentioned fears is hair loss; however, this side effect fortunately does not commonly occur, except in dogs with constantly growing haircoats, such as poodles and schnauzers.

Meeting the fears and concerns of each client head on with frank, open discussions before beginning to care for the cancer patient is absolutely vital to meeting the medical needs of the patient and the nonmedical needs of the client. It is often said that the more time the team invests at the beginning to make the client as knowledgeable about the disease and treatment as the rest of their pet's health care team, the less frustration and disappointment will follow. The net outcome is that the patient and client are cared for with compassion.

The Commandments

- **Do not let them hurt!**[1-4] Providing an active, preemptive, and ongoing pain management/prevention program for dogs with cancer is absolutely imperative. This reassures the client that the patient's quality of life is optimal. Management should begin with comfort care and then, when needed, be extended to include oral medications (e.g., morphine, codeine, piroxicam, carprofen), transdermal delivery systems (fentanyl patches), acupuncture, or more advanced analgesic delivery systems (e.g., constant-rate intravenous infusion, epidural catheters, intrathoracic pleural analgesia). To keep pain management consistent, it should be overseen

> **KEY POINT**
> *Preventing discomfort, nausea, and anorexia is not only the right thing to do medically for the patient but also the correct thing to do to meet the nonmedical needs of the client.*

> **Commandments of Cancer Care: Action Steps**
>
> - Put your veterinary technician/nursing team in charge of pain management.
> - Make the client aware that discomfort, nausea, or anorexia is not normal and that early intervention is recommended.
> - Make frequent follow-up calls to ensure that the patient is doing well.

> **Karnofsky's Performance Criteria**
>
> | Grade (Circle one) | Criteria |
> |---|---|
> | **0** (normal) | Fully active; able to perform at predisease level |
> | **1** (restricted) | Activity less than predisease level but able to function as an acceptable pet |
> | **2** (compromised) | Severely compromised activity level; ambulatory only to the point of eating, sleeping, and consistently urinating and defecating in acceptable areas |
> | **3** (disabled) | Completely disabled; must be force-fed; unable to control urination and defecation |
>
> Reprinted from Ogilvie GK, Fettman MJ, Mallinckrodt CH, et al: Effect of fish oil, arginine, and doxorubicin chemotherapy on remission and survival time for dogs with lymphoma: A double-blind, randomized placebo-controlled study. *Cancer* 88(8):1916–1928, 2000; with permission.

by a veterinary technician/nursing team (see the box "Commandments of Cancer Care: Action Steps" on this page). The most important principle is that the caregivers know in advance that the veterinary health care team will not tolerate the patient suffering any pain but will work together to recognize, prevent, and manage it. A more complete discussion of pain management can be found in Chapter 29.

- **Do not let them vomit or have diarrhea!**[1-4] This commandment strikes at the preconceived and unfounded fear that dogs on chemotherapy often experience significant bouts of nausea and diarrhea. This simply is not true. With recent advances in cancer care, nausea, vomiting, and diarrhea are no longer commonly associated with chemotherapy. Moreover, the introduction of a large number of antiemetics and antidiarrheals in clinical practice has made it possible to control these problems if they do occur. Dispensing an oral medication such as metoclopramide to the caregiver each and every time a potentially nauseating drug is administered empowers the client to prevent this clinical sign at home. In addition, we must be prepared to stop nausea and vomiting by ensuring that medications and supportive care are immediately available. Having access to drugs such as ondansetron hydrochloride and dolasetron mesylate, although costly, will provide this level of assurance for all members of the team. Some practitioners believe that tylosin, metronidazole, and loperamide hydrochloride can reduce the risk of small- and large-bowel diarrhea, so they often dispense these drugs to their cancer patients to prevent these problems. Increasing fiber intake can be of great value in enhancing bowel health. A more comprehensive discussion about the management of nausea and vomiting can be found in Chapter 30.

- **Do not let them starve!**[1-4] This final commandment is just as vital as the first two. In the minds of many caregivers, patients undergoing cancer care often appear cachectic and weak. Using the team approach and providing care that ensures our patients will eat are vitally important. The reality is that appetite and adequate nutritional support are absolutely dependent on the success of the treatment plan to prevent and treat discomfort and nausea. If the plan has not resolved the problem, then nursing care (e.g., warming food, providing aromatic foods and comfortable environments), medicinal appetite stimulants, and, when needed, assisted feeding techniques such as esophagostomy, gastrostomy, or jejunostomy tube placement should be employed. All of these components of nutritional care must be available early in the course of the disease, and weight loss must not be tolerated, particularly in dogs that have fewer reserves due to their small size. To our clients, appetite is a vital, objective assessment of quality of life that must not be overlooked or left to chance. A more complete description of nutritional care can be found in Chapter 31.

Quantitating Quality of Life

Employing the commandments to meet the needs of the patient and the client is one very important step toward the holy grail of cancer therapy: enhancing quality of life.[5-7] Despite the importance of this ultimate goal, very little has been written about the subject. Each and every veterinarian takes a personal and professional oath to alleviate the pain and suffering of animals, yet few published papers directly define and quantitate this most important and essential of all objectives. Factors that contribute to quality of life for all animals are subjective but often involve good relationships, mental stimulation, health, food consumption, low stress, and control over the environment.[5-7]

People define quality of life differently for themselves and their pets. Therefore, the veterinary health care team must understand how it is defined by each client for his or her pet. The team must concurrently dispel the myths and misperceptions associated with cancer therapy to ensure that they do not

Table 5-1 Modified Eastern Cooperative Oncology Group Evaluation
(Completely circle appropriate boxes or strike out with "NA")

	Grade 0	Grade 1	Grade 2	Grade 3	Grade 4
Leukopenia					
White blood cells (×10³/µl)	>5.5	3–<5.5	2–<3	1–<2	<1
Neutrophils (×10³/µl)	>2.5	1.5–<2.5	1–<1.5	0.5–<1	<0.5
Lymphocytes (×10³/µl)	>1.5	1–<1.5	0.5–<1	0–<0.5	0
Thrombocytopenia (platelets ×10³/µl)	>130	90–<130	50–<90	25–<50	<25
Anemia					
Hematocrit (%)	>25	20–<25	15–<20	10–<15	<10
Clinical	None	—	—	Seizure	Transfusion
Hemorrhage	None	Minimal	Moderately debilitating	Debilitating	Life-threatening
Infection	None	No treatment needed	Requires treatment	Debilitating	Life-threatening
Urinary					
Blood urea nitrogen (mg/dl)	<20	21–40	41–60	>60	Sympt
Creatinine (mg/dl)	<2	2.1–4	4.1–6	>6	Uremia
Proteinuria	None	1+	2+–3+	4+	
Hematuria	None	Microscopic	Gross	Gross-Clot	Urinary obstruction
Hepatic (× normal limit)					
Alanine aminotransferase	<1.5	1.5–2	2.1–5	>5	
Alkaline phosphatase	<1.5	1.5–2	2.1–5	>5	
Bilirubin	<1.5	1.5–2	2.1–5	>5	
Clinical	None			Precoma	Coma
Nausea and vomiting	None	Nausea	Continuous vomiting	Intractable	
Diarrhea	None	Loose	Dehydration	Bloody	
Pulmonary (clinical)	None	Mild	Moderate	Severe	Requires oxygen
Cardiac	None	Heart rate >200 bpm	Arrhythmia	Mild congestive heart failure	Severe congestive heart failure
Neurology					
Peripheral nerves	None	Mild	Moderate	Moderate to severe	Severe
Central nervous system	None	Depressed	Moderate ± tremor	Severe ± coma	Coma

Reprinted from Ogilvie GK, Fettman MJ, Mallinckrodt CH, et al: Effect of fish oil, arginine, and doxorubicin chemotherapy on remission and survival time for dogs with lymphoma: A double-blind, randomized placebo-controlled study. *Cancer* 88(8):1916–1928, 2000; with permission.

cause the client to make inappropriate decisions about cancer and cancer therapy for their pet (see Chapter 3). When most veterinarians, other members of the veterinary health care team, and clients initially describe cancer, chemotherapy, radiation therapy, and cancer surgery, they often do so with words such as pain, vomiting, diarrhea, starvation, and lack of hope. However, the reality is often perceived much more positively. In one study, clients whose dogs had lymphoma and were treated with multidrug chemotherapy were interviewed to assess the quality of their pet's life during treatment.[7] Most owners (68%) considered their dog's quality of life to be the same as before the lymphoma occurred, and the rest felt that their pet's quality of life was acceptable although poorer than before the lymphoma occurred. Most clients (92%) had no regrets about treating their dog with chemotherapy.

Converting the myriad of subjective parameters into objective, numeric data for analysis and comparison has been difficult in both human and veterinary medicine. Several investigators have tried to enumerate parameters of toxicity and performance (see the box "Karnofsky's Performance Criteria," on page 19, and Table 5-1).[8] More recent efforts, especially those in enumerating parameters associated with discomfort, have employed a scale of 0 to 100. The caregiver is asked to subjectively rate parameters such as quality of life, appetite, and nausea initially and at subsequent specified time points during treatment, then to compare the subsequent assessments with the initial findings (Figure 5-1). The veterinary health care team scores and records these assessments for later analysis.

There is little doubt that all therapies should be linked to their impact on the patient's and client's quality of life. This parameter is considered by many to be at least as important—if not more so—than duration of remission and quality of life.

At our care center, your pet's quality of life is very important to us. In order to help us help your pet, please have the same person subjectively mark the parameters noted below. Do it at the same time each week. Please bring this with you at the time of your next appointment.

How is your pet doing now?

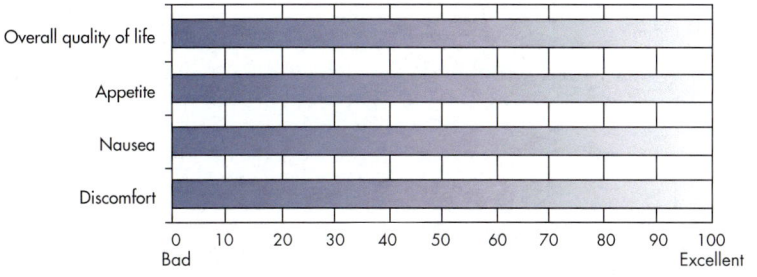

How is your pet doing at the end of the first week?

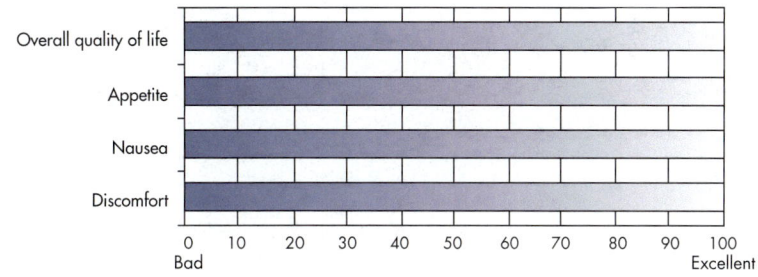

How is your pet doing at the end of the second week?

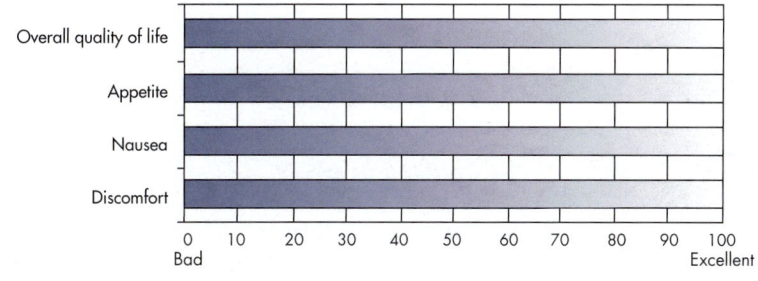

How is your pet doing at the end of the third week?

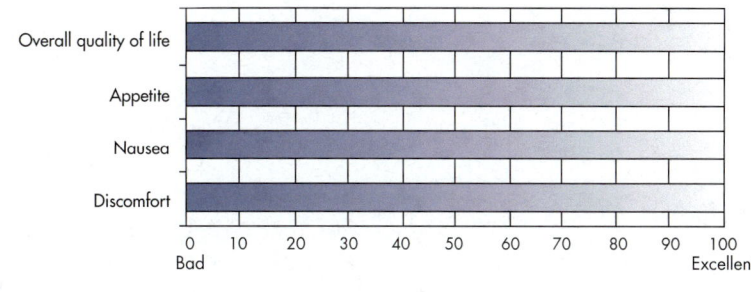

Figure 5-1. *Linear subjective assessment of each patient. Clients place a mark on the bar to assess their pet's quality of life. These are converted into numeric numbers (mm of bar, to a maximum of 100 mm) that can then be assessed.*

REFERENCES

1. Mitchener KL, Ogilvie GK: Rekindling the bond. *Vet Econ* 40:30–36, 1999.
2. Mitchener KL, Ogilvie GK: Giving cancer patients hope. *Vet Econ* 40:84–88, 1999.
3. Ogilvie GK, Moore AS: Compassionate care of the cancer patient, in Ogilvie GK, Moore AS (eds). *Feline Oncology: A Comprehensive Guide for Compassionate Care.* Yardley, PA, Veterinary Learning Systems, 2001, pp 1–6.
4. Ogilvie GK: The care of animals with cancer, in Lascelles BD, Dobson J (eds). *BSAVA Manual of Canine & Feline Oncology,* ed 2. Gloucester, UK, British Small Animal Veterinary Association, 2003, pp 68–72.
5. McMillan FD: Maximizing quality of life in ill animals. *JAAHA* 39(3):227–235, 2003.
6. McMillan FD: Quality of life in animals. *JAVMA* 216(12): 1904–1910, 2000.
7. Mellanby RJ, Herrtage ME, Dobson JM: Owners' assessments of their dog's quality of life during palliative chemotherapy for lymphoma. *J Small Anim Pract* 44(3): 100–103, 2003.
8. Ogilvie GK, Fettman MJ, Mallinckrodt CH, et al: Effect of fish oil, arginine, and doxorubicin chemotherapy on remission and survival time for dogs with lymphoma: A double-blind, randomized placebo-controlled study. *Cancer* 88(8): 1916–1928, 2000.

SETTING GOALS FOR COMPASSIONATE CARE

Gregory K. Ogilvie and Antony S. Moore

CLINICAL BRIEFING

Definitive (curative) care	• Elimination of all evidence of cancer for the normal life of the patient.
Palliative care	• Treatment of a patient to improve quality of life but not necessarily length of life.
Supportive care	• Implies treating the patient's clinical signs rather than the tumor itself. Supportive care is often used in combination with palliative care.
Hospice care	• Care to maintain quality of life, especially comfort in the terminal phases of a disease.
Euthanasia	• Termination of life.

Establishing Goals and Providing Care[1-8]

Once the myths have been dispelled, the team has been established (see Chapter 3), and the commandments have been initiated to enhance quality of life (see Chapter 5), the goals of therapy need to be defined so that the patient can be cared for. Patient care includes providing direct therapy for the underlying disease and providing compassionate care focused on accomplishing the goals set by the client in close cooperation with the veterinary health care team. Care to fulfill these goals is provided by using the appropriate tools at hand, such as supportive care, surgery, chemotherapy, or radiation therapy.

> **KEY POINT**
> *Cancer is the most curable of all chronic diseases in human and veterinary medicine.*

Some clients and members of the veterinary health care team think that if cure is not achievable, then "success" cannot be secured. This is simply not true, especially with the advent of more recent therapies that can control or arrest cancer for sustained periods. In addition, each client has his or her own goals for quality and length of life as well as his or her own limits for the possibility of adverse effects and cost of care. In short, all options should be given, from the very highest level of curative and palliative therapy to supportive and hospice care and finally to euthanasia. Each step should be made and supported by the whole veterinary health care team. However, this may require that the veterinary health care team define its limits and capabilities in advance. The following are a few of the many options that may be considered for each patient.

Definitive, Curative Intent[1-8]

Cancer is the most curable of all chronic diseases in human and veterinary medicine. Cure is the goal of every client and veterinary health care team and is often mistaken as the only goal. Most cures are accomplished through good surgical techniques and a clear understanding of cancer biology. Radiation therapy and chemotherapy may be key in the realization of some of these benefits, but to a lesser degree. The success rate of curative intent will increase by first knowing the name and extent of the disease and by planning to control or cure the cancer while maintaining quality of life (Figure 6-1). The definition of "cure" is elusive, as there is no absolute cutoff past which it can be guaranteed that the cancer is eradicated; however, some consider 2 years and others consider 5 years as the point to call the disease cured.

Palliative Care[1-8]

Palliative care is the treatment of a patient to improve quality of life but not necessarily length of life. For example, coarse fraction radiation to a site of bony metastasis is primarily designed to alleviate pain without curing or lengthening the life span of the patient. This is exactly what is done in many other, nonneoplastic, chronic diseases such as osteoarthritis and chronic renal failure. Indeed, cancer is being redefined in biomedical sciences as a chronic disease.

24 MANAGING THE CANINE CANCER PATIENT

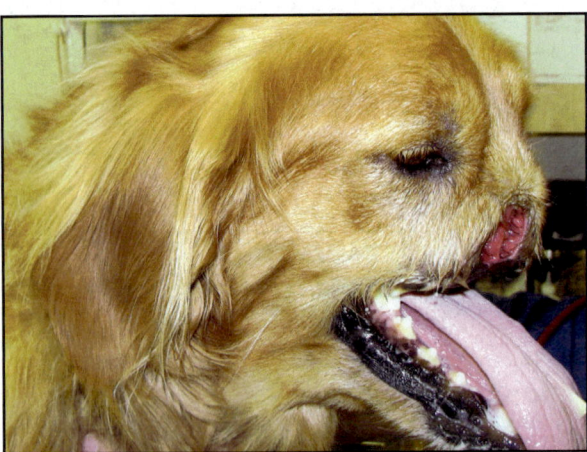

Figure 6-1. *Cancer can be cured or controlled, or the patient can be supported as long as possible. A rostral maxillectomy resulted in cure for this golden retriever with a soft tissue sarcoma. The client was willing to accept the cosmetic changes in trade for the pet's improved quality of life and increased length of life. The client was supported by the entire veterinary health care team and empowered with information before and after surgery. The result was complete resolution of the cancer, a happy client, and a dog that now lives a normal life.*

As molecular therapeutic agents, radiation therapy, and other treatments are developed and evaluated, veterinary medicine will have to go through a paradigm shift so that we can celebrate and be pleased with improving the quality of life despite the fact that the length of life may not be increased.

> **KEY POINT**
> *As molecular therapeutic agents, radiation therapy, and other treatments are developed and evaluated, veterinary medicine will have to go through a paradigm shift so that we can celebrate and be pleased with improving the quality of life despite the fact that the length of life may not be enhanced.*

Supportive and Hospice Care[1-8]

Little difference exists between palliative and supportive care. Both are defined as treatment to improve quality of life without necessarily increasing length of life. Supportive care often treats the patient's clinical signs rather than the tumor itself and often is used in combination with palliative care. Supportive care is provided by administering analgesics, antiemetics, appetite stimulants, and treatments for anemia and leukopenia. Hospice care, or care to maintain quality of life, is a type of supportive care; however, it is usually defined as comfort or supportive care at the end of life. Hospice care, especially comfort in the terminal phases of a disease, is a defined specialty in human medical care. This type of care is rapidly developing in veterinary medicine. Dignity and comfort until death, whether from euthanasia or natural causes, are rapidly becoming acceptable necessities in many practices.

The most common misconceptions—and the realities—about hospice care are as follows:

- **Patients have to be cared for 24 hours a day, 7 days a week.** With appropriate arrangements for patient care and safety, pets can be left alone for short periods.
- **Hospice care is not sophisticated.** The care of the animal patient in a hospice setting can be as complex as the client and the rest of the veterinary health care team wish. Oxygen cages, constant-rate infusion nutritional support, and epidural analgesia are always possible in a home environment with appropriate education and support.
- **Animals that enter a hospice care environment cannot be admitted to the hospital for routine care.** The level of care is totally up to the client and the veterinary health care team at all times.
- **Animals that enter a hospice care situation cannot be resuscitated.** Clients can ensure that resuscitation is possible if their pet has a cardiac or respiratory arrest.

Euthanasia[1-8]

An important aspect of many levels of care, including hospice care, is the process of euthanasia. Euthanasia is also often employed to alleviate pain, suffering, or unwanted aspects of care or the disease. The importance of performing euthanasia properly cannot be emphasized enough. More clients leave a practice as a result of an unpleasant experience over the loss of a pet than for any other reason. Managing this difficult aspect of compassionate care involves adequate preparation as well as ongoing dialogue between the entire veterinary health care team and the client both before and at the time of euthanasia and death. Because euthanasia is such an important part of veterinary medicine, a brief description of that process is included in Chapter 7.

REFERENCES

1. Ogilvie GK, Moore AS: Compassionate care of the cancer patient, in Ogilvie GK, Moore AS: *Feline Oncology: A Comprehensive Guide for Compassionate Care.* Yardley, PA, Veterinary Learning Systems, 2001, pp 1–6.
2. Ogilvie GK: Préservation de la santé des animaux âgés, in *Gériatrie vétérinaire. Les Editions du point vétérinaire*. Nantes, Intervet, 2004, pp 51–56.
3. Ogilvie GK: Pris en charge du cancer chez l'animal âgé, in *Gériatrie vétérinaire. Les Editions du point vétérinaire*. Nantes, Intervet, 2004, pp 61–66.
4. Ogilvie GK: The care of animals with cancer, in Dobson JM, Lascelles BD (eds): *BSAVA Manual of Canine & Feline Oncology*, ed 2. Gloucester, UK, British Small Animal Veterinary Association, 2003, 68–72.
5. Mitchener KL, Ogilvie GK: Rekindling the bond. *Vet Econ* 40:30–36, 1999.
6. Mitchener KL, Ogilvie GK: Giving cancer patients hope. *Vet Econ* 40:84–88, 1999.
7. Downing R: *Pets Living with Cancer: A Pet Owner's Resource*. Denver, American Animal Hospital Association, 2000, pp 1–8.
8. Ogilvie GK: Meeting the needs of patient and client through compassionate care, in Ettinger SJ, Feldman EC (eds): *Textbook of Veterinary Internal Medicine*, ed 6. Philadelphia, WB Saunders, 2005, pp 535–538.

PET LOSS AND BEREAVEMENT
Gregory K. Ogilvie and Antony S. Moore

CLINICAL BRIEFING

Key steps for a compassionate euthanasia process
- Discuss procedure, body care, and emotions in advance if possible.
- Prepare at the time of euthanasia by reviewing the procedure and the cascade of emotions that are likely to ensue.
- Preplace the catheter before the client enters the room or area for euthanasia.
- Administer euthanasia solutions.
- Follow up to allow grief to proceed normally.

The wisest veterinary health care teams often bring up the topic of euthanasia and the inevitable process of grieving and bereavement with their clients before they are imminent. This is a key part of preparing clients for this very important event. If clients consider the options facing their pet at a time when they are not fearful and grieving, they will be able to make clearer decisions that benefit them later. It is also a good idea for caregivers to make a list of the positive aspects of their pet's life at a time before treatment has started and before the cancer is advanced. This can be life-affirming and may also act as a "baseline" for future assessments of the impact of the cancer and treatment on quality of life.

Knowing When "It Is Time"

Most clients ask how they will know when it is time to euthanatize their pet. People base this decision on their own value systems, but the timing is often quite similar for most pet owners. While it is tempting to respond to the question, "What would you do if it were your dog, Doc?" most clinicians believe that the veterinarian and other members of the veterinary health care team should take the role of educator and leave the ultimate decision to the client.

The veterinary health care team can assist the client by defining objective parameters for quality of life, such as appetite, normal behavior patterns, and energy level that can be monitored and assessed at home. These definitions and measured observations allow the caregiver to objectively assess his or her pet's quality of life and to monitor changes. Unless there are extenuating circumstances, clients should be supported once they have come to the conclusion that euthanasia is the best option for them. This support can happen in a number of ways, such as validating the client's decision or assisting the client in understanding the euthanasia and bereavement processes. By supporting the caregivers and allowing them to be active decision makers, the veterinary health care team provides a sense of empowerment during a time that would otherwise be marked only by feelings of helplessness and defeat.

Preparing the Client and Staff

The success of the euthanasia process can be enhanced by preparing the client adequately about what will take place. Myths can be dispelled with an open, clear description of the euthanasia process and the impact that it may have on the pet owner for months or years in the future. The caregivers need to first understand how a patient is euthanatized. Empowering clients with information and the ability to select details such as the timing, location, and tempo of the euthanasia process can help them feel more in control. Each client will differ in his or her needs and wants, but examples include organizing the presence of family and friends, reading poetry or books, or reciting favorite stories about their beloved pet. When possible, a secluded, comfortable location in the clinic should be available with a private entrance and exit to avoid any embarrassing situations such as having the tearful client walk through a waiting room full of clients and their healthy pets.

The client is not the only one who will be affected by euthanasia. Indeed, each member of the veterinary health care team is likely to be impacted by the loss of the patient. Therefore, time should be set aside before and after the procedure not only for the client and his or her family but also for the health care team to say goodbye. Finally, the health care team should ensure that the client and all staff members who might be seriously impacted by the loss of the pet have thought in advance of how they will get home safely.

In families with children, the children are often involved in the decision to perform euthanasia. It is important that children not be sheltered from the decision-making process. Excluding children or making up stories (e.g., Fluffy ran

26 MANAGING THE CANINE CANCER PATIENT

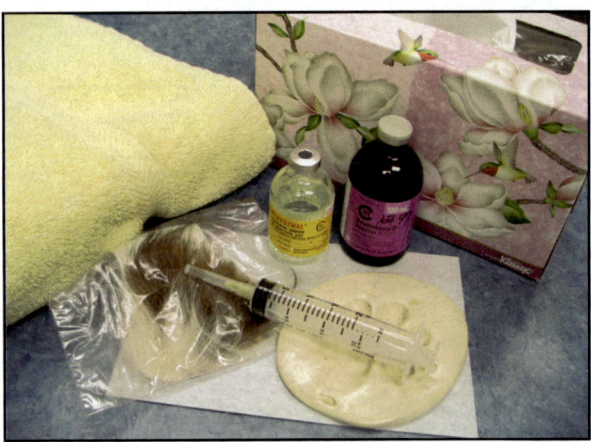

Figure 7-1. *Essential supplies for euthanasia should be known by the entire veterinary health care team to ensure that the process is efficient and that the experience is meaningful for the client. A towel or blanket is often helpful, especially if there is loss of bowel or bladder control. Facial tissues should always be plentiful and easily accessible. Thiopental sodium and the euthanasia solution should be drawn up before euthanasia into Luer-Lok syringes to prevent accidental loss of drug at the time of injection. Thiopental relaxes the patient and prevents unwanted movements, gasps, and trembles when the euthanasia solution is injected. Finally, transition objects to help grieving should also be available. A plastic bag and scissors for clipping fur and clay for making paw prints can help the family long after the euthanasia itself is complete.*

away) is destructive and can cause psychological damage that can affect the way people process grief or even the decision to bring another animal into the home. An open and honest discussion with children is imperative. They should be allowed the chance to say goodbye to their pet, too.

Finally, it is obviously very important to discuss openly, frankly, and compassionately what will be done with the dog's remains. Burial, cremation, and disposal by your facility are viable options. If burial or cremation is considered, a choice of coffins or urns may be important to some clients. Commercial cardboard coffins are available and affordable for most. Ideally, all of these decisions can be made early in the course of treatment, but for many clients the final details will have to wait until they are prepared to consider the choices.

When discussing the euthanasia process, what to expect, and body care before the time of euthanasia, the veterinary health care team should reinforce the following points for the client:

- A catheter will need to be placed before the procedure. Many clinics prefer to place the catheter in a back leg to allow caregivers to sit by the patient's head.
- Identifying a comfortable, quiet location that meets the wishes of the client is a vital aspect of a successful euthanasia. Include children, friends, and other family animals, and encourage full participation by everyone who wishes to be involved. Spending appropriate time with the pet before and after euthanasia is important.
- The euthanasia process is quick, and the injections will place the pet into a peaceful level of sleep that will then stop the heart forever, resulting in death. (Many veterinary health care teams ask their clients to sign an informed consent form for euthanasia.)
- At the time of death, the pet's eyes may not close, and there may be loss of bladder and bowel control. That is normal.
- Clients are encouraged to memorialize their pet in any way they prefer, such as clipping hair, making paw prints, or taking photographs at any time.
- Body care options may include cremation, burial, or disposal by the hospital and its associates.

The Procedure

If given the option, most clients wish to be present during the euthanasia process. This requires that the staff be trained and prepared during this emotional time, but it does not suggest that emotion should not be shared or that sadness, crying, or tears are ever unprofessional. If an owner decides not to be present, that decision should be supported as well.

To expedite the process, a catheter is often preplaced within the distal extremity. This reduces the need to acquire vascular access in a dog at a time when the client's expectations and tensions are highest. Some teams find that placement in the medial saphenous vein allows good access to a vein often not used for previous therapy. When the euthanasia solution is delivered, clients should not be restrained or discouraged from comforting or holding the pet, nor should they have to observe the needle and syringe.

As discussed above, the veterinarian and the health care team should review the process with the client regarding what to expect before, during, and after euthanasia. While euthanasia can be performed with a number of different drugs, many veterinarians are comfortable that thiopental (18 mg/kg IV over 10 to 30 seconds) followed immediately by pentobarbital (88 mg/kg IV over 10 seconds) results in a smooth, effortless transition to a state of death. Some believe it is ideal to premedicate certain patients with a tranquilizer before catheter placement. A towel or other absorbent object may be placed under the dog to capture any body excretions, and a towel covering the dog's rear end will prevent the owner from seeing any elimination that might occur (Figure 7-1).

After the process is reviewed with the client, the catheter is placed, the location, setting, and rituals are designed, and the time for euthanasia arrives. While every veterinarian has his or her own style and procedures, many feel it is important for

Support Resources for Grieving Pet Owners

University of California, Davis Pet Loss Hotline (staffed by veterinary students)
Phone: 800-565-1526
Web: www.vetmed.ucdavis.edu/petloss/index.htm

Cornell University Pet Loss Support Hotline (staffed by Cornell University veterinary students)
Phone: 607-253-3932
Web: http://web.vet.cornell.edu/public/petloss/

Tufts University Pet Loss Support Hotline (staffed by Tufts University veterinary students)
Phone: 508-839-7966
Web: www.tufts.edu/vet/petloss

Argus Institute for Families and Veterinary Medicine
Phone: 970-297-1242
Web: www.argusinstitute.colostate.edu

Washington State University Pet Loss Hotline
Phone: 509-335-5704
Web: www.vetmed.wsu.edu/PLHL/home/index.asp

Pet Loss Support
Web: www.pet-loss.net/resources/CA.html

Common Feelings, Behaviors, and Symptoms That May Be Seen in Clients after the Death of a Pet[1-5]

Feelings and Behaviors
Hope or hopelessness
Disbelief
Relief, especially with a prolonged illness or financial restrictions
Helplessness
Yearning
Tearfulness and crying
Confusion or inability to concentrate
Waves of mental pain
Feelings of separation or longing
Anger or guilt
Fear or anxiety

Physical Symptoms
Increased or decreased appetite with subsequent changes in body weight
Decreased energy, weakness
Nausea or diarrhea
Altered libido
Sleeplessness
Feeling that something is stuck in the throat
Tightness in the chest
Sensitivity to noise
Vivid dreams
Dry mouth

---

other team members to be present or at least say their goodbyes. The process may be reviewed briefly one more time before the catheter is checked for patency and the drugs are injected. It is very important for the attending veterinarian to listen to the heart for an appropriate period and then indicate when the heart has stopped and that the beloved dog has died. A gentle touch and an offer of facial tissues are appropriate, affirmative, supportive gestures. They tell a client that a display of emotion is accepted by everyone, including the attending clinician. At this point, the client and friends and family may wish to spend time alone with their dog. Many veterinarians do not have clients deal with paying bills at this time but prefer instead to mail them the charges.

Following Up

Follow-up communication can be very important for the client and the veterinary health care team alike. Cards, letters, or flowers sent by the staff can not only be important to the client but also help bring closure for the entire team. Adding a picture of the patient to a scrapbook or a bulletin board of beloved pets may also be of value in memorializing special patients.

There is no single way for clients or the team to work through their grief. Ideally, clients should be made aware of pet loss support groups, hotlines, and local specialists who are knowledgeable about loss and receptive to helping people who have lost a beloved pet (see box at top left). These support services, even if they are not used, provide a sense of validation for the caregiver's loss and grief and can be of lasting benefit to everyone involved.

Establishing a Smooth Process

Employing curative, palliative, supportive, hospice, and euthanasia care requires careful client communication in oral, written, and visual formats. The client and the veterinary health care team need to define goals and realistic expectations. Boundaries and limits must be set by both sides, with the intent being always to provide compassionate care for the patient. When there are philosophic differences between the veterinary health care team and the client regarding a decision to perform euthanasia or to continue care, referral to another center with the patient's complete records is important. If local support groups or counselors with specific training in pet loss and bereavement exist, they should be employed at the earliest possible moment to establish a relationship and a plan before a moment of crisis. In addition, creating a plan for a natural death or euthanasia is very important, preferably at moments of calm and support rather than during a crisis. Following are action steps for establishing a smooth euthanasia process:

- Review all possibilities for cure, palliation, support, terminal care, and euthanasia with the client. Include cost and time requirements as well as potential toxicity and probability of success of care.

- Educate clients that care is often a transition from palliation and support to hospice care and finally to euthanasia.
- Set milestones of time to review goals using medical information in combination with emotional support.

Helping Bereaved Clients

At the time of death, clients, their family members, and, in many cases, members of the veterinary health care team are in a state of shock. Some clients may be distraught to the point of being violent (see "Common Feelings" box on previous page). The veterinary health care team can help these families by openly sharing their grief, by sharing personal stories about the patient, and by celebrating what the family did to support and care for the patient that has passed away. The day after the pet's death, it is often very helpful to call the family to offer condolences and help. The key at this time is to be a good listener. Writing a condolence letter or penning a card of sympathy is often of profound importance to the family of a pet that has died. One to 2 months after the pet's death, another call or letter will show sincerity and sympathy and can be of great help to the family.

Clinicians and health care team members can support clients and other team members in their time of grief by doing the following[1-5]:

- Reassuring everyone involved that the pain will subside and that grief over the loss of a pet is normal.
- Encouraging clients to attend support groups that are sensitive to the importance of pets in the family.
- Encouraging bereaved clients to talk to others about their feelings and thoughts.
- Encouraging everyone involved to exercise regularly.
- Ensuring that each person has time alone for reflection and recovery.
- Reassuring everyone involved that it is normal to have negative feelings and that each person's grief is unique.
- Ensuring that everyone is allowed to feel their loss and to grieve in their own way.

REFERENCES

1. Ogilvie GK: The care of animals with cancer, in Dobson JM, Lascelles BD (eds): *BSAVA Manual of Canine and Feline Oncology*, ed 2. Gloucester, UK, British Small Animal Veterinary Association, 2003, pp 68–72.
2. Mitchener KL, Ogilvie GK: Rekindling the bond. *Vet Econ* 40:30–36, 1999.
3. Mitchener KL, Ogilvie GK: Giving cancer patients hope. *Vet Econ* 40:84–88, 1999.
4. Ogilvie GK: Meeting the needs of patient and client through compassionate care, in Ettinger SJ, Feldman EC (eds): *Textbook of Veterinary Internal Medicine*, ed 6. Philadelphia, WB Saunders, 2005, pp 535–538.
5. Lagoni L, Butler C, Hetts S: *The Human Animal Bond and Grief.* Philadelphia, WB Saunders, 1994.

COMPASSION FATIGUE
Gregory K. Ogilvie and Antony S. Moore

CLINICAL BRIEFING

Definition	• Inevitable consequence of empathy and caring from the heart; results from depletion of internal emotional resources; often confused with burnout.
Critical incident	• An emotional event can trigger the onset of compassion fatigue.
Clinical signs	• Loss of interest, decreased enthusiasm, and physical and psychological changes.
Prevention and therapy	• Recognition of condition; taking breaks; exercising; ensuring balanced nutrition.

The Cost of Caring: Compassion Fatigue

Providing care from both the heart and science requires the ability to express empathy. However, the empathetic response can lead to compassion fatigue.[1-8] When we find ourselves giving without adequately replenishing ourselves, it is only a matter of time before we experience a shortage of compassion and a sense of fatigue. Simply put, compassion fatigue occurs when we have depleted our emotional resources as we care for others.

Compassion fatigue is not a reflection of our character, professionalism, or skill level but is directly related to our willingness to be emotionally engaged with another being that is hurting. Compassion fatigue has or will strike every member of a caring health care team. The phenomenon is not limited to veterinary professionals but occurs in physicians, nurses, firemen, combat medics, and others in similar professions.[1-8]

Compassion fatigue is the reason many caring, compassionate veterinarians, nurses, receptionists, and other caregivers leave the profession. The desire to leave the veterinary profession can strike at any age but seems to occur most often when a person is at the height of his or her professional career as a caregiver. Awareness and understanding of this condition are essential in its prevention and treatment and in maintaining the health of the team.

Compassion Fatigue versus Burnout

Compassion fatigue is perhaps the greatest threat to the health and happiness of any member of the veterinary health care team. Although compassion fatigue is considered to be a form of burnout and has many of the same symptoms,[1] the two conditions are unique. The conditions must be distinguished because they have different causes and paths to recovery.

Compassion fatigue is not predictable; it results when one's internal emotional resources are depleted.[1] Sometimes a member of the veterinary health care team provides so much care and compassion to clients who are experiencing an emotional moment, such as when a diagnosis of cancer is being discussed, that they find themselves depleted. Compassion fatigue is triggered by one or more emotionally charged events (called *critical incidents*) at a time when one's emotional resources are exhausted. Members of the veterinary health care team often experience critical incidents when other people become emotionally distressed.

> **KEY POINT**
> *Compassion fatigue is perhaps the greatest threat to the health and happiness of any member of the veterinary health care team.*

Extreme examples are the experiences of those who identified or provided care to people or animals killed or injured in the September 11 World Trade Center disaster or to the search-and-rescue dogs involved in the recovery efforts; more commonplace examples include performing and experiencing euthanasia, helping an owner through the loss of a pet, informing a caregiver that his or her pet has cancer, providing terminal patient care, and discussing the financial affordability of care.[1-8] Each member of the veterinary health care team must be considered unique, and the way each person deals with critical incidents differs, often based on his or her individual experiences, beliefs, and values. In addition, compassion fatigue may intensify the emotional and physical symptoms in team members who are already experiencing burnout, and burnout can likewise intensify compassion fatigue.

> **Key Points in Mitigating Compassion Fatigue**
>
> - Educate the entire veterinary health care team about compassionate fatigue and its consequences.
> - Establish weekly debriefing sessions in which the entire staff can discuss needs, concerns, and cases that weigh on them.
> - Establish resources about compassion fatigue, including a library, for team members.
> - Use relaxation techniques both within the hospital and outside the workplace.
> - Take breaks during the day.
> - Define and preserve a sanctuary or comfort room where team members can be alone to meditate or relax.
> - Inform all team members about every case and allow them to have adequate closure at the end of any patient's life.
> - Whenever possible, work out sabbatical or continuing education opportunities for personal reward and growth.
> - Teach team members how to set limits and boundaries on interactions with clients and patients, especially when they are susceptible to compassion fatigue.
> - Employ humor when appropriate.
> - Find a friend or colleague who understands and appreciates the experience of providing empathy and compassion, and share with that person.
> - Eat right and exercise.
> - Get in touch with nature and the outdoors.
> - Interact with children and animals.

The following experiences are sometimes associated with compassion fatigue:[1-8]

- Avoiding thoughts, feelings, activities, or situations that remind one of a frightening experience.
- Feeling estranged from other members of the veterinary health care team or feeling that there is no one to talk to.
- Having difficulty falling or staying asleep, especially when loss of sleep is related to memories or experiences being played over and over in one's mind.
- Experiencing outbursts of anger or irritability with little provocation.
- Needing to "work through" a traumatic experience associated with a patient or client to get over the event.
- Being preoccupied with a previous critical incident or with specific patients or their caregivers.
- Losing concern about the well-being of coworkers, patients, and caregivers.
- Feeling trapped, hopeless, edgy, weak, tired, run down, or depressed.
- Wanting to avoid certain patients and their caregivers.
- Feeling disliked by clients and their families.
- Being unable to separate work and personal life.
- Feeling like one works more for the money than for personal fulfillment.
- Having feelings of failure.

Burnout is predictable and very common. It is not necessarily associated with the exhaustion of emotion or empathy but rather is a state of mental and/or physical exhaustion caused by excessive and prolonged stress. Two major causes of burnout are bureaucratic atmospheres and overwork. Burnout is not associated with the aforementioned critical incidents, but it is predictably associated with the stress of overwork, repetition, or the bureaucracy of seemingly less-important tasks, such as paying bills, reviewing reports, and endless paperwork without apparent value or worth.

Prevention and Therapy

So how do people provide compassionate care, meet the medical and nonmedical needs of patients and caregivers, and stay true to what brought them to a caring profession without experiencing fatigue and potentially devastating consequences? First, we must acknowledge that as a profession—by the very nature of what we do and who we are—we are at risk for compassion fatigue. Simply by acknowledging the condition and accepting that we are vulnerable, we can see the potential hazards, recognize likely inciting situations, and hopefully prevent devastating outcomes. We also must work with all staff members to experience and then celebrate the sense of achievement in the work in which we are involved. On a daily basis, veterinary health care teams intervene in the lives of clients and their pets to provide high-quality medical, surgical, and preventive care while offering emotional support and validating the bond that brings pets and people to our offices. This is compassionate care; to accomplish it well requires a great deal of emotional energy from every team member. In this manner, we provide for the needs of our patients and caregivers. The act of caring is the epitome of success in our profession, regardless of the emotional nature of the situation or the medical outcome. Although compassion fatigue cannot be completely avoided, there are many strategies to help team members mitigate its impact (see box on this page).

Conclusion

When we employ compassion in caring for our patients, we must do so by expressing empathy, yet the act of empathizing with our clients can lead to compassion fatigue. When any member of the veterinary health care team finds him- or herself giving without allowing him- or herself to be replenished emotionally, it is only a matter of time before there will be a shortage of compassion. Simply put, compassion fatigue results when there is a depletion of internal emotional resources as we care and provide compassion for others. This depletion is not a reflection of the character, professionalism, or skill level of the team member. Rather, one's strength and willingness to be emotionally engaged with another being is affected. All members of the veterinary health care team join the profession to provide care, which comes from both their minds (through medical and surgical skills) and their hearts (by supporting and providing for the emotional needs of caregivers). The success of veterinary care stems from providing this level of compassionate care and supporting the individuals who provide it. By appreciating the reality of compassion fatigue and providing mechanisms to mitigate its effects, a practice can thrive by providing the finest in compassionate care.

REFERENCES

1. Mitchener KL, Ogilvie GK: Understanding compassion fatigue: Keys for the caring veterinary health care team. *JAAHA* 38(4):307–310, 2002.
2. Collins S, Long A: Too tired to care? The psychological effects of working with trauma. *J Psychiatr Ment Health Nurs* 10(1):17–27, 2003.
3. Radziewicz RM: Self-care for the caregiver. *Nurs Clin North Am* 36(4):855–869, 2001.
4. Clark ML, Gioro S: Nurses, indirect trauma, and prevention. *Image J Nurs Sch* 30(1):85–87, 1998.
5. Vachon ML: Caring for the caregiver in oncology and palliative care. *Semin Oncol Nurs* 14(2):152–157, 1998.
6. Welsh DJ: Care for the caregiver: Strategies for avoiding "compassion fatigue." *Clin J Oncol Nurs* 3(4):183–184, 1999.
7. Thomas RB, Wilson JP: Issues and controversies in the understanding and diagnosis of compassion fatigue, vicarious traumatization, and secondary traumatic stress disorder. *Int J Emerg Ment Health* 6(2):81–92, 2004.
8. Boscarino JA, Figley CR, Adams RE: Compassion fatigue following the September 11 terrorist attacks: A study of secondary trauma among New York City social workers. *Int J Emerg Ment Health* 6(2):57–66, 2004.

SECTION 2

CANCER DIAGNOSTICS

Chapter 9   The Veterinary Oncologic Pathologist 35

Chapter 10   Clinical Chemistries and Tumor Markers 40

Chapter 11   Veterinary Cancer Imaging 44

Chapter 12   Biopsy, Biopsy, Biopsy! Theory and Practice 56

Chapter 13   Skin Biopsy 61

Chapter 14   Lymph Node Biopsy 66

Chapter 15   Respiratory Tract Biopsy 70

Chapter 16   Bone Marrow Aspiration and Biopsy 78

Chapter 17   Lower Urogenital Tract Biopsy 82

Chapter 18   Digestive System Biopsy 87

Chapter 19   Clinical Cytology and Neoplasia 96

THE VETERINARY ONCOLOGIC PATHOLOGIST

Gregory K. Ogilvie and Antony S. Moore

CLINICAL BRIEFING

Clinical vs anatomic pathology	• Clinical pathology is easily obtained, cost-effective, and easy to perform. • Anatomic pathology is more accurate, more reflective of the entire tissue involved, and considered the gold standard of cancer pathology.
Pathologist	• Key member of the veterinary health care team who must be given detailed information about history and clinical findings to enhance diagnostic accuracy.
Pathologist's obligation	• Accurate diagnosis, determination of metastatic potential and biologic behavior of a tumor, and completeness of excision.
Tumor grading	• Subjective determination of the histologic characteristics of a tumor that predicts its biologic behavior.
Determination of margins	• Evaluation of the completeness of tumor excision.
Response to therapy	• Determination of the degree of tumor killing or ablation.
Special stains	• Use of stains such as AgNOR, melanin bleach, alcian blue, mucicarmine, Masson's trichrome, and others to enhance the accuracy of diagnosis.
Immunohistochemistry	• Special stains for cytokeratin, desmin, actin, insulin, glucagon, factor VIII antigen, S100, HMB-45, chromogranin, neuron-specific enolase, α_1-antitrypsin, CD3, Ki67, p-glycoprotein, and others are helpful in determining tumor type and biologic behavior.
Flow cytometry	• Use of fluorochrome-labeled antibodies or fluorescent DNA-binding dyes to identify cellular proteins or DNA to characterize tumors.
Polymerase chain reaction	• Molecular biologic technique to identify the unique characteristics of the cell and the presence of neoplasias such as lymphoma.

The veterinary pathologist is an important member of the veterinary health care team. Pathologists, like every specialist, have strengths, weaknesses, and areas of interest and expertise (Figure 9-1). Some are superb in cancer pathology, while others are not as gifted in this unique area. There is almost no other specialty whose work is more pivotal in managing an animal with cancer. Therefore, identifying anatomic and clinical pathologists who excel in oncologic pathology is a very high priority when developing a first-class cancer care team.

Some pathologists specialize in clinical pathology, some specialize in anatomic pathology, and some have experience and training in both disciplines. Clinical pathologists examine indi-

> **KEY POINT**
> *There is almost no other specialist whose work is more pivotal in managing an animal with cancer than the pathologist.*

vidual cells to determine the identity of the disease. Anatomic pathologists examine intact tissue and associated architecture to determine the underlying pathologic process. Clinical pathologists should provide information about the cytologic diagnosis. Veterinary anatomic pathologists should provide not only a histologic diagnosis and classification of the cancer but also a grade and stage of the disease whenever possible.

36 MANAGING THE CANINE CANCER PATIENT

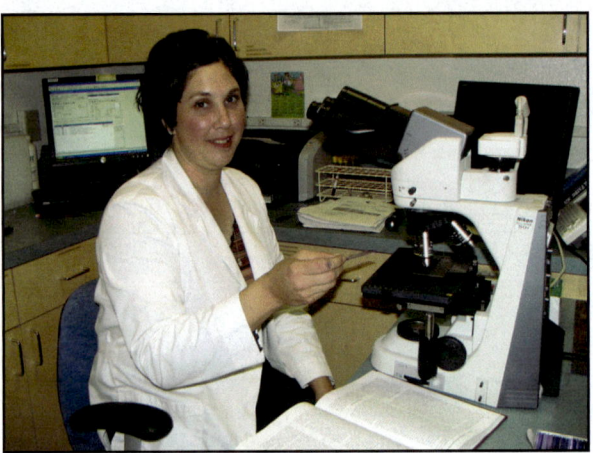

Figure 9-1. *Identifying a highly trained, confident, team-oriented pathologist and developing a close relationship with that person are crucial steps in securing accurate diagnoses for patients.*

The information each type of pathologist can provide depends on the tissue samples obtained by biopsy. Anatomic pathologists use surgically obtained samples, whereas clinical pathologists use samples collected by fine-needle aspiration or impression smears of tissues of interest. The advantages and disadvantages of these different samples include:

- Clinical pathology samples can be easily obtained preoperatively and can be used to screen patients for more intensive diagnostics.
- Fine-needle aspiration cytology is more cost-effective than surgical biopsy.
- The fine-needle aspiration cytology procedure is less likely than surgical biopsy to result in adverse effects.
- Fine-needle aspiration cytology is less accurate and less representative of the entire tissue of concern than is surgical biopsy.
- Fine-needle aspiration cytology does not provide information on tissue architecture compared with surgical biopsy.

In specially equipped centers, pathologists can direct the acquisition of appropriate diagnostic tissues and can identify tumor-free margins during surgery using frozen sections. Finally, the pathologist directs the tissue for specialized testing using advanced techniques to enhance diagnostic accuracy. These techniques may include special stains, immunohistochemistry, electron microscopy, flow cytometry, and polymerase chain reaction (PCR).

Including the Veterinary Oncologic Pathologist as Part of Your Team

Developing a comfortable relationship between the pathologist and allied staff is essential because initiating a dialogue enhances the diagnosis in many cases. The dialogue must begin at the time of sample submission to ensure that the pathologist has a complete, detailed, written description of the lesion and a history of the condition. For example, when a pathologist reviews a biologically high-grade yet histologically low-grade soft tissue sarcoma, he or she may be tempted to describe the lesion as a histopathologically benign condition. However, if the veterinary team informs the pathologist that the tumor comes from the maxilla of a golden retriever with a lesion that has been growing for months, has been unsuccessfully resected twice, and is causing some alteration in the radiographic appearance of the skull, the pathologist is equipped with information that allows him or her to consider more appropriate differentials. The dialogue should continue if the histopathologic description does not fit the clinical picture or the biologic behavior of the disease. If, as in the previous example, the pathologist renders a diagnosis of benign fibroma, it would be in the patient's best interest to enter into a discussion with the pathologist to obtain additional evaluations and even a second opinion. Pathologists, like all other specialists, are often comfortable obtaining second opinions to ensure that the patient receives the best treatment possible. Finally, giving the pathologist feedback on the outcome of the case is very important to allow him or her to determine the value and accuracy of the work and diagnosis.

> **KEY POINT**
> *While it is crucial to develop a dialogue with the pathologist, it is just as important to provide adequately obtained and prepared tissue or cells for review.*

While it is crucial to develop a dialogue with the pathologist, it is just as important to provide adequately obtained and prepared tissue or cells for review. Further information about obtaining appropriate tissue, fluid, or cells is found elsewhere in this section. Specific attention should be focused on obtaining appropriate samples and their fixation, if any, at the time of procurement. For example, PCR analysis is best done on fresh tissue, whereas immunohistochemistry is best conducted on tissue placed in Z-fix to preserve the proteins in question. Cells for cytology should never be exposed to formalin as it prevents subsequent adequate fixation.

What to Expect from a Veterinary Oncologic Pathologist

The management of a cancer patient is often directly dependent on the information obtained from a veterinary pathologist. The clinician should have knowledge of key definitions concerning the histopathologic or cytologic diagnoses[1,2] (see box on page 37). If the pathologist uses terms that are unfamiliar to the attending veterinarian, an open discussion should ensue.

The pathologist should always answer key questions about the sample, assuming adequate tissue is available for review. These include:

- Is it a tumor?
- What type of tumor is it?
- From where did the tumor likely arise?
- Has the tumor metastasized?
- What is this tumor's biologic behavior?
- Has the tumor been completely excised?

Tumor Grading and Staging

In addition to determining the type of neoplasm, the grading of tumors is one of the most important tasks of a veterinary pathologist. The biologic behavior of some tumors is not always predicted by the histologic grade, although the list of tumors for which this is applicable is growing. Grading results from a subjective evaluation of the histologic characteristics of the cancer and is often based on the degree of differentiation, mitotic index, degree of cellular or nuclear pleomorphism, amount of necrosis, invasiveness, stromal reaction, and lymphoid response. These characteristics can be used to grade the tumor as low grade (well differentiated, grade I), intermediate grade (moderately differentiated, grade II), or high grade (poorly differentiated, grade III). The subjective nature of grading can result in variability between pathologists, further defining why it is so important to identify highly skilled pathologists who have extensive experience and confidence in cancer pathology.

Section 5 provides many specific examples of tumors for which the grade is prognostic. Examples include mast cell tumors,[3-5] lymphoma,[6,7] dermal and ocular melanoma,[8,9] mammary gland carcinoma,[10] synovial cell sarcoma,[11] multilobular osteochondrosarcoma,[12] hemangiosarcoma,[13] non-lymphoid–nonangiomatous splenic sarcoma,[14] transitional cell carcinoma,[15] squamous cell carcinoma,[16] pulmonary carcinoma,[17] osteosarcoma,[18,19] and soft tissue sarcoma.[20]

The pathologist may assist in staging the tumor by determining its size, depth of invasion, and metastasis to regional lymph nodes or distant sites such as the lung. Staging is essential to direct therapy and to help provide an accurate prognosis.

Evaluation of Tumor Margins

One of the key tasks of the pathologist is to assess the success of surgical removal of a tumor, or obtaining "clean" margins. Clean margins are essential regardless of whether the tumor is benign or malignant. Margins must be checked for completeness in all directions, including width and depth. While it is not possible to check all margins, the pathologist should evaluate a tumor of concern in many different areas

---

Cancer Terminology: Pathology

Speaking the same language as your pathologist must begin with a common set of definitions. Following are a few of the most common oncology terms and their definitions[1,2]:

Adenocarcinoma: Malignant tumor of epithelial origin that is forming glands and ducts

Adenoma/papilloma: Benign tumor of epithelial origin

Anaplasia: Total loss of microscopic characteristics of cell differentiation

Carcinoma: Malignant tumor of epithelial origin

Dysplasia: Change in the microscopic characteristics of a tissue; may be a preneoplastic condition

Hyperplasia: Increase in the number of cells present

In situ: Malignancy that is restricted to the superficial tissue and has not yet invaded underlying tissue below the basement membrane

Metaplasia: Abnormal transformation of differentiated tissue of one type into differentiated tissue of another type

Neoplasia: Abnormal benign or malignant growth of cells that is not responsive to normal growth control

Pleomorphism: Presence of multiple shapes and forms of cells and nuclei

Sarcoma: Malignant tumor of mesenchymal origin

Scirrhous response: Abundant fibroblastic proliferation with collagen formation in response to invasive malignant tumors

Tumor: Mass or swelling that may or may not be neoplastic

---

to enhance confidence that the mass was removed completely. The more anaplastic the tumor, the less defined the margins become, requiring wider margins. As a general rule, 1-mm margins are considered incomplete whereas 1- to 3-cm margins are generally considered wide and clean. The margins in between have different connotations, depending on the type of tumor to be considered. For example, a well-differentiated mammary adenocarcinoma is unlikely to regrow with a 0.5-cm margin, whereas mast cell tumors and soft tissue sarcomas are at greater risk for recurrence because these tumors extend "fingers" into the surrounding tissue. To enhance the accuracy of determining the margins, different colored inks or sutures should be placed in the tissue edges or regions of interest to guide the pathologist. That said, the determination of complete or clean margins does not always ensure lack of disease recurrence.[21]

Assessment of Response to Therapy

In some cases, the pathologist's chief role is to determine the efficacy of therapy. This is not as common in veterinary medicine but is best exemplified with the histopathologic evaluation of osteosarcoma after radiation therapy. For example, when an osteosarcoma is irradiated, the tumor removed during limb-sparing surgery, and the irradiated tissue evaluated histopathologically, the percentage of tumor that is necrotic can be prognostic for tumor control.[1,2] In one study, tumor necrosis of 90% or greater had a local control rate of 91% after limb-sparing surgery, but an 80% tumor necrosis rate had a local control rate of 28% in response to radiation therapy.[22]

Tools of the Veterinary Oncologic Pathologist

SPECIAL STAINS

Most tumors are clearly identifiable via light microscopy. In some situations, however, the tumor is too undifferentiated to determine its cell of origin. The use of special stains can be helpful in determining the tissue of origin, which can be pivotal for treatment and hence outcome. For example, differentiating a mast cell tumor from a lymphoma—both round cell tumors—can be very important because their treatment is dramatically different. Poorly granulated mast cell tumors are best identified with toluidine blue or Giemsa stains.[1] Select examples of special stains include:

- Staining of nucleolar organizer regions (AgNORs) is prognostically significant in canine mammary gland tumors,[23] lymphoma,[24] and mast cell tumors.[25]
- Melanin bleach or iron stains are helpful in distinguishing melanin and hemosiderin to determine whether the patient has a melanoma.
- Alcian blue stain is helpful in determining whether the tumor in question is a neurofibrosarcoma or myxosarcoma.
- Mucicarmine or periodic acid–Schiff stain highlights mucus to identify poorly differentiated carcinomas.
- Masson's trichrome stain is helpful in identifing collagen fibrils to differentiate specific mesenchymal tumors derived from muscle (i.e., leiomyoma, leiomyosarcoma, rhabdomyoma, rhabdomyosarcoma) from matrix-derived tumors (fibrosarcomas).

IMMUNOHISTOCHEMISTRY

Immunohistochemistry is a specialized area of cancer pathology that uses antibodies directed toward specific epitopes such as intermediate filaments, secretory substances, hormones, and proteins of various types.[1,2] Formalin-fixed or fresh tissue can be evaluated; however, specialized fixatives such as Z-fix enhance the ability of the antibodies to bind specifically to the epitopes of interest. The antibodies used in these tests are specific for the proteins in question. Additional steps are taken to identify the primary antibodies, which are then linked to peroxidase or another substance for easy identification. These assays are variable in their specificity and sensitivity. Some examples of commonly stained epitopes and the conditions for which they are diagnostic include[1,2]:

- Intermediate filaments such as vimentin for tumors of mesenchymal origin
- Cytokeratin for tumors that originate from epithelial cells
- Desmin or actin for tumors that arise from muscle cells
- Insulin, glucagons, calcitonin, and similar substances to identify hormone-producing tumors
- Factor VIII antigens for endothelial cell tumors
- S100 and HMB-45 for melanomas
- Chromogranin for some neuroendocrine tumors
- Neuron-specific enolase for tumors of the nervous system
- Glial fibrillary acidic protein for astrocytic tumors
- α_1-Antitrypsin or lysozyme to identify macrophages or histiocytes
- T-cell markers (e.g., CD3) and B-cell markers (e.g., CD79a) for T- and B-cell lymphomas, respectively
- Ki67 as a cell proliferation rate marker to determine the speed of tumor progression
- p-Glycoprotein, a protein associated with resistance to naturally occurring chemotherapeutic agents

ELECTRON MICROSCOPY

This form of microscopy is ultrahigh resolution (600 angstroms) and is used to evaluate extremely small amounts of tissue for structural details at the cellular level.[1,2] The tissue is ideally fixed in glutaraldehyde, although formalin-fixed tissue can be assessed with some loss of detail. This ultrastructural microscopy can be used to identify the granules in mast cell tumors and hence identify these tumors and the viruses within some virally induced squamous cell carcinomas. Similarly, some specific cellular details can be used to confirm tumors of lymphoid origin. The resolution is so high that this methodology is not very effective at determining benign versus malignant tissue.

FLOW CYTOMETRY

This technique involves taking a single-cell suspension of a tumor, blood, or other tissue and then staining the cells with specific fluorochromes. Fluorescently conjugated antibodies or fluorescent DNA-binding dyes are used to identify cell surface or intracellular proteins or DNA, respectively, to enumerate or characterize cells and/or their contents. In this process, the stained cells are passed through the flow cytometry chamber and at least one laser beam. The laser light is then refracted and analyzed by various detectors based on the degree of laser light refraction. The cells can be counted or separated (sorted) by their unique characteristics.

The most common use of flow cytometry is to count the number of chromosomes in the cells in question. This determination of DNA content, or ploidy, can help determine whether the DNA count is normal (diploid) or abnormal (aneuploid). Malignant cells are more likely to be aneuploid, whereas normal cellular processes are more likely to be diploid. This can be used not only to determine whether the tissue in question is malignant, but it may be prognostic in some tumor types.

Flow cytometry can be used to determine the cell cycle characteristics of the cells in question.[1,26] For example, this method can determine the number of cells in the S-phase and the cell cycle time. The S-phase kinetics can be prognostic as they reflect the growth kinetics of the sample analyzed.

Other applications of flow cytometry in small animal oncology include immunophenotyping of hematopoietic malignancies.[1,26] Identifying T- versus B-cell lymphomas, for example, can be of prognostic significance. In addition, specific identification of the cell of origin of various leukemias is done by flow cytometry. This can direct specific therapy for the different diseases of bone marrow origin and can predict outcome.

Impending applications of flow cytometry include identification of acute leukemias; immunophenotyping of and molecular abnormalities associated with lymphomas, leukemias, and solid malignancies; and detection of residual disease and therefore direction of therapy for various cancers.

POLYMERASE CHAIN REACTION

PCR is a molecular biologic technique fairly recently employed to identify the unique characteristics of a cell. While the most common application is in the research laboratory, PCR is being used on a routine basis to assist in diagnosing lymphoma. In this method, PCR is used to amplify DNA encoding for a specific antigen-binding region of lymphocytes and a clonal rearrangement of cell surface proteins. With PCR, occult lymphoma can be identified accurately in 93% of cases. Blood, body fluids, bone marrow, fresh nodal tissue, and formalin-fixed tissue can be analyzed.

REFERENCES

1. Powers BE: The pathology of neoplasia, in Withrow SJ, MacEwen EG (eds): *Small Animal Clinical Oncology*, ed 3. Philadelphia, WB Saunders, 2001, pp 4–17.
2. Borowitz M, Westra W, Cooley LD, et al: Pathology and laboratory medicine, in Abeloff MD, Armigage JO, Niederhuber JE, et al (eds): *Clinical Oncology*, ed 3. Philadelphia, Elsevier, 2004, pp 299–339.
3. Patnaik AK, Ehler WJ, MacEwen EG: Canine cutaneous mast cell tumor: Morphologic grading and survival time in 83 dogs. *Vet Pathol* 21(5):469–474, 1984.
4. Bostock DE, Crocker J, Harris K, Smith P: Nucleolar organiser regions as indicators of post-surgical prognosis in canine spontaneous mast cell tumours. *Br J Cancer* 59(6):915–918, 1989.
5. Murphy S, Sparkes AH, Smith KC, et al: Relationships between the histological grade of cutaneous mast cell tumours in dogs, their survival and the efficacy of surgical resection. *Vet Rec* 154(24):743–746, 2004.
6. Carter RF, Valli VE, Lumsden JH: The cytology, histology and prevalence of cell types in canine lymphoma classified according to the National Cancer Institute Working Formulation. *Can J Vet Res* 50(2):154–164, 1986.
7. Teske E, van Heerde P, Rutteman GR, et al: Prognostic factors for treatment of malignant lymphoma in dogs. *JAVMA* 205(12):1722–1728, 1994.
8. Bostock DE: Prognosis after surgical excision of canine melanomas. *Vet Pathol* 16(1):32–40, 1979.
9. Wilcox BP, Peiffer RL: Morphology and behavior of primary ocular melanomas in 91 dogs. *Vet Pathol* 23(4):418–421, 1986.
10. Kurzman ID, Gilbertson SR: Prognostic factors in canine mammary tumors. *Semin Vet Med Surg (Small Anim)* 1(1):25–32, 1986.
11. Vail DM, Powers BE, Getzy DM, et al: Evaluation of prognostic factors for dogs with synovial sarcoma: 36 cases (1986–1991). *JAVMA* 205(9):1300–1307, 1994.
12. Dernell WS, Straw RC, Cooper MF, et al: Multilobular osteochondrosarcoma in 39 dogs: 1979–1993. *JAAHA* 34(1):11–18, 1998.
13. Ogilvie GK, Powers BE, Mallinckrodt CH, Withrow SJ: Surgery and doxorubicin in dogs with hemangiosarcoma. *J Vet Intern Med* 10(6):379–384 1996.
14. Spangler WL, Culbertson MR, Kass PH: Primary mesenchymal (nonangiomatous/nonlymphomatous) neoplasms occurring in the canine spleen: Anatomic classification, immunohistochemistry, and mitotic activity correlated with patient survival. *Vet Pathol* 31(1):37–47, 1994.
15. Valli VE, Norris A, Jacobs RM, et al: Pathology of canine bladder and urethral cancer and correlation with tumour progression and survival. *J Comp Pathol* 113(2):113–130, 1995.
16. Carpenter LG, Withrow SJ, Powers BE, et al: Squamous cell carcinoma of the tongue in 10 dogs. *JAAHA* 29:17–23, 1993.
17. McNeil EA, Ogilvie GK, Powers BE, et al: Evaluation of prognostic factors for dogs with primary lung tumors: 67 cases (1985–1992). *JAVMA* 211:1422–1425, 1997.
18. Straw RC, Powers BE, Klausner J, et al: Canine mandibular osteosarcoma: 51 cases (1980–1992). *JAAHA* 32:257–262, 1996.
19. Kirpensteijn J, Kik M, Rutteman GR, Teske E: Prognostic significance of a new histologic grading system for canine osteosarcoma. *Vet Pathol* 39(2):240–246, 2002.
20. Kuntz CA, Dernell WS, Powers BE, et al: Prognostic factors for surgical treatment of soft-tissue sarcomas in dogs: 75 cases (1986–1996). *JAVMA* 211(9):1147–1151, 1997.
21. Michels GM, Knapp DW, DeNicola DB, et al: Prognosis following surgical excision of canine cutaneous mast cell tumors with histopathologically tumor-free versus non-tumor-free margins: A retrospective study of 31 cases. *JAAHA* 38(5):458–466, 2002.
22. Powers BE, Withrow SJ, Thrall DE, et al: Percent tumor necrosis as a predicator of treatment response in canine osteosarcoma. *Cancer* 67(1):126–130, 1991.
23. Sarli G, Preziosi R, Benazzi C, et al: Prognostic value of histologic stage and proliferative activity in canine malignant mammary tumors. *J Vet Diagn Invest* 14(1):25–34, 2002.
24. Kiupel M, Teske E, Bostock D: Prognostic factors for treated canine malignant lymphoma. *Vet Pathol* 36(4):292–300, 1999.
25. Kravis LD, Vail DM, Kisseberth WC, et al: Frequency of argyrophilic nucleolar organizer regions in fine-needle aspirates and biopsy specimens from mast cell tumors in dogs. *JAVMA* 209(8):1418–1420, 1996.
26. Culmsee K, Nolte I: Flow cytometry and its application in small animal oncology. *Methods Cell Sci* 24(1–3):49–54, 2002.

CLINICAL CHEMISTRIES AND TUMOR MARKERS

Gregory K. Ogilvie and Antony S. Moore

CLINICAL BRIEFING

Clinical chemistry	• Biologically meaningful chemicals in body fluids that are often monitored to stage the patient and to monitor general health. • Some, but not all, chemistries are used as tumor markers. However, none is specific for cancer.
Tumor marker	• Substance present in the body that is associated with the presence of a tumor and is used clinically to identify the presence of a tumor, to determine the effectiveness of therapy, and to determine when occult cancer is recurring after treatment.
Clinical examples of tumor markers	• Bence Jones proteins: Multiple myeloma. • Hypercalcemia: Lymphoma, anal sac adenocarcinoma, parathyroid tumor. • Alkaline phosphatase: Osteosarcoma. • Hyperinsulinemia/hypoglycemia: Insulinoma, hepatic carcinoma, hepatoma. • V-BTA: Transitional cell carcinoma. • α_1-Acid glycoprotein: Many malignancies. • Matrix metalloproteinase: Many tumors. • Thymidine kinase: Lymphoma.

Veterinarians have searched for laboratory tests that can be used to help diagnose cancer and follow the success of therapy. Clinical chemistries are used worldwide in veterinary medicine to stage the patient with cancer and to monitor general health. These tests document serum, plasma, or urine levels of certain biologically meaningful chemicals. Although they have never been shown to be specific for the diagnosis of cancer (Table 10-1), they often contribute to a definitive diagnosis.

Some clinical chemistries have been used by veterinarians as tumor markers; however, this family of diagnostic tests is composed of a wide variety of substances also known as cancer markers, biomarkers, or, in rare circumstances, cancer-related antigens.[1] These tumor markers may be found in cells, tissues, and body fluids and are measured by a number of assay systems, including clinical chemistry methods, radioimmunoassay, or enzyme-linked immunosorbent assays. These markers are often enzymes, hormones, oncofetal antigens, carbohydrates, proteins, receptors, enzymes, electrolytes, genes, or gene-related proteins.[1] Because the canine genome has been sequenced, it is quite likely that specific cancer-associated gene sequences will be identified as tumor markers. This chapter focuses primarily on substances that may serve as tumor markers that are secreted and detected in the serum because they are likely to be the most widely used in the course of managing cancer.

> **KEY POINT**
>
> *Clinical chemistries are used worldwide to stage patients with cancer, monitor general health, and contribute to a definitive diagnosis; however, they have never been shown to be specific for the diagnosis of cancer.*

Serum and Urine Tumor Markers

The first tumor marker recognized in human or veterinary medicine was the Bence Jones protein, which is found in urine.[1] This monoclonal light chain of immunoglobulins was identified in 1847 as a marker for multiple myeloma or plasma cell myeloma. The test for Bence Jones proteinuria is commonly used to identify the same disease in dogs, although more up-to-date methods such as immunoelectrophoresis have replaced the original assay methodology.

Oncofetal antigens are very helpful in the management of human cancer,[1] but these markers have not been as help-

Table 10-1 Examples of Cancer-Related and Non–Cancer-Related Alterations in Select Clinical Chemistries (Other Than Laboratory Error)

Biochemical Parameter	Cancer-Related Etiology	Non–Cancer-Related Etiology
↑Alanine aminotransferase	Primary metastatic hepatic neoplasia	Drugs; endocrine diseases; hypoxia; inflammation; infection; toxicoses; hepatic trauma; regenerative hepatopathy
↓Alanine aminotransferase	None	Decreased hepatic mass
↑Albumin	None	Dehydration
↓Albumin	Cancer cachexia; multiple myeloma	Liver failure; proteinuria; malassimilation; maldigestion; severe skin damage; hemorrhage; malnutrition
↑Alkaline phosphatase	Osteosarcoma; functional adrenal tumor; pituitary hyperadrenocorticism; functional parathyroid tumor	Cholestasis; pancreatitis; drugs; Cushing's disease; hyperthyroidism; GI disease (minor)
↑Anion gap	Cancer-induced hyperlactatemia (lactic acidosis); hyperglobulinemia of multiple myeloma	Lactic, metabolic or hyperchloremic acidosis; diabetic ketoacidosis; kidney failure; toxins
↓Anion gap	None	Hypoalbuminemia
↑Bile acids	Diffuse hepatic neoplasia	Decreased liver function; icterus; cholestasis
↑Bilirubin	Biliary, metastatic neoplasia	Hemolytic anemia; cholestasis; ruptured gallbladder; ruptured duodenum
↑Blood urea nitrogen	Transitional cell carcinoma obstructing urinary tract; GI tumor bleed; mast cell–induced GI bleed	Dehydration; high-protein diet; heart failure; shock; GI bleed; fever; renal failure; urinary tract obstruction
↓Blood urea nitrogen	Hyperadrenocorticism	Diuresis; liver failure; low-protein diet; malnutrition
↑Calcium	Parathyroid tumor; lymphoma; multiple myeloma; anal sac adenocarcinoma; carcinoma with bone metastasis; C-cell thyroid tumor	Renal secondary hyperparathyroidism; toxins; dehydration; hyperalbuminemia; hypoadrenocorticism; chronic or acute renal failure; osteolysis; granulomatous disease; acidosis
↓Calcium	C-cell thyroid tumor	Eclampsia; renal secondary hyperparathyroidism; hypoalbuminemia; hypomagnesemia; hypoparathyroidism; pancreatitis; rhabdomyolysis diet; malabsorption; hypercalcitoninism; phosphate enemas; intravenous phosphate; alkalosis; ethylene glycol
↑γ-Glutamyltransferase	Primary, metastatic liver tumor	Cholestasis; steroids; anticonvulsants
↑Globulin	Monoclonal: multiple myeloma; polyclonal: neoplasia	Monoclonal: ehrlichiosis, dirofilariasis; polyclonal: chronic inflammation, dental disease, dermatitis, inflammatory bowel disease, parasites, immune-mediated disease
↓Globulin	None	Immunodeficiency; blood loss; protein-losing enteropathy
↑Glucose	Macroadenoma; adrenal or pituitary-induced hyperadrenocorticism; neoplasia-induced altered carbohydrate metabolism	Diabetes mellitus; pancreatitis; drugs; liver failure
↓Glucose	Hepatic carcinomas; β-cell tumor (insulinoma); leukemia; neoplasia-induced hypopituitarism	Liver failure; hypoadrenocorticism; starvation; hyperinsulinism; septicemia; glycogen storage disease

(Table continues)

Table 10-1 (continued)

Biochemical Parameter	Cancer-Related Etiology	Non–Cancer-Related Etiology
↑Lipase	Primary or metastatic pancreatic neoplasia	Pancreatitis; enteritis; renal disease; steroid therapy
↑Phosphorus	Functional thyroid tumor	Renal disease; dehydration; hemolysis; toxins; diet; osteolysis; hypoparathyroidism
↓Phosphorus	PTHrP–producing tumors; C-cell tumors; pituitary- or adrenal-induced hyperadrenocorticism	Insulin therapy; diabetic ketoacidosis; diet; eclampsia; hyperadrenocorticism
↑Potassium	Leukemia	Renal disease; postrenal disease; hypoadrenocorticism; acidosis; muscle damage; dehydration; drugs
↓Potassium	Cancer cachexia	Alkalosis; diet; drugs; GI loss; renal disease; periodic hypokalemic paralysis
↑Thyroxine, triiodothyronine	Functional thyroid neoplasia	Antithyroid antibodies
↓Thyroxine, triiodothyronine	None	Hypothyroidism; nonthyroidal illness; steroids; phenobarbitol

GI = gastrointestinal.
Adapted from Dunfort RM: Abnormal laboratory findings, in Ettinger SJ, Feldman EC (eds): *Textbook of Veterinary Internal Medicine: Diseases of the Dog and Cat*, ed 6. Philadelphia, WB Saunders, 2005, inside cover; with permission.

ful or effective in identifying or monitoring cancer in dogs. Common examples of oncofetal antigens in human oncology are human chorionic gonadotropin, cancer antigen (CA), α-fetoprotein, carcinoembryonic antigen (CEA), and prostate-specific antigen (PSA).[1] Food and Drug Administration–approved tumor marker assays used in human diagnostics, but not veterinary oncology, include[1]:

- **Breast cancer:** CA15-3, CA27.29, HER-2*neu*, CA 125, CA 19-9, CEA
- **Prostate cancer:** Total PSA, free PSA, prostatic acid phosphatase
- **Ovarian cancer:** CA 125
- **Lung cancer:** CEA

Veterinarians have used many assays, including the analyses of hormones, to assess the presence of cancer. For example, serum calcium and, more recently, factors that cause hypercalcemia, including parathyroid hormone (PTH) and PTH-related peptide (PTHrP), are commonly used to diagnose the presence of lymphoma and anal sac adenocarcinoma (PTHrP) or parathyroid tumors (PTH). Serum levels of cortisol or sex hormones such as estrogen have been used to diagnose and monitor adrenal or pituitary tumors. Urinary levels of metabolites of catecholamines are periodically used to help confirm the presence of a pheochromocytoma. Serum thyroid hormone levels may be elevated in the presence of carcinoma of the thyroid.

> **KEY POINT**
>
> *A bladder tumor antigen test kit, V-BTA, can be used to evaluate the urine of dogs to help screen for transitional cell carcinoma; however, proteinuria and hematuria may interfere with the accuracy of the test.*

A bladder tumor antigen test kit known as V-BTA (veterinary version of the bladder tumor antigen) is a good example of use of a tumor marker to help screen dogs for transitional cell carcinoma.[2] The sensitivity and negative predictive value of the test suggest that it is a practical screening test to rule out transitional cell carcinoma in geriatric patients or in patients with clinical signs related to the lower urinary tract.[2] The test has significant limitations in that proteinuria and hematuria may interfere with its accuracy.[2] The sensitivity and specificity of the test are outlined in the box on page 43.[2]

Acute-phase proteins have been found to be nonspecific but sensitive markers of cancer in dogs and people.[3] For example, serum α_1-acid glycoprotein concentrations were found to be elevated in dogs with previously untreated, histologically confirmed, high-grade lymphoblastic lymphoma and a variety of other histologically confirmed nonhematopoietic malignancies.[3] These levels decreased when remission was attained.

Sensitivity and Specificity of the V-BTA Bladder Tumor Antigen Test Kit[2]

Specificity (healthy subjects and urologic controls): 78%
Specificity (healthy subjects): 95%
Sensitivity (active transitional cell carcinoma): 90%
Positive predictive [value]
Negative predictive [value]

Molecular [text obscured] opment of many ne[text obscured] cancer in dogs and [text obscured] ne kinase activity [text obscured] and sensitive tu[text obscured]oma.[4] Dogs with [text obscured]m thymidine kin[text obscured] survival times. F[text obscured] concentrations [text obscured]ma.[4] Serum thymi[text obscured] predicting prognosis [text obscured]ally detectable disease [text obscured]oing chemotherapy.[1] [text obscured] polymerase chain reaction [text obscured] rearrangement.[5,6] PCR has [text obscured] for detecting and phenotyping [text obscured]ring response to therapy, identifying re[text obscured]ing breeds at risk.[5,6]

Clinical Application of Tumor Markers

The ideal cancer marker should be easily identified even at very small concentrations and be a substance that is very specific to one clinically important malignancy.[1] The ideal marker must be able to distinguish benign from malignant disease and be present even when microscopic amounts of cancer are present to allow early detection and monitoring of the efficacy of therapy. While the assay must be sensitive, repeatable, and quantitative, it should also have results that parallel the amount of cancer present.

Work is under way to develop cancer-screening assays to identify cancer before it becomes clinically evident. The impact of this worthy goal will be to reduce the morbidity and mortality of canine patients worldwide.[1] Few, if any, cancer screening tests exist today for routine use in veterinary medicine.

Because most tumor markers are not very sensitive or specific, they have limited application in cancer screening in the general canine population. They do have a role in the diagnosis of cancer and are used to render a prognosis for dogs with histologically proven cancer. For example, the concentrations of matrix metalloproteinases 2 and 9 in serum, plasma, and tumor tissue are directly related to the histologic grade of mast cell tumors.[7]

One key use of tumor markers is to monitor the treatment and progression of cancer. For example, serum levels of the tumor marker can be measured before, immediately after, and throughout the disease-free period to document the success of therapy and the recurrence of cancer. Pretreatment serum alkaline phosphatase levels can be very predictive of posttreatment disease-free intervals for dogs with osteosarcoma. Levels can decline after the tumor is removed and increase at the time of recurrence.[8,9]

> **KEY POINT**
> *The ideal marker must be able to differentiate benign from malignant disease and be present even when microscopic amounts of cancer are present to allow early detection and monitoring of the efficacy of therapy.*

REFERENCES

1. Sokoli LJ, Chan DW: Clinical chemistry: Tumor markers, in Abeloff MD, Armitage JO, Niedelhuber JE, et al (eds): *Clinical Oncology*, ed 3. Philadelphia, Elsevier, 2004, pp 329–339.
2. Borjesson DL, Christopher MM, Ling GV: Detection of canine transitional cell carcinoma using a bladder tumor antigen urine dipstick test. *Vet Clin Pathol* 28(1):33–38, 1999.
3. Ogilvie GK, Walters LM, Greeley SG, et al: Concentration of alpha 1-acid glycoprotein in dogs with malignant neoplasia. *JAVMA* 203(8):1144–1146, 1993.
4. von Euler H, Einarsson R, Olsson U, et al: Serum thymidine kinase activity in dogs with malignant lymphoma: A potent marker for prognosis and monitoring the disease. *J Vet Intern Med* 18(5):696–702, 2004.
5. Burnett RC, Vernau W, Modiano JF, et al: Diagnosis of canine lymphoid neoplasia using clonal rearrangements of antigen receptor genes. *Vet Pathol* 40(1):32–41, 2003.
6. Keller RL, Avery AC, Burnett RC, et al: Detection of neoplastic lymphocytes in peripheral blood of dogs with lymphoma by polymerase chain reaction for antigen receptor gene rearrangement. *Vet Clin Pathol* 33(3):145–149, 2004.
7. Leibman NF, Lana SE, Hansen RA, et al: Identification of matrix metalloproteinases in canine cutaneous mast cell tumors. *J Vet Intern Med* 14(6):583–586, 2000.
8. Garzotto CK, Berg J, Hoffmann WE, Rard WM: Prognostic significance of serum alkaline phosphatase activity in canine appendicular osteosarcoma. *J Vet Intern Med* 14(6):587–592, 2000.
9. Kirpensteijn J, Kik M, Rutteman GR, Teske E: Prognostic significance of a new histologic grading system for canine osteosarcoma. *Vet Pathol* 39(2):240–246, 2002.

VETERINARY CANCER IMAGING

Gregory K. Ogilvie and Antony S. Moore

CLINICAL BRIEFING

Anatomic methods	• Radiography. • CT. • Ultrasonography.
Functional/ anatomic methods	• MRI. • PET. • SPECT. • PET/CT. • SPECT/CT. • Color-flow Doppler.
Planar radiography	• Radiography is the simplest, most cost-effective diagnostic modality for evaluating cancer patients. • It is sensitive but has limited ability to assess contrast among tissues.
Computed tomography	• Rapidly becoming the cornerstone technology of oncologic imaging. • Provides rapid, high-resolution imagery in "slices" to visualize in three dimensions. • Essential for radiation planning.
Magnetic resonance imaging	• Diagnostic method of choice for imaging neoplasia of the CNS and musculoskeletal system. • Not ideal for imaging some bony structures.
Ultrasonography	• Cost-effective, sensitive diagnostic method with high sensitivity for imaging tumors within soft tissue structures. • Color-flow Doppler enhances the ability of ultrasonography to determine blood flow in tumors.
Planar scintigraphy	• Diagnostic method of choice for identifying bone metastases and for imaging thyroid neoplasia.
Single-photon emission computed tomography	• Nuclear medicine diagnostic tool to evaluate the functional characteristics of tumors. This diagnostic method is enhanced when combined with CT.
Positron emission tomography	• Nuclear imaging tool using ^{18}fluorodeoxyglucose is becoming useful in diagnosing and staging a wide variety of cancers. When combined with CT, the diagnostic value is enhanced.

Imaging has evolved over the past 20 years into a key tool for diagnosing and staging cancer.[1] Whereas veterinarians once relied exclusively on planar radiography, they now commonly have access to ultrasonography, nuclear medicine, computed tomography (CT), and magnetic resonance imaging (MRI). Positron emission tomography (PET), single-photon emission computed tomography (SPECT), MRI spectroscopy, and PET/CT are rapidly becoming more accessible to veterinarians; thus, their use in diagnosing the veterinary cancer patient is becoming more common. The primary purpose of radiography, MRI, CT, ultrasonography, and the combination of CT and PET is to document the presence of

Table 11-1 Resolution, Sensitivity, Specificity, and Functional Imaging Ability of the Most Common Cancer Imaging Methods

Modality[a]	Resolution	Sensitivity	Specificity	Functional Imaging Ability
MRI	3 mm	Moderate	Moderate	Moderate with spectroscopy
CT	2 mm	Moderate	Moderate	Low except with angiography
Radiography	2 mm	Low	Moderate	Very little
SPECT	1 cm	High	Moderate	Excellent
PET	5 mm	High	High	Excellent
Ultrasonography	5 mm	Low	Low	Some
Angiography	2 mm	Moderate	Moderate	Low

underlying anatomic and, in some cases, functional changes associated with diseases such as cancer.[1-3] The identification of metabolic changes and changes in the function and molecular characteristics of a tissue are best determined by PET/SPECT and PET/CT.[1-3] The use of these modalities has resulted in more rapid and accurate diagnoses, more precise delivery of therapy, and less morbidity and mortality. One example of the value of advanced diagnostics is the decline in the number of exploratory laparotomies, once a key diagnostic tool in more difficult cases.

> **KEY POINT**
>
> *The primary purpose of radiography, MRI, CT, ultrasonography, and the combination of CT and PET is to document the presence of underlying anatomic and, in some cases, functional changes associated with diseases such as cancer.*

The sensitivity and specificity of each diagnostic test must be taken into account (Table 11-1). Thoracic radiography, for example, is inexpensive but relatively insensitive for the visualization of pulmonary metastases compared with the more expensive and technically more demanding CT, which is the standard diagnostic test in human medicine.[2,3] Although CT is far superior to thoracic radiography at identifying the presence of a pulmonary lesion, both tests are poor at distinguishing the underlying histopathologic characteristics that separate a benign lesion, such as a pulmonary granuloma, from a metastatic lung lesion, as can occur with osteosarcoma. An absolute diagnosis can only be obtained by cytology or histopathology.

The purpose of this chapter is to introduce some of the more common cancer imaging techniques, their limitations, and their benefits. References dealing with the unique characteristics and capabilities of each modality are available for additional information.[1-47] Specific details of diagnostics in veterinary oncology are found in the chapters in this book that address specific diseases.

Planar Radiography

Standard planar radiography will always be the most important diagnostic tool in veterinary medicine because of its relative ease of operation, availability, and lower cost (Figures 11-1 and 11-2).[1] However, contrast is limited because planar radiography produces images that are the summation of all tissues rather than a special relationship of one tissue to another, as is determined by CT or MRI, although the introduction of phosphor screens has dramatically increased the resolution.

> **KEY POINT**
>
> *Standard planar radiography will always be the most important diagnostic tool in veterinary medicine because of its relative ease of operation, availability, and lower cost compared with other diagnostic methods.*

Mammography is a specialized form of standard radiography. It is the only screening test that is helpful in predicting breast cancer at an early stage in women, leading to rapid treatment and an increased cure rate.[1-3] The accuracy of this method has increased with the incorporation of digital technology with phosphor screens. Although breast cancer is the

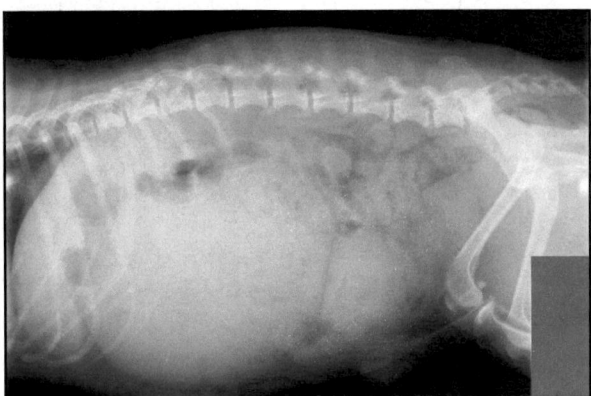

Figure 11-1. *Radiography is a readily available, cost-effective way of identifying changes in organ sizes, as can be seen in this dog with an enlarged spleen. (Courtesy of Lenore A. Mohammadian, DVM, California Veterinary Specialists, and Donald Thrall, DVM, North Carolina State University)*

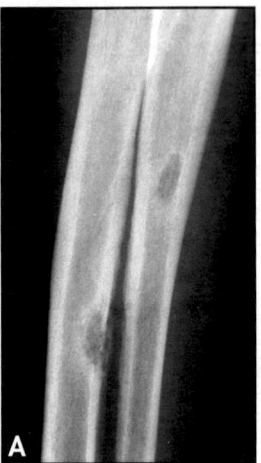 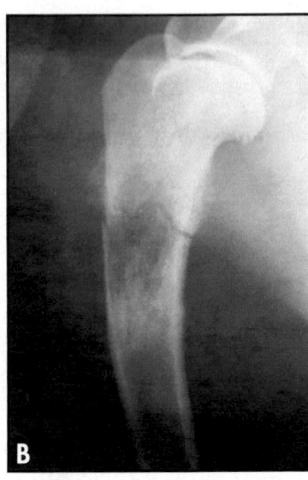

Figure 11-2. *Radiographs are ideal for rapidly identifying changes in bony structures such as the lytic metastatic lesions of the radius and ulna (**A**) and the proximal femoral osteosarcoma with a pathologic fracture (**B**). Note the lytic and proliferative pattern forming a "sunburst" pattern characteristic of a primary bone tumor. (Courtesy of L. A. Mohammadian and D. Thrall)*

most common malignancy in intact female dogs, mammography is not commonly used, presumably because of the cost and the facts that approximately half of mammary tumors are benign and most malignant tumors are cured with surgery alone.

Angiography has been used for decades to evaluate the vascular supply of organs or tissues in response to the presence of a tumor.[1-3] One common example is the evaluation of a potential pheochromocytoma before surgery via a vena cava portogram. The surgical approach and potential outcome may be dramatically different based on the presence of a tumor in the vena cava. Angiography has become far more valuable with CT contrast radiography (see below).

Computed Tomography

CT is the dominant diagnostic tool for staging and evaluating response to therapy in human cancer medicine and is becoming common in centers that provide advanced veterinary cancer care worldwide. CT is conducted with an x-ray tube and a detector to obtain planar or spiral "slices" of the patient's anatomy.[1-3] The information obtained from the detectors is reconstructed in 1- to 10-mm slices by a computer to give striking images that can be further reconstructed to make three-dimensional (3-D) images. The newer generation of CT units is able to obtain extremely thin slices of the anatomy in a short time. The newest generation of CT scanners obtains multislices, with each rotation further enhancing the speed and detail of every image. These helical or spiral CTs are ideal to conduct "breath-hold studies" to obtain rapid imaging of the lungs with continuous, rapid "orange peel" slices. This method is excellent for evaluating a patient for pulmonary metastases in less than a minute. Regardless of the type of CT obtained, this method requires that the patient be immobilized with anesthesia, especially during single breath-hold studies.

> **KEY POINT**
>
> *Helical or spiral CTs are ideal to conduct "breath-hold" studies to obtain rapid imaging of the lungs with continuous, rapid "orange peel" slices. Pulmonary metastases can be evaluated in less than a minute.*

The detail of each CT is enhanced when a contrast agent is injected intravenously and compared with noncontrast images. More recent software and units conduct dynamic "wash in" and "wash out" of contrast agents to help define the perfusion of tumors and vascular permeability.[1-3] Contrast-enhanced imaging via CT may identify small nodules within the liver, spleen, and musculature that are often not detectable via ultrasonography.

CT is superior to MRI when assessing bone and lung tissue.[1-3] Although MRI is excellent at providing information about soft tissue structures, including (and especially) the central nervous system (CNS), some anatomic distortion can occur with this modality, making the delineation of tumor margins difficult in some situations.[1]

CT is superior to planar radiography for imaging the nasal cavity, skull, cribriform plate, maxilla, mandible, pelvis, and vertebral bones (Figures 11-3 to 11-7).[1-3] 3-D imaging via computer reconstruction is often possible, making it ideal to define the extent of tumors within or on these structures and the destruction of the involved tissue. In addition, metastasis to regional lymph nodes and other nearby structures is often evident. CT has dramatically increased the sensitivity of identifying pulmonary metastases, especially when using

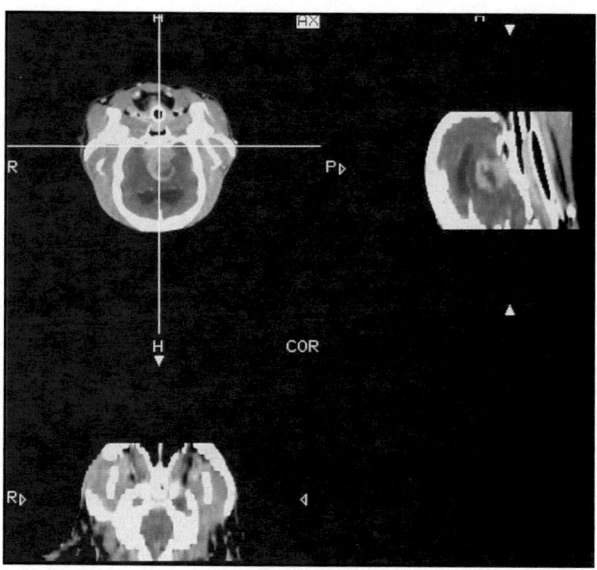

Figure 11-3. *CT with contrast enhancement provides excellent imaging of intracranial disease such as this cystic pituitary mass. The computer reconstructs available images for 3-D viewing. (Courtesy of L. A. Mohammadian and D. Thrall)*

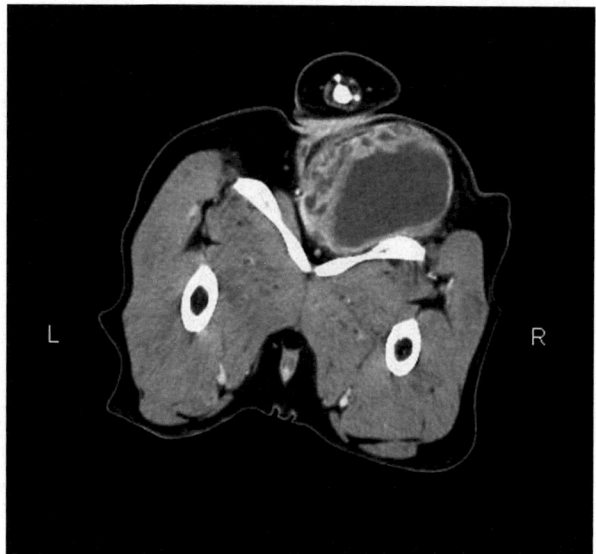

Figure 11-4. *CT can enhance cure rates by allowing surgeons to plan complex surgery, such as for complex tumors of the pelvis and nearby structures. (Courtesy of L. A. Mohammadian)*

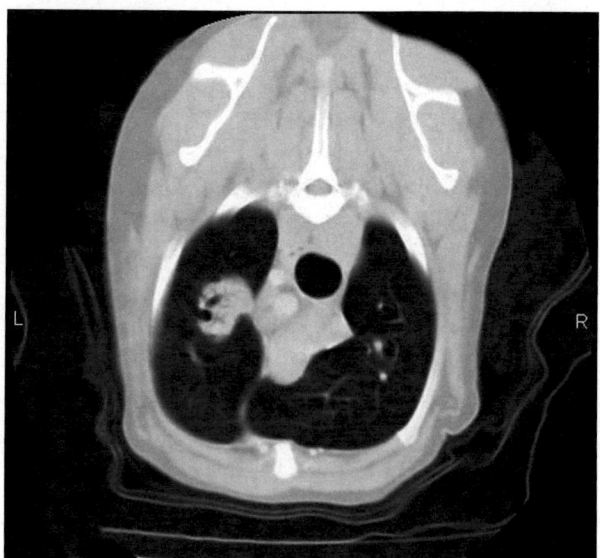

Figure 11-5. *Helical CT can provide striking images of pulmonary masses not easily seen on planar radiographs. This mass was located within the pulmonary parenchyma and was documented to be malignant histiocytosis. (Courtesy of L. A. Mohammadian)*

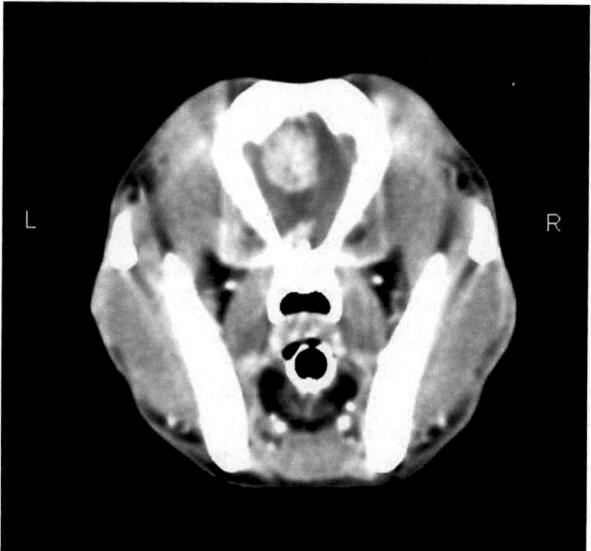

Figure 11-6. *Seizures in older dogs are often caused by brain pathology, including brain neoplasia. This CT documents the presence of a mass (meningioma) within the brain. (Courtesy of L. A. Mohammadian)*

breath-hold studies, although this increased sensitivity also means a decrease in specificity, which must be taken into account when evaluating images.

CT-guided biopsies are considered a standard of care in human medicine and are now becoming common in advanced veterinary centers.[1-3] This is especially helpful for deep-seated tumors, such as brain tumors. For example, in one study, investigators documented the efficacy of CT-guided stereotactic brain biopsies on 50 consecutive dogs using a modified Pelorus Mark III Stereotactic System.[4,5] The study conclusion was that this CT-guided biopsy procedure can provide an accurate pathologic diagnosis of brain lesions detected by CT and magnetic resonance neuroimaging. As the technique is refined, the complication rate currently seen in this procedure will likely be reduced.

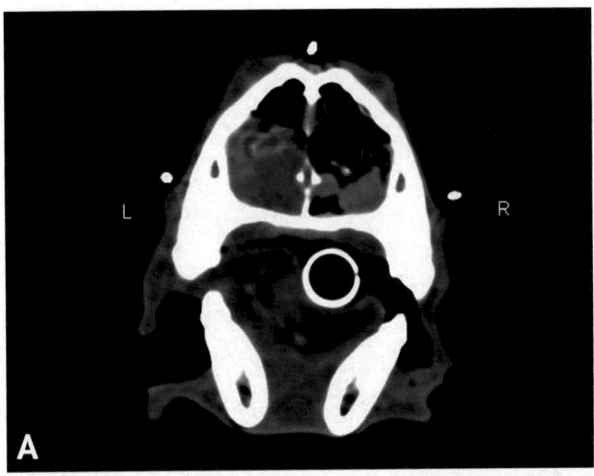 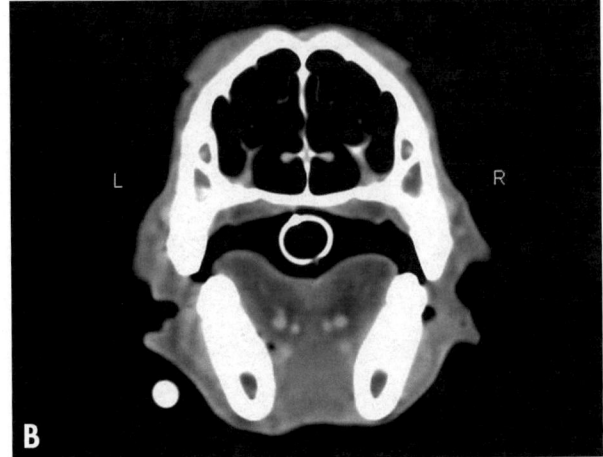

Figure 11-7. *CT has revolutionized the accuracy of diagnosing intranasal disease such as this nasal carcinoma in a dog (**A**). The efficacy of radiation therapy was documented by CT in this same dog 3 months after treatment was completed (**B**).*

CT can be a valuable tool in identifying the extent of cancer, thereby directing surgical removal of the tumor.[6,7] For example, 10 dogs with previously untreated appendicular osteosarcoma were treated by limb amputation.[6] Amputated limbs were imaged using radiography, CT, and MRI and examined microscopically to determine the longitudinal extent of neoplastic cell involvement and length of associated intramedullary fibrosis. In this group of dogs, CT was the most effective imaging modality in predicting tumor involvement compared with MRI and radiography.

CT has become essential in the planning of radiation therapy fields and in the delivery of radiation via radiosurgery.[1-3] Radiosurgery uses multiple noncoplanar stereotactically focused beams of radiation in a series of arcs to deliver a single dose to the target with extreme accuracy.[8] The large number of beams enhances the ability to deliver radiation precisely to the tumor while sparing the nearby normal tissue. CT with a stereotactic localizer secured to the skull allows generation of a 3-D image of the target and provides accurate spatial coordinates for computerized treatment planning and delivery of radiation via a linear accelerator.

> **KEY POINT**
> *CT is essentially always superior to planar radiography for imaging the nasal cavity, skull, cribriform plate, maxilla, mandible, pelvis, and vertebral bones.*

Ultrasonography

Ultrasonography is considered a vital diagnostic tool in veterinary medicine. The decreasing cost of sophisticated ultrasonography machines and easy access to training opportunities for veterinarians worldwide have made this modality a favorite of progressive practitioners. There is little doubt that this diagnostic tool has increased the speed and accuracy of the diagnosis of cancer and has reduced the need for more invasive diagnostic tools such as exploratory laparotomy (Figures 11-8 to 11-12). However, ultrasonography remains the most operator-dependent of all modalities, and considerable training and expertise are required to maximize its utility.

> **KEY POINT**
> *Although an experienced ultrasonographer is able to distinguish subtle changes within normal tissues and gain suspicion of neoplasia, an absolute diagnosis can only be obtained by cytology or histopathology.*

Ultrasonograms provide dynamic visualization of nonosseus or air-filled organs by the transmission of ultrasound energy through the body. The return of these pulses to the transducer is converted into an image that is visualized on a screen that can be recorded or paused for analysis. The use of contrast agents and color-flow Doppler, as well as 3-D and nonlinear imaging, has enhanced the ability to visualize different tissues.[1] Fortunately, the acoustic properties of tumors differ from those of normal tissues.

Ultrasonography is ideal for imaging all solid soft tissue structures, including abdominal contents; mediastinal structures, including the heart; and superficial tissues. Although an experienced ultrasonographer is able to distinguish subtle changes within normal tissues and gain suspicion of neoplasia, an absolute diagnosis can only be obtained by cytology or histopathology.

Ultrasonography has been used recently to characterize a wide variety of diseases. For example, investigators used

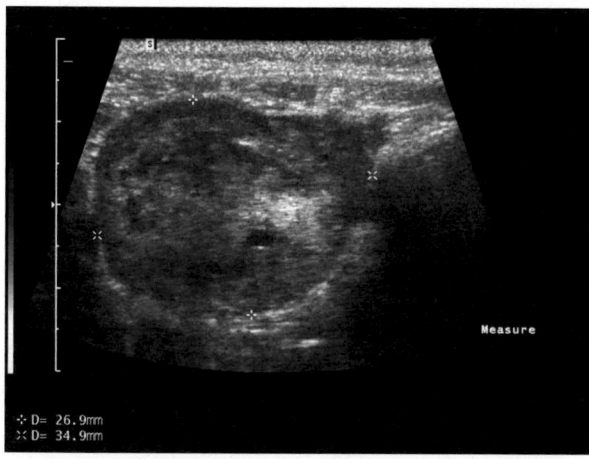

Figure 11-8. *Ultrasonography is ideal for identifying macroscopic structural changes in organs, and it can determine blood flow within the imaged organs. This ultrasound image shows a thyroid carcinoma located peritracheally. Color-flow Doppler confirmed a great deal of blood flow characteristic of thyroid tumors. (Courtesy of L. A. Mohammadian and D. Thrall)*

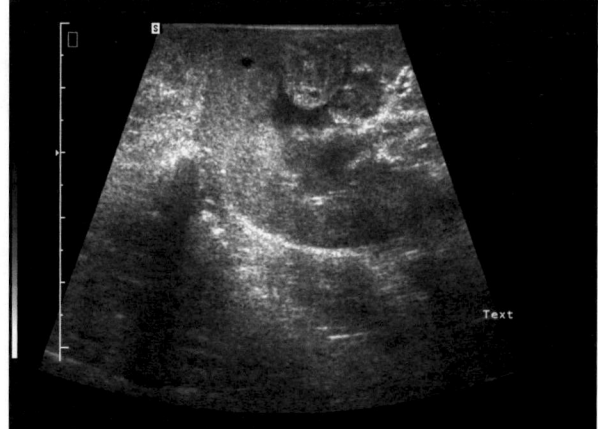

Figure 11-9. *The identification of intra-abdominal lesions that are suggestive of metastatic disease is commonly done by ultrasound imaging. The mass within this kidney was determined to be metastatic hemangiosarcoma. It is characterized by mixed echogenicity. (Courtesy of L. A. Mohammadian and D. Thrall)*

ultrasonography to characterize intestinal tumors in dogs.[9] These poorly echogenic lesions were transmural and associated with complete loss of wall layering. There is evidence that the experience and excellence of the ultrasonographer can profoundly impact the accuracy of diagnosing gastric and intestinal neoplasia.[9,10] However, not every disease has unique ultrasonographic findings. In one study, investigators characterized the ultrasonographic features of canine malignant histiocytosis and found nonspecific ultrasonographic features.[11] The anatomic changes associated with gastric carcinoma,[10] malignant mammary tumors,[12] laryngeal tumors,[13] ovarian tumors,[14] testicular tumors,[15] and urethral tumors[16] were easily visualized, although few ultrasonographic findings were pathognomonic for their respective histologic diagnoses.

Ultrasonography has dramatically enhanced the accuracy and speed of diagnosing endocrine diseases such as hyperadrenocorticism.[19-21] Pituitary-dependent hyperadrenocorticism (PDH) causes bilateral adrenomegaly, whereas an adrenal cortical tumor is almost always visible on ultrasonograms.[19-21] Ultrasonography has confirmed that the incidence of bilateral adrenocortical tumors occurs in approximately 20% of the dogs examined.[19] However, the ultrasonographic method used in this study was unable to discern a decrease in the size of contralateral glands.[19]

In many cases, ultrasonography can be helpful in guiding a needle-core biopsy instrument or needle directly into the tissue with minimal damage to surrounding tissue and a high degree of accuracy.[20,21] Care must be taken to ensure that neoplastic cells are not released into the surrounding tissues, thereby causing a "seeding" of tumor cells; this is rare except in malignancies such as transitional cell carcinoma.[22] Of particular note is the value of using ultrasonography to identify pathologic fractures and to direct needle aspiration through the cortex of cortical bone in dogs with osteosarcoma. This technique is surprisingly accurate and eliminates the need for anesthesia in many patients during a bone biopsy core. The use of analgesics, both systemic and locally applied, is essential to ensure patient comfort after the procedure.

> **When performing an ultrasound-guided biopsy or aspiration, care must be taken to ensure that neoplastic cells are not released into the surrounding tissues, thereby causing a "seeding" of tumor cells. This is rare except in malignancies such as transitional cell carcinoma.**

Ultrasonography is gaining popularity as a tool for guiding more accurate treatment of malignancies. Some centers use intraoperative ultrasonography to direct the surgical resection of lesions within tissue structures. Ultrasonographic guidance of the injection of chemicals such as ethanol within tumors or vasculature leading into tumors has been described in humans and animals.[23] The injection of ethanol and the direction of radiofrequency waves with ultrasonographic guidance for the treatment of parathyroid tumors in dogs has had some success.[23]

Although ultrasonography provides elegant details about various anatomic structures, it also provides functional information, especially about tumor vasculature, as with color-flow

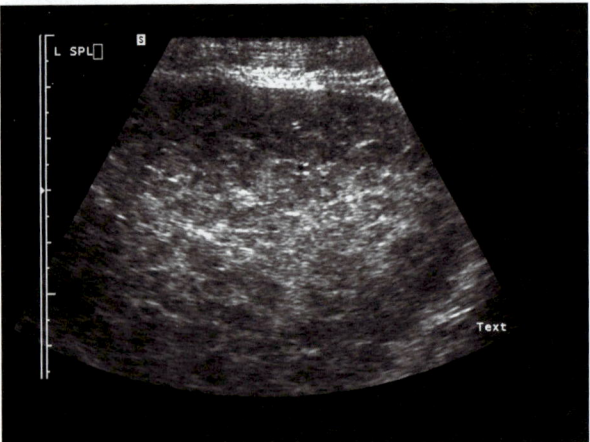

Figure 11-10. *The mixed echogenicity of this spleen led to ultrasound-guided aspiration of this organ and a diagnosis of lymphoblastic lymphoma. (Courtesy of L. A. Mohammadian and D. Thrall)*

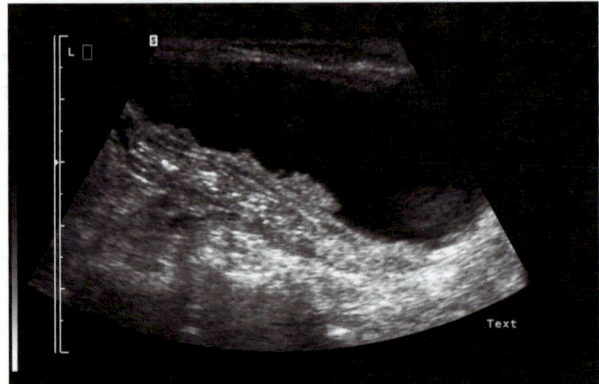

Figure 11-11. *Ultrasonography is often used to identify stones, hematomas, and tumors within the lumen of the bladder. The irregularity of the mucosal surface of the bladder and the thickened bladder wall was proven to be a transitional cell carcinoma via histopathology. (Courtesy of L. A. Mohammadian and D. Thrall)*

Doppler.[1–3] Doppler is based on the shift in sound frequencies that occurs when sound waves bounce off moving substances, such as blood cells in a blood vessel. It can be used to determine tissue vascularization and arteriovenous shunting.

Magnetic Resonance Imaging

The principal difference between MRI and CT is that whereas MRI detects differences in the chemical properties of tissue, CT detects differences in density between tissues.[1–3] In MRI, images are formed when water-hydrogen protons within an animal are aligned with the axis of a magnetic field produced by a very powerful magnet contained within an MRI machine.[1,3] This machine sends pulsed radiofrequency waves from the magnet to the patient, causing the hydrogen to "wobble." The hydrogen molecules then return to their normal position, releasing energy that is detected by a receiver and converted into an image by a computer. This is repeated in all three directions (x, y, and z axes), producing highly detailed definitions within tissues.[1–3] Contrast agents, such as gadolinium, enhance the ability to determine differences between tissues and chemicals within a tissue (Figures 11-13 to 11-19).

MRI has become the imaging modality of choice for evaluating the CNS. Although CT provides very good images, MRI often provides more detailed information about subtle changes within the brain. Brain tumors, strokes, and chemical changes within the brain after seizures are all commonly identified. More specifically, MRI has been successful in identifying and characterizing the features of tumors within the spine, spinal cord, and brain of dogs.[24–31] In these studies, meningiomas were usually extra-axial lesions that enhanced dramatically with gadolinium contrast agent.[28–30] Gliomas were intraaxial lesions that caused a significant mass effect, surrounding edema, and a wide variety of

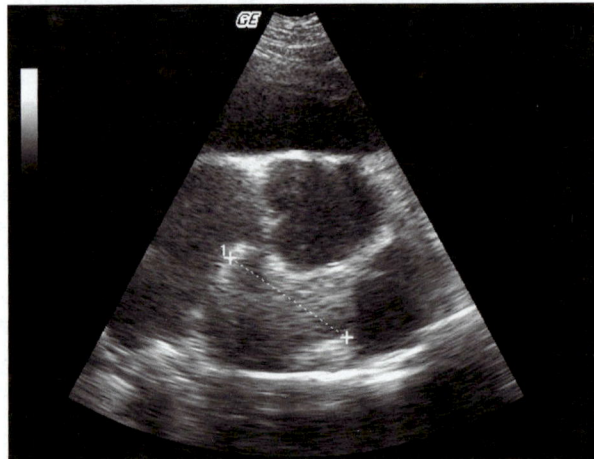

Figure 11-12. *Ultrasonography is ideal for identifying masses within or around the heart such as this heart-based tumor. (Courtesy of L. A. Mohammadian)*

enhancement patterns.[28–30] Choroid plexus tumors and pituitary tumors were identified by their location and marked gadolinium contrast enhancement.[27] A large mass identified on the MRI in the pituitary gland, suprasellar region, or both was consistent with a macroadenoma and often associated with hyperadrenocorticism.[31]

MRI is also used to evaluate tissues outside the CNS, such as soft tissue structures within the musculoskeletal system.[30–33] Peripheral nerve sheath tumors and the extent of osteosarcoma of the appendicular skeleton in dogs have been determined using MRI. Functional changes within the tissue can be determined by magnetic resonance spectroscopy, a technique in which the concentration of cell metabolites or chemicals is determined; the unique spectrum of chemical changes within a cell can be suggestive of certain malignancies.

VETERINARY CANCER IMAGING

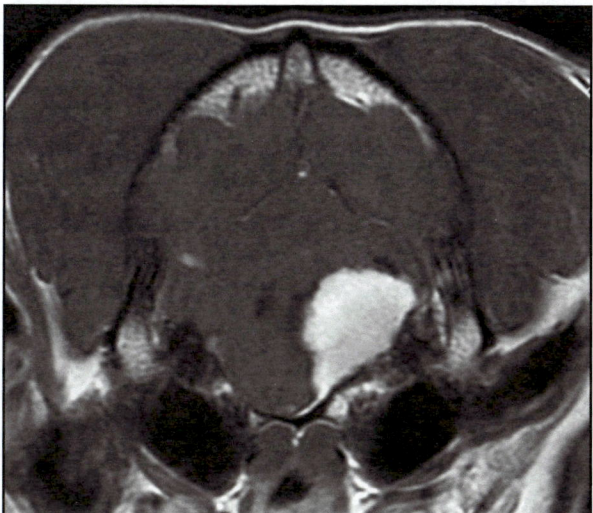

Figure 11-13. T_1-weighted postcontrast MRI of a dog's brain in the transverse plane. There is a large, intensely contrast-enhancing, extra-axial, space-occupying mass at the right cerebellopontine angle. The lesion is compressing the adjacent brain and fourth ventricle and exhibits a "dural tail sign." Findings were most consistent with a meningioma. (Courtesy of Susan L. Kraft, DVM, College of Veterinary Medicine and Biomedical Sciences, Colorado State University)

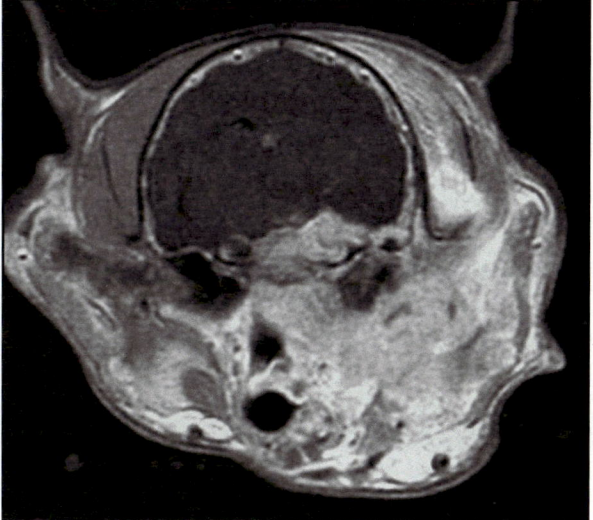

Figure 11-14. Postcontrast T_1-weighted MRI in the transverse plane of a carcinoma involving the right ear. The contrast-enhancing tumor has invaded the skull base and is compressing the ventral aspect of the brain. (Courtesy of S. L. Kraft)

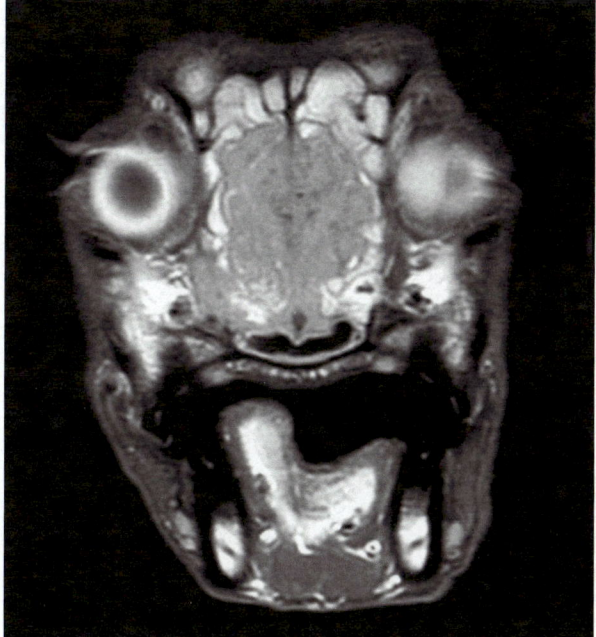

Figure 11-15. T_1-weighted postcontrast MRI in the transverse plane of a nasal carcinoma that has filled the caudal nasal passage bilaterally. (Courtesy of S. L. Kraft)

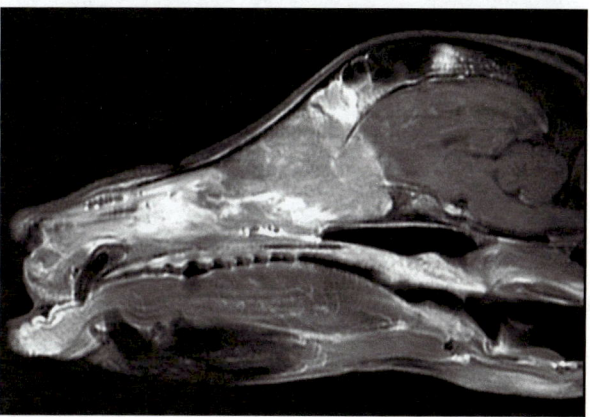

Figure 11-16. T_1-weighted postcontrast MRI in the sagittal plane of the same nasal carcinoma as in Figure 11-15 that extends around the cribriform plate. (Courtesy of S. L. Kraft)

Planar Scintigraphy

Nuclear medicine has been used in clinical veterinary and human oncology for decades. Scintigraphy uses a metabolically active molecule bound with a radioactive substance that is administered to the patient. The metabolically active substance distributes to the tissue of interest and is then detected by placing the patient on a gamma camera that has detectors to identify the presence of the radioactively tagged material within the body.[1–3] A computer then acquires the image obtained from the gamma camera for analysis, dynamic uptake and decay, and static anatomic images. Although the ability of this technique to form a detailed anatomic image is poor, its sensitivity to detect the radioactive substance is very high (Figures 11-20 to 11-22). The most common use of scintigraphy in veterinary medicine is in the detection of bone and thyroid tumors.[33–38] Bone scintigraphy is conducted using ^{99m}technetium [Tc]-methylene diphosphonate. Although bone scintigraphy seems to be a sensitive method,

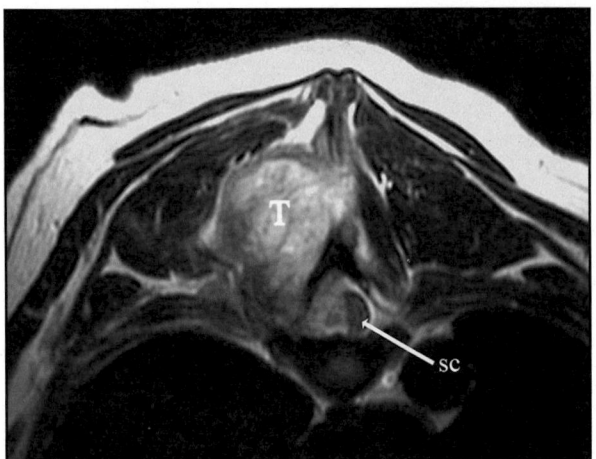

Figure 11-17. T_2-weighted MRI in the transverse plane of a spinal chondrosarcoma of the midthoracic spine. The tumor (T) involves the lamina and spinous process, with the extradural mass causing extradural spinal cord (sc) compression. (Courtesy of S. L. Kraft)

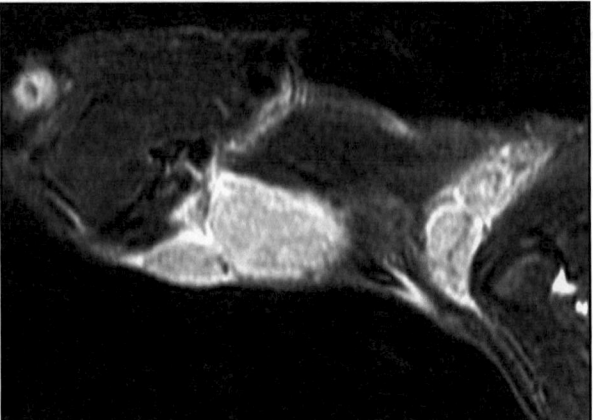

Figure 11-19. This is a sagittal short tau inversion recovery (STIR) MRI image of hyperintense enlarged mandibular, retropharyngeal, and superficial cervical lymph nodes due to malignant lymphoma. (Courtesy of S. L. Kraft)

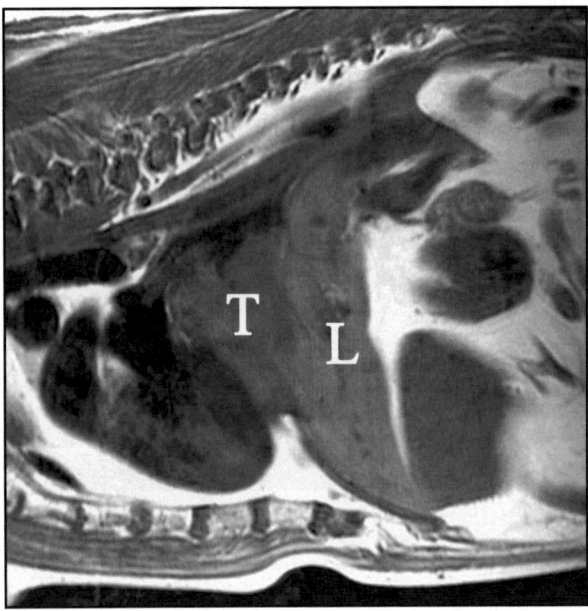

Figure 11-18. T_1-weighted MRI in the sagittal plane showing an accessory lung lobe tumor (T) between the heart and liver (L). (Courtesy of S. L. Kraft)

> **KEY POINT**
> **MRI is the diagnostic test of choice for neoplasia of the CNS.**

it is not specific for primary and metastatic bone tumors; additional diagnostics are essential to accurately identify abnormal bone lesions detected via scintigraphy.

Nuclear medicine has been helpful in diagnosing and staging thyroid neoplasia in dogs.[37-38] The most common scintigraphic appearance associated with thyroid cancer is a unilateral thyroid mass with increased radionuclide uptake relative to that of the parotid salivary glands. There is, however, no association between distribution of radionuclide

> **KEY POINT**
> *Bone scintigraphy using ^{99m}Tc-methylene diphosphonate is very sensitive, but not very specific, for determining bone metastases from diseases such as osteosarcoma.*

uptake and histologic diagnosis, although one investigator reported an association between distribution of uptake and histologic degree of capsular invasion.[37] Scintigraphy does not appear to be superior to standard thoracic radiography in identifying lung metastases from thyroid carcinomas. Nuclear imaging can be an important prelude to therapy with radioactive iodine.[37,38]

Newer radionuclides used to image the heart have been shown to be of value in staging certain cancers.[1-3,39] ^{99m}Tc methoxy-isobutyl-isonitrite (sestamibi) has been used to image malignant lymphoma. This methodology can not only detect lymphoma within organs of the body but also predict drug resistance to some chemotherapeutic agents. Therefore, sestamibi imaging has potential application in the management of patients to document response to treatment and to determine extent of disease.

Nuclear medicine has been helpful in diagnosing and staging β-cell tumors that produce insulin and cause hypoglycemia.[40,41] Scintigraphy conducted after the injection of 111 MBq of ^{111}In-pentetreotide is a useful method to identify insulinomas and associated metastases in selected patients. It is also useful in identifying the presence of the lesion and ruling out hepatic metastases.[40]

VETERINARY CANCER IMAGING

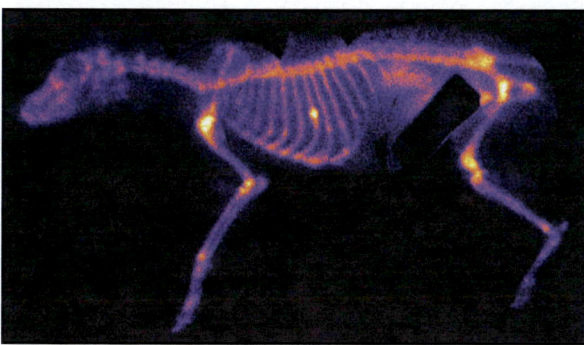

Figure 11-20. *Metastatic disease to the bone can be detected in some cases with bone scintigraphy before clinical signs are noted. In a bone scan, the radionuclide is bound to a material that is taken up where there is high bone turnover. This diagnostic procedure is sensitive but not specific for determining metastatic disease. (Courtesy of Gregory B. Daniel, DVM, American College of Veterinary Radiology, University of Tennessee)*

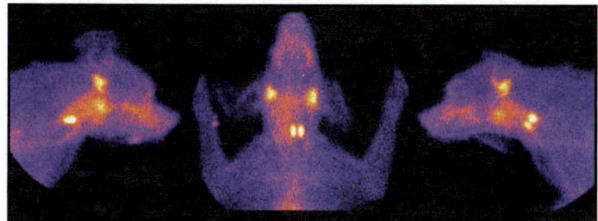

Figure 11-21. *Nuclear medicine is effective in diagnosing endocrine diseases, as in this dog with a carotid body tumor. Note that the radionuclide is taken up not only in the carotid body tumor but also within other tissues such as thyroid glands. (Courtesy of G. B. Daniel)*

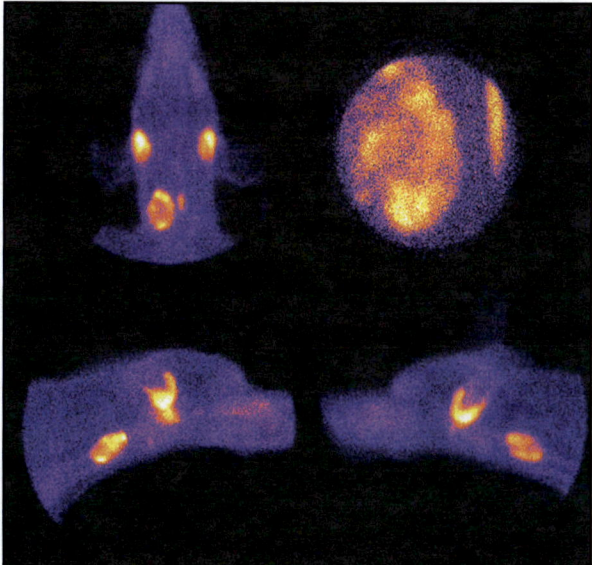

Figure 11-22. *Thyroid tumors and their metastases are often easily observable via nuclear scintigraphy. Radioactive iodine or technetium scintigraphy can be used to image thyroid neoplasia and their metastases. (Courtesy of G. B. Daniel)*

SPECT and SPECT/CT

SPECT uses the same approach as CT in creating slices of the body by detecting the single-photon emission of radiopharmaceuticals from radioactive tracers injected into the body.[1-3] A ring of detectors "senses" the emissions from the patient and counts the number of gamma rays from the area being imaged. This is then converted via a computer into a special image or "slice" of the patient. When the SPECT unit concurrently images the patient with a standard CT, the merged images not only give excellent anatomic resolution but also identify the tissue in question via SPECT imagery.

In veterinary medicine, most of the SPECT studies have been used to evaluate cardiac disease and cardiac function. A vitamin B_{12} analog, indium-111 (^{111}In)–labeled diethylenetriaminepentaacetate adenosylcobalamin (^{111}In DAC), has been used to image dogs and humans with malignancies using SPECT technology.[42] In one case, an 11-year-old, castrated Labrador retriever was imaged with ^{111}In DAC that resulted in significant uptake by both primary tumors and lung metastases. Thus, ^{111}In DAC may provide a useful differentiation technique for evaluation of masses because B_{12} is preferentially taken up by metabolically active tissues (such as tumors).[42]

> **SPECT uses the same approach as CT in creating slices of the body by detecting the single-photon emission of radiopharmaceuticals from radioactive tracers injected into the body.**

PET and PET/CT

PET is similar to CT, MRI, and SPECT in that it provides cross-sectional imagery by the administration of a β+ (positron)-emitting radionucleotide with a very short half-life of minutes to hours.[1-3] These positron-emitting particles are attached to a molecule of interest, such as glucose, that distributes to specific areas based on the unique aspects of that carrier. As with CT, MRI, and SPECT, a ring of detector is used to register the emission of the radioactive particle, and the end result is a computer-generated image of the patient. One radiotracer commonly used in PET imaging is ^{18}fluorodeoxyglucose (FDG), which accumulates in tissues of high metabolic activity such as tumors. As with SPECT and planar nuclear imaging, anatomic details of PET images are limited, but the specific identification of structures that take up the radiopharmaceutical is exquisite. In addition, the short half-life of FDG allows the patient to be discharged shortly after imaging with no risk to the client or caregivers. When PET imaging is combined with concurrent CT imaging, anatomic and functional detail is phenomenal, enhancing the value of this diagnostic modality.

PET imaging has been used to evaluate many canine tumors, including oral melanoma, lymphoma, osteosarcoma, soft tissue sarcoma, pheochromocytoma, and thyroid

> **KEY POINT**
>
> *PET is similar to CT, MRI, and SPECT in that it provides cross-sectional imagery by the administration of a β+ (positron)-emitting radionucleotide with a very short half-life of minutes to hours.*

carcinoma.[44,46,47] This methodology identifies occult malignancies and metastases with high sensitivity. The technology and the tracers used during imaging are expected to become more readily available and less costly in the near future.

Future Prospects in Imaging

"Functional imaging" is the watchword for the future of oncologic imaging. Anatomic imaging will always be important, but the greatest advances will be used to understand the molecular aspects of cancer, including apoptosis, proliferation, hypoxia, and the presence of proteins or other targets that can be used to direct therapy. Advanced imagery will determine whether drugs or molecular therapeutics, such as gene therapy, reach their biologic targets or induce their desired effects at the cellular level within a tumor. Further evaluations could determine whether the dosage of a treatment drug is adequate and whether a dog has an adequate response to therapy.

REFERENCES

1. Wisner ER, Pollard RE: Trends in veterinary cancer imaging. *Vet Comp Oncol* 2(2):49–74, 2004.
2. Wahl RL, Hapreet P: Imaging, in Abeloff MD, Armigage JO, Niederhuber JE, et al (eds): *Clinical Oncology*, ed 3. Philadelphia, Elsevier, 2004, pp 341–364.
3. Bragg DG, Rubin P, Hricak H: Imaging strategies for oncologic diagnosis and multidisciplinary treatment, in Bragg D, Rubin P, Hricak H (eds): *Oncologic Imaging*, ed 2. Philadelphia, WB Saunders, 2002, pp 3–20.
4. Koblik PD, LeCouteur RA, Higgins RJ, et al: Modification and application of a Pelorus Mark III stereotactic system for CT-guided brain biopsy in 50 dogs. *Vet Radiol Ultrasound* 40(5):424–433, 1999.
5. Koblik PD, LeCouteur RA, Higgins RJ, et al: CT-guided brain biopsy using a modified Pelorus Mark III stereotactic system: Experience with 50 dogs. *Vet Radiol Ultrasound* 40(5):434–440, 1999.
6. Davis GJ, Kapatkin AS, Craig LE, et al: Comparison of radiography, computed tomography, and magnetic resonance imaging for evaluation of appendicular osteosarcoma in dogs. *JAVMA* 220(8):1171–1176, 2002.
7. Samii VF, Nyland TG, Werner LL, Baker TW: Ultrasound-guided fine-needle aspiration biopsy of bone lesions: A preliminary report. *Vet Radiol Ultrasound* 40(1):82–86, 1999.
8. Wood EF, O'Brien RT, Young KM: Ultrasound-guided fine-needle aspiration of focal parenchymal lesions of the lung in dogs and cats. *J Vet Intern Med* 12(5):338–342, 1998.
9. Lester NV, Hopkins AL, Bova FJ, et al: Radiosurgery using a stereotactic headframe system for irradiation of brain tumors in dogs. *JAVMA* 219(11):1562–1567, 2001.
10. McEntee MC, Thrall DE: Computed tomographic imaging of infiltrative lipoma in 22 dogs. *Vet Radiol Ultrasound* 42(3):221–225, 2001.
11. Paoloni MC, Penninck DG, Moore AS: Ultrasonographic and clinicopathologic findings in 21 dogs with intestinal adenocarcinoma. *Vet Radiol Ultrasound* 43(6):562–567, 2002.
12. Kaser-Holz B, Hauser B, Arnold P: Ultrasonographic findings in canine gastric neoplasia in 13 patients. *Vet Radiol Ultrasound* 37(1):51–56, 1996.
13. Ramirez S, Douglass JP, Robertson ID: Ultrasonographic features of canine abdominal malignant histiocytosis. *Vet Radiol Ultrasound* 43(2):167–170, 2002.
14. Gonzalez de Bulnes A, Garcia Fernandez P, Mayenco Aguirre AM, Sanchez de la Muela M: Ultrasonographic imaging of canine mammary tumours. *Vet Rec* 143(25):687–689, 1998.
15. Rudorf H, Brown P: Ultrasonography of laryngeal masses in six cats and one dog. *Vet Radiol Ultrasound* 39(5):430–434, 1998.
16. Diez-Bru N, Garcia-Real I, Martinez EM, et al: Ultrasonographic appearance of ovarian tumors in 10 dogs. *Vet Radiol Ultrasound* 39(3):226–233, 1998.
17. England GC: Ultrasonographic diagnosis of non-palpable Sertoli cell tumours in infertile dogs. *J Small Anim Pract* 36(11):476–480, 1995.
18. Lamb CR, Trower ND, Gregory SP: Ultrasound guided catheter biopsy of the lower urinary tract: Technique and results in 12 dogs. *J Small Anim Pract* 37(9):413–416, 1996.
19. Chastain CB, Panciera D, Waters C: Use of endogenous ACTH concentration and adrenal ultrasonography to distinguish the cause of canine hyperadrenocorticism. *Small Anim Clin Endocrinol* 11(3):15, 2001.
20. Hoerauf A, Reusch C: Ultrasonographic characteristics of both adrenal glands in 15 dogs with functional adrenocortical tumors. *JAAHA* 35(3):193–199, 1999.
21. Besso JG, Penninck DG, Gliatto JM: Ultrasonographic evaluation of adrenal lesions in 26 dogs. *Vet Radiol* 38(6):448–455, 1997.
22. Hanson JA, Tidwell AS: Ultrasonographic appearance of urethral transitional cell carcinoma in ten dogs. *Vet Radiol* 37(4):293–299, 1996.
23. Pollard RE, Long CD, Nelson RW, et al: Percutaneous ultrasonographically guided radiofrequency heat ablation for treatment of primary hyperparathyroidism in dogs. *JAVMA* 218:1106–1110, 2001.
24. Mellema LM, Koblik PD, Kortz GD, et al: Reversible magnetic resonance imaging abnormalities in dogs following seizures. *Vet Radiol Ultrasound* 40(6):588–595, 1999.
25. Kippenes H, Gavin PR, Bagley RS, et al: Magnetic resonance imaging features of tumors of the spine and spinal cord in dogs. *Vet Radiol Ultrasound* 40(6):627–633, 1999.
26. Levitski RE, Lipsitz D, Chauvet AE: Magnetic resonance imaging of the cervical spine in 27 dogs. *Vet Radiol Ultrasound* 40(4):332–341, 1999.
27. Lipsitz D, Levitski RE, Chauvet AE: Magnetic resonance imaging of a choroid plexus carcinoma and meningeal carcinomatosis in a dog. *Vet Radiol Ultrasound* 40(3):246–250, 1999.
28. Hathcock JT: Low field magnetic resonance imaging characteristics of cranial vault meningiomas in 13 dogs. *Vet Radiol* 37(4):257–263, 1996.
29. Thomas WB, Wheeler SJ, Kramer R, et al: Magnetic resonance imaging features of primary brain tumors in dogs. *Vet Radiol* 37(1):20–27, 1996.
30. Kraft SL, Gavin PR, DeHaan C, et al: Retrospective review of 50 canine intracranial tumors evaluated by magnetic resonance imaging. *J Vet Intern Med* 11(4):218–225, 1997.
31. Duesberg CA, Feldman EC, Nelson RW, et al: Magnetic resonance imaging for diagnosis of pituitary macrotumors in dogs. *JAVMA* 206(5):657–662, 1995.
32. Platt SR, Graham J, Chrisman CL, et al: Magnetic resonance imaging and ultrasonography in the diagnosis of a malignant peripheral nerve sheath tumor in a dog. *Vet Radiol Ultrasound* 40(4):367–371, 1999.
33. Forest LJ, Thrall DE: Bone scintigraphy for metastasis detection in canine osteosarcoma. *Vet Radiol Ultrasound* 35(2):124–130, 1994.
34. Berg J, Lamb CR, O'Callaghan MW: Bone scintigraphy in the initial evaluation of dogs with primary bone tumors. *JAVMA* 196(6):917–920, 1990.
35. Lamb CR, Berg J, Bengtson AE: Preoperative measurement of canine primary bone tumors, using radiography and bone scintigraphy. *JAVMA* 196(9):1474–1478, 1990.
36. Hahn KA, Hurd C, Cantwell D: Single-phase methylene diphosphate bone scintigraphy in the diagnostic evaluation of dogs with osteosarcoma. *JAVMA* 196(9):1483–1486, 1990.
37. Marks SL, Koblik PD, Hornof WJ, et al: 99mTc-pertechnetate imaging of thyroid tumors in dogs: 29 cases (1980–1992). *JAVMA* 204(5):756–760, 1994.
38. Kintzer PP, Peterson ME: Nuclear medicine of the thyroid gland: Scintigraphy and radioiodine therapy. *Vet Clin North Am Small Anim Pract* 24(3):587–605, 1994.
39. Steyn PF, Ogilvie G: 99mTc-methoxy-isobutyl-isonitrile (sestamibi) imaging of malignant canine lymphoma. *Vet Radiol* 36(5):411–416, 1995.
40. Lester NV, Newell SM, Hill RC, Lanz OI: Scintigraphic diagnosis of insulinoma

in a dog. *Vet Radiol Ultrasound* 40(2):174–178, 1999.
41. Chastain CB, Panciera D, Walters C: Scintigraphic diagnosis of insulinoma in a dog. *Small Anim Clin Endocrinol* 9(3):14, 1999.
42. Whittemore JC, Gionfriddo JR, Steyn PF, Ehrhart EJ: Indium-111 labeled vitamin B_{12} imaging of a ciliary adenoma with concurrent grade 2 soft tissue sarcoma of the leg in a Labrador retriever. *Vet Ophthalmol* 7(3):209–212, 2004.
43. Nakamoto Y, Chin BB, Kraitchman DL, et al: Effects of nonionic intravenous contrast agents at PET/CT imaging: Phantom and canine studies. *Radiology* 227(3):817–824, 2003.
44. Berry CR, DeGrado TR, Nutter F, et al: Imaging of pheochromocytoma in 2 dogs using p-[18F] fluorobenzylguanidine. *Vet Radiol Ultrasound* 43(2):183–186, 2002.
45. Rine GP, Dewhirst MW, Cobb ED, et al: Feasibility of estimating the temperature distribution in a tumor heated by a waveguide applicator. *Int J Radiat Oncol Biol Phys* 23(5):1009–1019, 1992.
46. Larson SM, Weiden PL, Grunbaum Z, et al: Positron imaging feasibility studies. I: Characteristics of (3H)thymidine uptake in rodent and canine neoplasms: Concise communication. *J Nucl Med* 22(10):869–874, 1981.
47. Larson SM, Weiden PL, Grunbaum Z, et al: Positron imaging feasibility studies. II: Characteristics of 2-deoxyglucose uptake in rodent and canine neoplasms: Concise communication. *J Nucl Med* ss(10):875–879, 1981.

BIOPSY, BIOPSY, BIOPSY! THEORY AND PRACTICE

Gregory K. Ogilvie and Antony S. Moore

CLINICAL BRIEFING

Indications A biopsy should be performed before definitive therapy if the results will:
- Change the treatment.
- Influence the client's willingness to treat his or her dog.

Guidelines
- Biopsy should be performed only after consultation with the surgeon who will perform the definitive surgery.
- Obtain as large a sample as possible without significantly altering the benefits of the definitive therapy.
- *Do not* use electrocautery or surgical instruments that can potentially crush or otherwise damage tissues.
- Never "evaporate" a tumor with a laser.
- Place each biopsy sample in a separate, properly labeled container.
- Submit the entire lesion that has been resected and properly prepared in an adequate amount of fixative when possible.
- Consider submitting portions of the lesion for culture and sensitivity testing or other analyses before placing the sample in fixative.
- Submit the biopsy sample to a highly qualified veterinary pathologist. Samples are best analyzed by an anatomic pathologist and cytology samples by a clinical pathologist.
- Always have a plan to prevent and treat any discomfort with appropriate analgesics.

The first step in successfully managing a patient with cancer is to know which disease is being treated. Therefore, the three golden rules in oncology are biopsy, biopsy, and biopsy! To determine prognosis, treatment options, and palliative care, one must know the histopathologic diagnosis and, whenever biologically meaningful, the grade of the tumor.[1-5] These rules are the key to the successful management of any dog with cancer. A biopsy before the definitive procedure is critical in canine oncology because "salvage" procedures are often less successful and usually much more expensive. Consequently, the definitive treatment must be selected correctly the *first time*.

KEY POINT
The biopsy provides the entire veterinary health care team and the caregiver with the first vital piece of information in developing a plan of action. This is the first phase of reversing the sense of loss of power that accompanies a cancer diagnosis.

The biopsy is one of the most important procedures performed when evaluating a dog with cancer. Biopsy results must be interpreted carefully in conjunction with the results of other diagnostic procedures such as blood work, radiography, ultrasonography, computed tomography (CT), magnetic resonance imaging (MRI), and other imaging modalities. A biopsy specimen is of value only if it is properly collected and prepared and then interpreted by a highly trained pathologist who is willing to use all available clinical information to arrive at an accurate diagnosis.

Each biopsy should be performed with the assumption that the lesion is malignant. Therefore, the procedure should be performed so that the entire surgical field, including all tissues or tissue planes that may have been disturbed and any post-biopsy hemorrhage, seroma, or hematoma, can be removed during subsequent surgery. Second surgeries performed to remove the tumor and surrounding tissues should involve at least one fascial layer below the tumor and all tissues disturbed by previous surgery.

Several types of biopsies exist, including needle core, punch, incisional (wedge), and excisional biopsies. A small core of tissue is obtained with a needle core biopsy, whereas a portion of the tumor is removed with an incisional biopsy. Incisional biopsies are generally taken at the junction of normal and abnormal tissue and are preferred in cases in which

BIOPSY, BIOPSY, BIOPSY! THEORY AND PRACTICE

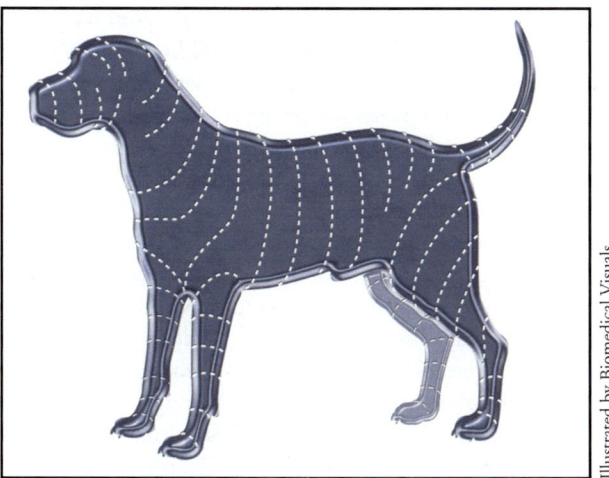

Figure 12-1. *When a biopsy or definitive procedure is performed, the incision should minimize tension on the skin. Generally, incisions are made like the stripes on a tiger to minimize skin tension and maximize the amount of tissue that can be removed around the tumor.*

a punch or needle biopsy cannot provide an adequate tissue sample for analysis. Regardless of the type, the biopsy procedure must be performed correctly to avoid compromising subsequent curative resection. An excisional biopsy, which removes the entire tumor, is preferred in cases in which knowledge of the tissue type will not influence the definitive procedure or treatment plan (e.g., a solitary lung mass, a splenic mass).

> **KEY POINT**
> *The biopsy is one of the most important procedures performed when evaluating a dog with cancer.*

The biopsy should be performed before definitive therapy if the results will alter the type of therapy to be employed or influence an owner's willingness to treat his or her dog.[1] For example, if biopsy results indicate a benign perianal adenoma, the clinician can confidently proceed with a conservative resection and castration, if indicated. If, however, the biopsy results reveal that the mass is a high-grade perianal adenocarcinoma, which is a more aggressive tumor, then wide surgical resection around the periphery of the tumor (after careful evaluation for metastatic disease) is required and adjunctive therapy may be recommended. For financial and/or emotional reasons, some owners may be more willing to treat a dog with a benign tumor than one with a more malignant/aggressive biologic behavior.

Biopsy Guidelines[1,2]
1. **When performed appropriately, biopsies do not negatively influence the survival of the patient.** The myth

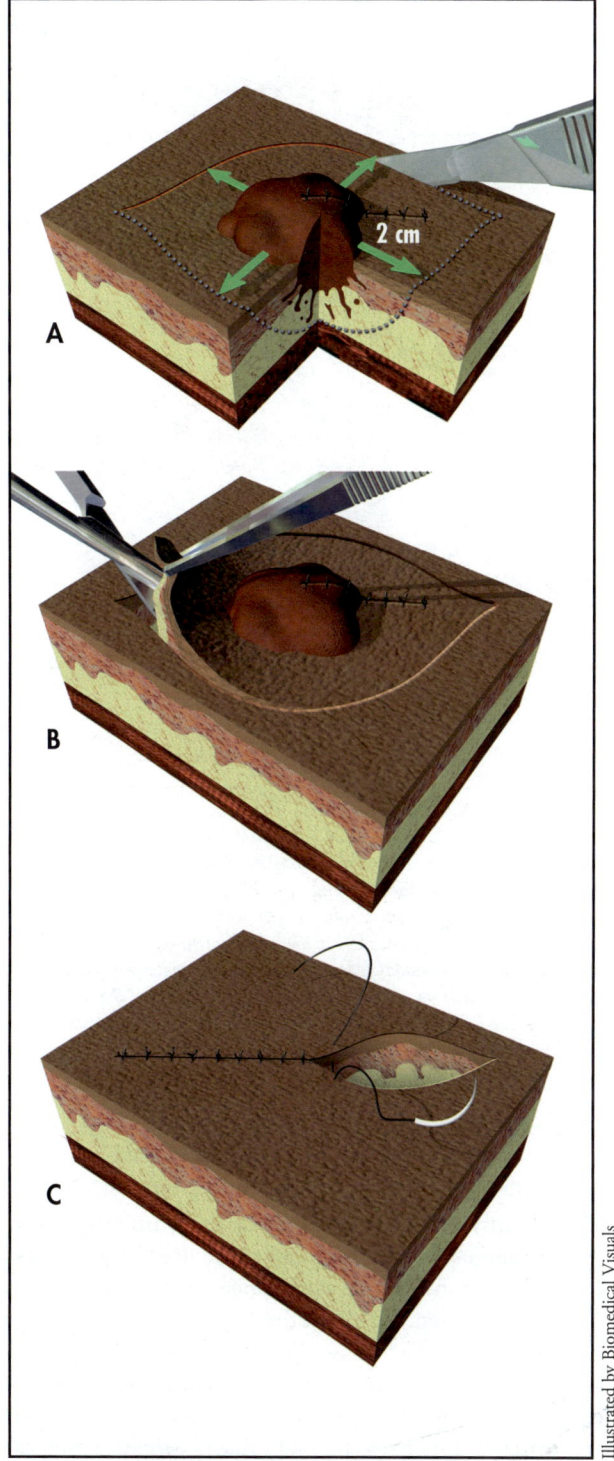

Figure 12-2. *Removal of the site of a previous biopsy. The entire previous surgical field, including all tissues or tissue planes that may have been disturbed (**A**), is removed by the definitive surgery. Note that this involves making an elliptical "bird's-eye" incision, going at least one fascial layer below the tumor, and obtaining wide surgical margins laterally (**B**). The surgeon should not leave any portion of the tumor or any tissue that was disrupted by the previous biopsy (**C**).*

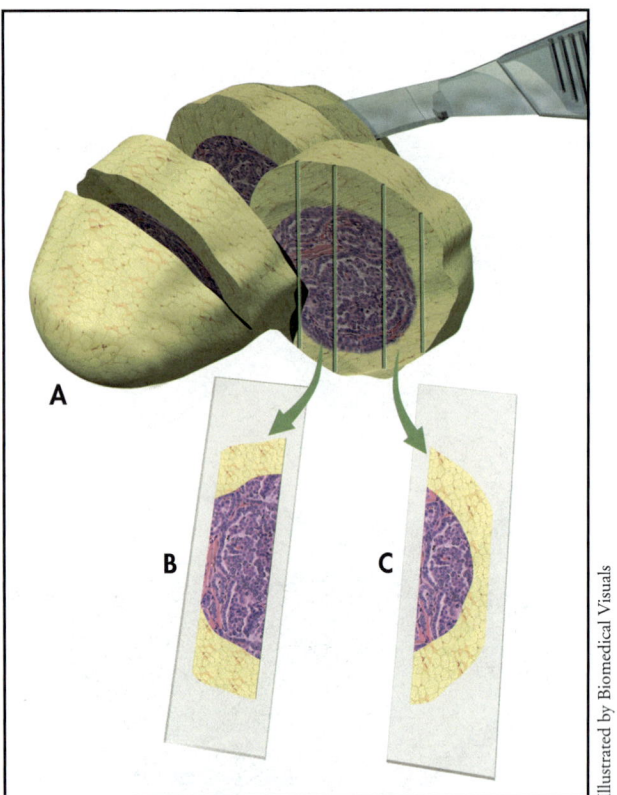

Figure 12-3. *Samples larger than 1 cm in diameter should be incompletely sliced like a loaf of bread, leaving one side uncut to retain the tumor's spatial relationship (**A**). The slices should be 1 cm apart to allow adequate fixation. Note that the ability of the pathologist to determine whether the margins are free of tumor (tumor noted as darkest area) may depend on where the representative sample was taken from the biopsy specimen (**B**) and how it was placed on a microscope slide (**C**). Therefore, the entire properly fixed and prepared biopsy specimen should be submitted with a detailed history and description for the most accurate results.*

that the biopsy procedure causes cancer cells to spread throughout the dog's body, resulting in early demise of the patient, is not supported in the scientific literature.

2. **A biopsy should be performed after consultation with the surgeon who will perform the definitive surgery.** This gives the surgeon the information needed to ensure that the lesion and the entire biopsy tract are removed without "spilling" or "seeding" tumor cells into the surgical field. In addition, the biopsy incision should be oriented to cause the least amount of tension on the skin, thereby simplifying any subsequent definitive surgical procedure(s). In general, incisions should be made like the stripes on a tiger (Figure 12-1) to minimize skin tension and maximize the amount of tissue that can be removed around the tumor. There are, however, some exceptions, such as the presence of odd-shaped tumors in areas where the skin is tight.

3. **To assist the pathologist in making a correct diagnosis, as large a sample as possible should be obtained.** With incisional biopsy, the juncture of normal and abnormal tissue is an ideal site for sampling the tumor. Tumors involving bone, such as osteosarcoma, are exceptions to this rule. When this tumor type is suspected, biopsy specimens should be taken from the *center* of the tumor because the periphery of the lesion is primarily composed of reactive bone. Ulcerated, necrotic tissue should not be collected unless absolutely necessary because secondary pathologic lesions may obscure the primary diagnosis. In addition, if needle core biopsies are performed, multiple samples (at least three to five) should be taken throughout the tumor. Regardless of the biopsy technique used, the entire biopsy field must be placed so that the biopsy tracts can be removed with the definitive procedure (Figure 12-2).

4. **The original architecture of the tissue sample should be maintained.** Therefore, electrocautery, lasers, or surgical instruments that burn, vaporize, crush, or otherwise damage tissues should not be used.

5. **Tissue must be adequately fixed in 10% buffered neutral formalin (one part tissue to 10 parts fixative).** Fresh tissue should be placed in fixative for 24 to 48 hours. Although most pathologists prefer 10% buffered formalin, other fixatives, such as Zenker's or Bouin's, can be used for special purposes (e.g., optic tissue). For best results and to ensure proper exposure to the fixative, tissue samples should not be thicker than 1 cm. If an excisional biopsy is performed and the entire sample is larger than 1 cm, it can be cut like a loaf of bread to allow proper exposure of the tissue to the fixative (Figure 12-3). The exception to this rule is brain tissue, which can be fixed intact without the bread-loaf technique. Very thin samples should be avoided because the fixation process can distort the tissue architecture. The tissue should not be exposed to heat, cold, or water at any time.

6. **Each biopsy specimen should be placed into a separate, properly labeled container.** The container should be labeled on its side rather than on the lid to prevent mix-ups in case the tops are switched. If multiple samples are collected, all containers should be labeled *before* the procedure to reduce the chance of confusing samples.

7. **When possible, all resected tissue should be properly prepared and submitted for appropriate analysis.** This enables the pathologist to examine the tissue for completeness of removal ("clean" or "dirty" margins) and architectural detail. Particularly when an excisional biopsy is performed, trimming the biopsy specimen or submitting only a small section means that this valuable information may be lost. However, if mailing costs must

be reduced, smaller, adequately fixed representative tissue samples can be sent in the minimum amount of formalin to keep them moist. Tissues that are adequately fixed in formalin can be placed in sealable plastic bags with a formalin-saturated paper towel or sponge. If only a portion of the sample is submitted, the original tissue should be kept by the attending clinician in the event that additional samples are needed. Overfixation may adversely affect future immunohistochemical examination of the tissue. All margins should be marked with ink or suture and submitted to determine the adequacy of surgical excision (Figure 12-4). Again, if decreasing the size of the submitted sample is necessary, margins may be submitted separately.

8. **Before the tissue sample is placed in fixative, consideration should be given to submitting portions for culture and sensitivity testing or alternative analysis (e.g., polymerase chain reaction).** For best results, it is essential to plan which types of samples are to be submitted and analyzed before preparing the biopsy sample. Once the tissue is in the formalin, other tests or analyses may not be possible.

9. **Biopsy specimens should be submitted to a highly qualified veterinary pathologist who is willing to work with the clinician.** In addition:
   — The pathologist should be given a detailed history and a complete account of all relevant clinical material.
   — When an excisional biopsy is performed, margins should be identified with ink or suture. The pathologist will then have all the information necessary to make an accurate diagnosis.
   — It is important for the clinician and pathologist to work together to help coordinate the clinical picture with the diagnosis. If the two do not match, then the clinician and pathologist should work together to reevaluate all case information, including histopathology. This cooperative interaction is essential for accurate diagnosis and optimum treatment of the dog's disease.
   — Board-certified, anatomic pathologists are best qualified to analyze histopathologic specimens, whereas board-certified clinical pathologists are the most appropriate specialists to evaluate cytology, hematology, and biochemical problems.

> **KEY POINT**
>
> *A plan to include pre- and postbiopsy analgesia must be determined before every procedure, taking into account the dog's history, vital signs, and any concurrent conditions.*

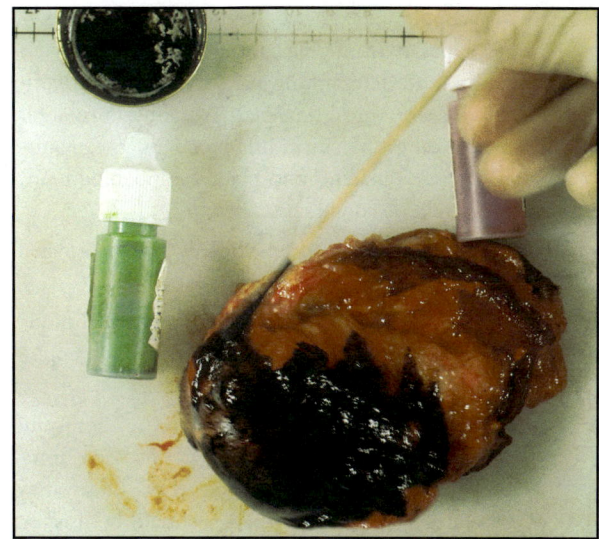

Figure 12-4. *Marking the margins of the sample to be submitted with various colored inks allows the pathologist to determine whether all abnormal tissue has been removed. Alternatively, sutures can be used to identify areas of interest or concern.*

Contraindications

The risks and benefits of the biopsy procedure should be evaluated and clearly described to the owner. In most cases, risks are minimal. Uncontrollable hemorrhage is the most common (but still rare) complication with all biopsy procedures, except possibly bone marrow aspiration. Therefore, hemostatic abnormalities caused by deficiencies in platelet numbers and function or coagulation disorders should be identified and, if possible, corrected before biopsy. Aseptic technique is critical to avoid the uncommon but serious complications of infection at the biopsy site and/or sepsis in the dog. Lastly, a biopsy should not be performed if it could potentially inhibit or jeopardize a definitive procedure. For example, an incisional biopsy of a primary lung tumor or mass on the spleen may contaminate the entire chest or abdominal cavity with tumor cells, which is why primary lung tumors or splenic masses are usually removed during the primary definitive surgical procedure (i.e., excisional biopsy). Note that diffuse enlargement of the spleen is most often caused by lymphoma or mast cell tumor, and diagnosis is often by transabdominal fine-needle aspiration cytology.

Sedation and Anesthesia for Biopsy

Cancer patients are often older and frequently have concurrent medical disorders that must be known before sedation or anesthesia is planned. In addition, because almost every procedure confers some degree of discomfort, an analgesic plan is essential.

- The risks and benefits of the sedation or anesthesia and the procedure itself should be carefully outlined with the dog's owner before obtaining written authorization.

- Each dog should be assessed before the procedure by obtaining a history from the client, performing a physical examination, and determining pain status. Also, a complete blood count (including platelet count), urinalysis, and biochemical profile, including blood glucose, alanine aminotransferase, alkaline phosphatase, and blood urea nitrogen, should be conducted.
- Placing an intravenous catheter is always encouraged. The following guidelines are recommended:
  — The catheter must be placed using aseptic technique, including washing hands and clipping and prepping catheter sites.
  — If the dog is suspected to be or is at risk for becoming volume contracted and anesthesia will be used, intravenous fluids should be administered via intravenous pumps or drip sets. Mini-drip sets should be used on patients weighing less than 5 kg.
  — Preemptive use of analgesics should be considered at this time.
  — If anesthesia is used, continuous monitoring should include evaluation of the following parameters: respiration, heart rate, arterial blood pressure, pulse pressure, palpebral reflex, eye position, jaw tone, and mucous membrane color. In addition, behavioral changes and signs of anxiety and/or pain should be monitored pre- and postoperatively.
  — If sedation is used, respiration, heart rate, mucous membrane color, and respiratory rate must be evaluated every 5 minutes until the patient is alert and responsive.

> **KEY POINT**
>
> *Plan all analyses of the tissue before the biopsy, particularly the required fixatives and tissue handling that may be necessary.*

Biopsy as a Prelude to Definitive Therapy

A palpable, persistent mass is the most common indication for biopsy as a prelude to definitive therapy.[1–4] As accuracy and sensitivity of diagnostic tests (e.g., ultrasonography, CT, MRI, positron emission tomography, single-photon emission axial tomography) improve, biopsies are being performed with increasing frequency to clarify the diagnosis of visualized, yet nonpalpable, masses.

When developing a diagnostic strategy for a dog with cancer, the clinician must consider subsequent disease management.[4] Advanced malignant disease is often diagnosed in dogs, and formulation of an appropriate diagnostic and therapeutic strategy early in the course of the disease is essential. The first step toward diagnosing most palpable lesions is fine-needle aspiration cytology. If the cytologic diagnosis strongly suggests a malignant condition or is highly suggestive of a particular condition (e.g., soft tissue sarcoma), a definitive procedure such as surgical removal can be planned. In addition, this tentative diagnosis can help guide the staging procedure ahead. Fine-needle aspiration cytology can also confirm the presence of a benign process, eliminating the need for further diagnostic steps.

If fine-needle aspiration cytology is not definitive, then an incisional biopsy should be performed or guided by the surgeon who will perform the definitive surgery. Before collecting a biopsy sample, standard diagnostic tests can be conducted to identify any concurrent disease or clinically evident metastatic disease.

Staging is accomplished through certain diagnostic tests that determine the extent of the neoplastic disorder. The staging schema differs for each neoplastic disease but should include a history, physical examination, complete blood count, biochemical profile, urinalysis, thoracic radiography, and cytologic evaluation of regional lymph nodes. Discussions regarding additional diagnostic steps in specific staging schemas are included in the review of each individual disease.

Conclusion

Each biopsy should be performed with the assumption that the lesion is malignant. Therefore, the biopsy should be done so that the entire surgical field, including all tissues or tissue planes that may have been disturbed as well as any postbiopsy hemorrhage/hematoma, can be removed by subsequent surgery. The definitive surgery should be performed to remove the tumor and surrounding tissues. This procedure frequently involves going at least one fascial layer below the tumor and all tissues disturbed by the previous surgery. Analgesics should be used to minimize the dog's discomfort.

REFERENCES

1. Ogilvie GK, Moore AS: *Managing the Veterinary Cancer Patient: A Practice Manual.* Yardley, PA, Veterinary Learning Systems, 1995, pp 1–47.
2. Ogilvie GK, Moore AS: *Feline Oncology: A Comprehensive Guide for Compassionate Care.* Yardley, PA, Veterinary Learning Systems, 2002, pp 7–12.
3. Withrow SJ: Biopsy principles, in Withrow SJ, MacEwen EG (eds): *Small Animal Clinical Oncology*, ed 3. Philadelphia, WB Saunders, 2001, pp 52–57.
4. Morrison WB, Hamilton TA, Hahn KA, et al: Diagnosis of neoplasia, in Slatter D (ed): *Textbook of Small Animal Surgery*, ed 2. Philadelphia, WB Saunders, 1993, pp 2036–2048.
5. Wolmark N: Biopsy as a prelude to a definitive operative therapy for breast cancer, in Wittes RE (ed): *Manual of Oncologic Therapeutics 1991/1992.* Philadelphia, JB Lippincott, 1991, pp 5–8.

SKIN BIOPSY

Gregory K. Ogilvie and Antony S. Moore

CLINICAL BRIEFING

Methods	Benefits
Punch biopsy	• Outpatient diagnostic procedure. • Quick and simple.
Incisional biopsy	• Diagnostic. • Allows surgeon to plan definitive procedure.
Excisional biopsy	• Diagnostic. • Potentially therapeutic.
Needle core biopsy	• Outpatient diagnostic procedure. • Allows surgeon to plan definitive procedure. • Rapid, simple, minimal recovery.

A skin biopsy is essential to diagnosing and evaluating potentially malignant skin conditions. *Punch, incisional, excisional,* and *needle core biopsies* are employed.[1-5]

Punch Biopsy[1-4]

Biopsy punches are available as expensive reusable instruments or inexpensive disposable units that may be reused after appropriate sterilization until they become dull. Punches are available in diameters ranging from 2 to 6 mm (Figure 13-1). Generally, taking a larger biopsy specimen is preferred so that the pathologist has an adequate sample from which to make a histologic diagnosis. When possible, multiple samples should be collected at the juncture between normal and abnormal tissue. Punch biopsies are usually inadequate to obtain tissue below the dermis.

Indication: Identification of any dermal or epidermal lesion of unknown etiology.

Contraindications/complications: Coagulopathies; lidocaine toxicities (unlikely).

Benefits: General anesthesia is not required; simple outpatient procedure.

Limitation: Small tissue samples may not be diagnostic.

Equipment: Sedation and analgesia should be considered (see box on page 62); 2% lidocaine and 8.4% bicarbonate (50:50) with or without NSAIDs; Baker's biopsy instrument; standard surgical instruments; suture material.

Technique (Figures 13-2 and 13-3):

1. Clip the hair and prepare the site with proper aseptic surgical technique.
2. Dilute 2% lidocaine 50:50 with 8.4% bicarbonate to reduce stinging on injection. Using a 25-gauge needle, inject approximately 0.25 to 1 ml of this local anesthetic agent around the lesion. It is important that injection of lidocaine does not distort or disturb the normal architecture of the tissue to be biopsied.
3. Surgically scrub the biopsy area a final time after the lidocaine is injected.

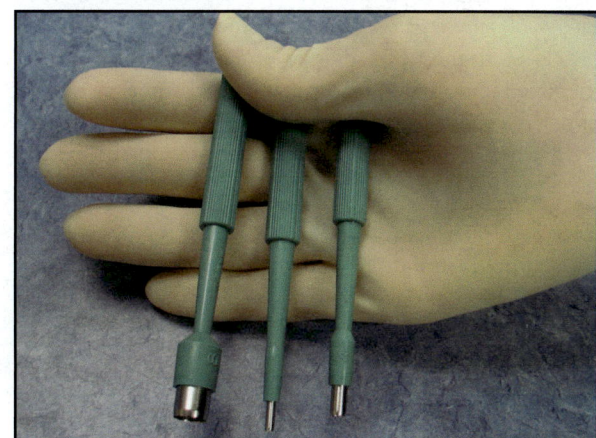

Figure 13-1. *Several sizes of punch biopsy instruments are available. Consideration should be given to obtaining as large a sample as possible from the margin of normal and abnormal tissue.*

62 MANAGING THE CANINE CANCER PATIENT

Selected NSAIDs for Simple Procedures
• Carprofen: 2.2 mg/kg PO q12h • Etodolac: 10–15 mg/kg PO q12h • Ketoprofen: 1–2 mg/kg IV, IM, or SC q24h or 1 mg/kg PO q24h • Meloxicam: 0.1–0.2 mg/kg IV, IM, or SC q24h; 0.1 mg/kg PO q24h • Piroxicam: 0.3 mg/kg PO q24–48h

4. Stretch the skin of the site to be biopsied between the thumb and index finger.
5. Place the biopsy punch at a right angle to the skin surface.
6. Rotate the punch in one direction while simultaneously applying firm downward pressure until the subcutis is reached.
7. Angle the punch almost parallel with the skin while still applying pressure along the long axis of the instrument.
8. Rotate the punch to sever at least part of the base of the biopsied tissue.
9. Remove the punch and gently elevate the core of tissue with the point of a needle; sever the base that is still attached with a scalpel blade or a pair of iris scissors.
10. Place one or two sutures as needed to close the defect, depending on the size of the punch taken.

Supportive Care: Oral analgesics; periodic cleansing of the surgery site; consider the use of an Elizabethan collar to prevent self-trauma.

Incisional Biopsy[1–4]

In some cases, an incisional biopsy is preferred to a punch biopsy because larger sections of tissue can be obtained for histologic diagnosis. In addition, if the lesion is biopsied at the junction of the normal and abnormal tissue, a "wedge" of tissue is obtained that retains a larger section of the tissue's architecture. This makes it easier for the histopathologist to see characteristics of malignancy, such as invasion into the normal tissue.

Indication: Identification of dermal, epidermal, or subcutaneous lesion of unknown etiology.

Contraindications: Coagulopathies; dogs that are at high risk during general anesthesia.

Benefit: Larger tissue sample often results in a more accurate diagnosis.

Limitations: General anesthesia is often needed; not a definitive procedure.

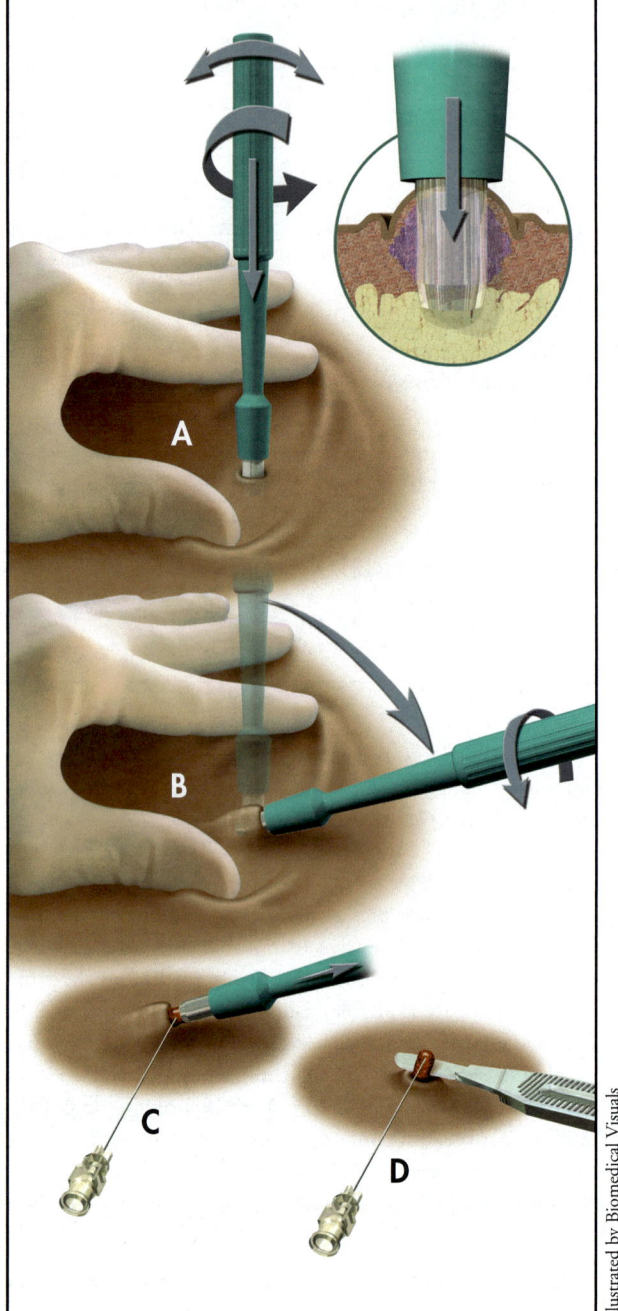

Figure 13-2. A punch biopsy procedure begins by injecting lidocaine around the area to be biopsied, being careful not to alter the tissue architecture of interest. (**A**) The skin is then stretched between the thumb and index finger, and the biopsy punch (e.g., Baker's biopsy punch) is placed at a right angle to the skin surface. The punch is rotated in one direction; at the same time, firm downward pressure is applied until the subcutis is reached. (**B**) The punch is then angled almost parallel with the skin while still applying pressure along the long axis of the biopsy punch. The punch is rotated to sever at least part of the base of the biopsied material. The punch is removed (**C**), and the core of tissue is gently elevated with the point of a needle and severed at the base with a scalpel (**D**).

SKIN BIOPSY

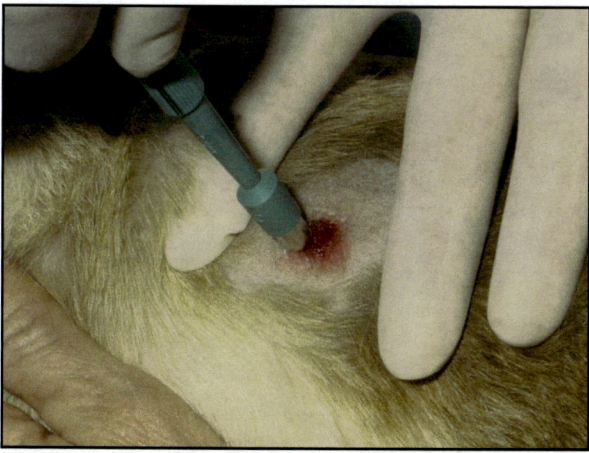

Figure 13-3. *After lidocaine is injected and the biopsy site prepared, the biopsy punch is placed at a 90° angle to the stretched skin. Note that the punch is located at the junction of normal and abnormal skin.*

Sample Protocol for Low to Moderately Painful Incisional Biopsy

Preemptive Analgesia
- Acepromazine: 0.02–0.04 mg/kg SC
- Atropine: 0.04 mg/kg SC
- Oxymorphone: 0.05–0.1 mg/kg SC

Anesthesia (as indicated)
- Propofol or thiopental induction followed by inhalant anesthesia

Postoperative Analgesia
- Ketoprofen: 2.2 mg/kg SC

Equipment: Sedation and general anesthesia (see box above); standard surgical instruments; suture material.

Technique (Figure 13-4A):

1. Conduct routine screening tests to identify problems such as coagulopathies and metabolic disease.
2. Place the dog under general anesthesia.
3. Surgically prepare the area with clipping and strict aseptic technique, then properly drape the site. Make an elliptic or wedge incision at the margin of normal and abnormal tissue. Take care to obtain adequate tissue and to ensure that subsequent definitive surgery can remove the tumor and the incisional biopsy area successfully.
4. Carefully identify and ligate vessels going to and from the tissue to be biopsied.
5. Lift the specimen and sever the connection at the base with either scissors or a scalpel blade.
6. Suture the incision closed.

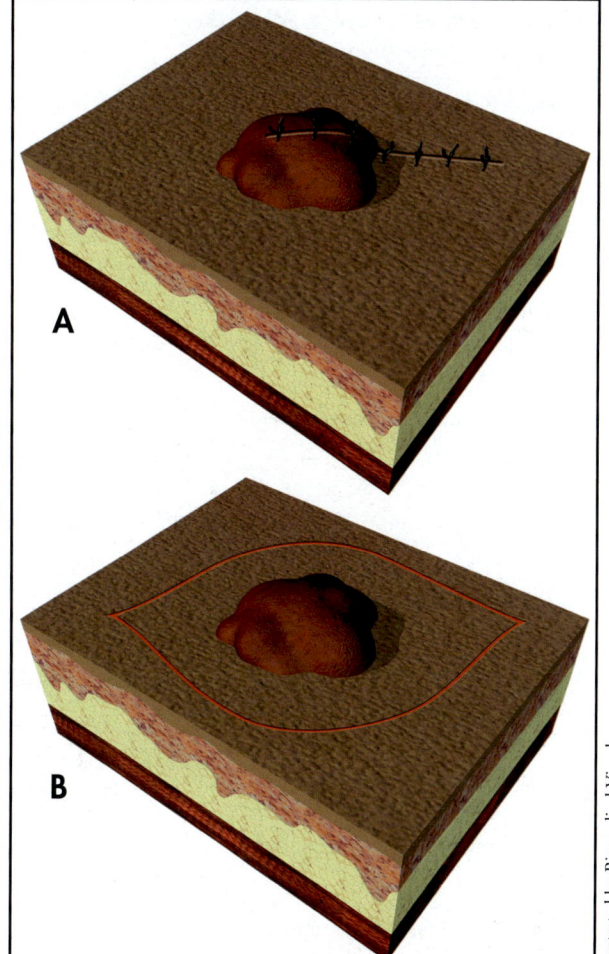

Figure 13-4. *(**A**) An incisional biopsy taken from the margin of normal and abnormal tissue. When performing an incisional biopsy, it should be kept in mind that the entire tumor and the biopsy tract will need to be removed in a subsequent definitive procedure. In definitive tumor removal after incisional biopsy (performed in the same manner as excisional biopsy), the entire tumor is removed. (**B**) With excisional biopsy, wide margins are obtained through the use of an elliptic "bird's-eye" incision, and the tissue removed includes one fascial plane below the tumor.*

Supportive Care: Oral or parenteral analgesics for several days to weeks; periodic cleansing of the surgery site.

Excisional Biopsy[1-4]

Excisional biopsy should be performed for histologic diagnosis of a small lesion located where wide surgical removal is

> **KEY POINT**
> *Excisional biopsy should be performed on a lesion that is small enough to be completely excised with adequately wide and deep surgical margins.*

> **Sample Protocol for Low to Moderately Painful Excisional Biopsy**
>
> **Preemptive Analgesia**
> - Acepromazine: 0.02 mg/kg SC
> - Atropine: 0.04 mg/kg SC
> - Morphine: 1 mg/kg SC
> - NSAIDs orally before and after surgery (ensure adequate hydration and renal function)
>
> **Anesthesia (as indicated)**
> - Propofol or thiopental induction followed by inhalant anesthesia
>
> **Postbiopsy Analgesia (choose one)**
> - Carprofen: 4 mg/kg SC
> - Ketoprofen: 2 mg/kg SC
> - Morphine: 0.5–1 mg/kg SC as needed q4–6h
> - Nalbuphine: 1 mg/kg SC as needed q4–6h
>
> **Home Analgesia (choose at least one)**
> - Carprofen: 2.2 mg/kg PO q12h
> - Etodolac: 10–15 mg/kg PO q12h
> - Ketoprofen: 1 mg/kg PO
> - Meloxicam: 0.1 mg/kg PO q24h
> - Morphine: 0.5 mg/kg PO q6–8h
> - Piroxicam: 0.3 mg/kg PO q24–48h
> - Transdermal fentanyl: 2–3 mg/kg/hr

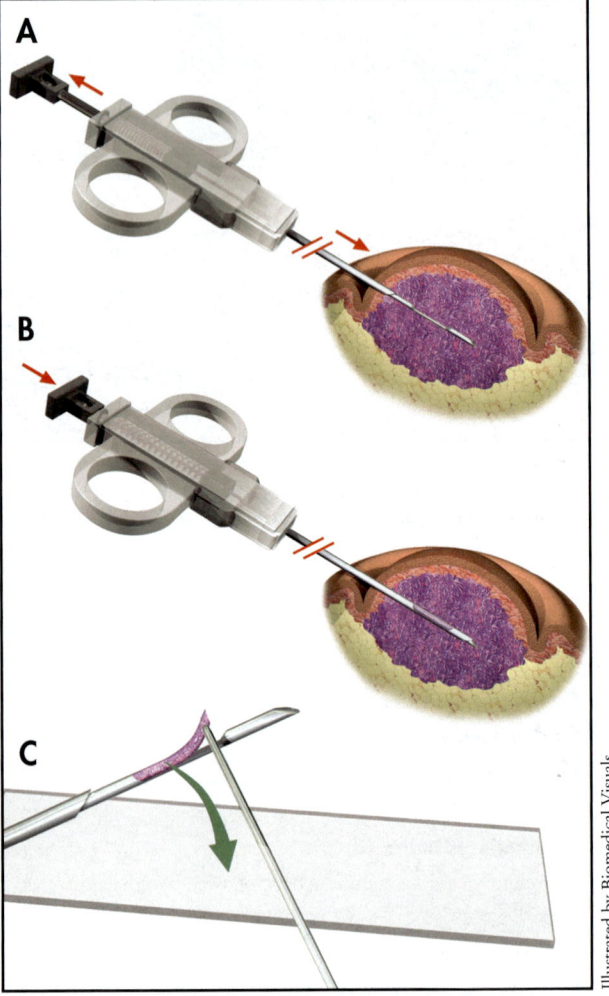

Figure 13-5. A needle core biopsy is accomplished by making a stab incision through the skin with a No. 11 surgical blade after the skin and underlying structures are anesthetized locally with 0.25 to 0.5 ml of lidocaine. A needle core biopsy instrument is then advanced through the skin to the periphery of the lesion. (**A**) The stylet is advanced into the tissue to be biopsied, and the outer cannula is advanced over the stylet to "cut" off the tissue left in the notch of the stylet (**B**). The entire instrument is removed from the incision, and the tissue is teased out of the stylet using a 22-gauge needle (**C**).

possible but will not compromise the normal tissue around it (e.g., a cutaneous, basal cell tumor <0.5 cm in diameter on the lateral abdominal wall). In nearly all dogs, an excisional biopsy is preceded by fine-needle aspiration cytology and/or incisional biopsy to give the surgeon as much information as possible about the characteristics of the tumor before removal. For example, a vaccine-associated sarcoma requires wide surgical margins (2 to 3 cm), whereas a benign basal cell tumor can be excised with smaller margins.

Indication: Identification of dermal, epidermal, or subcutaneous lesion of unknown etiology.

Contraindications: Coagulopathies; dogs that are at high risk during general anesthesia.

Benefit: Larger tissue sample often results in a more accurate diagnosis.

Limitations: Requires general anesthesia; may make a definitive second procedure more difficult to achieve.

Equipment: Sedation and general anesthesia (see box above); standard surgical instruments; suture material.

Technique (Figure 13-4B)**:** Performed in the same manner as incisional biopsy except that the lesion is excised completely with adequate margins.

Supportive Care: Oral or parenteral analgesics for days to weeks; periodic cleansing of the surgery site.

Needle Core Biopsy[1-4]

Needle core biopsy generally is safe and quick and can be performed on an awake, cooperative dog on an outpatient basis when appropriate analgesia and sedation are used.[1] Unless medically contraindicated, analgesics are used before and after the biopsy. Generally, histopathology results are more accurate than those of fine-needle aspiration cytology but are not as accurate as the results of an excisional or incisional biopsy because of the size of tissue sample obtained.

SKIN BIOPSY

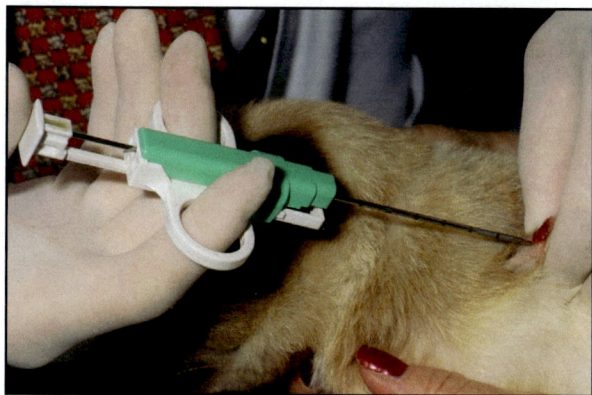

Figure 13-6. *A spring-loaded needle core biopsy instrument such as this one is placed through a stab incision, and the inner cannula is advanced through the tumor tissue. When the spring-loaded outer cannula is triggered, it will swiftly and automatically advance over the inner cannula, cutting the tissue in a fraction of a second and providing the tissue sample.*

> **KEY POINT**
>
> *Needle core or spring-loaded needle core biopsy generally is safe and quick and can be performed on an awake, cooperative dog as an outpatient using appropriate analgesia and, when indicated, sedation.*

Needle core biopsy instruments, especially the spring-loaded models that can be adjusted to obtain tissue from different depths, are preferred.

Indication: Identification of a skin or subcutaneous lesion of unexplained etiology.

Contraindications/complications: Coagulopathies; lidocaine toxicity (unlikely).

Benefit: General anesthesia is not required, so the procedure can be performed on an outpatient basis.

Limitation: The small tissue samples obtained may not be diagnostic.

Equipment: Sedation and analgesia should be considered (see box on page 62); No. 11 surgical blade; 2% lidocaine; needle biopsy instrument.

Technique (Figures 13-5 and 13-6):

1. Immobilize the cutaneous or subcutaneous lesion (usually done by an assistant), and prepare the biopsy site with surgical scrub for an aseptic procedure.
2. Inject approximately 0.25 to 1 ml of 2% lidocaine around the lesion to be biopsied while trying not to disturb the architecture of the tissue to be evaluated with the lidocaine. (The lidocaine will sting less on injection if diluted 50:50 with 8.4% bicarbonate.)
3. Using a No. 11 surgical blade, make a stab incision in the skin to allow easy entry of the needle core biopsy instrument.
4. Advance the needle core biopsy instrument through the incision to the outer portion of the lesion to be biopsied. In the case of the skin, the instrument is advanced just into the tissue to be biopsied.
5. Obtain three to five biopsy specimens from the suspect tissue through the same stab incision. This will allow the histopathologist to evaluate a sample of tissue from various portions of the mass, enhancing the probability of making an accurate diagnosis. These individual biopsies are best obtained by redirecting the needle within the mass.
6. Fix the needle biopsy specimens in 10% buffered formalin, as described previously. A separate container should be used for each lesion that is biopsied and should be labeled accordingly.
7. Suture the stab incision only if indicated by its size and depth.

Supportive Care: Oral analgesics for several days; periodic cleansing of the surgery site.

REFERENCES

1. Ogilvie GK, Moore AS: *Managing the Veterinary Cancer Patient: A Practice Manual.* Yardley, PA, Veterinary Learning Systems, 1995, pp 1–47.
2. Ogilvie GK, Moore AS: *Feline Oncology: A Comprehensive Guide for Compassionate Care.* Yardley, PA, Veterinary Learning Systems, 2002, pp 7–12.
3. Withrow SJ: Biopsy principles, in Withrow SJ, MacEwen EG (eds): *Small Animal Clinical Oncology,* ed 3. Philadelphia, WB Saunders, 2001, pp 52–57.
4. Sober AJ: Skin biopsy in the diagnosis and management of malignancy, in Wittes RE (ed): *Manual of Oncologic Therapeutics 1991/1992.* Philadelphia, JB Lippincott, 1991, pp 1–5.
5. Rosenberg SA: Principles of cancer management: Surgical oncology, in DeVita VT, Hellman S, Rosenberg SA (eds): *Cancer: Principles and Practice of Oncology,* ed 6. Philadelphia, JB Lippincott, 2001, pp 260–261.

LYMPH NODE BIOPSY

Gregory K. Ogilvie and Antony S. Moore

14

CLINICAL BRIEFING

Method	Benefits
Lymph node excision	• Most accurate method to evaluate complete nodal architecture.
Needle core biopsy	• Outpatient diagnostic procedure. • Quick and simple.

Lymph node biopsy is often important in the diagnosis, staging, and proper therapeutic management of the dog with cancer.[1-3] Excisional or needle core biopsy is frequently performed after fine-needle aspiration cytology suggests the presence of disease. Despite the accuracy of fine-needle aspiration cytology in determining the presence of diseases such as lymphoma, mast cell tumors, or metastatic solid tumors, a histopathologic diagnosis is always recommended before initiation of therapy. A completely excised lymph node is always preferable as it will allow the histopathologist to assess subtle architectural changes not always present in tissue obtained by needle core biopsy. Regardless, if an excisional lymph node biopsy is not possible, then fine-needle aspiration or needle core biopsy is a good substitute. In each case, adequate tissue must be obtained for histopathologic diagnosis and for special stains, if indicated.

If other lymph nodes are enlarged, the submandibular lymph nodes should be avoided; they are often reactive in the normal dog because they drain the oral cavity, where the bacterial count is usually quite high. This is especially true when lymphoma is suspected because reactive lymphocytes can look neoplastic and vice versa. When a malignancy is suspected, the biopsy should be planned so that the entire biopsy tract can be removed by the definitive surgery. This is because the biopsy procedure can "seed" the operative field with tumor cells if the principle of en bloc dissection is violated. The most vivid example is transitional cell carcinoma of the bladder, which can be transplanted all along a needle biopsy tract or incision after a biopsy. As with all biopsies, the surgeon who will perform the definitive surgery should be consulted before the biopsy to ensure that incisions are properly placed for a subsequent definitive procedure.

Lymph Node Excision[1-6]

The type of biopsy done on the lymph node will depend on each case; however, an excisional biopsy should be performed when possible[1-3] because this allows the pathologist to determine the architecture of the entire lymph node and to determine whether capsular invasion exists. This is especially valuable when lymphoma must be differentiated from lymph node hyperplasia.

> **KEY POINT**
> *Despite the accuracy of fine-needle aspiration cytology in determining the presence of diseases such as lymphoma, mast cell tumors, or metastatic solid tumors, a histopathologic diagnosis is always recommended before initiation of therapy.*

Lymph node excisions are performed commonly in dogs that have lymphadenopathy, especially when lymphoma, mast cell tumors, or other malignant conditions are suspected. It should be noted, however, that removal of a lymph node can be of great predictive value in other neoplastic conditions, such as oral malignant melanomas, in which metastatic disease can be detected in a normal-sized lymph node. A lymph node that is not easily seen or palpated by the casual observer should not be considered for removal. Hair should be clipped before surgery; however, the amount of hair clipped should not be excessive because dogs receiving chemotherapy often have slow hair regrowth. In addition, antineoplastic agents can cause alopecia, which makes the surgical site cosmetically noticeable for weeks to months after the procedure.

> **KEY POINT**
> *The submandibular lymph nodes should not be biopsied when lymphoma is suspected; they are often reactive because they drain the oral cavity, where the bacterial count is usually high.*

LYMPH NODE BIOPSY 67

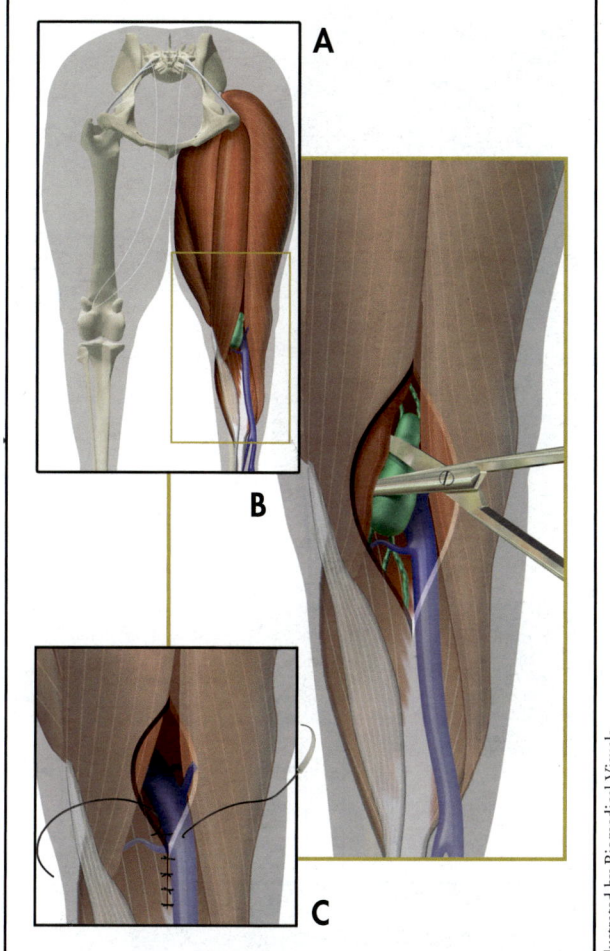

Figure 14-1. *Removal of the popliteal lymph node is accomplished by making an incision over the lymph node and then identifying the popliteal artery for ligation if necessary. Care is taken to avoid the saphenous vein (**A**). The lymph node in the capsule is bluntly dissected and removed (**B**). The subcutaneous tissue and skin are closed routinely (**C**).*

Options for Sedation, Anesthesia, and Analgesia for Lymph Node Biopsy

Preemptive Analgesia
- Acepromazine: 0.02 mg/kg SC
- Atropine: 0.04 mg/kg SC
- Morphine: 0.5 mg/kg SC
- NSAID orally pre- and postoperatively (ensure adequate hydration and renal function)

Anesthesia (as indicated)
- Propofol or thiopental induction followed by inhalant anesthesia

Postbiopsy Analgesia (choose one)
- Carprofen: 4 mg/kg SC
- Ketoprofen: 2 mg/kg SC
- Morphine: 0.5–1 mg/kg SC as needed q4–6h
- Nalbuphine: 1 mg/kg SC as needed q4–6h

Home Analgesia (choose at least one)
- Carprofen: 2.2 mg/kg PO q12h
- Etodolac: 10–15 mg/kg PO q12h
- Ketoprofen: 1 mg/kg PO
- Meloxicam: 0.1 mg/kg PO q24h
- Morphine: 0.5 mg/kg PO q6–8h
- Piroxicam: 0.3 mg/kg PO q24–48h
- Transdermal fentanyl: 2–3 mg/kg/hr

Indications: Lymphadenopathy of unexplained etiology; staging of tumor types when the risk of nodal metastasis is known to be high.

Contraindications: Coagulopathies; dogs that are at high risk for complications of anesthesia.

Benefit: An accurate histopathologic diagnosis can be obtained because the entire lymph node architecture is present.

Limitation: Requires general anesthesia.

Equipment: Sedation and general anesthesia (see box above); standard surgical instruments; suture material.

Technique (Figure 14-1):

1. Place the dog under general anesthesia after routine screening tests are conducted to identify problems such as coagulopathies and metabolic disease.
2. Clip the hair; prepare the surgical site using proper aseptic technique.
3. After the region is draped, make an incision over the enlarged lymph node.
4. Carefully identify and ligate the vessels going to and from the lymph node to be excised.
5. After the lymph node is removed, close the subcutaneous tissue with absorbable suture and close the skin with either absorbable or nonabsorbable suture.

Supportive Care: Oral or parenteral analgesics for days to weeks, periodic cleansing of the surgery site.

Needle Core Biopsy[1–6]

Needle core biopsy generally is safe and quick. It can be performed on an awake, cooperative patient.[1] The histopathologic results are generally more accurate than those of fine-needle aspiration cytology but not as accurate as the results of an excisional biopsy.

Indications: Lymphadenopathy of unexplained etiology; staging of tumor types when the risk of nodal metastasis is known to be high.

68 MANAGING THE CANINE CANCER PATIENT

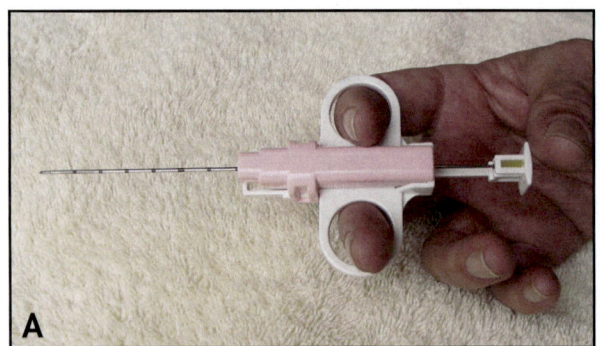

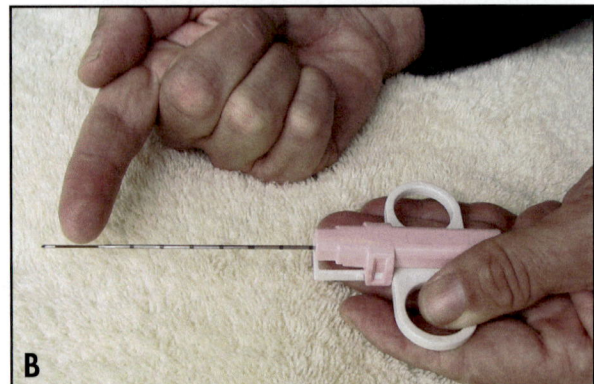

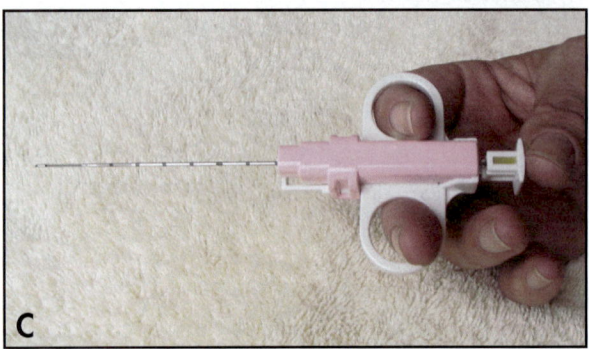

Figure 14-2. *Example of a needle core biopsy instrument. A spring-loaded biopsy instrument can be used with one or two hands. The instrument is first "cocked" by pulling back the handle; the inner cannula is advanced into the tumor by pushing on the "trigger" with the thumb (**A**) so that the notched portion of the stylet will fill with tissue (**B**). The spring-loaded outer portion of the biopsy instrument is then "fired" by continuing to press on the "trigger," resulting in quick advancement of the outer portion of the instrument over the piece of tumor that is within the recessed area of the inner stylet (**C**).*

Contraindication: Coagulopathies.

Benefit: General anesthesia is not required, so the procedure can be performed on an outpatient basis.

Limitation: The small tissue samples obtained may not be diagnostic.

Equipment: No. 11 surgical blade; 2% lidocaine; needle biopsy instrument.

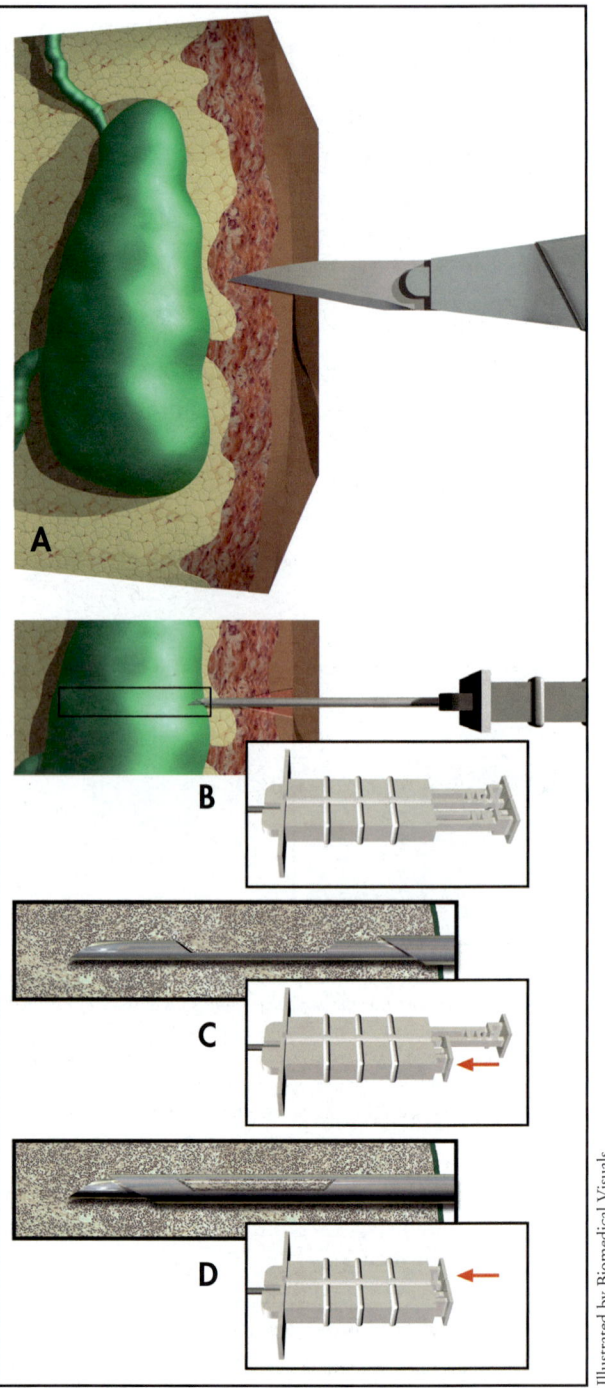

Figure 14-3. *Needle core biopsy of a lymph node is performed after the skin and nearby structures are anesthetized with approximately 2 to 3 ml of lidocaine. Using a No. 11 surgical blade, a stab incision is made in the skin to allow easy entry of the needle core biopsy instrument (**A**). The biopsy instrument is then advanced through the incision and into the capsule of the enlarged lymph node (**B**). The inner cannula is advanced first (**C**), followed by the outer portion, which cuts the tissue and leaves a biopsy sample in the needle (**D**). At least three to five biopsy specimens are taken through the same stab incision.*

Illustrated by Biomedical Visuals

Technique (Figures 14-2 and 14-3):

1. As an assistant grasps the lymph node and holds it firmly against the overlying skin, prepare the site for biopsy by clipping and applying surgical scrub as noted in Figures 14-1A and B for lymph node excision.
2. Inject approximately 2 to 3 ml of 2% lidocaine under the skin overlying the enlarged lymph node.
3. Using a No. 11 surgical blade, make a stab incision in the skin to allow easy entry of the needle core biopsy instrument.
4. Advance the biopsy instrument through the incision and into the capsule of the enlarged lymph node.
5. Take at least three to five biopsy specimens of the lymph node through the same stab incision.
6. Fix the biopsy specimens in 10% buffered formalin. A separate container should be used for each lesion that is biopsied.
7. Suture the stab incision only if indicated.

REFERENCES

1. Ogilvie GK, Moore AS: *Managing the Veterinary Cancer Patient: A Practice Manual.* Yardley, PA, Veterinary Learning Systems, 1995, pp 1–47.
2. Avis F: Lymph node biopsy, in Wittes RE (ed): *Manual of Oncologic Therapeutics 1991/1992.* Philadelphia, JB Lippincott, 1991, pp 8–9.
3. Ogilvie GK, Moore AS: *Feline Oncology: A Comprehensive Guide for Compassionate Care.* Yardley, PA, Veterinary Learning Systems, 2002, pp 7–12.
4. Withrow SJ: Biopsy principles, in Withrow SJ, MacEwen EG (eds): *Small Animal Clinical Oncology*, ed 3. Philadelphia, WB Saunders, 2001, pp 52–57.
5. Sober AJ: Skin biopsy in the diagnosis and management of malignancy, in Wittes RE (ed): *Manual of Oncologic Therapeutics 1991/1992.* Philadelphia, JB Lippincott, 1991, pp 1–5.
6. Rosenberg SA: Principles of cancer management: Surgical oncology, in DeVita VT, Hellman S, Rosenberg SA (eds): *Cancer: Principles and Practice of Oncology*, ed 6. Philadelphia, JB Lippincott, 2001, pp 260–261.

RESPIRATORY TRACT BIOPSY

Gregory K. Ogilvie and Antony S. Moore

▶ THORACIC CAVITY

CLINICAL BRIEFING

Methods	Benefits
Bronchoscopy	• Ideal for visualization, biopsy, and characterization of lesions, especially in airways.
Thoracoscopy	• Ideal for visualization, characterization, and collection of biopsy samples and removal of lung tumors and masses.
Transthoracic aspiration	• Quick, simple, and inexpensive method of diagnosing pleural and pulmonary lesions; accuracy improves with ultrasonographic, fluoroscopic, or CT guidance.
Transtracheal/ transendotracheal wash	• Relatively quick and simple method of diagnosing some lesions confined to the airways.

Bronchoscopy is commonly used to diagnose primary lung tumors in humans but not frequently in dogs,[1-5] possibly because tumors arising from the major airways are less common in animals than in people. In dogs, primary and metastatic lung tumors often arise in the pulmonary parenchyma; therefore, taking samples through transendotracheal tubes (small dogs) or performing transtracheal washes is often not successful in obtaining a sample of primary or metastatic tumors in this area. These tumors must be accessed via techniques that can sample pulmonary tissue from outside the airways. Bronchoscopy is helpful in the diagnosis of metastatic neoplastic conditions that shed tumor cells into the major airways but is usually of more value in nonneoplastic conditions of the lungs and major airways.[1-6] Transthoracic needle aspiration, with or without imaging guidance (ultrasonography, computed tomography [CT], or fluoroscopy), may be helpful in successfully obtaining cells or tissue samples from the peripheral pulmonary parenchyma when bronchoscopy is unproductive. Thoracoscopy is a method of visualizing the pleural spaces and associated structures and can be used to determine the extent of pulmonary masses as well as to obtain biopsy samples and, in specific cases, remove masses. Dogs occasionally have pleural effusion associated with primary or metastatic pulmonary neoplasia; therefore, thoracentesis and fluid cytology can be of diagnostic help. If these methods fail, an open biopsy via thoracotomy may be successful.

Bronchoscopy[1,2,4]

The flexible fiberoptic bronchoscope has proven to be superior to the rigid bronchoscope because the former does not limit lung visualization, permits visualization of the respiratory tract in a wide view, and is more effective in obtaining significant amounts of diagnostic tissue. In addition, a large variety of brushes, biopsy instruments, and grasping forceps can be introduced through the bronchoscope to obtain tissue or cytologic samples. It is estimated that more than 90% of all tumors located in the airways and 50% of peripheral lung tumors can be diagnosed with this modality when the procedure is performed by an experienced operator.[1-6] The benefits of imaging and biopsies guided by the bronchoscope include the ability to explore a large portion of the lungs and upper respiratory tract and to obtain tissue or cells from localized areas.[6] Disadvantages include the need for general anesthesia, the inability to obtain tissue samples larger than those that can be obtained through a 1- to 2-mm channel, and the complication of secretions from the respiratory tract obscuring visualization. When possible, multiple biopsy specimens should

> **KEY POINT**
> *Extreme care should be used to prevent overinflating the lungs or overdosing the dog with inhalant anesthetic gases during bronchoscopy.*

RESPIRATORY TRACT BIOPSY

> **Example of Sedation, Anesthesia, and Analgesia for Respiratory Tract Biopsy**
>
> **Preemptive Analgesia**
> - Morphine (1 mg/kg SC), acepromazine (0.02 mg/kg SC), and atropine (0.04 mg/kg SC) with an oral NSAID pre- and postoperatively (ensure adequate hydration and renal function)
>
> **Anesthesia (as indicated)**
> - Propofol or thiopental induction followed by inhalant anesthesia. Thoracoscopy is generally performed with a ventilator or ventilatory support. Note that if a lung lobe is of concern, a cuffed endotracheal tube is placed in the contralateral main stem bronchus to allow deflation of the lung lobe(s) in question.
>
> **Postbiopsy Analgesia (choose one)**
> - Carprofen: 4 mg/kg SC
> - Ketoprofen: 2 mg/kg SC
> - Morphine: 0.5–1 mg/kg SC as needed q4–6h
> - Nalbuphine: 1 mg/kg SC as needed q4–6h
>
> **Home Analgesia (choose one)**
> - Carprofen: 2.2 mg/kg PO q12h
> - Etodolac: 10–15 mg/kg PO q12h
> - Ketoprofen: 1 mg/kg PO
> - Meloxicam: 0.1 mg/kg PO q24h
> - Morphine: 0.5 mg/kg PO tid–qid
> - Piroxicam: 0.3 mg/kg PO q24–48h
> - Transdermal fentanyl: 2–3 mg/kg/hr

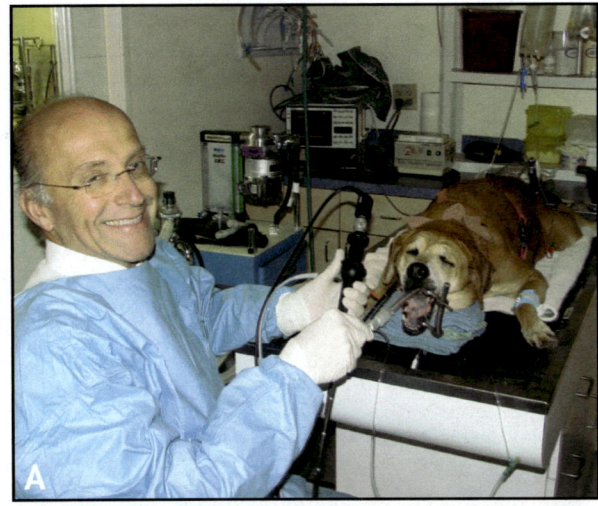

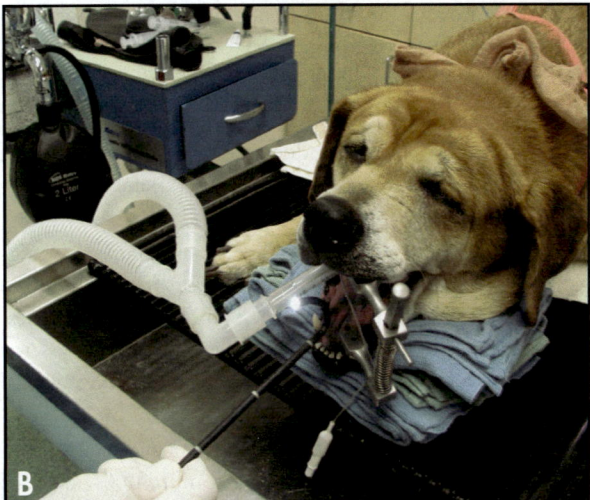

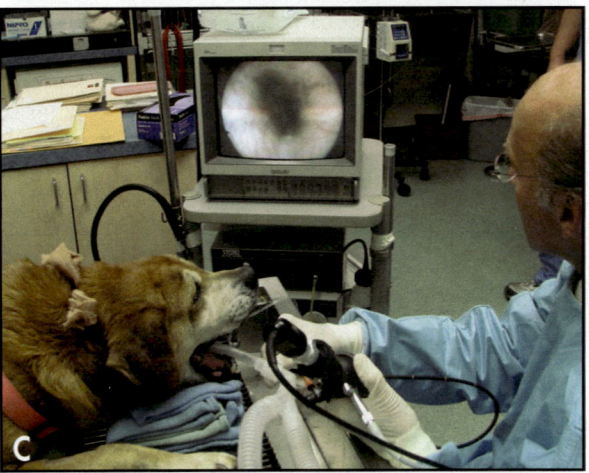

Figure 15-1. *(A) In the absence of a bronchoscope, a larger endoscope can be used to examine the upper respiratory tract. (B) Larger endoscopes are ideal for retroflexing the scope while (C) placing it over the soft palate to look for any abnormalities above that structure.*

be obtained to increase the probability of an accurate diagnosis. Large pieces of tissue should not be extracted through the biopsy channel of the endoscope; instead, the endoscope is removed from the trachea and endotracheal tube with the biopsy instrument still extended through the biopsy port.

Indications: Exploration of any disease that appears to involve the airways or alveoli, including primary or metastatic lung tumors.

Contraindications: Coagulopathies; dogs that are at high risk during general anesthesia, including patients with limited pulmonary or cardiac function.

Benefits: Relatively minimal risk; noninvasive procedure.

Limitations: Requires general anesthesia (see box above); the small tissue samples obtained may not be diagnostic.

Equipment (Figure 15-1): There are many fiberoptic endoscopes available for performance of bronchoscopy (see box on page 72); adapters can be used to pass the bronchoscope down into the respiratory tract with oxygen and inhalant anesthetic gases.

Complications: Rare; can include bleeding, which usually stops spontaneously. If brisk bleeding persists, a Fogarty

> **Selecting an Endoscope**
>
> Adult or pediatric endoscopes (5 mm in diameter) can be inserted into the trachea of dogs. The endoscope should:
> - Have an instrument port and channel
> - Be at least bidirectional
> - Bend more than 100° in at least one direction
> - Have an external light source
>
> Instruments that should be available and be able to pass through the instrument port of the endoscope:
> - Biopsy forceps
> - Cytology brushes
> - Graspers

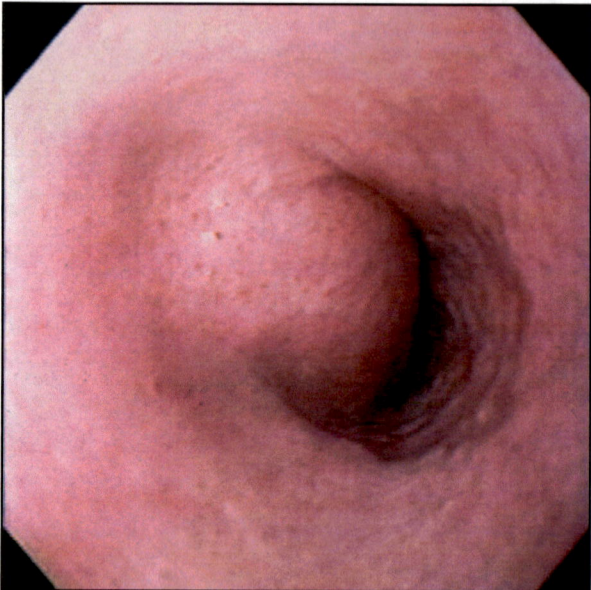

Figure 15-2. *Methodic examination of the respiratory tree can locate tumors, such as this bronchial adenocarcinoma compressing the terminal bronchioles. (Courtesy of David C. Twedt, DVM, Colorado State University)*

balloon catheter can be introduced to occlude the opening. In humans, the risk for pneumothorax is reported to be less than 1%; when it occurs, it is usually after a transbronchial biopsy of peripheral lymph nodes.

Technique:

1. After tests have been conducted to ensure the absence of life-threatening diseases, induce general anesthesia with endotracheal intubation.
2. Once the dog is well oxygenated, attach one end of a Y-piece adapter specifically designed for bronchoscopy to the endotracheal tube and fix the other end to the anesthesia machine. The open end is available to pass the bronchoscope through the Y-piece into the endotracheal tube and down the trachea.
3. Insert the bronchoscope through the Y-piece and down the trachea. If the bronchoscope compromises adequate endotracheal space for normal respiration, oxygen, with or without anesthetic gases, can be supplied through the bronchoscope. Perform a systematic exploration of the respiratory tree (Figure 15-2).

> **KEY POINT**
>
> *Transthoracic needle aspiration, with or without imaging guidance, may be helpful in successfully obtaining cells or tissue samples from the peripheral pulmonary parenchyma when bronchoscopy is unproductive.*

4. Sample suspect lesions first with the cytology brush, and then collect biopsy samples for histopathology. If a diffuse lesion is suspected, perform bronchoalveolar lavage. Introduce a catheter down the bronchoscope into the area to be sampled, and then inject 5 to 20 ml of 0.9% NaCl (depending on the size of the patient and the space to be lavaged) into the area and immediately withdraw the catheter for bacteriologic culture and cytologic evaluation of the tissue. This procedure can be repeated several times.

Supportive Care: Monitor respiration; oral analgesics are occasionally indicated.

Transthoracic Aspiration[2-6]

Transthoracic aspiration cytology and thoracentesis are procedures to remove or sample pleural fluid or tissue within the lung for diagnostic or therapeutic reasons. Fluoroscopy and occasionally ultrasonography are generally used to guide the biopsy of pulmonary, parenchymal, pleural, and mediastinal lesions. Ultrasonography is effective when the tissue to be examined is surrounded by fluid or other tissue but not if it is surrounded by air. In cases that cannot be clearly defined by fluoroscopy or ultrasonography, CT or magnetic resonance imaging (MRI) can be used to guide tissue sampling. In one study of human patients that included percutaneously collected biopsy samples from more than 400 pulmonary lesions, the accuracy of needle aspiration was determined to be 96.5%.[4] Ultrasound-guided fine-needle aspiration or blind aspiration was successful in obtaining

> **KEY POINT**
>
> *Dogs considered at high risk during general anesthesia, including patients with limited pulmonary function, should **not** undergo transthoracic aspiration or bronchoscopy.*

diagnostic samples from 20 of 25 dogs in one series.[5] Fluoroscopy- or CT-guided aspiration may be the most accurate for small or less peripheral lesions.

Indication: Investigation of any masses, lesions, or fluid accumulations within or around the pulmonary parenchyma that are not near or associated with the heart or blood vessels.

Contraindications: Coagulopathies, poor pulmonary reserve, and pulmonary arterial hypertension.

Benefit: Cells or fluid can be acquired with limited risk and without a thoracotomy.

Limitations: Requires general anesthesia or tranquilization (see box on page 71); may cause pneumothorax or hemothorax.

Equipment: 2% lidocaine; 3- to 12-ml syringe; 22-gauge, 1.5-inch needle.

Complications: Rarely (<10%), hemothorax and pneumothorax; placement of a chest tube may be required to resolve these problems.

Technique (Figure 15-3):

1. After routine screening tests have been conducted to identify such problems as coagulopathies, metabolic disease, or organ failure, place the dog under general anesthesia or tranquilization. An opiate or NSAID may be administered to reduce any discomfort.

2. Identify the lesions with fluoroscopy, ultrasonography, or CT. Clip the hair, and prepare the site with surgical scrub and aseptic technique. A surgical drape is sometimes placed to enhance sterility.

3. If tranquilization is used instead of general anesthesia, anesthetize the skin and underlying tissue, up to the pleura, with 0.5 (small dog) to 5 ml (large dog) of 2% lidocaine that has been diluted with 8.4% bicarbonate at a ratio of 50:50.

4. Advance a 22-gauge needle attached to a 3- to 12-ml syringe through the skin and intercostal muscles. This can be done blind but is best accomplished using additional imaging techniques, such as fluoroscopy, ultrasonography, or CT. Take care to avoid the heart and great vessels. Pneumothorax is always a potential complication but is not commonly a major concern if appropriate care is taken during the procedure. If fluid is to be sampled, attach a three-way stopcock between the syringe and needle to facilitate removal of large amounts of fluid.

5. Aspirate tissue while the needle is advanced through the lesion. To prevent injury to normal lung tissue, insert the needle and aspirate the mass over a relatively short period. The pressure is eliminated before removing the needle from the mass and chest cavity to prevent aspirating the acquired cells into the syringe, where they may be unre-

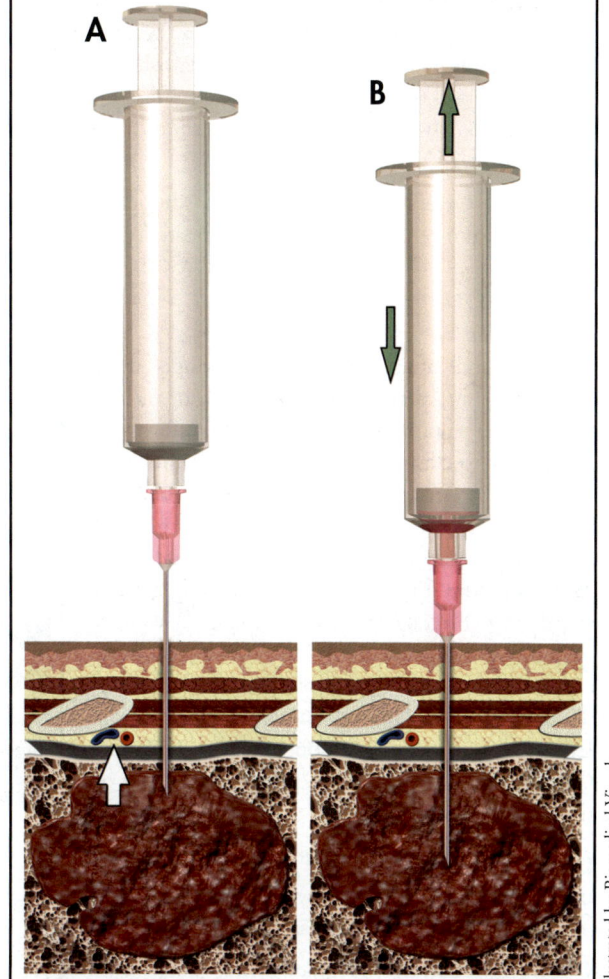

Figure 15-3. *Transthoracic lung aspiration is accomplished with a 22-gauge needle attached to a 3- to 12-ml syringe, which is advanced through the skin and intercostal muscles (**A**), ideally using fluoroscopic, ultrasonographic, or CT guidance. Care is taken to avoid the intercostal vein and artery caudal to the adjoining rib (white arrow). Tissue is quickly aspirated while the needle is advanced through the lesion (**B**). The pressure is eliminated before removing the needle from the mass and chest cavity. If fluid is to be sampled, a three-way stopcock is attached between the syringe and needle to facilitate removal of large amounts of fluid. In addition, it is advisable to use a 35- or 60-ml syringe.*

coverable. Then remove the syringe from the needle and fill it with air. Reattach the needle to the syringe, and forcefully expel the material in the needle onto a clean microscope slide. If indicated, gently spread the material over the slide to obtain a single layer of cells for subsequent analysis. If fluid or sufficient tissue is removed, make slides and save the fluid for culture and sensitivity testing. Save the remaining fluid in two tubes (an EDTA tube and a red-top tube without anticoagulant) for subsequent submission to a clinical pathologist for analysis.

6. Carefully observe the dog for several hours for signs of respiratory difficulty. Ideally, a thoracic radiograph is taken to ensure that hemothorax or pneumothorax has not developed after the procedure. In addition, the dog should be rested for 24 to 48 hours.

Supportive Care: Monitor respiration for hours to days; administer oral analgesics as indicated.

Thoracoscopic Lung, Pericardial, Mediastinal, or Pleural Biopsy

In the hands of an experienced endoscopist, thoracoscopic lung, pericardial, mediastinal, or pleural biopsy takes approximately 5 to 10 minutes from chest entry to closure. With this method, the chest cavity can be directly visualized for specific localization of lesions for subsequent biopsy. The method varies slightly depending on the equipment used. This procedure may be accomplished using general anesthesia or, in fragile patients, local anesthesia with tranquilizers and analgesics. The site for thoracoscope insertion can be paraxyphoid just to the left of the dog's midline, along the thoracic inlet for mediastinoscopy or, more commonly, between the ribs. Choosing the appropriate site depends on the area of the chest to be explored.

Indications: Evaluation and diagnosis of malignant and nonmalignant chest disease; determining the extent of the neoplastic processes.

Contraindications: Coagulopathies; dogs with significantly compromised cardiovascular or respiratory systems (because of the mild insufflation of the chest, venous return to the heart can be reduced, which can compress the diaphragm and lungs, thereby compromising the ability to inspire easily).

Benefits: Biopsy can be selectively performed to acquire tissue to analyze cellularity, architecture, and content. In selected cases, the procedure can be done with local anesthesia, systemic analgesia, and, if absolutely essential, tranquilization (see box on page 71). If there are any concerns about the dog's ability to lie quietly, however, general anesthesia should be administered.

Limitations: Small biopsy samples may not be representative of the entire lesion. Lung lobectomies can be performed, but large lesions may be difficult to exteriorize without doing at least a minithoracotomy. Because this procedure allows visualization of lesions only on the surface of vis-

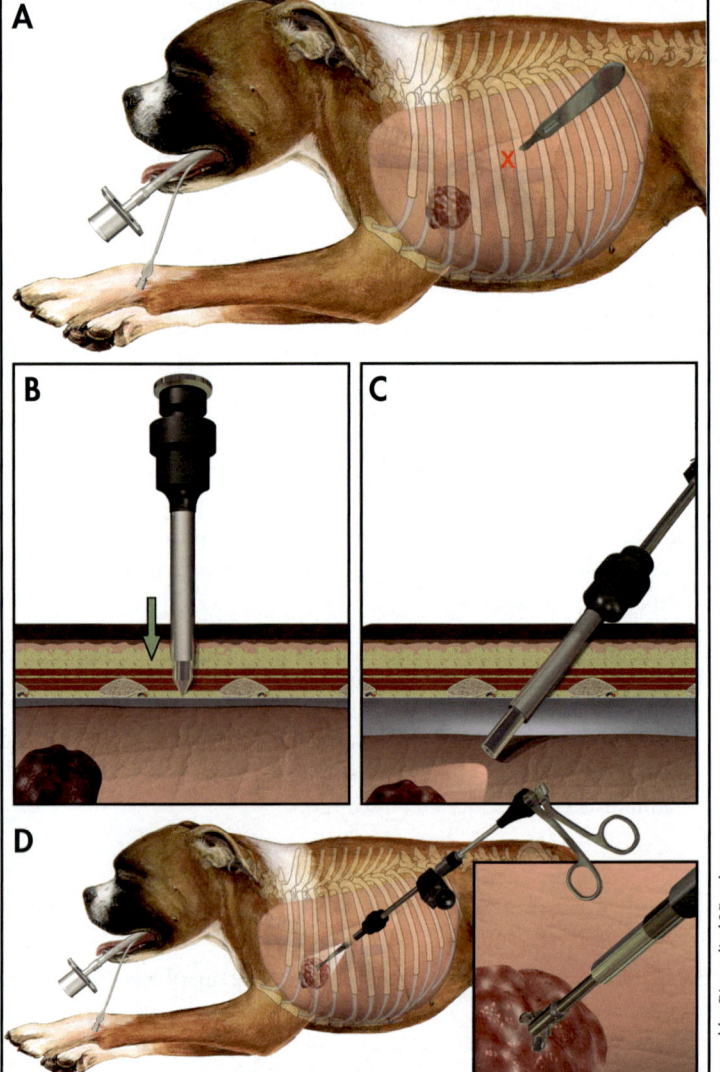

Figure 15-4. Intercostal thoracoscopy can be performed in an anesthetized patient. Ideally, the end of the endotracheal tube is inserted into the main stem bronchus opposite the side to be examined. Place the patient in left lateral recumbency and make a small incision (0.5–1 cm) in the skin between the fifth and sixth intercostal space at the midpoint of the ribs, where the trocar will be placed (**A**). Push the trocar and cannula assembly (**B**) through the incision, the intercostal muscles, and the pleura to enter the chest cavity. Remove the trocar, and advance the thoracoscope (in this example, attached to a carbon dioxide or nitrous oxide insufflator and a light source and video camera) through the cannula to visualize the heart, lung, mediastinum, diaphragm, and pleura (**C**). A small amount of air can be allowed into the chest to allow adequate visualization without compromising respiratory capability. Advance a biopsy instrument through a separate access port of the thoracoscope or through an identically but separately placed cannula and trocar and direct it to sites of interest by direct visualization (**C** and **D**). Take five to six biopsy specimens, and submit at least one for bacterial culture and sensitivity (**D**, inset). Methods exist for resecting and stapling or suturing lung lobes for subsequent removal. After observing the biopsy sites for several minutes for excessive bleeding, evacuate the carbon dioxide, remove the instrument from the chest cavity, and suture the small incision with absorbable material in a simple interrupted pattern.

ible organs, lesions below the surface may be overlooked.

Equipment: Standard surgical instruments; laparoscope/thoracoscope and thoracoscopic biopsy instruments; Verres needle; thoracoscopic scissors, graspers, staplers, and cautery instruments; trocar and cannula assembly.

Technique (Figure 15-4)**:**

1. Administer a general anesthetic with analgesic properties (e.g., butorphanol, fentanyl, morphine, oxymorphone). Care is optimal when pre- and postoperative analgesics are used to minimize discomfort.
2. If a lateral approach is used, place the dog with the area in question facing up. If the patient is tranquilized, apply gentle but firm restraint of the limbs so that the dog cannot change position during the procedure, ideally with an assistant nearby to calm the dog. Clip the hair, and prepare the skin with a surgical scrub. Drape the insertion site.
3. If tranquilization is used instead of general anesthesia, inject approximately 0.5 to 2 ml of lidocaine in and around the site where the thoracoscope and any biopsy needles are to be introduced. The 2% lidocaine stings less on injection if it is diluted 50:50 with 8.4% bicarbonate.
4. Insert a Verres needle to allow a slight introduction of air, or advance the trocar within the sleeve. After it is determined that the needle is not in a blood vessel, use carbon dioxide or nitrous oxide to insufflate the chest. Take extreme care to ensure that the dog is breathing properly.
5. Make a small incision (0.5–1 cm) between the ribs. Push the trocar and cannula assembly into the gas-filled abdomen through the incision. Remove the Verres needle. Remove the trocar, and advance the thoracoscope (attached to a carbon dioxide or nitrous oxide insufflator and a light source) through the cannula to visualize the heart, lung, mediastinum, diaphragm, and pleura. If blood or other material obscures visualization, remove the thoracoscope (but not the outer cannula) and clean it in a bowl of saline.
6. Advance a biopsy needle through the thoracoscope or a separate puncture site nearby. Direct the cup or needle biopsy instrument to sites of interest by direct visualization. Take five to six biopsy specimens, at least one of which is submitted for bacterial culture and sensitivity testing. Methods do exist for resecting and stapling or suturing lung lobes for subsequent removal.
7. Observe the biopsy sites for several minutes for excessive bleeding, then evacuate the carbon dioxide, remove the instrument from the chest cavity, and suture the small incision with absorbable material in a simple interrupted pattern.

Supportive Care: Oral or parenteral analgesics.

NASAL CAVITY

CLINICAL BRIEFING

Methods	Benefits
Rhinoscopy	• Visualization of lesion and collection of biopsy samples; especially valuable to differentiate tumor from infectious or inflammatory causes.
Cup biopsy	• Instruments allow collection of large samples, usually via blind biopsy approaches.
Cannula biopsy	• Large-core biopsy samples acquired, maximizing accurate diagnosis.
Curette biopsy	• Especially valuable for small dogs.

Nasal Biopsy[1,4]

A nasal biopsy should be considered for every dog with a facial deformity, unilateral or bilateral epistaxis, or epiphora of unknown etiology. A nasal tumor or rhinitis of fungal, viral, or bacterial origin must be suspected in many of these cases. A biopsy is always required before appropriate therapy can be recommended. Suspect tumors in dogs can be sampled using equipment that is relatively inexpensive and quite effective. Although fiberoptic examinations (Figure 15-5) and nasal flushes are valuable in some cases, they are not as rewarding as biopsy cup or curette techniques. Regardless of the procedure, general anesthesia is required for all dogs. To reduce discomfort, lidocaine can be diluted in saline and administered through a soft catheter placed in the rostral third of the nasal cavity with the nose directed upward. Lidocaine enhances comfort and decreases the need for anes-

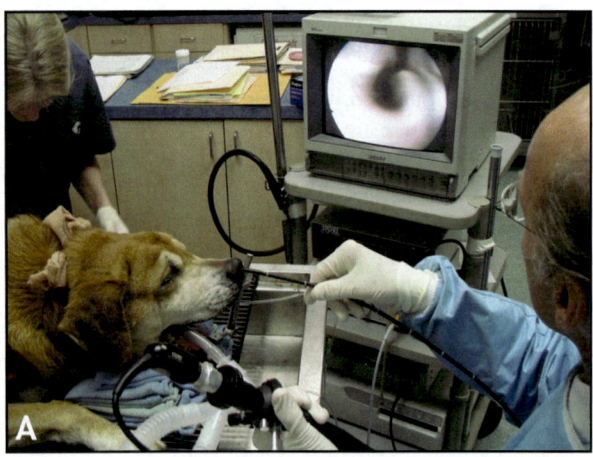
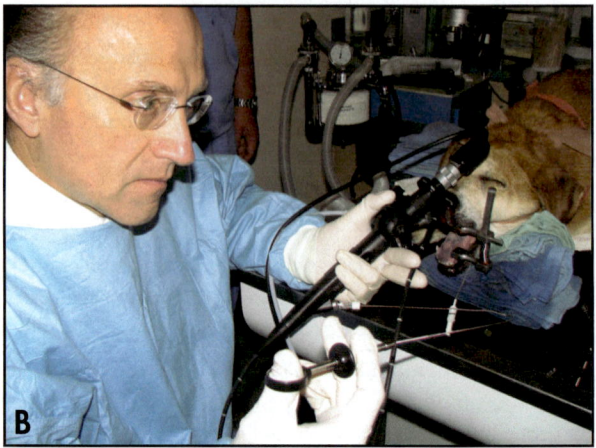

Figure 15-5. (**A**) Fiberoptic examination of the rostral nasal airways can provide information about the size, location, and nature of a tumor. Although this information is valuable, a biopsy specimen should be obtained during endoscopy (**B**) and submitted for histopathologic analysis.

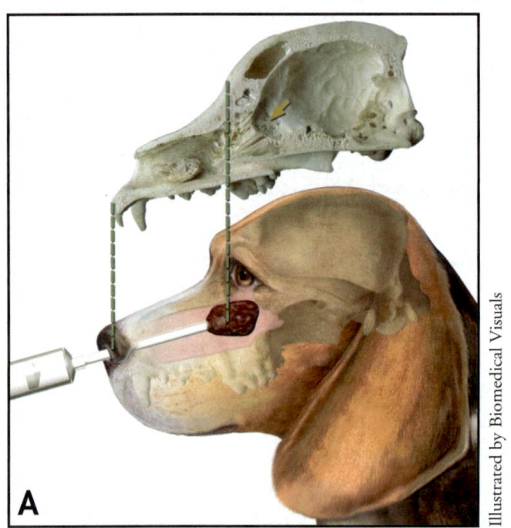
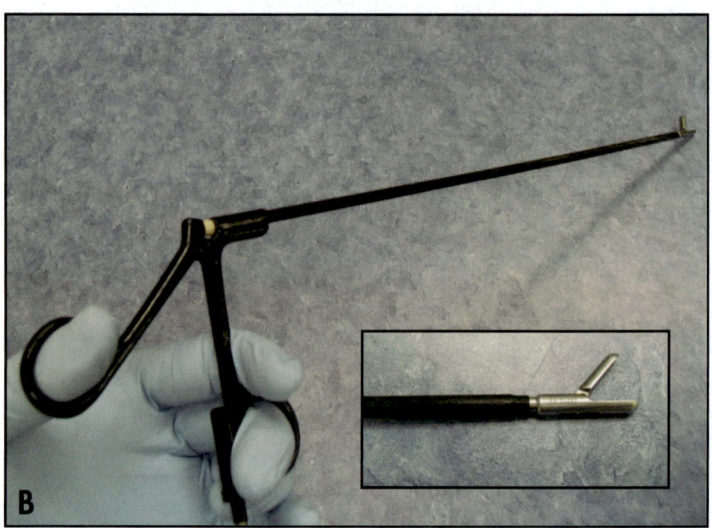

Figure 15-6. A nasal biopsy can be accomplished in medium to large dogs with a large-bore (3- to 5-mm) plastic cannula. (**A**) This cannula is fixed to the hub of a needle with the metal portion removed (with a knife or old scissors). The cannula/needle hub is then fixed to a 12-ml syringe, and the entire apparatus is passed up the nostril and into the tumor. The biopsy instrument should never pass farther caudal than the medial canthus of the eye (dotted line) to prevent it from entering the cribriform plate and brain (arrow). The tumor is entered forcefully, and suction is applied to core and aspirate the tumor effectively. The apparatus is removed from the nasal cavity, and the tumor is then ejected from the cannula by forcefully ejecting a syringe full of air or saline through the needle hub and cannula. The same landmarks and procedures can be used in small dogs, except that a small to medium bone curette is used to "scoop up" the tumor. (**B**) Alternatively, a mare uterine biopsy instrument can be used to "bite off" chunks of tumor.

thetic drugs. It should be recognized that some of the lidocaine can be absorbed systemically; therefore, the dosage should not exceed 2 mg/kg. Biopsy samples should be collected through the external nares rather than the skin to reduce surgical exposure, which could contaminate normal tissue with tumor cells from the nasal cavity. Biopsy of nasal tumors frequently involves the use of a bone curette, cannula, or a relatively small cup biopsy instrument (Figure 15-6). Although biopsy through a bronchoscope or a cystoscope is relatively easy to accomplish, the size of the tissue sample obtained is often inadequate for an accurate diagnosis. In part, this is because the tissue removed by these methods is superficial and the underlying true pathology is frequently obscured by septic inflammation. Note, however, that a flexible endoscope is ideal for identifying lesions in the trachea (Figure 15-7). In addition, the bronchoscope can be retro-

> **KEY POINT**
>
> *The biopsy instrument should never be passed farther caudal than the medial canthus of the eye to prevent it from entering the cribriform plate and brain.*

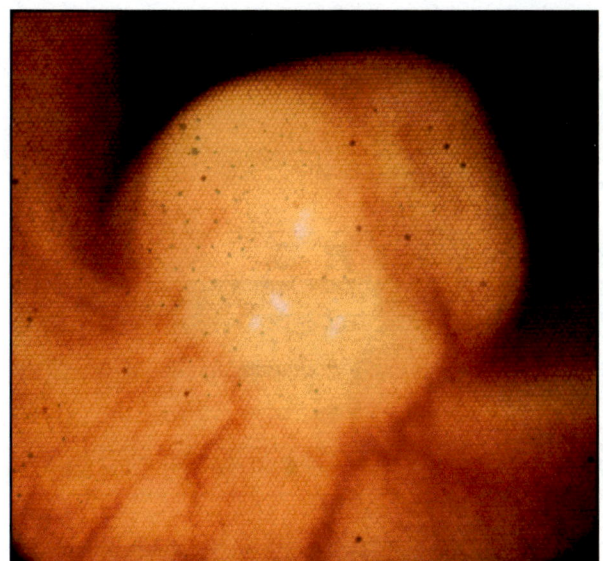

Figure 15-7. *Tracheal oncocytoma as noted on bronchoscopy, which is an excellent method for localizing lesions in the respiratory tract. The size and location of the tumor can be characterized, and a biopsy sample is readily obtainable. (Courtesy of D. C. Twedt)*

flexed over the soft palate to clearly visualize the caudal nasal airways (Figure 15-1).

Indication: Examination of any undiagnosed nasal problem, especially when the dog has epiphora, epistaxis, or facial deformity.

Contraindications: Coagulopathies; dogs that are at high risk during general anesthesia.

Benefit: The large tissue sample that can be obtained allows a more accurate diagnosis than the potentially smaller endoscopically obtained samples.

Limitation: Requires general anesthesia.

Equipment: Sedation, analgesia, and general anesthesia (see box on page 71); small- to medium-sized bone curette or "cup" biopsy instrument.

Technique (Figure 15-6):

1. Place the dog under general anesthesia after routine screening tests have been conducted to identify clinical problems, such as coagulopathies, metabolic disease, or organ failure.
2. Identify the nasal lesion with skull radiography or (preferably) CT. The most valuable skull radiograph is an intraoral exposure, which is best made with nonscreen film placed inside the mouth to allow imaging of the caudal aspect of the nasal cavity. General anesthesia is required for this procedure.
3. Flush a solution of 0.5 to 1 ml of 2% lidocaine diluted 50:50 with 8.4% bicarbonate into the biopsy site by placing a tomcat or soft catheter, without the needle, through the nasal passage to the level of the lesion. This may reduce local discomfort and allow a lighter plane of anesthesia.
4. Obtain biopsy samples from medium to large dogs with a large-bore (3- to 5-mm) plastic cannula. Fix the cannula to the hub of a needle with the metal portion removed; then attach this to a 12-ml syringe. Pass the entire apparatus up the nostril and direct it into the tumor. It is essential to premeasure the distance from the nares to the medial canthus of the eye and either cut the straw off at the proper length or mark it with tape. Enter the tumor forcefully, and apply suction to core and aspirate the tumor effectively. Remove the apparatus from the nasal cavity, and eject the tumor from the cannula by forcefully expelling a syringe full of air through the needle hub and cannula. Alternatively, and specifically for small dogs, measure the largest bone curette that can be passed up the opening of the nasal cavity and mark it with tape or a marking pen. Use the curette to scoop or scrape the tumor into the instrument. Small biopsy cup instruments can be used to pinch off portions of the tumor. Place the tumor in formalin for subsequent analysis.
5. Mild to moderate hemorrhage is expected but should subside within a relatively short period. If hemorrhage is excessive, ipsilateral carotid artery ligation should assist in reducing the bleeding. Monitor hematocrit levels hourly until all bleeding has stopped.

Supportive Care: Any crusting, dried material, or moist exudates should be removed from the nose regularly and barrier creams applied; oral or parenteral analgesics should be administered for days to weeks as needed.

REFERENCES

1. Ogilvie GK, Moore AS: *Managing the Veterinary Cancer Patient: A Practice Manual.* Yardley, PA, Veterinary Learning Systems, 1995, pp 1–47.
2. Ogilvie GK, Moore AS: Theory and practice of tumor biopsy, in Ogilvie GK, Moore AS (eds): *Feline Oncology: A Comprehensive Guide for Compassionate Care.* Yardley, PA, Veterinary Learning Systems, 2002, pp 7–12.
3. Martini N: Diagnostic procedures relating to the thorax, in Wittes RE (ed): *Manual of Oncologic Therapeutics 1991/1992.* Philadelphia, JB Lippincott, 1991, pp 9–10.
4. Westcott JL: Direct percutaneous needle aspiration of localized pulmonary lesions: Results in 422 patients. *Radiology* 137:31–35, 1980.
5. Withrow SJ: Biopsy principles, in Withrow SJ, MacEwen EG (eds): *Small Animal Clinical Oncology,* ed 3. Philadelphia, WB Saunders, 2001, pp 52–57.
6. Kurtz RC, Ginsberg RJ: Cancer diagnosis: Endoscopy, in DeVita VT, Hellman S, Rosenberg SA (eds): *Cancer: Principles and Practice of Oncology,* ed 6. Philadelphia, JB Lippincott, 2001, pp 736–739.

BONE MARROW ASPIRATION AND BIOPSY

Gregory K. Ogilvie and Antony S. Moore

CLINICAL BRIEFING

Methods	Benefits
Illinois or Rosenthal bone marrow needle aspiration	• Relatively quick and simple outpatient procedure for obtaining marrow for cytology.
Jamshidi needle biopsy	• Simple method of obtaining marrow core aspirates and biopsies in anesthetized dogs.

Bone marrow aspiration and biopsy are essential procedures for identifying cytologic and histologic abnormalities of the bone marrow caused by a wide variety of neoplastic, infectious, and myelodysplastic conditions.[1-3] Bone marrow aspiration and biopsy are indicated when an abnormality in the production of blood cells is suspected or when attempting to stage a dog with a hematopoietic malignancy.

Bone marrow aspiration is performed to acquire a monolayer of cells for individual evaluation.[1-3] Aspiration is therefore good for evaluating the cytology of the bone marrow, while a bone marrow biopsy is preferred for evaluating the undisturbed architecture. To identify a wide variety of malignant and nonmalignant disorders, Romanovsky (including Wright's and Giemsa) stains are preferred. When the cytologic diagnosis of a cell type is not certain, additional special stains (including myeloperoxidase, Sudan black, and periodic acid–Schiff) can be used. Bone marrow biopsies are beneficial in determining bone marrow cellularity, the presence and extent of fibrosis or granulomatous conditions, and the presence of nonhematopoetic malignancies.

> **KEY POINT**
>
> *Bone marrow aspiration and biopsy are essential procedures for determining cytologic and histologic abnormalities of the bone marrow caused by a wide variety of neoplastic, infectious, and myelodysplastic conditions. The accuracy and value of the information from these diagnostics are directly related to the experience and training of the pathologist.*

Indications: Blood cell production abnormality; staging procedure for a hematopoietic or nonhematopoietic malignancy.

Sedation, Anesthesia, and Analgesia for a Bone Marrow Aspirate or Biopsy

Preemptive Analgesia
- Morphine (1 mg/kg SC), acepromazine (0.02 mg/kg SC), and atropine (0.04 mg/kg SC) with an oral NSAID pre- and postoperatively (ensure adequate hydration and renal function)

Anesthesia (as indicated)
- Propofol or thiopental induction followed by inhalant anesthesia

Home Analgesia (choose one)
- Carprofen: 2.2 mg/kg PO q12h
- Etodolac: 10–15 mg/kg PO q12h
- Ketoprofen: 1 mg/kg PO
- Meloxicam: 0.1 mg/kg PO q24h
- Morphine: 0.5 mg/kg PO tid–qid
- Piroxicam: 0.3 mg/kg PO q24–48h
- Transdermal fentanyl: 2–3 mg/kg/hr

Contraindications: Coagulopathies.

Benefits: Aspiration can provide a sample for individual cell analysis, whereas a biopsy can provide tissue to analyze cellularity, architecture, and content; often, this can be done using local anesthesia in conjunction with systemic analgesia and/or tranquilization (see box above).

Limitation: A single sample may not be representative of the entire bone marrow.

Equipment: No. 11 surgical blade; 2% lidocaine; 6- to 12-ml syringe; 18-gauge Illinois, Rosenthal, or disposable bone marrow needle with a handle (Figure 16-1); microscope slides; EDTA container. Sedation or anesthesia is preferred with a local anesthesia.

BONE MARROW ASPIRATION AND BIOPSY

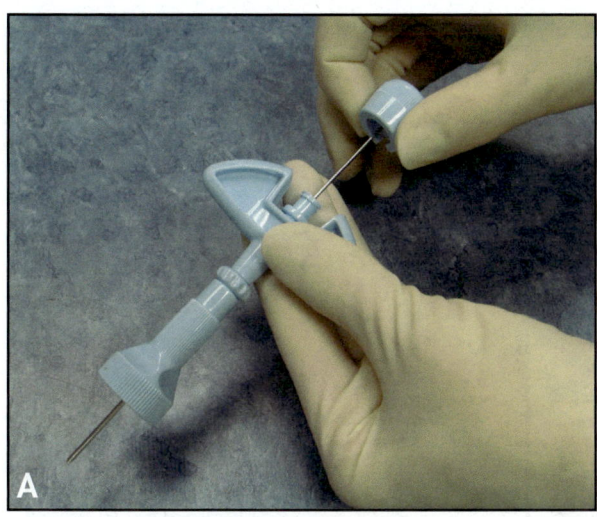
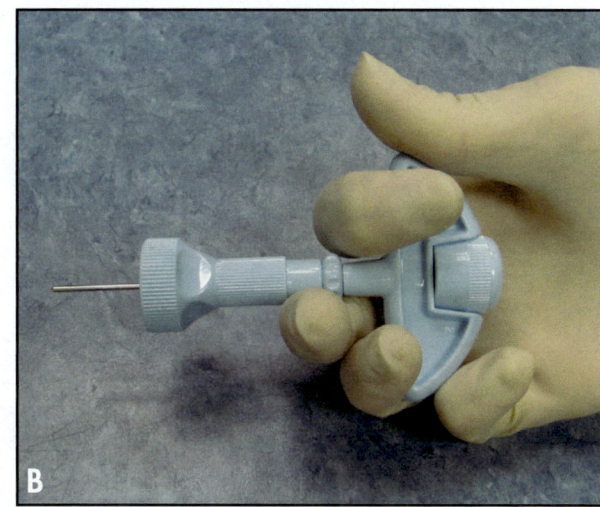

Figure 16-1. *(A) Bone marrow needle with the stylet removed. (B) The plastic handle on the needle allows better control and ease of placement.*

Technique[1–3] (Figure 16-2):

1. Clip the hair, clean and prepare the microscope slides for the sample (which will clot quickly) to be processed, and prepare the bone marrow aspiration site with a surgical scrub. Preferred sites and positioning in dogs include:
   —Dorsocranial or lateral aspects of the iliac crest (with the dog in sternal or lateral recumbency).
   —Greater trochanter of the femur (dog in lateral recumbency).
   —Rostral aspect of the greater tubercle of the humeral head (dog in lateral recumbency).
2. Using a 25-gauge needle, inject approximately 0.5 to 1 ml of lidocaine (2%) in and around the site where the bone marrow needle will be introduced. Take care to inject the lidocaine in and around all the tissue that extends from the skin to the periosteum. The lidocaine will sting less on injection if it is diluted 50:50 with 8.4% bicarbonate.
3. Scrub the biopsy area one more time after the lidocaine injection. Place a surgical drape for sterility.
4. Identify the bone marrow site, and stretch the skin between the thumb and index finger. Make a small stab incision with a No. 11 surgical blade in the area blocked with lidocaine.
5. Advance the bone marrow needle, with the stylet in place, into the stab incision and through the skin, subcutaneous tissue, and muscle all the way to the bone. It is crucial to keep the stylet in place because it has a tendency to back out during the procedure. An 18-gauge Illinois or Rosenthal needle is preferred for most dogs. After a sample is obtained for cytologic evaluation, use a 14-gauge Jamshidi (bone marrow biopsy instrument) needle to collect a biopsy specimen if required.
6. With the stylet in place, advance the bone marrow needle into the bone using a corkscrew motion. Do not allow the instrument to wobble, and fix it firmly into the bone like a nail that has been securely hammered into wood. When the needle is firmly fixed in the bone, remove the stylet and affix the syringe. Many clinical pathologists suggest rinsing the syringe and bone marrow needle with EDTA before the procedure to reduce clotting of the bone marrow sample. Heparin should never be used.
7. Briskly aspirate the bone marrow sample into the 5- to 12-ml syringe (0.5 to 1 ml of marrow is usually adequate). The aspiration may be accompanied by a few seconds of pain, but this can be prevented by the use of oral or parenteral analgesics such as fentanyl, butorphanol, morphine, or carprofen.
8. If a sample is not obtained, replace the stylet in the bone marrow needle and advance the instrument farther into the bone for a second attempt at aspirating marrow. Once marrow has been obtained, prepare smears. This can be done in the following ways (the first two of which may enhance the ability to evaluate the nucleated cell population of the bone marrow specimen):
   —Expel the marrow and blood into a small petri dish that contains a few drops of EDTA. Place the marrow-rich spicules on a slide or coverslip and then spread them between slides or coverslips to make a monolayer of cells. The slides must have been cleaned and readied for the sample to be processed, as it will clot quickly.
   —Place a portion of the marrow sample on the proximal portion of the slide; tip the slide downward to allow the blood to run down and off the slide. The spicules

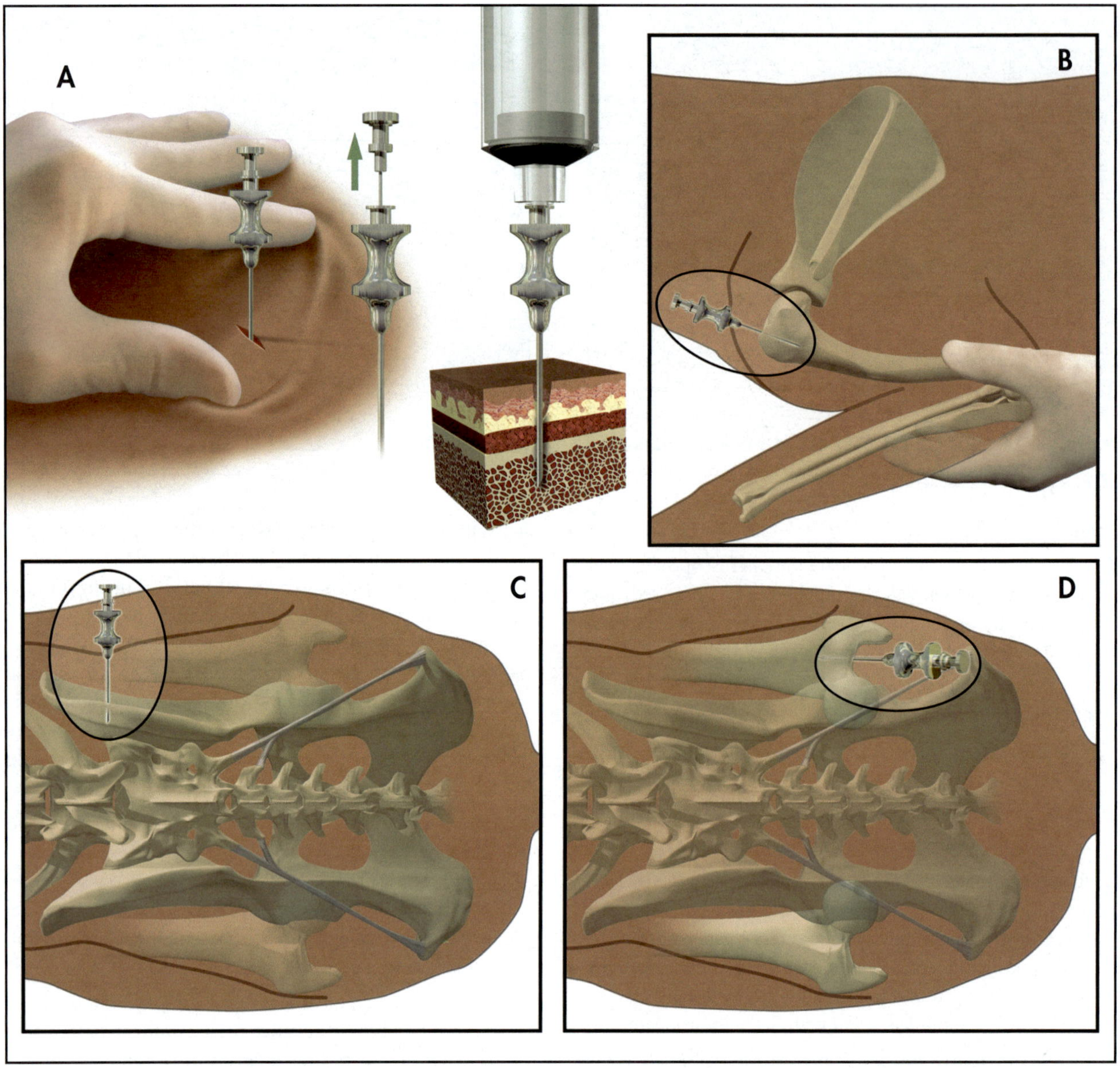

Figure 16-2. *A bone marrow sample is obtained by advancing a 1-inch, 18-gauge bone marrow needle, with the stylet in place, through a single stab incision in the skin and into the bone using a corkscrew motion. When the needle is fixed in the bone, the stylet is removed and the syringe is affixed (**A**). The bone marrow sample is then aspirated briskly into the 5- to 12-ml syringe and placed on slides and/or in a 1.5-ml EDTA tube. Ideal locations for bone marrow aspiration are the greater tubercle of the proximal aspect of the humeral head (**B**), the dorsocranial aspect of the iliac crest (**C**), and the greater trochanter of the femur (**D**).*

and heavier nucleated cells do not run off and are used for subsequent slide preparation.

—Spread marrow into a monolayer as in a routine blood smear.

A biopsy of a bone lesion or bone marrow can be obtained with the Jamshidi needle (Figure 16-3) or the bone marrow needle after aspiration is performed (Figure 16-4). For biopsy, the stylet is removed. After the aspiration, the instrument is advanced as described earlier. The needle is then rocked back and forth to sever the sample from its base. In humans, pain is usually minimal, so premedication often is not necessary if local anesthesia is adequate. The biopsy instrument is then removed, and a smaller wire obturator is used to retrograde the biopsy sample out of the top end of the biopsy instrument. Cytology and histopathology can then be conducted on this tissue. Direct pressure should be applied to the site for several

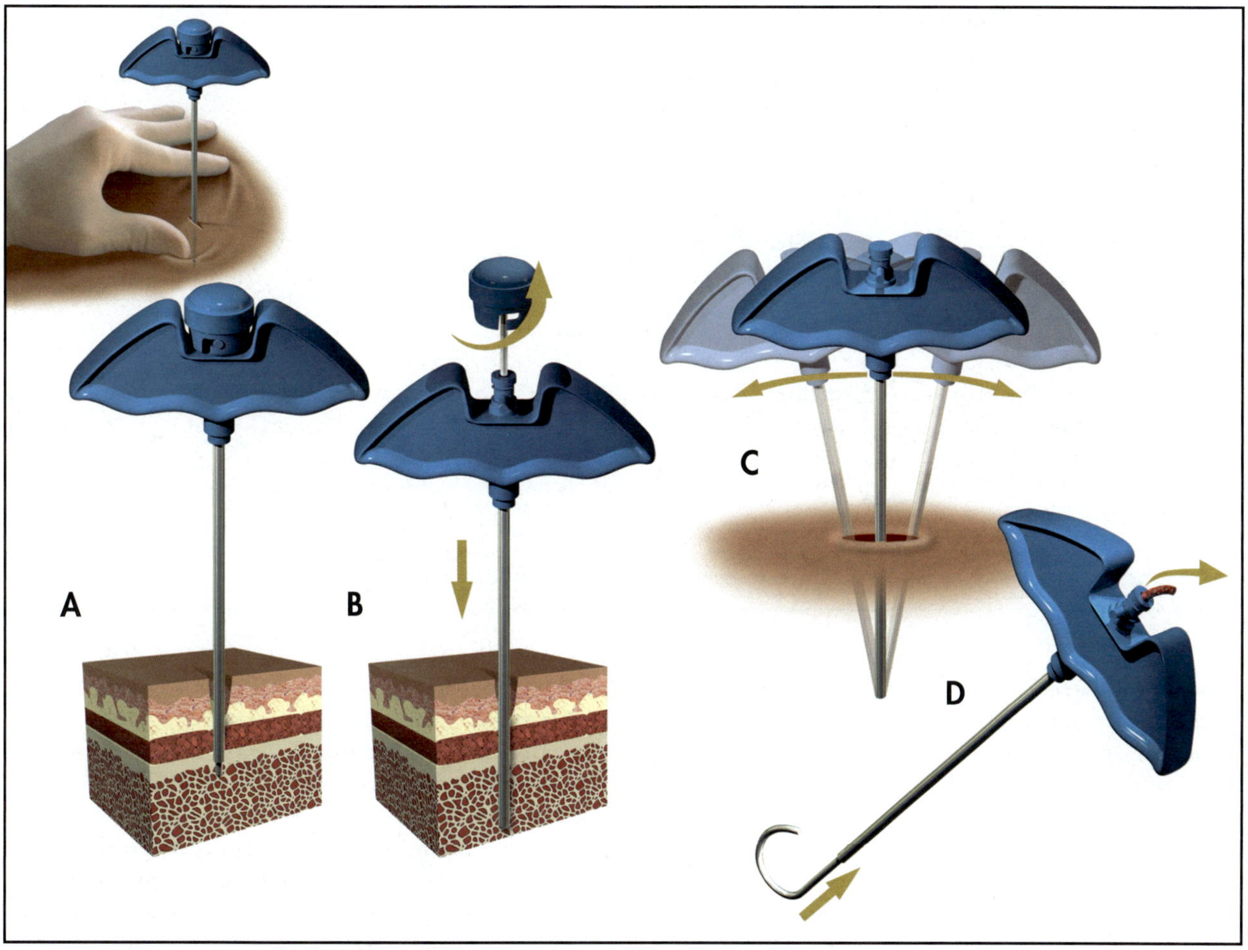

Figure 16-4. *Obtaining a bone marrow core biopsy. The stylet is kept in place until the needle is seated in bone (**A**). The stylet is removed, and the needle is advanced farther (**B**). The instrument is rocked back and forth to "break off" a biopsy specimen of bone at the base within the needle (**C**). The needle is removed, and the biopsy specimen is pushed out the top with the smaller wire obturator inserted through the end (**D**).*

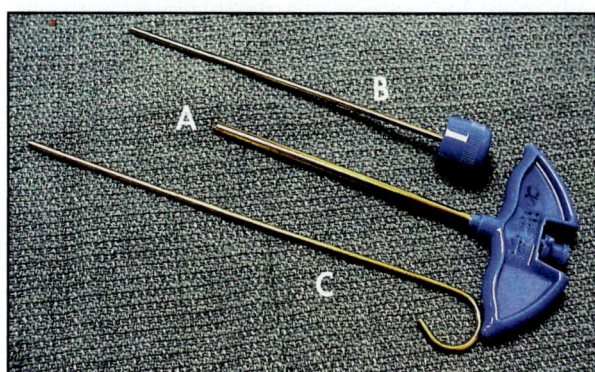

Figure 16-3. *A Jamshidi or bone marrow biopsy needle (**A**) with the stylet (**B**) removed from the instrument. The smaller wire (**C**) is used to push the biopsy specimen from the needle after the needle has been removed from the bone.*

minutes to prevent hematoma formation. The small incision may be sutured or glued closed.

Gentle rolling of the biopsy on a glass slide before fixation may provide a good cytologic sample. An adequate sample is 1 cm of cancellous bone.

Supportive Care: Oral or parenteral analgesics for hours to days may be indicated.

REFERENCES

1. Ogilvie GK, Moore AS: *Managing the Veterinary Cancer Patient: A Practice Manual.* Yardley, PA, Veterinary Learning Systems, 1995, pp 1–47.
2. Ogilvie GK, Moore AS: Bone narrow aspiration and biopsy, in Ogilvie GK, Moore AS (eds): *Feline Oncology: A Comprehensive Guide to Compassionate Care.* Yardley, PA, Veterinary Learning Systems, 2002, pp 26–29.
3. Lee EJ, Schiffer CA: Bone marrow aspiration and biopsy, in Wittes RE (ed): *Manual of Oncologic Therapeutics 1991/1992.* Philadelphia, JB Lippincott, 1991, pp 24–26.

LOWER UROGENITAL TRACT BIOPSY

Gregory K. Ogilvie and Antony S. Moore

CLINICAL BRIEFING

Methods	Benefits
Cystotomy bladder biopsy	• Surgical procedure allows most complete visualization, obtaining large biopsy specimens, and staging of tumor.
Open-ended catheter bladder biopsy	• Relatively inexpensive procedure for obtaining a biopsy specimen.
Flexible or rigid fiberoptic cystoscopy	• Visualization of lesion and direction of biopsy enhance diagnosis.
Transabdominal needle	• Not recommended because of risk for tumor seeding.

Biopsies of the lower urogenital tract are common procedures for practitioners. Bladder tumor biopsies can be performed via laparotomy or a less invasive procedure, such as using cystoscopy or an open-ended catheter.[1,2] Pediatric bronchoscopes, rigid cystoscopes, and arthroscopes of the smallest size are the instruments suitable for cystoscopy in dogs. Currently, most oncologists recommend caution when performing biopsies of the prostate if there is any chance that the underlying disease is a prostatic or transitional cell carcinoma that can recur along the biopsy tract. When a prostate biopsy cannot be performed via lower urinary tract fiberoptic cystoscopy or traumatic catheter biopsy, it can be performed transabdominally, transrectally, or via laparotomy.[1-4] Testicular biopsies can be performed by castration or through fine-needle aspiration cytology or biopsy.[1]

> **KEY POINT**
> *Care should be taken to prevent overinflation and rupture of the bladder. In addition, biopsy specimens should be taken with caution because the bladder wall is likely to be friable due to the presence of the underlying disease.*

Dogs with microhematuria or gross hematuria, with or without stranguria and dysuria, that cannot be resolved with antibiotic therapy must be evaluated for an underlying etiology, including a bladder tumor.[1,2] Transitional cell carcinoma is the most common bladder tumor in dogs. Other differentials causing the above clinical signs, including uroliths, must be ruled out. In each case, a biopsy is required to make an appropriate diagnosis. Before the biopsy, double-contrast cystography or bladder ultrasonography is essential to localize and characterize the lesion. The most common method for nonsurgical biopsy of the bladder is cystoscopy with a rigid or flexible fiberoptic endoscope. A more practical and less expensive method is to use an open-ended urinary catheter that is advanced against the tumor; the tumor is vigorously aspirated into the catheter and the entire instrument is then retracted, ideally with a piece of tumor held within the catheter lumen.

Catheter Biopsy of the Bladder[1-4]

Indication: Any undiagnosed persistent bladder mass, especially in a dog with cystitis or hematuria that does not respond to standard therapy.

Contraindications/complications: Coagulopathies; dogs that are at high risk during general anesthesia; this technique is understandably more challenging in smaller dogs.

Benefits: Tissue samples can be obtained without surgery and often result in an accurate diagnosis; no risk of tracking tumor cells through the abdomen.

Limitation: Requires general anesthesia or at least sedation and good analgesia.

Equipment: 12-ml syringe and open-ended canine urinary catheter; general anesthesia (see box on page 83) is preferred.

Technique (Figure 17-1):

1. After routine screening tests have been conducted to identify problems such as coagulopathies, metabolic dis-

LOWER UROGENITAL TRACT BIOPSY

> **Option for Sedation, Anesthesia, and Analgesia for Bladder Biopsy Using a Catheter**
>
> **Preemptive Analgesia**
> - Oxymorphine (0.05–0.1 mg/kg SC), acepromazine (0.02–0.04 mg/kg SC), and atropine (0.04 mg/kg SC)
>
> **Anesthesia (as indicated)**
> - Propofol or thiopental induction followed by inhalant anesthesia
>
> **Postoperative Analgesia**
> - Ketoprofen: 2.2 mg/kg SC

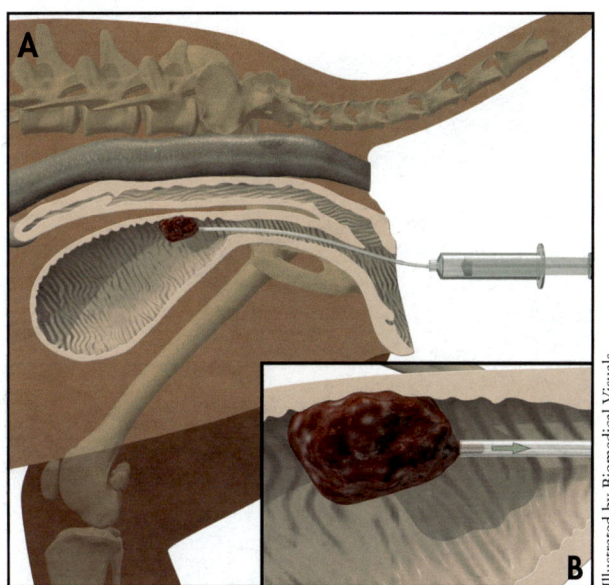

Figure 17-1. Biopsy of a bladder tumor can be accomplished by advancing a catheter with an open end into the tumor (**A**). Suction is applied to aspirate a plug of tumor into the catheter (**B**). The catheter is removed while suction is maintained to ensure that the tissue remains in the catheter.

ease, or organ failure, place the dog under general anesthesia or provide sedation and analgesia.

2. Identify the bladder or urethral lesion with ultrasonography or double-contrast cystography.

3. Premeasure the catheter so that the length to be advanced does not exceed the measurement from the area of the distal urethra to the level of the tumor, which generally is not farther forward than the caudal two mammary glands. This precaution reduces the risk for bladder perforation.

4. Advance the open-ended catheter through the urethra and then forcefully into the tumor. This is best accomplished with ultrasonographic or fluoroscopic guidance or by palpating the mass per abdomen. When possible, stabilize the tumor transrectally with digital or transabdominal palpation.

5. Once the tumor has been entered, apply suction while withdrawing the instrument. Expel tissue that has been suctioned into the catheter and torn off during catheter removal and place it in 10% buffered formalin for subsequent fixation and analysis. If impression smears are desired for cytology, take them before the tissue is formalinized. Formalin fumes will alter cytologic characteristics.

Suction Capsule Biopsy Instrument Technique: Suction capsule (e.g., Quinton) biopsy instruments are used in exactly the same way as described for the catheter biopsy method except that the biopsy port is on the side. Therefore, the operator must direct the instrument so that the biopsy port is directed toward the tumor. Once the biopsy port is against the tumor, apply suction to aspirate the tissue into the capsule. Then activate the self-contained wire that acts as a knife to sever the biopsied tissue from the main tumor for subsequent retrieval.

Supportive Care: Analgesics and possibly an antiinflammatory agent may be needed.

Flexible Fiberoptic or Rigid Cystoscopic Biopsy[1,2,4]

Indication: Any disease that appears to involve the urethra or bladder (Figures 17-2 and 17-3).

Contraindications: Coagulopathies; dogs that are at high risk during general anesthesia, including those with limited pulmonary or cardiovascular function (insufflation of the bladder can reduce venous return to the heart and compress the diaphragm, compromising the ability to inspire easily); procedure is restricted to medium to large female dogs or large males that have had a perineal urethrostomy.

Complications: Very rare but can include bleeding (which usually stops spontaneously) and bladder rupture.

Benefit: Relatively minimal risk.

Limitation: Requires general anesthesia and analgesia at the time of laparotomy (see box on this page).

Equipment: Few fiberoptic endoscopes are small enough for cystoscopy in dogs; pediatric bronchoscopes, rigid cystoscopes, and arthroscopes of the smallest size are often good choices. Pediatric bronchoscopes (<5 mm in diameter) can be inserted into the urethra of most large male dogs that have had a perineal urethrostomy. The endoscope should have an instrument port and channel, be at least bidirectional, bend more than 100° in at least one direction, and have an external light source; cytology brushes and biopsy forceps should be of a size and type

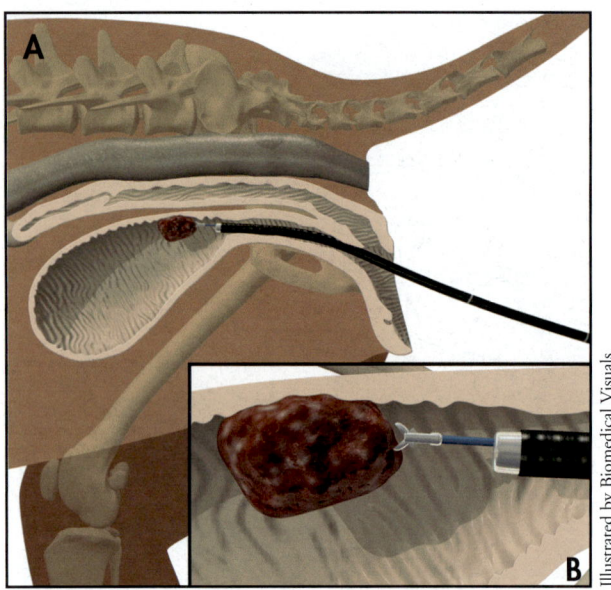

Figure 17-2. *A bladder tumor biopsy via flexible endoscopy is performed by first locating the tumor (**A**) and then taking several "pinch" samples through the endoscope (**B**).*

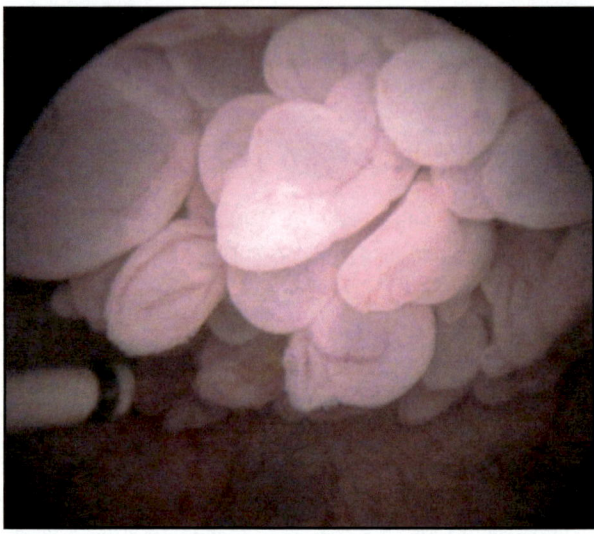

Figure 17-3. *Endoscopic view of a bladder tumor biopsy being performed. Several "pinch" samples should be taken from different locations within the lesion. This lesion was diagnosed histologically as transitional cell carcinoma. (Courtesy of David C. Twedt, DVM, Colorado State University)*

that will pass through the instrument port with the bronchoscope in a flexed position.

Technique (Figure 17-2):

1. After tests are done to ensure the absence of life-threatening diseases, administer general anesthesia or other chemical restraint.
2. Perform a routine laparotomy; identify and pack off the bladder; and make a small incision into the bladder to introduce the fiberoptic instrument.
3. Using aseptic technique, insert the rigid or flexible fiberoptic endoscope through a surgically created stoma in the bladder (or preferably through the urethra of a female or male dog with a perineal urethrostomy). In some large dogs, a very small, flexible fiberoptic scope can be passed through the os penis into the bladder for visualization purposes. Suction off any urine, and insufflate a judicious amount of carbon dioxide, air, or sterile water into the bladder to enhance visualization of any pathology.
4. Sample suspect lesions first with the cytology brush for cytologic evaluation and then obtain a biopsy sample for histopathology. If a diffuse lesion is suspected, acquire random samples. After biopsies are performed, suction off the air and remove the instrument; in the case of a laparotomy, close the bladder stoma and the abdomen routinely.

Supportive Care: Oral analgesics and antiinflammatory agents may be needed in some cases.

Biopsy of the Prostate[1]

Every attempt must be made to perform a biopsy of the prostate via the urethra (urethroscopy or traumatic urinary catheter biopsy). This can be accomplished by passing an open-ended catheter or a red rubber feeding tube to the level of the prostate, followed by repeated aspiration attempts using a syringe. Tissue "plugs" are often found in the collected urine. When these methods are not possible, a prostatic mass can be biopsied externally or transrectally after it is identified on abdominal or rectal examination or after prostatic ultrasonography or abdominal radiography. A tumor of the prostate should always be suspected in a male dog, especially if the prostate is firm, asymmetric, fixed to nearby tissues, and calcified on radiographs. Diagnosis can be made by fine-needle aspiration cytology; exploratory surgery and biopsy; transabdominal biopsy with a needle biopsy instrument, with or without ultrasonographic guidance; and transrectal needle biopsy methods. The latter two methods are outlined because they are easy to perform and are highly accurate.

NEEDLE CORE BIOPSY[1,2]

This type of biopsy is usually safe and quick. With proper analgesia and tranquilization, it can be performed on an awake, cooperative patient. The histopathologic results generally are more accurate than those of fine-needle aspiration cytology but less accurate than open biopsy.

Indication: Prostatomegaly of unexplained etiology.
Contraindications: Coagulopathies; prostatic abscess.

LOWER UROGENITAL TRACT BIOPSY

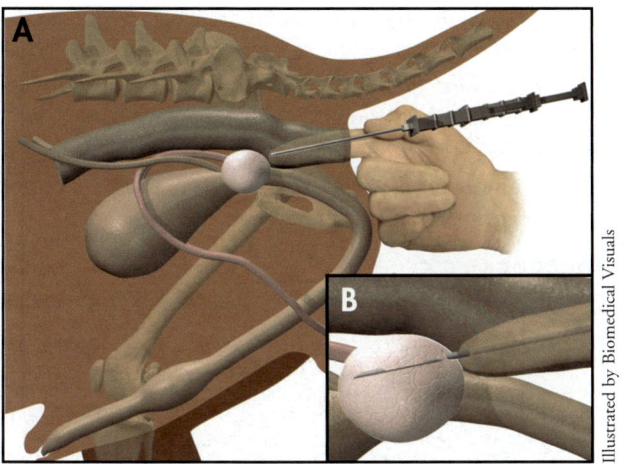

Figure 17-4. *A transrectal needle core biopsy is performed by placing a gloved index finger along the top of the biopsy needle tip; a finger cut from another glove is then drawn over the needle tip and the overlying index finger (so that the glove finger sheaths the needle and the operator's finger). The outer portion of this finger cover is lubricated, and the covered finger and needle tip are then inserted rectally (**A**). The prostate is pushed up and back by the operator or an assistant and held into position for biopsy. The needle core biopsy instrument is advanced through the glove cover, rectum, and outer capsule of the prostate (**B**). The inner stylet is then advanced into the tissue, and the outer cannula is advanced over the stylet to cut off the tissue. Several biopsy specimens of the prostate are taken through the same stab incision. The needle biopsy specimens are fixed in 10% buffered formalin, as described in the text.*

Benefit: General anesthesia is not routinely required; however, it should be considered for uncooperative patients.

Limitations: The small tissue samples that are obtained may not be diagnostic; perforation of the urethra or rupture of a prostatic abscess can lead to life-threatening complications.

Equipment: No. 11 surgical blade; 2% lidocaine; needle biopsy instrument.

Technique:

1. An assistant brings the prostate close to the nearby abdominal wall using abdominal palpation. Hold the organ firmly against the abdominal wall, and prepare the biopsy site for surgery.
2. Inject approximately 2 to 3 ml of lidocaine under the skin overlying the prostate. Systemic analgesia is as described in the box on this page.
3. Make a stab incision in the skin using a No. 11 surgical blade to allow easy entry of the needle core biopsy instrument.
4. Advance the needle core biopsy instrument through the incision and into the capsule of the prostate. The accuracy of the biopsy is enhanced by using an ultrasound probe covered with a sterile glove, lubricating the biopsy site with sterile ultrasound gel, and imaging the prostate to visualize and direct the biopsy.
5. Remove several biopsy specimens of the prostate through the same stab incision.
6. Fix the needle biopsy specimens in 10% buffered formalin in the manner described previously. Use separate containers for specimens of each different lesion that is biopsied.
7. Suture the stab incision if indicated.

Options for Sedation, Anesthesia, and Analgesia for Biopsy of the Urinary Tract

Preemptive Analgesia
- Morphine (1 mg/kg SC), acepromazine (0.02 mg/kg SC), and atropine (0.04 mg/kg SC) with oral NSAID before and after surgery (ensure adequate hydration and renal function)

Anesthesia (as indicated)
- Propofol or thiopental induction followed by inhalant anesthesia

Postbiopsy Analgesia (choose one)
- Carprofen (4 mg/kg SC)
- Ketoprofen (2 mg/kg SC)
- Morphine (0.5 to 1 mg/kg SC) as needed q4–6h
- Nalbuphine 1 mg/kg SC as needed q4–6h

TRANSRECTAL NEEDLE CORE BIOPSY

Like the transabdominal biopsy technique, the transrectal prostatic biopsy method is generally safe and quick. As mentioned previously, this method may result in seeding tumor cells along the biopsy tract. With proper analgesia and tranquilization, it can be performed on an awake, cooperative patient. The histopathologic results are generally more accurate than fine-needle aspiration cytology but less accurate than open biopsy. The rectum must be evacuated before the procedure. Surprisingly, abscess formation is not a common complication of this method.

Indication: Prostatomegaly of unexplained etiology.

Contraindications: Coagulopathies; prostatic abscess.

Benefit: General anesthesia is not routinely required, but it should be considered for uncooperative patients.

Limitation: The small tissue samples that are obtained may not be diagnostic.

Equipment: Surgical glove; a finger of a second surgical glove; 2% lidocaine; needle biopsy instrument.

Technique (Figure 17-4):

1. Inject approximately 2 to 3 ml of lidocaine into the distal rectum and colon using a lubricated syringe without

a needle attached. The patient should receive appropriate tranquilizers, analgesics, or general anesthesia.

2. Place the gloved index finger along the top of the biopsy needle tip; then draw the finger cut from another glove over the needle tip and the overlying index finger (so that the glove finger sheaths the needle and the operator's finger). Lubricate the outer portion of this finger cover, and then insert the covered finger and needle tip into the rectum. Push the prostate up and back and hold it in position for biopsy.

3. Advance the needle core biopsy instrument through the glove cover, rectum, and outer capsule of the prostate. The accuracy of the biopsy is enhanced by covering an ultrasound probe with a sterile glove, lubricating the biopsy site with sterile ultrasound gel, and imaging the prostate to visualize and direct the biopsy.

4. Take several biopsy specimens of the prostate through the same stab incision.

5. Fix the needle biopsy specimens in 10% buffered formalin as described previously. Use separate containers for specimens of each different lesion that is biopsied.

REFERENCES

1. Ogilvie GK, Moore AS: *Managing the Veterinary Cancer Patient: A Practice Manual.* Yardley, PA, Veterinary Learning Systems, 1995, pp 1–47.
2. Withrow SJ: Biopsy principles, in Withrow SJ, MacEwen EG (eds): *Small Animal Clinical Oncology,* ed 3. Philadelphia, WB Saunders, 2001, pp 52–57.
3. Herr HW, Shipley WU, Bajorin D: Cancer of the bladder, in DeVita VT, Hellman S, Rosenberg SA (eds): *Cancer: Principles and Practice of Oncology,* ed 6. Philadelphia, JB Lippincott, 2001, pp 1396–1400.
4. Ogilvie GK, Moore AS: *Feline Oncology: A Comprehensive Guide to Compassionate Care.* Yardley, PA, Veterinary Learning Systems, 2001, pp 30–32.

DIGESTIVE SYSTEM BIOPSY

Gregory K. Ogilvie and Antony S. Moore

Surgical exploration with biopsy remains the most complete method of exploring the digestive system in dogs. The oral cavity is readily accessible; however, planning for correct placement of the surgical biopsy tract is critical for long-term care of dogs with cancer. The biopsy is crucial not only to obtain a definitive diagnosis but also to ensure that definitive surgery can be performed subsequently with minimal cosmetic and functional alterations to the dog.[1] Surgical exploration of the abdomen and thorax is more invasive than fiberoptic endoscopy and may be associated with greater risks.

Although exploratory surgery has many benefits, endoscopic examination of the gastrointestinal (GI) tract is a common, effective, low-risk means of diagnosing malignant conditions of this organ system.[1–5] In addition, with endoscopy, benign conditions that mimic malignancy can be identified for subsequent treatment.[1,5] Flexible fiberoptic endoscopes can be used to examine all areas of the esophagus, stomach, proximal duodenum, rectum, and colon. Rigid endoscopes or proctoscopes can be used to examine portions of the esophagus, rectum, and most of the descending colon. Laparoscopy has the advantage of evaluating many organs of the abdomen with very little trauma to the dog. The techniques of oral cavity biopsy, upper and lower GI endoscopy, and abdominal laparoscopy will be discussed separately.

▶ ORAL CAVITY BIOPSY

CLINICAL BRIEFING

Methods	Benefits
Excisional biopsy	• Diagnostic and therapeutic; requires knowledge of the extent of disease before surgery, which is best obtained through high-detail radiography, CT, or MRI.
Incisional biopsy	• Diagnosis allows logical planning of definitive therapeutic procedure.

Biopsy of the oral cavity lesion is essential because almost all of the tumors in this area have different prognoses and treatments, despite similar gross appearances. Before an oral lesion biopsy is performed, high-detail images, including radiographs, should be obtained to determine the presence of bone invasion. (However, bone invasion may not be visible using radiography as more than 50% of mineral needs to be lost for radiographic lysis to be noticeable; computed tomography [CT] and magnetic resonance imaging [MRI] are more sensitive.)

High-detail imagery provides essential information to the pathologist and surgeon. For example, a pathologist would consider a diagnosis of a biologically high-grade yet histologically low-grade fibrosarcoma rather than fibrous connective tissue or a fibroma if radiographs suggest the presence of bone involvement, despite a biopsy finding consistent with a diagnosis of fibroma. Similarly, a mandibulectomy or maxillectomy would be the surgical approach if bone were involved. When a tooth is extracted in a dog, a biopsy should be considered to rule out the presence of cancer as an underlying cause of disease. Before biopsy, the surgeon who will perform the definitive procedure should be consulted to ensure that the biopsy will not compromise the success of the procedure or the health of the dog. If the biopsy involves tissue essential for closure or if the tumor is seated into an area that is too large to resect, a successful outcome of the definitive procedure may not be possible. Although excisional biopsy is an option, incisional biopsy is more frequently performed to determine what definitive procedure is needed.

> **KEY POINT**
>
> *Biopsy of an oral cavity lesion is essential because almost all of the tumors in this area have different prognoses and treatments, despite similar gross appearances.*

Indication: Identification of an oral mass of unexplained etiology.

Contraindications: Coagulopathies; dogs that are at high risk during general anesthesia.

Benefit: An accurate histopathologic evaluation can be obtained because part or all of the oral mass can be sampled.

Limitations: Any condition that would place the patient at risk for receiving anesthesia or sedation; coagulopathies.

Equipment: General anesthesia (see box at right); standard surgical instruments.

Technique:

1. After routine screening tests have been conducted to identify problems such as coagulopathies and metabolic disease, place the dog under general anesthesia. Place an endotracheal tube with a properly fitting cuff and secure it to prevent aspiration of blood or other oral contents.
2. Obtain images of the oral mass using radiography (along with other imaging methods when appropriate). Intraoral radiographs should be included in the views obtained. More specific details regarding oral tumors are outlined in Chapter 53.
3. After a nerve block is placed and/or parenteral analgesics are started, make an incision over the oral mass and remove a section of the lesion at the junction of normal and abnormal tissue. Be careful not to biopsy through normal lip or skin because this tissue may be needed for reconstructive surgical techniques. Options include excisional or incisional biopsy procedures.
4. Stop any bleeding with ligation, cautery, or, in the case of an open bone biopsy, bone wax. Bleeding usually subsides within 5 to 10 minutes.
5. After the oral mass is removed, suture the surrounding tissue if possible. Keep in mind that the oral cavity is a contaminated area.
6. Adequately fix the tumor in 10% formalin.

Supportive Care: Oral or parenteral analgesics may be indicated, and soft food should be offered for several days.

Options for Sedation, Anesthesia, and Analgesia for Oral Cavity Biopsy

Preemptive Analgesia
- Ketamine microdose constant-rate infusion (CRI) at 10 µg/kg/min after an IV bolus of ketamine (0.5 mg/kg) (can reduce the need for analgesics postoperatively)
- Local block for the oral cavity (see Chapter 29)
- Morphine (1 mg/kg SC), acepromazine (0.02 mg/kg SC), and nerve block if appropriate to local area

Anesthesia (as indicated)
- Propofol or thiopental induction followed by inhalant anesthesia

Postoperative Analgesia
- Fentanyl bolus (2 mg/kg IV) followed by 3–5 µg/kg/hr IV CRI by syringe pump or IV pump; bupivacaine nerve block and acupuncture

Home Analgesia (choose one or more)
- Carprofen: 2.2 mg/kg PO q12h
- Etodolac: 10–15 mg/kg PO q12h
- Ketoprofen: 1 mg/kg PO
- Meloxicam: 0.1 mg/kg PO q24h
- Morphine: 0.5 mg/kg PO tid–qid
- Piroxicam: 0.3 mg/kg PO q24–48h
- Transdermal fentanyl: 2–3 mg/kg/hr

▶ UPPER AND LOWER GASTROINTESTINAL BIOPSY

CLINICAL BRIEFING

Methods	Benefits
Surgical exploration and biopsy	• Allow visual determination of the extent of disease and directed biopsy.
Fiberoptic endoscopic biopsy	• Allows noninvasive visualization of the GI tract; useful for specifically directing biopsy.
Ultrasound-guided biopsy	• Allows visualization of the entire GI tract and other intraabdominal organs.

Upper Gastrointestinal Endoscopy[5]

Indications for upper GI endoscopy include regurgitation, dysphagia, retching, nausea, vomiting, hematemesis, diarrhea, melena, and any masslike lesions identified in the esophagus, stomach, or upper duodenum (Figure 18-1). The diagnostic accuracy of flexible endoscopic biopsies is approximately 95% in humans, but it may be lower in dogs. Accuracy is highest with intraluminal disease, regardless of

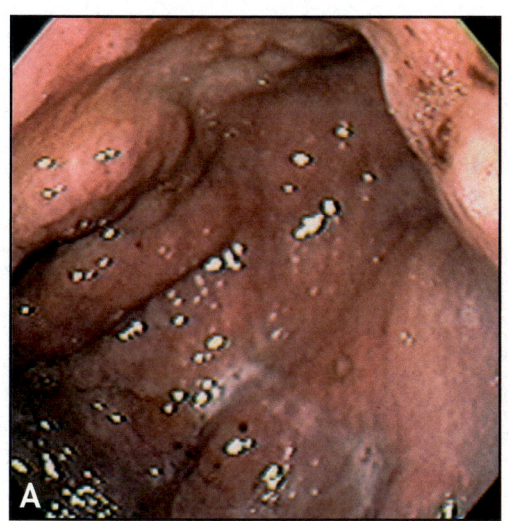 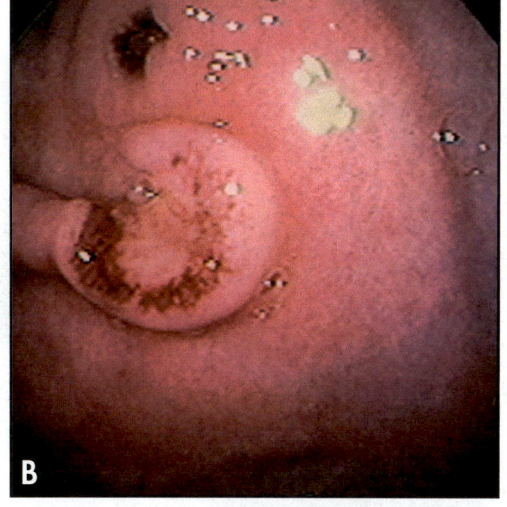

Figure 18-1. Systematic endoscopic evaluation of the gastric mucosa can allow visualization of lesions, such as these gastric (**A**) and pyloric (**B**) lymphomas. (Courtesy of David C. Twedt, DVM, Colorado State University)

whether it is focal or diffuse and regardless of malignancy. Less diagnostic accuracy is seen with infiltrating cancers such as lymphoma, in which a full-thickness biopsy is often ideal to make a diagnosis. Because dogs can have patchy distribution of lesions, multiple biopsies are indicated to maximize the chance of diagnosing the disease. In addition, endoscopy is ideal for the diagnosis and evaluation of intraluminal lesions. A veterinary pathologist who is interested and experienced in examining endoscopic biopsies is absolutely essential to the success of this type of diagnostic procedure.

> **KEY POINT**
>
> *Care must be taken to avoid overdistention of the patient's GI tract with gas when performing upper GI endoscopy, as this can result in compromised blood return to the heart and rupture of the stomach or intestines.*

Indications: Any disease that appears to involve the esophagus, stomach, or upper duodenum.

Contraindications: Coagulopathies; dogs that are at high risk during general anesthesia.

Complications: Very rare but can include bleeding, which usually stops spontaneously. If brisk bleeding persists, introducing a Fogarty balloon catheter to occlude the bleeding vessel is recommended. If perforation occurs, perform emergency surgery to repair the rent or resect the section of bowel (in humans, the risk for bowel perforation is reported to be <0.1%).

Benefits: Minimal risk; noninvasive.

Limitations: Requires general anesthesia (see box on page 223); biopsy samples are small and superficial and, therefore, may miss deeper pathology.

Equipment: There are many fiberoptic endoscopes on the market that can be used to perform upper GI endoscopy. The flexible fiberoptic endoscope should have an instrument port and channel, be at least bidirectional, bend more than 100° in at least one direction, and have an external light source, suction, and water insufflation capability. Cytology brushes, biopsy forceps, and graspers that will pass through the instrument port with the endoscope in a flexed position should be available. Adult or pediatric fiberoptic endoscopes 5 to 8 mm in diameter and at least as long as 150 cm can be inserted into the duodenum of most dogs.

Technique (Figure 18-2):

1. Dogs should be fasted for 6 to 8 hours before undergoing upper GI endoscopy. After tests are conducted to ensure the absence of life-threatening diseases, place the animal under general anesthesia with endotracheal intubation. Use a mouth gag to prevent the dog from biting the endoscope.

2. Insert the endoscope through the mouth and down into the esophagus. Insufflate carbon dioxide or air into the structure to be examined. If excessive fluid is encountered, aspirate it. Perform a systematic examination of the esophagus, lower esophageal sphincter, stomach, and proximal duodenum (Figure 18-3).

3. Sample suspect lesions first with the cytology brush for cytologic evaluation, then take multiple biopsy samples for histopathology. A minimum of five samples should be collected for histopathologic analysis.

Supportive Care: Antiemetics or intestinal protectants administered after the procedure may be helpful; in some cases, analgesics may be indicated.

90 MANAGING THE CANINE CANCER PATIENT

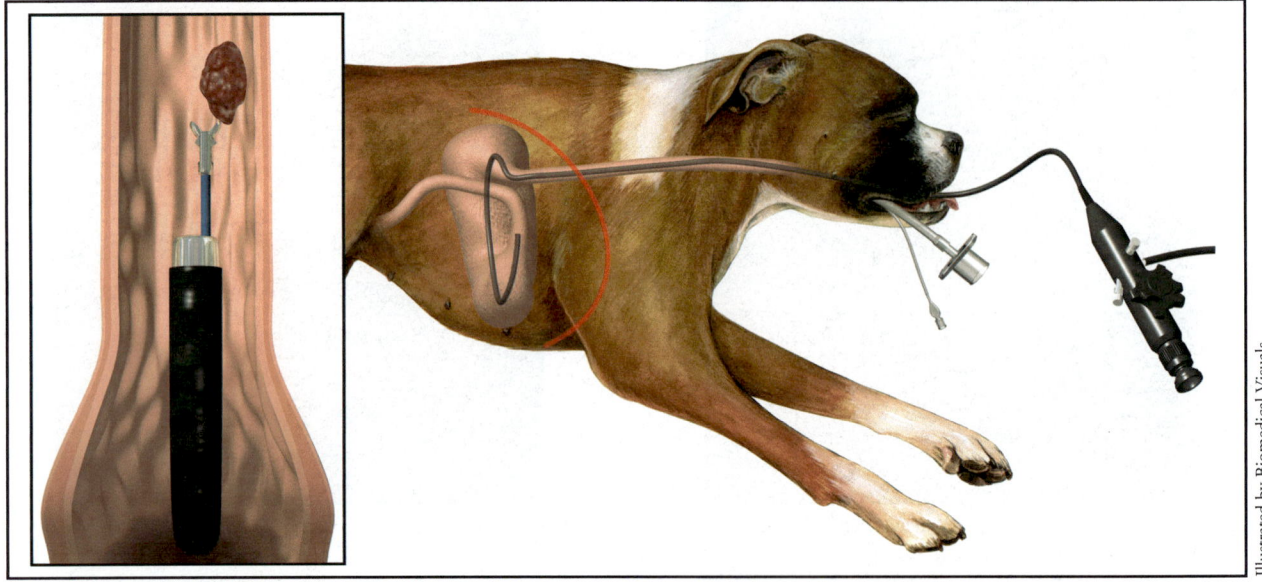

Figure 18-2. *A flexible endoscope can be used to localize, characterize, and biopsy esophageal, gastric, or upper duodenal tumors or lesions. The animal is given general anesthesia and placed on its right side. A mouth gag is used. In each case, multiple biopsy specimens should be obtained to ensure that an accurate diagnosis is made.*

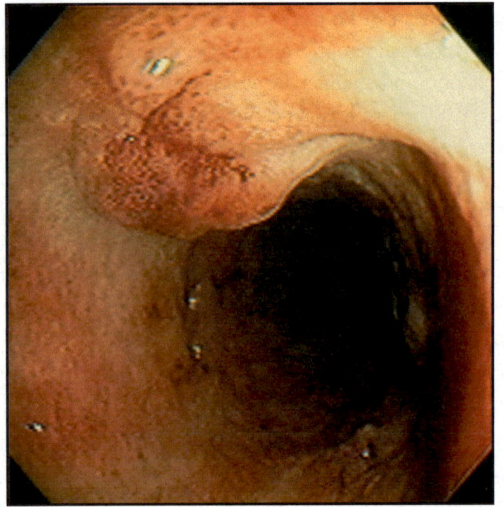

Figure 18-3. *Systematic endoscopic evaluation of the upper GI tract can allow visualization of lesions, such as this duodenal lymphoma. (Courtesy of D. C. Twedt)*

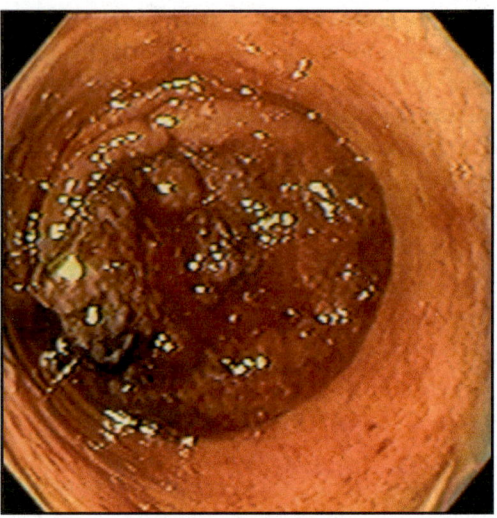

Figure 18-4. *Flexible fiberoptic endoscopic view of a colonic adenocarcinoma. (Courtesy of D. C. Twedt)*

Lower Intestinal Endoscopy[1,4]

Indications for endoscopic evaluation of the rectum, colon, and ileum include diarrhea, dyschezia, constipation, and a mass in the lower intestinal tract. Because it allows greater visualization of the colon (Figure 18-4) and rectum, lower intestinal flexible fiberoptic endoscopy is surpassing rigid sigmoidoscopy in popularity. The rigid scope is more effective in evaluating the large bowel. Both instruments provide a means of examining the mucosal surface of the entire large bowel in great detail. Pinch samples can be taken for subsequent evaluation by a veterinary histopathologist. Although the procedure is best accomplished with the dog under general anesthesia, chemical tranquilization with analgesia may be adequate for some dogs.

Indications: Any disease that appears to involve the colon or rectum, especially those of the mucosal surface.

Contraindications: Coagulopathies; dogs that are at high risk during general anesthesia or tranquilization. Dogs with fulminant, severe colitis may be at increased risk for perforation.

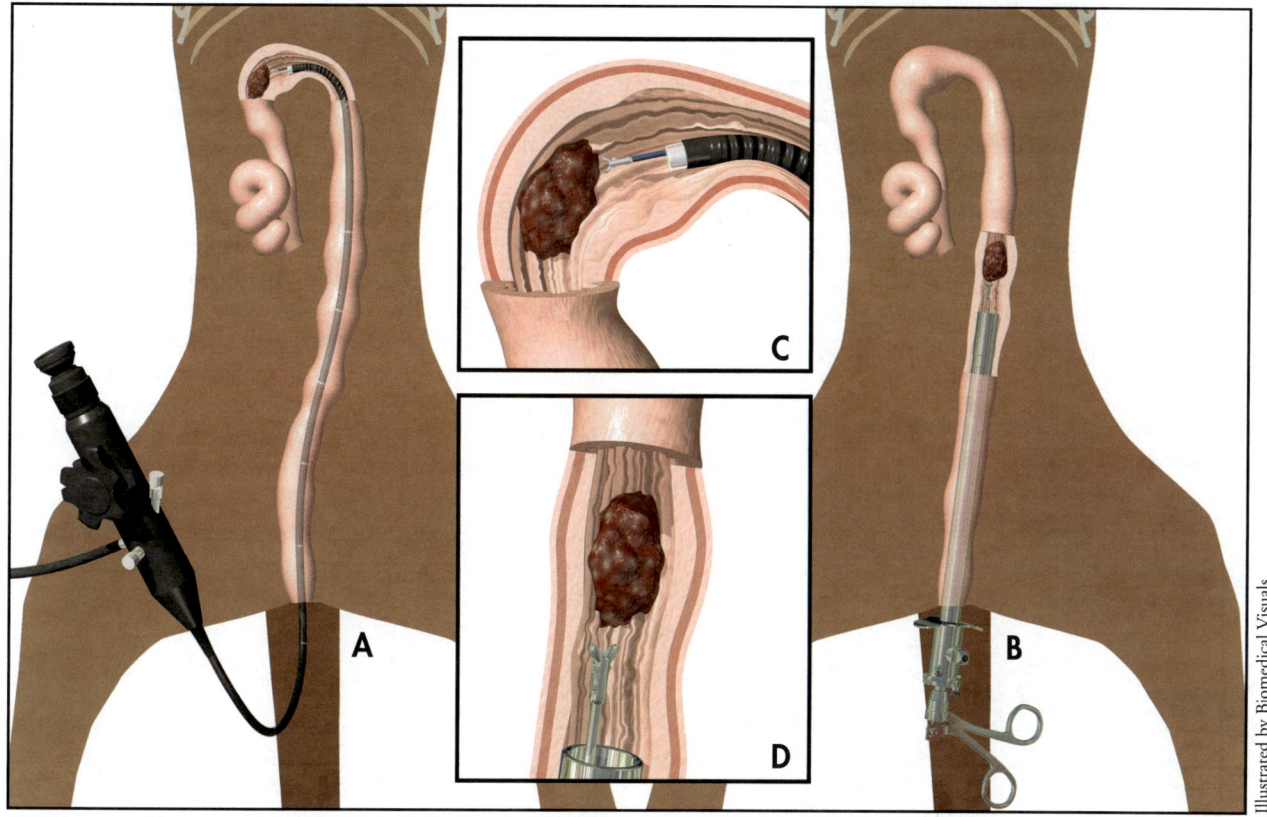

Figure 18-5. Colonoscopy can be performed with either a flexible endoscope (**A**) or a rigid proctoscope (**B**). The flexible fiberoptic endoscope is more effective for exploring the area of the ileocecocolic junction and the transverse colon. The biopsy instrument is extended through the biopsy port to take small pinch samples (**C**) in the transverse colon. The rigid endoscope may be more effective for draining the colon of blood and for introducing larger biopsy instruments. Larger biopsy specimens can be taken from the descending colon by extending rigid biopsy instruments (**D**) to the lesion to be biopsied.

Complications: Very rare but can include bleeding, which usually stops spontaneously. If brisk bleeding persists, introduction of a Fogarty balloon catheter to occlude the bleeding vessels is recommended. If bowel perforation occurs, perform emergency surgery to repair the rent or resect the section of bowel (in humans, the risk of perforating the bowel is reported to be <0.5%, which is higher than for the upper GI tract).

Benefits: Minimal risk; noninvasive.

Limitations: Requires general anesthesia or tranquilization with analgesia; the procedure is generally effective only for diagnosing diseases that affect the lumen of the colon or rectum.

Equipment: There are many fiberoptic endoscopes available for performing lower GI endoscopy. The flexible fiberoptic endoscope should have an instrument port and channel, be at least bidirectional, bend more than 100° in one direction, and have an external light source, suction, and water insufflator. Adult or pediatric fiberoptic endoscopes 5 to 8 mm in diameter and longer than 1 m can be inserted into the colon and advanced to the level of the cecum in most dogs. A skilled operator can occasionally pass the scope into the ileum. The rigid scope should be 25 cm in length and have a light source. Cytology brushes, biopsy forceps, and graspers that can pass through the instrument port with the flexible fiberoptic endoscope in a flexed position should be available; these same biopsy instruments can be used with a rigid scope. Mare uterine biopsy instruments should be used with extreme care because of the high risk of perforating the colon or rectum.

Technique (Figure 18-5):

1. Fast the dog for 24 to 36 hours, followed by a warm-water enema. In some cases, a GI lavage solution containing polyethylene glycol as the main nonabsorbable solute (e.g., Golytely, Braintree Laboratories, Braintree, MA; Colyte, Endlaw Preparations, Farmington, NY) may be used. Give the solution twice, each time at a dosage of 25 ml/kg via orogastric tube. The doses should be given 1 hour apart, 12 to 18 hours before the endoscopy procedure (giving metoclopramide 30 min before the solution

is administered may decrease distention and nausea). Phosphate-containing enemas (e.g., Fleet) are usually not adequate to allow the patient to void all fecal material. Give the dog the opportunity to eliminate all fecal material before the procedure is performed. After diagnostics are performed to ensure the absence of life-threatening disease, administer general anesthesia or tranquilization.

2. Insert the endoscope through the anus and into the colon. Insufflation of carbon dioxide or air allows adequate visualization of the colon and proximal rectum. If liquid material is present, suction it out. Examine the lower GI tract systematically.

3. Sample suspect lesions first with the cytology brush for cytologic evaluation, and then take biopsy samples for histopathology. A minimum of five biopsy samples should be collected for histopathologic analysis.

Supportive Care: Low-residue food may be helpful for some; analgesics may be indicated in select cases.

Intestinal Ultrasonography

Ultrasonography is often superior to contrast radiography in identifying a mass involving the intestinal wall, although it may be difficult to identify the specific area of the bowel where the lesion is present.[6-9] Ultrasonography may identify intraabdominal metastases, such as in the liver, that are not suspected on radiography. Ultrasonography may also identify enlarged regional lymph nodes and guide a needle biopsy for definitive diagnosis. An ultrasound-guided, automated, 18-gauge Tru-cut needle is available in 11- and 23-mm lengths, enabling biopsy of thickened intestinal wall with little risk of perforation. Limitations of ultrasonography include a poor ability to visualize peritoneal tumor seeding even in the presence of ascites. It is important to remember that barium will interfere with the diagnostic accuracy of ultrasonography. Ultrasonography is therefore best performed before barium administration. Despite these limitations, ultrasonography is probably the imaging modality of choice for intestinal tumors.

▶ LIVER BIOPSY[1-3]

CLINICAL BRIEFING

Methods	Benefits
Surgical exploration	• Allows visual determination of the extent of disease and directed biopsy.
Ultrasonography-guided biopsy	• Allows visualization of disease and directed biopsy.
Transabdominal percutaneous biopsy	• Relatively easy and safe method for obtaining liver tissue.
Keyhole liver biopsy	• Allows the liver to be isolated and stabilized for blind biopsy.
Laparoscopy	• Allows direct visualization of abdominal contents and visually directed biopsy.

Liver biopsy is a common procedure used to determine the histologic characteristics of a tumor or nonmalignant condition after laboratory work and routine imaging methods have determined that the liver is abnormal.[1-4] Liver biopsies are accurately performed with ultrasonographic or fluoroscopic guidance.[2,4] Biopsies are becoming even more accurate as CT imaging becomes more commonly used in canine practice. Other methods of obtaining a liver biopsy include direct visualization by laparoscopy or open surgical biopsy. An unguided (blind) percutaneous biopsy is generally not recommended because ultrasonography is so widely available and makes the procedure much safer. In all types of liver biopsies, the most common complication is bleeding from the biopsy site. Therefore, before a liver biopsy is performed, hematocrit, platelet count, activated clotting time or one-step partial thromboplastin time, and activated par-

> **KEY POINT**
> *Ultrasonography can be very helpful in guiding a liver biopsy to prevent laceration of the liver and underlying structures.*

DIGESTIVE SYSTEM BIOPSY

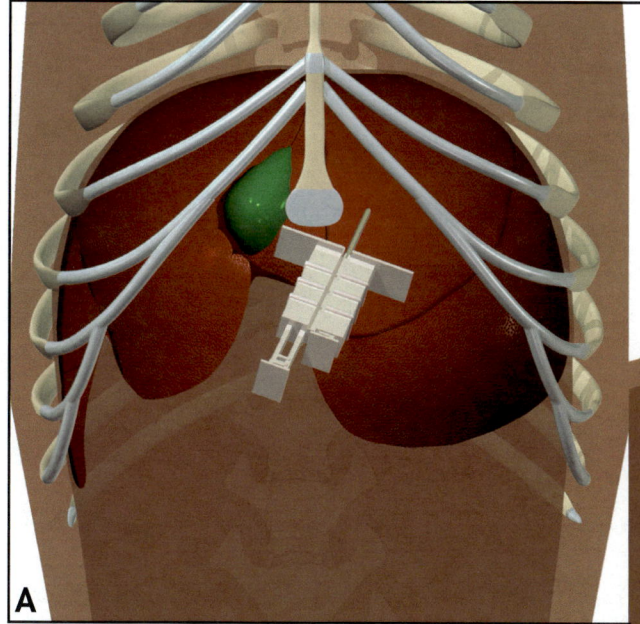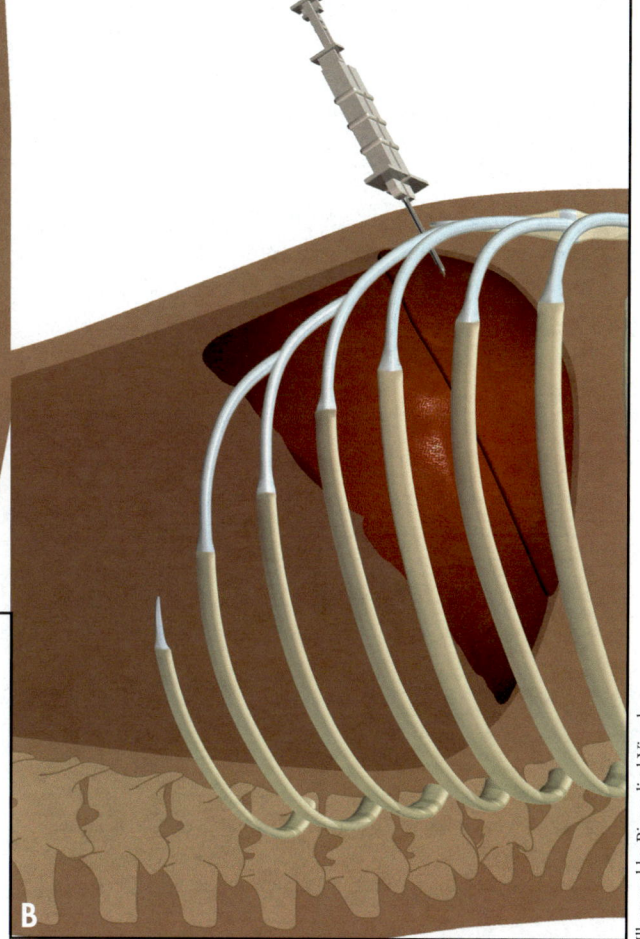

Figure 18-6. A liver biopsy can be performed with a needle core biopsy instrument, which is advanced through a skin incision, through the subcutaneous tissue, and then just through the abdominal wall. The biopsy needle is directed slightly craniad and to the animal's left (**A**). At this point, to prevent lacerating the liver and underlying structures, the biopsy instrument should be advanced no more than 1 to 3 cm into the abdomen to the liver (**B**). The inner stylet is then advanced into the liver, and the outer cannula is advanced over the stylet to cut off the tissue. If ultrasonography is available, it is used to direct the biopsy equipment. At least one biopsy specimen is obtained, and one piece of tissue is submitted for bacterial culture and sensitivity testing and the others for histopathology and for special analyses such as for copper.

tial thromboplastin time should be determined to identify dogs that may be at high risk for bleeding after the procedure. In addition, dogs should be kept quiet after the procedure, and a hematocrit should be measured to compare with that obtained before the procedure.

Transabdominal Percutaneous Liver Biopsy[1-3]

Indications: Evaluation and diagnosis of malignant and nonmalignant liver disease.

Contraindications: Coagulopathies; dogs that are at high risk during general anesthesia or tranquilization.

Benefits: Aspiration can only provide a sample for individual cell analysis, whereas a biopsy can provide tissue to analyze the cellularity, architecture, and content of the liver section; the procedure can often be done with local anesthesia, systemic analgesia, and tranquilization (see box on page 94); if there are any concerns about the dog's ability to lie quietly on its back, general anesthesia should be administered.

Limitation: Single samples taken may not be representative of the entire liver.

Equipment: Standard surgical instruments; needle core biopsy instrument.

Technique (Figure 18-6):

1. For the largest view of the liver, position the dog in dorsal recumbency with its right side tilted slightly down toward the table surface. Ideally, the caudal aspect of the dog should be lowered to allow the liver to "fall" caudally for easier access during the biopsy procedure. Clip an area of hair 4 to 6 cm in diameter, encompassing the xyphoid process and the ventral left costal arch, and prepare the liver biopsy site with a surgical scrub. A lateral approach is also possible to view or perform a biopsy of the extreme right or left lobe of the liver.

2. Using a 25-gauge needle, inject approximately 0.5 to 2 ml of lidocaine in and around the site where the biopsy needle is to be introduced. The lidocaine will sting less on injection if it is diluted 50:50 with 8.4% bicarbonate.

3. Scrub the area to be biopsied a final time after the lidocaine is injected. A surgical drape can be applied for sterility.
4. Using aseptic surgical technique, make a small stab incision with a No. 11 surgical blade at a point to be directed by ultrasonography.
5. Using ultrasonographic guidance, advance the needle core biopsy instrument into the subcutaneous tissue and then just through the abdominal wall.
6. Obtain at least five biopsy specimens; submit one piece of tissue for bacterial culture and sensitivity testing, and submit the others for histopathology and for special analyses such as for copper levels.
7. Place the dog in sternal recumbency, and observe for 24 to 48 hours for signs of bleeding or other complications. This technique has a very high likelihood of obtaining diagnostic-quality tissue and has a mortality rate of approximately 1% in humans.

Supportive Care: Oral or parenteral analgesics are indicated.

> **KEY POINT**
> *Providing the patient with compassionate care during a biopsy procedure means minimizing discomfort through the use of analgesia before and after surgery.*

Options for Sedation, Anesthesia, and Analgesia for Liver Biopsy

Preemptive Analgesia
- Morphine (1 mg/kg SC), acepromazine (0.02 mg/kg SC), and atropine (0.04 mg/kg SC) with oral NSAID before and after surgery (to ensure adequate hydration and renal function)

Anesthesia (as indicated)
- Propofol or thiopental induction followed by inhalant anesthesia

Postbiopsy Analgesia (choose one)
- Morphine (0.5–1 mg/kg SC) as needed q4–6h
- Nalbuphine 1 mg/kg SC as needed q4–6h
- Ketoprofen (2 mg/kg SC)
- Carprofen (4 mg/kg SC)

Keyhole Liver Biopsy[1-4]

In the keyhole method, after the dog is prepared using the same methods as noted above, a sterile gloved index finger is inserted through the abdominal musculature at the same site that is used for the percutaneous biopsy technique, and the abdominal wall is bluntly dissected. After the finger is introduced into the abdomen through this blunt dissection, the liver is palpated and stabilized against the abdominal wall for subsequent biopsy, as noted previously. Compassionate care is optimal when discomfort is minimized through the use of analgesia before and after surgery.

Laparoscopic Liver Biopsy[1-3]

In the hands of an experienced endoscopist, laparoscopic liver biopsy takes approximately 5 to 10 minutes from the time the abdomen is insufflated to the time of closure. With this method, the liver can be directly visualized for specific localization of lesions. The method is well described[1-3] and varies slightly, depending on the equipment used. This procedure may be accomplished using either general anesthesia or local anesthesia with tranquilizers and analgesics. The site for insertion of the laparoscope can be on the midline or, more commonly, the right lateral abdominal wall just caudal to the ribs and ventral to the lateral spinous processes. Choosing the appropriate site of insertion depends on the area of the abdomen that is to be explored and biopsied.

Indications: Evaluation and diagnosis of malignant and nonmalignant liver disease; determining the extent of the neoplastic processes.

Contraindications: Coagulopathies; dogs with significantly compromised cardiovascular or respiratory systems (because of insufflation of the abdomen, venous return to the heart can be reduced and compress the diaphragm, compromising the ability to inspire easily).

Benefits: Biopsy can be selectively performed to acquire tissue to analyze cellularity, architecture, and content. In selected cases, the procedure can be done with local anesthesia, systemic analgesia, and tranquilization (see box on this page). If there are any concerns about the dog's ability to lie quietly, however, general anesthesia should be administered.

Limitations: Small biopsy samples may not be representative of the entire liver. Because this procedure allows visualization of lesions on the surface of all visible organs, lesions below the surface of each organ may be overlooked.

Equipment: Standard surgical instruments, laparoscope and laparoscopic biopsy instruments, Verres needle, trocar and cannula assembly.

Technique (Figure 18-7):
1. Administer general anesthesia or tranquilizers with analgesic properties (e.g., butorphanol, fentanyl, morphine, oxymorphone). Compassionate care is optimal when discomfort is minimized through the use of analgesia before and after surgery.

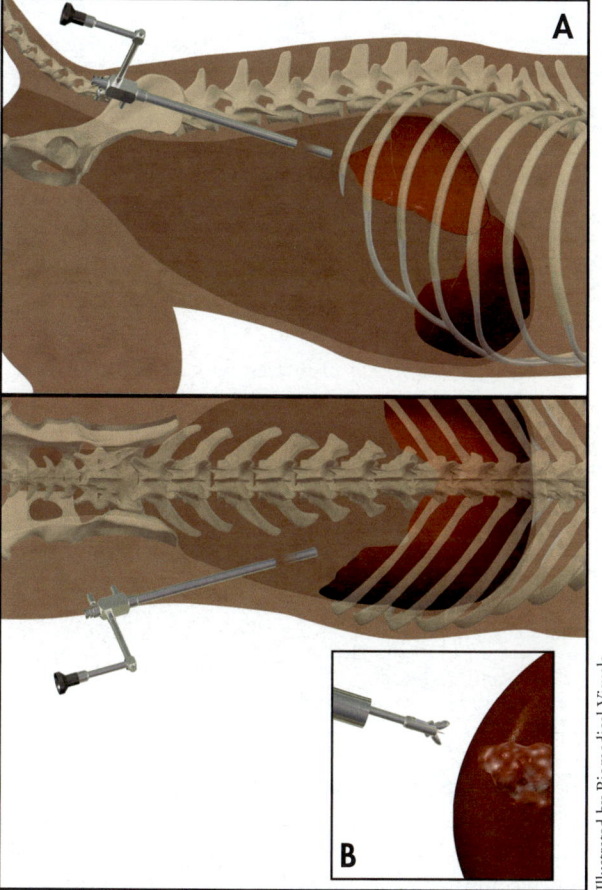

Figure 18-7. *Laparoscopy is ideal for visually characterizing the health and structure of many abdominal organs, including the liver. In addition, it is effective for directing a biopsy instrument to localized lesions. (**A**) The laparoscope is advanced through an area bordered on the right side below the lateral spinous processes of the lumbar vertebrae and caudal to the last rib. The liver is identified, and a biopsy instrument is advanced to acquire at least one sample (**B**).*

2. If a lateral approach is used, place the dog with its left side down. If the patient is tranquilized, apply gentle but firm restraint on the limbs so that the dog cannot change position during the procedure, ideally with an assistant nearby to calm the dog. Clip the hair and prepare the skin with a surgical scrub from the ninth rib to the caudal flank and from the dorsal to the ventral midline on the right side. Drape the insertion site.

3. If tranquilization is used instead of general anesthesia, inject approximately 0.5 to 2 ml of lidocaine in and around the site where the laparoscope and any biopsy needles are to be introduced. The 2% lidocaine will sting less on injection if it is diluted 50:50 with 8.4% bicarbonate.

4. Insert a Verres needle into the right side, below the lateral spinous processes of the lumbar vertebrae and caudal to the last rib into the peritoneal cavity. After it is determined that the needle is not in a hollow viscus or blood vessel, use carbon dioxide or nitrous oxide to insufflate the abdomen to 10 mm Hg. Injecting saline and aspirating material through the needle looking for blood, bowel contents, or urine can check the placement of the Verres needle. Take extreme care to make sure that the dog is breathing properly.

5. Make a small incision (0.5 to 1 cm) ventral to the lumbar muscles and caudal to the costal arch on the right side. Push the trocar and cannula assembly into the gas-filled abdomen through the incision. Remove the Verres needle. Remove the trocar and advance the laparoscope that is attached to the carbon dioxide or nitrous oxide insufflator and light source through the cannula to visualize the liver and other abdominal organs. If blood or other material obscures visualization, remove the laparoscope (but not the outer cannula) and clean it in a bowl of saline.

6. Advance a biopsy needle through the laparoscope or a separate puncture site nearby. Direct the alligator or needle biopsy instrument to the sites of interest by direct visualization. Take five to six biopsy specimens; submit at least one for bacterial culture and sensitivity, and submit another for copper stains if indicated.

7. After observing the biopsy sites for several minutes for excessive bleeding, evacuate the carbon dioxide, remove the instrument from the abdominal cavity, and suture the small incision with simple interrupted absorbable sutures.

Supportive Care: Oral or parenteral analgesics.

REFERENCES

1. Ogilvie GK, Moore AS: Digestive system biopsy, in *Managing the Veterinary Cancer Patient: A Practice Manual.* Yardley, PA, Veterinary Learning Systems, 1995, pp 29–36.
2. Lightdale CJ: Liver biopsy, in Wittes RE (ed): *Manual of Oncologic Therapeutics 1991/1992.* Philadelphia, JB Lippincott, 1991, pp 20–22.
3. Jones BD, Hitt M, Hurst T: Hepatic biopsy. *Vet Clin North Am Small Anim Pract* 15:39–64, 1985.
4. Withrow SJ: Biopsy principles, in Withrow SJ, MacEwen EG (eds): *Small Animal Clinical Oncology,* ed 3. Philadelphia, WB Saunders, 2001, pp 52–57.
5. Lightdale CJ7: Upper gastrointestinal endoscopy, in Wittes RE (ed): *Manual of Oncologic Therapeutics 1991/1992.* Philadelphia, JB Lippincott, 1991, pp 14–15.
6. Penninck DG, Nyland TG, Kerr LY, Fisher PE: Ultrasonographic evaluation of gastrointestinal diseases in small animals. *Vet Radiol* 31:134–141, 1990.
7. Penninck DG, Crystal MA, Matz ME, Pearson SH: The technique of percutaneous ultrasound guided fine-needle aspiration biopsy and automated microcore biopsy in small animal gastrointestinal diseases. *Vet Radiol Ultrasound* 34:433–436, 1993.
8. Crystal MA, Penninck DG, Matz ME, et al: Use of ultrasound-guided fine-needle aspiration biopsy and automated core biopsy for the diagnosis of gastrointestinal diseases in small animals. *Vet Radiol* 34:438–444, 1993.
9. Münster M: Effizienz der Endoskopie bei Magen-Darm-Erkrankungen von Hund und Katze. *Prakt Tierarzt* 4:309– 312, 1993.

CLINICAL CYTOLOGY AND NEOPLASIA 19
Gregory K. Ogilvie and Antony S. Moore

CLINICAL BRIEFING

Methods	Benefits
Fine-needle aspiration cytology	
"Needle-on" technique	• Inexpensive, easy, and rapid.
"Needle-off" technique	• Lack of negative pressure reduces chance for dilution of cells of interest with blood or fluid.
	• Ideal for vascular and very small lesions.
Impression smears	• Increase chances for obtaining many representative cells.
	• May indirectly reveal architecture and associated cells of the mass.
Tissue scrapings	• Potentially therapeutic and diagnostic.
Needle core biopsy	• Ideal for sarcomas and other tissues that exfoliate poorly.

Cytology is a practical, cost-effective, minimally invasive tool used for making a tentative diagnosis and directing the initial management and staging of dogs with cancer. It is also helpful in providing information and a tentative prognosis. Aspiration is a rapid screening test that gives the power of information quickly to the clinician, the team, and the caregiver. A histopathologic diagnosis is also important for the evaluation of dogs with cancer but is often interpreted with increased accuracy if the results are combined with cytologic findings obtained by the following method:

- First, a representative sample must be obtained by the attending clinician. Specialized analysis such as flow cytometry can be employed to determine ploidy or cell type, as in lymphoid malignancies.[1] Virtually every part of the body can be sampled, including the brain and pancreas.[2-9] Complications are rare but should be assessed in each situation.
- Next, the sample must be adequately prepared with appropriate stains. The quality of the sample must be protected from contaminants such as formaldehyde.
- Finally, the sample must be accurately interpreted. The attending clinician is responsible for ensuring that the sample is a high-quality, representative sample. A tentative diagnosis may be attempted by the attending clinician, but it is always advisable to obtain the interpretation of a board-certified veterinary cytopathologist.

Fine-Needle Aspiration
Fine-needle aspiration is used to acquire tissue or fluid quickly from almost any part of the body with minimal risk. When compared with histopathology, cytology of cutaneous tumors has been reported to have a sensitivity of 89%, a specificity of 100%, positive and negative predictive values of 100% and 96%, respectively, and an overall accuracy of 97%.[2] The accuracy of cytology and histopathology can be enhanced with the use of immunohistochemical stains. An overview of immunohistochemistry is provided in the box on page 97.

FINE-NEEDLE ASPIRATION OF SOLID TISSUES[2-8]

Indication: Any condition suspected to be benign or malignant.

Contraindications: Coagulopathies (rare); any abscessed or neoplastic tissue that may rupture, spill into, and contaminate a body cavity. Transitional cell carcinoma has been reported to be transplanted from the bladder through the body cavity and other tissues along a fine-needle aspirate tract.[9]

Benefits: Aspiration can be selectively performed to acquire cells to analyze cellularity and cell morphology, with or without the direction of imaging modalities such as ultrasonography or fluoroscopy. In most cases, the procedure can be done on an outpatient basis without any anesthe-

Immunohistochemistry

Histologic diagnosis can be made more accurate by the use of immunohistochemical staining for various cell-specific antigens or structural elements. A brief synopsis of the concepts of immunohistochemistry is noted below:

- **Intermediate filaments** are intracellular structural proteins that can be identified by staining in order to distinguish between epithelial tumors (such as carcinomas) and mesenchymal tumors (sarcomas). These structures also differ between types of mesenchymal cells. Stains to document the presence of intermediate filaments are most useful in distinguishing the histogenesis of poorly differentiated tumors. For example, an oral tumor may be so poorly differentiated that the pathologist cannot tell if it is an adenocarcinoma, a fibrosarcoma, or a melanoma. Overfixation of tissue (longer than a few days) in formalin may make it impossible to use these stains.
- **Cytokeratins** are found in a variety of epithelial tumors and are therefore a marker for carcinomas. There are different cytokeratins found in dog tissue, but they cannot easily distinguish between different types of carcinomas.
- **Vimentin** is found in all mesenchymal cells and is therefore a marker for sarcomas.
- **Desmin** is found in tissues of muscle derivation and may therefore be used to distinguish a rhabdomyosarcoma or a leiomyosarcoma from other vimentin-positive sarcomas.
- **Glial fibrillary acidic protein** is a marker of neuroectodermal tissue and may distinguish tumors of that histogenesis.
- **S-100** is a structural protein that is seen in some tissues of neuroectodermal origin as well as in melanomas and is therefore a good marker for poorly differentiated melanomas.
- **Melan A** is a more sensitive marker for melanoma cells than S-100.
- **Factor VIII** may be used to distinguish tumors with vascular endothelial derivation, such as hemangiosarcomas.
- **Lymphomas** can be distinguished from other tumors and subclassified into two groups by stains for antigens that distinguish B and T lymphocytes from each other. A common T-cell marker is CD3. Histiocytic cells may be distinguished using a CD68 stain.

sia. If there are any concerns about the dog's ability to lie quietly while a deep abdominal organ is being sampled, general anesthesia should be performed.

Limitation: Small samples may not be representative of the entire tissue of interest.

Equipment: A 3-, 6-, or 12-ml syringe; a 22-gauge needle with sufficient length to sample the tissue of interest; microscope slides; proper staining materials; and a microscope.

Technique:
1. Identify and immobilize the mass to be sampled.
2. Clean the skin with surgical soap and alcohol if an abdominal cavity is to be entered. Superficial skin lesions can be cleaned solely with alcohol.
3. Advance the needle into the tissue and partially withdraw it several times, with or without the syringe attached (Figure 19-1), in several different directions through the same entry point in the skin.
   — The *"needle-off"* method is ideal for vascular tissues such as thyroid tumors to avoid diluting the sample with blood and results in a higher probability of a diagnostic sample.[2]
   — The *"needle-on"* technique is ideal for tissues that do not exfoliate well, such as soft tissue sarcomas, because of the presence of negative pressure.[5] Apply suction as the needle is advanced through the tissue in several directions. Release all negative pressure before the needle is withdrawn from the tissue. The objective is to fill only the needle with cells; therefore, if blood or other tissue is noted in the hub of the needle or in the syringe, discontinue sampling.
4. Remove the needle from the syringe. Fill the syringe with air before it is reattached, and forcefully expel the cellular contents of the needle onto clean glass slides.
5. Make a "squash-prep" by placing two slides on top of each other in a parallel orientation so that only the weight of the upper slide "squashes" the cells as they are pulled apart.[5] The result is a smear of fluid or tissue on both slides.

   Alternatively, slides can be made by spreading a drop of fluid in the same manner as preparing a blood smear. First, place a small drop of fluid on the primary slide. Second, place a second slide on the first at a 45° angle so that the second slide is in front of the drop of fluid. Then back the slide that is at an angle into the sample so that the acute angle is facing it. Allow the fluid to flow down the edge of the angled slide. Then firmly and smoothly push the angled slide along the other slide until the entire sample is distributed. The best smears can be obtained when the volume of the sample is relatively small; this prevents making a thick smear.

Supportive Care: Short-term oral analgesics may be helpful but are usually not necessary.

> **KEY POINT**
> *The "needle-off" method is ideal for vascular tissues because it avoids the aspiration of blood into the sample, preventing dilution of the sample with blood.*

ABDOMINAL PARACENTESIS[2,5]

Indication: Evaluation of any fluid within the abdominal cavity.

Contraindications: Coagulopathies; any abscessed or neoplastic tissue that may rupture, spill into, and contaminate a body cavity. Fluid may leak into subcutaneous sites or completely through the skin after the aspiration procedure; injury to the bowel or other organs is rare but possible.

Benefits: Aspiration of the abdominal cavity can be selectively performed to acquire fluid but is best used with the direction of imaging modalities such as ultrasonography or fluoroscopy (which will also reduce the risk of penetration into organs such as the spleen). In most cases, the procedure can be done on an outpatient basis, with or without local anesthesia.

Limitation: Fluid analysis may not be diagnostic for an underlying malignancy.

Equipment: A 12-ml syringe, a 22-gauge needle, microscope slides, proper staining materials, and a microscope.

Technique:

1. To reduce the probability of accidentally aspirating the spleen, perform abdominal paracentesis at a site 3 to 5 cm caudal to the umbilicus and to the right of midline. Clip and prepare the area following aseptic techniques.
2. Local anesthesia (see Chapter 29) is preferred.
3. Fill the syringe with 1.5 ml of air, then slowly advance the needle on the syringe into the abdominal cavity. Gently apply negative pressure after the abdominal wall is penetrated. If no fluid is acquired, inject 0.5 ml of air into the abdomen to clear the needle of any blockage. Apply negative pressure once more. Repeat the procedure with the needle in different positions or depths within the abdominal cavity.

Supportive Care: Oral analgesics may be helpful for short-term discomfort.

THORACENTESIS[5]

Indication: Evaluation of any fluid within the thoracic cavity.

Contraindications: Coagulopathies; any abscessed or neoplastic tissue that may rupture, spill into, and contaminate a body cavity.

Complications: Fluid may leak into subcutaneous sites or completely through the skin. Alternatively, a pneumothorax may develop. Injury to the lung or heart is rare but possible.

Benefits: Aspiration of the thoracic cavity can be selectively performed to acquire fluid with or without the direction of imaging modalities such as ultrasonography or fluo-

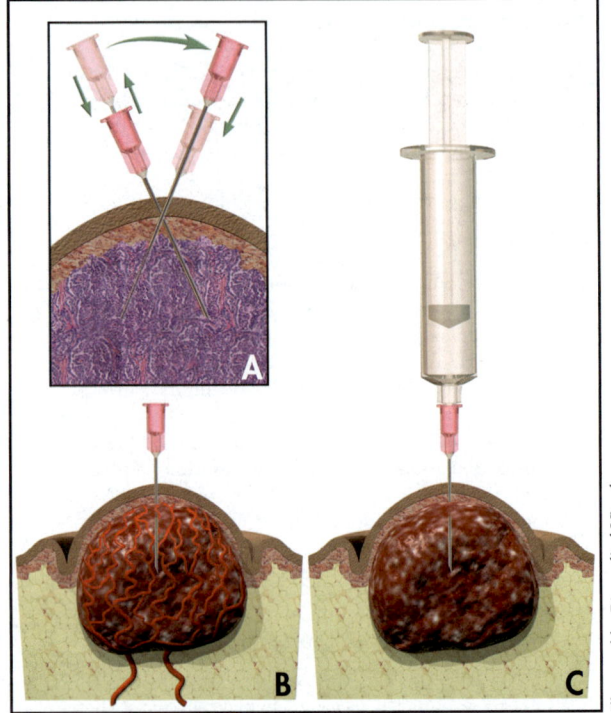

Figure 19-1. Fine-needle aspiration is performed by advancing the needle into the tissue and partially withdrawing it several times (**A**), with or without the syringe attached, in several different directions through the same entry point in the skin. The "needle-off" method (**B**) is ideal for vascular tissues, whereas the "needle-on" technique (**C**) is ideal for tissues that do not exfoliate well, such as soft tissue sarcomas. When using the needle attached to the syringe ("needle on"), suction is applied as the needle is advanced through the tissue in several directions. All negative pressure is then released before the needle is withdrawn from the tissue. The objective is to fill the needle with cells. The sampling is discontinued if blood or other tissue is noted in the hub of the needle or in the syringe. With both methods, the syringe is filled with air before the needle filled with cells is attached, and the cellular contents of the needle are forcefully expelled onto clean glass slides.

roscopy. In most cases, the procedure can be done on an outpatient basis, with or without local anesthesia.

Limitation: Fluid analysis may not be diagnostic for an underlying malignancy.

Equipment: A 12- to 60-ml syringe, a three-way stopcock, a 22-gauge needle, microscope slides, proper staining materials, and a microscope.

Technique:

1. Ideally, the dog should be standing and quiet. Administration of analgesics and/or tranquilizers is preferred. However, many of these drugs can depress respiration and place dogs with minimal respiratory reserve at risk. Local anesthesia is recommended in addition to analgesia and tranquilizers. To reduce the sting associated with the injection of 2% lidocaine, dilute the drug with

> **Types of Inflammation**
>
> **Acute:** >70% of inflammatory cells are neutrophils; neutrophils can be well preserved, hypersegmented, toxic, or lysed
>
> **Chronic active:** Approximately 30% to 50% of the inflammatory cell population is plasma cells and monocytes; neutrophils are also present in significant numbers
>
> **Chronic or granulomatous:** Mononuclear inflammatory cells and macrophages predominate

equal parts of 8.4% bicarbonate. The site for thoracentesis varies depending on the site of the fluid but is commonly around the seventh or eighth intercostal space. Clip the area and prepare it with surgical scrub and alcohol.
2. Slowly advance the needle on the syringe into the thoracic cavity just cranial to the nearby rib to prevent hitting the intercostal arteries, located just caudal to the ribs. The bevel should face the pleural lining. Gently apply negative pressure after the pleural space is entered. Use the three-way stopcock to prevent air from leaking into the chest while syringes are changed to drain the chest.
3. Once a sample is acquired, put it in EDTA and a culturette for bacterial culture and sensitivity testing, if indicated. Slides also can be made directly, or the fluid can be centrifuged to concentrate the cells for subsequent analysis.

Impressions and Scraping Techniques[2-8]

Cells can be acquired from masses or biopsy specimens once the tissue has been removed from the dog by taking impressions of the tissue or by scraping cells from the tissue. Impression smears are ideal for lymph nodes, whereas scrapings are optimal for tissues that do not exfoliate easily, such as soft tissue sarcomas.

Indications: Almost any potentially abnormal tissue that has been removed from the dog. Occasionally, an ulcerated mass on the dog can be sampled by making an impression or by scraping cells directly from its surface.

Contraindications: None known.

Benefits: An impression is ideal for indirectly acquiring information about the cell types involved as well as providing some idea of cellular architecture within the mass. If done correctly, the cells may be less traumatized than when aspirates and squash preps are made.

Limitation: Small samples may not be representative of the entire tissue of interest.

Equipment: A surgical blade, Brown-Adson forceps, microscope slides, proper staining materials, and a microscope.

Technique:
Impressions
1. Blot dry a freshly removed piece of tissue and transect it in half to obtain a flat surface for performing the impressions. The surface should be smaller than the slide to allow multiple impressions.
2. Blot the cut surface on an absorbent surface such as a paper towel.
3. Make several impressions on each slide.

Scrapings
1. Blot the tissue dry to allow any blood or fluid to be removed.
2. Gently scrape the surface of the tissue with a new surgical blade, and then gently smear the cells on the blade across the slide.

Supportive Care: Oral or parenteral analgesics may be needed.

Slide Preparation[5]

At least one slide from every site should be saved for submission to a clinical pathologist. In each case, slides should be prepared with the utmost care. Tumor cells often are very fragile and easily disrupted. After the slides are made, one representative slide should be stained and examined to ensure that it is likely to be diagnostic. The most frequently used stains in the clinic or laboratory are Wright's-Giemsa, new methylene blue, and Papanicolaou stains. An adaptation of the Wright's stain (Diff-Quik) is commonly used in canine practice; it can be done in a 15-second, three-step procedure. This stain is very effective in providing good cytoplasmic detail. The new methylene blue stain is also easy to use and provides good nuclear detail. The Papanicolaou stain is more labor-intensive and generally is used only in a clinical pathology laboratory, but it provides excellent cellular morphology.

> **KEY POINT**
>
> *The practitioner should call on the expertise of a clinical pathologist to confirm pivotal diagnoses and to help make subtle diagnoses.*

General Cytologic Interpretation[2-8]

Detailed interpretation of cytology requires considerable experience and knowledge of normal cellular morphology. The practitioner should call on the expertise of a clinical pathologist to confirm diagnoses. With practice, the clinician can determine whether a sample is likely to have adequate cellularity for subsequent diagnosis by an expert in the field. In addition, with experience, inflammation can be dif-

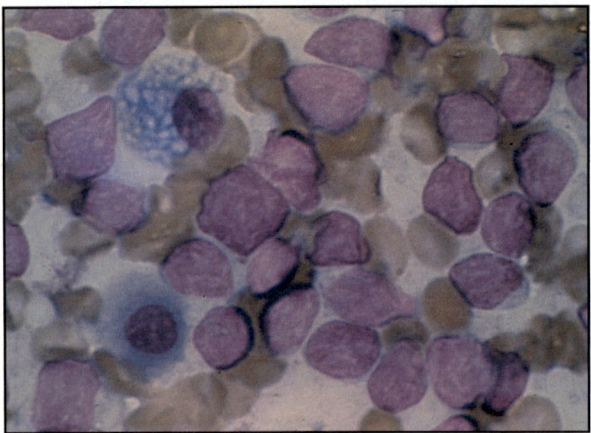

Figure 19-2. *Cytology from a normal lymph node. Lymph nodes—even reactive lymph nodes—have an orderly maturation of lymphocytes; however, small lymphocytes usually predominate.*

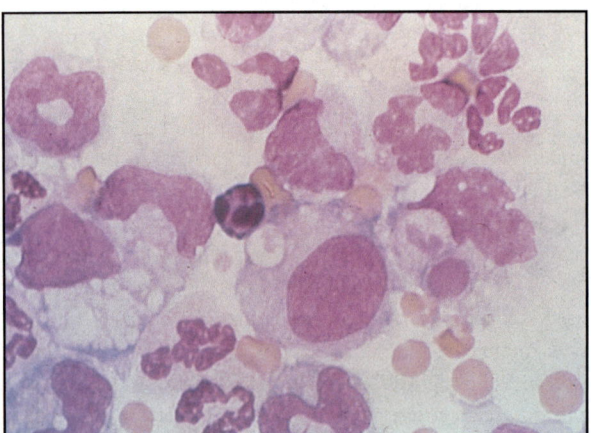

Figure 19-3. *Nondegenerate neutrophils, macrophages, and erythrocytes predominate in this lymph node aspirate that is diagnostic for an inflammatory condition. It is important to differentiate hyperplasia or inflammation from neoplasia. Hyperplasia principally differs from normal tissue in that hyperplastic cells exhibit the features of cytoplasmic activity and are cytologically immature. Therefore, reactive or hyperplastic cells may have more basophilic cytoplasm and the nuclei may be larger than in normal cells. One key differentiating feature is that hyperplastic cells have a fairly constant nuclear:cytoplasmic ratio, whereas neoplastic tissue does not.*

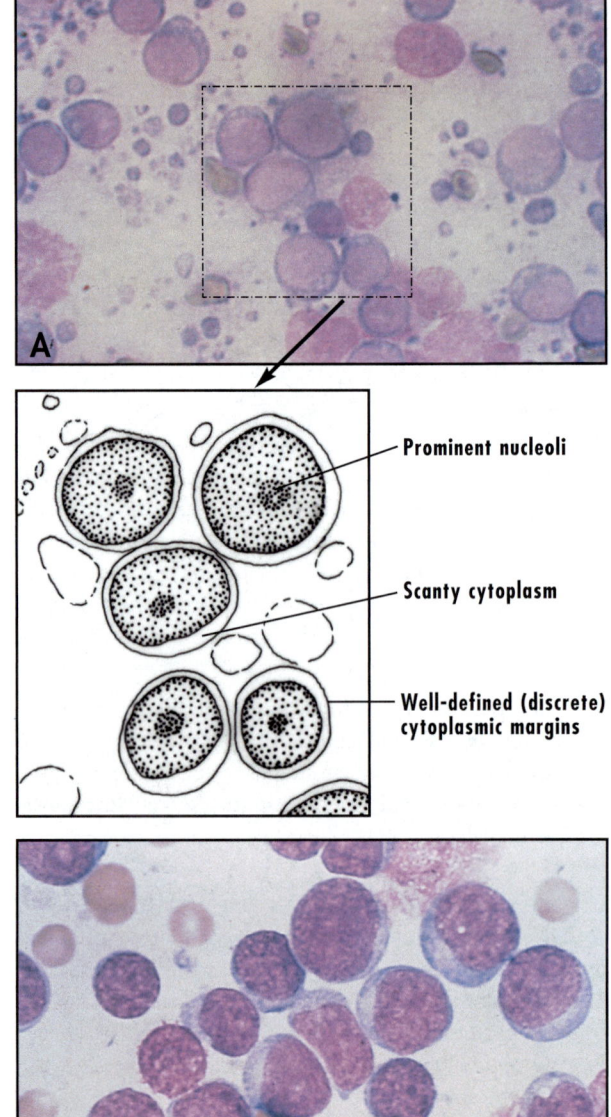

Figure 19-4. *(A and B) These photomicrographs are representative of lymphoma. Note the mitotic figures and the prominent nucleoli that are characteristic features of malignancy. The cells are characterized as being made up of a monotonous population of large, poorly differentiated lymphoid cells with scanty blue cytoplasm, dense nuclear margins, and round to slightly irregularly shaped nuclei, generally with at least one nucleolus. Some cells may have azurophilic granules. Lymphoma cells usually resemble lymphoblasts, although in a few rare cases they can be very well differentiated and resemble normal lymphocytes. A biopsy is required to confirm the diagnosis of each case of lymphoma, especially small-cell or well-differentiated lymphoma. In B, note the malignant lymphocytes with prominent nucleoli, a scanty rim of cytoplasm, well-defined or discrete borders, and a variable nuclear:cytoplasmic ratio.*

ferentiated from neoplasia, which can be of great value for directing other diagnostic tests. In any case, the cytology findings should be interpreted in combination with other clinical information to make an appropriate diagnosis.

Once all the slides are reviewed, representative clusters of cells are evaluated at 100× (oil immersion). The cells are then assessed to determine whether they represent normal tissue (Figure 19-2), an inflammatory process (Figure 19-3), hyperplasia, or neoplasia (Figures 19-4 through 19-19).

An inflammatory process can be divided somewhat arbitrarily into acute, chronic active, chronic, or granulomatous

CLINICAL CYTOLOGY AND NEOPLASIA 101

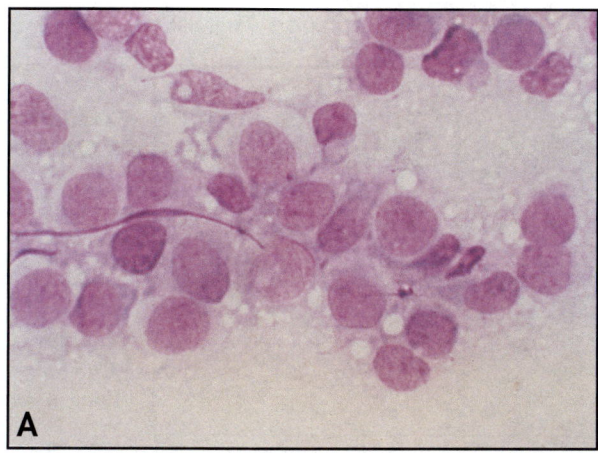 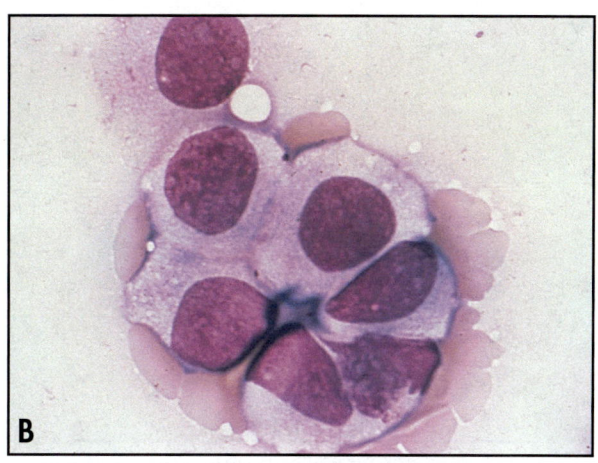

Figure 19-5. (*A* and *B*) Cytology from hairless, red, raised lesions from two young dogs, later diagnosed histopathologically as histiocytomas. Cytologically, these tumors are composed of a uniform population of round cells that resemble monocytes and epithelioid cells that are 10 to 25 μm in diameter. Nuclei appear benign cytologically, although they may vary in size and shape. The pale cytoplasm of these cells varies in amount from cell to cell and is surrounded by a distinct cytoplasm. Histiocytomas can resemble TVTs, but the former show more variation in nuclear and cytoplasmic shape.

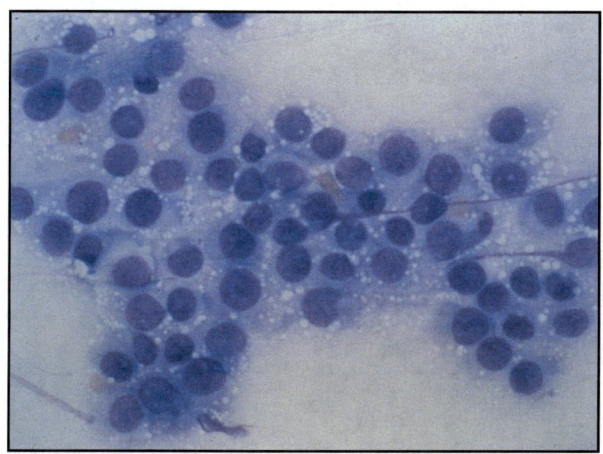

Figure 19-6. TVT cells are round, measure approximately 15 to 30 μm in diameter, and have round to oval nuclei that may be placed eccentrically within the cytoplasm. The nuclear chromatin generally is coarsely granular. A single prominent nucleolus often is present. The cytoplasm is distinguished as being relatively abundant, moderately basophilic, and, often, vacuolated. Plasma cells, lymphocytes, and macrophages often are seen within a TVT cell. TVT cells can be distinguished from lymphoma cells because they have more abundant cytoplasm. Compared with histiocytomas, TVTs have a more uniformly round nucleus and cytoplasm.

tory responses are those in which mononuclear inflammatory cells and macrophages predominate. If epithelial or inflammatory giant cells are present, the condition is considered to be granulomatous.

It is important to differentiate hyperplasia from neoplasia. Hyperplasia principally differs from normal tissue in that hyperplastic cells exhibit the features of cytoplasmic activity and are cytologically immature. Therefore, reactive or hyperplastic cells may have more basophilic cytoplasm and the nuclei may be larger than in normal cells. One key differentiating feature is that hyperplastic cells have a fairly constant nuclear:cytoplasmic ratio, whereas neoplastic tissue does not.

The diagnosis of neoplasia is made on the cytologic characteristics of nuclear, cytoplasmic, and structural features. On occasion, immunohistochemistry is needed to help differentiate cell types, enhancing the accuracy of diagnosis in clinical pathology and histopathology. In brief, the criteria for diagnosing malignancy include[2-5]:

- **Structural changes and appearance**

  Round cell tumors (Figures 19-4 through 19-9)
  — Round to oval cells
  — Easy exfoliation of individual cells
  — Well-defined cytoplasmic margins

  Epithelial cell tumors (Figures 19-10 through 19-16)
  — Easy exfoliation of cells in clusters, clumps, or sheets
  — Oval to round cells
  — Arranged in a ductular or acinar pattern around a central lumen
  — Cytoplasm may contain a secretory product

inflammation based on the presence or absence of neutrophils, monocytes, plasma cells, eosinophils, and differentiated macrophages (see the box on page 99).

Acute inflammation can be diagnosed when more than 70% of the inflammatory cells are neutrophils. The neutrophils can be well preserved, hypersegmented, toxic, or lysed. Chronic active inflammation can be diagnosed when 30% to 50% of the inflammatory cell population is composed of plasma cells and monocytes. Chronic inflamma-

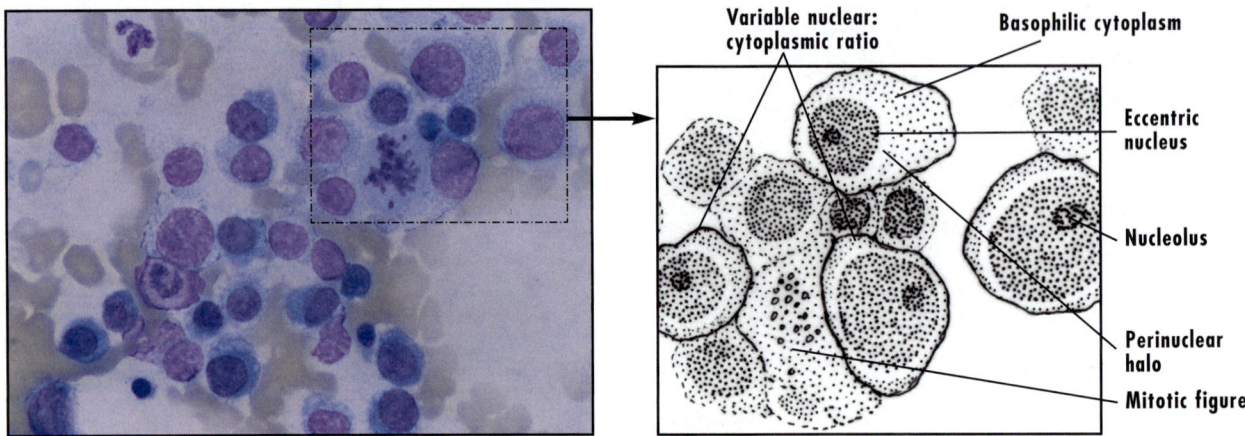

Figure 19-7. *Cytology from the bone marrow of a dog with a monoclonal gammopathy in the serum, Bence Jones proteins in the urine, and hypercalcemia consistent with a diagnosis of a plasma cell tumor, also known as multiple myeloma. Note the round cell tumor cells with eccentric nuclei. The cytoplasm of plasma cells often contains a perinuclear halo that is actually immunoglobulin before release from the cell. The cytologic features noted outline characteristics of a malignant plasma cell tumor, including an eccentric nucleus, a perinuclear halo, and a variable nuclear:cytoplasmic ratio.*

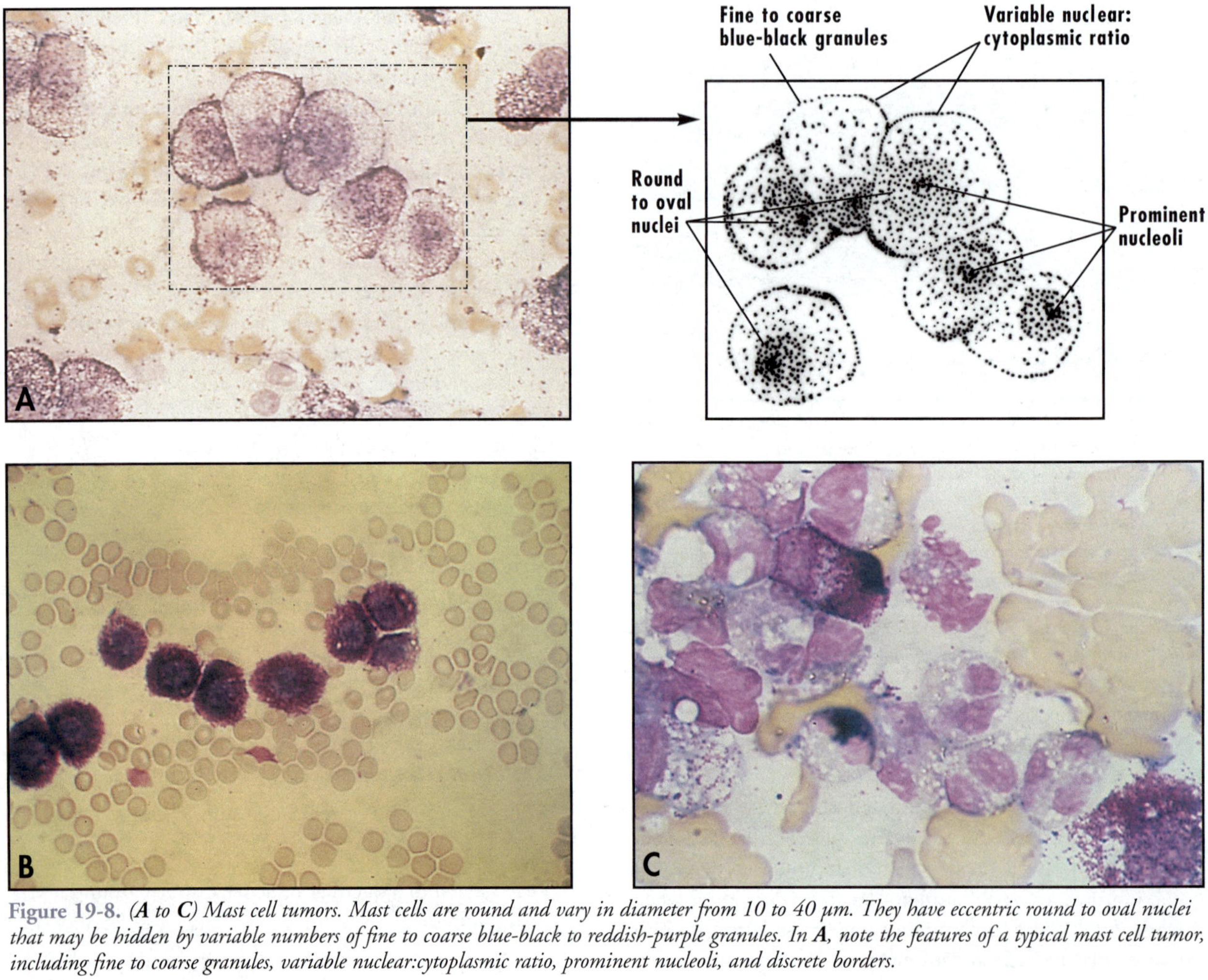

Figure 19-8. *(**A** to **C**) Mast cell tumors. Mast cells are round and vary in diameter from 10 to 40 μm. They have eccentric round to oval nuclei that may be hidden by variable numbers of fine to coarse blue-black to reddish-purple granules. In **A**, note the features of a typical mast cell tumor, including fine to coarse granules, variable nuclear:cytoplasmic ratio, prominent nucleoli, and discrete borders.*

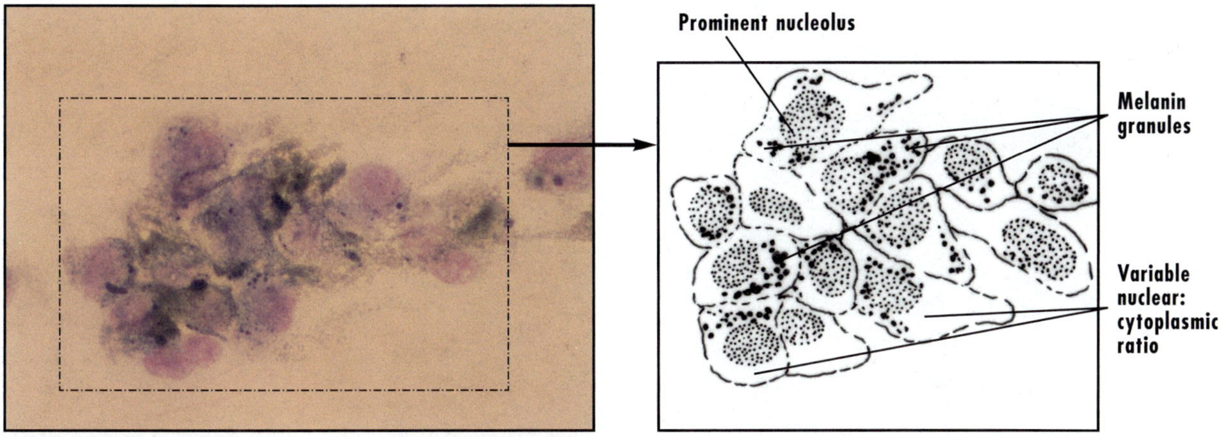

CLINICAL CYTOLOGY AND NEOPLASIA 103

Figure 19-9. *Melanomas are rare in dogs but are considered by some to be a discrete cell tumor. Others believe the tumor has characteristics of both epithelial and mesenchymal cells. Because melanomas often have intracytoplasmic granules, they must be differentiated from mast cell tumors. With most stains, the granules are black or brown and irregular in shape and size. They are usually small and appear dust-like. The granules are often noted extracellularly because they are released from some cells. The features depicted show typical prominent nucleoli, melanin granules, and variable nuclear:cytoplasmic ratio.*

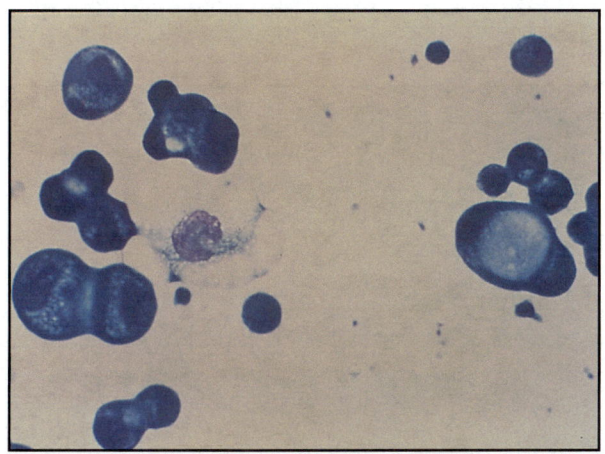

Figure 19-10. *Cytology from a mammary mass confirmed histologically to be a mammary adenocarcinoma. Note the secretory product within some cells and the attempt of some cells to maintain a duct-like arrangement. The secretory contents often make the cells resemble signet rings, which is characteristic of many carcinomas.*

Connective tissue tumors (Figures 19-17 through 19-20)
— Difficult to exfoliate
— Individual cells or disorganized clusters
— Spindle-shaped cells
— Cytoplasmic extensions with ill-defined cytoplasmic borders

• **Nuclear changes and appearance** (Figures 19-4, 19-7, 19-8, 19-9, 19-10, and 19-18)
— Marked variation in nuclear size
— Marked variation in nuclear:cytoplasmic ratio
— Irregular nuclear membrane

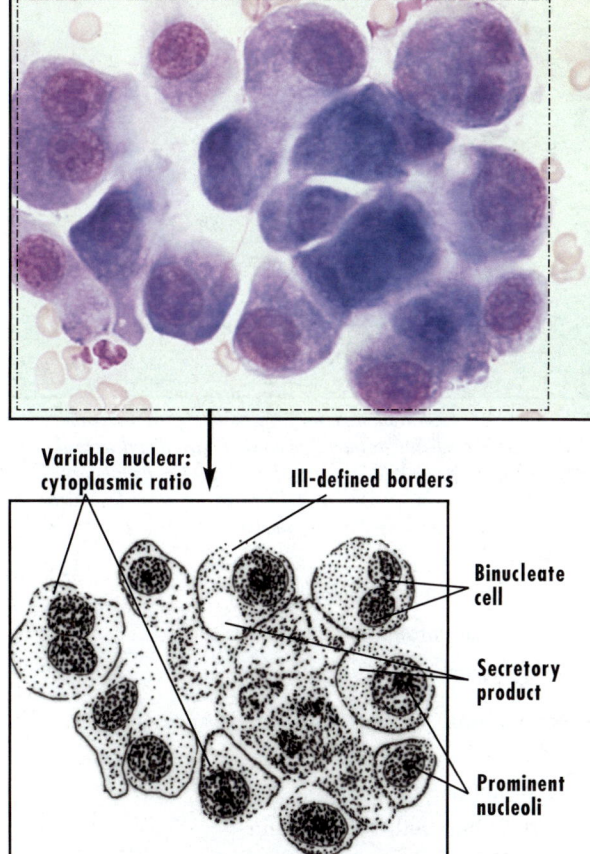

Figure 19-11. *Carcinoma from a dog with an intestinal tumor. Note the round cells, some with multiple nuclei, multinucleated cells, variable nuclear:cytoplasmic ratio, and other indications of malignancy as well as the ill-defined borders, binucleate cells, secretory product, prominent nucleoli, and variable nuclear:cytoplasmic borders.*

104 MANAGING THE CANINE CANCER PATIENT

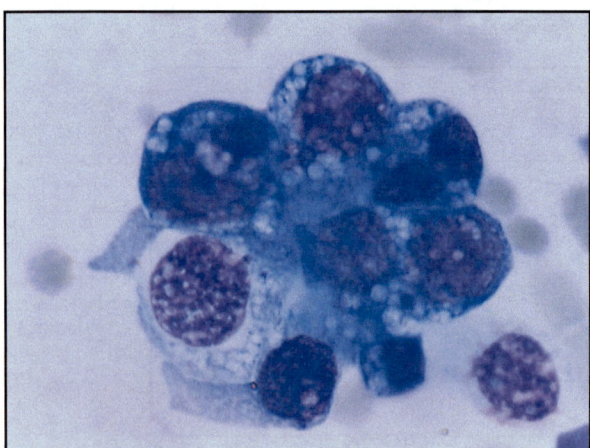

Figure 19-12. *Carcinoma cells from a transtracheal wash of a dog later determined to have a bronchogenic carcinoma. Note the large, round cells with prominent nucleoli that exhibit criteria of malignancy.*

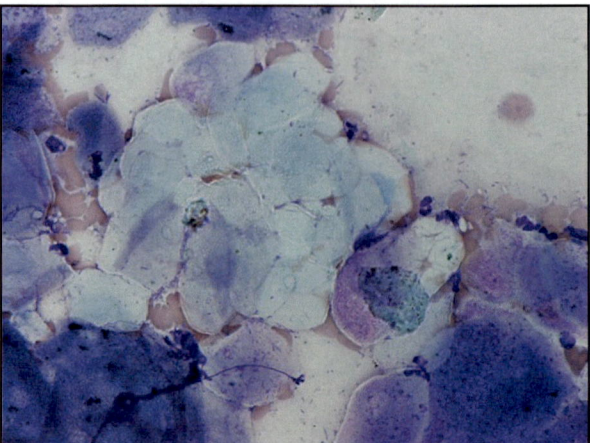

Figure 19-13. *High numbers of mature, keratinized, anucleated squamous epithelial cells are observed in small, thick clusters with low numbers of melanin granules and a small amount of peripheral blood in the background. Cytologic differentials include an epidermal inclusion cyst, a follicular cyst, a benign hair follicle tumor, and an intracutaneous cornifying epithelioma. (Courtesy of Kimberly Caruso, DVM, California Veterinary Specialists)*

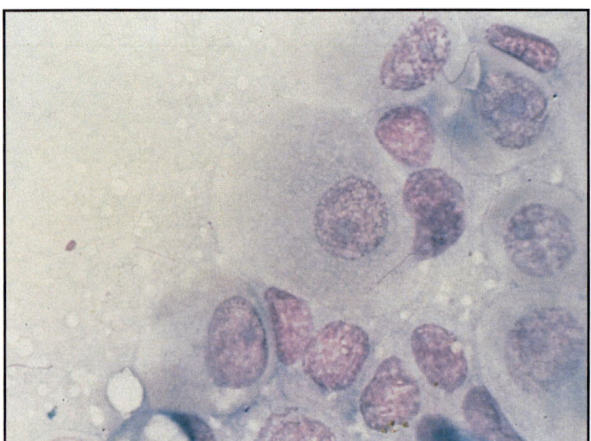

Figure 19-14. *Cells from a perianal adenoma of an intact male dog. These cells exfoliate readily into clusters, are often described as hepatoid in appearance, and are characterized as having an abundant, foamy pale cytoplasm and eccentric or centrally located round to oval nuclei that may vary in size.*

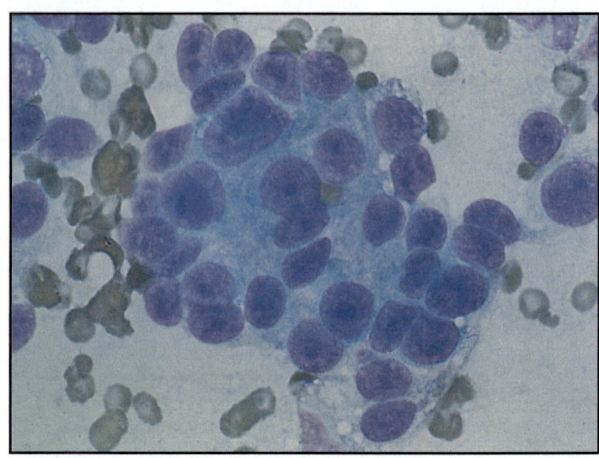

Figure 19-15. *Cytology from a poodle with small, raised, pedunculated fleshy masses determined histologically to be sebaceous adenomas. Note the sheets or clusters of round cells with abundant cytoplasm that are relatively uniform in size and shape with few mitotic figures.*

— Variably sized, irregular nucleoli
— Irregular chromatin that clumps
— Abnormal mitotic figures
- **Cytoplasmic changes and appearance** (Figures 19-7, 19-8, 19-11, 19-17, and 19-18)
  — Vacuolization
  — Basophilia with Wright's stain
  — Irregular and indistinct cytoplasmic boundaries
  — Variable cytoplasmic amount from cell to cell

Cytology of Specific Neoplasms

Once a neoplastic process is suspected using the above criteria, the cells are examined and categorized as follows:

- As benign or malignant
- As carcinomas, sarcomas, or discrete cell tumors
- By specific cell type
- By degree of differentiation

> **Hyperplasia is difficult to differentiate from neoplasia in many cases. Whenever there is a question, a biopsy should be performed.**

KEY POINT

CLINICAL CYTOLOGY AND NEOPLASIA **105**

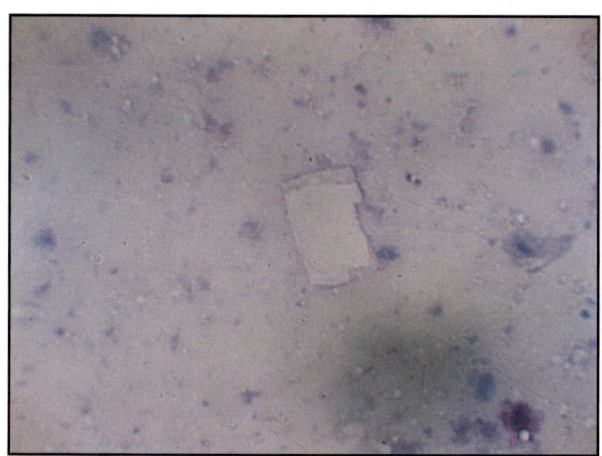

Figure 19-16. *This sample was obtained from a mass located in the skin and determined to be a sebaceous cyst. Note the amorphous debris and the unstained area in the center, characteristic of a cholesterol cleft commonly seen in these masses.*

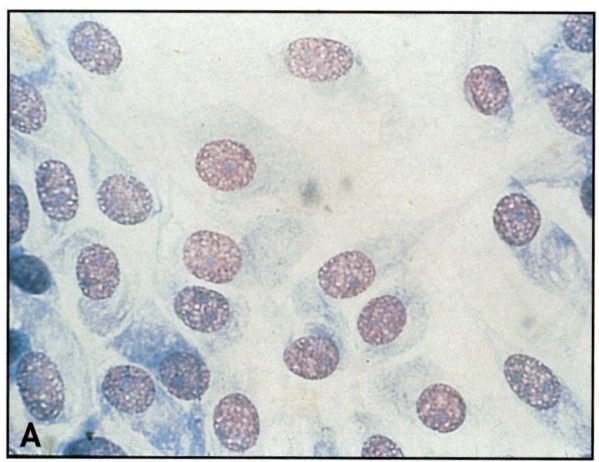

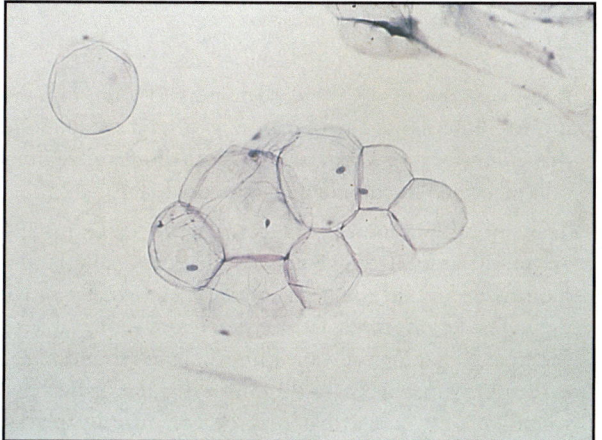

Figure 19-17. *Cytology from a lipoma. Adipocytes range from very large cells that are fully distended with fat to collapsed cells with lacy cytoplasm. This photomicrograph shows fully distended adipocytes with small, eccentric nuclei.*

Several excellent resources are available to aid the clinician in further understanding clinical veterinary cytology.[2-5] A brief description of some of the more common tumors diagnosed cytologically in veterinary medicine follows. In each case, a biopsy should be performed to confirm the cytologic diagnosis.

DISCRETE CELL NEOPLASMS: ROUND CELL TUMORS

Round cell tumors (Figures 19-4 through 19-9), commonly seen in canine medicine, have unique distinguishing cytologic features. On cytologic evaluation, the cells are all round, have well-defined cytoplasmic borders, and are easily exfoliated into single cells because of their lack of cell-to-

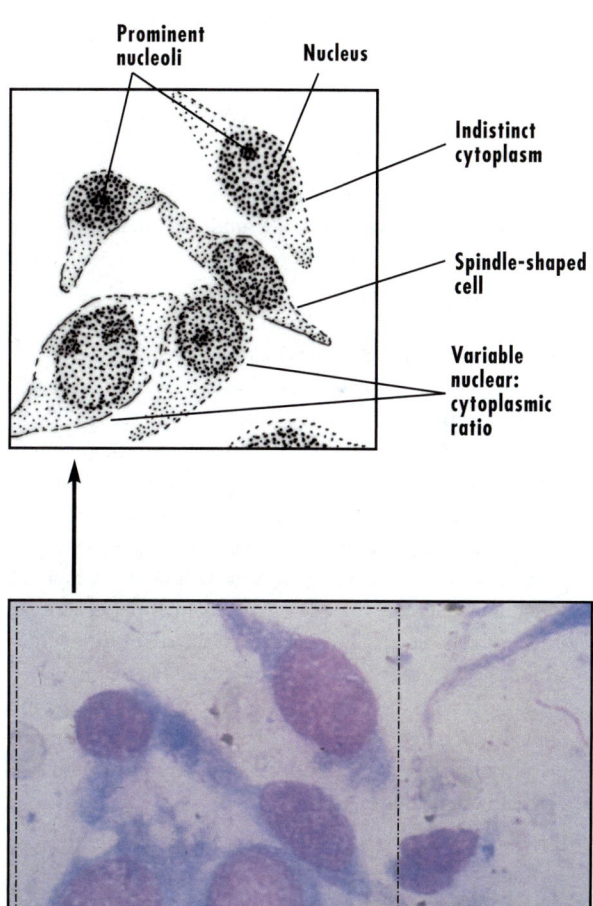

Figure 19-18. *Fine-needle aspiration cytology of an oral mass (**A**) and a submandibular lymph node (**B**) from a dog with an oral fibrosarcoma. The cells are usually seen alone or in disorganized clusters. The cytoplasm is often indistinct and spindle shaped.*

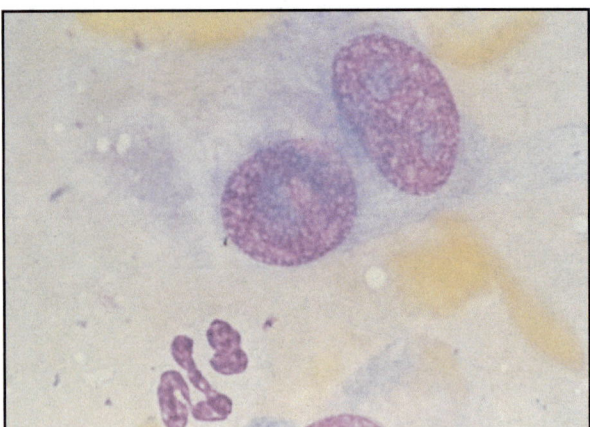

Figure 19-19. *Cells from a dog with a hemangiopericytoma. Note the poorly defined cytoplasmic borders, the nucleoli, and wispy, streaming cytoplasm. In some cases, some cells appear to form a whirling pattern that may distinguish them from other mesenchymal tumors.*

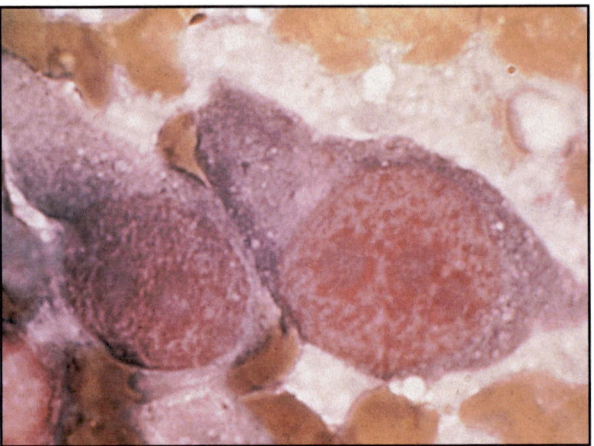

Figure 19-20. *Cells from a dog with osteosarcoma. The cells from an osteosarcoma are often spindle shaped and have abundant foamy basophilic cytoplasm surrounding a variably sized nucleus, with coarse chromatin and variable numbers of nuclei. Sometimes, these cells have an eosinophilic substance within the cytoplasm that occasionally may be noted extracellularly as an osteoid matrix. Normal osteoblasts may be seen in conjunction with the malignant cells.*

cell attachments. The following is a brief description of some distinguishing features of specific types of round cell tumors:

- **Lymphomas** (Figure 19-4) are usually found in the lymph nodes, liver, spleen, bone marrow, and extranodal sites such as the skin. The cells are composed of a uniform population of small to large, poorly differentiated lymphoid cells with scant blue cytoplasm, dense nuclear margins, and round to slightly irregularly shaped nuclei with generally at least one nucleolus. Some lymphoma cells may have azurophilic granules on staining. Lymphoma cells usually resemble lymphoblasts, although in many cases they can be very well differentiated and resemble normal lymphocytes. Therefore, a biopsy and histologic confirmation are required to confirm the diagnosis before initiation of therapy. In each case, lymphoma must be differentiated from lymphoid hyperplasia, which is characterized by the presence of lymphocytes in all stages of differentiation. However, immature cells such as lymphoblasts and lymphocytes are increased in numbers in lymphoma when compared with those in a normal lymph node. Mitotic figures may be increased in number in hyperplastic lymph nodes, but the appearance of mitotic figures is normal within a lymph node.
- **Histiocytomas** (Figure 19-5) are benign tumors that are commonly seen in young dogs. They are apparent clinically as hairless, raised lesions that may be ulcerated and/or inflamed. Cytologically, the tumor is composed of a uniform population of round cells, which resemble monocytes, and epithelioid cells that are 10 to 25 μm in diameter. Nuclei appear benign cytologically, although they may vary in size and shape. The pale cytoplasm of these cells varies in amount from cell to cell and is surrounded by a distinct cytoplasm. Histiocytomas can resemble transmissible venereal tumors (TVTs), but the former show more variation in nuclear and cytoplasmic shape. Histiocytomas can be difficult to differentiate from cells identified in chronic inflammatory lesions.
- **Transmissible venereal tumors** (Figure 19-6) usually are found around the genitalia and occasionally in the mouths or around the heads of younger, sexually active dogs. The lesions often are cherry red and very friable to the touch. Cytologically, the tumor cells are round, measure approximately 15 to 30 μm in diameter, and have round to oval nuclei that may be eccentrically placed within the cytoplasm. The nuclear chromatin generally is coarsely granular. A single prominent nucleolus is often present. The cytoplasm is distinguished as being relatively abundant in quantity and moderately basophilic; it is often vacuolated. Plasma cells, lymphocytes, and macrophages are often seen when these tumor cells are present. TVTs can be distinguished from lymphoma cells because they have more abundant cytoplasm. TVTs have a more uniformly round nucleus and cytoplasm than histiocytomas.
- **Plasma cell tumors** (Figure 19-7) contain cells that are oval to round with round nuclei and coarse, clumped chromatin. A single, relatively small nucleolus may be identified within each nucleus. The mitotic activity of these cells is generally low due to the benign nature of this condition. The amount of basophilic cytoplasm in these cells varies. Plasma cell tumors from dogs with multiple myeloma appear cytologically similar to immature plasma cells. The more mature cells may have an eccentric nucleus and a round to oval cyto-

plasm, which may have a perinuclear halo consistent with active production of immunoglobulin.

- **Mast cell tumors** (Figure 19-8) are found in the skin, spleen, liver, lymph node, and bone marrow of affected dogs. Mast cell tumors may contain eosinophils and fibroblasts. They are round and vary in size from 10 to 40 μm in diameter. Staining reveals eccentric round to oval nuclei that may be hidden by variable numbers of fine to coarse blue-black to reddish-purple granules. Diff-Quik may not stain the granules effectively; leaving the slide in the fix for at least 2 minutes may stain the granules more completely. Normal mast cells can be seen in a variety of inflammatory conditions. However, they are usually accompanied by neutrophils and macrophages in these cases.
- **Melanomas** (Figure 19-9) are considered by some to be discrete/round cell tumors. Others believe the tumor has characteristics of both epithelial and mesenchymal cells. This neoplastic process is common in dogs. The lesion may be pigmented or amelanotic. As expected, pigmented lesions are almost black in color, whereas amelanotic lesions may be pink or white. Because melanomas often have intracytoplasmic granules, they must be differentiated from mast cell tumors and pigmented basal cell tumors. With most stains, the granules are black or brown and irregular in shape and size. The granules are often noted extracellularly because they are released from some cells. The melanoma can be composed of round or epithelioid cells or cells can be spindle shaped; sometimes, there are cells of different shapes within the same tumor. Malignant melanomas must be differentiated from mast cell tumors, pigmented basal cell tumors, and macrophages that contain hemosiderin. The best method of distinguishing a melanoma is to submit a tissue biopsy for histopathologic evaluation.

ADENOMAS AND CARCINOMAS: EPITHELIAL CELL TUMORS

Epithelial cell tumors (Figures 19-10 through 19-16) are found throughout the body. Regardless of whether they originate from the lung (Figure 19-12), the intestine (Figure 19-11), or the mammary gland (Figure 19-10), they all have similar characteristics, including easy exfoliation of cells in clusters, clumps, or sheets; oval to round cells; ductular or acinar arrangement around a central lumen; and cytoplasm that may contain a secretory product. This secretory product may induce a "signet-ring" appearance because the nucleus is eccentrically located within the cytoplasm. A clinical pathologist may be able to determine the cell of origin. Following are some characteristic epithelial cell tumors commonly seen in canine practice:

- **Perianal gland adenomas** (Figure 19-14) are common tumors seen primarily in intact male dogs; they occasionally occur in female dogs with hyperadrenocorticism. These raised, hairless tumors of the perianal glands are often small and multiple, but they may become very large. Cytologically, perianal gland adenomas may resemble perianal gland adenocarcinomas; therefore, a biopsy using parameters such as invasion of the basement membrane is essential to differentiate between the two types. These cells exfoliate readily into clusters, often are described as hepatoid in appearance, and are characterized as having an abundant, foamy pale cytoplasm and eccentric or centrally located round to oval nuclei that may vary in size.
- Cells from **mammary adenocarcinomas** (Figure 19-10) are similar to those found in any adenocarcinoma. The cells often are arranged in clusters and exhibit cytoplasmic basophilia and variable nuclear:cytoplasmic ratios. Mitotic figures are common; some cells may be distended with a cytoplasmic product forming a signet-ring appearance.
- **Sebaceous gland tumors** (Figures 19-15 and 19-16) are small, fleshy tumors of the skin of older dogs that often are pedunculated, and they are almost always benign. The cells have a high nuclear:cytoplasmic ratio with a scant basophilic cytoplasm. The cells do not have criteria for malignancy. The nucleus usually is centrally located. The cytoplasm is abundant and foamy.
- **Squamous cell carcinomas** occur throughout the body in dogs and cats and often have a different biologic behavior depending on the location of the tumor. They may be ulcerated and therefore may have an inflammatory component mixed with a bacterial infection. Squamous cell carcinomas often exfoliate into clusters; however, they are just as likely to be individual cells. The cells of this tumor may vary morphologically depending on the degree of differentiation. The more anaplastic cells are small and round with a basophilic cytoplasm, which often contains hyperchromatic nuclei. Cells in an intermediate stage of differentiation are larger, with more abundant, paler cytoplasm. The nuclei generally are large and have marked clumps of chromatin. More mature cells actually show signs of forming keratin, which may be seen in the extracellular space. The more mature cells may have cytoplasmic borders that appear quite angular due to keratinization. An inflammatory response is often seen in conjunction with the tumor cells. As with all aspirates, a histologic sample is essential to confirm the diagnosis.
- **Intracutaneous cornifying epitheliomas** or **inclusions** are two benign conditions of the skin that often are cytologically indistinguishable (Figure 19-13). The intracutaneous cornifying epithelioma often occurs in Norwegian

elkhounds. Inclusion cysts can be seen in any breed. The tumors are actually cavities within the skin that contain keratinized cellular debris. They may open and drain to the outside. Cytologically, they are composed of epithelial cells, keratin debris, and cholesterol crystals or clefts (Figure 19-16).

CONNECTIVE TISSUE TUMORS

Connective tissue tumors (Figures 19-17 through 19-20) exfoliate poorly and therefore may be difficult to diagnose cytologically. Cytologic diagnosis of a sarcoma is reasonably straightforward; however, specifically distinguishing connective tissue tumors may not be possible. Types include:

- **Lipomas** (Figure 19-17) are very common tumors in dogs. They must be distinguished from invasive lipomas by histopathology. When a fine-needle aspiration sample is placed on a slide, the sample is oily and fails to dry. The sample will often rinse off the slide with alcohol. Adipocytes will appear to range from very large cells that are fully distended with fat to collapsed cells with lacy cytoplasm.

- **Soft tissue sarcomas** (Figure 19-18) may occur anywhere on the dog's body. In general, soft tissue sarcomas have a relatively low probability for metastasis and are locally invasive. The cells exfoliate poorly and usually are seen alone or in disorganized clusters. The cytoplasm often is indistinct and spindle shaped. Biopsy is required to distinguish hemangiopericytomas, fibrosarcomas, neurofibrosarcomas, fibromas, schwannomas, myxosarcomas, and myxomas. The fine-needle aspirate of a dog with hemangiopericytoma is pictured in Figure 19-19. Note the poorly defined cytoplasmic borders, the nucleoli, and wispy, streaming cytoplasm. In some cases, some cells appear to form a whirling pattern that may distinguish them from other soft tissue sarcomas. Practically speaking, all soft tissue sarcomas are highly locally invasive with a relatively low metastatic behavior.

- **Osteosarcomas** (Figure 19-20) may have sufficient distinguishable cytologic characteristics to allow the practitioner to make a tentative diagnosis based on fine-needle aspiration cytology, especially when combined with the history, physical examination, and radiographs. These tumors often occur in the metaphyses of long bones or in the axillary skeleton. Cytologically, the tumor may be composed primarily of osteoblasts that vary dramatically in size but are usually quite large. The cells are often spindle shaped and have abundant foamy basophilic cytoplasm that surrounds a variably sized nucleus, with coarse chromatin and variable numbers of nuclei. Some of these cells have an eosinophilic substance within the cytoplasm that occasionally may be noted extracellularly as an osteoid matrix. Normal osteoblasts may be seen in conjunction with the malignant cells.

REFERENCES

1. Culmsee K, Simon D, Mischke R, Nolte I: Possibilities of flow cytometric analysis for immunophenotypic characterization of canine lymphoma. *J Vet Med A Physiol Pathol Clin Med* 48(4):199–206, 2001.
2. Platt SR, Alleman AR, Lanz OI, Chrisman CL: Comparison of fine-needle aspiration and surgical-tissue biopsy in the diagnosis of canine brain tumors. *Vet Surg* 31(1):65–69, 2002.
3. Chalita MC, Matera JM, Alves MT, Longatto Filho A: Nonaspiration fine needle cytology and its histologic correlation in canine skin and soft tissue tumors. *Anal Quant Cytol Histol* 23(6):395–399, 2001.
4. Bennett PF, Hahn KA, Toal RL, Legendre AM: Ultrasonographic and cytopathological diagnosis of exocrine pancreatic carcinoma in the dog and cat. *JAAHA* 37(5):466–473, 2001.
5. Raskin RE, Denny J: *Meyer Atlas of Canine and Feline Cytology*. Philadelphia, WB Saunders, 2001.
6. Herring ES, Smith MM, Robertson JL: Lymph node staging of oral and maxillofacial neoplasms in 31 dogs and cats. *J Vet Dent* 19(3):122–126, 2002.
7. Cowell RL, Dorsey KE, Meinkoth JH: Lymph node cytology. *Vet Clin North Am Small Anim Pract* 33(1):47–67, 2003.
8. De Vico G, Sfacteria A, Maiolino P, Mazzullo G: Comparison of nuclear morphometric parameters in cytologic smears and histologic sections of spontaneous canine tumors. *Vet Clin Pathol* 31(1):16–18, 2002.
9. Nyland TG, Wallack ST, Wisner ER: Needle-tract implantation following US-guided fine-needle aspiration biopsy of transitional cell carcinoma of the bladder, urethra, and prostate. *Vet Radiol Ultrasound* 43(1):50–53, 2002.

SECTION 3

COMMON THERAPEUTIC AND SUPPORTIVE PROCEDURES

Chapter 20   Drug Handling and Administration 111

Chapter 21   Chemotherapy: Properties, Uses, and 126
             Patient Management

Chapter 22   Radiation Therapy: Properties, Uses, ... 148
             and Patient Management

Chapter 23   Biologic Response Modifiers: Properties, ... 167
             Uses, and Patient Management

Chapter 24   Surgical Oncology: Properties, Uses 174
             and Patient Management

Chapter 25   Complementary and Alternative 179
             Veterinary Medicine: Properties, Uses,
             and Patient Management

Chapter 26   Bone Marrow Transplantation 190

SECTION 3

COMMON THERAPEUTIC AND SUPPORTIVE PROCEDURES

Chapter 27 Hyperthermia, Cryotherapy, and 197
Photodynamic Therapy: Properties,
Uses, and Patient Management

Chapter 28 Emerging Cancer Therapies: Gene 204
Therapy, Cancer Vaccines, and
Molecularly Targeted Therapies

Chapter 29 Prevention and Treatment of Pain............. 213

Chapter 30 Prevention and Treatment of Nausea 225
and Vomiting

Chapter 31 Nutritional Support 230

Chapter 32 Transfusion Support........................ 246

Chapter 33 Hematopoietic Growth Factor Support 251

DRUG HANDLING AND ADMINISTRATION

Gregory K. Ogilvie and Antony S. Moore

CLINICAL BRIEFING

Procedures for handling chemotherapeutic agents must meet or exceed the guidelines outlined by OSHA and any state or local regulations.

Risk	Recommendations
Unsafe handling of chemotherapy	• Provide frequent training on guidelines regarding risks and methods to minimize exposure. • Store chemotherapy in a secure area per manufacturer's requirements. • Dilute, transport, and administer drugs using appropriate equipment and procedures. • Dispose of drug and all associated materials separately and as a biohazard. • Be prepared to safely handle spills.
Absorption via skin or mucous membranes	• Wear appropriate nonpowdered latex gloves, protective eyewear, and a protective disposable gown with long, cuffed sleeves. • Wash hands frequently. • Do not allow food in work area.
Inhalation	• Wear a respirator-type or high-dust mask.
Aerosol formation when reconstituting	• Use a hydrophobic filter (chemotherapy "pin") for removing liquid chemotherapeutic agents. • Use the PhaSeal system.
Metabolites or drug (e.g., carboplatin) in urine	• Wear appropriate latex gloves when handling waste.
Self-inoculation when recapping needles	• Do not recap needles.

The health and well-being of the veterinary health care team, including the client, is paramount regardless of whether one is dealing with anesthetic agents, antibiotics, or chemotherapeutic agents. Like all drugs, chemotherapeutic agents have potential risks if they are handled inappropriately. Fortunately, new, practical systems are available, such as the PhaSeal injectable drug mixing and administration system (Carmel Pharma, Mölndal, Sweden; distributed by Baxa Corp., Englewood, CO), that can reduce the risk associated with the handling of these agents.

As the benefits of anticancer drugs become more apparent, the use of these drugs is rapidly expanding, putting the veterinary health care team at increased risk for exposure during drug preparation and administration. All chemotherapeutic agents must be considered potentially toxic; most are mutagenic or teratogenic, and at least some are carcinogenic. Reliable information regarding the amount of drug exposure needed for any of these effects is difficult to obtain; however, some toxicities have been seen in caregivers who prepare and administer chemotherapy for human patients without appropriate protection and precautions, including[1,2]:

- **Chromosomal aberrations.** Some studies have found increases in chromosomal aberrations, including sister chromatid exchanges, structural aberrations (e.g., gaps, breaks, translocations), and micronuclei in peripheral blood lymphocytes; others have found decreases.[2–6] The biologic effects of these findings are unknown.
- **Reproductive effects.** Hemminki et al[7] found no difference in exposure between nurses who had spontaneous abortions and those who had normal pregnancies with regard to exposure to cytotoxic drugs, whereas Selevan et al[8] and others[9] found a relationship between cytotoxic drug exposure and adverse reproductive outcomes.
- **Hepatocellular damage.** Liver damage has been reported in nurses who work on human oncology wards.[10]

> **KEY POINT**
>
> *The health and well-being of the veterinary health care team, including the client, is paramount regardless of whether one is dealing with anesthetic agents, antibiotics, or chemotherapeutic agents. Safe handling techniques of all drugs must be employed at all times among a well-trained staff.*

When possible, the practitioner should minimize exposure to all workplace hazards, including chemotherapeutic agents. All institutional, local, regional, state, and national regulations and laws must be reviewed and followed to the letter. When possible, the team should contract the duties of preparing chemotherapeutic agents to institutional, local, or regional pharmacies that prepare chemotherapeutic agents routinely. All regulations and procedures for handling, mixing, and administering chemotherapeutic agents and other hazards should be readily available and followed during routine training periods for the entire team. Exposure to cytotoxic agents can occur in four ways:[1,11–13]

- Inhalation of drug aerosolized during mixing or administration
- Absorption of the drug through the skin
- Ingestion of contaminated food or contact with contaminated cigarettes
- Accidental inoculation

Common clinical examples of situations in which exposure may occur include:

- Withdrawal of a needle from a pressurized drug vial (the "pssst" as the needle is removed)
- Transfer of drugs between containers
- Opening of glass ampules

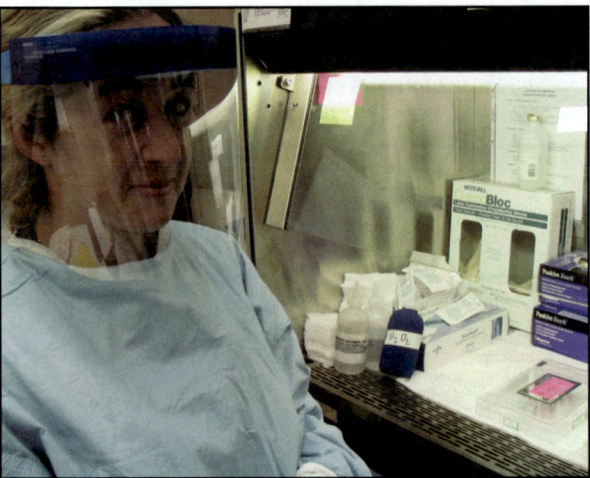

Figure 20-1. *A biologic safety cabinet should be used when handling chemotherapeutic agents. Latex gloves, a nonpermeable gown, and eye and face protection should be worn whenever chemotherapeutic agents are handled outside the hood or in case of spills.*

- Expulsion of air bubbles from drug-filled syringes
- Failure or improper setup of equipment
- Exposure to excreta from patients treated with certain cytotoxic drugs
- Crushing or breaking of tablets

> **KEY POINT**
>
> *All regulations and procedures for handling, mixing, and administering chemotherapeutic agents and other hazards should be readily available and used during actual incidents and routine training periods for the entire team.*

Safe drug handling in veterinary practice can be greatly aided by employing a biologic safety cabinet (Figure 20-1) or the PhaSeal system. Because of the relatively small doses of chemotherapy delivered by most practitioners, the risk for exposure is relatively low if the drugs are handled appropriately. Everyone who prepares or administers antineoplastic drugs should be appropriately trained and equipped and should undergo routine health examinations. Women of childbearing age should exercise extreme caution when handling cytotoxic agents, and pregnant women should not handle antineoplastic drugs at all. Procedures for handling chemotherapeutic agents must meet or exceed the guidelines outlined by the Occupational Safety and Health Administration (OSHA) and any state or local regulations. Clients and all personnel coming into contact with chemotherapeutic agents should wear personal protective equipment (see box on page 113). A chemotherapy logbook that includes identification of patients treated and personnel involved in treatments should be maintained in order to track exposures.

The risk for exposure can be greatly reduced by understanding the hazardous properties listed in the Material Safety Data Sheet (MSDS) for each drug and by using appropriate protective equipment. The information contained in each MSDS includes the specific health hazards, including carcinogenicity, primary routes of exposure, required protective equipment, treatment of personnel acutely exposed, chemical activators, solubility, stability, volatility, and specific procedures to be undertaken in case of a spill. The MSDS should be requested with the initial shipment of any chemotherapeutic agent and should be kept on file in an easily accessible location.

> **KEY POINT**
> *Procedures for handling chemotherapeutic agents must meet or exceed the guidelines outlined by OSHA and any state or local regulations. Both clients and clinic personnel coming into contact with chemotherapy agents should be protected to the best of the veterinarian's abilities.*

A Hazardous Drug Safety and Health Plan should be developed for each hospital and clinic that handles chemotherapeutic agents. This plan should include at least[1,11–13]:

- A standard operating procedure for the mixing and handling of hazardous drugs and an exposure response/control plan
- Control measures the employer will implement to reduce employee exposure to hazardous drugs
- A ventilation system and other protective equipment necessary to mix, administer, and clean up chemotherapeutic agents
- Provisions for information and training
- Provisions for medical examinations of exposed personnel
- Assignment of staff in leadership positions to ensure that personnel apply and adhere to all safety measures
- Establishment of a designated area to mix, handle, and administer chemotherapeutic agents
- Procedures to safely remove contaminated waste
- Decontamination procedures

Antineoplastic agents should be stored according to each manufacturer's directions. Drugs that require refrigeration should be kept in a separate refrigerator away from other medications and foodstuffs. If a reconstituted drug is stored, the vial should be placed in a sealable plastic bag labeled with the date of reconstitution.

Personal Protective Equipment for Use in Handling Chemotherapeutic Agents

Minimizing exposure to chemotherapy drugs requires the use of appropriate equipment. The following are considered the essentials of personal protective equipment[1,11–13]:

- Nonpowdered, appropriate-thickness latex gloves. Change them at least every hour.
- A protective disposable gown made of lint-free, low-permeability fabric with a closed front, long sleeves, and elastic or knit closed cuffs.
- A biologic safety cabinet, or, if one is not available, an approved respirator with a high-efficiency filter.
- Eye and face protection with an appropriate plastic face or splash shield in situations where splashes, sprays, or aerosols may be created.

Preparing Chemotherapeutic Agents

Chemotherapeutic agents must be mixed with care and respect because these drugs can be dangerous if they are not handled appropriately. The following are some guidelines on handling chemotherapeutic agents[1,11–13]:

- Wear a disposable, closed, moisture-barrier gown with elastic or knit cuffs, appropriate-thickness latex gloves, and safety glasses or a face shield.
- Use a class II or III biologic safety cabinet (Figure 20-1) that meets the current National Sanitation Foundation Standard, have the drugs mixed at an off-site facility that has the appropriate equipment, and/or use the PhaSeal system.
- Mix agents in a quiet area.
- Use absorbent plastic-backed liners to collect spills.
- Use hydrophobic filters (chemo pins) to air-vent vials, or use the PhaSeal system.
- Use Luer-Lok syringes.
- Have a pharmacy prepare injectable agents when possible.
- Wash hands before donning and after removing gloves. Immediately change gowns or gloves that become contaminated. (Employees should be trained in proper methods to remove contaminated gloves and gowns.) After use, gloves and gowns should be disposed of in accordance with standard recommendations.
- Observe infusion sets and pumps, which should have Luer-Lok fittings, for leakage during use. Place a plastic-backed absorbent pad under the tubing during administration to catch any leakage. Place sterile gauze around any push sites, and tape IV tubing connection sites.

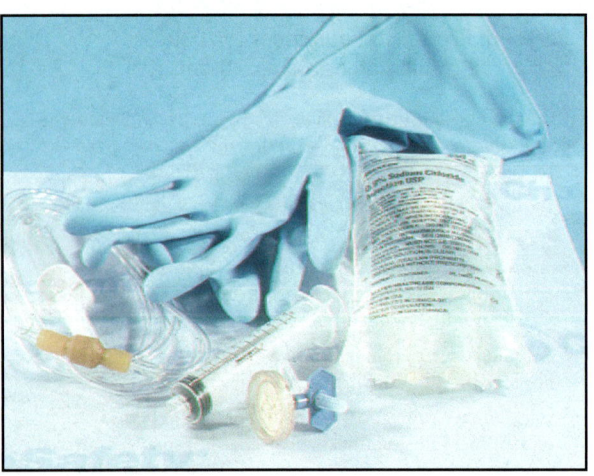

Figure 20-2. *Materials that should be on hand for preparing or handling chemotherapeutic agents include latex gloves, chemotherapy dispensing pins to prevent contamination of the bottle or exposure to the handler, Luer-Lok syringes, and prefilled IV drip sets. Everything must be clearly labeled.*

- Prime IV sets or expel air from syringes in a biologic safety cabinet, and/or use the PhaSeal system. If done at the administration site, prime lines with nondrug-containing solution or a backflow closed system. Do not use IV containers with venting tubes.
- Using sterile gauze, wipe syringes, IV bottles and bags, and pumps clean of any drug contamination. Do not crush or clip needles and syringes. Instead, place them in a puncture-resistant container and then into the chemotherapy disposal bag with all other contaminated materials.

> **KEY POINT**
> *Chemotherapeutic agents must be mixed with care and respect because these drugs can be dangerous if they are not handled appropriately.*

The ideal way to prepare cytotoxic agents is in a biologic safety cabinet—specifically, a class II, type A vertical laminar airflow cabinet that is exhausted outside the facility. The manufacturer of the PhaSeal system suggests that the system may preclude the need for a cabinet.[14] The biologic safety cabinet or hood is the preferred site for mixing chemotherapeutic agents and is essential for practices that handle large volumes of these drugs. Many pharmacies will prepare chemotherapeutic agents for a fee. Practitioners should take advantage of this option when possible. However, regardless of the quantity of drug and the system used, the safety principles involved in drug handling and reconstitution are the same.

Chemotherapeutic agents should be mixed in a designated quiet, low-traffic area. Eating, drinking, and smoking

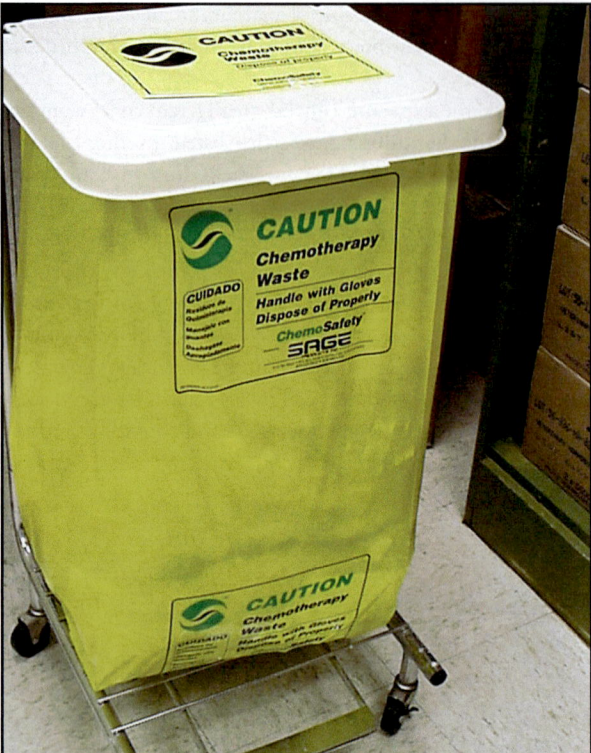

Figure 20-3. *Chemotherapeutic agents and all material that may be contaminated during chemotherapy must be disposed of appropriately.*

> **KEY POINT**
> *The ideal way to prepare cytotoxic agents is in a class II, type A vertical laminar airflow cabinet that is exhausted outside the facility.*

should not take place in this area. If a biologic safety cabinet is not available, then an approved respirator is essential. Materials that should be kept readily available in the mixing area include a plastic-backed absorbent liner to absorb any leaks and spills (the liner should be changed if it becomes contaminated with any drug and when the area is cleaned), heavy-duty latex gloves, hydrophobic filters (chemo pins), an infusion pump and IV lines prefilled with sodium chloride (NaCl) if appropriate, a stack of gauze squares, and alcohol-soaked cottonballs or swabs (Figure 20-2). A large, sealable plastic bag should be available for chemotherapy waste (Figure 20-3), and a puncture-proof container is needed for all contaminated sharps. If the PhaSeal system is used, then all of these materials should still be available.

All materials needed for drug preparation should be placed in the area before starting any work. Outer packages should be discarded to prevent accumulation of debris. Before reconstituting a drug, recommendations for the diluent should be verified. For most chemotherapy drugs, 0.9%

NaCl or sterile water is used; however, for some drugs (e.g., carboplatin), a solution of 5% dextrose in water is required.

When preparing cytotoxic agents, a gown with long sleeves, closed cuffs, and a closed front should be worn. The gown should be made of a disposable fabric with low permeability. Latex gloves should be pulled over the cuffs of the gown to protect the skin from drug exposure. Vinyl gloves should not be used—they are more permeable and thus more likely to allow skin contamination. Goggles and a mask are necessary. The use of a dust-and-mist respirator or a mask with a filter to prevent inhalation of aerosolized drugs is recommended. A conventional surgery mask does not provide adequate protection.

From this point, either a conventional approach is used to mix and administer drugs, or the PhaSeal system is used. Because the PhaSeal system may be safer, it is described first, followed by the standard approach.

PHASEAL SYSTEM APPROACH

PhaSeal, a closed, double-membrane system for ensuring leak-free transfer of drugs, has been shown to reduce environmental and personnel exposure compared with existing processes for the preparation and administration of antineoplastics. PhaSeal uses a dry-connection system for drug transfer, with each element sealed off with a membrane cover. The injectable drug is transferred via a specially cut injection cannula. When the components of the PhaSeal system are separated after transfer, the membranes act as tight seals, preventing leakage. In this way, the cytotoxic drugs have no contact with the atmosphere, and workers and all connections are kept dry. At present, the system cannot be deployed for use with ampules, and some vials are too small or large to accommodate the protector unit.

This system may be ideal for use in veterinary medicine. In a study at Ängelholm Hospital in Sweden, PhaSeal was tested for 1 year.[14] No safety cabinet was used during preparation of the drugs. When contamination levels were determined after 1 year, no cytotoxic drugs were found in the environment. This study suggests that the use of PhaSeal alone is sufficient to prevent environmental contamination.

The PhaSeal system has four basic components:

1. An infusion adapter with an inline spike to connect the bag to the external intravenous set. The adapter and set have a built-in connector to allow for sealed transfer of the medication to the bag.
2. A Luer-Lok connector to ensure a sealed connection between the injector and the IV administration set.
3. A Luer-Lok injector, an encapsulated, specially cut cannula that is permanently attached to a syringe and allows sealed transfer of the medication by means of a double membrane.
4. A protector unit, a pressure-equalizing device that permanently attaches to the medication vial. The expansion chamber makes sure that neither overpressure nor vacuum occurs during drug preparation. This effectively prevents vapor leakage. The drugs have no contact with the atmosphere, and hence no spreading of aerosols or vapor occurs.

To prepare the chemotherapeutic drug, the plastic lid is removed from the vial and the top of the vial is wiped with an alcohol swab. The vial is kept upright and placed into the PhaSeal clamping device provided. The plastic protector unit is then placed into the clamping device (Figure 20-4). The clamping device is closed to seal it permanently to the protector unit to ensure that pressure changes are contained within the system. The vial and protector are removed from the clamping device for reconstituting the drug or to withdraw the contents.

When reconstituting a drug, the syringe is prefilled with air or diluent to be added and is attached to an injector that has the needle guarded (Figure 20-5). The injector–syringe combination is then connected to the protector device, which is attached to the drug in question and rotated to the "locked" position. The safety latch of the injector is released, and the needle is advanced into the vial to inject air or diluent. The injector–syringe combination is then withdrawn from the vial so that the needle is no longer within the vial and is subsequently disconnected. The double-membrane system prevents the drug from ever coming into contact with the operator.

If the syringe contents are to be delivered into a bag of fluids, a Luer-Lok connector is placed between the IV bag and the tubing to ensure a sealed connection between the injector and the IV administration set (Figure 20-6). The IV tubing leading to the connector is then clamped off. This connector has a special adapter to receive the injector–syringe complex. The injector–syringe combination is advanced into the adapter and then rotated to fix it into place. The safety latch of the injector is released, and the needle is advanced into the connector to subsequently inject the drug into the bag. The needle is withdrawn from the injection port of the IV bag connector, and the injector is withdrawn.

If the drug is to be administered directly into the patient's IV line, a separate connector is attached to the IV catheter or associated tubing (Figure 20-7). The injector and its associated syringe containing the drug are then attached to the IV connector and injected and removed as before.

STANDARD APPROACH
Intravenous Agents

Chemo pins prevent both aerosolization of the drug and pressure from building in the vials when reconstituting drugs and are thus recommended when preparing injectable

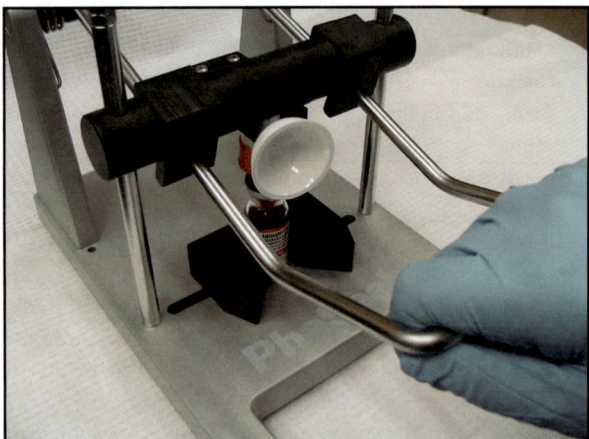

Figure 20-4. To prepare the chemotherapeutic drug using the PhaSeal system, the plastic lid is first removed from the vial and the top of the vial is wiped with an alcohol swab. The vial is kept upright and placed into the PhaSeal clamping device provided. The plastic protector unit is then placed into the clamping device, which is closed to seal the device permanently to the protector unit to ensure pressure changes are contained within the system. The vial and protector are removed from the clamping device for reconstituting the drug or to withdraw the contents.

drugs (Figure 20-8). Luer-Lok syringes (Figure 20-9) are recommended because they prevent the syringe from separating from the chemo pin or needle.

To prepare injectable drugs, the first step is to remove the plastic lid from the vial and aseptically wipe the top of the vial with an alcohol swab. The chemo pin is then inserted into the vial. The vial is kept upright while the syringe is attached to the chemo pin and twisted tight. When reconstituting a drug, diluent is slowly pushed into the vial, and the bottle is gently rolled or shaken. A Luer-Lok syringe can remain attached while mixing. After the drug is completely dissolved, the vial is turned upside down, and the drug is aspirated slowly into the syringe to avoid excess air bubbles (Figure 20-10). When the correct amount has been retrieved, any air or excess drug should be pushed back into the vial. The vial should then be turned upright and put down. An alcohol-moistened gauze square is wrapped around the top of the pin and syringe, and the syringe is gently removed from the pin. The gauze will trap any drug that leaks or aerosolizes. A covered needle should be placed on the syringe and the chemo pin capped after clearing the filter with an air-filled syringe. The labeled syringe should then be put into a sealable plastic bag (Figure 20-11). If the remaining drug is to be stored, the chemo pin is left inserted into the vial to allow access for multiple doses.

If chemo pins are not available, the diluent must be slowly added to the drug directly through the needle and the displaced air allowed to escape back into the syringe to avoid excess pressure in the vial. Once the drug has been

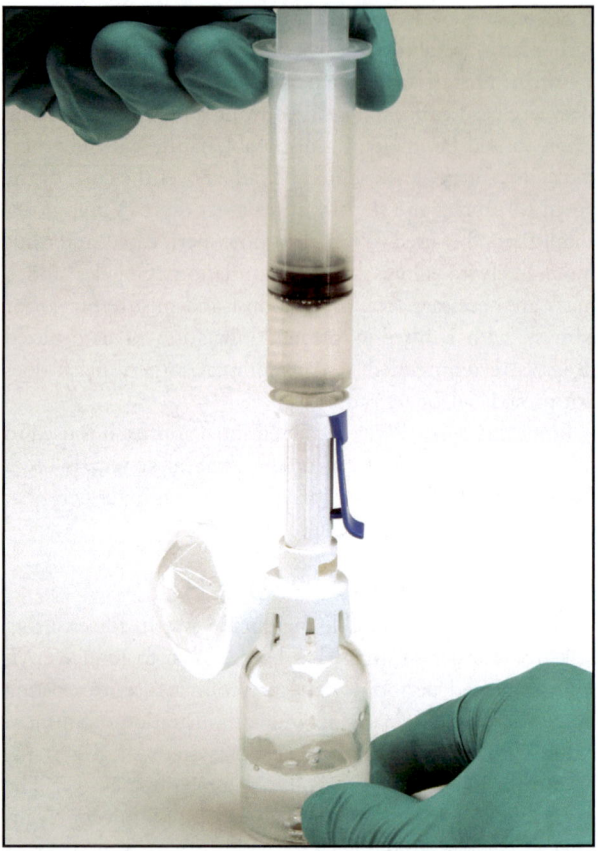

Figure 20-5. When reconstituting a drug with the PhaSeal system, the syringe is prefilled with air or diluent to be added and is attached to an injector that has the needle guarded. The injector–syringe combination is then connected to the protector device that is attached to the drug in question and rotated to the "locked" position. The safety latch of the injector is released, and the needle is advanced into the vial to inject air or diluent. The injector–syringe combination is then withdrawn from the vial so that the needle is no longer within the vial and is subsequently disconnected. Note that the double-membrane system prevents the drug from ever coming into contact with the operator.

reconstituted and the correct dose retrieved, an alcohol-moistened gauze square should be wrapped around the top of the vial and the needle. Then the needle should be slowly pulled out of the vial. Any air bubbles that are present should be injected into an alcohol-soaked cottonball and discarded in the appropriate waste container. The cap should be carefully placed on the needle and the syringe put into a sealable plastic bag and labeled. As a general rule, needles should not be recapped.

When preparing a drug to be delivered by IV drip infusion, it is a good idea to prime the administration set by filling the fluid lines with diluent from the bag before the chemotherapeutic agent is added. This reduces the risk for exposure when connecting the drip set to the patient. Once reconstituted, the drug should be slowly injected into the

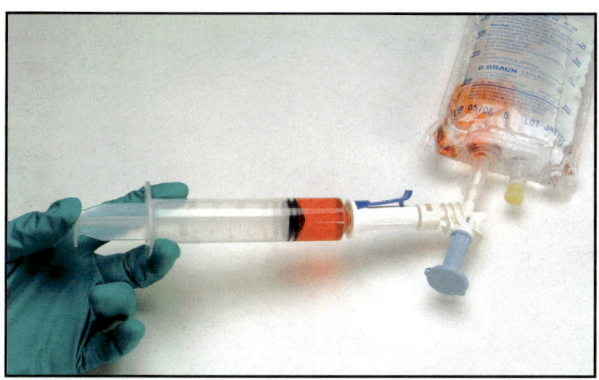

Figure 20-6. When using the PhaSeal system to deliver the contents of a syringe into a bag of fluids that will then be administered to a patient, a Luer-Lok connector is placed between the IV bag and the IV tubing to ensure a sealed connection between the injector and the IV administration set leading to the bag. The IV tubing leading to the connector is then clamped off. This connector has a special adapter to receive the injector–syringe complex. The injector–syringe combination is advanced into the adapter and then rotated to fix it into place. The safety latch of the injector is released, and the needle is advanced into the connector to subsequently inject the drug into the bag. The needle is withdrawn from the injection port of the IV bag connector, and the injector is withdrawn.

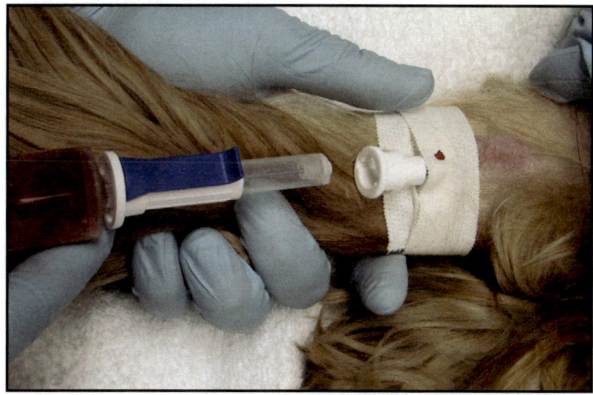

Figure 20-7. If the drug is to be administered directly into the patient's IV line with the PhaSeal system, a separate connector is attached to the IV catheter or associated tubing. The injector and its associated syringe containing the drug are then attached to the IV connector and injected and then removed as before.

bag. A gauze square wrapped around the injection port as the needle is withdrawn helps prevent aerosolization of the drug. The fluid that contains the drug should be stored in a labeled, sealable bag until it is administered. Again, materials should be discarded appropriately. An infusion pump will allow the rate of administration of any infusion to be constant and is preferred when the drug is diluted in a fluid bag.

Oral Agents

Some chemotherapeutic agents are prepared for oral administration. When preparing or administering pills, non-porous latex gloves are strongly recommended. Cytotoxic powder has been found as far as 12 inches away from where tablets are crushed or split; therefore, drugs are best dispensed in whole tablets only. When small quantities of some orally administered drugs are needed, they may be prepared from the injectable formulation for use as an elixir (rather than splitting tablets). When crushing or splitting of pills cannot be avoided—and especially if a safety hood is not available—gown, goggles, and a respirator mask are mandatory, and the preparation surface must be well cleaned afterward. Oral medications should be placed in clearly labeled containers with a warning label for dispensing to owners. Owners should wear latex gloves when administering oral agents to their pets and should return empty vials to the veterinarian for proper disposal. Detailed information about how owners should administer and dispose of these medications should accompany each prescription. Although the exposure risks from metabolized chemotherapeutics are low, latex gloves should be worn when handling bodily fluids or stool (including disposal of litter) from patients that have received chemotherapeutic agents. Caution should be employed to reduce aerosolization of bodily waste (e.g., high-pressure hosing should not be used as a cleaning method).

Intralesional Agents

Intralesional injections consisting of a cytotoxic agent mixed with a vehicle (i.e., bovine collagen matrix, sterile sesame oil, or some other biodegradable polymer or material that acts to slowly release the drug into the tumor) have been recommended by some for select localized cancers. The mixture is injected into a tumor, providing a very high drug concentration to the tumor cells but minimal systemic drug levels, thereby avoiding the risk for systemic toxicity. These mixtures are prepared in the biologic safety cabinet, but two Luer-Lok syringes, one containing the cytotoxic agent and one containing the vehicle, should be prepared. Each agent should be placed into a syringe with sufficient capacity to contain both liquids when combined (e.g., 5 ml of drug and 5 ml of vehicle in a 10-ml syringe). The syringes are attached to a three-way stopcock, and the two liquids can then be rapidly mixed between the syringes to create an oily emulsion. The syringe that now contains all of the mixture should be detached after covering the attachment with an alcohol-moistened gauze swab to prevent aerosolization, and a needle should be attached. The remaining syringe and stopcock should be discarded as contaminated waste.

It is preferable to mix multiple small volumes of drug in this way rather than a single large volume because separation of drug from vehicle may occur rapidly, thereby reducing the efficacy of the treatment. Likewise, the drug-vehicle mixture should be administered soon after preparation. If a delay is encountered, the drug can be remixed with its vehicle using

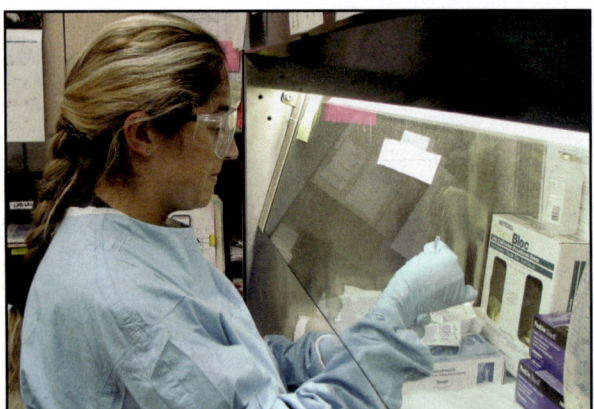

Figure 20-8. *Chemotherapeutic agents can be safely mixed if the handler wears latex gloves and uses hydrophobic filters (or uses the PhaSeal system).*

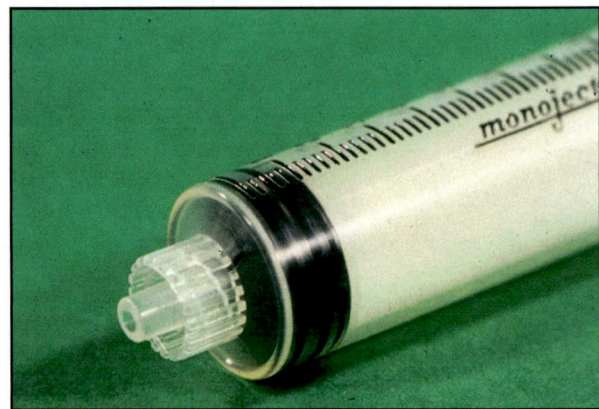

Figure 20-9. *Luer-Lok syringes should be used whenever possible because their screw-on ends allow a secure connection with the needle.*

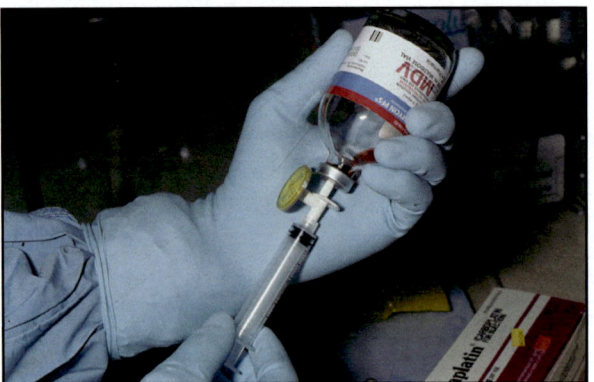

Figure 20-10. *To remove a quantity of drug from a vial, the Luer-Lok syringe can remain attached while mixing when not using the PhaSeal system. After the drug is completely dissolved, the vial is turned upside down and the drug is aspirated into the syringe slowly to avoid excess air bubbles. When the correct amount has been retrieved, any air or excess drug should be pushed back into the vial.*

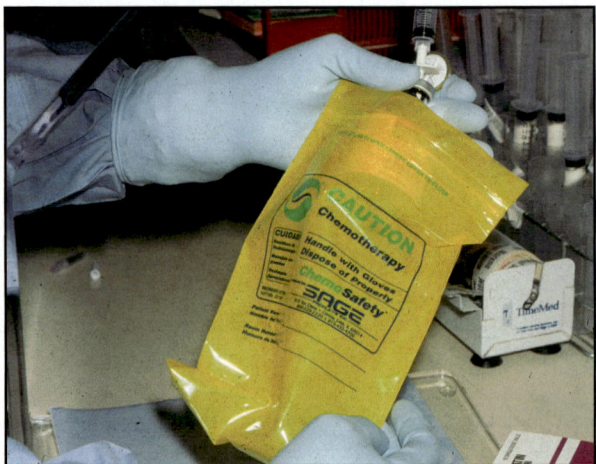

Figure 20-11. *Drugs and syringes should be placed in plastic bags to contain any inadvertent spills during transportation within the hospital.*

a new syringe and three-way stopcock; gloves, mask, goggles, and a gown must be worn. It may be wise to mix inside a sealable plastic bag. The needles on used syringes should not be recapped. All materials should be disposed of as contaminated waste. Note that some of the drugs reported for intralesional chemotherapy rely on reconstitution of the lyophilized drug to a higher concentration than would normally be administered systemically. Some of those drugs (e.g., cisplatin, carboplatin) are available as reconstituted drug, which is too dilute for intralesional use.

GENERAL PRECAUTIONS

Regardless of whether the PhaSeal system or the standard administration technique is used, it is extremely important to label all chemotherapeutic drugs. All syringes, fluid bags, pill bottles, and other containers must have a chemotherapy label listing the drug name, milligrams of drug, patient's name, and dose. The drug vial should be put into a sealable plastic bag to be stored in a refrigerator or discarded according to storage instructions. Every drug has a package insert that states the expiration date and storage conditions.

All nonsharp materials used in drug preparation should be placed into a large sealable plastic bag, and all sharps must be placed in a puncture-proof container. Once everything is discarded and all vials and syringes are inside sealable plastic bags, gloves should be removed by rolling them off the hands; they can then be placed in the plastic bag with the rest of the items. Care must be taken to avoid touching the outside of the gloves.

Bags containing the drugs should be sealed before protective gear is removed. If protective garments are contaminated during drug preparation, they should be discarded and replaced immediately. Thorough handwashing after drug preparation is strongly recommended to remove any potential drug residues. A large, clearly labeled barrel or chemotherapy waste container should be kept in the drug preparation area for full waste bags (e.g., containing contaminated gauze squares, cottonballs) and all contaminated safety gear (e.g., gowns, gloves, masks).

Safety and Disposal of Chemotherapeutic Agents

When administering chemotherapeutic agents, the same principles and care are followed as those used for mixing and handling of chemotherapeutic agents. Specifically, it is important to[1,11–13]:

- Wear personal protective equipment, including a disposable, closed, moisture-barrier gown with elastic or knit cuffs, appropriate-thickness latex gloves, and safety glasses or a face shield.
- Wear disposable, nonpowdered latex gloves.
- Use absorbent plastic-backed liners to catch spills.

> **KEY POINT**
> *When chemotherapeutic agents are spilled, or if there is elimination of any body excreta within 48 hours after the drug is administered, the contaminated area should be closed and traffic rerouted.*

When chemotherapeutic agents are spilled, or if there is elimination of any body excreta within 48 hours after the drug is administered, the contaminated area should be closed and traffic rerouted. Personal protective equipment must be used appropriately by all individuals involved. Commercially available "spill kits" should be used when possible. The following recommendations should be followed[1,11–13]:

- Wear two pairs of doubled, nonpowdered latex gloves.
- Wash skin with soap and water upon contact with drug.
- Clean minor spills with 70% isopropyl alcohol.
- Decontaminate large spills with a neutralizing agent or high-pH soap.
- Wear protective clothing when cleaning up fecal matter and urine for approximately 48 hours after the administration of chemotherapeutic agents.

Chemotherapeutic agents are considered a biologic hazard and therefore must be disposed of appropriately using the following guidelines[1,11–13]:

- Contaminated sharps and other contaminated materials must be appropriately discarded as soon as feasible in containers that are puncture resistant, closable, leakproof, and labeled.
- Containers for contaminated sharps should be replaced routinely and not be allowed to overfill.
- Containers for contaminated sharps should be easily accessible to personnel and located as close as feasible to the immediate area where sharps are used or can be reasonably anticipated to be found.
- Hazardous drug–related waste should be handled separately from other hospital trash and disposed of in accordance with applicable Environmental Protection Agency, state, local, and OSHA regulations for hazardous waste.

The Health Care Team

Cancer chemotherapy requires a team approach; team members include the veterinarian, who listens, diagnoses, and prescribes therapy; the veterinary technicians or nurses, who provide care, information, and technical expertise; and the receptionist, who informs, coordinates, and enables the caregiver and the health care team. The team approach also involves extended team members, such as the attending or consulting oncologist or internist, the pharmacist, and the radiologist; these members are vital links in the advanced care of the cancer patient, especially when it comes to chemotherapy.

The most important members of the team are the caregivers/clients. When the caregiver is recognized, enabled, and empowered with information and the ability to extend

> **KEY POINT**
> *Cancer chemotherapy requires a team approach; team members include the veterinarian, who listens, diagnoses, and prescribes therapy; the veterinary technicians or nurses, who provide care, information, and technical expertise; and the receptionist, who informs, coordinates, and enables the caregiver and the health care team.*

care to his or her best friend, compassionate care can truly be delivered. The process of caregiver education involves giving detailed oral and written information about the cancer and chemotherapy, providing ongoing intellectual and emotional support via the entire team, and ensuring that the caregiver understands and is able to provide continual and seamless care at home.

The following information summarizes the technical procedures associated with the administration of chemotherapy, yet the most important aspects of providing this type of care depend on the ability of the health care team to extend compassionate care to the patient and the caregiver.

> **KEY POINT**
>
> *Caregivers should be empowered with information about the disease and decisions regarding the treatment. They should be considered the most important members of the veterinary health care team.*

Dosing and Administration of Chemotherapeutic Agents

Chemotherapeutic agents can be administered via several routes: intravenous, intramuscular, intracavitary, subcutaneous, intralesional (with a vehicle to slow absorption), and oral (see box on this page). Intrathecal and intraarterial administration are used less commonly in canine medicine. Regardless of the route of administration or who is administering the drugs, protective apparel should be worn when handling cytotoxic agents.

DOSING

The dosing of chemotherapy also requires a team approach. Because many of the drugs used to treat cancer can have serious, potentially life-threatening side effects, and because the margin of safety is not as great as with other medications, team members must constantly check and recheck dosages, labels, and administration procedures. The safety of the patient, caregiver, and the veterinary health care team must be paramount.

There has recently been discussion in the literature about the validity of dosing chemotherapeutic agents using body surface area (BSA) in square meters.[1,11-13] Studies have shown that this dosing method may not be ideal for all veterinary patients, especially smaller animals, in which increased toxicity may be observed.[6] The best known example is doxorubicin: The standard dose of 30 mg/m² may be too high for very small dogs, and a dose of 1 to 1.1 mg/kg (or 20 to 25 mg/m²) is more routinely used. However, until a better dosing scheme is developed, many chemotherapeutic agents will continue to be dosed on a square-meter basis.

> **KEY POINT**
>
> *Chemotherapy drug doses should always be double-checked. Care should be taken with drugs for which milligrams do not equal milliliters (e.g., doxorubicin, which is 2 mg/ml). Chemotherapeutic drugs can be toxic enough at the correct dose! If there is a question about anything, stop, and do not proceed until all questions are answered. It is impossible to be too careful when dealing with chemotherapeutic agents.*

Methods of Chemotherapy Administration

- Intracavitary (e.g., cisplatin, carboplatin, mitoxantrone)
- Intralesional (e.g., carboplatin, cisplatin, 5-fluorouracil, bleomycin)
- Intramuscular (e.g., L-asparaginase)
- Intravenous
  — Butterfly catheter (e.g., vincristine, vinblastine)
  — Over-the-needle or indwelling catheter (e.g., doxorubicin, mitoxantrone, cisplatin)
- Oral (e.g., cyclophosphamide, chlorambucil, melphalan)
- Subcutaneous (e.g., bleomycin)

General Concepts in Calculating and Administering Doses

1. Convert weight in pounds to kilograms by dividing by 2.2. A 22-lb dog weighs 10 kg (22 ÷ 2.2 = 10).

2. Look up weight in kilograms on a weight–to–BSA conversion table (Table 20-1). If a conversion table is not available, the following formula can be used in dogs to calculate the BSA in square meters:

$$m^2 = \frac{10.1 \times \text{Weight (in grams)}^{2/3}}{10^4}$$

3. Determine the dose of a drug (in this example, vincristine) by multiplying the dosage (0.5 to 0.7 mg/m²) by the patient's BSA (m²). The patient's metabolic status should be evaluated by assessing the biochemical profile to help select the type of drug to be used (Table 20-2). The severity of chemotherapy-induced myelosuppression should also be considered (see box on page 121).

4. Before the quantity of drug is drawn up or obtained, check the concentration (mg/ml, mg/pill, or mg/capsule) of the chemotherapeutic agent. For example, doxorubicin has a concentration of 2 mg/ml, so it is necessary to divide the milligrams by 2 to determine how many milliliters to administer. If the drug is a pill or capsule, the amount to be administered is rounded down to the next whole tablet. To prevent inadvertent exposure of the handler to cytotoxic drugs and overdose of the patient, chemotherapy pills or capsules must never be split, crushed, reformulated, or repackaged.

5. Before the drug is administered, double-check the dose and results of the complete blood count (CBC). If the neutrophil count is below 3,000/µl, administration of myelosuppressive drugs (e.g., doxorubicin, cyclophosphamide) should be postponed and the CBC rechecked in 3 to 4 days.

6. A CBC is sometimes obtained 7 days after administering the first dose of any potentially myelosuppressive

Table 20-1 Conversion of Body Weight to BSA for Dogs[a]

Body Weight (kg)	Body Surface Area (m²)	Body Weight (kg)	Body Surface Area (m²)
0.5	0.06	26	0.88
1	0.10	27	0.90
2	0.15	28	0.92
3	0.20	29	0.94
4	0.25	30	0.96
5	0.29	31	0.99
6	0.33	32	1.01
7	0.36	33	1.03
8	0.40	34	1.05
9	0.43	35	1.07
10	0.46	36	1.09
11	0.49	37	1.11
12	0.52	38	1.13
13	0.55	39	1.15
14	0.58	40	1.17
15	0.60	41	1.19
16	0.63	42	1.21
17	0.66	43	1.23
18	0.69	44	1.25
19	0.71	45	1.26
20	0.74	46	1.28
21	0.76	47	1.30
22	0.78	48	1.32
23	0.81	49	1.34
24	0.83	50	1.36
25	0.85	51	1.38

[a]Most chemotherapeutic agents are dosed on a BSA basis.

Myelosuppressive Potential of Some Commonly Used Chemotherapeutic Agents in Veterinary Medicine

Highly Myelosuppressive
- Doxorubicin
- Vinblastine
- Cyclophosphamide
- Actinomycin D

Moderately Myelosuppressive
- Melphalan
- Chlorambucil
- 5-Fluorouracil
- Methotrexate

Mildly Myelosuppressive
- L-Asparaginase[a]
- Vincristine[a]
- Bleomycin
- Corticosteroids

[a]Myelosuppression can occur if these two drugs are administered concurrently.

drug (7–10 days is the neutrophil nadir for most drugs such as doxorubicin, mitoxantrone, and cyclophosphamide; refer to drug list in Chapter 21 for individual variation). If the neutrophil count is below 1,500/µl 7 days after treatment, the drug dose may be reduced by 25%, especially if the dog demonstrates clinical signs relating to neutropenia. The new dose can be administered subsequently, assuming the patient does well with the reduced dose. Doses can then be increased by increments of 10% until the originally calculated "full" dose is reached, provided the patient continues to tolerate the lower doses.

7. Anorexia is a common side effect of many chemotherapeutic agents in dogs. If anorexia is severe or accompanied by more than 10% loss of body weight, consider a dose reduction. A good rule of thumb is 25%, although the dose may subsequently be increased by increments of 10% if no further anorexia is observed.

> **KEY POINT**
> *If the neutrophil count is below 3,000/µl, the drug should not be given and the CBC should be checked again in 3 to 4 days. To ensure a neutrophil count above 1,500/µl, a CBC should be conducted 7 to 10 days after administration of any drug that has the potential to cause myelosuppression.*

Table 20-2 Possible Effect of Organ Dysfunction on Dosing of Select Chemotherapeutic Agents

Drug	Critical Organ	Dose Modifications
Bleomycin	Kidney	Decrease initial dose by as much as 50%–75% if creatinine clearance is <25 ml/min/m^2.
Carboplatin	Kidney	Dose reduction is directly proportional to creatinine clearance.
Cisplatin	Kidney	Do not use with clinically evident renal failure; use caution in animals with any renal problems.
Cyclophosphamide	Kidney, liver	Decrease initial dose by as much as 50%–75% if creatinine clearance is <25 ml/min/m^2; because the liver is needed to activate the drug, liver disease may warrant dose modification.
Doxorubicin	Liver	Initial dose reductions of as much as 50% when bilirubin is >1.5 mg/dl.
Methotrexate	Kidney	Dose reduction is directly proportional to creatinine clearance.
Vinblastine	Liver	Dose reduction is directly proportional to liver dysfunction.
Vincristine	Liver	Dose reduction is directly proportional to liver dysfunction.

8. For some drugs, the results of a biochemistry profile should be reviewed before the drug is administered. For example, lomustine (CCNU) can result in liver failure if not discontinued when serum alanine aminotransferase activity rises; carboplatin may be poorly excreted when renal dysfunction is present, resulting in more severe myelosuppression than would be predicted.

INTRAVENOUS ADMINISTRATION

Many chemotherapeutic agents are administered IV. Because some of these agents are vesicants or irritants, every attempt must be made to ensure that the veins are cared for and that catheters are placed as cleanly and atraumatically as possible. As a general rule, peripheral veins should be preserved for catheter placement only and should never be used for venipuncture to collect blood samples. Chemotherapeutic agents are usually administered by butterfly catheter, over-the-needle catheter, through-the-needle intracatheter (such as used for central venous access), or vascular access port. Vascular access ports can be placed subcutaneously and the catheter placed in a free-flowing vein such as the jugular.

Peripheral vessels are preferred for IV drug administration because of the ease of monitoring for drug extravasation. Regardless of the type of catheter used, certain preparatory steps should be taken. The leg to be used should be clipped at the site of injection and prepared using aseptic technique. When a drug is known to be a vesicant, an indwelling catheter or a vascular access device should be placed, particularly if the drug is not being administered as a bolus.

Drugs should never be administered when venipuncture is less than perfect (i.e., when the vein is entered more than once); another leg should be used instead. If another leg is unavailable, the first venipuncture site should be allowed to clot before another attempt is made proximal to that site. A second venipuncture should never be attempted distal to the site of a failed attempt. It is a good idea to alternate and record the veins being used to allow them to recover between administrations.

The catheter should be flushed with nonheparinized 0.9% NaCl (minimum, 10 ml) before and after each drug administration to determine patency. When multiple drugs are being given, the catheter should be flushed between agents. Nonheparinized 0.9% NaCl is recommended because heparin causes precipitates to form when mixed with some drugs (e.g., doxorubicin).

> **KEY POINT**
> *Any chemotherapeutic agent that is administered intravenously should be given through a "first-stick" patent catheter to prevent extravasation of the drug.*

The catheter and leg should be monitored constantly during drug administration to detect any extravasation. If the catheter is to be secured, use only one piece of tape and ensure that visualization of the injection site, the area surrounding the site, and the leg proximal to the site is not obscured.

It is important to check whether there is a specific rate at which a drug should be administered to minimize toxicity. For example, undiluted doxorubicin should be given at a maximum rate of 1 ml/min, whereas vincristine can be given as a bolus. Alternatively, doxorubicin can be placed in 35 ml of 0.9% NaCl and administered over 10 to 15 minutes. The drug should be injected slowly and evenly to prevent excessive pressure to the vein and leakage of drug around the needle or catheter.

After the drug has been administered and the catheter flushed, a piece of gauze or an alcohol-soaked cottonball should be placed (with a gloved hand) over the needle as it is withdrawn from the injection port or over the catheter as it is removed from the vein; this minimizes drug aerosolization. All of the drug should be flushed through the catheter without reaspirating the catheter, as reaspiration at this time allows diluted drug to remain in the catheter. A cottonball can be taped over the insertion site after the catheter is removed and pressure applied for several minutes.

All materials should be discarded into appropriate chemotherapy waste containers. Syringes and needles should be placed in a puncture- and leakproof container that is clearly marked as containing hazardous or chemotherapy waste. Even though latex gloves are always worn, it is important to wash hands thoroughly after every drug administration.

Butterfly Catheter

A butterfly catheter is generally recommended when administering a small amount (≤3 ml) of drug as a bolus. When using a butterfly catheter, all materials should be organized and readily available (within arm's reach) before starting. Equipment needed includes two to three 3- to 5-ml syringes of nonheparinized 0.9% NaCl for flushing the catheter, the labeled drug, an alcohol swab, the butterfly catheter with an injection port attached, and a pressure bandage. The labeled syringes should be placed on a pad or plastic bag and lined up in order of use. The needles should be removed (or the caps loosened) to help the administration proceed swiftly and smoothly.

When all of the drug has been delivered, the port and catheter should be flushed with saline.

Intravenous Over-the-Needle Catheter

Generally, drugs that are to be given as a bolus (but over a period of minutes) or in a volume greater than 3 ml are given through IV over-the-needle catheters. Over-the-needle catheters should be used for doxorubicin administration, for which a slow rate of delivery is important to prevent an allergic reaction. It is preferable to place the catheter while wearing latex gloves, but the catheter may be placed before drugs are prepared as long as patency is reconfirmed before drug administration.

For over-the-needle catheter administration, long, clear, male-adapter injection ports allow better viewing of the flashback of blood and the drug being administered. In addition, these plugs allow the person administering the drug to determine when all of the drug has been flushed out of the catheter at the end of the procedure.

Once the catheter has been placed, a 4 × 4–inch gauze square should be folded in half and slipped under the injection cap to absorb any drug that may leak out of the injection cap during administration. Needles should be inserted as far as possible into the injection port to allow easier flushing of residual drug after injection.

Continuous Intravenous Infusion

An indwelling catheter should be used when drugs (e.g., cytosine arabinoside, ifosfamide) are to be administered over a long period (6 to 48 hours)[1,11-13] or for saline diuresis that accompanies administration of nephrotoxic drugs such as cisplatin or streptozotocin. In these administrations, an infusion pump is recommended. Free-flowing fluid administration, even when monitored continuously, may not ensure continued diuresis or could result in uneven delivery of the drug dose. Both can affect the risk for toxicity. A calibrated infusion pump will allow predictable administration of the chemotherapy dose. The catheter site and all connections in the IV line should be monitored frequently for patency and leakage. The patient must be prevented from chewing on or disconnecting the IV line.

During long periods of drug administration, disposal of contaminated waste, particularly urine, becomes important. When the patient or any waste is handled, latex gloves, a gown, goggles, and a mask should be worn to reduce the risk for exposure to excreted active metabolites. Cages, runs, or excreta should not be hosed down because this aerosolizes the drug and distributes it more widely. All waste, including litter material, should be discarded as contaminated material.

Subcutaneous Infusion Port

Many veterinary patients are small, and their vascular integrity may be compromised by multiple anesthesias (surgery, radiation therapy) before chemotherapy. With the risk for extravasation reactions being high in these patients, an indwelling, subcutaneously located implantable vascular access port may ensure timely drug delivery and also reduce patient stress during restraint for catheter placement and administration of chemotherapy. Such a port may be maintained for the duration of the chemotherapy protocol and then removed. The implantable vascular access port must be placed surgically, in a similar manner to a tunneled catheter, with a subcutaneous pocket for positioning of the port. Ports for veterinary patients are available from Norfolk Vet Products, Skokie, Illinois.

INTRAMUSCULAR OR INTRALESIONAL ADMINISTRATION

IM injections are administered in the normal fashion, but latex gloves should be worn. Because L-asparaginase can cause an anaphylactic reaction when given intravenously, the syringe must be checked for blood to ensure that a vessel has not been inadvertently entered before injecting the drug intramuscularly. Preferred sites of injection include well-muscled areas such as the caudal thigh region or lumbar musculature.

> **KEY POINT**
>
> *Anaphylaxis caused by the administration of L-asparaginase can be reduced substantially if the drug is administered intramuscularly rather than intravenously or intraperitoneally.*

Intralesional chemotherapy is always administered as a suspension in oil or another vehicle, not as pure drug. Latex gloves, goggles, and a protective gown should be worn when administering intralesional chemotherapy, and it is important to watch the area carefully for any leakage of chemotherapeutic agent. If leakage occurs, the area should be swabbed and cleaned with soap and water and the cleaning materials disposed of as hazardous waste. When the needle is repositioned during intralesional therapy, there is often pressure on the syringe contents that will cause the mixture to leak out when the needle is withdrawn from the tumor. Negative pressure on the syringe when withdrawing will help reduce leakage.

ORAL ADMINISTRATION

Wearing latex gloves is necessary when administering pills. The patient is given the pills in the normal fashion. It is important to ensure that the patient has indeed swallowed the pill; it may be helpful to follow pill administration with water given via syringe. If owners are to administer oral chemotherapy, they must be instructed to wear disposable protective latex gloves and wash their hands immediately after administration.

INTRACAVITARY ADMINISTRATION

Some chemotherapeutic agents (e.g., cisplatin, carboplatin, mitoxantrone) can be administered into body cavities (thorax, abdomen, pericardial sac, urinary bladder).[1,4] Both the person administrating the drug and the one restraining the animal should wear gloves. As with IV administration, the IV line needs to be primed *before* the drug is added to the bag. The diluent should be warmed to body temperature or slightly above before the drug is added and the solution administered.

For thoracic and abdominal administration, and particularly for pericardial administration, ultrasonographic guidance may be very helpful in avoiding needle puncture of organs and other structures.

For thoracic administration, the patient is placed in lateral recumbency and the injection site is aseptically prepared. The right side is preferred, and the area of the cardiac notch provides the least risk of lung puncture. The area is infiltrated with lidocaine, and an 18-gauge rigid plastic IV cannula is inserted between the ribs and flushed with a minimum of 12 ml of warm saline to ensure a patent pathway. If there is resistance to the flush or if the dog appears uncomfortable or coughs, the cannula should be removed and a new one inserted.

For abdominal administration, the patient is placed in dorsal recumbency and a midline site caudal to the umbilicus is used. The site chosen should be caudal enough to avoid the spleen. Allowing the patient to urinate before administration reduces the risk of bladder puncture. The site is aseptically prepared and the catheter placed as described for thoracic administration.

Once patency is determined, the fluid line is attached and the drug is administered. A maximum volume of 250 ml/m^2 should be infused into the thoracic cavity and 1,000 ml/m^2 into the abdominal cavity to ensure adequate exposure of all surfaces with minimal discomfort to the patient. The fluid should flow fairly easily into the cavity. If the fluid drip slows or is intermittent, the cannula can be adjusted slightly. The area should be monitored constantly to make sure the fluid is not being administered SC. Once the bag is empty, the IV line should be turned off; a piece of gauze should be wrapped around the cannula and the cannula slowly removed. At this point, the person restraining the animal should hold an alcohol-moistened gauze square over the site and apply pressure to stop any bleeding or leakage that may occur. Finally, the patient should be allowed to move around for a few minutes to allow the drug to distribute through the entire cavity. All materials must be discarded as contaminated waste.

REFERENCES

1. *OSHA Work Practice Guidelines for Personnel: Dealing with Cytotoxic Drugs.* OSHA Instructional Publication 8-1.1, Washington DC, Office of Occupational Medicine, 1986.
2. Nikula E, Kiviniitty K, Leisti J, Taskinen P: Chromosome aberrations in lymphocytes of nurses handling cytostatic agents. *Scand J Work Environ Health* 10:71–74, 1984.
3. Norppa H, Sorsa M, Vainio H, et al: Increased sister chromatid exchange frequencies in lymphocytes of nurses handling cytostatic drugs. *Scand J Work Environ Health* 6:299–301, 1980.
4. Pohlova H, Cerna M, Rossner P: Chromosomal aberrations, SCE and urine mutagenicity in workers occupationally exposed to cytostatic drugs. *Mutat Res* 174:213–217, 1986.
5. Stiller A, Obe G, Bool I, Pribilla W: No elevation of the frequencies of chromosomal aberrations as a consequence of handling cytostatic drugs. *Mutat Res* 121:253–259, 1983.
6. Stucker I, Hirsch A, Doloy T, et al: Urine mutagenicity, chromosomal abnormalities and sister chromatid exchanges in lymphocytes of nurses handling cytostatic drugs. *Int Arch Occup Environ Health* 57:195–205, 1986.
7. Hemminki, K, Kyyronen P, Lindbohm ML: Spontaneous abortions and malformations in the offspring of nurses exposed to anaesthetic gases, cytostatic drugs, and other potential hazards in hospitals, based on registered information of outcome. *J Epidemiol Commun Health* 39:141–147, 1985.
8. Selevan SG, Lindbolm ML, Hornung RW, Hemminki K: A study of occupational exposure to antineoplastic drugs and fetal loss in nurses. *N Engl J Med* 313:1173–1178, 1985.

9. Stucker I, Caillard JF, Collin R, et al: Risk of spontaneous abortion among nurses handling antineoplastic drugs. *Scand J Work Environ Health* 16:102–107, 1990.
10. Rosner F: Acute leukemia as a delayed consequence of cancer chemotherapy. *Cancer* 37:1033–1036, 1976.
11. Chabner BA: Principles of cancer therapy, in Wyngaarden JB, Smith LH (eds): *Cecil Textbook of Medicine.* Philadelphia, WB Saunders, 1982, p 1032.
12. Takada S: Principles of chemotherapy safety procedures. *Clin Tech Small Anim Pract* 18(2):73–74, 2003.
13. Ogilvie GK: Principles of oncology, in Morgan RV (ed): *Handbook of Small Animal Internal Medicine.* Philadelphia, Churchill Livingstone, 1992, pp 799–812.
14. Wick C, Slawson MH, Jorgenson JA, et al: Using a closed-system protective device to reduce personnel exposure to antineoplastic agents. *Am J Health Syst Pharm* 60(22):2314–2320, 2003.

CHEMOTHERAPY: PROPERTIES, USES, AND PATIENT MANAGEMENT

Gregory K. Ogilvie and Antony S. Moore

CLINICAL BRIEFING

Common Drugs	Potential Toxicoses	Reported Indications
Alkylating Agents		
Chlorambucil	BAG, cerebellar toxicity	Chronic lymphocytic leukemia, lymphoma
Cyclophosphamide	BAG, sterile hemorrhagic cystitis	Lymphoma, sarcoma, mammary adenocarcinoma
Dacarbazine	BAG	Lymphoma, sarcoma
Hydroxyurea	BAG, anemia	Myelogenous leukemia, primary erythrocytosis
Ifosfamide	BAG, sterile hemorrhagic cystitis	Soft tissue sarcoma, lymphoma, hemangiosarcoma
Lomustine (CCNU)	Bone marrow suppression, alopecia, cumulative thrombocytopenia, hepatic and renal toxicity	Lymphoma, mycosis fungoides, mast cell tumor, brain tumor
Mechlorethamine (mustargen)	BAG, perivascular slough	Lymphoma
Melphalan	BAG	Multiple myeloma
Procarbazine	BAG	Lymphoma
Streptozocin (streptozotocin)	Nephrotoxicity, emesis, occasional hypoglycemic-induced weakness postinfusion, alanine aminotransferase elevation	Insulinoma
Thiotepa	BAG	Transitional cell carcinoma
Antibiotics		
Bleomycin	Pulmonary fibrosis, BAG	Squamous cell carcinoma, lymphoma
Dactinomycin	BAG, perivascular slough	Lymphoma
Doxorubicin	BAG, perivascular slough, allergic reaction during administration, anorexia and weight loss, renal failure (rare), cardiomyopathy	Lymphoma, sarcoma (including hemangiosarcoma), thyroid carcinoma, mammary adenocarcinoma
Idarubicin	BAG	Lymphoma
Mitoxantrone	BAG	Lymphoma, mammary adenocarcinoma, squamous cell carcinoma
Plicamycin (mithramycin)	BAG, vesicant	Hypercalcemia of malignancy
Antimetabolites		
Cytarabine	BAG	Lymphoma, leukemia
5-Fluorouracil	Neurotoxicity, BAG	?Skin tumors, GI malignancies
Gemcitabine	BAG, neurotoxicity	?Hepatic and pancreatic carcinomas, lymphoma, bladder tumors
Methotrexate	BAG	Lymphoma

Common Drugs	Potential Toxicoses	Reported Indications
Enzymes		
L-Asparaginase; pegaspargase	Anaphylaxis, disseminated intravascular coagulopathy, pancreatitis, pain on injection	Lymphoma
Hormones		
Prednisone/prednisolone	GI toxicity, iatrogenic Cushing's syndrome	Lymphoma, mast cell tumor
Plant Alkaloids		
Vinblastine	BAG, peripheral neuropathy, perivascular slough	Lymphoma, mast cell tumor
Vincristine[a]	BAG, peripheral neuropathy, perivascular slough	Lymphoma, sarcoma, mast cell tumor, thrombocytopenia
Vinorelbine	BAG, peripheral neuropathy, perivascular slough	Pulmonary carcinoma, lymphoma
Miscellaneous Agents		
Amifostine	Hypotension, nausea	To reduce cisplatin or radiation toxicity
Carboplatin	BAG, nephrotoxicity (rare), emesis (rare)	Osteosarcoma, squamous cell carcinoma, germinal cell tumor, transitional cell carcinoma
Cisplatin	BAG, nephrotoxicity, ototoxicity	Osteosarcoma, squamous cell carcinoma, transitional cell carcinoma
Dexrazoxane	GI toxicity	To reduce doxorubicin-induced cardiotoxicity
Epoetin alfa	Hypertension, fever, lethargy	Cancer-related anemia
Gallium nitrate	Nephrotoxicity, nausea, vomiting, diarrhea	Hypercalcemia of malignancy
Isotretinoin	Keratoconjunctivitis sicca, hypertriglyceridemia, hepatotoxicity	Cutaneous neoplasms such as sebaceous adenoma, mycosis fungoides
Mesna	GI toxicity	To prevent cystitis secondary to ifosfamide toxicity
Mitotane	Signs associated with hypoadrenocorticism	Adrenocortical carcinoma
Paclitaxel	BAG, diluent Cremophor EL and alcohol cause an acute allergic reaction, hypotension, and collapse on administration	Mammary adenocarcinoma, osteosarcoma, malignant histiocytosis (preliminary data)
Pamidronate disodium	Nephrotoxicity, emesis	Bone metastasis, osteosarcoma
Piroxicam	GI ulceration and nephrotoxicity	Transitional cell carcinoma, squamous cell carcinoma, pain relief
Thalidomide	Somnolence, fatigue, GI toxicity	Multiple myeloma, ?hemangiosarcoma

[a]Bone marrow suppression is dose dependent.

Unfortunately, most people are just as frightened of chemotherapeutic agents as they are of cancer itself. A great deal of this fear is due to preconceived, incorrect notions about the toxicity of chemotherapy and the danger involved in handling these drugs (see Chapter 20). To dispel the myths and misconceptions associated with chemotherapy, the entire veterinary health care team must be very aware of the properties, benefits, and risks associated with anticancer agents. When dealing with clients and outside members of the cancer care team, it is very important to discuss the preconceived notions they have about chemotherapy while outlining the real issues involved. By discussing and preventing the perceived toxicities associated with the use of chemotherapeutic agents, we can meet the nonmedical needs and fears of our clients. Preventing toxicities before they occur and aggressively treating them if they do occur are essential to meeting the medical needs of the patient.

General Principles of Cancer Therapy

Before a therapeutic strategy can be defined and instituted, the patient should be fully evaluated and stabilized and the tumor identified histologically and staged to determine the extent of disease. In addition, the client, the veterinarian, and the rest of the veterinary health care team need to be aware of the following:

- The potential benefits and toxicoses associated with the administration of chemotherapeutic agents. All parties should be committed to preventing toxicosis from developing and promptly resolving it if it does occur.
- The need to follow the treatment protocol, including timing, dosages, and treatment intervals, when possible.
- The expenses associated with chemotherapy (fortunately, many chemotherapeutic agents are becoming available as generic products at a fraction of the cost of the patented parent drug).
- The time and expertise required to provide optimal treatment.

When a practice decides to provide chemotherapy, the following management decisions must be made:

- Chemotherapy must be available for routine use.
- Ideally, localized solid malignancies should be removed surgically to the greatest extent possible before therapy.
- Adjuvant chemotherapy should begin as soon after surgery as possible while maintaining quality of life.
- Therapy should be given at appropriate dosages for limited periods of time.
- Procedures should be set up to manage urgent care situations 24 hours a day.
- Clients should be given oral and written information about the chemotherapeutic agents and protocol being used as well as medication that can prevent nausea, vomiting, diarrhea, and anorexia (e.g., metoclopramide).

Chemotherapeutic agents are used to induce remission and for intensification, consolidation, and maintenance therapy. The following definitions are important when discussing classical clinical chemotherapy:

- **Remission:** *Complete remission* exists when all clinical evidence of a tumor has disappeared. In contrast, the term *partial remission* is often used when the sum of the products of the two longest diameters of the tumor in question is reduced in size by at least 50% and there is no additional evidence of new tumors anywhere. Progressive disease occurs when the tumor increases in size by at least 50% of the sum of the products of the two largest diameters.
- **Adjuvant treatment:** After surgery, adjuvant chemotherapy may be given to slow the progress of metastatic disease or to potentially provide a cure. The optimum time to administer primary chemotherapy is when the patient has microscopic disease rather than when there are gross metastases. An example of successful adjuvant veterinary chemotherapy is the use of platinum compounds and doxorubicin after surgery for canine osteosarcoma.
- **Intensification,** which is introduced after remission has been obtained, involves the administration of chemotherapeutic agents with different mechanisms of action in an attempt to kill any resistant tumor cells.
- **Consolidation,** which also takes place after a patient is in remission, is the phase of treatment in which different drugs are administered to improve clinical response by reducing the microscopic tumor burden.
- **Maintenance therapy** refers to the drugs used to keep the patient in remission. Consolidation and maintenance therapies are more important in the treatment of hematopoietic tumors (e.g., lymphoma) than solid tumors (e.g., carcinoma, sarcoma). Chemotherapeutic agents also can be used as *adjuvant therapy* after another treatment modality to delay recurrence and increase survival time.
- **Neoadjuvant therapy** is used to decrease the bulk of primary tumors with chemotherapy before surgery or radiation.
- **Cancer prevention by delay** is defined as the use of treatments to enhance the disease-free interval, survival, and quality of life after surgery, chemotherapy, or radiation.[1] It is based on the use of treatments designed to reduce the rate of cancer development or incidence after surgery. While the ultimate goal for the treatment of high-grade malignancies is to eliminate all evidence of cancer, resulting in a cure, this goal is often not accomplished unless

Stages of a Combination Treatment Protocol[2-6]

Induction is the often intensely scheduled initial treatments during which a patient has a relatively higher risk of toxicity but usually also the greatest chance of response; (e.g., the first 12 weeks of VELCAP [vincristine, L-asparaginase, cyclophosphamide, doxorubicin, prednisone]).

Consolidation is sometimes used at the end of induction using unrelated, effective drugs to further reduce the proportion of surviving cancer cells (e.g., MOPP [mechlorethamine, vincristine, procarbazine, and prednisone] and lomustine with VELCAP).

Maintenance is a less intense (usually decreased frequency of administration) phase using drugs already given during induction. Maintenance therapy probably has little influence on whether an animal is cured but may prolong survival in animals by slowing the time to relapse.

Rescue is a term used for therapy given at a point when drugs used during the other three phases no longer result in remission. Unrelated drugs, often alkylating agents because they are less likely to show cross-resistance, are used in the rescue setting.

additional therapies can be initiated. Cancer prevention by delay is currently of great interest, in part because the National Cancer Institute is redefining cancer and cancer therapy. Cancer has traditionally been defined as a chronic disease. With many of the molecular cancer therapies available today, the goal is not to eliminate the cancer but to arrest its growth to prevent it from becoming a clinically evident problem. The importance of this approach is underscored by the fact that, despite decades of intense effort and billions of dollars of expenditure, the cure rate by traditional approaches (i.e., chemotherapy, radiotherapy, and surgery) has remained elusive in human and veterinary patients. Cancer prevention by delay is an important mechanism behind the successes of several therapeutic agents.[1] Studies have shown the following:

— **Tamoxifen** significantly diminishes the risk for breast cancer in humans, but this has not been documented in dogs.
— **Retinoids and interferon-α** reduce the risk for head and neck cancer in some human and rodent tumors. **Tretinoin** has been beneficial in treating mycosis fungoides in dogs.
— **NSAIDs** delay or reduce the development of colorectal cancer.
— **Polyunsaturated fatty acids of the n-3 series** decrease the risk for breast cancer recurrence in women and lymphoma in dogs.
— **Antiangiogenesis agents** reduce the risk for cancer recurrence.

The delay of cancer growth and development, also known as *clinical cancer chemoprevention*, is a valuable clinical tool until permanent or absolute cancer prevention can be achieved. Piroxicam may delay tumor regrowth after surgery or other traditional modalities used against transitional cell carcinoma and head and neck squamous cell carcinoma in dogs.

The beneficial effects of chemotherapy are inversely proportional to tumor size; therefore, when anticancer drugs are being used as adjuvants, the tumor should be reduced to its smallest volume and lowest number of cells, such as with surgery or radiation therapy, before chemotherapy is initiated. To use chemotherapeutic agents to their fullest advantage, clinicians should be knowledgeable about a drug's indications for use, doses, timing of administration, resistance, and toxicity. Chemotherapy should be considered for patients with such malignancies as leukemia, lymphoma, multiple myeloma, and other hematopoietic tumors or with highly malignant tumors that metastasize rapidly.

Drugs

Chemotherapy-induced cures are possible with combination chemotherapy protocols but almost never with single-agent protocols. Each drug in a combination protocol *must* be effective for the treatment of the cancer in question. Compared with multiple-drug regimens, single-drug regimens are less toxic, less expensive, and require less time for clients and the veterinary health care team. However, multiple-drug protocols are believed to be more effective—especially for lym-

> *Chemotherapy-induced cures are possible with combination chemotherapy protocols and almost never with single-agent protocols.*

phoid malignancies—because the drugs may have different mechanisms of action and resistance develops more slowly. Currently in veterinary medicine, however, few multiple-drug protocols have been shown to be more effective than single-agent protocols for the treatment of nonlymphoid malignancies. This is probably because the doses used to treat dogs with cancer are an order of magnitude lower than those used in human cancer patients. The stages of a combination treatment protocol are described in the box on this page.

When drugs are used in combination, several important points must be kept in mind[2-6]:

- Each drug must be effective when used alone to treat a specific malignancy.
- Combinations of drugs with overlapping toxicities should be avoided unless they are arranged in a protocol to prevent superimposition of toxicoses.

- Drugs should be used with an intermittent treatment schedule for maximum efficacy.
- Combined chemotherapeutics are most effective when they have different mechanisms of action and act at different stages of the cell cycle.

DOSES

With few exceptions, the most effective dose of chemotherapeutic agents is very close to the toxic dose. In addition, a given dose of a drug kills a constant fraction of cells regardless of the number of cells present at the start of therapy. Doses of chemotherapeutic agents are often given on the basis of metabolic rate, described as body surface area in square meters. All antineoplastic agents seem to be metabolized or excreted in a complex fashion and thus should be dosed on a square-meter basis. Table 20-1 provides a chart for converting weight in kilograms to body surface area. Be extremely cautious *not* to use the weight in pounds when reading the kilogram chart. This can result in serious toxicity.

> **KEY POINT**
>
> *The response to chemotherapy is inversely proportional to the amount of tumor present—the smaller the better! In addition, the success of therapy is directly related to appropriate drug selection, dosages, and timing of therapy.*

Dosing and toxicity can depend on many factors, including an animal's ability to metabolize and eliminate chemotherapeutic agents. Table 20-2 reviews organ dysfunction that would lead to altered drug metabolism and the way in which doses may need to be changed. While there are no established guidelines, it may be safest to reduce the dose of hepatically metabolized drugs by 50% if the serum bilirubin is greater than 1.5 mg/dl and by 75% if serum bilirubin is greater than 3.0 mg/dl. Doses can then be slowly increased following each cycle that occurs without toxicity.

> **KEY POINT**
>
> *The most effective dose of chemotherapeutic agents is often very close to the toxic dose, and thus careful client education and vigilant medical monitoring and care are essential. In some cases, as with paclitaxel and etoposide, the vehicle used to keep the drug into solution may result in as much or more risk of toxicity than the chemotherapeutic agent itself.*

Because carboplatin is renally excreted, the carboplatin dose should ideally be based on the glomerular filtration rate. If the glomerular filtration rate cannot be estimated, an arbitrary dose reduction of 50% to 75% should be followed for animals with renal azotemia, after which the dose can be increased after each cycle with no toxicity.

TIMING

The timing of administration of antitumor drugs is critical. Unlike many tumor cells, normal cells have repair mechanisms that are able to correct cellular damage. Therefore, cytotoxic drugs must be given at proper intervals to allow the tumor cells to die while normal cells recover. An improper administration schedule results in either excess toxicity or a lack of antitumor activity.

RESISTANCE

In contrast to normal cells, most tumor cells develop resistance to antitumor medicine. Resistance is one of the limiting factors in tumor chemotherapy. This resistance results from an acquired or induced phenomenon known as *multiple-drug resistance*, which is caused by a cell membrane protein that literally pumps out cellular toxins such as chemotherapeutic agents. Because chemotherapeutics diffuse into cells passively, the pump mechanism is able to prevent intracellular accumulation of these drugs. Certain anticancer drugs (e.g., doxorubicin, paclitaxel) are eliminated from the cell by this mechanism even though they have different molecular structures. Fortuitously, there seems to be little cross-resistance among alkylating agents (e.g., cyclophosphamide, chlorambucil, melphalan). Resistance to other drugs, such as the enzyme L-asparaginase, is induced when antibodies are formed against the drug, thereby causing a rapid destruction of the substance after administration.

> **KEY POINT**
>
> *Resistance of a tumor to chemotherapy is a consistent and ever-present threat. Use chemotherapeutic agents at appropriate doses and schedules from the outset to minimize resistance.*

TOXICITY

Select chemotherapeutic agents and their toxicities are noted in the Clinical Briefing at the beginning of this chapter and in Table 21-1. Most of these agents kill or damage rapidly dividing cells. The most clinically important toxicoses include bone marrow suppression, alopecia, and gastrointestinal toxicity. Together, they are referred to by the acronym *BAG*. Methods of identifying and treating some of the more common side effects follow.

Bone Marrow Toxicity

Many antitumor drugs cause a decrease in the number of blood cells present in the body days to weeks after administration (see the box on page 121, "Myelosuppressive Potential of Some Commonly Used Chemotherapeutic Agents in Veterinary Medicine"). Neutropenia and thrombocytopenia are early signs of bone marrow suppression. Clinical signs may include those related to sepsis, petechial and ecchymotic hemorrhages, pallor, and weakness. Many animals are physically normal despite low leukocyte and platelet counts; therefore, only patients exhibiting clinical signs should be treated. The treatment of clinically significant bone marrow toxicity includes using aseptic techniques when placing indwelling devices (e.g., catheters), minimizing trauma, and controlling any bleeding with prolonged application of direct pressure or cold packs.

If an animal develops a fever or becomes septic, urine, blood, and, if indicated, material obtained via transtracheal aspiration should be analyzed and cultured immediately before the initiation of therapy unless the delay is likely to be life threatening. The affected animal should be treated with broad-spectrum bactericidal antibiotics (e.g., cephalosporins, sulfamethoxazole–trimethoprim) until results of culture and sensitivity testing are available. Do not delay antibiotic treatment while awaiting culture results. In addition, the patient should be supported with fluids, warmth, and nutritional therapy and given transfusions of fresh whole blood (collected in plastic containers) or specific cell lines as needed.

The availability of recombinant human granulocyte colony-stimulating factor now makes it possible to treat bone marrow toxicity by boosting endogenous production of neutrophils. The drug(s) that induced the bone marrow suppression should be discontinued until blood counts have recovered, and subsequent doses should be reduced (e.g., decrease cyclophosphamide doses by 25%).

Administration of sulfamethoxazole–trimethoprim to dogs for 14 days from the day of treatment with doxorubicin markedly reduces the likelihood of gastrointestinal (GI) toxicity (vomiting or diarrhea), hospitalization, and lower quality of life (modified Karnofsky score). This effect was most marked in dogs with lymphoma[7] and may be due to reduced bacterial translocation in damaged intestinal epithelial layers.

Anemia may develop later in response to the administration of chemotherapeutic agents, but, unlike neutropenia, it is rarely acute or severe because red blood cells have a longer life span. It is not uncommon for dogs to present with mild anemia due to chronic disease before chemotherapy.

Recombinant human erythropoietin may be useful in treating dogs with nonregenerative anemia secondary to chemotherapy or the underlying malignancy. Human cancer patients treated with erythropoietin for anemia report that they have greater energy and a better quality of life while on chemotherapy. No similar data exist for dogs. Caution is advised when using recombinant human products because antibodies to these foreign proteins can develop in approximately 3 to 6 weeks and occasionally may react with the patient's own hematopoietic growth factors.

Alopecia

Alopecia is an uncommon complication of chemotherapy but often a major concern of caregivers. Dogs can lose their whiskers, but the development of generalized alopecia is relatively uncommon except in dogs with constantly growing hair coats, such as poodles, schnauzers, Old English sheep dogs, and terriers. Coat color and texture changes, however, are common during prolonged courses of chemotherapy. Light skin may turn dark, and dark skin may turn light.

Gastrointestinal Toxicity

The clinical signs of this relatively common side effect include vomiting, anorexia, and diarrhea. Diagnostics should proceed to eliminate non–chemotherapy-induced causes, such as internal parasites, giardiasis, and clostridial colitis. The treatment varies depending on the cause but may include antiemetics (e.g., metoclopramide, dolasetron, ondansetron), protectants and absorbents (e.g., bismuth-containing compounds [e.g., Pepto Bismol]), and broad-spectrum antibiotics, if indicated. In addition, support with

> **KEY POINT**
> *Signs of L-asparaginase hypersensitivity include urticaria, vomiting, diarrhea, hypotension, and loss of consciousness soon after administration.*

fluids, warmth, and nutritional therapy should be provided. As a preventive measure, some clinicians dispense metoclopramide to the client to initiate therapy at home when a medication with the potential to cause nausea is administered. Clients may be instructed to give metoclopramide, even if nausea and vomiting are not noted, both as a preventive measure and because nausea may be difficult for caregivers to assess accurately. Metoclopramide is preferred because of its overall efficacy and lack of systemic side effects; chlorpromazine may induce the clinically worrisome side effect of sedation. Serotonin antagonists, such as dolasetron and ondansetron, are superior to metoclopramide, but the cost of these drugs is greater.

Anorexia in dogs can often be resolved with antiemetics, adequate hydration, pain relief, and administration of the appetite-stimulating drugs cyproheptadine and megestrol acetate. Subsequent doses of the specific chemotherapy agent that caused the anorexia should be reduced by 25%.

Table 21-1 Toxicities Associated with Some Commercially Available Anticancer Drugs and Hormones

Drug	Acute Toxicity	Delayed Toxicity
L-Asparaginase	Anaphylaxis or hypersensitivity (less likely if given IM), nausea and vomiting, fever, chills, abdominal pain, and hyperglycemia leading to coma	CNS depression or hyperexcitability, acute hemorrhagic pancreatitis, coagulation defects, thrombosis, renal damage, hepatic damage (not reported in dogs but seen in other species)
Bleomycin	Nausea and vomiting, fever, anaphylaxis, and other allergic reactions	Pneumonitis and pulmonary fibrosis, rash, alopecia
Busulfan	Nausea and vomiting and, rarely, diarrhea	Bone marrow suppression, pulmonary infiltrates and fibrosis, hyperpigmentation, alopecia, leukemia
Carmustine	Nausea and vomiting and local phlebitis	Leukopenia and thrombocytopenia (may be prolonged), pulmonary fibrosis (may be irreversible), renal damage, reversible liver damage
Chlorambucil	Bone marrow suppression, pulmonary infiltrates and fibrosis, leukemia, hepatic toxicity, and hallucinations	None
Cisplatin	Acute nephrotoxicity, nausea, vomiting	Neutropenia, thrombocytopenia, alopecia, delayed nausea, diarrhea, neuropathy, deafness
Cyclophosphamide	Nausea and vomiting and type I (anaphylactoid) hypersensitivity	Bone marrow suppression, hemorrhagic cystitis, bladder fibrosis and cancer, sterility (may be temporary), pulmonary infiltrates and fibrosis, hyponatremia, leukemia
Cytosine arabinoside	Nausea and vomiting, diarrhea, and anaphylaxis	Bone marrow suppression, oral ulceration, hepatic damage, fever (not reported in dogs but seen in other species)
Dacarbazine	Nausea and vomiting, diarrhea, anaphylaxis, and pain on administration	Bone marrow suppression, renal impairment, hepatic necrosis, photosensitivity, alopecia
Dactinomycin	Nausea and vomiting, diarrhea, local reaction and phlebitis, and anaphylactoid reaction	Stomatitis, oral ulceration, bone marrow suppression, alopecia, folliculitis, dermatitis in previously irradiated areas
Daunorubicin	Nausea and vomiting, diarrhea, severe local tissue damage and necrosis on extravasation, transient ECG changes, and anaphylactoid reaction	Bone marrow suppression, cardiotoxicity (may be irreversible), alopecia, anorexia, diarrhea, fever and chills
Doxorubicin	Nausea and vomiting, severe local tissue damage and necrosis on extravasation, diarrhea and colitis, transient ECG changes, ventricular arrhythmia, anaphylactoid reaction, and urticaria and pruritus after one injection	Bone marrow suppression, renal damage, cardiotoxicity, stomatitis, anorexia, diarrhea, fever, alopecia
Etoposide (VP16)[a]	Nausea and vomiting, profound hypotension, anaphylaxis, cutaneous reactions, diarrhea, and fever	Bone marrow suppression, peripheral neuropathy, allergic reactions, hepatic damage, alopecia
5-Fluorouracil[b]	Seizures and other neurotoxicity	Bone marrow suppression, alopecia, nausea
Hydroxyurea[c]	Nausea and vomiting	Bone marrow suppression, stomatitis, dysuria, alopecia
Lomustine (CCNU)	Nausea and vomiting	Delayed leukopenia and thrombocytopenia (may be prolonged), transient elevation of aminotransferase activity, neurologic reactions, pulmonary fibrosis
Mechlorethamine	Nausea and vomiting, local reaction, and phlebitis	Bone marrow suppression, diarrhea, oral ulcers, pulmonary infiltrates and fibrosis, leukemia, alopecia

Table 21-1 (continued)

Drug	Acute Toxicity	Delayed Toxicity
Melphalan	Mild nausea and hypersensitivity reactions	Bone marrow suppression (especially platelets), pulmonary infiltrates and fibrosis, leukemia
Mercaptopurine	Nausea and vomiting, diarrhea	Bone marrow suppression and cholestasis, hepatic necrosis (rare), oral and intestinal ulcers, pancreatitis
Methotrexate	Nausea and vomiting, diarrhea, fever, and anaphylaxis	Oral and GI ulcers, bone marrow suppression, hepatic toxicity (including cirrhosis)
Mitotane	Nausea and vomiting, diarrhea	Adrenal insufficiency, CNS depression, rash, albuminuria, hypertension
Mitoxantrone	Nausea and vomiting	Bone marrow suppression
Thiotepa	Nausea and vomiting, local pain and perivascular slough with extravasation	Bone marrow suppression, pulmonary infiltrates and fibrosis, leukemia
Vinblastine	Nausea and vomiting, local reaction and phlebitis with extravasation	Bone marrow suppression, stomatitis, loss of deep tendon reflexes, jaw pain, muscle pain, paralytic ileus, inappropriate ADH secretion, alopecia
Vincristine	Local slough with extravasation	Peripheral neuropathy, mild bone marrow suppression, constipation, paralytic ileus, inappropriate ADH secretion, hepatic damage, jaw pain, seizures, alopecia

[a]Not reported to be used in dogs.
[b]Not recommended in dogs.
[c]Still investigational in dogs.
ADH = antidiuretic hormone; *CNS* = central nervous system; *ECG* = electrocardiogram.
Adapted from Ogilvie GK: Principles of oncology, in Morgan RV (ed): *Handbook of Small Animal Internal Medicine.* Philadelphia, Churchill Livingstone, 1992, pp 799–812; with permission.

Allergic Reactions

Signs of L-asparaginase hypersensitivity include urticaria, vomiting, diarrhea, hypotension, and loss of consciousness soon after administration. These signs can essentially be eliminated by administering the medication intramuscularly. Doxorubicin- or paclitaxel-induced allergic reactions include cutaneous hyperemia, intense pruritus, head shaking, and vomiting during administration. These reactions are due to histamine release from mast cells and can be reduced substantially by slowing the infusion rate (e.g., give the entire dose over approximately 20 to 30 minutes). Other drugs that can induce allergic reactions include bleomycin, cytosine, and procarbazine. Both etoposide and paclitaxel induce dramatic cutaneous reactions and hypotension during administration, not because of the medication itself but rather the vehicle that keeps each drug in solution.

Treatment of allergic reactions includes immediately discontinuing drug administration and giving epinephrine, diphenhydramine, and glucocorticoids for acute allergic reactions. Premedication with diphenhydramine, cimetidine, and glucocorticoids may prevent or reduce allergic reactions to doxorubicin, paclitaxel, or etoposide; for doxorubicin, simply slowing the infusion rate is often sufficient to prevent allergic reactions during administration.

Cardiac Toxicity

Doxorubicin has been shown to induce dose-dependent dilated (congestive) cardiomyopathy and transient dysrhythmias during administration in dogs. Both can occur in dogs predisposed to cardiac disease or with underlying acquired myocardial disease. Until more is known, most oncologists limit the cumulative dose of doxorubicin to 180 to 240 mg/m^2 (six to eight treatments) during a dog's lifetime.

> **KEY POINT**
>
> *Anaphylaxis caused by the administration of L-asparaginase can be reduced substantially if the drug is administered intramuscularly rather than intravenously or intraperitoneally.*

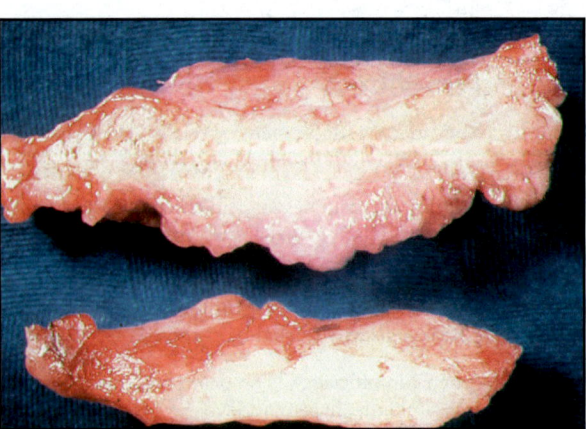

Figure 21-1. *Thickened bladder wall after cyclophosphamide administration. This adverse effect may be reduced by giving furosemide to enhance urine production and eliminate the amount of cyclophosphamide metabolites in the urine with increased urination.*

While the relative prevalence of doxorubicin-induced cardiotoxicity in dogs is unknown, routine echocardiograms and electrocardiograms should be conducted on dogs given more than 180 mg/m² of doxorubicin. Doxorubicin should be given with great caution in breeds that are predisposed to cardiomyopathy (e.g., Doberman pinscher, boxer).

> **KEY POINT**
>
> *Anaphylaxis caused by the administration of L-asparaginase can be reduced substantially if the drug is administered intramuscularly rather than intravenously or intraperitoneally.*

Cystitis

Cyclophosphamide and ifosfamide have been reported to induce sterile chemical cystitis in dogs (Figure 21-1). Cyclophosphamide and ifosfamide are hepatically metabolized to their active forms as well as to compounds that can cause urothelial damage (acrolein). Prolonged contact time between the bladder wall and acrolein results in hemorrhagic cystitis. Clinical signs include stranguria, hematuria, and dysuria. Furosemide given as a single dose (2 mg/kg) at the time of cyclophosphamide administration almost completely abrogates this toxicity and is recommended even in dogs receiving concurrent prednisone. Allowing ample opportunity for the dog to void urine is equally important, and cyclophosphamide is preferably administered in the morning rather than late in the day. Mesna is a thiol drug that is active only in urine, binding to acrolein and avoiding the toxicity of urothelial damage. The cost of mesna is high, which usually limits its use to dogs receiving ifosfamide that have a much higher risk of urothelial damage.

Treatment of cystitis includes replacing cyclophosphamide with another alkylating agent (e.g., chlorambucil) or discontinuing the ifosfamide to prevent exacerbation of the condition. Secondary infections are common, so urine should be collected for culture and sensitivity testing any time cystitis is suspected. Appropriate antibiotics must be administered if cystitis becomes septic. If renal function is normal, piroxicam (0.3 mg/kg PO q24–48h) may be helpful in reducing adverse effects, and for prolonged cases, intravesicular dimethyl sulfoxide may accelerate recovery. Most cases resolve with time but may take several weeks to subside; therefore, this is a toxicity best prevented. The risk of developing cystitis can be decreased by administering cyclophosphamide in the morning (thereby allowing the animal maximum opportunity to urinate during the day), encouraging fluid intake (e.g., salting food), and, if a combination protocol that includes prednisone is being used, giving cyclophosphamide at the same time as the glucocorticoid (steroids tend to induce polydipsia and secondary polyuria). In addition, the administration of furosemide has been suggested to reduce cyclophosphamide-induced cystitis.

Nephrotoxicity

Cisplatin, streptozocin, and, less commonly, lomustine, doxorubicin, methotrexate, and carboplatin have been associated with the development of nephrotoxicity in dogs, especially those with preexisting renal disease. Identifying animals with evidence of kidney disease, ensuring adequate hydration, and eliminating the concurrent administration of nephrotoxic agents are essential steps to limit this problem.

Neurotoxicity

Cisplatin, vincristine, vinblastine, lomustine, and 5-fluorouracil are most commonly linked directly or indirectly to neurotoxicity in dogs. Peripheral neuropathy is associated with vincristine and vinblastine in humans but is rare in dogs; 5-fluorouracil has been shown to cause severe seizures and disorientation in dogs. Cisplatin can cause ototoxicity. Chlorambucil, when used at high dosages for prolonged periods, may be linked to central neurotoxicity. Lomustine and many other drugs may cause hepatotoxicity and subsequent disorders of the central nervous system.

> **KEY POINT**
>
> *Doxorubicin, dactinomycin, mechlorethamine, vincristine, and vinblastine have been known to cause severe localized cellulitis if they are extravasated.*

> **KEY POINT:** *Any chemotherapeutic agent administered intravenously should be given through a "first-stick" patent catheter to prevent drug extravasation.*

Local Dermatologic Toxicity

Doxorubicin, dactinomycin, mechlorethamine, vincristine, and vinblastine have been known to cause severe localized cellulitis if they are extravasated. Many other drugs are classified as irritants if administered perivascularly. These reactions and their prevention are discussed in detail in Chapter 39. Treatment includes stopping the injection, aspirating the drug and 5 ml of blood back into the syringe, and then withdrawing the syringe. For perivascular injections of vincristine and vinblastine, infiltrating the area with 4 to 6 ml of saline and approximately 8 mg of dexamethasone and then applying warm compresses may be helpful. In contrast, if doxorubicin is the extravasated agent, the area is *not* infused with saline, as this will enlarge the affected area. Cold packs should be applied to areas of doxorubicin extravasation and hot packs to areas of vincristine and vinblastine administration. Aggressive surgical debridement and skin grafts may be necessary for deep, ulcerative lesions.

Pulmonary Toxicity

Bleomycin has rarely been associated with the development of severe pulmonary fibrosis.

▶ SPECIFIC DRUGS USED IN VETERINARY CHEMOTHERAPY

Chemotherapeutic drugs can be classified as alkylating agents, antimetabolites, antibiotics, cytokines and hematopoietic growth factors, enzymes, hormones, plant alkaloids, topoisomerase-1 inhibitors, and other agents.

Alkylating Agents

Alkylating agents are cell-cycle–nonspecific drugs that act by cross-linking DNA.

BUSULFAN

Dose supplied: 2-mg tablets.

Dosage: 2 mg/m^2/day.

Route of administration: PO.

Storage: Room temperature.

Mechanism of action: Alkylating agent.

Metabolism: Well absorbed orally; metabolites are excreted in urine.

Toxicity: Myelosuppression is the major toxicity; thrombocytopenia may be particularly dangerous. Prolonged bone marrow suppression may occur. Pulmonary fibrosis has been reported in humans.

Note: Busulfan has been reported to be effective in the treatment of chronic myelogenous leukemia and polycythemia.

CHLORAMBUCIL

Dose supplied: 2-mg coated tablets.

Dosage: 6–8 mg/m^2/day; 0.1 mg/kg/day and 20 mg/m^2 PO q1–2wk.

Route of administration: PO.

Storage: Refrigerated.

Mechanism of action: Alkylating agent similar to mechlorethamine.

Metabolism: Well absorbed from the GI tract, but information on metabolism is incomplete.

Toxicity: BAG (alopecia primarily seen as whisker loss).

Note: Chlorambucil is used to treat lymphoma (especially when substituted for cyclophosphamide in patients with chemotherapy-induced sterile hemorrhagic cystitis) and chronic lymphocytic leukemia. Remission exceeding 1 year has often been reported in patients with chronic lymphocytic leukemia treated with chlorambucil.

CYCLOPHOSPHAMIDE

Dose supplied: 25- and 50-mg tablets; 100-, 200-, 500-mg and 1- and 2-g vials.

Dosage: 50 mg/m^2/day PO q3wk for 4–5 days or 250 mg/m^2 PO or IV q3wk. Adjust actual dose by rounding down to the next whole tablet based on tablet size. For example, a calculated total dose of 220 mg may result in a dosing regimen of approximately 50 mg PO q24h for four doses, or giving the exact dosage IV.

Route of administration: PO or IV, preferably in morning. May be mixed with any volume of saline for IV administration: If using the powdered form, shake well, allow to stand for 10–15 minutes so that crystals dissolve completely, and administer over 20–30 minutes. Concurrent administration of furosemide or glucocorticoids may decrease the occurrence of chemical-induced sterile hemorrhagic cystitis.

Storage: Vials of unreconstituted drug can be stored at room temperature; reconstituted solution should be used within 24 hours if stored at room temperature or 6 days if refrigerated.

Mechanism of action: Alkylating agent; prevents cell division by cross-linking strands of DNA.

Metabolism: Requires in vivo activation by enzymes (phosphamidase) in the liver and serum. Cyclophosphamide and its metabolites are excreted by the kidney. The dose should be reduced if serum creatinine levels are elevated and may require modification in the presence of liver disease.

Toxicity: Anorexia and vomiting occur frequently with IV administration and may begin 6 hours after drug administration. Oral administration may reduce the incidence of vomiting. Alopecia may be noted. Leukopenia (nadir: 7–14 days) may be the dose-limiting toxicity; recovery occurs 7–10 days after the nadir. Thrombocytopenia is usually not a problem. Sterile chemical cystitis may occur in some dogs treated with IV and PO cyclophosphamide as a result of chemical irritation of the bladder by cyclophosphamide metabolites; chemical irritation has been associated with the development of bladder tumors in dogs and humans. The risk of cystitis can be reduced by maintaining high fluid intake, frequent urination, morning administration, and concurrent use of a single dose of furosemide (2 mg/kg) as well as maintaining corticosteroids if they are part of the protocol. If cyclophosphamide-induced hemorrhagic cystitis occurs, the drug should be discontinued indefinitely and chlorambucil (6–8 mg/m^2/day PO) should be substituted.

Note: Cyclophosphamide is one of the most common and effective antineoplastic agents used in veterinary medicine. It is effective in treating lymphoma, soft tissue sarcomas (when combined with vincristine and/or doxorubicin), mammary neoplasia (when combined with doxorubicin), and other sarcomas.

DACARBAZINE (DTIC)
Dose supplied: 100- and 200-mg vials.

Dosage: 800 mg/m^2 q3–4 wk or 200 mg/m^2/day for 5 consecutive days q3wk.

Route of administration: IV infusion over 5 hours.

Storage: Refrigerated.

Mechanism of action: Nonclassic alkylating agent.

Metabolism: Metabolized by the liver; some excreted unchanged in urine.

Toxicity: Nausea and vomiting at administration controlled by single dose of dolasetron before drug is administered; diarrhea may occur. Myelosuppression (neutropenia) is seen.

Note: Dacarbazine has shown efficacy against lymphoma in dogs, particularly when administered with doxorubicin.

HYDROXYUREA
Dose supplied: 500-mg capsules.

Dosage: 50–80 mg/kg q3d. Rather than splitting capsules to meet dosing requirements, this drug may be prepared at a compounding pharmacy.

Route of administration: PO.

Storage: Room temperature.

Mechanism of action: Inhibits DNA synthesis.

Metabolism: Rapidly absorbed from the GI tract and excreted in urine.

Toxicity: Myelosuppression is often rapid and marked; thus, frequent monitoring of the leukocyte count is required and doses may need to be adjusted. This drug can cause anemia in dogs.

Note: Hydroxyurea has been used to treat chronic myelogenous leukemia and polycythemia (primary erythrocytosis).

IFOSFAMIDE
Dose supplied: 1- and 3-g vials (mesna is included in the package).

Dosage: 350 (dogs <10 kg) to 375 mg/m^2 q3wk.
- 1-g vial: Reconstitute with 20 ml 0.9% NaCl = 50 mg/ml.
- 3-g vial: Reconstitute with 30 ml 0.9% NaCl = 100 mg/ml.

Route of administration: IV as continuous infusion diluted in 0.9% NaCl and given over 30 minutes. Must be preceded (for 30 minutes) and followed (for 5 hours) by fluid diuresis (with 0.9% NaCl) at a rate of 18.3 ml/kg/hr. To help prevent hemorrhagic cystitis, mesna should be administered in three doses, each equal to 20% of the ifosfamide dose. Mesna is given as an IV bolus at the start of pretreatment diuresis and 2 and 5 hours after ifosfamide infusion.

Storage: Store unopened vials at room temperature. Reconstituted solution is chemically stable for 7 days at room temperature and for 6 weeks when refrigerated.

Mechanism of action: Alkylating agent.

Metabolism: Hepatic metabolism to active form (as for cyclophosphamide).

Toxicity: Myelosuppression (neutropenia; nadir: 1 week). Monitor serum creatinine and urinalysis before each treatment because hemorrhagic cystitis may occur; renal toxicity has been seen in humans.

Note: Ifosfamide has shown efficacy against soft tissue sarcoma and lymphoma in dogs.

LOMUSTINE (CCNU)
Dose supplied: 10-, 40-, and 100-mg capsules.

Dosage: 60–90 mg/m^2 q4–6wk.

Route of administration: PO.

Storage: Room temperature.

Mechanism of action: Alkylating agent.

Metabolism: Rapidly absorbed from the GI tract and metabolized by the liver.

Toxicity: Myelosuppression (neutropenia) can be rapid and marked (nadir: approximately 1 week but often 2–5 weeks). This drug can cause a cumulative thrombocytopenia. Hepatic and renal toxicities are possible and can be severe.

Note: CCNU has shown efficacy in the treatment of lymphoma and mast cell tumors in dogs. Because it is lipophilic, it has been effective in treating brain tumors in dogs.

MECHLORETHAMINE (MUSTARGEN)

Dose supplied: 10-mg vials.

Dosage: 3 mg/m^2 as per protocol (usually MOPP protocol; see Chapter 47).

Route of administration: Slow IV push. (Note: this is a strong vesicant when administered extravascularly.) Reconstitute vial with 10 ml 0.9% NaCl to concentration of 1 mg/ml.

Storage: Store unopened vials at room temperature; discard unused reconstituted material.

Mechanism of action: Nitrosourea alkylating agent.

Metabolism: Rapidly metabolized through spontaneous hydrolysis.

Toxicity: Myelosuppression (neutropenia) can be rapid and marked (nadir: 1 week). Nausea and vomiting may occur 30 minutes to 2 hours after administration and last for up to 8 hours. This drug is a strong vesicant and can cause tissue necrosis and sloughing if extravasated.

Note: Mechlorethamine has shown efficacy against lymphoma in dogs when used in combination protocols (e.g., MOPP).

MELPHALAN

Dose supplied: Scored 2-mg tablets; 500-mg vials.

Dosage: PO dose—0.1 mg/kg/day for 10 days, then 0.05 mg/kg/day; 2 mg/m^2/day for 7–10 days, then no therapy for 2–3 weeks (Note: Because of the tablet size, it may be necessary to have the drug compounded to an appropriate dose size).

Route of administration: PO or IV.

Storage: Refrigerate tablets; injectable solution must be used within 60 minutes of reconstitution.

Mechanism of action: Alkylating agent; cytotoxic action produced by cross-linking of DNA.

Metabolism: Absorption from GI tract; erratic metabolism.

Toxicity: Myelosuppression can be marked, and recovery may take up to 4 weeks. IV product may cause severe slough if injected perivascularly. Alopecia and GI signs may also be noted.

Note: Melphalan has been used for several years to treat multiple myeloma (also known as plasma cell myeloma). Remissions exceeding 1 year have frequently been reported.

PROCARBAZINE

Dose supplied: 50-mg capsules (10-mg capsules can be reformulated by a compounding pharmacy).

Dosage: 50 mg/m^2/day for 14 days.

Route of administration: PO.

Storage: Room temperature.

Mechanism of action: Nonclassic alkylating agent.

Metabolism: Rapidly absorbed from the GI tract and metabolized by the liver.

Toxicity: Myelosuppression (neutropenia) is seen in other species, but whether this occurs in dogs is uncertain because the drug is usually given concurrently with mechlorethamine. Nausea and vomiting occur commonly and can be dose limiting; diarrhea and anorexia also occur frequently. If these side effects are noted, cease drug administration and reinstitute when resolved with antinausea medications or at an every-other-day schedule; use prophylactic antinausea medications for future administration.

Note: Procarbazine has shown efficacy against lymphoma in dogs when used in combination protocols (e.g., MOPP).

STREPTOZOCIN (STREPTOZOTOCIN)

Dose supplied: 1-g vials.

Dosage: 500 mg/kg IV q2–3wk; IV saline at 18.3 ml/kg/hr for 7 hours. The dose of streptozocin is included in the infusion during hours 3 and 4. Butorphanol tartrate 0.4 mg/kg IM may be given at the end of the streptozocin portion of the infusion as an antiemetic, although ondansetron or dolasetron may be more effective.

Route of administration: IV.

Storage: Room temperature.

Mechanism of action: Nitrosourea alkylating agent. Selective toxicity for β cells.

Metabolism: Liver.

Toxicity: Nephrotoxicity, emesis, occasional hypoglycemia-induced weakness postinfusion, alanine aminotransferase elevation (usually resolves on discontinuing drug), diabetes.

Note: Streptozocin is used to treat insulinomas.

THIOTEPA
(TRIETHYLENE THIOPHOSPHORAMIDE)

Dose supplied: 15-mg vials.

Dosage: Maximum systemic dose is largely unknown but is thought to be 9 mg/m^2. Bladder instillation: 30 mg/m^2 q3–4wk; remove after 1 hour.

Route of administration: For intravesicular administration into the bladder, dilute 5–10 mg powder in 30 ml 0.9% NaCl. For systemic administration, give IM or SC. Drug may be administered into the pleural or abdominal cavity.

Storage: Refrigerated. The reconstituted solution is stable at 4°C for 5 days.

Mechanism of action: Alkylating agent; multiple cross-linking of DNA.

Metabolism: Unknown; 20% of the dose introduced into the bladder is absorbed systemically.

Toxicity: Myelosuppression is the dose-limiting toxicity; leukopenia and thrombocytopenia reach their nadir at 7–28 days; alopecia and GI signs may also be seen.

Note: Thiotepa has been used intravesicularly to treat transitional cell carcinoma of the bladder and intracavitarily for malignant pleural or peritoneal effusions.

Antibiotics

Antibiotics form stable complexes (intercalate) with DNA and therefore inhibit DNA or RNA synthesis.

BLEOMYCIN

Dose supplied: 15-U vials (1 U = 1 mg).

Dosage: 0.3–0.5 U/kg/wk IM or SC to total cumulative dose of 125–200 U/m^2. IV push over at least 10 minutes.

Route of administration: IM, SC; may be used intralesionally. May cause pain at injection site. IV administration should be slow (1 U/min).

Storage: Can be stored for 24 hours at room temperature, 1 to 2 months if refrigerated, and 2 years if frozen. Should not be used with heparin.

Mechanism of action: Antitumor antibiotic; inhibits DNA synthesis and, to a lesser extent, RNA and protein synthesis.

Metabolism: Rapidly excreted by the kidney. Dose should be decreased if serum creatinine level is elevated because of renal disease.

Toxicity: Pulmonary fibrosis has been reported in some species and seems to be dose related. A maximum cumulative dose of 200 mg/m^2 is recommended. Allergic reactions (fever) have been reported.

Note: Bleomycin has been suggested as a treatment for squamous cell carcinoma and, intralesionally, for acanthomatous epulis.

DACTINOMYCIN

Dose supplied: 0.5-mg vials.

Dosage: 0.5–0.9 mg/m^2 slow IV infusion q2–3wk.

Route of administration: Slow IV (over a minimum of 20 minutes); may cause pain at injection site.

Storage: Use within 24 hours of reconstitution because of the absence of preservatives.

Mechanism of action: Antitumor antibiotic that inhibits DNA synthesis and, to a lesser extent, RNA and protein synthesis.

Metabolism: Excreted by the liver.

Toxicity: BAG and extravasation reactions can occur.

Note: Dactinomycin has been used to treat lymphoma.

DOXORUBICIN

Dose supplied: 10-, 20-, 50-, 150-, and 200-mg vials.

Dosage: 30 mg/m^2 or 1 mg/kg or 25 mg/m^2 for small (<10 kg) dogs IV q3wk; total cumulative dose of up to 240 mg/m^2.

Route of administration: Dilute with 30 ml of 0.9% NaCl and administer IV over 15–30 minutes, or give undiluted drug IV at a rate of 1 ml/min. (Do not heparinize because this will cause precipitation. Doxorubicin hydrochloride is reportedly physically incompatible with aminophylline, cephalothin sodium, dexamethasone sodium phosphate, diazepam, fluorouracil [as an IV additive only], furosemide, heparin sodium, and hydrocortisone sodium succinate.)

Storage: Store at room temperature. Reconstituted solution is stable for months if refrigerated. Avoid storing with aluminum-hub needles.

Mechanism of action: Antitumor antibiotic; inhibits DNA and RNA synthesis.

Metabolism: Metabolized predominantly by the liver. Approximately 50% of the drug is excreted in bile. In animals with bilirubin levels above 2 mg/dl, the dose should be decreased by 50% to reduce toxicity. The drug is also excreted in urine and causes a red color in urine for up to 2 days after administration.

Toxicity: Leukopenia and thrombocytopenia (nadir: 7–10 days). GI toxicity, anorexia, vomiting, and hemorrhagic colitis are possible (2–5 days after administration). GI toxicity and quality of life improve when administered concurrently with sulfamethoxazole–trimethoprim.[7] The cumulative dose likely to cause cardiotoxicity in dogs has not been clearly elucidated, but most oncologists limit this agent to 180–240 mg/m^2. Extravasation causes severe tissue necrosis. Immediately apply ice or cold compresses to the area of extravasation for 6–10 hours. The drug has been reported to cause renal toxicity in dogs. Allergic reactions occur occasionally but may be eliminated by slowing the infusion or by pretreating with antihistamines. Alopecia may be seen in some dogs.

Note: Doxorubicin is used to treat lymphoma, thyroid carcinoma, sarcoma, and mammary carcinoma. This antineoplastic agent seems to have a broad spectrum of activity against a variety of tumors.

IDARUBICIN

Dose supplied: 2-mg capsules; 5- and 10-mg vials.

Dosage: Investigational, advise checking for updated recommendations from oncologists.

Route of administration: PO, IV.

Storage: Store at room temperature. Injectable form is stable for 7 days if refrigerated. Incompatible with heparin.

Mechanism of action: Antitumor antibiotic; inhibits DNA and RNA synthesis.

Metabolism: Metabolized predominantly by the liver.

Toxicity: BAG.

Note: Orally administered idarubicin may be effective in treating lymphoma. Limited availability worldwide.

LIPOSOMAL DOXORUBICIN

Dose supplied: 20- and 50-mg vials.

Dosage: 1 mg/kg IV q3wk.

Route of administration: Administer IV over 15–30 minutes or give undiluted drug IV at a rate of 1 ml/min. (Do not heparinize because this will cause precipitation. Doxorubicin hydrochloride is reportedly physically incompatible with aminophylline, cephalothin sodium, dexamethasone sodium phosphate, diazepam, 5-fluorouracil [as an IV additive only], furosemide, heparin sodium, and hydrocortisone sodium succinate.)

Storage: Store at room temperature. Avoid storing with aluminum-hub needles.

Mechanism of action: Antitumor antibiotic; inhibits DNA and RNA synthesis. The liposomal preparation can decrease toxicity and may, in some cases, enhance efficacy.

Metabolism: Metabolized predominantly by the liver. Approximately 50% of the drug is excreted in bile. In animals with bilirubin levels above 2 mg/dl, the dose should be decreased by 50% to reduce toxicity. The drug is also excreted in urine and causes a red color in urine for up to 2 days after administration.

Toxicity: Leukopenia and thrombocytopenia. Less cardiotoxicity than with native doxorubicin. Extravasation causes severe tissue necrosis. Immediately apply ice or cold compresses to the area of extravasation for 6–10 hours. The drug may cause renal toxicity in dogs. Allergic reactions occur occasionally but may be eliminated by slowing the infusion or by pretreating with antihistamines. Alopecia may be seen in some dogs. More importantly, palmar–plantar erythrodysesthesia syndrome is possible and may be reduced by administering concurrent pyridoxine.

Note: Doxorubicin is used to treat lymphoma, thyroid carcinoma, sarcoma, and mammary carcinoma. This antineoplastic agent seems to have a broad spectrum of activity against a variety of tumors but may not be more efficacious than native doxorubicin in many patients.

MITOXANTRONE

Dose supplied: 20-, 25-, and 30-mg multidose vials.

Dosage: 5.5 mg/m^2 IV (dogs <10 kg) (administered over at least 3 minutes) q3wk.

Route of administration: IV.

Storage: Room temperature. The drug is incompatible with heparin. Do not freeze.

Mechanism of action: Intercalates DNA; inhibits DNA and RNA synthesis.

Metabolism: Liver.

Toxicity: Unlike doxorubicin, this drug does not readily cause allergic reactions, cardiomyopathy, cardiac arrhythmias, or severe tissue damage at the site of extravasation. It is more myelosuppressive than doxorubicin and can cause alopecia and GI disturbances.

Note: Mitoxantrone is moderately effective for the treatment of lymphoma, squamous cell carcinoma, transitional cell carcinoma, mammary gland tumors, and a number of other neoplastic conditions.

PLICAMYCIN (MITHRAMYCIN)

Dose supplied: Lyophilized powder in vials containing 2.5 mg of drug.

Dosage: 0.1 mg/kg/wk for 2 weeks for the treatment of hypercalcemia of malignancy.

Route of administration: Slow IV (over a minimum of 20 minutes).
Storage: Room temperature.
Mechanism of action: Antitumor antibiotic.
Metabolism: Metabolized by the liver.
Toxicity: BAG and extravasation reactions can occur.
Note: Mithramycin has been suggested as a treatment of hypercalcemia of malignancy, and it may have anticancer properties.

Antimetabolites

Antimetabolites interfere with the biosynthesis of nucleic acids. They substitute for normal metabolites and inhibit normal enzymatic reactions. The dosing of each drug varies by protocol.

CAPECITABINE
Dose supplied: 150- and 500-mg capsules.
Dosage: Investigational; advise checking for updated recommendations from oncologists.
Route of administration: PO.
Storage: Room temperature.
Mechanism of action: Antimetabolite.
Metabolism: Metabolized in vivo to fluorouracil in the liver and then in the peripheral and tumor tissues to thymidine phosphorylase.
Toxicity: Neurotoxicity is theoretically possible. Myelosuppression and the canine equivalent of palmar–plantar erythrodysesthesia syndrome.
Note: Capecitabine may have efficacy in the treatment of lymphoma.

CYTOSINE ARABINOSIDE
Dose supplied: 100- and 500-mg and 1- and 2-g vials.
Dosage: 100 mg/m^2/day continuous IV infusion for 4 days; if no toxicity, increase to 150 mg/m^2/day for 4 days or 10 mg/m^2 SC once or twice daily. Can be administered intrathecally.
Route of administration: IV, SC. If administered IV, infuse via a Buretrol over 10–20 minutes or as continuous infusion.
Storage: Room temperature. Reconstituted solution is stable at room temperature for 48 hours. Discard solution if a slight haze develops.
Mechanism of action: Antimetabolite; pyrimidine analogue; inhibits DNA synthesis.
Metabolism: The drug is activated and inactivated by liver enzymes.
Toxicity: Myelosuppression is the major toxicity. Leukopenia and thrombocytopenia (nadir: 7–14 days in dogs) frequently occur and apparently are related to the dose and frequency of administration. Fever and thrombophlebitis are rarely seen. Alopecia may be seen.
Note: Cytosine arabinoside has been used alone or in combination with other agents to treat lymphoreticular neoplasms and myeloproliferative disorders. It has been administered intrathecally to dogs to treat lymphoma of the CNS. The efficacy of this drug as a single agent is not clear.

5-FLUOROURACIL (5-FU)
Dose supplied: 500-mg, 5-g ampules or vials; 1% or 2% topical ointment or solution.
Dosage: 5–10 mg/kg weekly IV.
Route of administration: IV push; topical.
Storage: Room temperature; protect from light.
Mechanism of action: Pyrimidine antimetabolite; blocks methylation reaction of deoxyuridylic acid to thymidylic acid, interfering with synthesis of DNA and, to a lesser extent, RNA.
Metabolism: The drug is metabolized by the liver and partially excreted by the kidneys.
Toxicity: This drug is neurotoxic. Myelosuppression (neutropenia and thrombocytopenia) reaches a nadir in 9–14 days. Nausea, alopecia, and GI toxicity are possible.
Note: This drug has had limited use in veterinary medicine because of its neurotoxicity. It is reportedly effective for the treatment of tumors of the GI tract. It is available as a topical cream and has been used to treat superficial malignancies, including cutaneous lymphoma and squamous cell carcinoma, with varying results.

GEMCITABINE
Dose supplied: 200-mg and 1-g vials.
Dosage: 250–300 mg/m^2 IV weekly for 4 weeks with a 1-week rest. Toxicity and, probably, efficacy depend on the rate the drug is infused. Preliminary studies suggest that the drug should be infused over 30–90 minutes.
Route of administration: IV, SC. If administered IV, infuse via a Buretrol over 10–20 minutes or as continuous infusion. Note that longer infusions will increase the effective dose proportionally.
Storage: This drug has a very short half-life. Discard unused solution.
Mechanism of action: Antimetabolite; cell phase specificity, primarily killing cells undergoing DNA synthesis

(S phase) and also blocking the progression of cells through the G1/S-phase boundary.

Metabolism: The drug is metabolized by the liver and kidneys.

Toxicity: Myelosuppression is the major toxicity. Leukopenia and thrombocytopenia (nadir: 3–5 days in dogs) frequently occur and apparently are related to the dose and frequency of administration. Alopecia may be seen. Pulmonary toxicity is reported in humans.

Note: Gemcitabine has been used to treat a wide variety of tumors; however, consensus on which tumors are best treated with this agent has yet to be reached. In humans, pancreatic, bladder, and breast cancers are successfully treated with this drug.

LIPOSOMAL CYTOSINE ARABINOSIDE

Dose supplied: 50-mg vials.

Dosage: Investigational; advise checking for updated recommendations from oncologists.

Route of administration: Intrathecal administration results in prolonged effect with minimal systemic effects.

Storage: Refrigerated.

Mechanism of action: Antimetabolite; pyrimidine analogue; inhibits DNA synthesis.

Metabolism: The drug is activated and inactivated by liver enzymes; however, liposomes prolong half-life dramatically.

Toxicity: Myelosuppression is the major toxicity. Leukopenia and thrombocytopenia may theoretically occur and may be related to the dose and frequency of administration; however, intrathecal therapy should minimize systemic effects.

Note: Applications are primarily for CNS lymphoma.

MERCAPTOPURINE

Dose supplied: 50-mg tablets.

Dosage: 50 mg/m^2/day. (Note: Because of the tablet size, may need to be recompounded or dosed at 50 mg q48–72h.)

Route of administration: PO.

Storage: Room temperature.

Mechanism of action: Purine antimetabolite; inhibits nucleotide synthesis required for RNA and DNA synthesis.

Metabolism: Metabolized by the liver and degraded by the enzyme xanthine oxidase. Xanthine oxidase is inhibited by allopurinol, so concurrent use of other drugs that use this enzyme necessitates a 75% dose reduction.

Toxicity: Myelosuppression.

Note: Mercaptopurine has been suggested as a treatment for leukemia and lymphoma; results are varied.

METHOTREXATE

Dose supplied: 2.5-mg tablets; 5-, 20-, 50-, 100-, 200-, and 250-mg and 1-g vials for injection.

Dosage: 2.5 mg/m^2/day PO.

Route of administration: PO, IV, IM, SC.

Storage: Room temperature. The drug must be protected from light. Vials may be frozen.

Mechanism of action: Antimetabolite; inhibits the conversion of folic acid to tetrahydrofolic acid by binding to the enzyme dihydrofolate reductase, which inhibits synthesis of thymidine and purines essential for DNA synthesis.

Metabolism: A large percentage of the drug is excreted unchanged in the urine. The drug is bound to serum albumin, so simultaneous administration of drugs that displace methotrexate from the plasma protein (e.g., sulfonamides, aspirin, metoclopramide, chloramphenicol, phenytoin, tetracycline) should be avoided to prevent excessive toxicity. Daily dose should be reduced if serum creatinine level is elevated.

Toxicity: Anorexia and vomiting occur frequently but may be prevented by premedication with antiemetics. The nadir of myelosuppression is 6–9 days in some species but has not been documented in dogs. Alopecia (whisker loss) may also be seen.

Note: Methotrexate has been used in combination with other drugs to treat lymphoma. It is a folic acid inhibitor and can be given at a very high dose and then reversed ("rescued") with leucovorin calcium to prevent potentially fatal toxicities. Its efficacy as a single agent is in question.

Cytokines, Hematopoietic Growth Factors

EPOETIN ALFA (ERYTHROPOIETIN)

Dose supplied: Vials of 2,000, 4,000, and 10,000 U as a human or canine recombinant protein.

Dosage: 100 U/kg three times weekly as needed for anemia.

Route of administration: IV, IM, or SC route results in measurable levels for 24 hours.

Storage: Refrigerated.

Mechanism of action: Acts as a hematopoietic growth factor specifically to increase the production of red blood cells.

Metabolism: Proteolysis within the serum is common. If the recombinant human product is used, antibodies are possible, resulting in destruction by the reticuloendothelial system.

Toxicity: Hypertension and flu-like syndrome seen in humans. If antibodies are directed against the protein, this may cross-react against the native erythropoietin, resulting in severe nonregenerative anemia that may be permanent.

Note: Erythropoietin can be used to resolve anemia.

FILGRASTIM (GRANULOCYTE COLONY-STIMULATING FACTOR)

Dose supplied: Single-dose vials of 300 and 480 mg in solution as a human or canine (not commercially available) recombinant protein.

Dosage: 5 mg/kg/day until neutropenia has resolved.

Route of administration: SC.

Storage: Vials should be kept refrigerated.

Mechanism of action: Acts as a hematopoietic growth factor specifically to increase the production of neutrophils.

Metabolism: Proteolysis within the serum is common. If the recombinant human product is used, antibodies are possible, resulting in destruction by the granulocytes.

Toxicity: Hypertension and flu-like syndrome seen in humans. If antibodies are directed against the protein, this may cross-react against the native granulocytes, resulting in serious neutropenia.

INTERFERON-α

Dose supplied: 3 million–50 million U per vial.

Dosage: Investigational; advise checking for updated recommendations from oncologists. Three million U/m^2 three times per week.

Route of administration: IV, IM, or SC.

Storage: Vials should be kept refrigerated.

Mechanism of action: Biologic response modifier, immunostimulant.

Metabolism: Proteolysis throughout the body.

Toxicity: Fatigue, fever, chills, anorexia, lethargy, diarrhea, and weight loss.

INTERLEUKIN-2

Dose supplied: 18 million U per vial.

Dosage: Investigational; advise checking for updated recommendations from oncologists.

Route of administration: IV, SC.

Storage: Vials should be kept refrigerated.

Mechanism of action: Biologic response modifier, immunostimulant.

Metabolism: Proteolysis.

Toxicity: Fatigue, fever, chills, anorexia, lethargy, diarrhea, weight loss, capillary leak syndrome, and hypotension. CNS and hepatic toxicity possible.

Note: Intralesional or systemic therapy may have efficacy for solid tumors.

Enzymes

The enzyme most commonly used in veterinary and human medicine is L-asparaginase.

L-ASPARAGINASE

Dose supplied: 10,000-U vials.

Dosage: 10,000–20,000 U/m^2 or 400 U/kg weekly or less frequently.

Route of administration: IM.

Storage: Refrigerated. Reconstituted drug may be active for up to 7 days. Do not use if cloudy.

Mechanism of action: Enzyme; inhibits protein synthesis by depriving tumor cells of the amino acid asparagine.

Metabolism: Not completely understood.

Toxicity: Allergic and anaphylactic reactions are seen, especially after several doses have been given. The incidence of anaphylaxis is minimal when administered IM. If administered IV, the potential for inducing an acute anaphylactic reaction is high. Pretreatment with antihistamines and steroids may reduce the risk for reactions. If anaphylaxis occurs, L-asparaginase should be discontinued indefinitely. Other toxicities include fever and vomiting shortly after administration. The drug has been associated with acute pancreatitis in dogs and humans. Myelosuppression may occur if this drug is administered concurrently with vincristine.

Note: The drug is used to treat lymphoma and lymphoblastic leukemia and may be combined with other antineoplastic agents. L-Asparaginase does not induce a sustained remission when used alone in the treatment of lymphoma.

PEGASPARGASE

Dose supplied: 750 U/ml in a 5-ml vial. No reconstitution or dilution necessary.

Dosage: 10,000–20,000 U/m^2 or 400 U/kg weekly or less frequently.

Route of administration: IM.

Storage: Refrigerate. Reconstituted drug may be active for up to 7 days. Do not use if cloudy.

Mechanism of action: Enzyme; inhibits protein synthesis by depriving tumor cells of the amino acid asparagine.

Metabolism: Polyethylene glycol added to naturally occurring enzyme to prolong half-life.

Toxicity: The drug is less immunogenic than native L-asparaginase. Toxicity similar to L-asparaginase, although specific toxicity in the dog is not clearly described in the literature. Coagulopathies, hypercholesterolemia, fever, chills, anorexia, lethargy, confusion, and tachycardia all theoretically possible.

Note: Pegaspargase can be effective in the treatment of lymphoma when L-asparaginase may be effective but cannot be used.

Hormones

Hormones are believed to interfere with the cellular receptors that stimulate growth. The most common examples of hormones used to treat cancer are the corticosteroids used to treat lymphoma and mast cell tumors.

PREDNISONE

Dose supplied: 5-, 10-, 20-, and 50-mg tablets; 1 mg/ml syrup; injectable solution.

Dosage: 30–40 mg/m^2/day or every other day or 1 mg/kg/day for 4 weeks; 1 mg/kg every other day thereafter, as long as the tumor is in remission and the patient is doing well.

Route of administration: PO, IV.

Storage: Room temperature.

Mechanism of action: Binds to cytoplasmic receptor sites, which then interact with DNA and prevent cell division.

Metabolism: Metabolized by the liver and excreted in the urine. Prednisone is activated by the liver to its active form, prednisolone; severe liver disease, however, does not significantly affect activation.

Toxicity: Polydipsia and polyuria are the major side effects. Long-term use may be associated with development of alopecia and other signs of iatrogenic Cushing's syndrome.

Note: Active in the treatment of lymphoma and mast cell tumors. Prednisone does not induce a sustained remission when used alone in the treatment of lymphoma.

Plant Alkaloids

Plant alkaloids disrupt the cell-division cycle.

ETOPOSIDE (VP-16)

Dose supplied: 50-mg capsules (erratic absorption in the dog), 100-mg multidose vials.

Dosage: 40 mg/m^2 reportedly results in profound hypotension during administration due to carrier.

Route of administration: IV slow infusion or PO (poor and erratic bioavailability). Due to acute and potentially fatal degranulation of mast cells upon administration, diphenhydramide, cimetidine, and dexamethasone must be administered 20 minutes before slow infusion of etoposide.

Storage: Vials of unreconstituted drug can be stored at room temperature.

Mechanism of action: Topoisomerase II inhibitor.

Metabolism: Metabolized by the liver and excreted in the urine.

Toxicity: Hypotension and death are possible during IV administration due to carrier polysorbate 80. Bone marrow suppression, alopecia, and nausea and vomiting can occur.

VINBLASTINE

Dose supplied: 10-mg vial.

Dosage: 2 mg/m^2/wk.

Route of administration: Potent irritant, avoid extravasation. Administer through a patent IV catheter; follow with adequate saline flush (10 ml).

Storage: Refrigerated reconstituted drug is stable for 30 days. Protect from light.

Mechanism of action: Vinca alkaloid. Causes metaphase arrest by binding to microtubular protein used in the formation of mitotic spindle.

Metabolism: Rapidly cleared from plasma; excreted in bile. A 50% decrease in dose is recommended in animals with bilirubin levels above 2 mg/dl.

Toxicity: Unlike vincristine, vinblastine may cause severe bone marrow suppression (neutrophil nadir: 4–7 days after administration). Neurotoxicity and mild peripheral neuropathies occur but are less severe than with vincristine. Extravasation can cause severe tissue irritation and necrosis. If extravasation occurs, immediately pack with warm compresses and infiltrate the area with saline and dexamethasone.

Note: Vinblastine is used to treat lymphoma and mast cell tumors.

VINCRISTINE

Dose supplied: 1-, 2-, and 5-mg vials; Hyporets (1- and 2-mg/ml disposable syringes).

Dosage: 0.5–0.75 mg/m^2 weekly.

Route of administration: Administer through a patent IV catheter; follow with adequate saline flush (10 ml).

Storage: Refrigerate. Protect from light until immediately before injection.

Mechanism of action: Vinca alkaloid. Causes metaphase arrest by binding to microtubular protein used in formation of mitotic spindle.

Metabolism: Rapidly cleared from plasma and excreted in bile. Decrease dose by 50% in animals with bilirubin levels above 2 mg/dl.

Toxicity: Can cause neurotoxicity and resultant paresthesia, constipation, and paralytic ileus. Anorexia in treated dogs may be due to ileus. This drug is a potent irritant that can cause severe tissue irritation and necrosis if extravasated; if extravasation occurs, apply warm compresses immediately and infiltrate with saline and 8 mg dexamethasone. Myelosuppression is dose related and uncommon unless drug is given in combination with L-asparaginase. Vincristine causes a marked increase in peripheral platelet counts in animals with adequate megakaryocytes.

Note: Vincristine is most commonly used to treat lymphoma, sarcomas, and immune-mediated thrombocytopenia.

VINORELBINE
Dose supplied: 10-mg vial.

Dosage: 15–18 mg/m²/wk.

Route of administration: Potent irritant, avoid extravasation. Administer through a patent IV catheter; follow with adequate saline flush (10 ml).

Storage: Refrigerated reconstituted drug is stable for 30 days. Protect from light.

Mechanism of action: Vinca alkaloid. Causes metaphase arrest by binding to microtubular protein used in the formation of mitotic spindle.

Metabolism: Rapidly cleared from plasma; excreted in bile. A 50% decrease in dose is recommended in animals with bilirubin levels above 2 mg/dl.

Toxicity: May cause severe bone marrow suppression. Neurotoxicity and mild peripheral neuropathies may be seen. Extravasation can cause severe tissue irritation and necrosis. If extravasation occurs, immediately pack with warm compresses and infiltrate the area with saline and dexamethasone.

Note: Vinorelbine has been suggested as an effective treatment for primary lung tumors.

Topoisomerase-I Inhibitors

9-AMINOCAMPTOTHECIN (9-AC)
Dose supplied: Investigational vials.

Dosage: 3.35–3.69 mg/m² IV.

Route of administration: As a continuous 72-hour IV infusion q3wk.

Storage: Use within 24 hours of reconstitution because of the absence of preservatives.

Mechanism of action: Inhibition of topoisomerase-I interferes with DNA synthesis.

Metabolism: Metabolized by the liver.

Toxicity: Bone marrow suppression, mild GI toxicity.

Note: This drug has been used to treat lymphoma in investigational trials.

Other Agents

AMIFOSTINE (WR-2721)
Dose supplied: 500-mg vial.

Dosage: Investigational; advise checking for updated recommendations from oncologists.

Route of administration: Poorly absorbed orally. IV administration is preferable.

Storage: Vials of unreconstituted drug can be stored at room temperature.

Mechanism of action: Cytoprotectant and free-radical scavenger. Documented as an agent to reduce bone marrow, kidney, and nerve toxicity during concurrent administration of radiation and cisplatin.

Metabolism: Metabolized to active metabolites that are excreted in the urine.

Toxicity: Hypotension when administered IV. Nausea, vomiting, somnolescence, and hypocalcemia are occasionally seen.

Note: Amifostine may protect against radiation- and cisplatin-induced toxicity to the bone marrow and kidney.

CARBOPLATIN
Dose supplied: 50-, 150-, and 450-mg vials.

Dosage: 250–300 mg/m² q3wk.

Route of administration: IV; must be diluted with 5% dextrose in water. Intralesional administration as a suspension in oil or collagen matrix. Intracavitary.

Storage: Dry powder is stable at room temperature for 2 years. Reconstituted solution is stable at room temperature for 8 hours.

Mechanism of action: Similar to alkylating agents and other heavy metals. Binds to DNA and causes cross-linkage.

Metabolism: Metabolized by the liver and kidney. Dose should be reduced if serum creatinine level is increased because of renal disease.

Toxicity: Myelosuppression is the most significant toxicity (neutrophil nadir: 17–21 days, may be prolonged). Carboplatin should not be administered without the current neutrophil count being known. Unlike with cisplatin, nephrotoxicity and emesis are rare.

Note: Carboplatin is used in treatment of squamous cell carcinoma and possibly other carcinomas and sarcomas.

CISPLATIN
(*CIS*-DIAMMINE-DICHLOROPLATINUM II)

Dose supplied: 10-, 50-, and 100-mg vials.

Dosage: 70 mg/m^2 with a fluid diuresis at 18.3 ml/kg/hr 3 hours before and 1 hour after the administration of cisplatin. Because aluminum causes precipitation, do not use aluminum needles.

Route of administration: IV or intracavitary; intralesional administration as a suspension in oil or collagen matrix only.

Storage: Dry powder is stable at room temperature for 2 years. Reconstituted solution is stable at room temperature for 20 hours. The reconstituted solution should not be refrigerated because a precipitate will form.

Mechanism of action: Similar to alkylating agents and other heavy metals. Binds to DNA and causes cross-linkage.

Metabolism: When given IV to dogs, cisplatin is rapidly distributed to liver, intestine, and kidneys; less than 10% is in plasma after 1 hour, and 50% of the administered dose is excreted in urine in 24–48 hours.

Toxicity: Myelosuppression with a nadir at days 5 and 16; alopecia, vomiting, nephrotoxicity, and neurotoxicity, including ototoxicity.

Note: Cisplatin is effective for the intralesional treatment of squamous cell carcinoma and soft tissue sarcomas.

DEXRAZOXANE

Dose supplied: 500-mg vial with diluent.

Dosage: 30 mg for every 1 mg of doxorubicin.

Route of administration: 15- to 30-minute IV infusion in 30 minutes before the administration of doxorubicin.

Storage: Vials of unreconstituted drug can be stored at room temperature.

Mechanism of action: Free-radical scavenger and chelating agent.

Metabolism: Metabolized by the liver and excreted in the urine.

Toxicity: Slight potentiation of doxorubicin toxicity reported in other species. Mild nausea, vomiting, diarrhea, and anorexia can occur.

Note: Dexrazoxane can be used to reduce the risk of doxorubicin cardiotoxicity.

DOCETAXEL

Dose supplied: 80 mg/2 ml vials with separate diluent.

Dosage: 30 mg/m^2 (investigational).[8]

Route of administration: IV. Must dilute with 0.9% NaCl to a concentration of 0.6–0.7 mg/ml. Prepare in a glass container; administer through a 0.22-µm inline filter using non-PVC tubing. Pretreat with corticosteroids, diphenhydramine, and H$_2$-receptor antagonists.

Storage: Refrigerate vials before use. Reconstituted solution is stable at room temperature for 24 hours.

Mechanism of action: Inhibits microtubule disassembly.

Metabolism: Metabolized by the liver and kidney.

Toxicity: Myelosuppression and anaphylactoid reactions (due to the diluent polysorbate 80) and somnolence (due to alcohol in the diluent) are the most significant toxicities.

Note: Docetaxel is a relatively new chemotherapeutic agent. Studies are under way to define its usefulness in veterinary medicine. Preliminary results are available for mammary carcinoma and lymphoma.[8]

GALLIUM NITRATE

Dose supplied: 500-mg vials.

Dosage: Investigational; advise checking for updated recommendations from oncologists.

Route of administration: Continuous IV infusion.

Storage: Vials should be kept refrigerated.

Mechanism of action: Heavy metal that antagonizes iron metabolism in cancer cells. Causes hypocalcemia by similar mechanism.

Metabolism: Not metabolized.

Toxicity: Nephrotoxicity, nausea, vomiting, diarrhea, and mild bone marrow suppression.

Note: Gallium is used to treat hypercalcemia of malignancy.

ISOTRETINOIN

Dose supplied: 10-, 20-, and 40-mg capsules.

Dosage: 1–3 mg/kg/day.

Route of administration: PO.

Storage: Room temperature.

Mechanism of action: Induces apoptosis. Derivative of vitamin A that binds to nuclear receptors and changes gene expression.

Metabolism: Metabolized by the liver and kidney.

Toxicity: Keratoconjunctivitis sicca, hypertriglyceridemia, hepatotoxicity, pruritus, conjunctivitis, xerostomia.

Note: This drug has been shown to be effective in treating a variety of cutaneous neoplasms and dysplasias.

MEGESTROL ACETATE

Dose supplied: 5-, 20-, 40-mg tablets and 40-mg/ml solution.

Dosage: 0.05 mg/kg/day for 3–5 days, then q48–72hr thereafter to enhance appetite.

Route of administration: PO.

Storage: Room temperature.

Mechanism of action: Appetite stimulant.

Metabolism: Metabolized by the liver and eliminated via the kidney.

Toxicity: Edema, weight gain, anxiety, sleep disturbances.

Note: Megestrol is used in humans and dogs to enhance weight gain and to reduce toxicity associated with chemotherapy, surgery, and radiation therapy.

MESNA

Dose supplied: Solution of 100 mg/ml as uroprotectant for cyclophosphamide and ifosfamide to prevent hemorrhagic cystitis.

Dosage: 60% of the daily ifosfamide dosage in milligrams.

Route of administration: IV bolus before and 2 and 5 hours after chemotherapy with ifosfamide, or as a constant-rate infusion.

Storage: Room temperature.

Mechanism of action: Inactivates highly reactive metabolite of cyclophosphamide and ifosfamide (acrolein).

Metabolism: Filtered by the kidneys.

Toxicity: Nausea, vomiting, diarrhea.

Note: Mesna is used to prevent cystitis attributable to ifosfamide and cyclophosphamide.

MITOTANE

Dose supplied: 500-mg tablet.

Dosage: Initially, 50–75 mg/kg PO in daily divided doses for 10–14 days. May supplement with predniso(lo)ne at 0.2 mg/kg/day. If basal or post-ACTH serum cortisol values are decreased but still above the therapeutic end point (<1 mg/dl), repeat therapy for an additional 7–14 days and repeat testing. If post-ACTH serum cortisol values remain greatly elevated or unchanged, increase mitotane to 100 mg/kg/day and repeat ACTH-stimulation test at 7- to 14-day intervals. If serum cortisol continues to remain greatly elevated, increase dosage by 50 mg/kg/day every 7–14 days until response occurs or drug intolerance ensues. Once undetectable or low-normal post-ACTH cortisol levels are attained, continue mitotane at 100–200 mg/kg/wk in divided doses with glucocorticoid supplementation.

Route of administration: PO.

Storage: Room temperature.

Mechanism of action: Adrenal cortical cytotoxin.

Metabolism: Metabolized by the liver and eliminated via the kidney.

Toxicity: Hypoadrenocorticism and associated clinical signs in addition to nausea, vomiting, diarrhea, and alteration of metabolism and clearance of other drugs.

Note: Mitotane has been shown to be effective for the treatment of adrenal cortical carcinomas.

OXALIPLATIN

Dose supplied: 50- and 100-mg vials of lyophilized powder.

Dosage: 35 mg/m^2 q3wk (investigational).

Route of administration: IV.

Storage: Dry powder is stable at room temperature for 2 years. Reconstituted solution is stable at room temperature for 8 hours.

Mechanism of action: Similar to alkylating agents and other heavy metals. Binds to DNA and causes cross-linkage.

Metabolism: Unchanged in circulation until excreted by the kidney. Dose should be reduced if serum creatinine level is increased because of renal disease.

Toxicity: Myelosuppression is the most significant toxicity (thrombocytopenia; neutropenia nadir: 7–10 days). Vomiting and depression are rare. Unlike with cisplatin, nephrotoxicity is rare.

Note: Lobaplatin, an investigational drug similar to oxaliplatin, has been reported in the treatment of osteosarcoma.[9]

PACLITAXEL

Dose supplied: 50 mg/5 ml vials.

Dosage: 132 mg/m^2 q3wk.[8]

Route of administration: IV. Must dilute with 0.9% NaCl to a concentration of 0.6–0.7 mg/ml. Prepare in a glass container; administer through a 0.22-μm inline filter using non-PVC tubing. Pretreat with corticosteroids, diphenhydramine, and H$_2$-receptor antagonists.

Storage: Refrigerate vials before use. Reconstituted solution is stable at room temperature for 24 hours.

Mechanism of action: Inhibits microtubule disassembly.

Metabolism: Metabolized by the liver and kidney.

Toxicity: Myelosuppression and anaphylactoid reactions (due to the diluent Cremophor EL) and somnolence (due to alcohol in the diluent) are the most significant toxicities.

Note: Paclitaxel is a relatively new chemotherapeutic agent. Studies are under way to define its usefulness in veterinary medicine. Preliminary results are available for mammary carcinoma, histiocytosis, and osteosarcoma.[9]

PAMIDRONATE

Dose supplied: 30- and 90-mg vials.

Dosage: 1 mg/kg IV over 2 hours 3 hours after and 1 hour before a saline diuresis at 18.3 ml/kg/hr.

Route of administration: IV.

Storage: Room temperature.

Mechanism of action: Bisphosphonate inhibitor of bone metastasis and hypercalcemia.

Metabolism: Excreted by the kidneys.

Toxicity: Nausea, fever, constipation, hypocalcemia.

Note: Pamidronate is used to treat metastatic bone lesions and hypercalcemia of malignancy.

PIROXICAM

Dose supplied: 10- and 20-mg capsules.

Dosage: 0.3 mg/kg/day PO; may need to be reformulated by a compounding pharmacy.

Route of administration: PO. Avoid other GI irritants and nephrotoxins.

Storage: Room temperature.

Mechanism of action: Unknown; possible biologic response modifier.

Metabolism: Metabolized by the liver and kidney.

Toxicity: Nephrotoxicity and GI irritation. Do not administer with other nonsteroidal or corticosteroid drugs. Administration with piroxicam may lead to worsening of renal toxicity.

Note: This NSAID has been shown to cause measurable regression in transitional cell carcinoma of the urinary bladder and squamous cell carcinoma in dogs and therefore may be of value in dogs.

THALIDOMIDE

Dose supplied: 50-mg tablets.

Dosage: Investigational, advise checking for updated recommendations from oncologists.

Route of administration: PO.

Storage: Room temperature.

Mechanism of action: Novel antiangiogenic and immunomodulatory agent.

Metabolism: Unknown.

Toxicity: Profound somnolence, fatigue, nausea, vomiting, diarrhea.

Note: Thalidomide is an antiangiogenic agent with at least theoretical benefit in the treatment of hemangiosarcoma and other malignant diseases.

ZOLEDRONIC ACID

Dose supplied: Vials of 4 mg of drug in powder form.

Dosage: Investigational; advise checking for updated recommendations from oncologists.

Route of administration: IV.

Storage: Store at room temperature.

Mechanism of action: Bisphosphonate inhibitor of bone metastasis and hypercalcemia.

Metabolism: Excreted by the kidneys.

Toxicity: Nausea, fever, constipation, hypocalcemia, and renal insufficiency.

Note: This drug is used to treat bone metastases and hypercalcemia of malignancy.

REFERENCES

1. Lippman SM, Hong WK: Cancer prevention by delay. Commentary re: JA O'Shaughnessy et al., Treatment and prevention of intraepithelial neoplasia: An important target for accelerated new agent development. *Clin Cancer Res* 8(2):305–313, 2002.
2. Simon D, Schoenrock D, Ueberschaer S, Nolte I: Adjuvant chemotherapy with docetaxel and doxorubicin in canine invasive mammary gland tumors: First results. *Proc 19th Annu Conf Vet Cancer Soc*:74, 1999.
3. Perry MC, Anderson CM, Donehower RC: Chemotherapy, in Abeloff MD, Armitage JO, Niedenhuber JE, et al (eds): *Clinical Oncology*, ed 3. Philadelphia, Elsevier Churchill Livingston, 2004, pp 483–535.
4. Chabner BA: Principles of cancer therapy, in Wyngaarden JB, Smith LH (eds): *Cecil Textbook of Medicine*. Philadelphia, WB Saunders, 1982, p 1032–1045.
5. Ogilvie GK: Principles of oncology, in Morgan RV (ed): *Handbook of Small Animal Internal Medicine*. Philadelphia, Churchill Livingston, 1992, pp 799–812.
6. Moore AS, Kitchell BE: New chemotherapy agents in veterinary medicine. *Vet Clin North Am Small Anim Pract* 33(3):629–649, 2003.
7. Chretin JD, Shaw NA, Hahn KA, et al: Prophylactic trimethoprim sulfadiazine during chemotherapeutic induction: A double blind, placebo controlled study. *Proc 20th Annu Conf Vet Cancer Soc*:47, 2000.
8. Poirier VJ, Hershey AE, Burgess KE, et al: Efficacy and toxicity of paclitaxel (Taxol) for the treatment of canine malignant tumors. *J Vet Intern Med* 18(2):219–222, 2004.
9. Kirpensteijn J, Teske E, Kik M, et al: Lobaplatin as an adjuvant chemotherapy to surgery in canine appendicular osteosarcoma: A phase II evaluation. *Anticancer Res* 22(5):2765–2770, 2002.

RADIATION THERAPY: PROPERTIES, USES, AND PATIENT MANAGEMENT

Antony S. Moore and Gregory K. Ogilvie

CLINICAL BRIEFING

Types of radiation therapy

Teletherapy	• External-beam radiation therapy delivered by orthovoltage or megavoltage machines. Intensity-modulated radiation therapy is a type of teletherapy designed to "sculpt" the radiation to the treatment volume.
Brachytherapy	• Radiation with shallow penetration applied using an external applicator or as implants.
Systemic therapy	• Administration of radioactive substances that preferentially localize within specific tissues in the body.

Possible tissues injured and possible therapy

General	• Long-chain polyunsaturated fatty acids such as DHA may reduce radiation damage to many normal tissues.
Skin	• Clean with mild soap and water; prevent self-mutilation. Other possible treatments include vitamin E and hydrogen peroxide or saline lavages as well as selected systemic therapy.
Ear canals	• Can be treated with dimethyl sulfoxide or steroid-containing medication.
Oral cavity, pharynx	• Feed palatable food and consider gastrostomy tube feeding early; provide oral rinses with saline or tea. Lidocaine viscous solution may help animals that experience pain when swallowing.
Colon, rectum	• Low-residue diet with a stool softener may alleviate painful defecation. Steroid enemas and a high-fiber diet may be helpful for nonresponsive colitis.
Eye	• Artificial tears for keratoconjunctivitis sicca and steroid ophthalmic solution or ointment for selected nonerosive conditions after fluoroscein staining.
Bone	• Bone sequestra should be removed.

Selected indications • Local control of oral tumors, nasal tumors, soft tissue sarcomas, mast cell tumors, brain tumors, and thyroid tumors. Can be palliative for primary or metastatic bone disease.

Radiation therapy has been used for decades in veterinary and human oncology. The equipment is readily available in the United States to large segments of the veterinary profession (primarily through referral centers) and, to a lesser degree, throughout the rest of the world. Radiation therapy is effective for controlling a wide range of tumors in domesticated animals. This treatment modality is used alone or in combination with other cancer therapies, including surgery and chemotherapy.

Radiation therapy is a local treatment; therefore, care should be taken to ensure that the animal is staged properly to delineate the extent of the neoplastic process. Dogs with metastatic disease may not be good candidates for an intensive course of radiation therapy. Consultation with an oncologist, and specifically a radiation oncologist, is essential to determine whether a particular patient with a malignancy is likely to benefit from radiation therapy.

Properties and Uses of Radiation Therapy

Before the practitioner can understand the potential benefits and risks of radiation therapy, a brief review of the properties and uses of radiation therapy is warranted.

Ionizing radiation can be electromagnetic or particulate. Electromagnetic radiation is a wave and a packet of energy (a photon). There are two types of electromagnetic radiation: roentgen rays made by electrical machines (orthovoltage, linear accelerator) and gamma radiation produced intranuclearly, most commonly by decay of radioactive isotopes such as cobalt-60 (^{60}Co) or cesium-137 (^{137}Cs).

Ionizing radiation may kill cells directly, primarily through its effects on DNA and, to a lesser extent, on membranes. Alternatively, radiation may interact with water in the cells and intracellular matrix to form cytotoxic free radicals. Cells damaged by ionizing radiation may be killed directly through apoptosis; they may later attempt to divide and then die; or they may divide aberrantly. Some cells remain functional but do not divide. These cells may be either terminally differentiated or sterile. Some tumor cells will have minimal damage that is repairable. These cells are the source of tumor relapse. Radiation-resistant tumors may have increased capacity to repair potentially lethal damage.

Radiation-induced apoptosis occurs at low doses for lymphocytes, bone marrow, and germ cells as well as tumors derived from those tissues. For tumors derived from other tissues, the proportion of cells undergoing apoptosis may be important in determining the response of that tumor to radiation therapy. Loss of apoptotic response may result in radiation resistance, so cells that have mutations in the pro-apoptotic genes, *bcl*-2 and *p53*, may be resistant to radiation therapy.

Cellular killing by radiation is by a constant proportion (rather than a constant number); hence, tumor killing is exponential. Because some of the initial damage done by radiation is sublethal and repairable, there is a threshold dose that needs to be delivered before cell killing becomes exponential.

The cell cycle can be divided into four phases: G_1, S, G_2, and M. The distribution of tumor cells throughout the cell cycle may affect radiation response. As cells proceed through G_1, they become more resistant to radiation damage, with cells in late S phase (and those in resting phase G_0) the most resistant. Cells that are in mitosis (M) or G_2 are the most sensitive to radiation damage. Depending on the proportion of cells in each phase, there may be alterations of the threshold dose and exponential killing rate. Radiation therapy may cause some degree of cell cycle synchronization, but as a practical matter, this is difficult to take advantage of before cells rapidly redistribute in the cell cycle.

Oxygen is critical to the clinical responsiveness of tumors to radiation therapy; greater doses of radiation are required under hypoxic conditions than under oxic conditions to provide equivalent cell killing. The enhanced cell killing occurs when oxygen is present because oxygen reacts with DNA lesions, rendering them permanent. If there is less oxygen available, then there is an increased chance of repair before the damage is made permanent. Between well-oxygenated and necrotic zones in the tumor are hypoxic cells. Larger tumors are more likely to have an abnormal blood supply and therefore more hypoxic cells; for this reason, radiation is most effective when treating small tumors or residual microscopic tumor tissue after surgery. Fractionation of the radiation dose may allow hypoxic cells to become reoxygenated between fractions after oxygenated cells are killed. Drugs that act as hypoxic-cell sensitizers (oxymimetics such as nitroimidazoles) may improve the efficacy of radiation therapy by increasing susceptibility of the resistant hypoxic cells.

Interactions may occur between drugs and radiation therapy. For example, the antineoplastic drugs doxorubicin, cisplatin, and dactinomycin may enhance radiation damage to both tumor and normal cells, primarily by reducing the threshold for damage. Doxorubicin administered even long after a course of radiation therapy may cause recurrence of acute effects of radiation (radiation recall). Hydroxyurea kills cells in S phase, when they are most resistant to radiation therapy. Radioprotective agents (sulfhydryl compounds) make cells more resistant by reducing the lifespan of oxygen free radicals.

Teletherapy, Brachytherapy, and Systemic Radiation Therapy

TELETHERAPY

The dose of radiation absorbed is the most biologically relevant factor influencing tumor control and toxicity. The unit of measurement of radiation-absorbed dose is the gray (Gy). A course of radiation therapy is described in terms of the total dose, the number of fractions in which the total dose is delivered, and the time course over which it is delivered (e.g., 60 Gy, given in 3-Gy fractions 5 days a week for 4 weeks). Most tumors in veterinary medicine receive a total dose of 40 to 60 Gy delivered in nine to 30 treatments over 3 to 6 weeks.

The delivery of radiation therapy from a machine to the patient is called *teletherapy* or *external-beam radiation therapy*. In veterinary medicine, external-beam radiation therapy is primarily delivered by linear accelerators, radioactive ^{60}Co or ^{137}Cs source units, or orthovoltage radiation therapy machines (Figure 22-1).

Because the source of radiation is external to the patient, teletherapy does not make the patient radioactive. Therefore, no period of isolation or quarantine is required for patients treated with teletherapy.

Radiation is absorbed by two major mechanisms: photoelectric effect (which is the radiation effect responsible for diagnostic radiographs) and Compton absorption.

Orthovoltage Teletherapy

Radiation produced by orthovoltage machines undergoes mainly photoelectric absorption. During photoelectric absorption, a photon interacts with tissue in the radiation field, causing ejection of an orbital electron. During this interaction, most of the energy is lost. Photoelectric absorption varies with the atomic number of the tissue. This means that the distance through tissue that radiation produced by an orthovoltage machine can travel is limited and, furthermore, that when dense materials such as bone are within the treatment field, the radiation travels an even shorter distance. In practical terms, penetration of orthovoltage radiation is limited to superficial tissues; the maximum dose is delivered to the skin, and deep-seated tumors do not receive an adequate dose when orthovoltage is used. In addition, areas of tumors that are surrounding or surrounded by bone may be "protected" due to absorption of the radiation dose. However, orthovoltage is valuable in treating superficial tumors (e.g., mast cell tumors, soft tissue sarcomas) and tumors within air-filled cavities (e.g., nasal tumors).

Acute side effects are seen mostly in the superficial tissues where the highest dose is delivered. In addition, because bone absorbs higher radiation doses than do surrounding tissues, late tissue effects are more common in bone when orthovoltage rather than megavoltage is the source of radiation.

Megavoltage Teletherapy

Radiation produced by megavoltage machines (^{60}Co and linear accelerator) mostly undergoes Compton absorption. During Compton absorption, an incident photon dislodges an electron with low binding energy. Much of the energy is released as a secondary photon, which travels farther in the tissue. Because Compton absorption is not dependent on the atomic number of the tissue, penetration is not affected by tissue density, and deeper structures can be irradiated than when using an orthovoltage source. The maximum dose is not achieved in tissues until a depth of approximately 0.5 cm below the surface; therefore, megavoltage radiation is "skin sparing." Irradiation of superficial tumors is achieved by placing a layer of tissue-equivalent bolus material over the tumor that allows buildup of the dose so the tumor is no longer "spared."

ELECTRON-BEAM THERAPY

Electron-beam therapy is available using certain linear accelerators. With electrons, the maximum dose is reached and then followed by a prompt decrease, so the dose is delivered to a much narrower volume. Because electrons can be given different energies, the distance they travel before energy reduces varies. With higher electron energies, penetration is greater and dose fall-off is not as steep. Lower-energy electrons are very useful in treating superficial tumors because deeper tissue is spared by a prompt decrease in radiation dose (e.g., a mast cell tumor on the thoracic wall of a small dog where underlying lung must be spared).

One disadvantage of electron-beam therapy is the same as for orthovoltage: Bone may shield underlying tissues.

PROTON-BEAM THERAPY

Proton-beam radiation is available for treatment of veterinary cancer patients at a few select sites. Protons have much

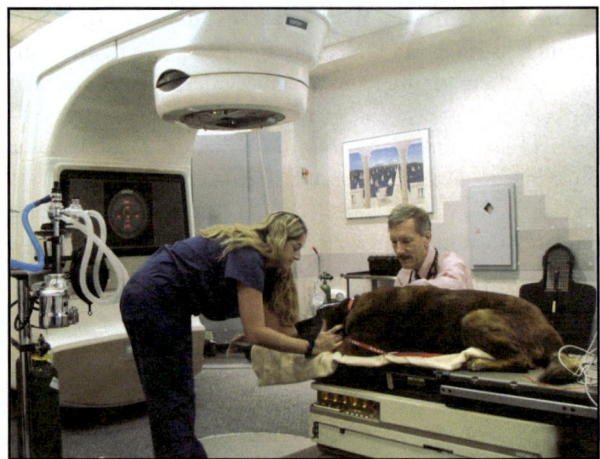

Figure 22-1. *Megavoltage radiation is the preferred treatment for many neoplastic conditions. This linear accelerator, like all other megavoltage radiation therapy units, has excellent penetrating capability and is able to reach deep-seated tumors while minimizing injury to overlying tissues.*

greater mass than electrons, travel more slowly, and are more likely to give up all their energy in a narrow tissue volume.

BRACHYTHERAPY

Radiation therapy is administered not only from external sources of energy but also from implanted radiation sources within or around the tumor (brachytherapy). Brachytherapy has a rapid decrease in intensity with increasing distance from the source and is therefore very effective for delivering extremely high doses very specifically to a local site, with normal tissue damage usually being restricted to immediately surrounding tissues. The amount of normal tissue injured is directly proportional to the energy of the radiation implanted as well as the time that the implant (radioactive source) is left in place.

Interstitial brachytherapy involves implanting "seeds" or "straws" of radioactive materials within the tumor. Interstitial brachytherapy seeds are often implanted in a removable package (e.g., Silastic tubing) and removed after the calculated dose has been delivered (Figure 22-2). Radiation therapy with a strontium-90 (^{90}Sr) handheld source delivers a very high dose of β-particle radiation that only penetrates 3 to 5 mm below the skin surface. Radioactive sources can also be administered into body cavities. Sources of radiation vary depending on the tissue to be implanted (e.g., cesium or radium for intracavitary placement, iridium for interstitial implants).

Because the source of radiation is implanted in the patient, interstitial or intracavitary brachytherapy makes the patient radioactive. Therefore, a period of isolation or quarantine is required for patients treated with interstitial brachytherapy.

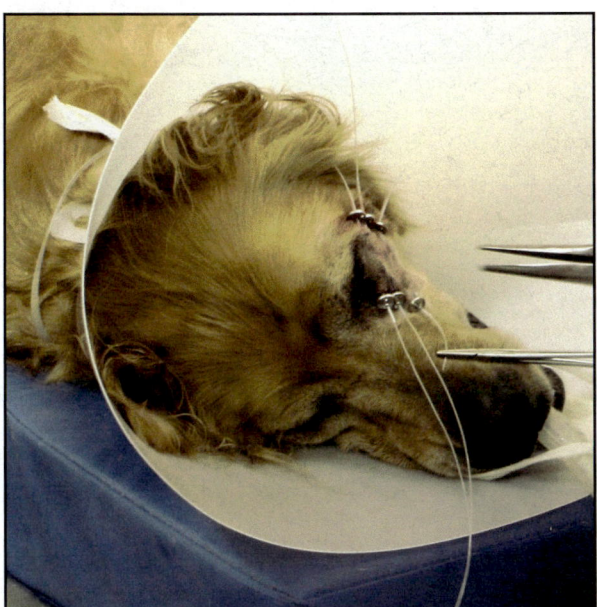

Figure 22-2. *This dog has a mast cell tumor that is to be treated with iridium-192 brachytherapy. The leaders are placed in the tumor bed, and iridium seeds are then introduced for the specified time to provide an adequate dosage. (Courtesy of Nicole Northrup, DVM, University of Georgia College of Veterinary Medicine)*

SYSTEMIC THERAPY

Radiation can be targeted to a specific tissue by use of a radionuclide with special affinity for the tumor cells. Examples in veterinary medicine include iodine-131 (^{131}I) for treatment of thyroid carcinoma and samarium-153 (^{153}Sm) targeted to bone for treatment of bone tumors in dogs.[1,2] Radionuclides such as these emit β particles that give up all their energy within a few millimeters of their source. It is therefore theoretically possible to deliver a very high dose to the tumor while restricting radiation of surrounding normal tissue.

Recently, radionuclides have been linked to monoclonal antibodies that "seek out" specific tumor tissues; this technique is also known as *radioimmunotherapy*.

Because the source of radiation is targeted to tissue within the patient, systemic radiotherapy makes the patient radioactive. Therefore, a period of isolation or quarantine is required for patients treated with systemic radiotherapy.

CONFORMAL RADIATION

Intensity-modulated radiation therapy or conformal radiation is an advanced mode of high-precision radiation therapy used in a few select veterinary centers. This technique utilizes computer-controlled linear accelerators to deliver precise radiation doses to a tumor. The radiation dose is designed to conform to the three-dimensional shape of the tumor by modulating the intensity of the radiation beam to focus a higher radiation dose to the tumor while minimizing damage to the nearby surrounding tissue. Many beams are directed to the treatment area from many different directions, producing a sculpted radiation dose that maximizes tumor dose while protecting adjacent normal tissues.

Intensity-modulated radiation therapy has been suggested to be so accurate that tissue more than 4 mm outside the beam has minimal radiation exposure. This is a great improvement over conventional radiation therapy but is not as accurate as one-session intracranial radiosurgery, which can obtain a precision of 0.33 to 1 mm.

Radiosurgery allows precise delivery of a single high dose of radiation in a single treatment. Stereotactic radiosurgery is used in human patients with head and neck tumors and requires that the patient be immobilized with skeletal fixation devices that allow the most accurate treatment. A linear accelerator mounted on a rotating gantry that is centered on the brain tumor provides accurate results, allowing a single large dose (10–15 Gy) of radiation to be delivered. The linear accelerator–based machines use one high-dose radiation beam that is redirected in many "arcs" to lessen the effect on surrounding healthy tissue. The exposure is brief, and only the tumor receives a significant radiation dose; the surrounding tissue remains unexposed.

Experience with this modality in veterinary patients is limited, but there are encouraging preliminary reports of radiosurgery for palliation of osteosarcoma and brain tumors.[3-5]

Palliative or Definitive Radiation Therapy

One of the most important decisions is whether a patient should be treated with curative or palliative intent. This decision influences not only the course of treatment but also the expectations of the caregiver for his or her pet.

Treatment with curative intent (definitive therapy) is often complicated, requiring frequent travel and multiple anesthesias. The total dose of radiation is usually higher than that required for palliation, and consequently the risks for unfavorable sequelae are greater. Such treatment is likely to be prolonged and expensive; however, for many patients, the chance of long-term tumor-free survival (>3 years) is high.

Palliative radiation therapy should have a specific and often short-term goal, usually to relieve pain or signs of cancer. It is often performed when a specific site is causing a problem to the patient but the rest of the cancer is unlikely to respond to any treatment (e.g., a painful digital metastasis from a pulmonary tumor that is not causing signs at any other site). For this reason, palliative therapy should minimize cost, inconvenience, discomfort, and risk for side effects and should be completed in the shortest reasonable time.

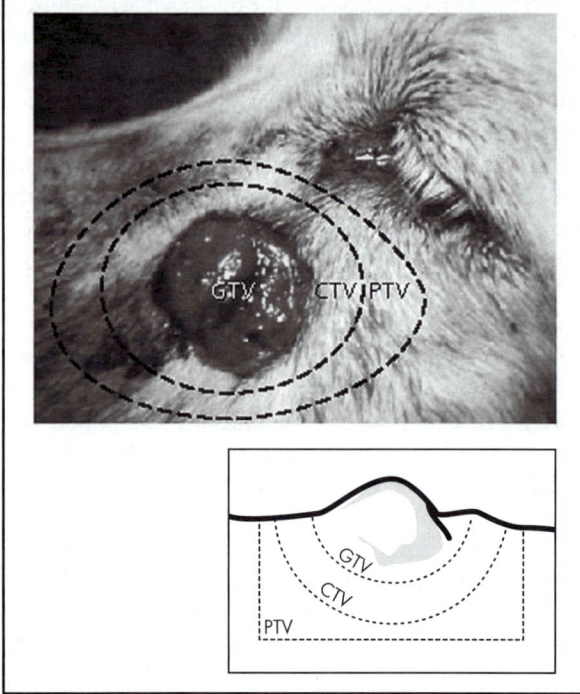

Figure 22-3. Gross tumor volume (GTV) is the clinically evident tumor based on palpation. Clinical tumor volume (CTV) is the gross tumor volume plus microscopic extension. The planning tumor volume (PTV) is the final volume irradiated and consists of the CTV plus a margin that allows for physiologic movement that could result in a geographic "miss." (From Moore AS: Radiation therapy for the treatment of tumours in small companion animals. Vet J 164:176–187, 2002; with permission)

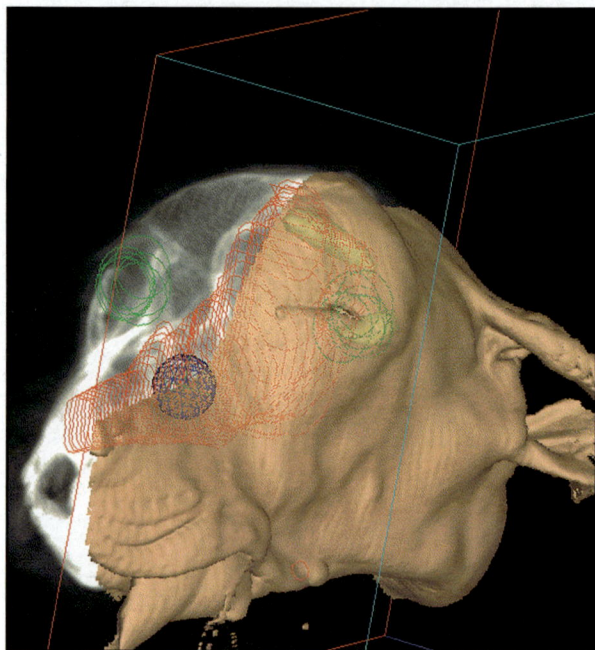

Figure 22-4. Reconstructed image of a patient undergoing radiation therapy, with the gross tumor volume (blue) and planning tumor volume (red) outlined. This allows the radiation oncologist to make adjustments to the field to protect normal tissue and to ensure that all tumor is treated.

Treatment Methods

A major component of successful radiation therapy is treatment planning. The importance of planning is illustrated by a study in which all recurrences of soft tissue sarcomas were seen at the edge of, or beyond, the treatment field, implying that the field may have not been properly planned. Dogs that did not have local recurrence lived a median of 5 years after treatment, emphasizing the importance of these marginal failures.[6]

Planning integrates beam distribution and homogeneity of dose within the target volume (tumor) while taking steps to minimize the dose to transit volume (normal tissue surrounding the tumor). This is achieved by using port films, patient immobilization, marking techniques using tattoos and laser localization, and detailed computed tomography (CT)–based treatment planning. Gross tumor volume is the clinically evidenced tumor based on imaging. More relevant is the clinical tumor volume, which is the gross tumor volume plus the volume at risk for tumor extension. If only the clinical tumor volume is irradiated, margins that contain tumor cells may receive an insufficient dose because of patient movement during treatment and inhomogeneity of the beam at the edge of the field. The planning tumor volume is the final volume irradiated and consists of the clinical tumor volume plus a margin that allows for physiologic motion and beam variation (Figure 22-3). CT-based radiation therapy planning also has the advantage of producing multiple images that can predict normal tissues that will be irradiated, allowing the radiation oncologist to block sensitive structures and to adjust the number and direction of the radiation fields (Figure 22-4).

The beam of radiation can be altered to make the dose conform to a specific target volume. Electrical machines deliver a beam that tends to have greater intensity in the center than on the sides. Wedges of a highly radiation-absorptive material such as lead may allow a more uniform dose to be delivered to the patient. Lead may also be used to block sensitive structures within the radiation field, where blocking will not protect tumor tissue (e.g., eyes can be blocked when irradiating a brain tumor).

After the treatment plan has been devised, a dosage is prescribed and the least toxic method of administering the energy determined. The dosage generally is limited by the tolerance of nearby normal tissues. The goal is to have less than 5% of patients experiencing significant toxicity.

Port films are radiographs made by the therapy machine to define the anatomic structures exposed to radiation and to assess the accuracy of treatment delivery (Figure 22-5). They

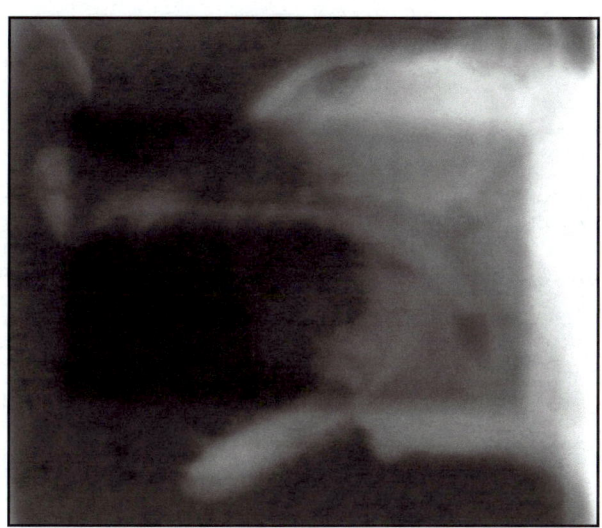

Figure 22-5. *Port films, such as this one of a dog with an oral tumor, help to determine whether radiosensitive structures need to be blocked.*

also help to determine whether radiosensitive structures need to be blocked. One study used port films to assess the accuracy of planned treatment in animals treated with radiation.[7] Port films taken on day 1 identified a reason to move or change the size of the radiation field in 53% of cases.

Much of the accuracy problem in veterinary radiation results because skin marks are mobile and therefore difficult to use. Fields defined by palpable structures such as lymph nodes or bony landmarks give more consistency to radiation planning and treatment. Patients are best immobilized using anesthesia. Short-acting injectable agents such as propofol are suitable before endotracheal intubation and isoflurane anesthesia because radiation treatments are usually completed in minutes and there are no painful stimuli. Repeatable positioning is important to reduce variation in dosing. In a study of pets with head tumors, animals positioned using a head holder attached to the table and an inflatable pillow for the thorax and neck had the most repeatable positioning.[8] Similar immobilization strategies may be used for animals with tumors at other body sites.

Timing of Radiation Therapy

Radiation is most effective at the periphery of a tumor where there are small numbers of cells that are well vascularized. In contrast, surgery is limited by preservation of normal tissues adjacent to the tumor and therefore fails microscopically and peripherally due to residual tumor cells. Surgery and radiation therapy are therefore complementary.

Most radiation therapy in veterinary practice is delivered postoperatively to the residual microscopic tumor. Postoperative (adjuvant) radiation therapy has the advantage that it is possible to histologically identify patients with residual disease that would benefit most from radiation therapy. The major disadvantage is that surgery may reduce tumor vascular supply. Tumor cells along the surgical scar may survive radiation therapy because they are protected in a relatively hypoxic environment. In addition, a large surgical scar will increase the size of the radiation field and hence the risk for side effects (Figure 22-6).

One study evaluated the effect of starting radiation therapy the day after surgery compared with delaying until 1 or 3 weeks after surgery. This study found that the strength of tissues was significantly less when radiation was started immediately after surgery, but healing was unaffected when the delay was 1 week or longer.[9]

Preoperative (neoadjuvant) radiation therapy has the advantage of sterilizing well-oxygenated cells at the periphery of a tumor before the vascular supply to these cells is compromised by surgery. Cells in the periphery that could be dislodged and seeded at the time of surgery are also irradiated. Preoperative radiation therapy may also reduce tumor volume in unresectable tumors, but this should not be used as a reason to reduce the size of the surgical field any more than is absolutely necessary to preserve normal structures. Disadvantages of preoperative radiation therapy include a delay of surgery while acute effects resolve; however, if peripheral cells are sterilized, this wait is not compromising the patient. A reduction in gross tumor size may lull the surgeon into attempting a less aggressive surgery. Another potential disadvantage is that fatally irradiated tumor cells may not die until they attempt mitosis, which can make histologic interpretation of surgical margins difficult.

> *The best tumor control for all malignancies is achieved if radiation is used early in the course of disease rather than after multiple surgeries.*

Whether radiation is used pre- or postoperatively, irradiation of a large volume of tissue leads to a poor outcome. When large areas are irradiated, planning is made more difficult and a larger volume of normal tissue is irradiated. This leads to a decreased chance of tumor control and an increased risk for complications. The earlier in the course of cancer that radiation is used, the more likely it is to result in a successful outcome and the less likely it is to result in severe toxicity.

Adverse Effects

The goal of radiation therapy is to increase tumor cell killing without increasing the adverse effects of radiation. This therapeutic index should be as wide as possible.

The dose (and therefore effectiveness) of radiation therapy is limited by the tolerance of normal tissues surrounding the tumor to the effects of radiation therapy. Differences in radiation response by normal tissues are determined not only by

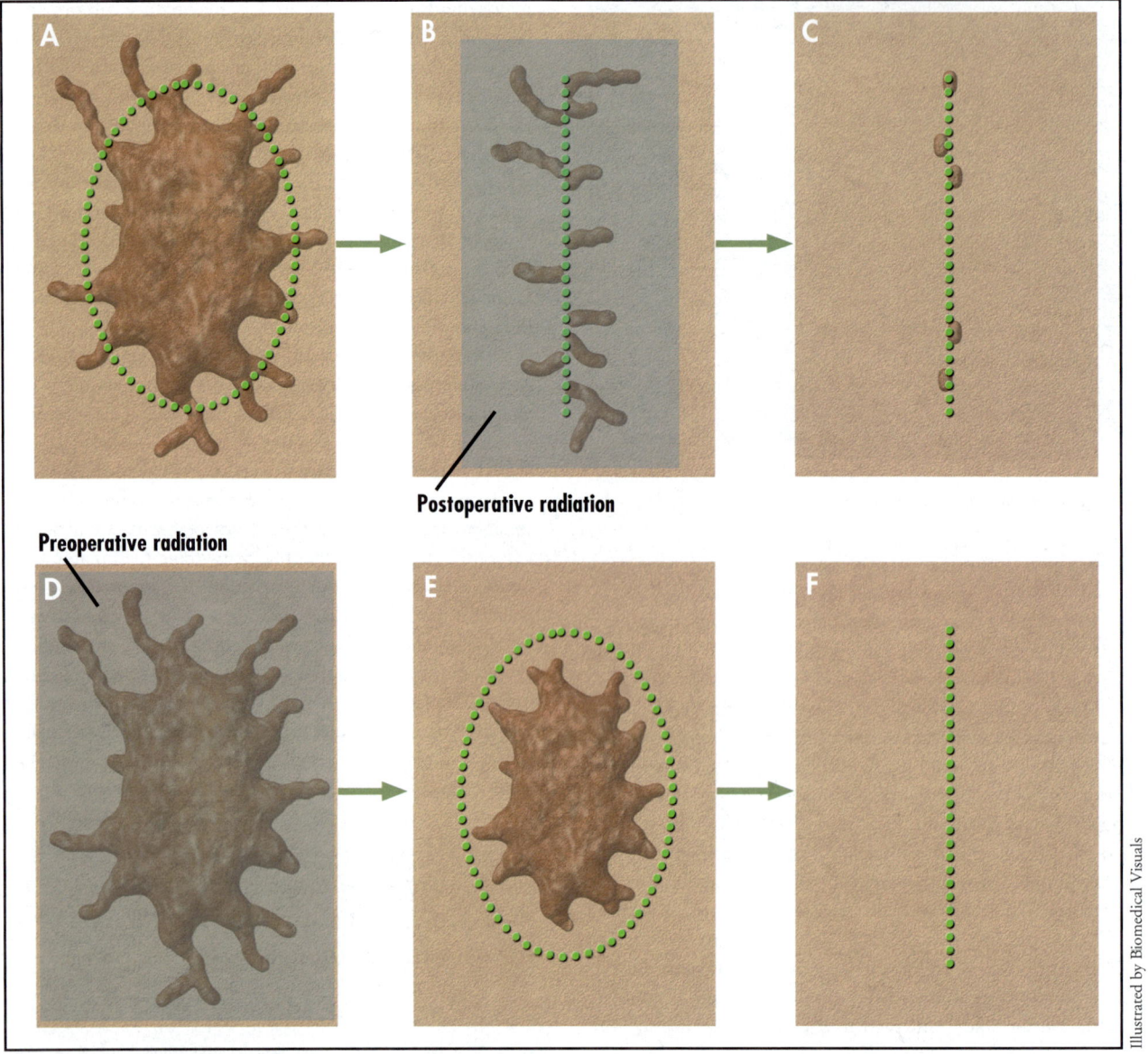

Figure 22-6. Surgery may leave hypoxic and hence radiation-resistant cells in the surgical scar. These are a source of failure. Preoperative radiation may affect the well-oxygenated periphery, thereby "sterilizing" margins and reducing the risk of failure. Despite the theoretic advantages of preoperative radiation therapy, neither preoperative nor postoperative radiation has clinically shown a marked advantage. (**A**) The surgical excision (dotted line) fails at the edges due to microscopic extensions (shown along the surgical scar). Postoperative radiation therapy (blue shaded area; **B**) to the scar may fail due to hypoxia at the scar line, allowing tumor regrowth (**C**). (**D**) Preoperative radiation therapy (blue shaded area) is most effective for the microscopic tissue, leaving only the hypoxic bulk of the tumor that is surgically excised (dotted line; **E**). Surgical excision will leave no residual tumor as long as the original surgical field is not reduced (**F**).

the actual cell type but also, and more importantly, by the proliferative requirement for tissue maintenance. If the proliferative requirement is high, the tissue is termed *radiosensitive*; if the proliferative requirement is low, it is termed *radioresistant*. For example, liver and bone undergo little or no proliferation in steady state, but there can be a problem if there is damage that requires cellular proliferation to reconstitute normal tissue, such as a bone fracture or liver damage. Tissues that are constantly renewing, such as skin, gastrointestinal mucosa, bone marrow, glands, and reproductive tissues, are considered radiosensitive, and these are the *acutely responding* tissues, in which the acute effects of radiation are most commonly seen. During radiation therapy, there may be differential recruitment of cells from unirradiated adjacent areas in order to replace and repair acutely damaged tissue. This may be the major difference between tumor and normal tissues because there is little opportunity for tumors to recruit new cells.

Most normal acutely responding tissues (except bone marrow stem cells) have a large threshold dose (see Properties and Uses of Radiation Therapy, above), so dividing the total radiation dose into multiple smaller dose fractions may preserve these tissues by allowing repair between subthreshold fractions. Increasing the size of each fraction means that a biologically higher equivalent dose will be given to late-responding tissues than to acutely responding tissues, and therefore the likelihood of late effects of radiation increases.

ACUTE EFFECTS

Acute effects of radiation are common and should be expected with clinically relevant doses of radiation toward the end of the treatment course and for days to weeks afterward. These effects arise in rapidly proliferating normal cells and may be exacerbated by release of catabolic products. Common acute side effects include mucositis, moist epidermal inflammation, and keratitis, depending on the tumor site and surrounding field irradiated. The occurrence of acute effects is thought to be acceptable because healing is usually rapid and complete. Acute effects will be worsened when there is insufficient time between radiation fractions for recruitment of new normal tissue cells and for repair of sublethal damage. Shorter radiation courses with larger fractions of radiation increase the severity of acute side effects compared with the same total dose given over a more protracted period in smaller dosages per fraction. For these reasons, excessive acute reactions can be ameliorated by a small decrease in fraction size or a short treatment break. This allows rapid resolution due to reconstitution of normal tissue. Small breaks, such as over weekends, may ameliorate acute effects and allow reoxygenation of tumor tissue. However, it is also possible that the same scheduling may protect rapidly proliferating tumors. Treatment of acute effects is usually symptomatic preceding repair or replacement of the damaged normal cells (see below).

LATE EFFECTS

Late effects of radiation are less common than acute effects in veterinary medicine. Common limitations on all organ systems may be based on radiosensitivity of vascular connective tissue and endothelial cells. Tissues in which functional activity does not require cell renewal, such as muscle and nervous tissue, are more resistant to the acute side effects of radiation. However, these tissues have vascular and connective tissue stromal cells, which may be required to divide and thereby show damage that translates into late effects of radiation. Radiation may also directly damage cell membranes and thus interrupt membrane transport, leading to edema. This process may be important in the development of central nervous system damage.

Second malignancies are an uncommon late effect of radiation and are more likely at lower total doses because at higher doses the risk falls, presumably due to cell killing. The latent period for carcinogenesis is measured in years, so there may be an increased risk of a second, radiation-induced malignancy when patients are treated at a younger age for tumors that are potentially curable by radiation therapy (Figure 22-7).

Unlike acute effects, late effects of radiation occur months to years after a course of radiation therapy and are irreversible. Examples of late effects are necrosis, fibrosis, nonhealing ulceration, central nervous system damage, and blindness. The occurrence of late effects depends on the size of each radiation fraction dose and somewhat on the total dose of radiation. The likelihood of late radiation effects is highest with large doses per treatment fraction. For example, late effects are higher with so-called *hypofractionated* or palliative treatment protocols, such as 8 Gy per fraction given weekly, than with small doses (e.g., 3 Gy) given daily. Protraction of the total treatment course by taking breaks in treatment will probably not help to avoid late radiation effects. Late effects of radiation are considered to be dose limiting, and considerable emphasis is placed on their avoidance in the design of radiation protocols. In human patients, aggressive therapy results in a high cure rate. A long life expectancy, even in older patients, means that effects seen 5 years after therapy may still result in considerable morbidity. In veterinary medicine, patient lifespan is shorter, and—particularly for older animals—survival times, even in cured patients, may be insufficient to see late radiation effects.

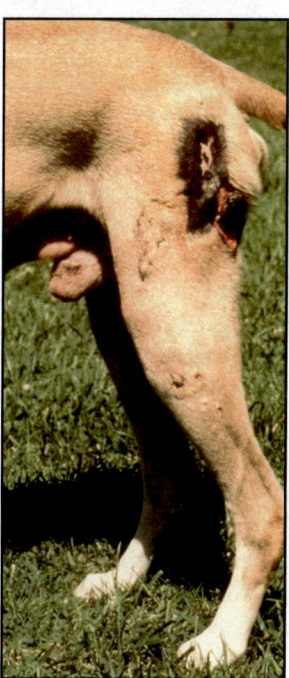

Figure 22-7. Second malignancies are very rare sequelae of radiation therapy but are more likely with coarsely fractionated protocols. This sarcoma occurred at the edge of the radiation field for a mast cell tumor treated with 4-Gy fractions 6 years previously. Many veterinary patients do not live long enough for this sequela to occur. (Courtesy of Bruce R. Madewell, VMD, University of California, Davis)

OTHER EFFECTS

Other effects of radiation are less common. Local radiation may cause a decreased immune response, presumably by irradiating circulat-

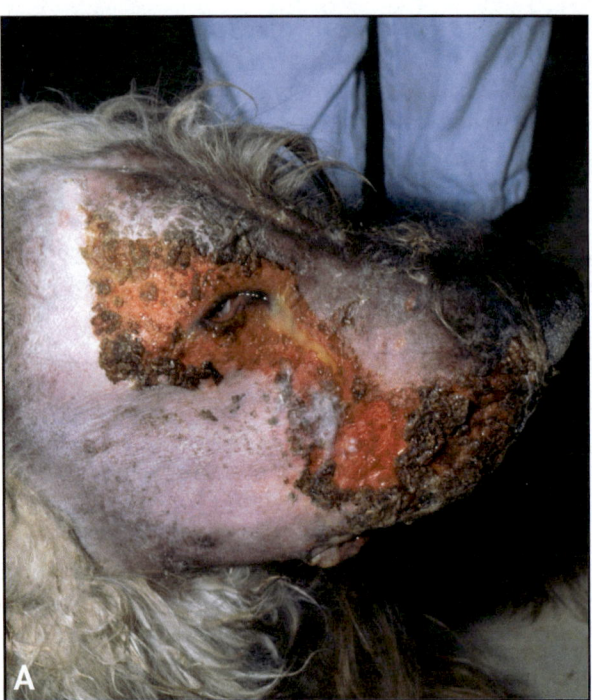 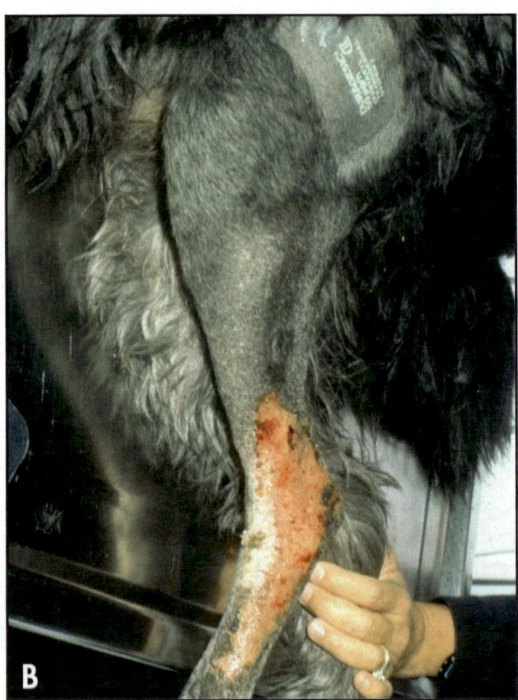

Figure 22-8. Acute reactions generally appear toward the end of radiation therapy; they include erythema, dry desquamation with pruritus, and moist desquamation. These dogs were treated with radiation therapy for a nasal tumor (**A**) and a mast cell tumor of the hind leg (**B**). In both dogs, acute adverse effects started in the third week of radiation therapy and worsened to this point 2 weeks later. Generally, the best treatment of these cutaneous injuries includes cleansing the area with mild soap and water, if symptomatic. A Water-Pic or hydropulsion with a 60-ml syringe may help clean the lesion. If self-mutilation is a problem, an Elizabethan collar, sidebars, or bandages should be employed. Note the fentanyl patch on the dog with the irradiated leg (**B**), placed to enhance comfort. Pain relief is essential to enhance quality of life in these cases. Both patients recovered uneventfully.

ing lymphocytes as they pass through irradiated volume or due to cytokine release. This rarely appears to be clinically significant. Mutagenesis is an uncommon problem. Even if germ-line cells are affected, most radiation-induced mutations are recessive and so rarely lead to abnormal births.

> **KEY POINT**
>
> *Generally, the acute effects of radiation therapy start toward the end of the treatment period, may substantially worsen 1 to 3 weeks after treatment is discontinued, and may last for several weeks. Late effects may occur 6 months to years after the end of treatment.*

Radiation therapy is a local treatment; therefore, side effects are confined to the area being treated. The only exception is when the entire body is irradiated, as with bone marrow transplantation, which is an uncommon procedure in veterinary medicine. It is important to educate clients about the ways different tissues respond to radiation therapy and the timing of the appearance of adverse effects.

Acute effects of radiation are to be expected, but in nearly all cases, such side effects resolve without limiting protocols. Protocols that use smaller doses per fraction (definitive or coarse) have a lower risk of late effects, thereby allowing higher total doses to be delivered, which leads to higher tumor control rates. In contrast, late effects of radiation are dose limiting and are more likely with higher doses per treatment fraction (hypofractionated or palliative). The higher risk of late effects is an excellent reason not to use a palliative protocol in a dog that has a radiosensitive tumor and a high likelihood of long survival.

Patient Management
SKIN

The skin is often injured in external-beam radiation therapy, particularly with orthovoltage and electron-beam sources (Figures 22-8 and 22-9). Acute reactions that generally appear toward the end of radiation therapy include erythema, dry desquamation with pruritus, and moist desquamation. The best treatment of these cutaneous injuries involves cleansing the area with mild soap and water, if symptomatic. A Water-Pic or hydropulsion with a 60-ml syringe may help clean the lesion. If self-mutilation is a problem, an Elizabethan collar,

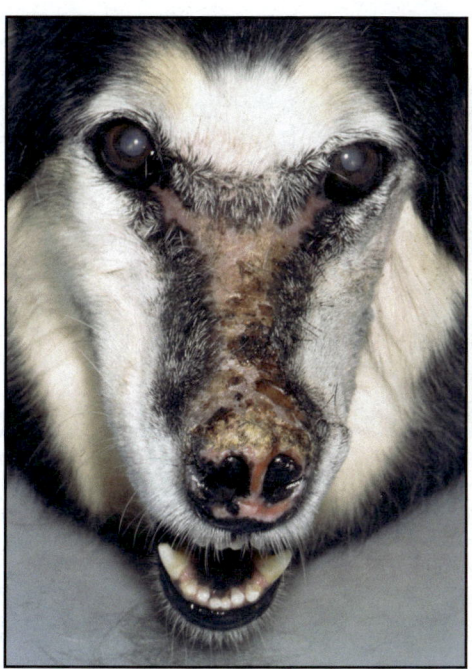

Figure 22-9. *These lesions demonstrate the hypopigmentation, hyperpigmentation, and alopecia that can occur months to years after the completion of radiation therapy. The lesions on this dog occurred weeks to months after a nasal chondrosarcoma was treated with megavoltage radiation therapy.*

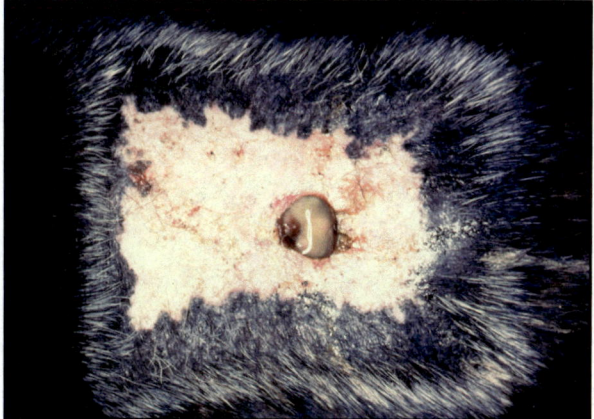

Figure 22-10. *Late effects of depigmentation, skin fibrosis, and ulceration with full-thickness necrosis in a dog treated with a high dose of orthovoltage radiation. The area delineating the periphery of the field is hyperpigmented, and the hair coat has changed color. Orthovoltage deposits most of the energy in the superficial layers of the skin, so high doses have the potential for late effects such as these. By contrast, megavoltage is "skin sparing."*

sidebars, or bandages should be employed. Non–petroleum-based vitamin E ointments have been used. Although controversial, some suggest that pets with severe pruritus or moist desquamation may benefit from cleansing the area with a 1:1 solution of hydrogen peroxide and normal saline and may require treatment with a topical or oral corticosteroid. If a topical corticosteroid is used, a non–petroleum-based product is recommended. Combining cleansing with a wetting solution such as Cara-klenz with subsequent application of aloe vera gel extract (Carrington Dermal Wound Gel) has been suggested. Telfa pads should be used when the area needs to be covered. Occasionally, a patient may develop a pruritic rash that originates from the area of treatment and spreads to areas outside the treatment field. Systemic antihistamines, such as diphenhydramine, or topical corticosteroids may be indicated for these patients. Late adverse effects include changes in pigmentation, telangiectasia, ulceration, and fibrosis, which, if extensive, can be painful (Figure 22-10). Debilitating late skin changes, which are extremely rare, can be repaired with reconstructive techniques using well-vascularized tissue.

ORAL CAVITY AND PHARYNX

Damage to the oral cavity and pharynx is very common in dogs that receive radiation therapy for nasal and oral tumors (Figure 22-11). This area can be very frustrating to treat because radiation-induced oral mucositis may result in anorexia and secondary debilitation. Placing a gastrostomy tube before initiating radiation therapy is recommended in any animal that does not have a good plane of nutrition and any time the oral cavity is to be included in the radiation field (e.g., oral melanoma in older small dogs). Oral mucositis and anorexia are common in the acute phase of radiation therapy, and xerostomia and dental caries may be seen in the chronic phase. Because oral damage can be so debilitating, care should be taken to ensure that all necessary dental work is completed before the start of radiation therapy. During treatment, owners may want to rinse their pet's mouth with a solution of salt and water (1 teaspoon of salt in 1 quart of water). Some recommend adding Maalox to this saltwater solution to coat the mouth. Cool tea solutions can be used to lavage the mouth three to six times per day (Figure 22-12), which may reduce the discomfort of the oral cavity and freshen the breath. If the patient experiences pain when swallowing, 5 to 15 ml of 2% lidocaine (xylocaine viscous solution) may be squirted into the mouth several times a day. Because oral and nasal damage from radiation therapy may reduce smell and taste sensations, more palatable, warmed, aromatic foods should be prescribed. Increasing the amount of liquids given may help overcome xerostomia brought on by salivary gland radiation. Artificial saliva preparations, such as a mixture of sorbitol, sodium, carboxymethyl cellulose, and methylparaben (Salivart; Gebauer, Cleveland, OH), may be beneficial in these patients. Some investigators have recommended oral glutamine supplementation to reduce the severity of oral mucositis. However, in one study, although changes in

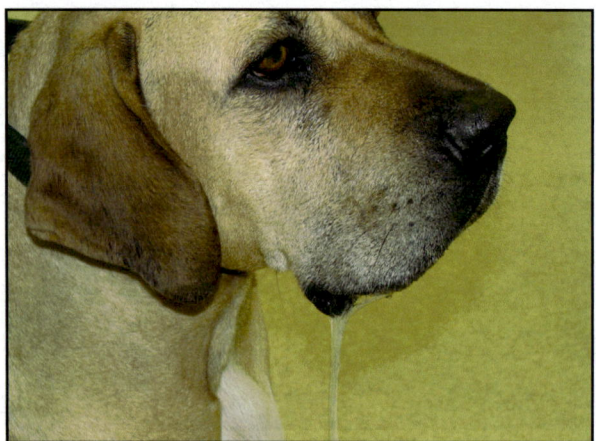

Figure 22-11. *Profuse salivation may occur toward the end of radiation therapy and may persist for several weeks after treatment is completed. The saliva is thick and tenacious and is associated with bad breath and significant oral mucositis. The mucositis can be profound enough to cause anorexia and weight loss. A gastrostomy or esophagostomy tube can allow enteral feeding to maintain a good plane of nutrition, which enhances quality of life and decreases morbidity and mortality.*

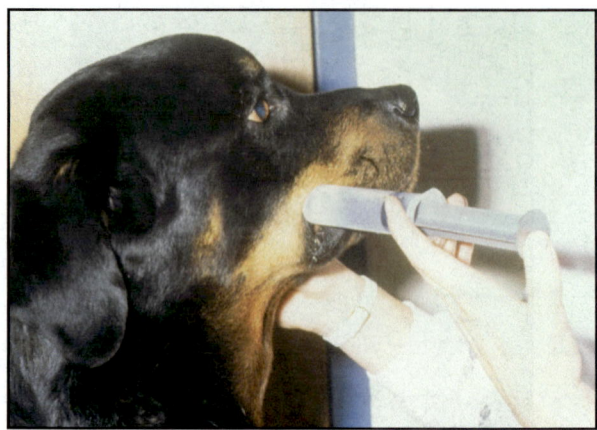

Figure 22-12. *Oral mucositis can be treated by lavaging the mouth frequently with a variety of liquids, including tea. The tea contains astringents and can decrease oral discomfort, decrease the bacterial count in the mouth, and reduce the viscosity of the saliva. This improves quality of life and reduces morbidity and mortality.*

prostaglandin levels appeared less pronounced in supplemented dogs than in dogs not receiving glutamine, clinical mucositis did not differ.[10] Mucositis usually resolves within 3 weeks after radiation therapy is completed.

Late effects are rare; occasionally, bone necrosis of the mandible or maxilla may be seen years after irradiation of an oral tumor.

COLON AND RECTUM

Occasionally, the colon and rectum are in the radiation therapy field. Irritation to these areas can be manifested by bleeding, tenesmus, and pain. A low-residue diet and a stool softener may provide relief. Steroid enemas (e.g., Proctofoam) may be beneficial in select patients. When the anus and perianal areas are injured by radiation therapy, the area should be kept clean using soap and water and dried thoroughly.

If radiation therapy is to be used for tumors of the caudal abdomen, small, frequent fractions are more likely to avoid complications. In one study, dogs receiving more than 3.3 Gy per fraction to the pelvic area had an increased risk of developing severe colitis, and 60% of these dogs had intestinal perforation. In contrast, dogs treated with fractions of 2.7 Gy or less had only mild to moderate self-limiting complications.[11]

EYE

The eye is often in the field of radiation therapy in dogs with nasal tumors (Figure 22-13). The lens of the eye is considered sensitive to relatively low doses of radiation therapy, which can result in cataract formation months to years after radiation therapy is completed. In addition, retinal hemorrhages may result in blindness. Conjunctivitis or keratoconjunctivitis sicca may occur acutely, and it is important to monitor tear production in animals during and after therapy. For keratoconjunctivitis sicca, artificial tear preparations may be beneficial. It is important to confirm that no corneal ulcers are present before prescribing steroid-containing ophthalmic ointments.

BLOOD

If a significant amount of the bone marrow is included in the radiation therapy field, bone marrow damage may occur. This may be a concern when large fields are irradiated and chemotherapy is also planned; myelosuppression may be enhanced in these patients. In addition, all lymphocytes that pass through the radiation field are lysed.

BONE

If bone is included in the radiation therapy field, a bone sequestrum due to necrosis may result. This late effect is much more likely to occur after orthovoltage radiation therapy than after megavoltage radiation (Figure 22-14). Bone necrosis occurs many months to years after therapy. Removal of the sequestrum is indicated in such cases. When brachytherapy is used to deliver radiotherapy to localized areas, radiation from these local sources can damage surrounding structures, including bone.

LUNG

If lung tissue is included in the radiation therapy field, radiation pneumonitis may result, even at relatively low radiation doses. Pneumonitis can cause decreased respiratory tidal volume if a large enough volume of lung is irra-

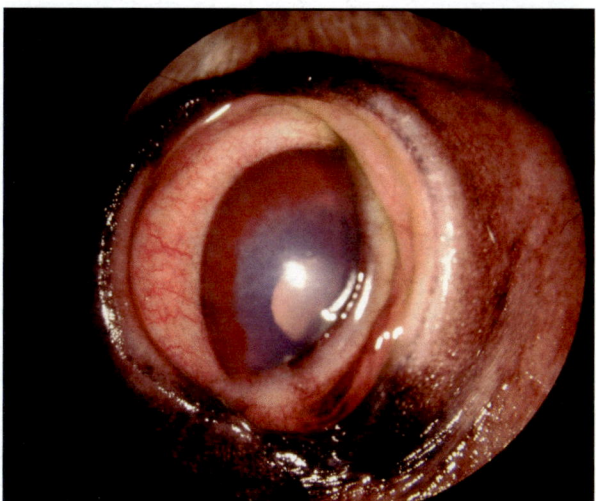

Figure 22-13. *The eye is often in the field of radiation therapy for dogs with tumors of the head. The lens of the eye is considered sensitive to relatively low doses of radiation therapy, which can result in cataract formation months to years after radiation therapy is completed. Conjunctivitis or keratoconjunctivitis sicca may also occur. This dog was treated for a nasal tumor 2 weeks before this picture was taken and developed conjunctivitis and keratitis that resolved 3 weeks after radiation therapy was completed.*

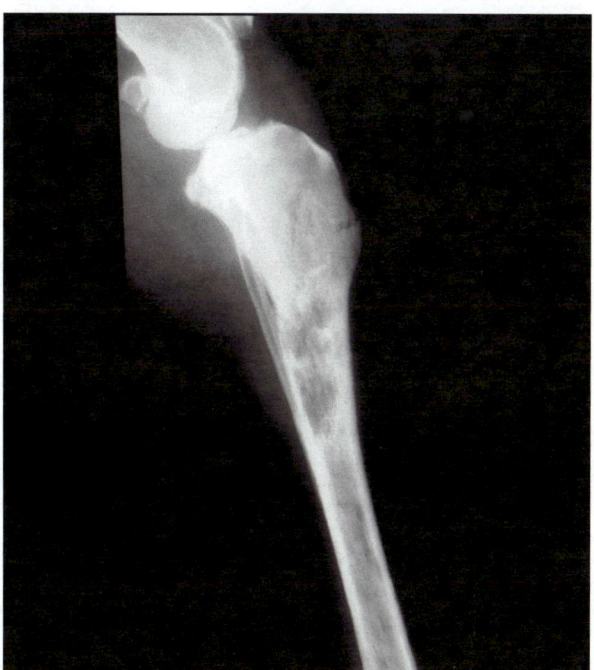

Figure 22-14. *Evidence of bone necrosis in a Bouvier des Flandres 3.5 years after orthovoltage radiation therapy for a cutaneous mast cell tumor. Orthovoltage deposits a greater amount of energy into bone than does megavoltage, but this side effect is still a rare occurrence.*

diated. Small volumes may not cause clinical problems, although pneumonitis can still occur. The use of electron-beam radiation therapy can reduce the risk of this toxicity because electrons give up most of their energy in a narrow depth so lung tissue underlying the irradiated tumor can be spared (Figures 22-15 and 22-16).

MISCELLANEOUS SITES

Other areas that can be damaged include the esophagus, stomach, small intestine, and liver.

The **endocrine system**, including the pituitary and thyroid glands, may be injured when radiation therapy of the head and neck is performed.

When the **heart** is included in the radiation therapy field, pericarditis and resultant pericardial effusion may be identified 4 to 6 months after radiation therapy is complete. A pericardectomy may be necessary to treat these animals.

When the **urinary bladder** is in the radiation therapy field, high single doses of radiation, such as those used in intraoperative radiation therapy, can result in severe fibrosis and lack of elasticity. Fibrosis may also occur as a late effect of fractionated external-beam radiation therapy.

Cranial radiation therapy occasionally results in headache, nausea, vomiting, and papilledema. Steroid therapy is generally indicated for these patients and should be considered during and after treatment. The most severe effect of radiation therapy to the brain includes brain necrosis, which can result in severe neurologic problems.

FATTY ACIDS AND RADIATION

Tumor sensitization to radiation by polyunsaturated fatty acids (PUFAs) has been investigated. One group studied the in vitro response of a chemically induced rat malignant astrocytoma cell line to radiation after the cell culture medium was supplemented with either γ-linoleic acid or the long-chain n-3 PUFAs eicosapentaenoic acid or docosahexaenoic acid (DHA) and found that n-3 PUFAs enhanced radiation-induced cell cytotoxicity.[12,13]

Another study documented the radiosensitivity-enhancing effect of dietary DHA on rat autochthonous mammary tumors.[14] Whether dietary n-3 PUFAs can lead to enhanced sensitivity of tumor tissue in the absence of a similar increase in the radiosensitivity of nontumor tissue remains a critical issue. Several studies have suggested that PUFAs do not sensitize normal tissues to radiation. For example, because ionizing radiation generates reactive oxygen species, a study was initiated to determine whether dietary DHA might sensitize mammary tumors to irradiation using a model in which mammary tumors were induced by *N*-methylnitrosourea in Sprague-Dawley rats.[14] In the study, it was shown that dietary DHA sensitized mammary tumors to radiation. The addition of vitamin E inhibited the beneficial effect of DHA, suggesting that this effect might be mediated by oxidative damage to the peroxidizable lipids.

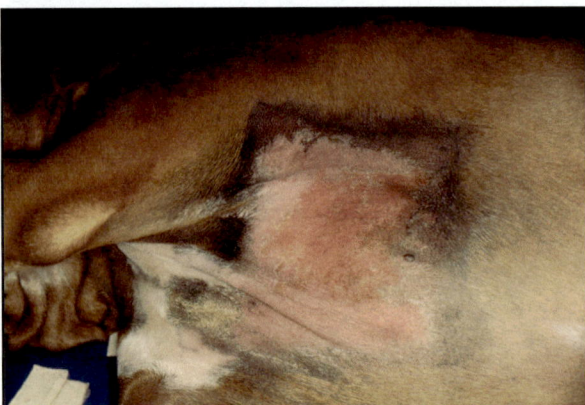

Figure 22-15. *This dog was treated with orthovoltage radiation for an axillary mast cell tumor; the field is outlined by alopecia and moist desquamation.*

Clinical Use of Radiation Therapy

Radiation is becoming widely available to treat tumors in animals. Orthovoltage machines capable of delivering low-energy external-beam radiation are less versatile than linear accelerators and ^{60}Co machines that deliver megavoltage radiation. In addition, electron-beam capabilities that are available with some linear accelerators allow more targeted treatment in smaller patients. With the increased availability of computerized treatment planning and the delineation of the extent of the disease by CT and magnetic resonance imaging, the beneficial effects of radiation therapy are bound to increase substantially. The future of radiation therapy will be tied into the use of radiobiologic and tumor biology information to enhance the beneficial effects of radiation therapy. In addition, the combination of radiation therapy with surgery and chemotherapy may result in substantial improvement in the efficacy of this treatment modality.

Differences in control rates between studies of treatment of the same tumor type may depend on the total dose, the size of each fraction, and the protraction of the course of radiation. Veterinary radiation protocols can be broadly characterized as definitive, coarse, hypofractionated (palliative), and hyperfractionated (accelerated):

- **Coarse fractionation:** Many reports of radiation therapy in veterinary medicine have used relatively high doses per fraction (≥4 Gy) delivered on an alternate-day schedule (Monday, Wednesday, and Friday) to a modest total dose (40–48 Gy). This relatively coarse fractionation would be expected to result in good control of radiation-sensitive tumors and a modest prevalence of late effects. In Great Britain, radiation has been delivered weekly with very large doses per fraction.

- **Definitive fractionation:** Recent studies using higher total dosages (usually 2.7–3.0 Gy per fraction daily to a total

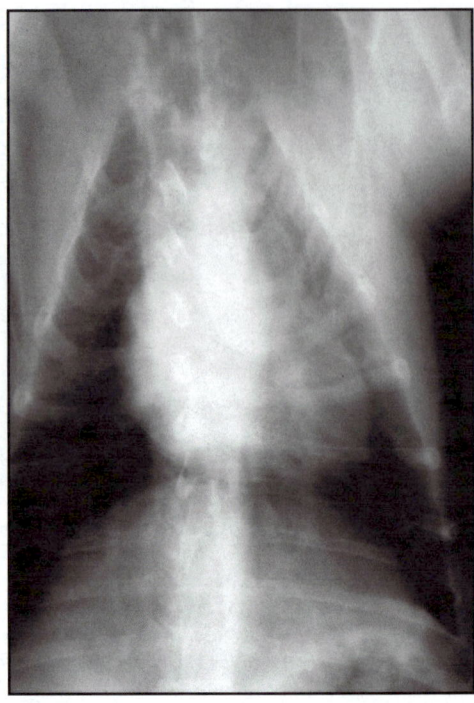

Figure 22-16. *A radiograph of the dog seen in Figure 22-15. There is a focal area of pneumonitis in the left cranial lung field, and the dog was coughing. The pneumonitis resolved with no residual problems, but if electron-beam radiation therapy is available, it is preferred for sites that overlie radiation-sensitive structures such as the lung.*

dose of 51–60 Gy), and long-term follow-up have reported durable control of a variety of tumor types. Using these definitive fractionation protocols, cures are possible in dogs with certain oral tumors, mast cell tumors, and brain tumors and in dogs with soft tissue sarcomas.

- **Hypofractionation:** The use of very large fractions (8–10 Gy per fraction) to a moderate total dose (16–30 Gy) has been employed for palliation in pets that have a short life expectancy and, therefore, little risk of late radiation side effects.

- **Hyperfractionation:** Rapid proliferation of tumor cells has a number of potential consequences. There is a higher risk of tumor escape through accelerated repopulation during the intertreatment interval of alternate-day treatment. In addition, the delay from surgery to treatment may allow regrowth in tumors with a high proliferative fraction. Tumors with a high proliferative component are probably not treated adequately using a coarse fractionation scheme. It has been thought that some tumors, particularly those of the nasal cavity in dogs, could have short doubling time, so shortening the time to deliver radiation may hinder repopulation by tumor cells. Accelerated fractionation protocols may be more effective when the tumor contains a large percentage of proliferating cells.

Despite the assumption that tumors are rapidly proliferating, few studies have directly measured the proliferative fraction of cells in tumors of cats and dogs. Proliferating cell nuclear antigen (PCNA) is expressed primarily during the S phase of the cell cycle, during which tumor cells are most resistant to radiation therapy. The proportion of cells expressing PCNA reflects the proliferative rate of tumors and is measured by immunohistochemical staining of tumor biopsy samples. Unfortunately, most clinical publications have not addressed the proliferative fraction of the tumors they are treating. Ideally, the variation in proliferative capacity between tumors should be exploited on an individual basis rather than devising radiation protocols based on information from tumors in human patients. Pretreatment measurement of proliferative fraction is feasible and would allow accelerated fractionation to be reserved for patients that could benefit the most and for whom the higher risk of side effects is balanced by an improved chance of tumor control.

It is possible to provide long-term tumor control in dogs using radiation therapy, particularly for mast cell tumors, soft tissue sarcomas, oral tumors, and brain tumors. Radiation therapy is also effective for the control of nasal, rectal, perianal, and anal tumors. When possible, individualizing treatment of tumors based on tumor staging and proliferative fraction should be considered rather than making blanket assumptions about the behavior of histologically determined tumor types.

The variability in response to radiation therapy of these various tumor types may also depend on the amount of radiation therapy delivered, the method by which radiation therapy is given, and the course and scheduling of radiation therapy.

When comparing results from veterinary studies that use radiation therapy, readers should note not only the median survival times and tumor control rates but also the long-term survival rates and acute and late complication rates. The low total doses used in early veterinary studies meant that, with few exceptions, long-term tumor control was rare, survival was short, and, therefore, late effects of radiation were rarely seen. The treatment schedule was determined by the difficulties of repeated anesthesia rather than by radiobiological necessity, and reported acute effects were relatively mild and short lived. More recently, safe short-acting anesthetics have allowed more frequent treatments with smaller doses per fraction, and the ability to deliver higher total doses has increased as fraction size has decreased. The recent radiation therapy literature is certainly more encouraging to veterinary practitioners.

ORAL TUMORS

The most common oral tumors in dogs are malignant melanoma, squamous cell carcinoma (SCC), fibrosarcoma, and epulides. Radiation therapy is effective for local control of many of these oral tumors.

Coarse fractionation: In one study, 105 dogs were treated for malignant oral tumors using megavoltage for a total dose of 48 Gy.[15] Acute reactions in the final week of treatment were considered severe enough to result in premature treatment cessation in 8% of dogs. A similar percentage of dogs developed late effects of bone necrosis or fistula. Late effects tended to occur after irradiation of large tumors and in dogs that had severe acute reactions involving contiguous bone. Dogs with SCC and oral melanoma had high early local recurrence rates when compared with dogs with fibrosarcoma, but all tumors had a similar late recurrence rate.[15] This emphasizes the need for longer periods of evaluation in the reporting of veterinary studies. Survival rates 3 years after treatment were 55% for SCC, 40% for fibrosarcoma, and 20% for oral melanoma. Large tumors of any histologic type were more likely to progress at an earlier time, and oral melanomas were more likely to metastasize.

The same protocol was used to treat 47 dogs with epulides.[16] These dogs were on average younger and had longer survival times than dogs with malignant oral tumors because of successful long-term control by radiation. Survival rates 3 years after treatment were more than 80%. In this study, 11% of dogs had late effects. Long-term survival in this group of dogs gives reliable information on late effects for this fractionation protocol.[16] It is possible that a lower dose per fraction may reduce the risk of late effects in dogs with oral tumors, but this has not yet been reported in the veterinary literature.

Hypofractionation: Traditionally, melanomas have been considered to be radioresistant. Recent research suggests that melanomas may be one of the few tumors for which large-dose fractions are necessary to cause death of tumor cells. Therefore, high dose-per-fraction schedules may be warranted in patients with malignant melanomas. Oral melanomas have a high metastatic rate, especially when the tumor is large, restricting the beneficial results of radiation therapy for this tumor.

In one study, 36 dogs with oral melanoma received 36 Gy in four weekly fractions of 9 Gy. Tumor size was reduced in all dogs, and 25 of them had complete remission. Median survival was 21 weeks, and acute radiation effects were predictably mild. Only 10 dogs survived for longer than 1 year, but late effects of bone necrosis or second malignancy were seen in five of these dogs.[17] Such hypofractionated protocols may not be ideal when long-term survival is possible, such as for dogs with small (early-stage) oral melanomas, because late effects of radiation should be of concern.

SQUAMOUS CELL CARCINOMA OF NONORAL SITES

Tonsillar SCCs typically have a poor response to therapy, primarily because of the high metastatic rate. In a study involving eight dogs with tonsillar SCC, median survival time was 4 months when radiotherapy was combined with surgical excision.[18] Another study used orthovoltage radiation therapy, cisplatin, and doxorubicin to treat tonsillar SCC in six dogs; the median disease-free interval was 8 months, and median survival was approximately 10 months.[19] SCC of the nasal planum in dogs has been reported to be refractory to the beneficial effects of radiotherapy.[20] The reason for this difference in response rate for the same tumor type at different sites is unknown.

CERUMINOUS GLAND CARCINOMA

Ceruminous gland carcinomas are frequently incompletely excised. Megavoltage radiation therapy (48 Gy in 12 fractions) was used to treat five dogs with ceruminous gland carcinoma.[21] Some dogs had been treated surgically with incomplete margins; therefore, radiation was adjuvant. One dog with recurrence received additional radiation treatment and survived another 20 months. Three dogs were alive and free of disease between 2 and 5 years after treatment.[21]

NASAL TUMORS

There is little doubt that radiation therapy is the treatment of choice for dogs with nasal tumors, but there is much variation within the literature regarding response to therapy. The prognostic factors that may influence response to therapy include tumor histology, clinical stage, tumor size, type of radiation therapy, and dose of energy delivered, as well as whether surgery was performed before radiation therapy.

Definitive and coarse fractionation: Nasal tumors in dogs are conventionally treated with radiation therapy. In the past, if megavoltage was used, surgical debulking was not recommended because it was thought that the air-filled nasal cavity would result in inconsistent dosing due to the sparing of 0.5 cm of tissue as radiation absorption builds. This assumption has recently been challenged.[22] If orthovoltage is used, surgical debulking is necessary to enable dosing of residual tissue by the lower-energy beam. Survival times for this tumor type are modest, ranging from 8 to 16 months depending on the study.[23–26] There is no difference between orthovoltage and megavoltage, and many dogs have residual nasal signs. The poor response has led to studies that have attempted to improve control by dose or schedule manipulation.

Hyperfractionation: Two studies[27,28] investigated an accelerated radiation course for nasal tumors (see Chapter 51 for study details). Radiation was delivered in daily fractions over 11 to 13 days or twice a day over 21 days. Acute toxicities were common, including mucositis that was severe and protracted (≤5 weeks); skin necrosis occurred in one dog. Few dogs lived longer than 6 months, and late effects were seen in nearly every dog. Unilateral or bilateral blindness occurred 6 months after treatment. Osteonecrosis was seen in three dogs and seizures in one. Five dogs died from acute or late tissue reactions. Theoretically, these protocols should have resulted in equivalent or better tumor control and a reduced risk of late effects. However, there was no reduction in recurrence rate compared with standard protocols, and survival times were actually worse.[29] In addition, the high incidence of late effects and the high rate of acute side effects made these approaches unacceptable.

Hypofractionation: Four doses of 9 Gy given once a week was used to treat 56 dogs with nasal tumors.[30] Clinical signs improved in most dogs by the end of the treatment schedule. Mild acute radiation side effects were observed in most dogs, but late radiation side effects were rare. The median survival time after the final dose of radiation was 7 months. The 1- and 2-year survival rates were 45% and 15%, respectively, which is little different than results with more conventional dosing schemes.[30] Some radiation oncologists now believe that hypofractionated protocols may offer a reasonable alternative for dogs with nasal carcinoma.

SOFT TISSUE SARCOMAS

Soft tissue sarcomas frequently recur after incomplete surgical excision because they have many "fingers" that extend into surrounding tissues. Often, the tumor is excised only around the area that can be palpated, which ensures that disease will recur. Soft tissue sarcomas have been considered to be radiation resistant; however, higher total dosages provide long-term control of this tumor in most dogs.

Coarse fractionation: Radiation therapy is frequently used postoperatively for incompletely excised sarcomas. In addition, radiation therapy seems to be effective for treating gross evidence of malignant soft tissue sarcomas (Figure 22-17). For example, one study reported that 50% of dogs with soft tissue sarcomas had their disease controlled 1 year after receiving radiation therapy dosages ranging from 45 to 50 Gy delivered in 10 fractions.[31] Predictably, smaller tumors responded better to radiation therapy; 60% to 75% of such tumors were controlled at 1 year when treated with 52 Gy of radiation therapy.[32,33] When radiation therapy was used to treat soft tissue sarcomas after incomplete surgical excision, 41% of dogs were disease-free 2 years after treatment.[33]

Currently, if complete excision cannot be attained, debulking down to the level of microscopic disease followed by radiation therapy is the recommended treatment for all soft tissue sarcomas.

Definitive fractionation: Smaller dose per fraction is an important factor in determining late effects in dogs. Treatment protocols utilizing 3-Gy fractions appear to have a low risk of causing late effects and allow high total doses to be administered. A protracted course of radiation to a total dose of 63 Gy in 3-Gy fractions on alternate days was given postoperatively to 48 dogs with soft tissue sarcomas.[6] By 1 and 5 years after treatment, 87% and 76% of dogs were alive,

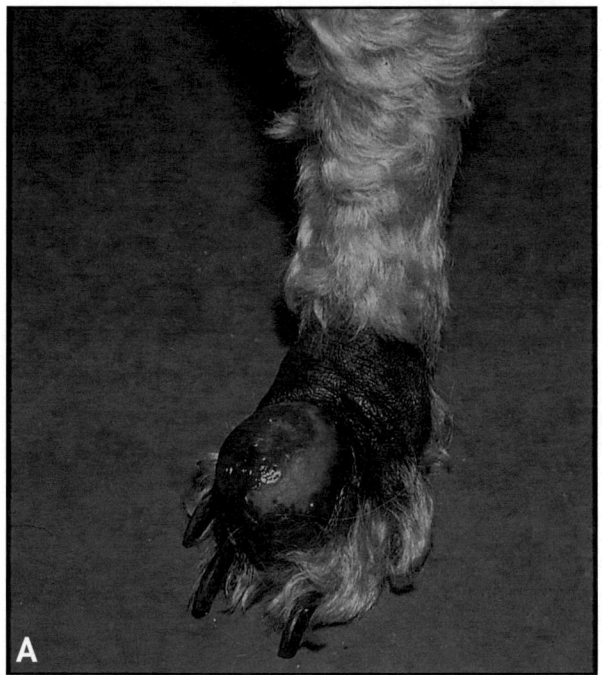 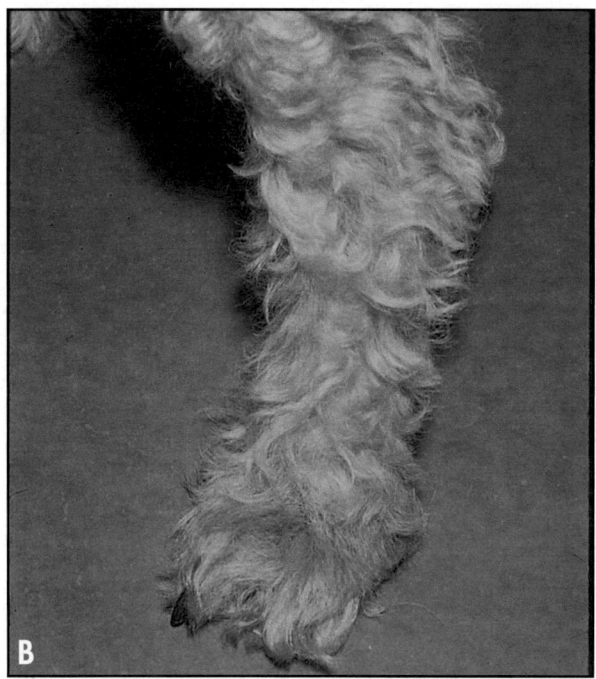

Figure 22-17. *This dog had a soft tissue sarcoma of the distal extremity that was treated with radiation therapy. Radiation therapy is an ideal alternative in the treatment of tumors that cannot be completely excised. The tumor was large before therapy (**A**) but was not palpable 2 months after therapy was completed (**B**).*

respectively; most deaths were unrelated to the tumor. Acute effects were mild, and no treatment delays were reported. The only late effect reported was a dog that developed osteosarcoma in the treatment field 6 years after radiation.

Doxorubicin is believed to be a radiation sensitizer and may increase the effect of radiation on cancer cells when given at low dosages. In a recent study, doxorubicin (10 mg/m^2 IV) was given once weekly 1 hour before a 3-Gy fraction of orthovoltage radiation (total dose: 51 Gy) to 39 dogs with incompletely excised soft tissue sarcomas.[34] Seven dogs (18%) developed local recurrences a median of 7 months after treatment, and this was more likely in dogs with grade 2 or 3 tumors. Six dogs (15%) developed distant metastases, two without local recurrence. The 1-, 2-, and 4-year survival rates were 85%, 79%, and 72%, respectively. Tumor control and patient survival were longer in dogs that had grade 1 tumors.[34] This control was similar to that seen with higher doses of radiation therapy.

MAST CELL TUMORS

Definitive and coarse fractionation: Long-term control is likely in dogs with incompletely excised grade 1 mast cell tumors after radiation therapy. Approximately 90% of dogs with this tumor treated to a total dose of 48 to 54 Gy in 3- or 4-Gy fractions given three times a week postoperatively were still alive and tumor-free 3 years after radiation.[35,36] This treatment is clearly the best choice for this tumor regardless of the protocol. Acute effects are the same as those reported for similar protocols and schedules. Late effects were seen in only one dog.[35,36]

Some investigators have recommended prophylactic irradiation of the regional lymph node in dogs with grade 2 mast cell tumors that have mast cells observed on cytologic examination of a lymph node needle aspirate.[37] Because of the difficulties in determining whether mast cells seen on cytology are inflammatory or neoplastic, most radiotherapists now include the regional lymph node adjacent to a mast cell tumor in the radiation field regardless of whether mast cells are present on cytology.

Radiation therapy (52.2 Gy in 2.9-Gy fractions given three times a week) was used to treat 31 dogs that had only residual microscopic disease after surgery for grade 3 mast cell tumor.[38] In all cases, the regional lymph node was irradiated as well. Local control of the mast cell tumor was excellent, with a median remission time of 28 months. More than half of the dogs (16 of 31) eventually developed lymph node metastases, underscoring the need for systemic therapy in this disease.[38]

Hypofractionation: Hypofractionated radiation therapy (four weekly 8-Gy fractions) was used to treat 35 dogs with nonresectable mast cell tumors of all grades on the head or limbs; 17 dogs had cytologic evidence of lymph node metastasis.[39] All dogs received concurrent prednisolone (40 mg/m^2/day) for 10 to 14 days before radiation therapy and at half that dose for 2 months after. A complete response was seen in 12 dogs and a partial response in 19. The median tumor control was 34 months, with 1- and 2-year control rates of 60% and 52%, respectively.

BRAIN TUMORS

Radiation therapy has been delivered to dogs either alone or after incomplete surgical removal of a brain tumor. Meningiomas and hypophyseal macroadenomas appear to be the most radioresponsive; however, responses have been seen in dogs with other types of malignant disease.

Coarse fractionation: In a study of 20 dogs with meningiomas treated with megavoltage radiation to a total dose of 48 Gy in 4-Gy fractions on alternate days, PCNA was high in seven dogs and low in nine.[40] The 2-year progression-free survival was 42% for dogs with rapidly proliferating tumors and 91% for those with slowly proliferating tumors. Late effects were seen in 20% of long-term survivors: of 14 dogs that lived longer than 12 months, two had presumed radiation-induced brain signs and one developed a radiation-induced glioma. In another study, the median survival for 65 dogs with brain tumors was 13.5 months.[41]

Definitive fractionation: Late effects were not seen in 29 dogs with brain tumors that received 48 Gy in 16 daily fractions of 3 Gy; however, the median survival was 8 months; therefore, the population at risk may have been low.[42]

Hypofractionation: Recent studies have adapted hypofractionated protocols for treatment of tumors when long-term survival is possible and when late effects of radiation should be of concern. In one study, 83 dogs with brain tumors were treated using a total of 38 Gy in five weekly fractions of 7.6 Gy.[43] Median survival was 11 months, although 12 dogs died due to late effects of treatment. Hypothetically, if 40 dogs lived longer than 1 year after receiving this treatment, treatment-related mortality would be 30% of patients at risk.[43]

Radiosurgery: In a preliminary report, control of tumors for more than 1 year was seen in three dogs that underwent radiosurgery, despite the relatively low total dose of radiation.[4] A preliminary report indicated that radiosurgery may be more effective in treating pituitary macroadenomas than other brain tumors.[5]

THYROID TUMORS

Radioisotopes: Radiation therapy using ^{131}I has been used to treat thyroid tumors in dogs even when they are not actively secreting hormone.

Coarse fractionation: Radiation to a dose of 48 Gy was reported for treatment of 25 dogs with unresectable thyroid carcinomas.[44] Of those, 72% were free of disease 3 years after treatment. Acute toxicities were common and resulted from mucositis in the larynx, trachea, and esophagus. Late effects, including chronic tracheitis, hypothyroidism, and hypoparathyroidism, were seen in 30% of 20 dogs that lived longer than 1 year.[44]

Hypofractionation: Another study reported four once-weekly fractions of 9 Gy to treat 13 dogs with invasive thyroid carcinoma; most responses were partial, with only one complete remission. Four of the dogs died from progression of the primary disease and four from metastatic spread. The median survival time for all dogs was 22 months (range: 2–57 months).[45] Side effects were similar to those described above. Radiation therapy for this disease may be more effective when given in small fractions rather than in larger "coarse" fractions.

In a compilation of three studies, metastases occurred in 14 of 46 dogs (30%), indicating a need for adjunctive chemotherapy in addition to radiation therapy (see Chapter 57 for study details).

THYMOMA

Coarse fractionation and hypofractionation: Radiation therapy is important in the treatment of thymoma in humans. In dogs, radiation may reduce tumor size to a point at which surgical excision is feasible, but risks of radiation toxicity to lungs and myocardium are dose limiting. In one report, 13 dogs were treated for thymoma with megavoltage radiation therapy. The radiation protocol varied but mostly consisted of 3- to 4-Gy fractions given daily or three times a week to 21 to 54 Gy (definitive) or weekly 5-Gy fractions to 15 Gy through parallel opposed portals. Three dogs had complete and five had partial (>50%) reduction in tumor size for a median of 3 to 6 months.[46]

TRANSITIONAL CELL CARCINOMA OF THE URINARY BLADDER

Coarse fractionation: A pilot study in two dogs using ^{60}Co teletherapy (44 and 48 Gy) and preradiation cisplatin chemotherapy (50 mg/m^2 twice, divided into three doses before the first three and last three radiation treatments) found a minor shrinkage in tumor volume but few severe side effects.[47] Survival times were 6 and 7 months, respectively.[47] Eight dogs in a group of 15 treated with mitoxantrone and piroxicam also received radiation therapy. The response rate was higher in the group receiving radiation therapy than in the group treated with chemotherapy alone, although survival times were not different.[48]

Hypofractionation: In another pilot study of 10 dogs, the addition of once-weekly coarsely fractionated radiation therapy (six fractions of 5.75 Gy weekly) to mitoxantrone and piroxicam did not improve on survival times seen with mitoxantrone and piroxicam chemotherapy alone.[49]

MAMMARY TUMORS

Radiation therapy has a role to play in preservation of breast tissue in women with mammary cancer, but its use in the treatment of canine mammary cancer has not been reported. It is possible that radiation therapy may play a role in reducing the risk of local recurrence for aggressive tumors such as inflammatory carcinomas or for tumors that cannot be completely removed.

OTHER TUMORS

Rectal, colonic, and prostate tumors have been treated successfully with radiation therapy. In each case, the extent of the disease must be clearly defined and the animal appropriately staged with at least abdominal radiography, ultrasonography or CT, hemogram, biochemical profile, and urinalysis. When radiation therapy is delivered to these particular sites, problems such as dysuria, colitis, and prostatitis must be expected. If radiation therapy is to be used for tumors of the caudal abdomen, small, frequent fractions are more likely to avoid complications (see discussion of the effects on the colon and rectum above). Whenever possible, radiation therapy should be combined with other treatment modalities to enhance their beneficial effects.

PALLIATIVE THERAPY

Radiation therapy can be given to alleviate the pain and discomfort of a wide variety of malignancies, especially those that involve bone. The risk of late effects is acceptable in terminal patients in which the chance of a cure, or even long-term tumor control, is considered remote and improvement in quality of life for a short period outweighs the higher risks of late effects and tumor recurrence.

Despite the risks of late effects, a German study using radiation therapy to a total dose of 32 to 48 Gy delivered once a week in 8-Gy fractions found that there were no significant acute side effects. Late side effects did not occur within the follow-up period, and 88% of the owners were satisfied with this kind of treatment and would choose it again.

OSTEOSARCOMA

Palliative radiation therapy of osteosarcoma is a logical and often effective mode of improving quality of life for patients in which surgical removal or amputation is not an option.

Hypofractionation: Radiation delivered in weekly fractions of 8 to 10 Gy has been reported as a palliative treatment for dogs with pain from osteosarcoma or other clinical signs related to the tumor. Improved limb function was seen in approximately 75% of the dogs treated with either 10 Gy on days 0, 7, and 21 or 8 Gy on days 0 and 7. Improvement lasted for a median of 2 months regardless of the protocol, and toxicities were rare and acute.[50,51]

Some radiation therapists believe that a reasonable clinical approach may be to deliver a single large dose to the affected site and then to repeat a single dose as necessary to maintain pain control. Others administer two doses 24 hours apart to the affected site until discomfort returns, when the treatment may be repeated.

Radioisotopes: [153]Sm-ethylenetetramethylene phosphate ([153]Sm-EDTMP) emits β particles and accumulates in areas of increased bony activity, thereby providing high-dose localized radiation therapy. This compound was given to 28 dogs with osteosarcoma of the appendicular (n = 20) or axial (n = 8) skeleton.[1] Many dogs showed functional improvement; however, the average survival of the 20 dogs with appendicular osteosarcoma was 240 days. This treatment may palliate in a manner similar to external-beam radiation. Another study found that, with the exception of one dog that had a long-lasting complete response, pain relief was poor in a series of nine dogs with presumed osteosarcoma; survival was for a median of 4 months.[52] There are anecdotal reports of long-term survival after surgery and [153]Sm-EDTMP.[2,53]

Other techniques: Targeted stereotactic radiosurgery may offer some advantages in delivering a single high dose of 30 Gy to the tumor alone. Preliminary results are encouraging.[3]

Other Radiation Techniques

Whole-body irradiation has been little used in the clinical setting in dogs. In normal dogs, the highest tolerated whole-body irradiation dose was 2.6 Gy, but 50% of the dogs were dead within 30 days.[54] More recently, clinical use of whole-body irradiation doses of 1.0 Gy to treat lymphoma resistant to chemotherapy in dogs resulted in infrequent biochemical changes consistent with tumor lysis syndrome, transient partial responses, and unexpected long-term thrombocytopenia.[55]

Another clinical technique using half-body irradiation has been reported: half the body receives 7 Gy of megavoltage radiation on day 1, and 28 days later, the other half is irradiated. In one study, acute radiation sickness was seen in all eight normal dogs when they received caudal irradiation.[56] The second treatment, regardless of anatomy, was more likely to cause bone marrow toxicity, and platelets were more affected. Pneumonitis was common, and there was permanent bone marrow atrophy (cellularity <20%) 1 year after radiation, implying that combining this technique with chemotherapy would be risky. Similar toxicities were seen when 14 dogs with failed lymphoma were treated; five dogs had a complete or partial response.[57] Again, acute radiation sickness was seen in 30% of dogs after cranial irradiation and in 80% of dogs after caudal irradiation. Deaths occurred in four dogs due to acute tumor lysis, thrombocytopenia, and gastrointestinal signs ascribed to parvovirus. Pneumonitis was seen in six dogs and was progressive until death in two. Clearly, this technique has toxicities that are difficult to justify.

In contrast, when half-body radiation therapy was given in two consecutive daily 4-Gy fractions (instead of a single dose), toxicities were mainly mild and self-limiting. Dogs in remission from lymphoma after chemotherapy appeared to benefit from the addition of radiation as a consolidation phase.[58]

REFERENCES

1. Lattimer JC, Corwin LA, Stapleton J, et al: Clinical and clinicopathologic response of canine bone tumor patients to treatment with samarium-153-EDTMP. *Nucl Med* 31:1316–1325, 1990.
2. Moe L, Boysen M, Aas M, et al: Maxillectomy and targeted radionuclide therapy with 153Sm-EDTMP in a recurrent canine osteosarcoma. *J Small Anim Pract* 37:241–246, 1996.
3. Farese JP, Milner R, Thompson M, et al: Stereotactic radiosurgery for the treatment of lower extremity canine appendicular osteosarcoma [abstract]. *Proc 23rd Annu Conf Vet Cancer Soc*:69, 2003.
4. Lester NV, Hopkins AL, Bova FJ, et al: Radiosurgery using a stereotactic headframe system for irradiation of brain tumors in dogs. *JAVMA* 219:1562–1567, 2001.
5. Fidel J, Kippenes-Skogmo H, Gavin PR, et al: Radiosurgery for selected canine and feline brain tumors, a retrospective analysis [abstract]. *Proc 23rd Annu Conf Vet Cancer Soc*:48, 2003.
6. McKnight JA, Mauldin GN, McEntee MC, et al: Radiation treatment for incompletely resected soft-tissue sarcomas in dogs. *JAVMA* 217:205–210, 2000.
7. McEntee MC, Thrall DE: Use of portal radiography to increase accuracy of dose delivery in radiation therapy. *Vet Radiol Ultrasound* 36:69–77, 1995.
8. Kippenes H, Gavin PR, Sande RD, et al: Comparison of the accuracy of positioning devices for radiation therapy of canine and feline head tumors. *Vet Radiol Ultrasound* 41: 371–376, 2000.
9. Henry C, Stoll MR, Higginbotham ML, et al: Effect of timing of radiation initiation on post-surgical wound healing in dogs [abstract]. *Proc 23rd Annu Conf Vet Cancer Soc*:52, 2003.
10. Lana SE, Hansen RA, Kloer L, et al: The effects of oral glutamine supplementation on plasma glutamine concentrations and PGE2 concentrations in dogs experiencing radiation-induced mucositis. *J Appl Res Vet Med* 1:259–265, 2003.
11. Anderson CR, McNiel EA, Gillette EL, et al: Late complications of pelvic irradiation in 16 dogs. *Vet Radiol Ultrasound* 43:187–192, 2002.
12. Vartak S, Robbins ME, Spector AA: Polyunsaturated fatty acids increase the sensitivity of 36B10 rat astrocytoma cells to radiation-induced cell kill. *Lipids* 32:283–292, 1997.
13. Vartak S, McCaw R, Davis CS, et al: Gamma-linolenic acid (GLA) is cytotoxic to 36B10 malignant rat astrocytoma cells but not to 'normal' rat astrocytes. *Br J Cancer* 77:1612–1620, 1998.
14. Colas S, Paon L, Denis F, et al: Enhanced radiosensitivity of rat autochthonous mammary tumors by dietary docosahexaenoic acid. *Int J Cancer* 109:449–454, 2004.
15. Théon AP, Rodriguez C, Madewell BR: Analysis of prognostic factors and patterns of failure in dogs with malignant oral tumors treated with megavoltage irradiation. *JAVMA* 210:778–784, 1997.
16. Theon AP, Rodriguez C, Griffey S, Madewell BR: Analysis of prognosis factors and patterns of failure in dogs with periodontal tumors treated with megavoltage irradiation. *JAVMA* 210:785–788, 1997.
17. Blackwood L, Dobson JM: Radiotherapy of oral malignant melanomas in dogs. *JAVMA* 209:98–102, 1996.
18. MacMillan R, Withrow SJ, Gillette EL: Surgery and regional irradiation for treatment of canine tonsillar squamous cell carcinoma: Retrospective review of eight cases. *JAAHA* 18:311–314, 1982.
19. Brooks MB, Matus RE, Leifer CE, et al: Chemotherapy versus chemotherapy plus radiotherapy in the treatment of tonsillar squamous cell carcinoma in the dog. *J Vet Intern Med* 1988; 2:206–211, 1988.
20. Lascelles BDX, Parry AT, Stidworthy MF, et al: Squamous cell carcinoma of the nasal planum in 17 dogs. *Vet Rec* 147:473–476, 2000.
21. Theon AP, Barthez PY, Madewell BR, Griffey SM: Radiation therapy of ceruminous gland carcinomas in dogs and cats. *JAVMA* 205:566–569, 1994.
22. Cohen M, Brawner WR, Henderson R, et al: Use of a soft tissue equivalent material inside the canine nasal cavity to maximize megavoltage dose distribution to the floor [abstract]. *Proc 22nd Annu Conf Vet Cancer Soc*:18, 2002.
23. Northrup NC, Etue SM, Ruslander DM, et al: Retrospective study of orthovoltage radiation therapy for nasal tumors in 42 dogs. *J Vet Intern Med* 15:183–189, 2001.
24. Evans SM, Goldschmidt M, McKee LJ, Harvey CE: Prognostic factors and survival after radiotherapy for intranasal neoplasms in dogs: 70 cases (1974–1985). *JAVMA* 194:1460–1463, 1989.
25. Theon AP, Madewell BR, Harb MF, Dungworth DL: Megavoltage irradiation of neoplasms of the nasal and paranasal cavities in 77 dogs. *JAVMA* 202:1469–1475, 1993.
26. Henry CJ, Brewer WG Jr, Tyler JW, et al: Survival in dogs with nasal adenocarcinoma: 64 cases (1981–1995). *J Vet Intern Med* 12:436–439, 1998.
27. Adams WM, Miller PE, Vail DM, et al: An accelerated technique for irradiation for malignant canine nasal and paranasal sinus tumors. *Vet Radiol Ultrasound* 39:475–481, 1998.
28. Thrall DE, McEntee MC, Novotney C, et al: A boost technique for irradiation of malignant canine nasal tumors. *Vet Radiol Ultrasound* 34:295–300, 1993.
29. LaDue TA, Dodge R, Page RL, et al: Factors influencing survival after radiotherapy of nasal tumors in 130 dogs. *Vet Radiol Ultrasound* 40:312–317, 1999.
30. Mellanby RJ, Stevenson RK, Herrtage M, et al: Long-term outcome of 56 dogs with nasal tumours treated with four doses of radiation at intervals of seven days. *Vet Rec* 151:253–257, 2002.
31. McChesney SL, Withrow SJ, Gillette EL, et al: Radiotherapy of soft tissue sarcomas in dogs. *JAVMA* 194:60-63, 1989.
32. McChesney SL, Gillette EL, Dewhirst MW, Withrow SJ: Influence of WR 2721 on radiation response of canine soft tissue sarcomas. *Int J Radiat Oncol Biol Phys* 12:1957–1963, 1986.
33. Evans SM: Canine hemangiopericytoma. A retrospective analysis of response to surgery and orthovoltage radiation. *Vet Radiol Ultrasound* 28:13–16, 1987.
34. Simon D, Ruslander DM, Rassnick KM, et al: Combination of orthovoltage radiation therapy and weekly low-dose doxorubicin for incompletely excised soft tissue sarcomas in 39 dogs. *Vet Rec* 2005 (in press).
35. Frimberger AE, Moore AS, LaRue SM, et al: Radiotherapy of incompletely resected, moderately differentiated mast cell tumors in the dog: 37 cases (1989–1993). *JAAHA* 33:320–324, 1997.
36. Al Sarraf R, Mauldin GN, Patnaik AK, Meleo KA: A prospective study of radiation therapy for the treatment of grade 2 mast cell tumors in 32 dogs. *J Vet Intern Med* 10: 376–378, 1996.
37. Chaffin K, Thrall DE: Results of radiation therapy in 19 dogs with cutaneous mast cell tumor and regional lymph node metastasis. *Vet Radiol Ultrasound* 43: 392–395, 2002.
38. Hahn KA, King GK, Carreras JK: Efficacy of radiation therapy for incompletely resected grade-III mast cell tumors in dogs: 31 cases (1987–1998). *JAVMA* 224:79–82, 2004.
39. Dobson J, Cohen S, Gould S: Treatment of canine mast cell tumours with prednisolone and radiotherapy. *Vet Comp Oncol* 2:132–141, 2004.
40. Théon AP, LeCouteur RA, Carr EA, Griffey SM: Influence of tumor cell proliferation and sex-hormone receptors on effectiveness of radiation therapy for dogs with incompletely resected meningiomas. *JAVMA* 216:701–707, 2000.
41. LaRue SM, Gillette EL: Recent advances in radiation oncology. *Compend Contin Educ Pract Vet* 15:795–804, 1993.
42. Spugnini EP, Thrall DE, Price GS, et al: Primary irradiation of canine intracranial masses. *Vet Radiol Ultrasound* 41:377–380, 2000.
43. Brearley MJ, Jeffery ND, Phillips SM, Dennis R: Hypofractionated radiation therapy of brain masses in dogs: A retrospective analysis of survival of 83 cases (1991–1996). *J Vet Intern Med* 13:408–412, 1999.
44. Theon AP, Marks SL, Feldman ES, Griffey S: Prognostic factors and patterns of treatment failure in dogs with unresectable differentiated thyroid carcinomas treated with megavoltage irradiation. *JAVMA* 216:1775–1779, 2000.
45. Brearley MJ, Hayes AM, Murphy S: Hypofractionated radiation therapy for invasive thyroid carcinoma in dogs: A retrospective analysis of survival. *J Small Anim Pract* 40:206–210, 1999.
46. Smith AN, Wright JC, Brawner WR Jr, et al: Radiation therapy in the treatment of canine and feline thymomas: A retrospective study (1985–1999). *JAAHA* 37:489–496, 2001.
47. McCaw DL, Lattimer JC: Radiation and cisplatin for treatment of canine urinary bladder carcinoma: A report of two case histories. *Vet Radiol Ultrasound* 29:264–268, 1998.
48. Turner AI, Hahn KA, King GK, Carreras JK: Mitoxantrone, piroxicam and external-beam radiation therapy in the treatment of canine bladder tumors, 15 cases (2001–2003) [abstract]. *Proc 23rd Annu Conf Vet Cancer Soc*:20, 2003.
49. Poirier VJ, Forrest LJ, Adams WM, Vail DM: Piroxicam, mitoxantrone, and coarse fraction radiotherapy for the treatment of transitional cell carcinoma of the bladder in 10 dogs: A pilot study. *JAAHA* 40:131–136, 2004.
50. McEntee MC, Page RL, Novotney C, Thrall DE: Palliative radiotherapy for canine appendicular osteosarcoma. *Vet Radiol Ultrasound* 34:367–370, 1993.
51. Ramirez O III, Dodge RK, Page RL, et al: Palliative radiotherapy of appendicular osteosarcoma in 95 dogs. *Vet Radiol Ultrasound* 40:517–522, 1999.
52. Milner RJ, Dormehl I, Louw WK, Croft S: Targeted radiotherapy with Sm-153-EDTMP in nine cases of canine primary bone tumours. *J S Afr Vet Med Assoc* 69:12–17, 1998.
53. Cooper S, Black AP, Smith BA, et al: Low grade osteosarcoma in a dog. *Aust Vet Pract* 32:104–111, 2002.
54. von Zallinger C, Tempel K: The physiologic response of domestic animals to ionizing radiation: A review. *Vet Radiol Ultrasound* 39:495–503, 1998.
55. Frimberger AE, Ruslander DM, Moore AS, et al: Low-dose whole body irradiation for dogs with chemoresistant lymphoma relapse. *Proc 20th Annu Conf Vet Cancer Soc*:28, 2000.
56. Laing EJ, Fitzpatrick PJ, Norris AM, et al: Half-body radiotherapy. Evaluation of the technique in normal dogs. *J Vet Intern Med* 3:96–101, 1989.
57. Laing EJ, Fitzpatrick PJ, Binnington AG, et al: Half-body radiotherapy in the treatment of canine lymphoma. *J Vet Intern Med* 3:102–108, 1989.
58. Williams LE, Johnson JL, Hauck ML, et al: Chemotherapy followed by half-body radiation therapy for canine lymphoma. *J Vet Intern Med* 18:703–709, 2004.

BIOLOGIC RESPONSE MODIFIERS: PROPERTIES, USES, AND PATIENT MANAGEMENT

Gregory K. Ogilvie and Antony S. Moore

CLINICAL BRIEFING

Definition	• Agents that reconstitute or enhance the immune system to fight malignancy using endogenous biologic processes.
Agents	• **Biologic agents:** Actively stimulate the immune system to get a nonspecific response. • **L-MTP-PE:** BCG derivative shown to be effective against canine osteosarcoma, hemangiosarcoma, and oral malignant melanoma. • **Acemannan:** Aloe vera extract with nonspecific anticancer properties. • **Cimetidine:** Potentiates the immune system with reports of anticancer effects. • **NSAIDs:** Antiinflammatory drugs with efficacy against TCC, oral squamous cell carcinoma, and oral melanoma. • **Interleukin-2:** Inhalation of IL-2 is effective against pulmonary neoplasia. • **MMP inhibitors:** Theoretic benefit against a wide variety of cancers. • **Bisphosphonates:** Analgesic, anticancer properties; effective in the treatment of hypercalcemia of malignancy. • **Tetracyclines:** Theoretic benefit in cancer therapy. • **Thalidomide:** Antiangiogenic agent with potential anticancer effects. • **TALL-104:** Irradiated effector cells with anticancer effects against osteosarcoma, mammary neoplasia, and malignant histiocytosis. • **Specific monoclonal antibodies:** Efficacy versus lymphoma documented.

Biologic response modifiers (BRMs) or biologic therapies are rapidly becoming a key component of cancer therapy. Defining this type of therapy can be difficult because of the many ways these agents prevent, reduce, or eliminate cancer growth and survival. Simplistically, in this type of therapy, the immune system is reconstituted or enhanced to fight the malignancy using endogenous biologic processes. This can be done with a wide variety of substances, including biologic products, chemicals, lymphokines, cytokines, hematopoietic growth factors, antibodies, gene therapy, and vaccines.[1-3] Gene therapy, cancer vaccines, and hematopoietic growth factors are covered elsewhere in this book (see Chapters 28 and 33). A few of the substances used as BRMs are listed in the box on page 168. This chapter focuses on a few key agents that are likely to be of clinical use to veterinary practitioners for the treatment of dogs with cancer, either now or in the near future.

> **KEY POINT**
> *Biologic agents and chemical immunopotentiators are nonspecific immunotherapeutic agents that actively stimulate the immune system to respond to substances that may harm the body, including cancer.[1-3]*

Nonspecific Immunomodulators

Biologic agents (e.g., *Serratia marcescens, Streptococcus pyogenes, Corynebacterium parvum* [also known as *Proprionibacterium acnes*], bacillus Calmette-Guérin [BCG]), liposome-encapsulated muramyl tripeptide-phosphatidylethanolamine (L-MTP-PE), and chemical immunopotentiators (e.g., Acemannan, levamisole, cimetidine) are categorized as active nonspecific immunotherapeutic agents. These agents actively stimulate the immune system to respond to a wide

Substances Used as Biologic Response Modifiers
Nonspecific Immunomodulators
Bacillus Calmette-Guérin *C. parvum*
Staphage lysate L-MTP-PE
Levamisole Cimetidine
Piroxicam Acemannan
Regressin-V Retinoids
Vitamin C Folic acid
Zinc Selenium
Vitamin E
Lymphokines/Monokines
Interleukin-1 Interleukin-2
Interferon Tumor necrosis factor
Adoptive Cellular Therapy
Lymphokine-activated killer cells
Tumor-infiltrating lymphocytes
Antibody Therapy
Antibody directed to lymphoma cells
Growth Factors
Granulocyte colony-stimulating factor (filgrastim)
Granulocyte–macrophage colony-stimulating factor (sargramostim)
Macrophage colony-stimulating factor

variety of substances that may harm the body, including cancer.[1-3]

BACTERIA AND BACILLUS CALMETTE-GUÉRIN

Studies involving the anticancer properties of various forms of *S. marcescens*, *S. pyogenes*, and *C. parvum* have resulted in responses in dogs with a wide variety of tumors; however, little interest persists today concerning the use of these agents. Mycobacterial cell wall fractions have resulted in the development of a commercially available product (Regressin-V), the manufacturer of which suggests that there is some efficacy against mammary tumors in dogs and against sarcoids in horses. More intense interest has focused on the use of the more active component of *Mycobacterium* bacteria, BCG.

BCG has been evaluated extensively in a variety of neoplastic diseases in humans and animals.[1-3] The active subunit of BCG is muramyl dipeptide, which is a potent macrophage activator that also has been used therapeutically.[4] Recently, derivatives of BCG have been described as effective agents for the treatment of some early cases of transitional cell carcinoma (TCC) of the bladder in humans.

L-MTP-PE

Several recent studies have shown that L-MTP-PE has potent antitumor properties.[5,6] L-MTP-PE is a nonspecific activator of monocytes and macrophages that results in anticancer effects. In one randomized, double-blind study involving dogs with osteosarcoma, those that received L-MTP-PE after amputation had a median survival time of 7.4 months, whereas dogs that underwent amputation and received empty liposomes (control) had a median survival time of 3 months.[5] Although this study clearly showed that L-MTP-PE was very important for increasing survival time, 70% of the dogs developed metastatic disease, which prompted the initiation of a second double-blind, randomized study.

In this second study, 40 dogs with osteosarcoma of the extremity without evidence of metastatic disease were treated with amputation followed by four doses of cisplatin.[6] They were randomized to receive either L-MTP-PE or empty liposomes. Of 14 dogs in the placebo group, 13 died as a result of metastases; the median survival time was 10 months, and the median disease-free interval was 7.6 months. The dogs that received L-MTP-PE had a median survival time of 14.6 months and a median disease-free interval of 12 months; eight of the 11 dogs developed metastases.

A related trial showed that there is no survival advantage of administering L-MTP-PE concurrently with cisplatin. These studies clearly show that L-MTP-PE is an important BRM for the treatment of osteosarcoma. Despite this efficacy, L-MTP-PE is not commercially available.

> **KEY POINT**
>
> *L-MTP-PE has been shown to be effective for the adjuvant treatment of osteosarcoma, hemangiosarcoma, and oral malignant melanoma.*

Other studies have been completed to determine whether L-MTP-PE is effective for the treatment of canine hemangiosarcoma and melanoma, but not necessarily mammary carcinoma. Specifically:

- In one prospective, randomized, double-blind, clinical study, the antitumor activity of L-MTP-PE was evaluated as an adjuvant immunotherapy in dogs with simple mammary carcinoma.[7] Dogs were randomized after surgery to one of two groups in which they were treated with either L-MTP-PE (n = 13) or empty liposomes (n = 14) according to the same protocol. The difference in disease-free interval between dogs treated with L-MTP-PE (median: 165 days; range: 15–905 days) and dogs in the placebo group (median: 133 days; range: 27–659 days) was not significant.

- In another study, 32 dogs with hemangiosarcoma without gross evidence of metastases were treated with splenectomy, stratified by clinical stage, and randomized to receive doxorubicin–cyclophosphamide chemotherapy and either L-MTP-PE immunotherapy or placebo liposomes.[6] Dogs receiving L-MTP-PE had significantly prolonged disease-free survival ($P = .037$) and overall survival ($P = .029$) times compared with dogs receiving placebo.
- In a third study, 48 dogs with histologically confirmed, clinically staged oral melanoma were entered into a randomized, double-blind, surgical adjuvant trial and stratified on the basis of clinical stage and extent of surgery (simple resection or radical excision).[8] Dogs were treated with L-MTP-PE twice a week and randomized to receive recombinant canine granulocyte–macrophage colony-stimulating factor (rcGM-CSF, sargramostim) or saline (placebo) daily for 9 weeks. This study documented that, after surgery, L-MTP-PE administered alone or combined with rcGM-CSF showed no significant antitumor activity in advanced-stage oral melanoma. In early-stage oral melanoma, L-MTP-PE was shown to result in prolonged survival time.

ACEMANNAN

Acemannan, an extract from the aloe vera plant, is a nonspecific immunostimulator that has been shown to be taken up by macrophages and to enhance the release of interferon (IFN), interleukin (IL)-1, tumor necrosis factor (TNF), and prostaglandin E_2.[1,9,10] It has direct immunostimulatory effects and, apparently, direct antiviral activity against HIV-1. The commercially available product has been reported to delay the development of clinical signs in cats infected with FeLV. Acemannan has been promoted to have antitumor properties against fibrosarcoma in dogs and cats.[10] There is some controversy about this effect. This polymer is the only BRM that is approved for commercial use as an antitumor agent for the treatment of solid tumors in veterinary medicine. One study involved a small number of patients (eight dogs and five cats) with histopathologically confirmed fibrosarcomas that were treated with acemannan in combination with surgery and radiation therapy.[10] Seven of the 13 animals were reportedly alive and tumor free at the time of data analysis, with a median survival time of 372 days. These data are similar to reports of surgery plus radiation therapy alone. The authors concluded that acemannan might be a valuable adjunct for the treatment of fibrosarcomas.

LEVAMISOLE

Levamisole is an imidazole compound that has immunorestorative properties.[9–12] At least three veterinary studies involving this particular agent have been conducted, two of them in dogs. One study evaluated 144 dogs with mammary neoplasia.[9] In this study, there was no difference in survival between dogs that received levamisole and those that were treated with a placebo after surgery. In another study, 154 dogs with lymphoma were divided into two groups.[12] The first group received chemotherapy and levamisole, and the second group received chemotherapy and a placebo. No significant difference was noted in the remission or survival times in these groups. Recently, levamisole has been shown to be beneficial for the treatment of colon carcinoma in humans. Additional studies in veterinary medicine will be needed to explore the potential benefit of this agent in animals.

CIMETIDINE

Cimetidine is an H_2-receptor antagonist that potentiates the immune system.[1,13] As a single agent, it has been shown to alter the activity level of suppressor cells. Some studies have shown that cimetidine is synergistic with interferon for the treatment of oral malignant melanoma in humans. One study demonstrated that this drug is effective in treating cutaneous malignant melanomas in horses.[13] The therapeutic value of this drug in small animal medicine has not been defined.

NONSTEROIDAL ANTIINFLAMMATORY DRUGS

Aspirin, indomethacin, sulindac, and piroxicam are NSAIDs that have been shown to have anticancer effects.[14–23] Great efforts are being made to determine whether the plethora of new NSAIDs on the market have similar effects. The exact mechanism of action of these agents is unclear; however, their antiinflammatory effect is induced by inhibition of prostaglandins that influence cell functions such as cellular adhesion and apoptosis. Each of these factors is important in cancer survival and proliferation. NSAIDs also inhibit cyclooxygenase, carcinogens, angiogenesis, and platelet aggregation, an essential step in metastasis.

> *Aspirin, indomethacin, sulindac, and piroxicam are NSAIDs that have been shown to have anticancer effects against several malignancies, including TCC.*

Several studies have confirmed that piroxicam is effective for the treatment of TCC. In one study, 34 dogs with histopathologically confirmed, measurable, nonresectable TCC of the urinary bladder were treated with piroxicam.[15] Tumor responses included two complete remissions, four partial remissions, 18 patients with stable disease, and 10 patients with progressive disease. The median survival of all dogs was 181 days.

The efficacy of this NSAID-anticancer effect can be enhanced with the concurrent use of cisplatin, carboplatin, or mitoxantrone. For example, cisplatin was combined with piroxicam to determine whether this combination would induce remission more frequently than cisplatin alone in dogs with invasive TCC. After eight dogs had been evaluated in each treatment group, a significant difference in remission rate was noted in the cisplatin–piroxicam group, which included two complete responses, four partial responses, two patients with stable disease, and no patients with progressive disease. Tumor responses to cisplatin alone in eight dogs were no complete or partial responses, four patients with stable disease, and four patients with progressive disease. However, when piroxicam and cisplatin are given concurrently, significant nephrotoxicity can occur because both are nephrotoxins.

Some oncologists favor the combination of mitoxantrone and piroxicam. In one study, 48 dogs with histologically confirmed TCC were treated with mitoxantrone and piroxicam.[20] Results included one complete response, 16 partial responses, 22 patients with stable disease, and nine patients with progressive disease, for an overall measurable response rate of 35.4%. Subjective improvement occurred in 75% of treated dogs. Median time to treatment failure and median survival time were 194 and 350 days, respectively.

> **KEY POINT**
> *Piroxicam has been shown to be effective for the treatment of TCC of the bladder, oral squamous cell carcinoma, and oral malignant melanoma.*

The efficacy of piroxicam appears to extend beyond TCC in dogs. Piroxicam has been used for the treatment of measurable oral squamous cell carcinoma in 17 dogs.[18] One dog had a complete response, and two dogs had partial responses. An additional five dogs had stable disease. Median and mean times to treatment failure for the three dogs that had a remission were 180 and 223 days, respectively. Median and mean times to failure for the five dogs with stable disease were 102 and 223 days, respectively. Rectal tubulopapillary polyps were diagnosed in eight dogs, seven of which were treated with piroxicam suppositories and one with oral piroxicam.[17] The extent of hematochezia, tenesmus, and fecal mucus production was reduced in all cases. The owners of seven of the dogs considered the improvement in clinical signs to be good or excellent. The antitumor activity and toxicity of cisplatin combined with piroxicam in 11 dogs with oral malignant melanoma and nine dogs with oral squamous cell carcinoma were explored.[23] Remission occurred in five of nine dogs with squamous cell carcinoma and in two of 11 dogs with oral malignant melanoma. The most common abnormality observed was renal toxicosis, as observed in the dogs treated with the same combination for TCCs of the bladder.

INTERLEUKINS AND INTERFERONS

Cytokines are soluble mediators secreted by a variety of cell types that regulate several aspects of the immune system.[1–3] Biotechnology has resulted in the development of production methods to provide health care professionals with large quantities of cytokines for therapeutic uses. TNF and IL-2 are examples of these therapeutic cytokines.

TNF is secreted from macrophages in response to a number of substances, including lipopolysaccharides. TNF results in the death of tumor cells by a variety of mechanisms, such as by causing changes in the cell membrane that result in the development of cytopathic pores and by inhibiting protein and RNA synthesis. TNF-α combined with IL-2 results in positive responses in dogs with oral malignant melanoma and cutaneous mastocytoma.[24] Theoretically, the efficacy of TNF can be enhanced by removing soluble or insoluble TNF receptors.

Recombinant human IL-2 has been shown to be effective in stimulating canine peripheral blood mononuclear cells and is effective at stimulating canine lymphokine-activated killer cells.[1–3,25] Liposome-encapsulated IL-2 appears to be effective for treating cancer, especially if inhaled. Seven dogs with pulmonary metastases from osteosarcoma and two dogs with primary lung carcinoma were treated with aerosols of IL-2 liposomes.[25] Two of four dogs with metastatic pulmonary osteosarcoma had complete regression of metastases; the regression remained stable for more than 12 and 20 months, respectively. One of two dogs with primary lung carcinoma had stabilization of disease for more than 8 months. Toxicity was minimal.

Although IFN-α has been used for the treatment of a number of human malignancies, no such product exists for canine cancers.[1–3] IFN-α has been shown to be effective for the treatment of human melanoma, hairy cell leukemia, chronic myelogenous leukemia, basal cell carcinoma, renal cell carcinoma, and genital warts (papilloma virus). IFN-α has been shown to enhance the efficacy of cisplatin, carboplatin, doxorubicin, etoposide, and other drugs. Canine veterinary cancer studies have not yet resulted in conclusions on the efficacy of this agent.

Antiangiogenesis Therapy

A wide variety of agents inhibit cancer growth and metastasis by inhibiting angiogenesis, the process of blood vessel ingrowth into tissue. These include inhibitors of matrix metalloproteinase (MMP) enzymes, fatty acids, tetracycline inhibitors, and thalidomide. Most of these agents have many other mechanisms of action and can be considered pharmacologic agents as easily as they can be considered BRMs.

MATRIX METALLOPROTEINASES AND THEIR INHIBITORS

MMPs are a family of zinc-dependent enzymes that are produced by multiple tissues throughout the body and are involved in the degradation of extracellular matrix and basement membrane components.[26] MMPs are active during normal tissue remodeling processes, including cancer metastasis and invasion, and angiogenesis.[26] An investigation was launched to evaluate the presence of MMP-2 and MMP-9 in the tumor, serum, and plasma, to correlate levels of MMP-2 and MMP-9 with the presence of canine malignancies, and to determine how these levels correlate with histologic tumor grade.[27] In this study, tumor, plasma, serum, and stromal tissue were harvested from dogs with various histologically confirmed and graded malignancies before therapy. Samples were analyzed by gelatin zymography to detect MMP-2 and MMP-9 activity. Dogs with measurable levels of active form MMP-9 were more than three times more likely to come out of remission than subjects that had undetectable levels. Dogs with the active form of MMPs present were, in general, significantly more likely to come out of remission by 90 days than were subjects with no active form of MMPs present. This was especially true when active MMPs were present in dogs with lymphoma. In general, dogs with stage IV lymphoma had the highest levels of MMPs and the poorest outcome compared with dogs with stage III disease. These data allow some to draw the conclusion that MMP inhibitors (which have antiangiogenic properties) may be of value in treating dogs with cancer.

> **KEY POINT**
>
> *MMPs are key enzymes that enhance cancer growth and metastases. Inhibitors of these enzymes may be of great value in controlling cancer.*

In a focused study involving dogs with mast cell tumors, the presence of MMP-2 and MMP-9 was determined in canine mast cell tumor tissue and normal stromal tissue from 24 dogs with spontaneously occurring cutaneous mast cell tumors.[28] Seventeen of the mast cell tumors were of histologic grade 2, and seven were of histologic grade 3. Gelatin zymography and computer-assisted densitometry image analysis were used to quantify MMP concentration. There was dramatically more proenzyme MMP-9 activity in histologic grade 3 mast cell tumors compared with grade 2 tumors. There was also dramatically more active enzyme MMP-2 and MMP-9 activity in tumor tissue compared with stromal tissue. This study demonstrates that the proenzyme and active enzyme forms of MMP-2 and MMP-9 are present in canine mast cell tumors. This appears to be related to the degree of histologic malignancy.

Several MMP inhibitors that appear to reduce the degree of MMP-induced angiogenesis are being developed for the treatment of cancer.[26] The most extensively studied class of MMP inhibitors includes collagen peptidomimetics and nonpeptidomimetic inhibitors of the MMP active site, tetracycline derivatives, thalidomide, and bisphosphonates.[29-35] Batimastat and its orally bioavailable analogue marimastat have been studied in detail. Marimastat is currently being studied in randomized clinical trials. Other MMP inhibitors such as Bay-129566 have been synthesized in an attempt to improve the oral bioavailability and pharmaceutical properties of the peptidic inhibitors. Several members of this class of compounds are undergoing evaluation in phase III clinical trials. The tetracyclines, particularly the nonantibiotic chemically modified tetracyclines, interfere with several aspects of MMP expression and activation and inhibit tumor growth and metastases in preclinical models.[29,30] An example of this group is COL-3 (CMT-3, Metastat), which is currently undergoing phase I clinical trials.

Antiangiogenic drugs such as minocycline may provide therapeutic benefits in canine cancer patients. A prospective study was done to evaluate the efficacy of chemotherapy with doxorubicin and minocycline, an antiangiogenic agent, in 18 dogs with hemangiosarcoma treated with doxorubicin, cyclophosphamide, and minocycline.[30] The authors concluded that there was no statistically significant difference in survival between the dogs treated with chemotherapy and minocycline and the historical controls (dogs that received chemotherapy alone). The statistical power of the study was extremely limited.

Inhibitors of MMPs and n-3 polyunsaturated fatty acids (PUFAs) have been shown to inhibit the growth and metastasis of cancer in animals, although their pathogenesis remains obscure. Diets supplemented with n-3 PUFAs have been shown to decrease serum lactate concentrations.[31] One blinded, randomized study was designed to evaluate the hypothesis that short-term supplementation with n-3 PUFAs can decrease serum, plasma, and tumor concentrations of MMP-2 and MMP-9, vascular endothelial growth factor (VEGF), prostaglandin E_2, lactate, and cyclooxygenase-2 and enhance concentrations of tissue inhibitor of metalloproteinase-2 (TIMP-2).[31] Nineteen dogs with osteosarcoma and soft tissue sarcomas were randomized to receive one of two diets identical in all ways except that the experimental diet was supplemented with menhaden fish oil while the control diet was supplemented with soybean oil. Diets were fed before biopsy and for 2 to 3 weeks until the tumor was biopsied again. Dogs fed the experimental diet had higher median serum levels of the n-3 PUFAs docosahexaenoic acid (C22:6) and eicosapentaenoic acid (C20:5) and lower concentrations of the n-6 PUFAs linoleic acid (18:2) and arachidonic acid (20:4) compared with controls.

Dogs fed the control diet had higher glucose concentrations and lower plasma concentrations of proenzyme and active MMP-2 and lactate. In addition, the concentration of proenzyme MMP-9 and active MMP-2 decreased in the experimental group and increased in the control group. Concentrations of TIMP-2 and VEGF increased in both groups. These data suggest that MMPs can be modulated, at least in part, via n-3 PUFAs.

Bisphosphonates such as alendronate, clodronate, and pamidronate are being used in veterinary and human medicine to treat hypercalcemia of malignancy and are being recognized by some as an effective treatment for metastatic bone pain and possibly the growth of cancer.[32,33] Bisphosphonates have an anticancer effect by inducing apoptosis in *in vitro* cultures, inhibiting angiogenesis, inhibiting MMP, and affecting cytokine and growth factors; they are also immunomodulatory.

Thalidomide is a potent drug that exerts its effects in part because of its antiangiogenic properties. This drug has enhanced the health and wellness of a number of human cancer patients, especially those with multiple myeloma and prostate carcinoma.[34,35] Specific veterinary studies are under way despite the difficulty in obtaining this drug.

TALL-104 CELLS

TALL-104 cells, lethally irradiated effector cells derived from a clonal human T-cell line (CD 16-, CD56+, CD8+, CD3+), exert potent antitumor effects in animal models with induced and spontaneous cancers.[36,37] They induce these effects through the release of cytostatic and cytotoxic mediators such as TNF-α, TNF-β, IFN-γ, and tumor-derived growth factor. One study was completed to determine the ability of systemically delivered TALL-104 cells to induce durable clinical remissions in four dogs with malignant histiocytosis.[36] Each dog received multiple injections of lethally irradiated TALL-104 cells. Three of the four dogs achieved complete remission. This same human cytotoxic T-cell line TALL-104 was investigated to determine the efficacy of TALL-104 cells given in an adjuvant setting to 23 dogs with appendicular osteosarcoma after surgery and

> **KEY POINT**
> *TALL-104 cells have induced remission in dogs with malignant histiocytosis.*

chemotherapy. Of the 23 dogs treated, the overall median survival time was 11.5 months, and the median disease-free interval was 9.8 months. The researchers concluded that this was an improvement over historical median survival and disease-free interval times of 9 and 7.5 months, respectively. Adoptive transfer of these human TALL-104 killer cells into a dog with metastatic mammary adenocarcinoma resulted in 50% reduction of the largest lung metastasis and stabilization of the other lesions for 10 weeks.[37]

Specific Monoclonal Antibodies

Specific monoclonal antibodies developed against tumor-specific or tumor-associated transformation antigens may prove to be an important therapeutic modality.[1,38,39] These monoclonal antibodies can be used for therapeutics and diagnostics. Using hybridomas, large quantities of monoclonal antibodies can be developed for a wide variety of malignant cells. These antibodies can be used to mediate antitumor cytotoxicity through either complement-mediated cytotoxicity or antibody-dependent cellular cytotoxicity. In addition, the antibodies can be "tagged" with a radioactive material to identify the presence of malignancies within the body. One potential problem is the difficulty in identifying a "cancer-specific" antigen that is not present on normal cells.

One monoclonal antibody developed for the treatment of cancer in humans or animals is canine lymphoma/monoclonal antibody 231 (CL/MAb 231, Synbiotics Corporation, San Diego), which recognizes canine lymphoma cells.[38,39] CL/MAb 231 mediates antibody-dependent cellular cytotoxicity against a canine lymphoma cell line and has been reported to prolong remission duration when used in combination with chemotherapy in dogs with lymphoma.[39] The median survival time of dogs treated with the monoclonal antibody and chemotherapy was 591 days compared with historical controls, which had a median survival time of 189 days. Additional studies are needed to further understand the clinical utility of this treatment modality.

REFERENCES

1. MacEwen EG, Helfand SC: Recent advances in the biologic therapy of cancer. *Compend Contin Educ Pract Vet* 15:909–922, 1993.
2. Elmslie RE, Dow SW, Ogilvie GK: Interleukins: Biological properties and therapeutic potential. *J Vet Intern Med* 5:283–293, 1991.
3. MacEwen EG: Approaches to cancer therapy using biological response modifiers. *Vet Clin North Am Small Anim Pract* 15:667–688, 1985.
4. Meyer JA, Dueland RT, Rosenthal RC, et al: Canine osteogenic sarcoma treated by amputation and MER. *Cancer* 49:1613–1616, 1982.
5. MacEwen EG, Kurzman ID, Rosenthal RC, et al: Therapy for osteosarcoma in dogs with intravenous injection of liposome-encapsulated muramyl tripeptide. *J Natl Cancer Inst* 81:935–938, 1989.
6. Vail DM, MacEwen EG, Kurzman ID, et al: Liposome-encapsulated muramyl tripeptide phosphatidylethanolamine adjuvant immunotherapy for splenic hemangiosarcoma in the dog: A randomized multi-institutional clinical trial. *Clin Cancer Res* 1(10):1165–1170, 1995.
7. Teske E, Rutteman GR, vd Ingh TS, et al: Liposome-encapsulated muramyl tripeptide phosphatidylethanolamine (L-MTP-PE): A randomized clinical trial in dogs with mammary carcinoma. *Anticancer Res* 18(2A):1015–1019, 1998.
8. MacEwen EG, Kurzman ID, Vail DM, et al: Adjuvant therapy for melanoma in dogs: Results of randomized clinical trials using surgery, liposome-encapsulated muramyl tripeptide, and granulocyte macrophage colony-stimulating factor. *Clin Cancer Res* 5(12):4249–4258, 1999.
9. Harris C, Pierce K, King G, et al: Efficacy of acemannan in treatment of canine and feline spontaneous neoplasms. *Mol Biother* 3:207–213, 1991.
10. King GK, Yates KM, Greenlee PG, et al: The effect of Acemannan immunostimulant in combination with surgery and radiation therapy on spontaneous canine and feline fibrosarcomas. *JAAHA* 31(5):439–447, 1995.

11. MacEwen EG, Harvey HJ, Patnaik AK, et al: Evaluation of effect of levamisole after surgery on canine mammary cancer. *J Biol Response Mod* 4:418–426, 1985.
12. MacEwen EG, Hayes AA, Mooney S, et al: Levamisole as adjuvant to chemotherapy for canine lymphosarcoma. *J Biol Response Mod* 4:427–433, 1985.
13. Goetz T, Ogilvie GK: Cimetidine for the treatment of malignant melanoma in 3 horses. *JAVMA* 196:449–452, 1990.
14. Knapp DW, Richardson RC, Bottoms GD, et al: Phase I trial of piroxicam in 62 dogs bearing naturally occurring tumors. *Cancer Chemother Pharmacol* 29(3):214–218, 1992.
15. Knapp DW, Richardson RC, Chan TC, et al: Piroxicam therapy in 34 dogs with transitional cell carcinoma of the urinary bladder. *J Vet Intern Med* 8(4):273–278, 1994.
16. Knapp DW, Glickman NW, Widmer WR, et al: Cisplatin versus cisplatin combined with piroxicam in a canine model of human invasive urinary bladder cancer. *Cancer Chemother Pharmacol* 46(3):221–226, 2000.
17. Knottenbelt CM, Simpson JW, Tasker S, et al: Preliminary clinical observations on the use of piroxicam in the management of rectal tubulopapillary polyps. *J Small Anim Pract* 41(9):393–397, 2000.
18. Schmidt BR, Glickman NW, DeNicola DB, et al: Evaluation of piroxicam for the treatment of oral squamous cell carcinoma in dogs. *JAVMA* 218(11):1783–1786, 2001.
19. Mohammed SI, Bennett PF, Craig BA, et al: Effects of the cyclooxygenase inhibitor, piroxicam, on tumor response, apoptosis, and angiogenesis in a canine model of human invasive urinary bladder cancer. *Cancer Res* 62(2):356–358, 2002.
20. Henry CJ, McCaw DL, Turnquist SE, et al: Clinical evaluation of mitoxantrone and piroxicam in a canine model of human invasive urinary bladder carcinoma. *Clin Cancer Res* 9(2):906–911, 2003.
21. Mohammed SI, Craig BA, Mutsaers AJ, et al: Effects of the cyclooxygenase inhibitor, piroxicam, in combination with chemotherapy on tumor response, apoptosis, and angiogenesis in a canine model of human invasive urinary bladder cancer. *Mol Cancer Ther* 2(2):183–188, 2003.
22. Knapp DW, Glickman NW, Mohammed SI, et al: Antitumor effects of piroxicam in spontaneous canine invasive urinary bladder cancer, a relevant model of human invasive bladder cancer. *Adv Exp Med Biol* 507:377–380, 2002.
23. Boria PA, Murry DJ, Bennett PF, et al: Evaluation of cisplatin combined with piroxicam for the treatment of oral malignant melanoma and oral squamous cell carcinoma in dogs. *JAVMA* 224(3):388–394, 2004.
24. Khanna C, Anderson PM, Hasz DE, et al: Interleukin-2 liposome inhalation therapy is safe and effective for dogs with spontaneous pulmonary metastases. *Cancer* 79(7):1409–1421, 1997.
25. Moore AS, Theilen GH, Newell AD, et al: Preclinical study of sequential tumor necrosis factor and interleukin-2 in the treatment of spontaneous canine neoplasms. *Cancer Res* 51:233–238, 1991.
26. Hidalgo M, Eckhardt SG: Development of matrix metalloproteinase inhibitors in cancer therapy. *J Natl Cancer Inst* 93(3):178–193, 2001.
27. Lana SE, Ogilvie GK, Hansen RA, et al: Identification of matrix metalloproteinases in canine neoplastic tissue. *Am J Vet Res* 61(2):111–114, 2000.
28. Leibman NF, Lana SE, Hansen RA, et al: Identification of matrix metalloproteinases in canine cutaneous mast cell tumors. *J Vet Intern Med* 14(6):583–586, 2000.
29. Tolomeo M, Grimaudo S, Milano S, et al: Effects of chemically modified tetracyclines (CMTs) in sensitive, multidrug resistant and apoptosis resistant leukaemia cell lines. *Br J Pharmacol* 133(2):306–314, 2001.
30. Sorenmo K, Duda L, Barber L, et al: Canine hemangiosarcoma treated with standard chemotherapy and minocycline. *J Vet Intern Med* 14(4):395–398, 2000.
31. Ogilvie GK, Lana S, Mitchener KM, et al: Effect of short term fish oil supplementation on MMP concentrations in canine osteosarcoma and soft tissue sarcoma: A blind, randomized study [abstract]. *Proc 21st Vet Cancer Soc*:12, 2001.
32. Teronen O, Heikkila P, Konttinen YT, et al: MMP inhibition and downregulation by bisphosphonates. *Ann NY Acad Sci* 30:453–465, 1999.
33. Milner RJ, Farese J, Henry CJ, et al: Bisphosphonates and cancer. *J Vet Intern Med* 18(5):597–604, 2004.
34. Rajkumar SV: Current status of thalidomide in the treatment of cancer. *Oncology* (Williston Park) 15(7):867–874, 2001.
35. Figg WD, Dahut W, Duray P, et al: A randomized phase II trial of thalidomide, an angiogenesis inhibitor, in patients with androgen-independent prostate cancer. *Clin Cancer Res* 7(7):1888–1893, 2001.
36. Visonneau S, Cesano A, Jeglum KA, Santoli D: Adjuvant treatment of canine osteosarcoma with the human cytotoxic T-cell line TALL-104. *Clin Cancer Res* 5(7):1868–1875, 1999.
37. Visonneau S, Cesano A, Jeglum KA, Santoli D: Adoptive therapy of canine metastatic mammary carcinoma with the human MHC non-restricted cytotoxic T-cell line TALL-104. *Oncol Rep* 6(6):11811–11818, 1999.
38. Rosales C, Jeglum KA, Obrocka M, et al: Cytolytic activity of murine anti-dog lymphoma monoclonal antibodies with canine effector cells and complement. *Cell Immunol* 115:420–428, 1988.
39. Jeglum KA: Monoclonal antibody treatment of canine lymphoma. *Proc East States Vet Conf*: 222–223, 1992.

SURGICAL ONCOLOGY: PROPERTIES, USES, AND PATIENT MANAGEMENT

Gregory K. Ogilvie and Antony S. Moore

CLINICAL BRIEFING

Oncologic surgeon	• Member of a multidisciplinary team who must understand tumor biology and the natural history of cancer to use unique surgical skills to diagnose and treat cancer in concert with medical and radiation oncologists. Practitioners can emulate these characteristics and provide excellent surgical care for dogs with cancer.
Cancer prevention	• Surgery to reduce the risk of cancer (e.g., ovariohysterectomy for mammary and vaginal tumors, castration for testicular tumors, removal of polyps to prevent colon carcinoma).
Diagnosis	• Surgery to obtain a representative sample from the tissue in question. Aspiration, punch, needle core, incisional, and excisional biopsy procedures are vital tools for obtaining a diagnosis. In each case, the biopsy should be performed in close consultation with the surgeon who will perform the definitive surgery. Pre- and postbiopsy analgesia should be used.
Definitive treatment	• The surgical plan should include therapy for the primary tumor and, if indicated, for residual and metastatic disease. The client should be informed of all risks and benefits, and the patient must be supported to ensure that pain, nausea, and intra- and postoperative fluid and nutritional needs are met.
Emergencies	• Surgery to preserve or save a life is relatively common and includes pericardiectomy for pericardial effusion and tamponade as well as surgical excision of a variety of tumors causing respiratory distress, abdominal hemorrhage, or urinary tract obstruction.
Palliation	• Surgery for pain or other symptomatic relief. Providing information to and support of the client is absolutely essential during palliative care.
Rehabilitation	• Reconstructive surgical techniques followed by physical and other supportive therapies allow rapid return to normal function.
Supportive care	• Analgesia and nutritional support are essential concerns.

Surgery is the oldest form of cancer therapy in human and canine oncology and has been responsible for the cure of more patients than any other treatment modality. The increasing success of surgical oncology is mainly related to the development of new surgical techniques, the integration of surgery with other cancer therapies, and a greater understanding of the biologic behavior of malignancies.[1-9] Indeed, the development of comparatively new adjunctive treatments, such as chemotherapy, radiation therapy, and biologic response modifiers, has enhanced the control of microscopic disease and prompted surgeons to reassess the type of surgery performed and the probability for long-term control of the disease. Despite advances in these fields, the surgeon continues to play an important role in the prevention, diagnosis, definitive treatment, palliation, and rehabilitation of the canine cancer patient. The surgeon who treats cancer must have a strong command of the principles of surgical oncology as well as the aforementioned modalities. The most successful surgeons understand that they must not

> **KEY POINT**
>
> *The most successful surgeons understand that they must not only meet the surgical needs of the cancer patient but also support the family during this process.*

only meet the surgical needs of the cancer patient but also support the family during this process.

Whenever possible, a biopsy should be performed before definitive surgery or other therapy. The adverse effects of the cancer and treatment modality must be known and fully explained to the client in oral and written format. Cure of the cancer must be a top priority, as long as the patient's quality of life is improved in the process. The surgery must be carefully thought out, and all alternative options must be explored with the client.

The Oncologic Surgeon[1–5,9]

An oncologic surgeon essentially uses the same techniques and procedures as any other surgeon but thinks differently. Cancer is different than any other disease that faces humans or animals and thus requires a different approach. The oncologic surgeon must understand the emotions connected with cancer and the importance of assembling a unique team of like-minded people who have a unified purpose of supporting the patient and family through a difficult emotional and physical ordeal.

> **KEY POINT**
>
> *An oncologic surgeon essentially uses the same techniques and procedures as any other surgeon but thinks differently. He or she recognizes that cancer is different than any other disease that faces humans or animals: It is a disease that conjures up feelings of fear in all of us.*

There are very few true oncologic surgeons in veterinary medicine, but there are many gifted surgeons who have evolved into gifted cancer surgeons. These surgeons have taken many paths to get where they are today, but they all have several things in common. The foremost cancer surgeons are members of health care teams that collaborate to defeat cancer using the most appropriate and effective therapy possible. Successful oncologic surgeons must have broad knowledge of cancer biology as well as extensive experience with the technical procedures needed to accurately diagnose and treat cancer with the highest probability of success and the least amount of cost and morbidity. In addition, the very best surgeons are those who do not operate needlessly and, when necessary, refer patients to other surgeons who have better skills or more experience.

The training programs available for cancer surgeons focus on:

- Training the surgeon in the art of meeting the nonmedical needs of the client while meeting the medical and surgical needs of the patient
- Educating the surgeon on the specifics of tumor biology and cellular and molecular cancer medicine, which are the underpinnings of cancer control and therapy, as well as mechanisms of cancer growth, survival, and metastasis
- Giving the surgeon extensive experience in the unique surgical skills associated with the treatment of cancer among exceptionally skilled surgeons
- Making the surgeon intimately aware of the principles and specifics of chemotherapy and radiation therapy
- Endorsing the team approach to provide comprehensive and compassionate care for the cancer patient
- Educating the surgeon in the specifics of clinical research and of the details of such essentials as trial design and statistical analysis
- Enhancing awareness of the specific capabilities of diagnostic tests to determine the type and extent of the cancer

Roles of Surgery
PREVENTION OF CANCER[1–5,9]

Prevention of cancer with ovariohysterectomy and orchiectomy in dogs is well defined. These surgical procedures can be critical to preventing not only malignant diseases (e.g., uterine, ovarian, and vaginal neoplasia in females; testicular neoplasia in males) but also nonneoplastic conditions (e.g., pregnancy, pyometra, prostatomegaly-related behavioral problems). Therefore, surgery is important for reducing the risk of cancer development in dogs.

STAGING AND DIAGNOSIS OF CANCER[1–5,9]

The veterinarian who performs the surgery plays an important role in staging and determining the extent of malignant disease.[1–4] The patient and its cancer must be fully assessed before treatment can begin. This assessment must include the tumor type and grade and disease stage. A surgical biopsy is often required to make a definitive diagnosis. The biopsy methods that the surgeon can use to diagnose the malignant condition or extent of the disease are aspiration, needle core, punch, incisional, and excisional biopsy.[1–4] It is exceedingly important to know the histologic diagnosis of a malignancy before performing definitive pinvolving this particular agent, involving this particular agent, rocedures. For example, knowing whether a tumor is a benign sebaceous

> **KEY POINT**
>
> *It is important to know the histologic diagnosis of a malignancy before performing most definitive procedures. This information helps the surgeon plan the appropriate surgery and also improves the chance for a cure.*

adenoma or a malignant soft tissue sarcoma is extremely important. This is because even though they may have the same outward appearance, the latter requires extensive surgical resection and additional diagnostic procedures (i.e., abdominal and thoracic radiographs, lymph node aspiration or biopsy) to determine the extent of disease. In contrast, a benign adenoma may only require a simple resection.

The following principles should be kept in mind when a surgical biopsy is performed[1-4]:

- Needle tracts or biopsy incisions should be placed with careful thought so that the entire biopsy tract can be removed when the definitive surgical procedure is performed. A tract is composed of tissue that is in contact with, or is disturbed by, the biopsy instrument. When the veterinarian who performs a diagnostic biopsy is unlikely to perform the definitive surgery, the surgeon who will perform the definitive procedure should be consulted before the biopsy.

- Extreme care should be taken to not spread cancer cells to surrounding tissue or through tissue planes during the biopsy procedure. For example, avoiding the formation of a hematoma or seroma is important because either one might allow cancer cells to spread as it dissects between fascial planes, requiring a more extensive definitive resection.

- When multiple biopsy specimens are taken from different sites, care should be taken to change instruments so the surgeon does not transplant tumor cells from one site to another.

- Biopsy techniques should be carefully selected to allow the acquisition of sufficient tissue to make a histopathologic diagnosis. Laser surgery should not be used because it can significantly alter the tissue, which will preclude a diagnosis and an adequate description of tissue margins. Additionally, tissues should be prepared in such a manner as to allow adequate evaluation by different procedures, such as immunohistochemistry. Taking multiple biopsy specimens increases the likelihood of an accurate diagnosis if an excisional biopsy is not planned.

- The biopsy specimen should be handled with extreme care to prevent crushing or altering the orientation of the tissue specimen or creating tissue artifacts. Specimens should be placed in enough preservative to allow complete fixation (a good rule is one part tissue to 10 parts formalin); however, prolonged fixation or storage in formalin may reduce the chances for future successful immunohistochemical staining. Using inked margins or sutures may give the pathologist information regarding the orientation of biopsy tissue within the body. The surgeon should check with the pathologist to determine his or her preferred method of marking tissue.

- The surgeon should have an acute awareness of the biologic behavior of malignant conditions to ensure that all possible sites of metastases are evaluated before a definitive procedure is performed.

TREATMENT OF CANCER

Surgical treatment of cancer can be divided into six areas:

- Definitive surgical treatment of primary cancer
- Surgery to reduce the bulk of residual disease
- Surgical resection of metastatic disease
- Surgery for treatment of oncologic emergencies
- Surgery for palliation
- Surgery for reconstruction and rehabilitation

Definitive Surgery for Primary Cancer[1-5,9]

Definitive surgery to cure primary cancer is the most common use of surgery for veterinary cancer patients. Before the definitive procedure, the patient must be completely staged to determine the extent of the cancer. The surgeon should have an acute awareness of the biologic behavior of malignant conditions to ensure that all possible sites of metastases are evaluated. In addition, he or she must consider all options and alternatives when planning the procedure. For example, a relatively conservative surgery may result in a 90% cure rate for a basal cell tumor.[4] A soft tissue sarcoma, however, must be treated with a wide surgical excision that should extend at least one fascial layer below the detectable margins of the tumor. Therefore, it is important to know the specific tumor type being treated and the biologic behavior of the tumor so that the client can be educated about the prognosis and amount of surgery that is necessary for a satisfactory outcome. It is equally vital that the surgeon know his or her own limits and abilities. For example, referring a patient with an invasive soft tissue sarcoma to a board-certified specialist for appropriate therapy may offer the best chance for a positive outcome. Finally, other options such as radiation therapy can be suggested to the client instead of or as an adjunct to surgery if appropriate.

Examples of some of the most important recent advances in canine cancer surgery include:

- Craniotomy to remove canine meningiomas
- Hemipelvectomy to remove pelvic or proximal femoral lesions
- Mandibulectomy or maxillectomy to remove oral tumors
- Orbitectomy to remove tumors of the ocular area and surrounding structures
- Tracheotomy or partial trachiectomy to remove tracheal tumors
- Chest wall resection to remove rib or other thoracic wall tumors

- Scapulectomy to remove tumors of the scapula or surrounding structures
- Plastic surgery techniques to repair soft tissue defects
- Liver lobectomy for hepatocellular carcinomas
- Hypophysectomy for pituitary adenomas
- Nasal plane resection for squamous cell carcinomas

> **KEY POINT**
>
> *Before surgery, the best surgeons and their clients know the diagnosis of the cancer, its biologic behavior, the potential for a cure, the amount or "dose" of surgery needed for a cure, and what alternatives or adjunctive therapies are necessary to enhance the patient's quality and quantity of life.*

Definitive surgery requires the use of basic surgical principles that are logical, yet often forgotten. Before performing surgery, the patient's age, nutritional and metabolic status, degree of tissue oxygenation, immune status, healing potential, and concurrent diseases should be assessed. An intra- and postoperative analgesia and nutritional plan should be designed. Once the tumor type is known, the tumor should be removed en bloc so that the entire tumor is successfully removed without the lateral or deep margins of the tumor being revealed. Marginal resections invite recurrence. During the removal process, the venous and lymphatic drainage should be ligated early on to prevent shedding of tumor cells. When possible, lymph nodes should be removed and examined histologically for any evidence of tumor metastases. Removal of nodes is not known to improve the outcome, but knowledge of node status can direct adjuvant therapy and influence the prognosis.

The surgeon must do everything possible to cure the cancer during the first surgery. Untreated tumors tend to have normal surrounding tissues, making the success of the first surgery more likely. When a tumor recurs, it is far more likely to have invaded the tissue planes disrupted by the previous surgery and therefore to be unresectable. Recurrent tumors also have a much higher probability of metastasizing, thereby dramatically reducing the probability of long-term tumor control. The most viable tumor is one that is well vascularized. Leaving behind microscopic tissue that may have a greater blood supply causes the cancer to accelerate its rate of growth and potential for metastasis. Finally, in a day and age in which finances and emotions play a big role in the intent and ability to proceed with expensive therapy, curing the disease with the first surgery is ultimately the least expensive and emotionally the most pleasing situation for both the client and the surgeon.

> **KEY POINT**
>
> *The best chance for cure is with the first definitive surgery.*

Surgery for Residual Disease[1–5,9]

The best opportunity to cure a dog with malignant disease is the first surgery. However, tumors are sometimes incompletely resected during a first surgery, so subsequent therapy is required. In many cases, surgery will not be adequate to treat the remaining disease, requiring the integration of other treatment modalities, such as radiation therapy and chemotherapy.[1–3] For example, resection of a soft tissue sarcoma on the distal extremity may result in significant morbidity if the tumor is completely resected, whereas if the tumor is removed until only microscopic disease remains and the surgical field is irradiated postoperatively, morbidity is usually minimal and the probability of long-term control is very good. "Debulking" (cytoreductive) surgery alone is rarely an acceptable form of therapy, and it should not be used inappropriately to reduce the bulk of the tumor without anticipating the use of another effective modality to control residual disease.[1] Except in cases of palliative surgery, there is no role for cytoreductive surgery when other effective therapies are available.

Surgery for Metastatic Disease[1–5,9]

Resection of metastases might be considered in select cases when it is obvious that the malignant disease is not progressing rapidly and that the metastatic disease is restricted to a single site or to a few sites that are amenable to surgical excision. This is especially true when the surgery will improve quality of life or serve as a diagnostic tool for the management of the patient. For example, pulmonary metastases from osteosarcoma can be removed to enhance and improve the patient's quality of life. However, there should be fewer than three lesions, the primary tumor should have been under control for at least a year, and the tumor should be slow growing as evidenced by minimal growth over at least 4 weeks. Another example is the removal of abdominal sublumbar lymph node metastases in dogs with anal sac adenocarcinoma. In most instances, however, the only role surgery has in metastatic disease is in palliation of bulky disease.

Surgery for Oncologic Emergencies[1–5,9]

The most common applications of oncologic surgery in an emergency setting include the treatment of hemorrhage, perforation, or obstruction of organs or the drainage of abscesses.[1–3] An example is an intestinal resection and anastomosis to treat a perforated malignancy of the gastrointestinal tract. The presence of pericardial effusion and tamponade may require a surgical procedure or thoracoscopy to remove the pericardial sac and the tumor that caused the effusion. A tracheal or thoracic wall tumor may cause respiratory distress, and an emergency resection of the tumor may be the fastest way to relieve that distress. A bleeding tumor within the abdominal organ (such as a splenic hemangiosarcoma) may need to be resected to prevent a fatal hemorrhage. A transabdominal Foley catheter may need to be placed or a tube urethrostomy performed in cases of total urethral obstruction.

Surgery for Palliation[1-5,9]

When a tumor or its metastasis results in significant discomfort for the veterinary cancer patient, surgery can be employed to improve or maintain quality of life.[1-4] In these patients, surgery should be used only if the client is clearly aware that this procedure will not be curative. An example may be mastectomy in a dog with a bleeding, abscessed mammary adenocarcinoma that also has pulmonary metastatic disease. The mastectomy may improve quality of life by reducing pain, even though the overall survival time may not be substantially increased.

Transurethral tumor tissue resection performed through a cystoscope was found to give palliative results in male dogs with obstructive urinary disease.[10] Based on this evidence, tumor tissue resection may be considered for rapid relief of urethral obstruction in male dogs.

Amputation alone may be considered palliative for dogs with osteosarcoma; however, the procedure may actually prolong life indirectly by relieving pain related to the cancer and thereby delaying euthanasia.

Surgery for Reconstruction and Rehabilitation[1-5,9]

Very wide resection of a malignancy is now possible because of the development of plastic surgery techniques, including free flap and microvascular anastomotic methods. These techniques can be used to rehabilitate areas that have been irradiated or in which substantial tissue injury is noted. An example would be a vascular flap to cover a defect after a tumor has been surgically removed from a distal extremity.

REFERENCES

1. Lascelles BD: Principles of oncological surgery, in Dobson JM, Lascelles BD: *BSAVA Manual of Canine and Feline Oncology*, ed 2. Gloucester, British Small Animal Veterinary Association, 2003, pp 73–86.
2. Niederhuber JE: Surgical interventions in cancer, in Abeloff MD, Armitage JO, Niederhuber JE, et al: *Clinical Oncology*, ed 3. Philadelphia, Elsevier, 2004, pp 579–590.
3. Withrow SJ: Surgical oncology, in Withrow SJ, MacEwen EG (eds): *Small Animal Clinical Oncology*, ed 3. Philadelphia, WB Saunders, 2001, pp 70–76.
4. Ogilvie GK, Moore AS: Surgical oncology—Properties, uses, and patient management, in Ogilvie GK, Moore AS (eds): *Feline Oncology: A Comprehensive Guide to Compassionate Care*. Yardley, PA, Veterinary Learning Systems, 2002, pp 88–90.
5. Aiken SW: Principles of surgery for the cancer patient. *Clin Tech Small Anim Pract* 18(2):75–81, 2003.
6. Powers BE, Dernell WS: Tumor biology and pathology. *Clin Tech Small Anim Pract* 13(1):4–9, 1998.
7. Szentimrey D: Principles of reconstructive surgery for the tumor patient. *Clin Tech Small Anim Pract* 13(1):70–76, 1998.
8. O'Brien MG: Principles of oncologic abdominal surgery. *Clin Tech Small Anim Pract* 13(1):42–46, 1998.
9. Soderstrom MJ, Gilson SD: Principles of surgical oncology. *Vet Clin North Am Small Anim Pract* 25(1):97–110, 1995.
10. Liptak JM, Brutscher SP, Monnet E, et al: Transurethral resection in the management of urethral and prostatic neoplasia in 6 dogs. *Vet Surg* 33(5):505–516, 2004.

COMPLEMENTARY AND ALTERNATIVE VETERINARY MEDICINE: PROPERTIES, USES, AND PATIENT MANAGEMENT

Gregory K. Ogilvie and Antony S. Moore

CLINICAL BRIEFING

Acupuncture	• Stimulation of specific anatomic points on the body for therapeutic purposes using needles, heat, pressure, friction, suction, or impulses of electromagnetic energy.
Chiropractic science	• Method that concerns itself with the relationship between biomechanics, structure, and function or impulses of electromagnetic energy in the body.
Massage therapy	• Manipulation of soft body parts to achieve a state of normalcy.
Biofield therapy	• Ancient art of the laying on of hands.
Homeopathic medicine	• Treatment with extreme dilutions of remedies made of naturally occurring substances from plants, animals, and minerals.
Pharmacologic/biologic treatments	• Treatment with drugs and vaccines that are not currently accepted by mainstream medicine and surgery.
Herbal/botanical medicine	• Treatment with herbs and other plants.
Nutritional therapy	• Treatment with nutrients to prevent and treat disease as well as to support individuals in the face of disease.

The inclusion of a chapter on complementary and alternative veterinary medicine (CAVM) is designed to ensure that this book is comprehensive and meets the needs of the progressive practicing veterinarian. In theory, in oncology—where we attempt to judge therapies using the tenets of evidence-based medicine—this chapter should not exist. Rather, therapies should be identified as effective, investigational, or ineffective. In reality, more and more clients, physicians, and veterinarians recognize CAVM as a unique discipline.[1-17] Clients are using complementary therapies for their dogs and themselves despite limited data on efficacy and toxicity. People around the world use the words "complementary," "alternative," "integrative," or "holistic" interchangeably to mean non–Western-style therapies. While many Westerners remain skeptical about some of these therapies, it is useful to keep in mind that approximately 4 billion people—80% of the world's population—use at least one form of alternative medicine, and many people seek this type of care for their pets when they become ill.[1-17] Conservative estimates indicate that one-third of all Americans routinely use alternative and complementary therapies, especially as a supplement to conventional health care methods.[14] In fact, Americans visit alternative practitioners more often than they visit their physicians, at a cost of more than $14 billion per year.[14] A recent survey showed that total out-of-pocket (i.e., not covered by insurance) expenditures related to alternative therapies were estimated at $27 billion, which was comparable with the projected out-of-pocket expenditures for all physician services.

> *Although many Westerners remain skeptical about some of these therapies, approximately 80% of the world's population uses at least one form of alternative medicine. Many also seek this type of care for their pets when they become ill.*

Another marker that documents that CAVM has become mainstream is the establishment of official research programs such as those at the Shipley Natural Healing Center at Colorado State University and the Center for Alternative Medicine Research in Cancer at the University of Texas—Houston Health Science Center. Additionally, the National Cancer Institute has established a link with the National Institutes of Health National Center for Complementary and Alternative Medicine.[15,16] In 1999, the American Society of Clinical Oncology and the American Cancer Society hosted their first symposium on CAVM.[16] Several large drug companies have developed herbal and nutraceutical products obtainable over the counter; some of these are promoted specifically for the prevention of cancer.[17,18]

> **KEY POINT**
> *Complementary therapy has never been shown to cure cancer when used alone; its potential value is to enhance the cancer patient's quality of life.*

The interest in CAVM is increasing dramatically in veterinary health care. There is a growing demand among clients for complementary medical treatments for their pets. This is true especially in the treatment of cancer patients for whom traditional options are rarely curative and potentially toxic. Until recently, there have been few Western-style studies to document the efficacy of CAVM as a useful adjunct in treating cancer patients. Scientists have undertaken and published studies using traditional research methods to discover the efficacy of certain treatments. With the results of each new study, the comfort level of some veterinarians in using some of these treatments grows. Despite the increased use of complementary or alternative medical treatments, however, none has ever been documented to cure a cancer patient. The potential place of CAVM in canine oncology and medicine is to support the patient.

To be a knowledgeable, progressive practitioner, it is important to first know the definition of these alternative modalities in order to be at least conversant with interested clients. Second, clinicians should be aware that while little is known

> **KEY POINT**
> *The veterinary health care team should understand that confrontation over or complete rejection of complementary therapy may alienate some clients and prevent their pets from receiving appropriate and comprehensive care.*

about the efficacy and toxicity of complementary therapies in canine medicine, there are some documented efficacies and toxicities in other species. We have noted some of these studies, particularly those that are relevant to cancer treatment, in this chapter.

The veterinary health care team should understand that confrontation over or complete rejection of complementary therapy may alienate some clients and prevent their pets from receiving appropriate and comprehensive care. On the other hand, the team and the client must clearly understand the strengths and limitations of this care. Few can disagree that CAVM is becoming an important aspect of palliative and supportive cancer care, but there is not a single complementary intervention that has been demonstrated to constitute an effective cure for cancer. Therefore, it seems prudent to state that it is unethical to promote CAVM as a cancer cure in canine medicine. False promotion of CAVM can misguide clients into giving up effective conventional treatments, it can raise false hopes, and it can financially exploit caring clients who seek any kind of help for their dog with cancer.

Despite the limitations of CAVM and the scarcity of data on this type of care, there is little doubt that patients can be helped in the palliative and supportive setting. CAVM in palliative or supportive care is directed at providing comfort and increasing the quality of life of dogs with cancer. Goals include promoting relaxation; decreasing fear, anxiety, and stress; relieving pain and nausea; enhancing appetite; and improving sleep. The end goal is improving the patient's quality of life through comprehensive, compassionate care.

> **KEY POINT**
> *While little is known about the efficacy and toxicity of complementary therapies in canine medicine, some efficacies and toxicities have been documented in other species.*

The objectives of this chapter are to simply introduce and define some complementary therapeutics that have been used in the treatment of cancer and other diseases in animals and humans. Due to space limitations, readers are encouraged to seek additional information in the references provided. Entire books have been written on each of the subjects introduced below.

Ethics and CAVM

A recent article in *JAVMA*[19] noted that "more inquiries and complaints are directed to the American Veterinary Medical Association [AVMA] about alternative and complementary therapies than any other issue." Credibility of the practitioner was a major concern. The article reinforced that practitioners who use complementary therapies should be licensed doctors of veterinary medicine who are specifically trained and experienced in their complementary discipline. In the article, the AVMA stated, "The veterinary profession wants to assure the public that, when alternative and complementary modalities are being used, they are being used by persons rendered capable and responsible through education and regulation, and that, as a result, these practitioners will 'do no harm.'"[19] It went on to state that there is a specific danger to clients and patients if they seek care from unlicensed nonprofessionals or if licensed individuals have not received adequate education or do not submit themselves to a required standard of practice in these modalities. Furthermore, the AVMA encourages the use of these modalities within the context of a valid veterinarian–client–patient relationship.[19]

Methods to appropriately care for the patient and the client and therefore minimize risk for legal steps against the attending veterinarian include the following[19]:

- Become knowledgeable about CAVM through continuing education courses, books, and journals
- Become familiar with the safety and efficacy of CAVM therapies
- Completely inform clients about the known risks and potential consequences if they forgo known, proven care
- Ensure that your referral to a CAVM practitioner does not delay, prevent, or minimize the opportunity for the patient to receive necessary care via conventional means and does not subsequently cause the patient to suffer
- Document discussions with the client about the pros and cons of pursuing CAVM
- Refer prudently and only to trained CAVM providers who are ethical and responsible
- Follow your best medical judgment

Acupuncture

Acupuncture involves the stimulation of specific anatomic points on the body for therapeutic purposes with needles, heat, pressure, friction, suction, or impulses of electromagnetic energy.[2-46] This ancient healing art is generally well accepted and widely used by human and veterinary health care professionals to treat a variety of ailments, including discomfort, nausea, and xerostomia.

> **KEY POINT**
> *Sound scientific data have shown that the stimulation of specific points in the body via acupuncture alters the body's chemical neurotransmitters, thereby inducing beneficial effects.*

MECHANISM OF ACTION

Acupuncture is used worldwide to normalize or correct the flow of *Qi* (pronounced "chee"), which refers to the body's life-giving force, to restore health.[2,4] Acupuncture points are very specific areas that can be stimulated by such implements as needles, lasers, heat, and beads to result in an intended effect, often at a distant site. Many of these points are related or linked through "meridians." The acupuncture points of dogs have been defined, but this healing art is best delivered by a practitioner who is highly trained by one of a handful of certifying or educating organizations for veterinarians such as the American Academy of Veterinary Medical Acupuncture or the International Veterinary Acupuncture Society (IVAS). Sound scientific data have shown that the stimulation of specific points alters the body's chemical neurotransmitters. Acupuncture is one of the most commonly used complementary therapies in human and veterinary medicine.

INDICATIONS

Well-designed studies in humans show efficacy of acupuncture for the treatment of osteoarthritis, chemotherapy-induced nausea, asthma, back pain, and headache, among other conditions (Table 25-1).[23-46] The most dramatic reports of the efficacy of acupuncture have been on its use in surgical analgesia.[2,22,35-45] In 1973, up to 25% of all human surgeries in mainland China were performed using acupuncture analgesia, with efficacy reported in up to 90% of the cases.[2,3] These numbers are estimated to be at least that high today. Acupuncture surgical anesthesia is not widely used in the United States in human or canine medicine. This modality obviously has the potential to benefit canine cancer patients for whom surgery is the mainstay of therapy.[4] Acupuncture is commonly used to prevent and reduce postsurgical and radiation-induced discomfort and to enhance the well-being of canine patients receiving cancer care of all types. In addition, chemotherapy-induced nausea is commonly treated with acupuncture.

To become minimally qualified in veterinary acupuncture, a veterinarian should take specific courses offered by qualified groups such as the IVAS. Certification is one mark of training for minimal competence.

Chiropractic Science

Chiropractic science is a healing method that concerns itself with the relationship between structure and function.[1-17] The structure of the spine and the function of the nervous system are the primary areas of interest in chiropractic therapy.

MECHANISM OF ACTION

Healing occurs via manipulative procedures and interventions, not surgical or chemotherapeutic treatments. The orthopedic structures in question are altered or aligned into

Table 25-1 Cancer-Related Ailments That May Benefit from Acupuncture[2–46]

Ailment	Evidence of Acupuncture Effects
Cancer-related breathlessness	70% reported marked symptomatic benefit, with significant improvements in breathlessness, relaxation, and anxiety.[25]
Chemotherapy- and opioid-induced nausea	Shows consistent results in reducing emetic effects of chemotherapy and opioids.[27–30]
Circulatory problems	Reduces edema in the extremities.[2]
Immune hypofunction	• Enhances natural killer cell cytotoxicity.[32] • Increases percentage of peripheral blood T lymphocytes.[3] • Enhances production of circulating interferon and interleukin-2.[31,32]
Malignant pain (e.g., postradiation fibrosis, muscle spasm, vascular problems, hyperesthesia, dysesthesia, resistant bone pain)	• A combination of herbal drugs and electroacupuncture markedly reduced the amount of analgesic and sedative medication needed by 212 patients with bone metastasis.[35] • Auricular stud acupuncture provided pain relief in terminally ill patients with neuropathic, soft tissue, bone, and malignant pain in whom pain remained uncontrolled by conventional means.[36] • Controls intractable and malignant pain.[38–41]
Phantom limb pain of amputees	62% of patients had marked improvement in phantom limb pain, and 23% had moderate improvement.[42]
Poorly healing wounds	Acupuncture treatment with electrical stimulation and laser facilitated wound healing in horses with granulomatous, ulcerating, poorly healing wounds.
Postoperative ileus	Acupuncture group had restoration of gastrointestinal motility.[2]
Postoperative pain	In combination with Chinese herbs and epidural morphine, acupuncture relieved pain in postoperative patients with liver cancer and reduced untoward side effects from morphine.[44]
Preoperative anxiety	Human patients who received acupuncture experienced less palmar sweating before anesthesia.[45]
Radiation-induced xerostomia	• 68% of patients receiving classical acupuncture and 50% of patients receiving superficial acupuncture had increased salivary flow rates.[45] • Acupuncture stimulation significantly increased the release of calcitonin gene-related peptide, vasoactive intestinal peptide, and neuropeptide Y in patients with xerostomia.[46]
Toxic side effects of radiation and chemotherapy	Helps increase patient participation in conventional treatment by reducing leukopenia and gastrointestinal and systemic reactions.

Modified from Robinson NG, Ogilvie GK: Complementary and alternative veterinary medicine and cancer, in Withrow SJ, MacEwen EG (eds): *Small Animal Clinical Oncology*. Philadelphia, WB Saunders, 2001, pp 183–197; with permission.

a normal relationship with the rest of the body to restore health and wellness. In some cases, this will result in spinal alignment and alleviate nerve compression. Chiropractic care involves integration of the disciplines of radiology, sports medicine, neurology, osteopathy, and orthopedics.

INDICATIONS

Research on the beneficial effect of chiropractic therapy within the veterinary profession is still very much in its infancy. Few data exist concerning the efficacy of this treatment discipline in canine medicine. Studied areas of efficacy in humans include back and other orthopedic pain and somatovisceral disorders such as hypertension. Chiropractic care of the canine cancer patient primarily seeks to improve general comfort, lameness, and mobility, especially in areas of orthopedic or neurologic disorders. Veterinarians who wish to become minimally qualified to perform chiropractic procedures should take a set of manipulative courses.

Massage Therapy

Massage therapy is the manipulation of soft body parts to achieve a state of normalcy.[1–17,47–55]

MECHANISM OF ACTION

This modality incorporates the use of fixed or movable pressure, rubbing, stroking, tapping, or kneading the body with a view toward treating physical or emotional conditions. This ancient healing art affects the musculoskeletal, circulatory, lymphatic, and nervous systems. Healing by touch in massage therapy involves *vis medicatrix naturae* (helping the body heal itself). When massage therapy is performed by a highly trained and experienced therapist, there is no doubt that the procedure results in intensive and pleasant relaxation to the body and mind (as reflected in improved attitude, appetite, and actions in the case of a dog). Techniques include Swedish massage, deep-tissue massage, neuromuscular massage, manual lymphatic massage, reflexology, zone therapy, tui na, acupressure, Rolfing, Trager, the Feldenkrais method, and the Alexander technique. Various adaptations of these techniques in human medicine are being used in veterinary medicine, although few data exist documenting their efficacy in dogs.

INDICATIONS

Trials in humans have shown efficacy in acute and chronic pain, acute and chronic inflammation, chronic lymphedema, nausea, muscle spasm, various soft tissue dysfunction, generalized tonic–clonic (grand mal) seizure, anxiety, and depression.[47-55] Massage has also been shown to stimulate the body's ability to control pain naturally by producing endorphins.[24] Some suggest that massage therapy is contraindicated in cancer patients because increased blood flow may result in increased metastases, but this theory has never been convincingly documented. Applications of massage therapy for canine cancer patients may revolve around relieving pain and discomfort and maintaining function. Some oncology centers combine massage with acupuncture or use massage alone to relieve lameness or discomfort that is not exclusively due to orthopedic disease. For example, massage therapy can be used to prevent or reduce deterioration of the use of a limb being treated with radiation or surgery for a soft tissue sarcoma of the extremity. Special training in manipulative techniques is available for veterinarians to become minimally qualified to practice in this area.

Biofield Therapy

Biofield therapy or spiritual healing is the ancient art of the laying on of hands. The earliest records of this healing method date between 2,500 and 5,000 years ago.[1-17,56,57]

MECHANISM OF ACTION

Healing is said to come from two sources.[56,57] The first is a source other than the therapist, such as God, the cosmos, or another supernatural entity. A second source is the practitioner of the modality, who modifies or amplifies the patient's biofield. During this type of healing, the therapist places his or her hands on or near the patient's body to improve general health or a disease condition. Practitioners of this therapy note that a biofield emanates for a distance beyond the physical body and that the strength, distance, and color of the field depend on the health and emotional state of the individual. Three forms of biofield therapeutics are used: healing touch (Reiki), therapeutic touch, and SHEN therapy.[56,57] Reiki originated from Japan in the 1800s and has a theoretical basis in channeling energy from an external source (e.g., God) through the healer to the patient to enhance well-being. In Reiki, the spiritual body is healed and is then expected to heal the physical body. Therapeutic touch involves a practitioner who restores the correct vibrational component to the patient's universal, unitary field. In SHEN therapy, healing is reported to occur through a biofield conforming to the natural laws of physics with a discernible pattern throughout the body. There are few if any published data documenting the efficacy of these modalities in dogs.

INDICATIONS

One review of 23 placebo-controlled studies in humans showed that 57% of these studies arrived at a positive conclusion about biofield therapy.[58] However, no good studies document the efficacy of biofield therapy in canine medicine. Until further data are known, this treatment approach should be used with caution and obviously never in place of a modality that is known to be effective.

Homeopathic Medicine

Homeopathic medicine is the use of extreme dilutions of substances to treat diseases or disorders. It is practiced worldwide, especially in Europe, Latin America, and Asia.[59,60] Homeopathic remedies are made of naturally occurring substances from plants, animals, and minerals that are diluted to as low as 10^{-30} to $10^{-20,000}$. These homeopathic substances are recognized and regulated by the Food and Drug Administration; however, this regulation does not suggest endorsement of the efficacy of homeopathic remedies.

MECHANISM OF ACTION

Diseases or disorders are treated with extreme dilutions of "like" substances.[59-62] For example, radiation illness could be treated with extreme dilutions of radium. Critics of homeopathy suggest that such extreme dilutions of compounds preclude any probability for efficacy. Scientists who have not rejected the potential benefits of homeopathy suggest that the efficacy can be explained by quantum physics, which says the electromagnetic energy of these remedies may interact with the body for beneficial purposes. A phenomenon known as the *memory of water* is used to explain how extreme dilutions can result in retained efficacy. In this theory, the structure of a water and alcohol solution is altered during the procedure of making the remedies so that the structure of the molecule is retained even after none of the actual substance remains.

Table 25-2 **Homeopathic Remedies That May Benefit Cancer Patients**[60–67]

Remedy	Potential Advantages and Indications	Potential Adverse Effects
Cadmium sulphuricum 30c	Intense nausea accompanied by chills and debilitating exhaustion, especially after chemotherapy	None known
Cantharis 6c	Eases skin discomfort and other dermatologic sequelae to radiation	None known
Gelsemium 6c	Calms nervousness and anticipatory anxiety; aids weak trembling	None known
Ipecac 30c	Eases persistent nausea and vomiting	None known
Nux vomica 6c	Eases nausea and vomiting accompanied by sensitivity to loud noises, strong odors, and bright lights	None known

Modified from Robinson NG, Ogilvie GK: Complementary and alternative veterinary medicine and cancer, in Withrow SJ, MacEwen EG (eds): *Small Animal Clinical Oncology*. Philadelphia, WB Saunders, 2001, pp 183–197; with permission.

INDICATIONS

The *British Medical Journal* presented a metaanalysis on 96 published reports of 107 controlled trials on homeopathic medicine.[63] Trials were scored using a predefined system, and 22 were designated as well-designed clinical trials involving homeopathy. Fifteen of 22 showed positive results. These rarely included any cancer patients. The types of ailments in human patients that were improved included allergic diseases and arthritis. Therefore, homeopathy may be of benefit in supporting cancer patients (Table 25-2[60–67]), but few data exist to suggest that it can be used to directly treat or prevent a malignant process. These homeopathic remedies are often available in grocery stores and are therefore easily obtained and frequently used by clients.

Pharmacologic and Biologic Treatments

Pharmacologic and biologic treatments use a wide variety of drugs and vaccines that are not currently accepted by mainstream medicine and surgery. There are no published data documenting the efficacy of these agents in canine medicine. Some of the more common agents being used in human and veterinary medicine include the following[1,22–33]:

- **Antineoplastons**, peptide fractions originally derived from blood and urine, are being used to treat a wide variety of malignancies in humans. This controversial treatment is often cited, but data regarding its efficacy are limited or nonexistent.

> **KEY POINT**
> *To date, there have been no well-controlled clinical trials documenting the efficacy of shark cartilage as an anticancer agent for any species, including dogs.*

- **Cartilage products**, especially those from sharks and cattle, are very popular despite the lack of evidence of efficacy and the decline in the shark population. Cartilage has been shown to have antiangiogenic properties. In addition, it contains tissue inhibitors of metalloproteinases (TIMPs) that inhibit tumor metastasis. Shark cartilage has become very popular because of reports of studies in Mexico and Cuba suggesting that this product resulted in the effective treatment of cancer in humans. These original studies were soundly criticized because of faulty study design, lack of controls, and failure to confirm that patients had a malignancy.[64] Despite the fact that every year, 50,000 Americans spend $7,000 each on cartilage products, few data exist to document the efficacy of cartilage. No clinical study reported to date has shown efficacy associated with shark cartilage therapy.[64,65]

- **EDTA chelation therapy** has been used to treat a number of conditions; however, the mechanism for treating cancer has not been clearly stated. It is interesting that metalloproteinases, especially those of gelatinase capability, are indeed inhibited by EDTA. Metalloproteinases 2 and 9 are critical for tumor growth and invasion. Therefore, there may be a reasonable explanation for the potential value of this therapy.

- **Immunoaugmentive therapy** is an experimental form of cancer therapy consisting of treatment with substances that enhance the immune system. More details of this approach can be found in Chapter 23.

Herbal and Botanical Medicine

Approximately 4 billion people, or 80% of the world's population, use herbal and botanical medicine.[67–74] Almost every system of native medicine around the world uses herbal treatments. Despite this widespread use, acceptance differs throughout the world. In the United States, herbal remedies

Table 25-3 Botanical Compounds That May Be Beneficial for Cancer Patients[67-85]

Botanical Medicine	Reported Beneficial Effects and Uses in Cancer Patients	Adverse Effects and Precautions	Interactions with Other Herbs or Drugs
Aloe vera	Increases immune function; stimulates production of interleukin-1 and TNF by macrophages; may inhibit metastasis	Avoid in pregnant patients and those with intestinal obstruction; may cause diarrhea	Caution is advised when used in conjunction with cardiac glycosides; aloe vera gel applied topically along with hydrocortisone acetate may enhance antiinflammatory activity
Ashwagandha	Adaptogen[a]; general immune stimulant	None reported	None reported
Asian ginseng (*Panax ginseng*)	Adaptogen[a]; chemotherapy support to improve mental and physical vitality; enhances hypothalamic–pituitary–adrenal cortical function and benefits immune function; restores hematopoietic function of bone marrow	None reported; considered safe at recommended dosages but may cause overstimulation and insomnia; caution is advised with hypertensive patients	Avoid concomitant use with heparin, aspirin, and NSAIDs; increases antibody levels and improves immune function after vaccination
Astragalus (*Astragalus membranaceus*)	Cancer prevention; immunomodulator; chemotherapy support; may enhance secretion of TNF; may potentiate activity of chemotherapeutic agents, inhibit recurrences, prolong survival time, and reduce adverse toxicities of antineoplastic agents	None reported	None reported
Garlic (*Allium sativum*)	Antibacterial; antifungal; antiplatelet; antiviral; cancer preventive	Discontinue use before surgery because of antiplatelet effects; large dosages may cause Heinz body anemia in small animals	No known drug interactions; caution advised when used in conjunction with other agents possessing antiplatelet effects (ginger, ginkgo, vitamin E, pharmaceuticals)
Ginger (*Zingiber officinale*)	Antiemetic, antiinflammatory, digestive tract tonic[b]; chemotherapy support; reduces postoperative and chemotherapy-induced nausea and vomiting; protects stomach from ulceration; inhibits platelet aggregation	Rare; sensitive individuals may experience gastrointestinal irritation; caution is advised in patients with clotting disorders	Avoid use with other antiplatelet agents, including herbs such as garlic, ginkgo, and vitamin E; anticoagulant activity may be additive with that of chemotherapy agents
Green tea	Antibacterial; antioxidant; stimulates production of immune cells; may decrease cancer risk (including in the upper digestive system); may inhibit metastasis	None reported	May interfere with orally administered codeine, theophylline, and atropine because of the high amount of tannins; stimulant effects from caffeine may be additive with other sympathomimetics
Ligustrum (*Ligustrum lucidum*)	Cancer protective; immune stimulant; immunomodulator; chemotherapy support	None reported with normal dosing; signs of overdose may include vomiting and dizziness	None reported
Maitake mushroom (*Grifola frondosa*)	Adaptogen[a]; antitumor immunomodulator; tonic[b]; immune enhancement; tumor inhibition	None reported	None reported

(Table continues)

Table 25-3 (continued)

Botanical Medicine	Reported Beneficial Effects and Uses in Cancer Patients	Adverse Effects and Precautions	Interactions with Other Herbs or Drugs
Milk thistle	Silymarin, a collection of complex flavonoids found in milk thistle seeds, is hepatoprotective and aids in liver regeneration	None reported	Silymarin has shown synergistic effects with cisplatin and doxorubicin in vitro, reduction of nephrotoxicity from cisplatin, and lack of interference with chemotherapy in cases of acute promyelocytic leukemia
Reishi mushroom (*Ganoderma lucidum*)	Hepatoprotective; chemotherapy support to treat general fatigue and weakness; immune activation; tumor and histamine inhibition	Rare; after continuous use over several months, dizziness, dry mouth and throat, epistaxis, and abdominal upset may appear; may increase bleeding time	Not recommended for those taking anticoagulant medications
Schisandra (*Schisandra chinensis*)	Adaptogen[a]; antioxidant; hepatoprotective	Uncommon; include gastrointestinal upset, anorexia, and dermatitis; signs of overdose include agitation, insomnia, and dyspnea[47]	Hepatoprotective
Shiitake mushroom (*Lentinan edodes*)	Antimicrobial; antiparasitic; antitumor; antiviral; cancer preventive; hepatoprotective; immune regulating	High dosages may cause diarrhea and bloating	None reported
Siberian ginseng (*Eleutherococcus senticosus*)	Strong adaptogen[a]; anabolic; antitumor; tonic[b]; minimizes side effects of radiation, chemotherapy, and surgery; promotes healing	Very uncommon; include headache, increased blood pressure, insomnia, and hypoglycemia; avoid use in febrile and hypertensive patients and in those experiencing myocardial infarction	May cause falsely elevated digoxin levels on laboratory tests while not actually increasing blood levels of digoxin; may reduce the risk of postvaccination reactions
Ten significant tonic decoction (*Shi-quan-da-bu-tang*); also known as Juzen-taiho-to, or TJ-48; a Japanese herbal (Kampo) medicine	Biologic response modifier (reduces side effects from chemotherapy and radiation and improves general condition of patients); tumor inhibitor; stimulates immune function and hematopoiesis; protects against renal and hepatic toxicity and bone marrow suppression caused by cisplatin; reduces leukopenia, thrombocytopenia, and weight loss associated with mitomycin	Generally rare when herbs are properly prescribed; acute interstitial pneumonitis and hypokalemia occasionally reported	None reported

[a]Adaptogens are substances that provide a nonspecific increase in the resistance of an organism to a wide range of physical, chemical, biologic, and psychologic stressors.
[b]A tonic is a remedy that is used to restore strength and vigor.
TNF = tumor necrosis factor
Modified from Robinson NG, Ogilvie GK: Complementary and alternative veterinary medicine and cancer, in Withrow SJ, MacEwen EG (eds): *Small Animal Clinical Oncology*. Philadelphia, WB Saunders, 2001, pp 183–197; with permission.

are considered to be without efficacy by many regulatory bodies, although many drugs we routinely use today are derived from plants. European governments, especially in Germany and France, have formally approved herbs for therapeutic purposes. Indeed, some of the best studies on the efficacy of these herbs have been done in Europe.

MECHANISM OF ACTION

The mechanism of action depends on the active ingredient of the individual herb or botanical agent. In many cases, the mechanism is unknown. Agents used in China include sesquiterpenes, diterpenes, triterpenes, quinones, podophyllotoxins, taxol, and alkaloids.[67–74] Many of these,

> **KEY POINT**
>
> *In China and elsewhere in the world, herbs and other plant derivatives have been used to treat a number of disorders, including cancer, chemotherapy-induced nausea, and depression associated with the diagnosis of cancer.*

such as paclitaxel, vincristine, and etoposide, have been adapted for Western-style cancer therapy.

INDICATIONS

In China and elsewhere in the world, herbs and other plant derivatives have been used to treat a number of disorders, including cancer, chemotherapy-induced nausea, and depression associated with the diagnosis of cancer (Table 25-3[67–85]). Discussion of all of the herbs and other plant-based materials used therapeutically is beyond the scope of this chapter. As an example of the potential benefit of these agents, in 1981, the US Department of Agriculture, in conjunction with the National Cancer Institute, concluded a 25-year study of plants with anticancer properties. The work includes 365 folk medicinal species and identifies more than 1,000 pharmacologically active phytochemicals.[36]

Few data clearly define the therapeutic benefit of most herbs in the treatment of cancer. These substances can have an impact on the pharmacokinetics of other prescription drugs in dogs. Similarly, because dogs have a different metabolism than cats and humans, extreme care should be taken when extrapolating the dosage and efficacy of these substances to canine medicine.

Postgraduate courses exist in the field of herbal and botanical medicine. The use of these substances is akin to using pharmaceutical agents. Extreme care should be exercised when considering their dosage, toxicity, efficacy, and drug interactions. When these data do not exist, as is often true for dogs, caution should be employed and the patient should be carefully monitored.

Nutritional Therapy

Nutritional therapy revolves around the notion that nutrients, other than those noted above, can be used to prevent, support, and treat humans and animals with cancer and a wide variety of other diseases.[1–11] See Chapter 31 for additional details.

GARLIC

Epidemiologic studies have suggested a correlation between high garlic consumption and reduced risk of cancer development.[1–11] Garlic extracts and several thioalkyl compounds from garlic have been shown to inhibit the activation of carcinogens and the bonding of polyarene thiol epoxide to DNA bases, which causes DNA lesions and initiates a chemically induced carcinogenic process. Garlic and the thioalkyl compounds inhibit carcinogen-induced aberrations in the cell nucleus. In addition, garlic extracts have an antipromotion effect in animals exposed to carcinogens. Also, garlic exerts direct cytolytic effects against cancer-cultured human breast cancer cells and human melanoma cells. Concentrations of garlic used in these studies arrested cancer cell growth, with no effect on normal cells. Pretreatment of rodents with garlic protects against subsequent induction of tumors by a variety of carcinogens. There are no studies demonstrating the safety and efficacy of garlic in the prevention or treatment of cancer in people or animals.

TEA

Although it may be a while before dogs acquire a taste for tea, there are compelling data that suggest that green and black teas may have anticancer properties.[70,72,73] Many clients ask about the potential efficacy of teas or tea extracts for their pets. Green tea extracts contain catechin, and black tea contains fermentation products, thioflavine, and thearubigins. These active agents inhibit cancer-promoting agents, protect against oxidative damage, and enhance antioxidant enzymes. Black tea seems to have soothing properties to reduce the discomfort associated with radiation-induced oral mucositis. The tannic acid and other ingredients act as an astringent and a local anesthetic agent when the oral cavity of affected dogs is lavaged two to three times a day.

> **KEY POINT**
>
> *Caution needs to be employed when assessing the efficacy of complementary therapies; however, data suggest that some of these modalities may be helpful in supporting and enhancing the canine cancer patient's quality of life.*

Conclusion

Caution needs to be employed when assessing the efficacy of complementary therapies; however, data suggest that some of these modalities may be helpful in treating canine cancer patients. Well-controlled studies must be encouraged and conducted because they are essential to document efficacy and toxicity. The expanding postgraduate opportunities for practicing veterinarians and the incorporation of didactic and clinical programs at key leading veterinary schools are important steps toward the logical use of CAVM. The greatest concern for veterinary practitioners may be that unproven therapies may be used instead of known treatments. Therefore, the client should be informed of all the benefits and risks associated with "traditional" and "nontraditional" therapies alike.

REFERENCES

1. Eisenberg DM, Kessler RC, Foster C, et al: Unconventional medicine in the United States: Prevalence, costs, and patterns of use. *N Engl J Med* 328(4):246–252, 1993.
2. Helms JM: *Acupuncture Energetics: A Clinical Approach for Physicians.* Berkeley, CA, Medical Acupuncture Publishers, 1995, pp 42–57.
3. Diamond EG: Acupuncture analgesia: Western medicine and Chinese traditional medicine. *JAMA* 218:1558–1561, 1971.
4. Robinson NG, Ogilvie GK: Complementary and alternative veterinary medicine and cancer, in Withrow SJ, MacEwen EG (eds): *Small Animal Clinical Oncology.* Philadelphia, WB Saunders, 2001, pp 183–197.
5. Ernst E: A primer of complementary and alternative medicine commonly used by cancer patients. *Med J Aust* 174(2):88–92, 2001.
6. Deng G, Cassileth BR, Yeung KS: Complementary therapies for cancer-related symptoms. *J Support Oncol* 2(5):419–426, 2004.
7. Weiger WA, Smith M, Boon H, et al: Advising patients who seek complementary and alternative medical therapies for cancer. *Ann Intern Med* 137(11):889–903, 2002.
8. Benjamin SA, Simone CH, Traub M: Part 3, Cancer treatment: Beyond the conventional. *Patient Care* 6(1):53–69, 1998.
9. Risberg T, Lund E, Wist E, et al: Cancer patients use of nonproven therapy: A 5-year follow-up study. *J Clin Oncol* 16(1):6–12, 1998.
10. Wynn SG: Wherefore complementary medicine? [commentary]. *JAVMA* 209(7):1228–1233, 1996.
11. Ernst E, Resch KL, Mills S, et al: Complementary medicine—A definition. *Br J Gen Pract* 45:506, 1995.
12. Crocetti E, Crotti N, Feltrin A, et al: The use of complementary therapies by breast cancer patients attending conventional treatment. *Eur J Cancer* 34(3):324–328, 1998.
13. Borkan J, Neher JO, Anson O, Smoker B: Referrals for alternative therapies. *J Fam Pract* 39:545–550, 1994.
14. Eisenberg DM, Davis RB, Ettner SL, et al: Trends in alternative medicine use in the United States, 1990-1997: Results of a follow-up national survey. *JAMA* 280:1569–1575, 1998.
15. Henkel G: The status of oncology research in complementary and alternative medicine. *Oncol Times* May:55–60, 1999.
16. Norton A: Oncologists acknowledge public clamor for alternative medicine. *Med Tribune* June 10:7–8, 1999.
17. Larkin M: Big drug companies joining dietary supplement bandwagon. *Oncol Times* May:61–62, 1999.
18. Adler SR, Fosket JR: Disclosing complementary and alternative medicine use in the medical encounter: A qualitative study in women with breast cancer. *J Fam Pract* 48(6):453–458, 1999.
19. House approves guidelines on alternative, complementary medicine. *JAVMA* 209(6):1026–1028, 1996.
20. Vickers AJ, Straus DJ, Fearon B, Cassileth BR: Acupuncture for postchemotherapy fatigue: A phase II study. *J Clin Oncol* 22(9):1731–1735, 2004.
21. Collins KB, Thomas DJ: Acupuncture and acupressure for the management of chemotherapy-induced nausea and vomiting. *J Am Acad Nurse Pract* 16(2):76–80, 2004.
22. Alimi D, Rubino C, Pichard-Leandri E, et al: Analgesic effect of auricular acupuncture for cancer pain: A randomized, blinded, controlled trial. *J Clin Oncol* 21(22):4120–4126, 2003.
23. Wong RK, Jones GW, Sagar SM, et al: A phase I-II study in the use of acupuncture-like transcutaneous nerve stimulation in the treatment of radiation-induced xerostomia in head-and-neck cancer patients treated with radical radiotherapy. *Int J Radiat Oncol Biol Phys* 57(2):472–480, 2003.
24. Zhou J, Li Z, Jin P: A clinical study on acupuncture for prevention and treatment of toxic side-effects during radiotherapy and chemotherapy. *J Tradit Chin Med* 19(1):16–21, 1999.
25. Filshie J, Penn K, Ashley S, Davis CL: Acupuncture for the relief of cancer-related breathlessness. *Palliat Med* 10:145–150, 1996.
26. Dundee JW, Ghaly RG, Fitzpatrick KT, et al: Acupuncture prophylaxis of cancer chemotherapy-induced sickness. *J R Soc Med* 82(5):268–271, 1989.
27. al-Sadi M, Newman B, Julious SA: Acupuncture in the prevention of postoperative nausea and vomiting. *Anaesthesia* 52(7):658–661, 1997.
28. Parfitt A: Acupuncture as an antiemetic treatment. *J Altern Complement Med* 2(1):167–173, 1996.
29. Vickers AJ: Can acupuncture have specific effects on health? A systematic review of acupuncture antiemesis trials. *J R Soc Med* 89:303–311, 1996.
30. McMillan C, Dundee JW, Abram WP: Enhancement of the antiemetic action of ondansetron by transcutaneous electrical stimulation of the P6 antiemetic point, in patients having highly emetic cytotoxic drugs. *Br J Cancer* 64:971–972, 1996.
31. Sato T, Yu Y, Guo SY, et al: Acupuncture stimulation enhances splenic natural killer cell cytotoxicity in rats. *Jpn J Physiol* 46(2):131–136, 1996.
32. Jianguo Y, Rongxing Z, Mingsheng Z, Qimei G: Effect of acupuncture on peripheral T lymphocytes and their subgroups in patients with malignant tumors. *Int J Clin Acup* 4(1):53–58, 1993.
33. Chin TF, Lin JG, Wang SY: Induction of circulating interferon in humans by acupuncture. *Am J Acupunct* 16(4):319–322, 1988.
34. Yu Y, Kasahara T, Sato T, et al: Enhancement of splenic interferon-γ, interleukin-2, and NK cytotoxicity by S36 acupoint acupuncture in F344 rats. *Jpn J Physiol* 47:173–178, 1977.
35. Guo R, Zhang L, Gong Y, Zhang B: The treatment of pain in bone metastasis of cancer with the analgesic decoction of cancer and the Acupoint Therapeutic Apparatus. *J Tradit Chin Med* 15(4):262–264, 1995.
36. Dillon M, Lucas C: Auricular stud acupuncture in palliative care patients. *Palliat Med* 13(3):253–254, 1999.
37. Omura Y, Losco BM, Omura AK, et al: Common factors contributing to intractable pain and medical problems with insufficient drug uptake in areas to be treated, and their pathogenesis and treatment: Part I. Combined use of medication with acupuncture, (+) Qi Gong energy-stored material, soft laser or electrical stimulation. *Acupunct Electrother Res* 17(2):107–148, 1992.
38. Nordenström BEW: An electrophysiologic view of acupuncture: Role of capacitive and closed circuit currents and their clinical effects in the treatment of cancer and chronic pain. *Am J Acupunct* 17(2):105–117, 1989.
39. Filshie J: The non-drug treatment of neuralgic and neuropathic pain of malignancy. *Cancer Surv* 7(1):161–193, 1988.
40. Filshie J, Redman D: Acupuncture and malignant pain problems. *Eur J Surg Oncol* 11(4):389–394, 1985.
41. Liaw M, Wong AM, Cheng P: Therapeutic trial of acupuncture in phantom limb pain of amputees. *Am J Acupunct* 22: 205–213, 1994.
42. Xunshi W, Zhaolin Z, Chenrang S, et al: Clinical study on the use of second metacarpal holographic acupoints for re-establishing gastrointestinal motility in patients following abdominal surgery. *Am J Acupunct* 22(4):353–356, 1994.
43. Li QS, Cao SH, Xie GM, et al: Combined traditional Chinese medicine and Western medicine; relieving effects of Chinese herbs, ear-acupuncture and epidural morphing [*sic*] on postoperative pain in liver cancer. *Chin Med J* 107(4):289–294, 1994.
44. Lewis GBH: An alternative approach to premedication: Comparing diazepam with auriculotherapy and a relaxation method. *Am J Acupunct* 15(3):205–214, 1987.
45. Blom M, Dawidson I, Fernberg JO, et al: Acupuncture treatment of patients with radiation-induced xerostomia. *Eur J Cancer B Oral Oncol* 32B(3):182–190, 1996.
46. Kirschbaum M: Using massage in the relief of lymphoedema. *Prof Nurse* 11(4):230–232, 1996.
47. Martin LA, Hagen NA: Neuropathic pain in cancer patients: Mechanisms, syndromes, and clinical controversies. *J Pain Symptom Manage* 14(2):99–117, 1997.
48. Ferrell-Torry AT, Glick OJ: The use of therapeutic massage as a nursing intervention to modify anxiety and the perception of cancer pain. *Cancer Nurs* 16(2):93–101, 1993.
49. Burke C, Macnish S, Saunders J, et al: The development of a massage service for cancer patients. *Clin Oncol (R Coll Radiol)* 6(6):381–384, 1994.
50. Field T: Massage therapy for infants and children. *J Dev Behav Pediatr* 16(2):105–111, 1995.
51. Francke AL, Luiken JB, Garssen B, et al: Effects of a pain programme on nurses' psychosocial, physical, and relaxation interventions. *Patient Educ Couns* 28(2):221–230, 1996.
52. Smith M, Stallings MA, Mariner S, Burrall M: Benefits of massage therapy for hospitalized patients: A descriptive and qualitative evaluation. *Altern Ther Health Med* 5(4):64–71, 1999.
53. Ironson G, Field T, Scafidi F, et al: Massage therapy is associated with enhancement of the immune system's cytotoxic capacity. *Int J Neurosci* 84(1–4): 205–217, 1996.
54. Cornish BH, Bunce IH, Ward LC, et al: Bioelectrical impedance for monitoring the efficacy of lymphoedema treatment programmes. *Breast Cancer Res Treat* 38(2):169–176, 1996.
55. Mortimer PS: Therapy approaches for lymphedema. *Angiology* 48(1):87–91, 1997.
56. Hibdon SS: Biofield considerations in cancer treatment. *Semin Oncol Nurs* 21(3):196–200, 2005.
57. Mehl-Madrona L: Integrative tumor board: Recurrent breast cancer or new primary? Mind-body-spirit medicine. *Integr Cancer Ther* 2(3):283–289, 2003.
58. Astin JA, Harkness E, Ernst E: The efficacy of "distant healing": A systematic review of randomized trials. *Ann Intern Med* 132(11):903–910, 2000.

59. Cook CA, Guerrerio JF, Slater VE: Healing touch and quality of life in women receiving radiation treatment for cancer: A randomized controlled trial. *Altern Ther Health Med* 10(3):34–41, 2004.
60. Rosser C: Homeopathy in cancer care: Part I—An introduction to "like curing like." *Clin J Oncol Nurs* 8(3):324–326, 2004.
61. Lee CO: Homeopathy in cancer care: Part II—Continuing the practice of "like curing like." *Clin J Oncol Nurs* 8(3):327–330, 2004.
62. Benjamin SD: Homeopathy: Can like cure like? *Patient Care* 16(1):16–27, 1999.
63. Wynn SG: Studies on use of homeopathy in animals. *JAVMA* 212(5):719–724, 1998.
64. Cucherat M, Haugh MC, Gooch M, Boissel JP: Evidence of clinical efficacy of homeopathy. A meta-analysis of clinical trials. Homeopathic Medicines Research Advisory Group (HMRAG). *Eur J Clin Pharmacol* 56(1):27–33, 2000.
65. Ostrander GK, Cheng KC, Wolf JC, Wolfe MJ: Shark cartilage, cancer and the growing threat of pseudoscience. *Cancer Res* 64(23):8485–8491, 2004.
66. Roudebush P, Davenport DJ, Novotny BJ: The use of nutraceuticals in cancer therapy. *Vet Clin North Am Small Anim Pract* 34(1):249–269, 2004.
67. Lin JH, Rogers PA, Yamada H: Chinese herbal medicine: Pharmacological basis, in Schoen AM, Wynn SG (eds): *Complementary and Alternative Veterinary Medicine*. St. Louis, Mosby, 1998, pp 379–404.
68. Lien EJ, Bensen DR, Li WY: *Structure Activity Relationship Analysis of Chinese Anticancer Drugs and Related Plants*. Taiwan, Oriental Healing Arts Institute, 1985, pp 1–140.
69. Duke JA, Ayensu ES: *Handbook of Medicinal Herbs*. Boca Raton, FL, CRC Press, 1985.
70. Weisburg JH: Interactions of nutrients in oncogenesis. *Am J Clin Nutr* 53:2265, 1991.
71. National Academy of Sciences: *Diet, Nutrition and Cancer*. Washington, DC, National Academy Press, 1982.
72. Wang ZY, Agarwal R, Khan WA, Mukhtar H: Protection against benzo(a)pyrene- and N-nitrosodiethylamine-induced lung and forestomach tumorigenesis in A/J mice by water extracts of green tea and licorice. *Carcinogenesis* 13(8):1491–1494, 1992.
73. Khan SG, Kartiyar SK, Agarwal R, Mukhtar H: Enhancement of antioxidant and phase II enzymes by oral feeding of green tea polyphenols in drinking water to SKH-1 hairless mice: Possible role in cancer chemoprevention. *Cancer Res* 52(14):4050–4052, 1992.
74. Wang ZY, Hong JY, Huang MT, et al: Inhibition of N-nitrosodiethylamine and 4-(methylnitrosamino)-1-(3-pyridyl)-1-butanone-induced tumorigenesis in A/J mice by green tea and black tea. *Cancer Res* 52(7):1943–1947, 1992.
75. Boik J: *Cancer and Natural Medicine*. Princeton, MN, Oregon Medical Press, 1996, p 121.
76. Sinclair S: Chinese herbs: A clinical review of Astragalus, Ligusticum, and Schizandrae. *Altern Med Rev* 3(5):338–344, 1998.
77. Chu DT, Wong WL, Mavligit GM: Immunotherapy with Chinese medicinal herbs: I. Immune restoration of local xenogeneic graft-versus-host reaction in cancer patients by fractionated *Astragalus membranaceus* in vitro. *J Clin Lab Immunol* 25(3):119–123, 1988.
78. Chu DT, Wong WL, Mavligit GM: Immunotherapy with Chinese medicinal herbs: II. Reversal of cyclophosphamide-induced immune suppression by administration of fractionated *Astragalus membranaceus* in vivo. *J Clin Lab Immunol* 25(3):125–129, 1988.
79. Yamahara J, Rong HQ, Naitoh Y, et al: Inhibition of cytotoxic drug-induced vomiting in sincus by a ginger constituent. *J Ethnopharmacol* 27(3):353–355, 1989.
80. Jones CLA: Allies in the breast cancer battle: Herbs for prevention, treatment, and healing. *Herbs Health* Jan–Feb:28–33, 1998.
81. Holzman D: Canada promotes research on alternative treatments for breast cancer. *Alt Comp Ther* 8:8–12, 1998.
82. Sun Y, Hersh EM, Lee SL, et al: Preliminary observations on the effects of the Chinese medicinal herbs *Astragalus membranaceus* and *Ligustrum lucidum* on lymphocyte blastogenic responses. *J Biol Response Mod* 2(3):227–237, 1983.
83. Zee-Cheng, RK: Shi-quan-da-bu-tang (ten significant tonic decoction), SQT. A potent Chinese biological response modifier in cancer immunotherapy, potentiation and detoxification of anticancer drugs. *Methods Find Exp Clin Pharmacol* 14(9):725–736, 1992.
84. Hisha H, Yamada H, Sakurai MH, et al: Isolation and identification of hematopoietic stem cell-stimulating substances from Kampo (Japanese herbal) medicine, Juzen-taiho-to. *Blood* 90(3):1022–1030, 1997.
85. Mizushima H, Kanba S: The use of Japanese herbal medicine in the treatment of medically unexplained physical symptoms. *J Psychosom Res* 46(6):531–535, 1999.

BONE MARROW TRANSPLANTATION
Angela E. Frimberger, Antony S. Moore, and Gregory K. Ogilvie

CLINICAL BRIEFING

Potential indications	• Cancers (mainly lymphomas, leukemias, and some solid tumors). • Severe congenital and acquired hematologic diseases (e.g., X-linked severe combined immunodeficiency, aplastic anemia). • Autoimmune diseases. • Experimental: Inborn errors of metabolism (lysosomal storage diseases), as preparation for solid organ transplantation, and for gene therapy.
Donor types	• Autologous: Patient's own cells. • Allogeneic: Other donor of the same species, generally major histocompatibility complex matched. • Syngeneic: Monozygotic twin.
Graft sources	• Bone marrow. • Adult peripheral blood. • Umbilical cord or placental blood.
Transplant types	• Myeloablative (conventional). • Nonmyeloablative ("mini-transplant").
Main complications	• Graft failure or rejection. • GVHD. • Disease relapse.

Hematopoietic stem cell transplantation (HSCT), or bone marrow transplantation (BMT), has become an increasingly important component of therapy for lymphoma, leukemia, and other malignancies as well as some nonmalignant bone marrow diseases in humans.[1,2] HSCT was developed primarily as a strategy to allow intensification of myelosuppressive anticancer therapies, such as chemotherapy and radiotherapy, by providing a hematopoietic rescue. The subsequent replacement of damaged or destroyed bone marrow allows patients to receive higher doses of chemotherapy, radiotherapy, or both. Clinical evidence such as improved cure rates in a variety of cancers clearly indicates that using HSCT to increase therapeutic dose intensity does impart an anticancer benefit in humans, and new data support this concept in dogs as well. Therefore, the goal of HSCT is often different from that of a traditional transplantation, in which a diseased organ is removed and replaced with a healthy one; rather, in many cases, the cancer patient's marrow is normal at the outset, but transplantation is needed as a rescue from the side effects of treating the disease of other organs. An obvious exception is HSCT for leukemia or a nonmalignant bone marrow disease, in which the bone marrow being replaced is the primary site of the disease.

The current availability of HSCT in veterinary medicine is extremely limited, but new developments may allow it to become more widely available in the coming years. Even so, it will still likely be restricted to the referral oncology setting. As with any other referral-based treatment modality, however, it is helpful for general practitioners to have a basic understanding of the procedure, related terms, and potential indications.

Indications

HSCT is used in the treatment of humans with both hematopoietic and solid tumors such as breast cancer[3]; nonmalignant bone marrow diseases, including congenital hemoglobinopathies,[4,5] myelodysplasia,[6] and aplastic anemia[7]; and various autoimmune diseases.[8,9] In the experimental stage, HSCT is also being explored to establish an immunologic platform for solid organ transplantation,[10] as a vehicle for gene therapy,[11,12] and for the treatment of lysosomal storage diseases, in which experimental transplantation in dogs and cats has been a major field of research.[13] Probably the main setting in which HSCT can be considered well established at this time is in the treatment of lymphomas and leukemias, but even in this area, the best approaches are not yet defined and clinical study and refinement are ongoing.

> **KEY POINT**
>
> *HSCT is most established for the treatment of hematopoietic cancers. Approaches are constantly being refined, and new applications are being developed.*

The Transplantation Process

There are many different permutations of HSCT (which are discussed in more detail below); however, there are several common points in the process. A recipient is identified as a candidate for the procedure based on diagnosis, overall relatively stable clinical condition, and the absence of major concurrent diseases. The graft is harvested from the patient or donor and may be enriched (discussed below). If necessary, the graft is stored until transplantation is performed; for storage longer than 36 to 48 hours, cells are normally cryopreserved, which involves suspending the graft in cryoprotective medium such as serum and dimethyl sulfoxide and gradually reducing its temperature to freezing at $-80°C$ in liquid nitrogen. The patient undergoes high-dose chemotherapy or chemotherapy in combination with total-body radiotherapy, also called *chemoradiotherapy*. This treatment is also referred to as the *conditioning regimen*; its function is to kill cancer cells and, in the case of allogeneic transplantation, to suppress the recipient's immune system. After the conditioning regimen is complete, the graft is infused intravenously and homes to the patient's bone marrow.

The patient usually goes through a period of myelosuppression caused by the conditioning regimen before engraftment takes place. The severity of myelosuppression depends on the type of transplant as well as patient-dependent factors. All conventional HSCT patients require hospitalization and substantial nutritional, transfusion, and antimicrobial support; however, newer HSCT approaches are making the procedure much less toxic. Engraftment can be identified by the return of normal levels of circulating blood cells and cessation of any clinical signs caused by myelosuppression. In allogeneic transplantation, patients often require posttransplant immunosuppressive medication to prevent immunologic complications (see Complications section, below).

Donor Selection

From an immunologic standpoint, there are several potential relationships between the donor and recipient, and these can affect the rate of different complications. In clinical practice, the main types of transplantation are autologous and allogeneic.

Autologous transplantation uses the patient's own cells, which are normally harvested and stored before high-dose chemotherapy, radiotherapy, or both begin. Autologous transplantation provides the most immunologically compatible graft possible, so complications of immune incompatibility (see Complications section, below) are rare, although other factors can still cause graft failure. In addition, there is no need to search for a donor.

The main disadvantages of autologous transplantation are:

- It requires the patient to have healthy marrow, which cancer patients do not always have.

- Undetectable numbers of malignant cells could be harvested with the graft and cause a relapse after transplantation.

- The patient's immune system could fail to recognize the cancer as foreign, in which case it will probably continue to do so after transplantation.

To address the problem of malignant cell contamination of an autologous graft, various approaches to "purging" have been employed: positively selecting hematopoietic stem cells (HSCs; hopefully leaving cancer cells behind); negatively selecting out cancer cells in which there is a known cancer antigen; or "chemical purging," which involves incubating the graft with a cytotoxic agent ex vivo. Any of these strategies could negatively affect engraftment, however, and purging is still an area that faces significant difficulties.[14]

Allogeneic transplantation uses cells from a donor, and because the cells can be harvested to coincide with the timing of the actual transplantation, they might not need to be stored. The donor most immunologically compatible with the recipient is always sought. To minimize complications of immune incompatibility, donors are matched with patients based on their respective alleles of the class I and class II genes of the major histocompatibility complex (MHC)—also known as the *dog leukocyte antigen (DLA)* or *human leukocyte antigen (HLA) profile*—to the largest extent possible. The DLA is now well defined,[15–22] and two highly polymorphic microsatellite markers can be used to easily match dogs within families.[23] A match between donor and recipient at all the loci of the DLA or HLA is termed *identical* or *matched*; a match at some of the loci is called *haploidentical, partially matched*, or *partially mismatched*; and a lack of matching is termed *mismatched* or *nonidentical*. The best chance of finding a DLA- or HLA-identical donor is among the recipient's siblings, each with a 25% chance of being a complete match. Barring the availability of siblings, unrelated volunteer donors are screened for a match (a matched unrelated donor), but the chances are much lower. Unrelated dogs of the same breed have a much better chance of matching than dogs of different breeds,[24,25] just as members of the same ethnic group have a better chance of matching than humans in different ethnic groups.

Even in a fully DLA- or HLA-identical transplant, some degree of incompatibility is inevitable. Antigens outside the MHC can contribute to incompatibility and its complications and are referred to as *minor transplantation antigens*. Because these minor antigens are outside the MHC, they are not tested for in the DLA or HLA matching process. This is another reason that related donors are often preferred, as the familial relation maximizes the chance of compatibility at the minor and major antigens. However, it is still unclear whether it is preferable to use a partially mismatched related donor or a matched unrelated donor.

Clinical investigators are constantly making progress with the permutations of allogeneic transplantation from donors matched to varying degrees; this allows more patients to undergo transplantation and even capitalizes on some immunologic differences. Recipients of an allogeneic graft are less likely to suffer from disease relapse than are patients who receive an autologous graft. This is true not only because graft contamination with tumor cells is not an issue in allogeneic transplantation but also because some immune incompatibility may assist the newly generated immune system in recognizing the cancer cells as foreign, termed the *graft-versus-tumor (GVT) effect*. The GVT effect is now understood to be a major component of the clinical effectiveness of allogeneic transplantation. It is the crux of the mechanism of action of mini-allotransplantation (discussed below) and can exert a powerful antitumor effect.[26]

The benefit of reduced relapse rates (see Complications section, below) in allogeneic compared with autologous HSCT is balanced by the morbidity and mortality associated with immunologic complications. Therefore, in the treatment of lymphoma in humans, the overall survival of allogeneic and autologous recipients is largely equivalent. For autologous transplantation, investigators are now focusing on procedures that will hasten or strengthen engraftment to reduce the period of immunosuppression immediately following transplantation. For allogeneic transplantation, the focus of investigation is to learn how to control the impact of immunologic complications without negating any GVT effect.

Syngeneic transplantation uses cells harvested from an identical twin, which, in theory, should be perfectly compatible. However, this may not be the case if the immune system of cancer patients is altered, as some investigators believe. If the immune system of the cancer patient is altered, the immunologic change imparted by syngeneic transplantation may actually be of benefit to the patient as a "return to normal." Rare instances of clinical incompatibility in syngeneic transplantation have been reported.[27]

The term *xenogeneic* refers to a graft from a member of another species. Such grafts are not currently in clinical use.

Graft Source

HSCs can be harvested from several different anatomic sources. Those in clinical use are bone marrow, peripheral blood, and umbilical cord blood. The term *bone marrow transplantation* has now been generalized to refer to transplantation from all these sources; however, *hematopoietic stem cell transplantation* is probably more correct to use as an umbrella term.

As the primary residence of normal HSCs, bone marrow is the source used in original studies in dogs as well as clinically in humans. Bone marrow has the advantage of providing the richest source of HSCs in their resting state. The main disadvantage from the standpoint of the donor is that the harvesting procedure is painful and requires general anesthesia and analgesia. In addition, resting bone marrow cells are not the quickest engrafting cell population. In humans, marrow is harvested from the iliac crests. In dogs, the humerus is the best site of harvest, with the femur being the second best site.

A very small number of HSCs circulate in the peripheral blood,[28,29] but the number is insufficient for clinical transplantation. However, the number in circulation can be increased to a clinically harvestable level using mobilization techniques.[30–32] The administration of hematopoietic colony-stimulating factors such as granulocyte colony-stimulating factor (G-CSF) and granulocyte–macrophage colony-stimulating factor, as well as stimulating activity in the marrow itself, causes an increased number of HSCs to mobilize into the circulation. Likewise, the recovery phase after a myelosuppressive insult results in increased circulating HSCs; therefore, chemotherapeutic drugs are often used to mobilize HSCs for peripheral blood harvest, even in allogeneic donors.

Once HSCs are mobilized, the peripheral blood mononuclear cells are harvested by leukapheresis, and this cell fraction contains the HSCs. This is significantly more involved and uncomfortable than simple blood donation, and the mobilization is not without side effects; however, most clinicians believe that the donation of mobilized peripheral blood HSCs (PBSCs) affects donors less than the donation of bone marrow does. Because mobilized HSCs are by definition stimulated, they provide faster engraftment than does resting bone marrow, although some investigators argue that cytokine-primed bone marrow also engrafts quickly.[33,34] Some research has suggested that, although stimulated HSCs provide faster engraftment than resting HSCs, their long-term engraftment capability may be less stable.[35] Nevertheless, because of their perceived advantages in terms of donor experience and rapid engraftment, PBSCs are now used for most transplantations in humans.[2] PBSCs can be used in dogs as well[36,37]; however, marrow is still used in most laboratory studies of HSCT in dogs. The clinical utility of PBSCs for transplantation in dogs is limited by the availability of hemapheresis equipment and by the extracorporeal volume of the pheresis in patients of varying size.

HSCs circulate in the blood of fetuses in greater numbers than in adults. Umbilical cord blood is the blood remaining in the placenta and cord after delivery and is rich in primitive stem cells, which are largely differentiated toward the hematopoietic lineage.[38] Some researchers suggest that these primitive cells may still have greater multiple lineage potential than do the HSCs of adults. Regardless, they have excellent hematopoietic potential and may be more immune tolerant than adult HSCs.[39–41] The great advantage of umbilical cord blood stem cells is their availability with every normal birth. One disadvantage is the relatively low number of cells owing to the small volume of cord blood. This led to early pessimism that umbilical cord blood would only be useful for transplantation in infants and small children; however, small- and medium-sized adults have now undergone successful transplantations from umbilical cord blood stem cells.[41] The other disadvantage is the cost of storing the cells until they are needed. A number of companies offer private storage of cord blood stem cells to act as a potential resource for the individual or family members in the case of future illness. Several public cord blood banks accept donations of cord blood so that even if private storage is too expensive, this resource need not be wasted. In dogs, umbilical cord blood is not normally available unless pups are delivered by cesarean section, and this source of HSCs has not been investigated.

In the fetus, one of the primary sites of normal hematopoiesis is the liver, and at specific times during gestation, the fetal liver is a rich source of HSCs.[42] This source is still sometimes used in experimental studies in mice but is not used clinically in humans or dogs.

Cell Population

Knowledge of the exact characteristics and potential of the true HSC is still evolving.[43] The basic definition is a cell that can engraft and give rise to all lymphoid and hematopoietic cell lines. While there is some disagreement about its precise phenotype, the true HSC is generally thought to be a relatively rare cell. Thus, whether the cell source used is bone marrow or mobilized peripheral blood, the majority of cells harvested are not true HSCs but a range of committed and partially differentiated progenitors. In certain settings, it is possible that cells other than HSCs may also benefit patients; for instance, partially committed progenitors will not engraft and provide an ongoing source of cells, but they may help to protect the patient during short-term myelosuppression. Whole bone marrow or peripheral blood mononuclear cells may be chosen in these circumstances. The main disadvantages to doing so in the autologous setting are the large volume of the resultant infusion and the slightly increased risk of malignant cell contamination. In the allogeneic setting, however, the number of T lymphocytes infused with the graft appears to be an important determinant of engraftment capability, graft-versus-host disease (GVHD), and the GVT effect and is therefore considered an important variable.[44]

In many cases, partially purified or enriched harvest products are used rather than whole bone marrow or peripheral blood mononuclear cells. Most commonly, the enrichment involves positive selection for CD34 immunopositivity because most investigators believe this marker denotes a population that includes the true HSC. This antigen has also been defined in dogs, and CD34-selected cells have been used successfully in canine transplantation.[45–48] In addition, T lymphocytes are sometimes depleted from allogeneic grafts to reduce the risk or intensity of GVHD.

Complications

Although for selected patients this intensified therapy can offer a hope for cure that would not be achievable using standard chemotherapy, the associated toxicity can be significant and is naturally the first concern for many pet owners. The main types of complications following HSCT include graft failure, GVHD, and cancer relapse.

Graft failure is usually immune mediated and results from disparity between the recipient and graft, so it is largely limited to the allogeneic setting. All conventional (myeloablative) HSCT patients require transfusion and antimicrobial support during engraftment, regardless of whether the graft is autologous or allogeneic; but graft failure, graft rejection, or delayed recovery can result in significant morbidity or death in recipients of allogeneic grafts because of immunosuppression, bleeding, and anemia. The risk of graft rejection is reduced by the presence of T lymphocytes in the graft and by posttransplantation immunosuppressive medication.

In GVHD, the transplanted marrow engrafts successfully and generates a new immune system, but the new system recognizes the recipient's tissues as foreign.[44,49,50] GVHD is acute or chronic and varies from mild to fatal. It is probably the most important cause of morbidity and mortality following allogeneic HSCT. The disease can be partially prevented or reduced by T-lymphocyte depletion of the graft, but a reduction in T lymphocytes increases the risk of graft failure, so this important variable in an allogeneic graft must be carefully balanced. Some degree of GVHD is nearly universal following allogeneic HSCT, but the disease is usually controllable with posttransplant immunosuppression. GVHD and the GVT effect are closely associated in function, and, despite efforts, the two processes have not yet been successfully separated. As a result, measures that reduce GVHD tend to result in somewhat reduced antitumor efficacy as well.

As noted previously, the risk of relapse is greater in autologous transplantation because of the absence of the GVT effect and the risk of graft contamination with cancer cells.

Nonmyeloablative HSCT

Initially, HSCT was developed as a rescue from myeloablative anticancer treatment. That is, after the patient's bone marrow is completely destroyed by chemotherapy or radiotherapy, HSCT provides for regeneration of the marrow. At that time, it was believed that allogeneic engraftment could not take place without completely destroying the patient's marrow, regardless of whether such destruction was actually needed from an antitumor standpoint; therefore, all allogeneic transplantations were necessarily myeloablative. More recently, it was discovered that allogeneic engraftment could take place without myeloablation, and recipient and donor marrow could coexist in a state of chimerism (bone marrow representing a mixture of recipient-origin and donor-origin cells). Investigators began to explore the use of nonmyeloablative transplantation ("mini-transplant"), the goal of which is to reduce the toxicity of the transplantation regimen while still providing the antitumor benefit of HSCT.

When used in the autologous setting, this approach could prove valuable for patients. Its advantages would include ameliorating other toxicities of the preparative regimen and reducing or even eliminating the period of immunosuppression compared with myeloablative transplantation while still exposing tumor cells to a higher-than-standard dose intensity of chemotherapy.

Mini-allotransplantation is probably the fastest-progressing field in HSCT at this time.[51–54] The initial goal is to establish stable chimerism, which will, in theory, generate a mutually tolerant immune system, reducing GVHD while hopefully allowing a GVT effect to proceed. This approach relies on the immune effect of transplantation rather than high-dose chemotherapy or radiotherapy to impart the antitumor effect. Stable chimerism can be converted to complete donor phenotype by infusion of donor lymphocytes, providing more robust GVT. The toxicity of the conditioning regimen is greatly reduced, and GVHD can be greatly diminished using this approach. However, because the functions of GVHD and the GVT effect have not been completely separated, GVHD cannot be completely eliminated without losing efficacy. A mini-allotransplantation regimen has been developed in laboratory dogs[37,55–58]; however, the results of those studies suggest that the current regimen appears to be too toxic for clinical use in tumor-bearing dogs.

Hematopoietic Stem Cell Transplantation in Dogs

Early in the development of HSCT, laboratory dogs were adopted as a preclinical experimental model[59–68] and are still used by some. Spontaneous lymphoma in dogs has been particularly useful as a therapeutic model.[36,60,64,68–75] Marrow engraftment and prolonged survival were seen in some of these dogs; however, a large percentage of dogs died because of complications following myeloablation. In addition, lymphoma relapses were common among transplantation survivors. In studies during the 1980s, preparative chemotherapy regimens were used to improve the clinical condition of dogs by inducing objective clinical remission before myeloablative radiation therapy and transplantation. Although improvement in long-term survival rates was achieved, recurrence of lymphoma was still a common problem, and early deaths occurred in approximately one-third of dogs undergoing transplantation. Although results of transplantation in the veterinary setting show better survival rates,[76] probably because of better supportive care, myeloablative transplantation has not been generally adopted in veterinary oncology as a therapeutic modality.

We have investigated nonmyeloablative autologous G-CSF–primed bone marrow transplantation for support of high-dose chemotherapy at the end of a 12-week, five-drug protocol for dogs with lymphoma.[77] Twenty-eight dogs were treated at three escalating dose levels of chemotherapy, with 13 dogs in the highest-dose group. All dogs were treated on an outpatient basis. Even at the highest chemotherapy dose used in the study, toxicity was comparable with that seen with standard chemotherapy, with only one of 13 dogs developing a fever, which responded to routine management within 24 hours. For the high-dose group, the median remission time was 54 weeks, with four (30%) of the dogs still in remission more than 3 years later (likely cured). Clearly, HSCT has a role to play in the treatment of dogs with lymphoma. For further discussion, see Chapter 47.

Current Recommendations

The availability of HSCT in veterinary medicine is extremely limited, but new developments may allow it to become more widely available in the coming years. The area in which this treatment modality holds the most immediate promise for dogs is in the treatment of lymphoma, although new indications relating to other diseases or in conjunction with gene therapy are on the horizon. For selected patients that may have an indication for HSCT, the veterinarian can investigate referral to an oncologist with an interest in this treatment modality.

REFERENCES

1. Thomas ED: Bone marrow transplantation: A review. *Semin Hematol* 36(4 suppl 7):95–103, 1999.
2. Goldman JM, Horowitz MM: The international bone marrow transplant reg-

istry. *Int J Hematol* 76(suppl 1):393–397, 2002.
3. Tartarone A, Romano G, Galasso R, et al: Should we continue to study high-dose chemotherapy in metastatic breast cancer patients? A critical review of the published data. *Bone Marrow Transplant* 31(7):525–530, 2003.
4. Souillet G: Indications and results of progenitor cell transplant in congenital haemopathies (except Fanconi anaemia). *Bone Marrow Transplant* 21(suppl 2):S28–S33, 1998.
5. Apperley JF: Bone marrow transplant for the haemoglobinopathies: Past, present and future. *Baillieres Clin Haematol* 6(1):299–325, 1993.
6. Giralt S: Bone marrow transplant in myelodysplastic syndromes: New technologies, same questions. *Curr Hematol Rep* 3(3):165–172, 2004.
7. Horowitz MM: Current status of allogeneic bone marrow transplantation in acquired aplastic anemia. *Semin Hematol* 37(1):30–42, 2000.
8. Furst DE: Stem cell transplantation for autoimmune disease: Progress and problems. *Curr Opin Rheumatol* 14(3):220–224, 2002.
9. Burt RK, Traynor AE, Craig R, Marmont AM: The promise of hematopoietic stem cell transplantation for autoimmune diseases. *Bone Marrow Transplant* 31(7):521–524, 2003.
10. Chiang KY, Lazarus HM: Should we be performing more combined hematopoietic stem cell plus solid organ transplants? *Bone Marrow Transplant* 31(8):633–642, 2003.
11. Kohn DB: Gene therapy for hematopoietic and immune disorders. *Bone Marrow Transplant* 18(suppl 3):S55–S58, 1996.
12. Vollweiler JL, Zielske SP, Reese JS, Gerson SL: Hematopoietic stem cell gene therapy: Progress toward therapeutic targets. *Bone Marrow Transplant* 32(1):1–7, 2003.
13. Haskins M: Bone marrow transplantation therapy for metabolic disease: Animal models as predictors of success and in utero approaches. *Bone Marrow Transplant* 18(suppl 3):S25–S27, 1996.
14. Alvarnas JC, Forman SJ: Graft purging in autologous bone marrow transplantation: A promise not quite fulfilled. *Oncology (Huntingt)* 18(7):867–876, 2004.
15. Vriesendorp HM, Epstein RB, D'Amaro J, et al: Polymorphism of the DL-A system. *Transplantation* 14(3):299–307, 1972.
16. Vriesendorp HM, Westbroek DL, D'Amaro J, et al: Joint report of 1st International Workshop on Canine Immunogenetics. *Tissue Antigens* 3(2):145–163, 1973.
17. Vriesendorp HM, Albert ED, Templeton JW, et al: Joint report of the Second International Workshop on Canine Immunogenetics. *Transplant Proc* 8(2):289–314, 1976.
18. Vriesendorp HM, Bijnen AB, Westbroek DL, van Bekkum DW: Genetics and transplantation immunology of the DLA complex. *Transplant Proc* 9(1):293–296, 1977.
19. Graumann MB, DeRose SA, Ostrander EA, Storb R: Polymorphism analysis of four canine MHC class I genes. *Tissue Antigens* 51(4 pt 1):374–381, 1998.
20. Kennedy LJ, Altet L, Angles JM, et al: Nomenclature for factors of the dog major histocompatibility system (DLA), 1998: First report of the ISAG DLA Nomenclature Committee. *Anim Genet* 31(1):52–61, 2000.
21. Kennedy LJ, Angles JM, Barnes A, et al: Nomenclature for factors of the dog major histocompatibility system (DLA), 2000: Second report of the ISAG DLA Nomenclature Committee. *Tissue Antigens* 58(1):55–70, 2001.
22. Wagner JL, Sarmiento UM, Storb R: Cellular, serological, and molecular polymorphism of the class I and class II loci of the canine major histocompatibility complex. *Tissue Antigens* 59(3):205–210, 2002.
23. Wagner JL, Burnett RC, DeRose SA, et al: Histocompatibility testing of dog families with highly polymorphic microsatellite markers. *Transplantation* 62(6):876–877, 1996.
24. Kennedy LJ, Carter SD, Barnes A, et al: Interbreed variation of DLA-DRB1, DQA1 alleles and haplotypes in the dog. *Vet Immunol Immunopathol* 69(2–4):101–111, 1999.
25. Kennedy LJ, Barnes A, Happ GM, et al: Extensive interbreed, but minimal intrabreed, variation of DLA class II alleles and haplotypes in dogs. *Tissue Antigens* 59(3):194–204, 2002.
26. Feinstein L, Sandmaier B, Maloney D, et al: Nonmyeloablative hematopoietic cell transplantation. Replacing high-dose cytotoxic therapy by the graft-versus-tumor effect. *Ann N Y Acad Sci* 938:328–337, 2001.
27. Latif T, Pohlman B, Kalaycio M, et al: Syngeneic graft-versus-host disease: A report of two cases and literature review. *Bone Marrow Transplant* 32(5):535–539, 2003.
28. Epstein RB, Graham TC, Buckner CD, et al: Allogeneic marrow engraftment by cross circulation in lethally irradiated dogs. *Blood* 28(5):692–707, 1966.
29. Debelak-Fehir KM, Catchatourian R, Epstein RB: Hemopoietic colony forming units in fresh and cryopreserved peripheral blood cells of canines and man. *Exp Hematol* 3(2):109–116, 1975.
30. Abrams RA, McCormack K, Bowles C, Deisseroth AB: Cyclophosphamide treatment expands the circulating hematopoietic stem cell pool in dogs. *J Clin Invest* 67(5):1392–1399, 1981.
31. Debelak-Fehir KM, Epstein RB: Restoration of hematopoiesis in dogs by infusion of cryopreserved autologous peripheral white cells following busulfan-cyclophosphamide treatment. *Transplantation* 20(1):63–67, 1975.
32. Kessinger A, Sharp JG: The whys and hows of hematopoietic progenitor and stem cell mobilization. *Bone Marrow Transplant* 31(5):319–329, 2003.
33. Arai S, Klingemann HG: Hematopoietic stem cell transplantation: Bone marrow vs. mobilized peripheral blood. *Arch Med Res* 34(6):545–553, 2003.
34. Elfenbein GJ, Sackstein R: Primed marrow for autologous and allogeneic transplantation: A review comparing primed marrow to mobilized blood and steady-state marrow. *Exp Hematol* 32(4):327–339, 2004.
35. Habibian HK, Peters SO, Hsieh CC, et al: The fluctuating phenotype of the lymphohematopoietic stem cell with cell cycle transit. *J Exp Med* 188(2):393–398, 1998.
36. Appelbaum FR, Deeg HJ, Storb R, et al: Cure of malignant lymphoma in dogs with peripheral blood stem cell transplantation. *Transplantation* 42(1):19–22, 1986.
37. Takatu A, Nash RA, Zaucha JM, et al: Adoptive immunotherapy to increase the level of donor hematopoietic chimerism after nonmyeloablative marrow transplantation for severe canine hereditary hemolytic anemia. *Biol Blood Marrow Transplant* 9(11):674–682, 2003.
38. Newburger PE, Quesenberry PJ: Umbilical cord blood as a new and promising source of unrelated-donor hematopoietic stem cells for transplantation. *Curr Opin Pediatr* 8(1):29–32, 1996.
39. Mogul MJ: Unrelated cord blood transplantation vs matched unrelated donor bone marrow transplantation: The risks and benefits of each choice. *Bone Marrow Transplant* 25(suppl 2): S58–S60, 2000.
40. Moscardo F, Sanz GF, Sanz MA: Unrelated-donor cord blood transplantation for adult hematological malignancies. *Leuk Lymphoma* 45(1):11–18, 2004.
41. Benito AI, Diaz MA, Gonzalez-Vicent M, et al: Hematopoietic stem cell transplantation using umbilical cord blood progenitors: Review of current clinical results. *Bone Marrow Transplant* 33(7):675–690, 2004.
42. Gale RP: Fetal liver transplants. *Bone Marrow Transplant* 9(suppl 1):118–120, 1992.
43. Quesenberry PJ, Colvin GA, Abedi M, et al: The marrow stem cell: The continuum. *Bone Marrow Transplant* 32(suppl 1):S19–S22, 2003.
44. Ferrara JL, Cooke KR, Teshima T: The pathophysiology of acute graft-versus-host disease. *Int J Hematol* 78(3):181–187, 2003.
45. Bruno B, Nash RA, Wallace PM, et al: CD34+ selected bone marrow grafts are radioprotective and establish mixed chimerism in dogs given high dose total body irradiation. *Transplantation* 68(3):338–344, 1999.
46. Bruno B, Goerner MA, Nash RA, et al: Purified canine CD34+Lin− marrow cells transduced with retroviral vectors give rise to long-term multi-lineage hematopoiesis. *Biol Blood Marrow Transplant* 7(10):543–551, 2001.
47. Niemeyer GP, Hudson J, Bridgman R, et al: Isolation and characterization of canine hematopoietic progenitor cells. *Exp Hematol* 29(6):686–693, 2001.
48. Suter SE, Gouthro TA, McSweeney PA, et al: Isolation and characterization of pediatric canine bone marrow CD34+ cells. *Vet Immunol Immunopathol* 101(1–2):31–47, 2004.
49. Storb R, Thomas ED: Graft-versus-host disease in dog and man: The Seattle experience. *Immunol Rev* 88:215–238, 1985.
50. Vogelsang GB, Lee L, Bensen-Kennedy DM: Pathogenesis and treatment of graft-versus-host disease after bone marrow transplant. *Annu Rev Med* 54:29–52, 2003.
51. Sandmaier BM, McSweeney P, Yu C, Storb R: Nonmyeloablative transplants: Preclinical and clinical results. *Semin Oncol* 27(2 suppl 5):78–81, 2000.
52. Mielcarek M, Sandmaier BM, Maloney DG, et al: Nonmyeloablative hematopoietic cell transplantation: Status quo and future perspectives. *J Clin Immunol* 22(2):70–74, 2002.
53. Hogan WJ, Storb R: Clinical developments in reduced intensity haematopoietic stem cell transplantation. *Expert Opin Biol Ther* 2(7):703–714, 2002.
54. Georges GE, Storb R: Review of "minitransplantation": Nonmyeloablative allogeneic hematopoietic stem cell transplantation. *Int J Hematol* 77(1):3–14, 2003.
55. Storb R, Yu C, Zaucha JM, et al: Stable mixed hematopoietic chimerism in dogs given donor antigen, CTLA4Ig, and 100 cGy total body irradiation before and pharmacologic immunosuppression after marrow transplant. *Blood* 94(7):2523–2529, 1999.
56. Zaucha JA, Yu C, Lothrop CD Jr, et al: Severe canine hereditary hemolytic anemia treated by nonmyeloablative marrow transplantation. *Biol Blood Marrow Transplant* 7(1):14–24, 2001.
57. Maris M, Storb R: Outpatient allografting in hematologic malignancies and nonmalignant disorders—Applying lessons learned in the canine model to humans. *Cancer Treat Res* 110: 149–175, 2002.
58. Niemeyer GP, Boudreaux MK, Goodman-Martin SA, et al: Correction of a large animal model of type I Glanzmann's thrombasthenia by nonmyeloablative bone

marrow transplantation. *Exp Hematol* 31(12):1357–1362, 2003.
59. Thomas ED, Storb R, Epstein RB, Rudolph RH: Symposium on bone marrow transplantation: Experimental aspects in canines. *Transplant Proc* 1(1):31–33, 1969.
60. Epstein RB, Graham TC, Storb R, Thomas ED: Studies of marrow transplantation, chemotherapy, and cross-circulation in canine lymphosarcoma. *Blood* 37(3):349–359, 1971.
61. Bodenberger U, Kolb HJ, Rieder I, et al: Fractionated total body irradiation and autologous bone marrow transplantation in dogs: Hemopoietic recovery after various marrow cell doses. *Exp Hematol* 8(4):384–394, 1980.
62. Epstein RB, Sarpel SC: Autologous bone marrow infusion following high dose chemotherapy of the canine transmissible venereal tumor (TVT). *Exp Hematol* 8(6):683–689, 1980.
63. Vriesendorp HM, Klapwyk WM, Heidt PJ, et al: Factors controlling the engraftment of transplanted dog bone marrow cells. *Tissue Antigens* 20(1):63–80, 1982.
64. Appelbaum FR, Deeg HJ, Storb R, et al: Marrow transplant studies in dogs with malignant lymphoma. *Transplantation* 39(5):499–504, 1985.
65. Szer J, Deeg HJ, Appelbaum FR, Storb R: Failure of autologous marrow reconstitution after cytolytic treatment of marrow with anti-Ia monoclonal antibody. *Blood* 65(4):819–822, 1985.
66. Deeg HJ, Beckham C, Huss R, et al: Rescue from anti-MHC class II antibody-mediated marrow graft failure by c-kit ligand. *Blood* 83(8):2352–2359, 1994.
67. Greinix HT, Ladiges WC, Graham TC, et al: Late failure of autologous marrow grafts in lethally irradiated dogs given anti-class II monoclonal antibody. *Blood* 78(8):2131–2138, 1991.
68. Ladiges WC, Storb R, Thomas ED: Canine models of bone marrow transplantation. *Lab Anim Sci* 40(1):11–15, 1990.
69. Weiden PL, Storb R, Lerner KG, et al: Treatment of canine malignancies by 1200 R total body irradiation and autologous marrow grafts. *Exp Hematol* 3(2):124–134, 1975.
70. Weiden PL, Storb R, Shulman H, Graham TC: Dimethyl myleran and autologous marrow grafting for the treatment of spontaneous canine lymphoma. *Eur J Cancer* 13(12):1411–1415, 1977.
71. Weiden PL, Storb R, Deeg HJ, Graham TC: Total body irradiation and autologous marrow transplantation as consolidation therapy for spontaneous canine lymphoma in remission. *Exp Hematol* 7(suppl 5):160–163, 1979.
72. Weiden PL, Storb R, Deeg HJ, et al: Prolonged disease-free survival in dogs with lymphoma after total-body irradiation and autologous marrow transplantation consolidation of combination-chemotherapy-induced remissions. *Blood* 54(5): 1039–1049, 1979.
73. Bowles CA, Lucas D: Clinical and immunological response of lymphoma dogs following chemotherapy and irradiation. *Comp Immunol Microbiol Infect Dis* 3(3):317–326, 1980.
74. Bowles CA, Bull M, McCormick K, et al: Autologous bone marrow transplantation following chemotherapy and irradiation in dogs with spontaneous lymphomas. *J Natl Cancer Inst* 65(3):615–620, 1980.
75. Deeg HJ, Appelbaum FR, Weiden PL, et al: Autologous marrow transplantation as consolidation therapy for canine lymphoma: Efficacy and toxicity of various regimens of total body irradiation. *Am J Vet Res* 46(9):2016–2018, 1985.
76. Rosenthal RC: The treatment of multicentric canine lymphoma. *Vet Clin North Am Small Anim Pract* 20(4):1093–1104, 1990.
77. Frimberger AE, Moore AS, Rassnick KM, et al: A combination chemotherapy protocol with dose intensification and autologous bone marrow transplant (VELCAP-HDC) for canine lymphoma. *J Vet Intern Med*, in press.

HYPERTHERMIA, CRYOTHERAPY, AND PHOTODYNAMIC THERAPY: PROPERTIES, USES, AND PATIENT MANAGEMENT

Gregory K. Ogilvie and Antony S. Moore

CLINICAL BRIEFING

Equipment

Local hyperthermia	• Generally applied with a handheld radiofrequency device. More sophisticated computer-controlled ultrasound or radiofrequency multisector units are being used to treat cancer more uniformly and precisely.
Whole-body hyperthermia	• Labor-intensive procedure to increase core temperature of an anesthetized, paralyzed dog to approximately 42°C. Hyperthermia treatment is usually done in combination with radiation or chemotherapy.
Cryotherapy	• Liquid nitrogen is applied to the tumor and tissue immediately surrounding the mass using probes or spray applicators; nitrous oxide is applied using probes.
Photodynamic therapy	• Fiberoptic cables direct laser light of a unique frequency (usually infrared) into the tumor; this light interacts with a previously administered photosensitizing agent and causes tumor cell death.

Indications

Local hyperthermia	• Most effective for the treatment of localized tumors. Best efficacy when combined with radiation therapy or chemotherapy; handheld hyperthermia devices are effective for the treatment of small (<1 cm diameter) benign and malignant superficial tumors, such as cutaneous hemangiomas, basal cell tumors, or melanomas.
Whole-body hyperthermia	• Therapy used to treat primary cancer and metastatic disease (e.g., lymphoma, osteosarcoma). Most effective when combined with chemotherapy or radiation therapy.
Cryotherapy	• Used in the treatment of small (<1 cm diameter) benign and malignant superficial tumors (e.g., basal cell tumors, meibomian gland adenomas, cutaneous hemangiomas) of such areas as the eyelid, nose, oral cavity, and skin. Adrenal tumors may also be effectively treated.
Photodynamic therapy	• Same indications as for local hyperthermia and cryotherapy; in addition, PDT may be useful in treating esophageal and bladder tumors.

Supportive care

• Analgesics are essential during and several days after these procedures; patients receiving PDT should be kept away from direct sunlight for some time after therapy because certain photosensitizers make dogs susceptible to sunburn.

Hyperthermia, cryotherapy, and photodynamic therapy (PDT) have been used for decades in some veterinary centers to treat specific benign and malignant tumors. These therapies have very specific applications and require equipment and expertise that may not be available to the general practitioner. Dogs have served as models for human cancer therapy, and a great deal of information that benefits clinical cancer patients has been generated from these studies.

Hyperthermia

Hyperthermia is not commonly used in private practice despite the decades of research spent to understand its efficacy and optimal application.[1–19] The biggest obstacles that

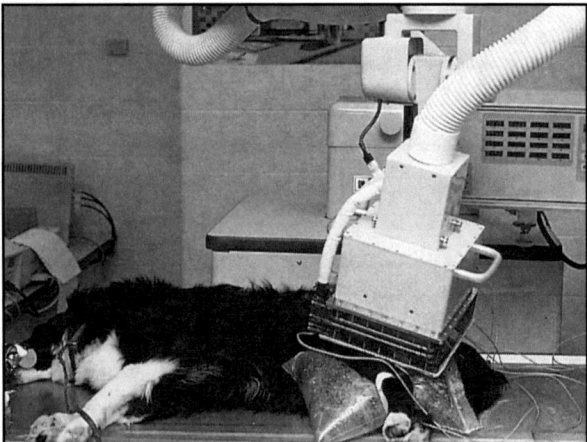

Figure 27-1. *Computer-controlled multisector ultrasound hyperthermia devices are effective at providing uniform heating to a relatively large localized area. Although the equipment used in this type of local hyperthermia is much more effective than handheld devices, it is expensive and relatively complex to operate.*

> **KEY POINT**
>
> *The concept of thermal dosage is critical regardless of whether hyperthermia is applied to a localized region of the body or systemically.*

exist for hyperthermia are the lack of affordable equipment that can deliver a uniform thermal dosage to target tissue and enhance tumor cell killing and the lack of data consistently confirming its efficacy.[1,2,12] The concept of thermal dosage is critical, regardless of whether hyperthermia is applied to a localized region of the body or systemically (e.g., whole-body hyperthermia).[1,2,12]

Local hyperthermia is most often used in veterinary practice, primarily with the use of handheld radiofrequency devices.[1,2] These devices allow the delivery of heat to a fairly small area (<2 cm) with each application. Local hyperthermia can also be delivered with isolated limb perfusion, lasers, and complex multisector or coiled ultrasound hyperthermia devices.[1–18] Efficacy is greatest when local hyperthermia is performed in conjunction with radiation or chemotherapy.[3–9] A wide variety of feline and canine tumors have been treated with hyperthermia, usually in conjunction with radiation or chemotherapy. These include soft tissue sarcomas, squamous cell carcinomas, melanomas, and meibomian gland adenomas.

Whole-body hyperthermia units are used to raise the dog's overall body temperature to approximately 42°C.[19] Dogs must be anesthetized and paralyzed for this procedure.[1,2] Whole-body hyperthermia appears to enhance the efficacy of chemotherapy for the treatment of lymphoma, soft tissue sarcoma, and osteosarcoma.[1–19] As with local

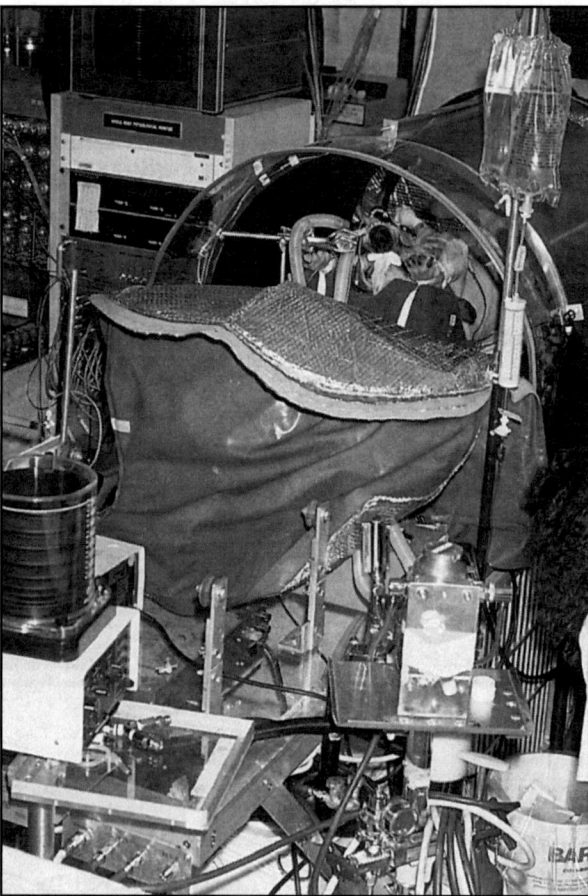

Figure 27-2. *Whole-body hyperthermia can involve the use of a radiant heat device. The patient is placed under general anesthesia, chemically paralyzed to ablate any panting during heating, and then placed in a semienclosed chamber during intensive physiologic monitoring. Whole-body hyperthermia (42°C) is used in conjunction with radiation and chemotherapy to control malignancies.*

hyperthermia, whole-body hyperthermia has been studied to document its ability to enhance the therapeutic index of radiation therapy.[17]

EQUIPMENT

Local hyperthermia techniques involve the use of external or internal heating sources.[1,2] External hyperthermia uses microwave, ultrasound (Figure 27-1), or radiofrequency energy sources to deposit energy within the tissue from an external applicator. Microwaves and radiofrequency methods deposit adequate energy to a depth of approximately 3 to 4 cm, whereas ultrasound energy can penetrate to a depth of 6 to 14 cm. Radiofrequency and microwave energy sources can also be inserted directly into the targeted tissue to produce interstitial hyperthermia.

Whole-body hyperthermia can be achieved by raising a patient's core body temperature to 41.8°C to 42.0°C using

HYPERTHERMIA, CRYOTHERAPY, AND PHOTODYNAMIC THERAPY

> **KEY POINT**
>
> *External hyperthermia uses microwave, ultrasound, or radiofrequency energy sources to deposit energy within the tumor and normal tissue from an applicator that is placed over or near the area being treated.*

various energy sources, including a radiant heat device (Figure 27-2), or extracorporeal heating techniques.[1,2] Although whole-body hyperthermia is available only in specific research institutions, it generally results in a more uniform temperature increase within tumor tissue compared with local treatment techniques, in which areas of both extreme heat and relatively normal temperatures may reduce the efficacy of hyperthermia.

GENERAL TECHNIQUE[1,2,19]

Whole-body hyperthermia is a complicated technique involving intensive measurement of a wide variety of physiologic parameters during treatment. Very few academic centers use whole-body hyperthermia because of the cost and the need for extensive, labor-intensive monitoring.

Handheld radiofrequency hyperthermia units are used in some small animal practices (Figure 27-3) as follows:

1. Ideally, the lesion to be treated should be smaller than 1 cm in diameter.
2. Place the dog under general anesthesia, and administer a systemic analgesic to minimize discomfort. Inject local anesthetic (0.25–2.00 ml of 2% lidocaine mixed 50:50 with sodium bicarbonate) around the lesion.
3. After obtaining a biopsy specimen, place radiofrequency tips on either side of the lesion. If the lesion is suspected to extend more than 0.2 cm below the skin's surface, place invasive radiofrequency tips through the skin and down to the level of the deepest portion of the tumor.
4. Heat the lesion at least twice; if nearby tissue is to be treated, reposition the applicator probes as needed. It is important to remember that both the tumor and a surrounding "cuff" of normal tissue should reach therapeutic temperatures (>42°C).
5. The heated area will become indurated and be somewhat painful for the first 24 to 48 hours after therapy. A scab may form and later fall off, revealing a bed of granulation tissue. The lesion gradually shrinks, leaving a small, hairless area or an area where the hair and skin are a different color.
6. Prescribe oral or transdermal analgesics for several days postoperatively.

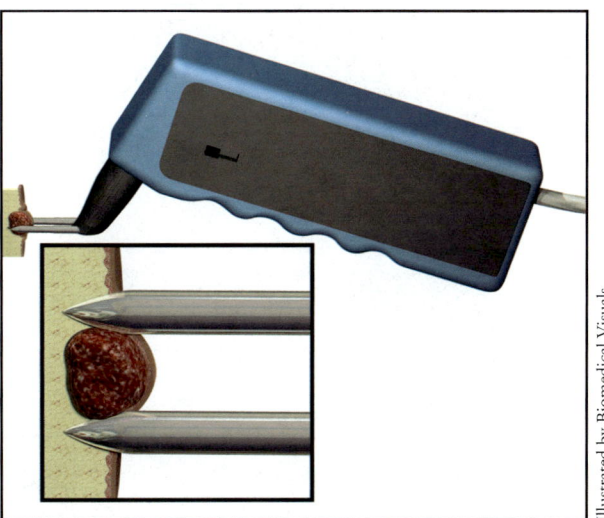

Figure 27-3. *Handheld local radiofrequency hyperthermia unit. Lidocaine is first injected around the lesion to be treated so that a biopsy specimen can be obtained. In this case, a handheld radiofrequency hyperthermia unit is used so that the applicator tips are placed on either side of the lesion. Because this lesion is suspected to be more than 0.2 cm below the skin's surface, the invasive radiofrequency tips are placed through the skin, down to the level of the deepest portion of the tumor. The lesion is heated at least twice; the applicator probes are used again if nearby tissue is to be treated. The tumor and a surrounding cuff of normal tissue should reach therapeutic temperatures (>42°C).*

CLINICAL APPLICATION

Hyperthermia alone provides only marginal control of local disease. In combination with radiation therapy or chemotherapy, however, the synergy enhances tumor control and subsequent survival. Local hyperthermia is not a commonly used modality.

Cryotherapy[20-24]

Cryotherapy kills tumor cells by using very cold temperatures to rapidly freeze tumors two to three times, with a very slow thawing process between the freezing cycles. This tech-

> **KEY POINT**
>
> *Cryotherapy kills tumor cells by using very cold temperatures to rapidly freeze tumors two to three times, with a very slow thawing process between the freezing cycles.*

nique was initially used to treat a variety of types and sizes of malignant and nonmalignant tumors. The greatest efficacy is seen when treating select, relatively small tumors such as squamous cell carcinomas, cutaneous papillomas, meibomian gland adenomas, cutaneous melanomas, and dermal hemangiomas.[20-22] More advanced techniques have been explored to treat dogs with adrenal and prostatic tumors.[22,23]

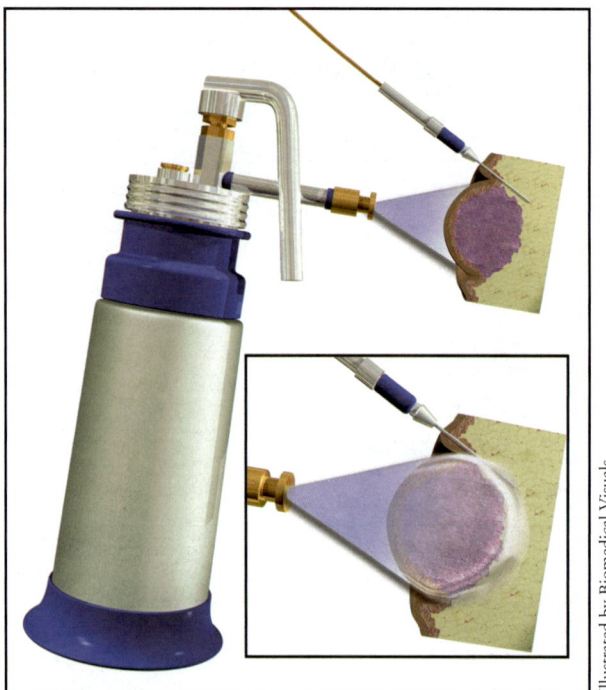

Figure 27-4. *Liquid nitrogen cryotherapy for a nasal squamous cell carcinoma. After the area is prepared and a local anesthetic is injected around the treatment area, the tumor is debrided and the tissue submitted for histopathology. Each tumor should be rapidly frozen and slowly thawed at least twice. In this figure, liquid nitrogen is applied with a contact probe directly to the tumor to form an iceball. Adequate temperatures (lower than –20°C) are reached at the peripheral margins of the tissue surrounding the tumor. Once the freezing is discontinued, the entire lesion is allowed to thaw; the target tissue is then frozen and allowed to thaw a second (and possibly a third) time. Tumors less than 1 cm in diameter are ideal for this type of therapy.*

This treatment modality is fast, relatively inexpensive, and can be employed with local and systemic anesthesia. It remains a standard treatment for a variety of localized small tumors in canine medicine.

EQUIPMENT[20–24]

Cryotherapy is a valuable tool in the treatment of a number of superficial dermal and oral lesions. It is ideal for cutaneous squamous cell carcinomas in such locations as the face and hairless underside and is helpful in treating other tumors, including basal cell tumors and sebaceous adenomas. Liquid nitrogen and nitrous oxide are the cryogens used most often in cryotherapy. Liquid nitrogen evaporates slowly and requires careful monitoring; nitrous oxide tanks are the same as those used for anesthetic purposes, and the gas does not evaporate between uses. Costs are similar regardless of which cryogen is used. Nitrous oxide has limited depth of penetration but is effective for lesions smaller than 1 cm in diameter; it cannot be used in spray applicators. Liquid nitrogen is much more effective for larger lesions or lesions with a rich blood supply that need to be frozen faster or that would be better treated with a spray applicator. Regardless of the cryogen used, temperature-monitoring devices (e.g., thermocouple needles) should be used to ensure that the tumor is frozen to critical temperatures (below –20°C).

> **KEY POINT**
> *When cryotherapy and hyperthermia are used, the tumor itself and a cuff of normal tissue around the tumor must be frozen or heated to the appropriate temperature to adequately control the tumor.*

GENERAL TECHNIQUE (Figure 27-4)

1. Cryotherapy should be restricted to small tumors (<1 cm in diameter) of the skin and other external areas.
2. Place the dog under general anesthesia, administer a systemic analgesic, and inject a local anesthetic (0.25–1.00 ml of 2% lidocaine mixed 50:50 with sodium bicarbonate) around the area to be frozen.
3. Part the surrounding hair or minimally clip and clean it.
4. Debride the tumor and submit the tissue for histopathology.
5. Coagulate the tissue with silver nitrate or a caustic agent or apply a purse-string suture to reduce bleeding at the site to be frozen. Restrict blood flow when possible to increase the freezing rate and decrease the warming rate.
6. Rapidly freeze and slowly thaw each tumor at least twice. When using a probe, make sure it is approximately the same size as the lesion. Apply warm probes to a warm, moist tumor surface. When freezing is initiated, the tumor freezes to the applicator and is maintained in that position throughout the process, which can last from seconds to several minutes.
7. Once the first iceball forms and adequate temperatures (–20°C or lower) are reached at the peripheral margins of the tissue surrounding the tumor, discontinue freezing and allow the probe to thaw until it detaches from the lesion. Allow the entire lesion to thaw, and then initiate a second (and possibly a third) freezing. Liquid nitrogen can be used as a spray, especially for larger tumors.
8. Warn owners that a scab will form at the site of freezing and then fall off in approximately 10 to 21 days, exposing a pink bed of epithelium or granulation tissue. This area will contract and epithelialize, leaving a small hairless area. Tell owners that the surrounding hair may change color. If bone is frozen, it may need to be debrided 2 to 3 months after cryotherapy. General hygiene is all that is required for the freezing site.

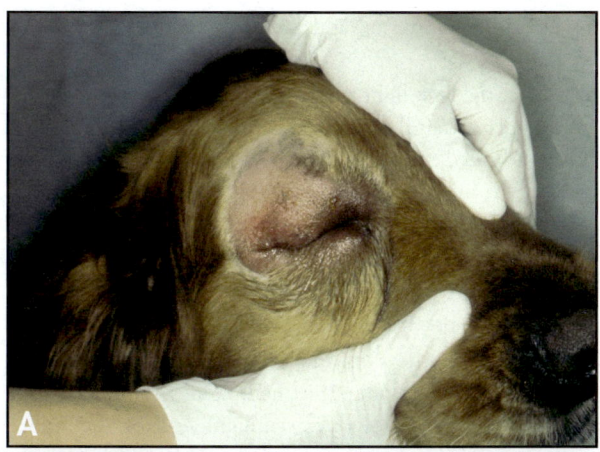 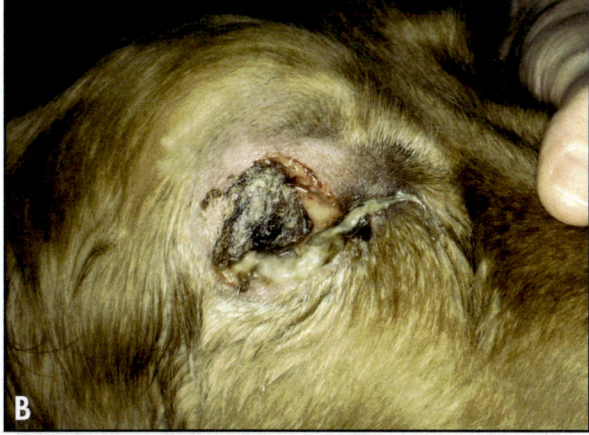
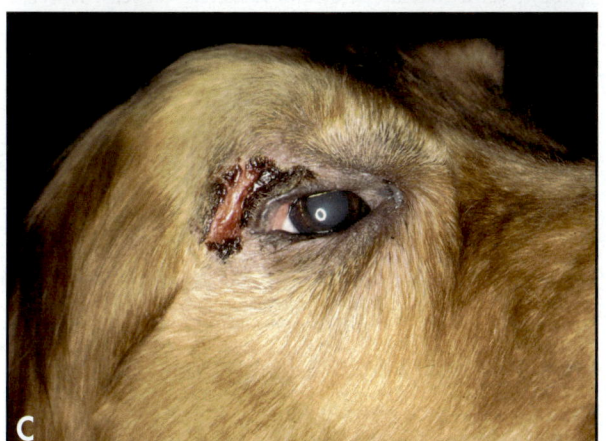 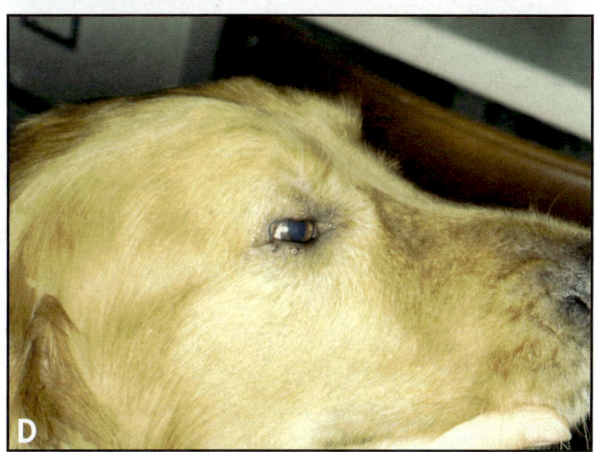

Figure 27-5. *PDT in a dog with a mast cell tumor in the eyelid. (**A**) Note marked edema of entire treatment field with some erythema 24 hours after treatment. (**B**) Six days later, there is a large, thick, devitalized scab in the area of the tumor (larger than the apparent tumor but not covering the entire treatment field). (**C**) Fourteen days after treatment, the ulcer is contracting and healing rapidly. (**D**) Four months after PDT, the eyelid is fully healed with a slight external rolling defect. (Courtesy of Angela E. Frimberger, VMD, Veterinary Oncology Consultants)*

9. If the dog appears to be uncomfortable, prescribe oral or transdermal analgesics for several days postoperatively.

CLINICAL APPLICATION[20–24]

Cryotherapy has been successfully used for decades to control localized tumors in humans and dogs. Best results occur with small (<1 cm diameter), localized, benign tumors.

Eyelid Tumors

Benign tumors of the eyelid, such as meibomian gland adenomas, papillomas, and melanomas, generally are treated very effectively with cryotherapy. The tumor should be submitted for histopathology before freezing. Recurrence rates are less than 5% if the tumor is smaller than 1 cm in diameter and adequately frozen.

Oral Tumors

Cryotherapy is effective in treating very small lesions of the oral cavity that invade bone, especially such benign lesions as epulides. After freezing, the tissue will slough rapidly as a result of abrasion within the oral cavity. A superficial area of dead bone may be exposed and become necrotic. If a sequestrum forms, it must be removed.

Skin Tumors

Small skin tumors are commonly treated with cryotherapy.[20] For example, cutaneous melanomas, basal cell tumors, squamous cell carcinomas, sebaceous adenomas, and papillomas smaller than 1 cm in diameter can be frozen with an excellent response. Squamous cell carcinomas are probably the only malignant tumors for which cryotherapy should be offered. As a general rule, tumors larger than 1 cm in diameter should be treated using other therapeutic modalities.

Photodynamic Therapy[25–39]

PDT involves the administration of a tumor-localizing photosensitizing agent, which may require metabolic synthesis (i.e., a prodrug), followed by activation of the agent

> **KEY POINT**
>
> *PDT involves the administration of a tumor-localizing photosensitizing agent, which may require metabolic synthesis (i.e., a prodrug), followed by activation of the agent using a specific wavelength of light (usually generated by a laser) that results in tissue death.*

using a specific wavelength of light (usually generated by a laser).[25-39] This therapy results in a sequence of photochemical and photobiologic processes that irreversibly damage tumor tissue. Results from preclinical and clinical studies conducted worldwide over a 25-year period in human and canine medicine have established PDT as a useful treatment approach for some cancers. Common applications in canine medicine have been in the treatment of cutaneous squamous cell carcinomas, transitional cell carcinomas, prostatic neoplasias, and nasal tumors, among others. Because of the significant equipment costs and limited application of this treatment modality, PDT is available in only a few—mostly academic—sites around the world.

EQUIPMENT[25]

The equipment required for PDT includes a laser to produce a specific wavelength of light (usually infrared), a fiberoptic delivery system, and a photosensitizing agent. Because the wavelength of laser light currently in use cannot pass through more than 2 cm of tissue, PDT is mainly used to treat tumors on or just under the skin or on the lining of internal organs (Figure 27-5). A photosensitizing agent is injected into the bloodstream and absorbed by cells throughout the body; the agent remains in cancer cells longer than in normal cells. When the treated cancer cells are exposed to laser light, the photosensitizing agent absorbs the light and produces an active form of oxygen that destroys the cancer cells. An advantage of PDT is that it causes minimal damage to healthy tissue. This treatment modality is available in only a few institutions in the United States, Europe, and Japan.

GENERAL TECHNIQUE

1. PDT should be restricted to small tumors (<1 cm in diameter) of the skin or on the lining of internal organs.
2. Administer the photosensitizing agent 6 to 48 hours (depending on the agent used) before treatment.
3. Place the dog under general anesthesia, cover its eyes, administer a systemic analgesic, and inject a local anesthetic (0.25–1.00 ml of 2% lidocaine mixed 50:50 with sodium bicarbonate) around the treatment site.
4. Part the surrounding hair or minimally clip and clean it.
5. Debride the tumor and submit the tissue for histopathology.
6. Direct the laser light through a fiberoptic conduit (a very thin glass strand) positioned close to the cancerous lesion. If indicated, pass the conduit through a bronchoscope into the lungs or through an endoscope into the esophagus to treat lung or esophageal cancer, respectively.
7. Time the light exposure carefully so that it occurs when most of the photosensitizing agent has left healthy cells but is still present in cancer cells.
8. PDT makes the skin and eyes sensitive to light for 6 weeks or longer after treatment. Dogs should be kept indoors and out of direct sunlight and bright indoor light until they are less photosensitive (at least 6 weeks for most drugs).
9. If the dog appears to be uncomfortable, prescribe oral or transdermal analgesics for several days postoperatively.

REFERENCES

1. Gillette EL: Hyperthermia effects in animals with spontaneous tumors. *Natl Cancer Inst Monogr* 61:361–364,1982.
2. Page RL, Thrall DE: Therapeutic hyperthermia: Contribution from clinical studies in dogs with spontaneous neoplasia. *In Vivo* 8(5):851–858, 1994.
3. Frew DG, Dobson JM, Stenning SP, Bleehen NM: Response of 145 spontaneous canine head and neck tumours to radiation versus radiation plus microwave hyperthermia: Results of a randomized phase III clinical study. *Int J Hyperthermia* 11(2):217–230, 1995.
4. Gillette SM, Dewhirst MW, Gillette EL, et al: Response of canine soft tissue sarcomas to radiation or radiation plus hyperthermia: A randomized phase II study. *Int J Hyperthermia* 8(3):309–320, 1992.
5. Denman DL, Legorreta RA, Kier AB, et al: Therapeutic responses of spontaneous canine malignancies to combinations of radiotherapy and hyperthermia. *Int J Radiat Oncol Biol Phys* 21(2):415–422, 1991.
6. Vujaskovic Z, Poulson JM, Gaskin AA, et al: Temperature-dependent changes in physiologic parameters of spontaneous canine soft tissue sarcomas after combined radiotherapy and hyperthermia treatment. *Int J Radiat Oncol Biol Phys* 46(1):179–185, 2000.
7. Theon AP, Madewell BR, Moore AS, et al: Localized thermo-cisplatin therapy: A pilot study in spontaneous canine and feline tumours. *Int J Hyperthermia* 7(6):881–892, 1991.
8. Ikenaga M, Ohura K, Kotoura Y, et al: Hyperthermic treatment of canine tibia through RF inductive heating of an intramedullary nail: A new experimental approach to hyperthermia for metastatic bone tumours. *Int J Hyperthermia* 10(4):507–516, 1994.
9. Hoekstra HJ, Meutstege FJ, Oosterhuis JW, et al: Effect of isolated limb perfusion with cisplatin (CDDP) on canine osteosarcoma. *Cancer Treat Res* 62:245–249, 1993.
10. Ogilvie GK, Reynolds HA, Richardson BC, et al: Performance of a multi-sector ultrasound hyperthermia applicator and control system: In vivo studies. *Int J Hyperthermia* 6(3):697–705, 1990.
11. Suzuki T, Kurokawa K, Higashi H, et al: Transurethral balloon laser enhanced thermotherapy in the canine prostate. *Lasers Surg Med* 21(4):321–328, 1997.
12. Page RL, Thrall DE, Dewhirst MW, Meyer RE: Whole-body hyperthermia: Rationale and potential use for cancer treatment. *J Vet Intern Med* 1(3):110–120, 1987.
13. Page RL, Macy DW, Ogilvie GK, et al: Phase III evaluation of doxorubicin and whole-body hyperthermia in dogs with lymphoma. *Int J Hyperthermia* 8(2):187–197, 1992.
14. Novotney CA, Page RL, Macy DW, et al: Phase I evaluation of doxorubicin and whole-body hyperthermia in dogs with lymphoma. *J Vet Intern Med* 6(4):245–249, 1992.
15. Page RL, McEntee MC, Williams PL, et al: Effect of whole body hyperthermia on carboplatin disposition and toxicity in dogs. *Int J Hyperthermia* 10(6):807–816, 1994.
16. Page RL, Lee J, Riviere JE, et al: Absence of whole body hyperthermia effect on cisplatin distribution in spontaneous canine tumors. *Int J Radiat Oncol Biol Phys*

32(4):1097–1102, 1995.
17. Thrall DE, Prescott DM, Samulski TV, et al: Radiation plus local hyperthermia versus radiation plus the combination of local and whole-body hyperthermia in canine sarcomas. *Int J Radiat Oncol Biol Phys* 34(5):1087–1096, 1996.
18. Hauck ML, Price GS, Ogilvie GK, et al: Phase I evaluation of mitoxantrone alone and combined with whole body hyperthermia in dogs with lymphoma. *Int J Hyperthermia* 12(3):309–320, 1996.
19. LaRue SM, Fox MH, Ogilvie GK, et al: Tumour cell kinetics as predictors of response in canine lymphoma treated with chemotherapy alone or combined with whole body hyperthermia. *Int J Hyperthermia* 15(6):475–486, 1999.
20. Farris Jr HE, Vestre WA: Veterinary cryosurgery. *Cryobiology* 19(3):228–230, 1982.
21. Munver R, Sosa RE: Cryosurgery of the adrenal gland. *Technol Cancer Res Treat* 3(2):181–185, 2004.
22. Butts K, Daniel BL, Chen L, et al: Diffusion-weighted MRI after cryosurgery of the canine prostate: Magnetic resonance imaging. *J Magn Reson Imaging* 17(1):131–135, 2003.
23. Collier LL, Collins BK: Excision and cryosurgical ablation of severe periocular papillomatosis in a dog. *JAVMA* 204(6):881–883, 1994.
24. Ward DA, Latimer KS, Askren RM: Squamous cell carcinoma of the corneoscleral limbus in a dog. *JAVMA* 200(10):1503–1506, 1992.
25. Lucroy MD: Photodynamic therapy for companion animals with cancer. *Vet Clin North Am Small Anim Pract* 32(3):693–702, viii, 2002.
26. Huang Z, Chen Q, Trncic N, et al: Effects of Pd-bacteriopheophorbide (TOOKAD)-mediated photodynamic therapy on canine prostate pretreated with ionizing radiation. *Radiat Res* 161(6):723–731, 2004.
27. Gloi AM, Beck E: Evaluation of porfimer sodium in dogs and cats with spontaneous tumors. *Vet Ther* 5(1):26–33, 2004.
28. Gloi AM, Beck E: Threshold dose of three photosensitizers in dogs with spontaneous tumors. *Vet Ther* 4(3):269–278, 2003.
29. Gloi AM, Beck E: Biodistribution of three photosensitizers in dogs with spontaneous tumors. *Vet Ther* 4(2):155–165, 2003.
30. Lucroy MD, Long KR, Blaik MA, et al: Photodynamic therapy for the treatment of intranasal tumors in 3 dogs and 1 cat. *J Vet Intern Med* 17(5):727–729, 2003.
31. Ridgway TD, Lucroy MD: Phototoxic effects of 635-nm light on canine transitional cell carcinoma cells incubated with 5-aminolevulinic acid. *Am J Vet Res* 64(2):131–136, 2003.
32. Chen Q, Huang Z, Luck D, et al: Preclinical studies in normal canine prostate of a novel palladium-bacteriopheophorbide (WST09) photosensitizer for photodynamic therapy of prostate cancers. *Photochem Photobiol* 76(4):438–445, 2002.
33. Lucroy MD, Bowles MH, Higbee RG, et al: Photodynamic therapy for prostatic carcinoma in a dog. *J Vet Intern Med* 17(2):235–237, 2003.
34. Cheli R, Addis F, Mortellaro CM, et al: Hematoporphyrin derivative photochemotherapy of spontaneous animal tumors: Clinical results with optimized drug dose. *Cancer Lett* 23(1):61–66, 1984.
35. Cheli R, Addis F, Mortellaro CM, et al: Photodynamic therapy of spontaneous animal tumors using the active component of hematoporphyrin derivative (DHE) as photosensitizing drug: Clinical results. *Cancer Lett* 38(1–2):101–105, 1987.
36. Frimberger AE, Moore AS, Cincotta L, et al: Photodynamic therapy of naturally occurring tumors in animals using a novel benzophenothiazine photosensitizer. *Clin Cancer Res* 4(9):2207–2218, 1998.
37. McCaw DL, Pope ER, Payne JT, et al: Treatment of canine oral squamous cell carcinomas with photodynamic therapy. *Br J Cancer* 82(7):1297–1299, 2000.
38. Roberts WG, Klein MK, Loomis M, et al: Photodynamic therapy of spontaneous cancers in felines, canines, and snakes with chloro-aluminum sulfonated phthalocyanine. *J Natl Cancer Inst* 83(1):18–23, 1991.
39. Peavy GM, Krasieva TB, Tromberg BJ, et al: Variation in the distribution of a phthalocyanine photosensitizer in naturally occurring tumors of animals. *J Photochem Photobiol B* 27(3):271–275, 1995.

EMERGING CANCER THERAPIES: GENE THERAPY, CANCER VACCINES, AND MOLECULARLY TARGETED THERAPIES

Gregory K. Ogilvie and Antony S. Moore

CLINICAL BRIEFING

Gene therapy
Definition	• Introduction of a gene or genes into a cell to treat or prevent cancer.
Vector	• System to deliver genes to replace defective genes or to insert antisense, suicide, or immunomodulatory genes.

Cancer vaccines
Definition	• Initiation of an immune response to recognize and destroy cells that have transformed or will transform into malignant or premalignant states.
Tumor antigens	• Tumor-specific macromolecules or molecules that support tumor growth.
Adjuvants	• Magnify tumor response to antigens; the most commonly used are aluminum or oil in water emulsions, although microorganisms have also been used.
Dendritic cell vaccines	• Vaccines that stimulate cells that are more potent stimulators of naïve T cells than any other antigen-presenting cells, such as B cells or macrophages.

Monoclonal antibodies and immunologic conjugates
Definition	• Immunoproteins that induce cytotoxicity through receptor binding and antibody-dependent cytotoxicity and by subsequently blocking the receptor's functions.
Radioimmunoconjugates	• Monoclonal antibodies that target and destroy or define tumors with radioisotopes.
Immunocytokines	• Monoclonals conjugated with cytokines such as IL-2 that activate the anticancer defense mechanism.
Immunotoxins	• Fusion of a monoclonal with a toxin such as ricin or diphtheria toxin to be directed against specific epitopes of tumor cells, thereby enhancing tumor selectivity and minimizing toxicity.

Molecularly targeted therapy
Definition	• Agents that target pathways activated in cancer cells.
Tyrosine kinase inhibitors	• Drugs that interfere with cell communication and growth and may prevent tumor growth.
Matrix metalloproteinase inhibitors	• Drugs that inhibit the family of zinc-dependent enzymes that are produced by multiple tissues throughout the body and are involved in the degradation of extracellular matrix and basement membrane components that are associated with cancer growth and metastasis.
Thalidomide	• Drug with anticancer effects in part because of its antiangiogenic effects.
L-MTP-PE	• Liposome-encapsulated substance with potent antitumor properties because of its nonspecific action to activate monocytes and macrophages.
Recombinant proteins	• Synthesized proteins designed to have the same effect, structure, and function of biologic proteins, such as IL-2 and IFN-α, that have anticancer properties.

EMERGING CANCER THERAPIES

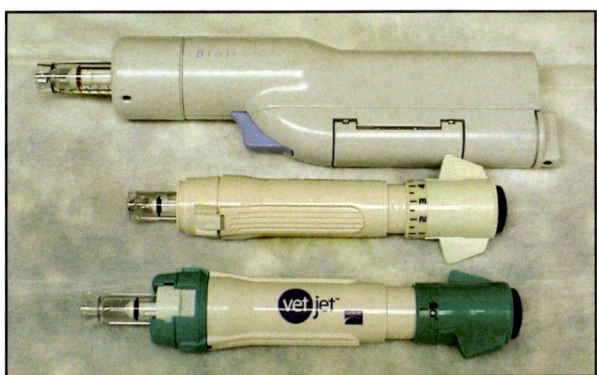

Figure 28-1. *The Biojector* (top), *Vitajet* (middle), *and VetJet* (bottom) *needle-free gene injector devices. The Biojector is an FDA-approved CO_2-powered device, while the Vitajet and VetJet are spring-powered. (Courtesy of Philip J. Bergman, DVM, Donaldson-Atwood Cancer Clinic)*

Traditional cancer therapies, including surgery, radiation, and chemotherapy, have not advanced nearly as fast as the treatments that capitalize on discoveries and new advances in molecular cancer biology. In fact, new advances in cancer therapy will revolve almost exclusively around the recent advances in gene therapy, cancer vaccines, and molecularly targeted cancer therapeutics. The purpose of this chapter is to introduce these subjects and to give some examples of the application of these principles in canine medicine. Readers are cautioned to remember that these therapies are evolving; therefore, the efficacy and toxicity of each are still the subjects of intense research. References are provided to direct interested readers to more comprehensive information.

> **KEY POINT**
>
> *The ideal vector specifically and precisely targets the gene to the tissue in question; is nontoxic, noninflammatory, and nonimmunogenic; and is capable of incorporating a large transgene.*

Gene Therapy

Gene therapy has been around, at least conceptually, for 40 years. It has evolved rapidly in recent years primarily due to the development of new vectors, enhanced vector targeting, improved transgene expression, and the rapid evaluation of these methods in outbred species with spontaneously occurring cancer. This therapeutic approach has been limited because of the lack of efficient, targeted, noninflammatory, and nonimmunogenic vectors and the identification of ideal cancers to test this modality. Ongoing research will address all these issues.

In its simplest definition, *gene therapy* is the introduction of a gene or genes into a cell to treat or prevent cancer. In order for gene therapy to be successful, it is necessary to[1-3]:

1. Understand the role of the gene(s) in question in controlling or preventing cancer
2. Be able to deliver the gene(s) in large enough numbers to the target tissue to get a biologically meaningful effect using a vector or other means
3. Ensure that the gene(s) can express themselves in a large enough amount and for a significant enough duration to affect the cancer in question

VECTORS

A vector is a system to deliver genes to a tumor or normal tissue. The ideal vector specifically and precisely targets the gene to the tissue in question; is nontoxic, noninflammatory, and nonimmunogenic; and is capable of incorporating a large transgene.[1-3] Gene therapy can be performed by removing cells from the patient and then delivering the gene to the cells by a vector before the modified cells are returned to the patient. More commonly, the genes are delivered to the patient in vivo using one of the following vectors[1-3]:

- **Naked DNA,** which is plasmid DNA injected directly into the tumor. The gene of interest is associated with a promoter that is then taken up by the tissue and incorporated into its own DNA. This method has poor yield.
- **A gene gun,** which delivers naked DNA on a plasmid that is adhered to gold particles and then "shot" through the overlying skin and into the underlying tissue with forced helium (Figure 28-1).
- **Liposomal-encapsulated DNA conjugates** that are then taken up by endocytes.
- **Ligand–DNA conjugates** that are used to target DNA to specific tumor tissue.
- **Retroviruses** that have the gene packaged into the virus for subsequent insertion into specific tissues.
- **Adenoviruses** that are replication incompetent but can infect tissues of interest for insertion of the gene that is packaged within the virus vector.
- **Adeno-associated viruses** that are potentially safer than, but as effective and at least safe as, adenoviruses, yet are capable of infecting and inserting the virus-packaged gene with great efficiency.
- **Recombinant lentiviruses** that infect actively and nonactively dividing cells and are stable.
- **Recombinant herpes simplex viruses** that target primarily neuronal tissue.
- **Recombinant vaccinia viruses** that are highly attenuated and host restricted and do not create productive infections.

- **Recombinant alphavirus vectors** that have rapid production of titers against the virus, a broad host range, and high transgene expression.

These vectors deliver genes to prevent or treat cancer in a number of ways, including by replacing defective genes or by inserting antisense, "suicide," or immunomodulatory genes.[1-3] The use of viruses has raised issues over the safety of these methodologies. These viruses have been documented to cause a number of clinical problems in human patients, from abnormal inflammatory responses to malignant transformation.[1-4] In addition, the use of exogenous genes has also been shown to cause problems, including autoimmunity and the induction of the desired anticancer effect within normal tissues (the so-called *bystander effect*).[1-4]

TYPES OF GENE THERAPY

A number of novel approaches to treat cancer exist, including gene therapy to replace defective genes, to modulate the immune system via cytokines and hormones, and to protect normal cells from the toxic effects of chemotherapy.[1-3]

Replacing Defective Genes

The tumor suppressor gene, *p53*, prevents the development of a number of cancers. When this gene is missing or is mutated, the risk of cancer increases. The gene is switched on when the cell is not working appropriately, causing the cell to undergo terminal cell death or apoptosis. This approach, while theoretically quite promising, has not yielded significant gains for dogs with cancer.

Delivering Suicide Genes

Gene therapy has been used to deliver genes that have the ability to convert relatively harmless prodrugs to active anticancer compounds within the cancer cell. For example, in a study in which dogs with experimentally induced gastric cancer underwent in situ transfer of a suicide gene into both the gastric cancer and regional lymph nodes that contained metastatic cancer, followed by intravenous administration of the prodrug ganciclovir, there was almost complete tissue degeneration of the tumor in the stomach and regional lymph nodes.[5] Another group studied the properties of toxic gene therapy using the prostate-specific antigen promoter–driving herpes simplex virus thymidine kinase suicide gene to induce highly selective molecular ablation of epithelial cells with minimal systemic toxicity in the canine prostate.[6] The goal of the study was to develop a novel gene therapy for the effective treatment of benign prostatic hyperplasia. The investigators showed that prostate-specific antigen promoter–based suicide gene therapy induced highly selective and definite ablation of epithelial cells in benign canine prostates. While this was not directed to cancer, it did prove the viability of this therapeutic approach.

Immunomodulation

It has been noted by many scientists that cytokines such as interleukin (IL)-2, interferon (IFN)-γ, IL-12, and IL-18 have anticancer effects in vitro in very small amounts.[1-3] Many of these effects are through the modulation of the immune system. When these cytokines are administered systemically, they often cause limiting, severe toxicities without the beneficial effect of controlling or eliminating the cancer.

Several veterinary studies have been conducted to test the hypothesis that gene therapy directed to induce the production of these cytokines might result in an anticancer or supportive effect in vivo without the concurrent systemic effects. Examples include:

- A study was conducted to evaluate the safety and efficacy of intratumoral injections of lipid-complexed plasmid DNA encoding for a bacterial superantigen with a cytokine gene for granulocyte–macrophage colony-stimulating factor (GM-CSF) or IL-2 in dogs with malignant melanoma.[5] Superantigens have been shown to induce a primary T-cell response with an anticancer effect caused by the expression of IL-2, tumor necrosis factor (TNF)-α, and IFN-γ. This effect is magnified with cytokines such as GM-CSF and IL-2. Survival times for dogs with stage III oral malignant melanoma treated by intratumoral gene therapy were prolonged significantly compared with those in animals treated by surgical tumor excision only. Thus, this study showed that local tumor transfection with superantigen and cytokine genes was capable of inducing both local and systemic antitumor immunity in an outbred animal with a spontaneously developing malignant tumor.

- Another study documented that an intramuscular injection of a plasmid that expressed growth hormone–releasing hormone is both safe and capable of stimulating the release of growth hormone and insulinlike growth factor I in dogs.[6] The observed anabolic responses to a single dose of this therapy are being further evaluated to determine if this approach is beneficial for the treatment of cancer cachexia in animals.

- A study demonstrated that cats and dogs with cancer treated with surgery, radiotherapy, and repeated local injections of xenogeneic Vero cells that secreted high levels of human IL-2 relapsed less frequently and survived longer than control animals treated by surgery and radiotherapy alone.[7] This confirmed the safety and therapeutic potential of a gene transfer strategy in animals with spontaneous metastatic and nonmetastatic tumors.

- Research was conducted to determine the gene expression and short-term effects of intralesional lipid-complexed immunogene therapy with constructs encoding *Staphylo-*

EMERGING CANCER THERAPIES

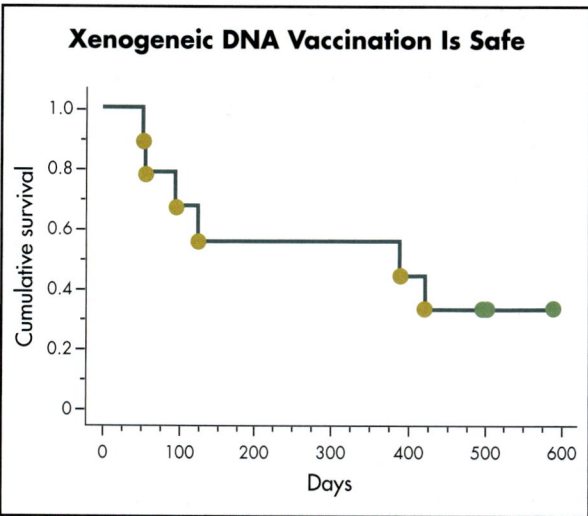

Figure 28-2. *In a study of xenogeneic DNA vaccination in nine dogs with advanced oral malignant melanoma using the human tyrosinase gene, the Kaplan-Meier median survival time for all nine dogs was 389 days, with some of the dogs having stabilization of disease or reduction in the size of the cancer. Green data points represent dogs that are still alive. (Courtesy of P. J. Bergman)*

coccus aureus enterotoxin A and canine IL-2 (L-SEA/cIL-2) in dogs with several tumor types.[8] The research was expanded to assess the safety and efficacy of repeated L-SEA/cIL-2 injections in dogs with spontaneous soft tissue sarcomas. The results of this translational research confirmed that this intralesional immunotherapy is well tolerated. They also confirmed transgene expression in canine tumors and, most interestingly, that there was antitumor activity in dogs with spontaneous soft tissue sarcomas.

> **KEY POINT**
>
> *A novel approach using xenogeneic DNA vaccination in canine advanced oral malignant melanoma using the human tyrosinase gene has been shown to be effective.*

- A trial to assess xenogeneic DNA vaccination in canine advanced oral malignant melanoma using the human tyrosinase gene was conducted.[9] This novel approach using a gene from another species elegantly and simply induced a good immune response against the malignant melanoma but not the patient's own tissue. The Kaplan-Meier median survival time for all nine dogs in this study was 389 days, with some of the dogs having stabilization of disease or reduction in the size of the cancer (Figure 28-2). The investigators concluded that xenogeneic DNA vaccination of dogs with advanced malignant melanoma is a safe and potentially therapeutic modality.

Chemoprotection

The gene that codes for multiple drug resistance has been the subject of intense research.[1-3] The *mdr* gene carries the codes for a protein complex that actively pumps certain chemotherapeutic agents out of the cell, resulting in cellular protection. Because this protects the cancer cell, it also has been hypothesized to be a mode to protect the patient's own bone marrow from the effects of chemotherapy when used at higher, potentially more cancer-cytodestructive dosages. The problem with this approach is that it does not necessarily transfer protection to other tissues within the body and may inadvertently transfer resistance to the cancer.

Cancer Vaccines

Controlling or eliminating cancer through the use of a vaccine has been the dream of many who study the hypothesis of cancer immunosurveillance.[2,3,9–12] This hypothesis suggests that the immune system recognizes and destroys cells that spontaneously transform into malignant or premalignant cells. This hypothesis was not uniformly accepted for decades, until studies showed that immunocompromised animals had a higher risk of developing cancer. The successes of monoclonal antibodies against canine and human lymphoma (CL/MAb 231, rituximab) and human breast cancer (Her2-neu) reaffirmed the importance of the immune system in controlling cancer.

> **KEY POINT**
>
> *Cancer vaccines are based on the immunosurveillance hypothesis, which suggests that the immune system recognizes and destroys cells that spontaneously transform into malignant or premalignant cells.*

The development of cancer vaccines has had to take into account that cancer cells are antigenic but poorly immunogenetic. This has resulted in the development of vaccines that have not only a vital tumor antigen but also an adjuvant to magnify the response to the antigen. Tumor antigens are often tumor-specific macromolecules such as k-Ras or fusion proteins such as bcr-abl. Tumor-specific antigens such as MAGE, GAGE, BAGE, or tyrosinase are also the focus of vaccine research.[2,3,10] Other targeted antigens have nothing to do with the tumor but are targeted to control tumors by disrupting tumor support, such as tumor-induced angiogenesis.

A huge number of clinical trials are under way to evaluate the efficacy of cancer vaccines. The greatest task for these studies is to document efficacy and vaccine safety. There is no question that antitumor immunity exists and that it can be induced.

CHOOSING ANTIGENS

Antigens come from whole tumor, tumor cell lysates, and defined antigens. Despite the fact that tumor vaccines directed against whole tumor or tumor cell lysates have engendered delayed-type hypersensitivity responses in human patients with melanoma, no randomized, controlled clinical studies have documented clinical benefit. In dogs, this approach has shown some benefit. For example, 30 dogs with histologically confirmed lymphoma were treated with combination chemotherapy followed by intralymphatic autochthonous tumor cell vaccines as maintenance therapy.[11] All dogs received two cycles of chemotherapy and at least three vaccine infusions. The median survival was 13 months. In a similar study,[12] 58 dogs with lymphoma were treated with combination chemotherapy. Twenty-eight of the dogs were also treated with intralymphatic autochthonous tumor cell vaccine. Dogs treated with chemotherapy and the vaccine had a significantly longer first remission than those that were treated with chemotherapy alone. These early studies affirmed the importance of cancer vaccines and became the basis of the development of defined antigen vaccines that have theoretic and actual advantages, in part because antigens can be relatively inexpensively produced in large quantities through DNA technology. Defined antigen vaccines serve as the basis of many current vaccine approaches.

CHOOSING ADJUVANTS

The choice of an adjuvant is crucial. Several types of adjuvants exist.[2,3,10] The most common traditional particulate vaccines incorporate aluminum salts and oil in water emulsions to enhance efficacy.[2,3,10] These adjuvants enhance dendritic cell maturation and stimulate cytokines that generate the immune response to the associated antigens. As discussed below, dendritic cells are vital for a good response. Microorganisms have also been used as adjuvants, including oncolytic viruses (e.g., poxviruses, vaccinia virus) and cell wall fractions from bacteria. *Listeria monocytogenes* and *Bacillus anthracis* are two bacteria that have been employed in the development of cancer vaccines. Dendritic cell vaccines represent one of the most promising areas of research.

DENDRITIC CELL VACCINES

Dendritic cells stimulate naïve T cells in a way that is far more potent than that of any other antigen-presenting cells, such as B cells or macrophages.[2,3,10,13,14] Dendritic cells are found everywhere in the body and are critical in the initiation of a protective immune response against a wide variety of antigen sources, including cancer.[13] They can be induced to form an immune response in the presence of lipopolysaccharides, viral RNA, mechanical stress, inflammation, and inflammatory mediators such as IL-1 and TNF-α.[13] Dendritic cell–based vaccines represent a very powerful way of initiating a response to a model antigen or tumor antigen.

> **KEY POINT**
> *Vaccines with dendritic cell bases represent a very powerful way of initiating a response to a model antigen or tumor antigen.*

Dendritic cell immunization had been shown to be of value for dogs with oral malignant melanoma.[2,3,10] For example, one study documented that canine blood–derived dendritic cells can be generated in vitro.[13] This was followed by another study in which therapeutic vaccines were developed from ex vivo acquisition of dendritic cells from the bone marrow of dogs with oral malignant melanoma.[14] The vaccine was made by first obtaining mononuclear cells from the bone marrow of three dogs with melanoma and one healthy dog. These cells were placed in media supplemented with recombinant human GM-CSF, stem cell factor, TNF, and Flt-3 ligand. Dendritic cells were transduced with an adenovirus vector encoding a xenoantigen, human melanoma antigen gp100. One dog developed an appropriate response and had no recurrent melanoma 48 months after initial injection of the dendritic cells. Another dog relapsed 22 months after vaccination.

Monoclonal Antibodies and Immunologic Conjugates

The use of hybridomas to develop monoclonal antibodies against specific tumor epitopes has increased the number and diversity of antibodies used to diagnose and treat cancer.[2,3,15] There are several mechanisms by which monoclonal antibodies induce their effects. For example, naked monoclonal antibodies kill tumors by receptor blockade or by inducing terminal cell death (apoptosis).[2,3,15] Other antibodies bring about tumor-induced cytotoxicity through receptor binding and antibody-dependent cytotoxicity. Alternatively, monoclonal antibodies can block receptors such as EGF-R, HER-2, and VEGF-R and subsequently their functions.[2,3,15]

Monoclonal antibodies are classified as naked monoclonal antibodies or immunoconjugates, including radioimmunoconjugates, immunocytokines, immunotoxins, antibody-directed enzyme prodrug therapy, and immunoliposomes.[2,3,15] Naked monoclonal antibodies gained great popularity when the anti-CD20 chimeric antibody rituximab was first approved for use by the US Food and Drug Administration for the treatment of non-Hodgkin's lymphoma. The treatment was well tolerated and is now accepted as first-line therapy in combination with chemotherapy for most B-cell–derived lymphomas. It has not shown efficacy in dogs, probably because of species selectivity. Other examples include tositumomab and ibritumomab for non-Hodgkin's lymphoma, alemtuzumab for chronic lymphocytic leukemia, trastuzumab for breast cancer, and gemtuzumab for acute myelogenous leukemia.[2,3,15] Other naked monoclonal antibodies against human solid tumors have also been developed.

The only monoclonal antibody that was approved but is no longer marketed for the treatment of cancer in dogs is CL/MAb 231 (Synbiotics Corporation, San Diego, California), which recognizes canine lymphoma cells.[16,17] It mediates antibody-dependent cellular cytotoxicity against a canine lymphoma cell line and has been reported to prolong remission duration when used in combination with chemotherapy in dogs with lymphoma.[17] The median survival time of dogs treated with the monoclonal antibody and chemotherapy was 591 days. Historical controls had a median survival time of 189 days. Additional studies are needed to further understand the clinical utility of this treatment modality.

> **KEY POINT**
> *Monoclonal antibodies used in cancer therapy induce cytotoxicity through receptor binding and antibody-dependent cytotoxicity and by subsequently blocking the receptors' functions.*

Monoclonal antibodies that target and destroy or define tumors with radioisotopes are called *radioimmunoconjugates*. The use of these radiolabeled immunoconjugates allows the use of single-photon emission computed tomography or positron emission tomography to define the tumor as well as its location and biology. This approach has been used to diagnose or treat lymphoma, leukemia, and solid tumors.[15]

Immunocytokines work in the same way as radioimmunoconjugates except that in this approach, monoclonals are conjugated with cytokines such as IL-2 to activate the anticancer defense mechanism.[15] Similarly, doxorubicin, melphalan, methotrexate, and vinca alkaloids have been conjugated to monoclonal antibodies to target specific tumor types. Immunotoxins are the fusion of a monoclonal with a toxin such as ricin or diphtheria toxin to be directed against specific epitopes of tumor cells, thereby enhancing tumor selectivity and minimizing toxicity.[15]

The use of monoclonal antibodies has great potential to selectively and precisely target and define cancer while minimizing adverse effects to normal tissues. The conjugation of chemotherapeutic agents, toxins, enzymes, and other substances has the potential to enhance diagnostic and therapeutic accuracy without enhancing toxicity. Continued development of these modalities is essential to bring them to the point of routine use.

Molecularly Targeted Therapy

Advances in cancer biology have allowed scientists to understand the molecular pathways that cancer cells employ to regulate their growth, survival, and angiogenesis.[18] Agents that target these pathways in cancer cells are called *molecularly targeted therapeutics*.[18] These targeted agents are best divided into those that target genetically defined abnormalities in cancer and those that target pathways activated by these genetic defects. Examples of agents that target genetically defined abnormalities in cancer include all-transretinoic acid for the treatment of promyelocytic leukemia and imarab for the treatment of chronic myeloid leukemia and other malignancies.[18]

> **KEY POINT**
> *Tyrosine kinase inhibitors are drugs that interfere with cell communication and growth and have been shown to prevent tumor growth in dogs with cancer.*

TYROSINE KINASE INHIBITORS

Fundamentally, tyrosine kinase inhibitors are drugs that interfere with cell communication and growth and may prevent tumor growth. Imarab and Gleevec are examples of tyrosine kinase inhibitors.[2,3,18] Imarab inhibits Abl, platelet-derived growth factor receptor, and Kit. This inhibitor has been shown to be beneficial for the treatment of acute B-cell leukemia, chronic myelogenous leukemia, chronic myelomonocytic leukemia, and gastrointestinal stromal tumors in human patients.

A unique receptor tyrosine kinase inhibitor was specifically evaluated in 57 dogs with a variety of cancers. The dogs were enrolled to orally receive a novel multitargeted indolinone receptor tyrosine kinase inhibitor (SU11654).[19] Ten of these dogs experienced progressive disease within the first 3 weeks. Six dogs achieved a complete response, primarily those with mast cell tumors (n = 1), mixed mammary carcinomas (n = 2), soft tissue sarcomas (n = 2), and multiple myeloma (n = 1). Stable disease longer than 10 weeks in duration was seen in an additional 15 dogs. This was enough for the authors to conclude that the orally administered kinase inhibitors exhibited activity against a variety of spontaneous malignancies.

ANTIANGIOGENESIS THERAPY

There are a wide variety of agents that inhibit cancer growth and metastasis by inhibiting angiogenesis, the process of blood vessel ingrowth into tissue. These agents include[2,3,18,19–29]:

- Inhibitors of matrix metalloproteinase (MMP) enzymes
- Inhibitors of endothelial cell proliferation
- Antagonists of angiogenic growth factors
- Inhibitors of endothelial cell matrix interactions

- Copper chelators
- Fatty acids
- Tetracycline inhibitors
- Thalidomide

Most of these agents have many other mechanisms of action and can be considered pharmacologic agents as easily as they can be considered biologic response modifiers (see Chapter 23).

MMPs are a family of zinc-dependent enzymes that are produced by tissues throughout the body and are involved in the degradation of extracellular matrix and basement membrane components.[20-27] MMPs are active during tissue remodeling processes, including cancer metastasis and invasion and angiogenesis.[26] An investigation was launched to evaluate whether the presence of MMP-2 and MMP-9 in the tumor, serum, and plasma correlated with the presence of canine malignancies and whether the MMP levels correlated with histologic tumor grade.[26] In this study, tumor, plasma, serum, and stromal tissue were harvested from dogs with various histologically confirmed and graded malignancies before therapy and analyzed by gelatin zymography to detect MMP-2 and MMP-9 activity. Dogs with measurable levels of MMP-9 were more than three times more likely to come out of remission than subjects that had no MMP levels. In most cases, dogs with the active form of MMPs were significantly more likely to come out of remission by 90 days than subjects with no active form of MMPs. This was especially true when the active form of MMPs was present in dogs with lymphoma. In general, dogs with stage IV lymphoma had the highest levels of MMPs and the poorest outcome compared with dogs with stage III disease. These data allow some to draw the conclusion that MMP inhibitors, which have antiangiogenic properties, may be of value in treating dogs with cancer.

In another study involving dogs with mast cell tumors, the presence of MMP-2 and MMP-9 was determined in canine mast cell tumor tissue and normal stromal tissue from 24 dogs with spontaneously occurring cutaneous mast cell tumors.[27] Seventeen tumors were of histologic grade 2, and seven were of histologic grade 3. Gelatin zymography and computer-assisted densitometry image analysis were used to quantify MMP concentration. There was dramatically more proenzyme MMP-9 activity in histologic grade 3 mast cell tumors compared with grade 2 tumors. There was also dramatically more active enzyme MMP-2 and active enzyme MMP-9 activity in tumor tissue compared with stromal tissue. This study demonstrates that the proenzyme and active enzyme forms of MMP-2 and MMP-9 are present in canine mast cell tumors. This appears to be related to the degree of histologic malignancy.

Many inhibitors of MMPs exist, including such nonspecific inhibitors as marimastat and specific inhibitors such as Bay-12-9566. Their efficacy as anticancer agents has not yet met expectations. The nonspecific inhibitors are associated with serious toxicity and therefore have limited clinical use. Specific inhibitors like Bay-12-9566 have less toxicity and have been evaluated in a large study involving over 400 dogs with lymphoma with positive results, especially in older dogs with measurable MMP levels in their tumor.[26]

Thalidomide is a potent drug that works in part because of its antiangiogenic effects.[28,29] This drug has enhanced the health and wellness of a number of human cancer patients, especially those with multiple myeloma and prostate carcinoma.[28,29] Specific veterinary studies are under way despite the difficulty in obtaining this drug.

MURAMYL TRIPEPTIDE–PHOSPHATIDYLETHANOLIMINE

Several studies have shown that liposome-encapsulated muramyl tripeptide–phosphatidylethanolamine (L-MTP-PE) has potent antitumor properties (see Chapter 23).[2,3,30-34] Unfortunately, this compound is not yet commercially available. L-MTP-PE is a nonspecific activator of monocytes and macrophages that results in anticancer effects. In one randomized, double-blind study involving dogs with osteosarcoma, those that received L-MTP-PE after amputation had a median survival time of 7.4 months, whereas those that had an amputation and empty liposomes (control) had a median survival time of 3 months.[30] Although this study clearly showed that L-MTP-PE was very important in increasing survival time, 70% of the dogs developed metastatic disease, which prompted the initiation of a second double-blind, randomized study.

> **KEY POINT**
>
> *L-MTP-PE is a nonspecific activator of monocytes and macrophages that results in anticancer effects against a wide number of canine malignancies.*

In this second study, 40 dogs with osteosarcoma of the extremity without evidence of metastatic disease were treated with amputation followed by four doses of cisplatin.[31] They were randomized to receive L-MTP-PE or empty liposomes. Of 14 dogs in the placebo group, 13 died of metastases; median survival time was 10 months, and median disease-free interval was 7.6 months. The dogs that received L-MTP-PE had a median survival time of 14.6 months and a median disease-free interval of 12 months; eight of the 11 dogs developed metastases. A related trial showed that there is no survival advantage of administering L-MTP-PE concurrently with cisplatin. These studies clearly show that L-MTP-PE is an important biologic response modifier for the treatment of osteosarcoma. Despite this efficacy, L-MTP-PE is not commercially available.

Other studies have been completed to determine whether L-MTP-PE is effective for the treatment of other canine cancers. For example, in one prospective, randomized, double-blind clinical study, the antitumor activity of L-MTP-PE was evaluated as adjuvant immunotherapy in dogs with simple mammary carcinomas.[33] Dogs were randomized after surgery to one of two groups in which they were treated with either L-MTP-PE (n = 13) or empty liposomes (n = 14). The difference in disease-free interval between dogs treated with L-MTP-PE (median: 165 days: range, 15–905 days) and dogs in the placebo group (median: 133 days; range: 27–659 days) was not significant. In another study, 32 dogs with hemangiosarcoma without gross evidence of metastases were treated with splenectomy, stratified by clinical stage, and randomized to receive doxorubicin–cyclophosphamide chemotherapy and either L-MTP-PE immunotherapy or placebo liposomes.[32] Dogs receiving L-MTP-PE had significantly prolonged disease-free survival ($P = .037$) and overall survival ($P = .029$) compared with dogs receiving placebo. In a third study, 48 dogs with histologically confirmed, clinically staged oral melanoma were entered into a randomized, double-blind, surgical adjuvant trial and stratified on the basis of clinical stage and extent of surgery (simple resection or radical excision), treated with L-MTP-PE twice a week, and randomized to recombinant canine GM-CSF or saline (placebo) given daily for 9 weeks.[33] This study documented that after surgery, L-MTP-PE administered alone or combined with recombinant canine GM-CSF showed no significant antitumor activity in treating advanced-stage oral melanoma. In early-stage oral melanoma, L-MTP-PE was shown to result in a prolongation of survival time.

RECOMBINANT PROTEINS

Recombinant proteins are synthesized to have the same effect, structure, and function of biologic proteins that have anticancer effects. Recombinant human IL-2 has been shown to be effective in stimulating canine peripheral blood mononuclear cells and is effective at stimulating canine lymphokine-activated killer cells.[2,3,35] Liposome-encapsulated IL-2 appears to be effective for treating cancer, especially if inhaled. Seven dogs with pulmonary metastases from osteosarcoma and two dogs with primary lung carcinoma were treated with aerosols of IL-2 liposomes.[34] Two of four dogs with metastatic pulmonary osteosarcoma had complete regression of metastases that remained stable for more than 12 and 20 months, respectively. One of two dogs with lung carcinoma had stabilization of disease for more than 8 months. Toxicity was minimal.

IFN-α has been used for the treatment of a number of human malignancies, although no such product exists commercially for canine cancers.[2,3] IFN-α has been shown to be effective for the treatment of human melanoma, hairy cell leukemia, chronic myelogenous leukemia, basal cell carcinoma, renal cell carcinoma, and genital warts. IFN-α has been shown to enhance the efficacy of cisplatin, carboplatin, doxorubicin, etoposide, and other drugs. Canine veterinary cancer studies have not yet come to a conclusion about the efficacy of this agent.

Conclusion

Therapeutics that take advantage of our knowledge of cancer cell survival and growth are a key area for future cures and control. Some therapies such as MMP inhibitors have not met expectations, but others are broadening opportunities beyond those that chemotherapy, radiation, and surgery can provide. Additional research is under way to explore molecular therapeutics.

REFERENCES

1. Talmadge JE, Cowan KH: Gene therapy in oncology, in Abeloff MD, Armitage JO, Niederhuber JE, et al (eds): *Clinical Oncology*, ed 3. Philadelphia, Elsevier, 2004, pp 603–622.
2. Argyle D: Gene therapy, in Dobson JM, Lascelles BDX (eds): *BSAVA Manual of Canine and Feline Oncology*, ed 2. Gloucester, England, BSAVA, 2003, pp 120–125.
3. Hogge GS, MacEwen EG: Immunology and biologic therapy of cancer, in Withrow SJ, MacEwen EG (eds): *Small Animal Clinical Oncology*, ed 3. Philadelphia, WB Saunders, 2001, pp 138–168.
4. Kiem HP, Sellers S, Thomasson B, et al: Long-term clinical and molecular follow-up of large animals receiving retrovirally transduced stem and progenitor cells: No progression to clonal hematopoiesis or leukemia. *Mol Ther* 9(3):389–395, 2004.
5. Dow SW, Elmslie RE, Willson AP, et al: In vivo tumor transfection with superantigen plus cytokine genes induces tumor regression and prolongs survival in dogs with malignant melanoma. *J Clin Invest* 101(11):2406–2414, 1998.
6. Draghia-Akli R, Hahn KA, King GK, et al: Effects of plasmid-mediated growth hormone-releasing hormone in severely debilitated dogs with cancer. *Mol Ther* 6(6):830–836, 2002.
7. Quintin-Colonna F, Devauchelle P, Fradelizi D, et al: Gene therapy of spontaneous canine melanoma and feline fibrosarcoma by intratumoral administration of histincompatible cells expressing human interleukin-2. *Gene Ther* 3(12):1104–1112, 1996.
8. Thamm DH, Kurzman ID, Macewen EG, et al: Intralesional lipid-complexed cytokine/superantigen immunogene therapy for spontaneous canine tumors. *Cancer Immunol Immunother* 52(8):473–480, 2003.
9. Bergman PJ, McKnight J, Novosad A, et al: Long-term survival of dogs with advanced malignant melanoma after DNA vaccination with xenogeneic human tyrosinase: A phase I trial. *Clin Cancer Res* 9(4):1284–1290, 2003.
10. Milone MC, June CH: Cancer vaccines, in Abeloff MD, Armitage JO, Niederhuber JE, et al (eds): *Clinical Oncology*, ed 3. Philadelphia, Elsevier, 2004, pp 677–694.
11. Jeglum KA, Young KM, Barnsley K, et al: Intralymphatic autochthonous tumor cell vaccine in canine lymphoma. *J Biol Response Mod* 5(2):168–175, 1986.
12. Jeglum KA, Young KM, Barnsley K, et al: Chemotherapy versus chemotherapy with intralymphatic tumor cell vaccine in canine lymphoma. *Cancer* 61(10):2042–2050, 1988.
13. Catchpole B, Stell AJ, Dobson JM: Generation of blood-derived dendritic cells in dogs with oral malignant melanoma. *J Comp Pathol* 126(2–3):238–241, 2002.
14. Gyorffy S, Rodriguez-Lecompte JC, Woods JP, et al: Bone marrow-derived dendritic cell vaccination of dogs with naturally occurring melanoma by using human gp100 antigen. *J Vet Intern Med* 19(1):56–63, 2005.
15. Cheung NK: Therapeutic antibodies and immunologic conjugates, in Abeloff MD, Armitage JO, Niederhuber JE, et al (eds): *Clinical Oncology*, ed 3. Philadelphia, Elsevier, 2004, pp 661–676.
16. Rosales C, Jeglum AK, Obrocka M, et al: Cytolytic activity of murine anti-dog lymphoma monoclonal antibodies with canine effector cells and complement. *Cell Immunol* 115:420–428, 1988.
17. Jeglum AK: Monoclonal antibody treatment of canine lymphoma. *Proc NAVC*:222–223, 1992.
18. Druker BJ: The present and future of molecularly targeted therapy, in Abeloff MD, Armitage JO, Niederhuber JE, et al (eds): *Clinical Oncology*, ed 3. Philadelphia, Elsevier, 2004, pp 623–639.
19. London CA, Hannah AL, Zadovoskaya R, et al: Phase I dose-escalating study of

SU11654, a small molecule receptor tyrosine kinase inhibitor, in dogs with spontaneous malignancies. *Clin Cancer Res* 9(7):2755–2768, 2003.
20. Handsley MM, Edwards DR: Metalloproteinases and their inhibitors in tumor angiogenesis. *Int J Cancer* 115(6):849–860, 2005.
21. Durko M, Brodt P: The metalloproteinases and their inhibitors, in Brodt P (ed): *Cell Adhesion and Invasion in Cancer Metastasis.* London, R.G. Landes Company, 1996, pp 113–150.
22. Cawston TE: Metalloproteinase inhibitors and the prevention of connective tissue breakdown. *Pharmacol Ther* 70:163–182, 1996.
23. Wojtowicz-Praga SM, Dickson RB, Hawkins MJ: Matrix metalloproteinase inhibitors. *Invest New Drugs* 15:61–75, 1997.
24. Liotta LA, Steeg PS, Stetler-Stevenson WG: Cancer metastasis and angiogenesis: An imbalance of positive and negative regulation. *Cell* 64:327–336, 1991.
25. MacDougall JR, Martisian LM: Contributions of tumor and stromal matrix metalloproteinases to tumor progression, invasion, and metastasis. *Cancer Metastasis Rev* 14:351–362, 1995.
26. Lana SE, Ogilvie GK, Hansen RA, et al: Identification of matrix metalloproteinases in canine neoplastic tissue. *Am J Vet Res* 61(2):111–114, 2000.
27. Leibman NF, Lana SE, Hansen RA, et al: Identification of matrix metalloproteinases in canine cutaneous mast cell tumors. *J Vet Intern Med* 14(6):583–586, 2000.
28. Rajkumar SV: Current status of thalidomide in the treatment of cancer. *Oncology* 15(7):867–874, 2001.
29. Figg WD, Dahut W, Duray P, et al: A randomized phase II trial of thalidomide, an angiogenesis inhibitor, in patients with androgen-independent prostate cancer. *Clin Cancer Res* 7(7):1888–1893, 2001.
30. Meyer JA, Dueland RT, Rosenthal RC, et al: Canine osteogenic sarcoma treated by amputation and MER. *Cancer* 49:1613–1616, 1982.
31. MacEwen EG, Kurzman ID, Rosenthal RC, et al: Therapy for osteosarcoma in dogs with intravenous injection of liposome-encapsulated muramyl tripeptide. *J Natl Cancer Inst* 81:935–938, 1989.
32. Vail DM, MacEwen EG, Kurzman ID, et al: Liposome-encapsulated muramyl tripeptide phosphatidylethanolamine adjuvant immunotherapy for splenic hemangiosarcoma in the dog: A randomized multi-institutional clinical trial. *Clin Cancer Res* 1(10):1165–1170, 1995.
33. Teske E, Rutteman GR, vd Ingh TS, et al: Liposome-encapsulated muramyl tripeptide phosphatidylethanolamine (L-MTP-PE): A randomized clinical trial in dogs with mammary carcinoma. *Anticancer Res* 18(2A):1015–1019, 1998.
34. MacEwen EG, Kurzman ID, Vail DM, et al: Adjuvant therapy for melanoma in dogs: Results of randomized clinical trials using surgery, liposome-encapsulated muramyl tripeptide, and granulocyte macrophage colony-stimulating factor. *Clin Cancer Res* 5(12):4249–4258, 1999.
35. Khanna C, Anderson PM, Hasz DE, et al: Interleukin-2 liposome inhalation therapy is safe and effective for dogs with spontaneous pulmonary metastases. *Cancer* 79(7):1409–1421, 1997.

PREVENTION AND TREATMENT OF PAIN

Gregory K. Ogilvie and Antony S. Moore

CLINICAL BRIEFING

General concepts of pain management	• Assess each patient for discomfort. • Believe the client's perception about quality of life. • Choose optimal analgesics. • Deliver the drugs in the most appropriate fashion. • Empower clients to directly participate in patient care. • Use analgesics preventively for maximum benefit. • Compassionate care, gentle handling, and a comfortable environment should be accompanied by local and systemic analgesics to anticipate discomfort and to treat ongoing pain.
Mild pain	• Eliminate the underlying cause. • Use nonopioids, including NSAIDs, with or without acupuncture and local anesthetic agents, as indicated. • Constantly reassess the patient's need for analgesia.
Moderate pain	• Eliminate the underlying cause. • Use nonopioids, including NSAIDs and opiate analgesics, with or without acupuncture and local anesthetics, as indicated. • If needed, consider α_2-adrenergic agonists and anxiolytics; changing the route of administration (e.g., oral to IV, SC, or IM) may be beneficial. • Constantly reassess the patient's need for analgesia.

Severe pain	• Eliminate the underlying cause.
	• Nonopioids, including NSAIDs, with increasing dosages of opiate analgesics, should be combined as needed with local analgesia (local, regional, intracavitary, or epidural analgesia), acupuncture, or sustained-release patches.
	• The above can also be combined with:
	  — CRI of fentanyl.
	  — Microdose ketamine.
	  — Palliative procedures (e.g., radiation therapy, surgery).
	• Maximize blood levels of analgesics with systemic administration.

Compassionate care is the watchword of canine oncology, and pain control is the cornerstone of the caring process. Unfortunately, pain control in dogs has only recently begun to be investigated and applied seriously. Canine pain management can be difficult because many signs of discomfort may be mistaken by clients and the rest of the veterinary health care team to be components of other disorders. The key to compassionate pain control is anticipating the onset of discomfort, thereby allowing timely intervention with analgesics. For optimal pain control, analgesics should be given prophylactically, before pain receptors ever identify discomfort. Educating the entire veterinary health care team, especially veterinary nurses, is key to ensuring that patient comfort is paramount. The following "ABCs" of pain management must be followed for each case[1,2]:

- **A**ssess each patient for discomfort; always think ahead to anticipate and prevent discomfort from diagnostics, therapeutics, and the disease itself.
- **B**elieve and respond to the client's perception about the pet's pain level and quality of life.
- **C**hoose optimal analgesics to treat and prevent discomfort or pain.
- **D**eliver the drugs in the most appropriate fashion to optimize analgesic effects, such as selecting constant-rate infusions (CRIs) over on-demand oral therapy.
- **E**mpower clients to directly participate in patient care by ensuring they understand as much about the disease, treatment, and philosophy of pain management as the rest of the veterinary health care team.

> **KEY POINT**
>
> *The key to compassionate pain control is anticipating the onset of discomfort, thereby allowing timely intervention with analgesics. For optimal pain control, analgesics should be given prophylactically, before pain receptors ever identify discomfort.*

The best assumption is that all patients with cancer have pain and that some sort of intervention is necessary. In addition, it is important to realize that each dog's need for analgesics is dynamic and that constant assessment by the entire veterinary health care team must be a priority. In many veterinary centers, the nursing team is best at recognizing discomfort and advocating the use of analgesics. Many excellent reviews exist for those seeking additional details of pain prevention, control, and management that are beyond the scope of this chapter.

> **KEY POINT**
>
> *Educating the entire veterinary health care team, especially veterinary nurses, is key to ensuring that patient comfort is paramount.*

Mechanisms of Cancer Pain

The most common mechanism of cancer pain is associated with tumor invasion and subsequent tissue damage that causes activation of pain receptors.[1-5] Some forms of therapy can induce pain as well. For example, surgery and radiation therapy may ultimately relieve pain and suffering but almost always cause short-term discomfort that must be minimized. Similarly, although chemotherapy can help control the underlying malignant process, chemotherapeutic drugs, albeit uncommonly, may be associated with discomfort. Cisplatin, vincristine, and vinblastine have caused painful polyneuropathy in a small percentage of human cancer patients. This adverse effect is suspected to occur in a relatively small number of dogs and can decrease the patient's quality of life.

Although very little is known about canine pain, a basic understanding of the types of discomfort may help increase awareness of how dogs with cancer can be managed with compassion and understanding. The types of pain associated with cancer include visceral pain, inflammatory and somatic pain, neuritis, and neuropathic pain.[1-5]

VISCERAL PAIN

Human patients describe this type of pain as a dull, deep, constant, aching pain. Visceral pain is poorly defined; patients with significant visceral pain may respond to opioid or nonopioid analgesics. It is suspected that this type of pain results in decreased activity, anorexia, and behavioral changes in dogs.

INFLAMMATORY AND SOMATIC PAIN

Frequently described in human medicine but rarely in canine medicine, this type of pain is well-localized, constant, and aching.[5] Common sources of inflammatory and somatic pain include bone metastasis, tissue damage, and musculoskeletal, dental, and integumental pain. Dogs may lick or bite at an area or may exhibit signs of discomfort in subtle ways, such as by decreasing their activity or limping if a limb is affected.

NEURITIC PAIN (NEURITIS)

Inflammation of nerves or nerve roots causes neuritic pain and can present as part of a paraneoplastic syndrome or as a direct effect of tumor compression. Human patients describe it as a constant, dull, aching pain that may have periods of burning, "shock-like" sensations. In dogs, these shock-like sensations can result in sudden, unexplained behavioral changes, such as aggression or scratching and biting at an area, often to the point of self-mutilation.

NEUROPATHIC PAIN

Neuropathic pain occurs when a segment of the nervous system that normally transmits pain stimuli is damaged. It arises from metabolic, immunologic, or direct physical effects on the nervous system. Neuropathic pain is difficult to control with standard analgesics.

Recognizing Pain

The goal of quality care is to prevent any pain from occurring. Realistically, many pets do have pain, stress, distress, and discomfort, and these patients must be identified early and reevaluated often in the course of the disease and its treatment. Dogs are quite variable in expressing discomfort. Some hide most outward and measurable manifestations of pain and rarely exhibit signs until discomfort is advanced. In these dogs, the only clinical indicator of pain and discomfort may be increased systolic blood pressure. Other dogs are demonstrative when in pain. Experienced practitioners and caregivers should watch for subtle changes in activity level, appetite, and movement. Vocalization, although not a specific indicator of pain, is noted in some dogs, especially when discomfort is significant. Some dogs become more reclusive; others, especially younger animals, pace and may thrash around. Tachypnea, tachycardia, and dilated pupils can be used to assess pain in dogs, even when they are stuporous.

The best veterinary practitioners anticipate and intervene early rather than waiting for clinical signs associated with discomfort. Caregivers need to be aware of which procedures are likely to cause discomfort, and preemptive analgesia should be practiced when possible.

Table 29-1 **General Approach to Pain Management**

Degree of Pain	Clinical Approach[a]
Mild	Nonopioid[b] ± acupuncture
Mild to moderate	Nonopioid ± acupuncture + opioids
Moderate	Nonopioid ± acupuncture + opioids (low-dose) ± anxiolytics
Moderate to severe	Nonopioid ± acupuncture + opioids (dose escalation, different route of administration) ± anxiolytics
Severe	Nonopioid ± acupuncture + opioids (dose escalation, different route of administration) ± anxiolytics + other palliative procedures (e.g., radiation, surgery)

[a]In each case, treat the underlying disease.
[b]NSAIDs and acetaminophen. Use with caution in patients with renal disease.

> **KEY POINT**
>
> *Many dogs with cancer have pain, stress, distress, and discomfort. These patients must be identified early and reevaluated often in the course of the disease and its treatment.*

Comprehensive management of pain involves careful evaluation and treatment of each dog.[1-5] To maximize quality of life, response to therapy, and survival time for canine patients, adequate pain control must be the highest goal for the veterinary practitioner and the associated veterinary health care team. Pain control in canine medicine has come to the forefront of attention primarily because of inappropriate attitudes of clinicians and nurses, lack of knowledge about analgesic medications, and lack of skill in assessing pain and appropriate therapeutic methods.[2,3] Client demand has also been an important force in bringing pain control to the forefront of compassionate care. In many cases, analgesics have been withheld because of fear of associated adverse side effects and because research demonstrating the beneficial effects of pain relief in dogs is scant. However, patient needs and client concerns require that pain relief and compassionate care become priorities in veterinary medicine.

General Concepts of Pain Therapy

The choice of analgesics and procedures to prevent, reduce, and eliminate discomfort differs depending on the cause and duration of the pain stimulus (Table 29-1). Pain control for an abdominal exploratory procedure differs from chronic pain management in a dog with metastatic bone disease. Discomfort associated with inflammatory conditions differs from that induced by nerve damage. Other factors that may influence the approach to treating the cancer patient include[1-3]:

- **Body condition:** In obese patients, drugs may be redistributed into fat stores, leading to overdosing. Metabolic derangements associated with cancer cachexia may result in altered pharmacokinetics and analgesic toxicity.

- **Age:** Some analgesics and anxiolytics that affect the central nervous system (CNS) may have a pronounced sedative or calming effect in very young and old animals.

- **Breed:** Unique breed differences should be considered when selecting pain therapeutics. For example, Labrador retrievers and other dogs may be more sensitive to a rare hepatopathy associated with the administration of drugs such as carprofen. Doberman pinschers may be more likely to exhibit extrapyramidal side effects of some opiate drugs. Boxers may be very sensitive to the effects of acepromazine and opiates.

- **Underlying concurrent diseases:** Cancer patients are often older, and they almost always have a metabolic or organ disorder that may influence their degree of, and sensitivity to, discomfort and their response to analgesics. Dogs with renal or hepatic insufficiency should be treated with care because this organ dysfunction will change the toxicity and efficacy profile of drugs metabolized or eliminated by these organs. Obtaining a minimum database of complete blood count, biochemistry profile, and urinalysis will help the clinician anticipate any potential problems.

- **Individual variation:** Some patients respond unpredictably and repeatedly to the effect of drugs. Nervous,

Table 29-2 Procedures and Associated Discomfort (and Associated Pain Management)

Degree of Pain	Clinical Procedures
None	Physical examination, restraint, radiography, bandage change
Mild	Suturing, debridement, fine-needle aspiration, needle core biopsy (nonopioid[a] ± acupuncture)
Moderate	Abdominal exploratory, skin tumor removal, liver biopsy, laparoscopy, thoracoscopy (nonopioid ± acupuncture + opioids [low-dose] ± anxiolytics)
Severe	Hemipelvectomy, limb-sparing surgery, thoracotomy, chest wall excision, limb amputation, ear canal ablation (nonopioid ± acupuncture + opioids [dose escalation, different route of administration] ± anxiolytics + other palliative procedures [e.g., radiation, surgery])

[a]NSAIDs and acetaminophen. Use with caution in patients with renal disease.

hyperexcitable, small indoor pets may be more expressive than sedate Labrador retrievers that are occasionally used for hunting. Keeping a careful drug history in these patients is critical, especially when many clinicians and nurses are involved in the care of each patient.

- **Duration of discomfort:** The use of a local analgesic agent may be all that is needed for short-term pain management; the same form of analgesia would be inappropriate for long-term chronic pain control.
- **Severity of discomfort:** Mild discomfort is clearly treated differently than severe discomfort (Tables 29-1 and 29-2).

Recent research has demonstrated that once pain is elicited, the pain response is magnified. Preventive therapy is therefore preferable to suppression of established pain. Premeditated, judicious use of analgesics is likely to increase patient comfort, decrease the need for hospitalization (and the associated costs), and reduce the amount of pain medication needed to achieve the same level of comfort.[2,4-6]

> **KEY POINT**
> *Cancer patients are often older and almost always have a metabolic or organ disorder that may influence their degree of, and sensitivity to, discomfort and their response to analgesics.*

The management of pain begins with high-quality, compassionate care by every member of the veterinary health care team. Careful nursing, gentle handling, and provision of a comfortable and relaxing environment are of great benefit to dogs. Local anesthesia should be employed to alleviate discomfort, and systemic analgesia should be used when local analgesia may be insufficient.

SELECTION OF MEDICATION TO MANAGE PAIN[5]

Effective selection of analgesics depends on consideration of their mechanism of action, potency, duration of efficacy, effect on the CNS, antiinflammatory effects, toxicity, metabolism, drug interactions, and price. Table 29-3 lists some selected analgesics and their dosing recommendations. The best practitioners gain experience with a set number of drugs, allowing them to prescribe maximum

> **KEY POINT**
> *Effective selection of analgesics can only be accomplished by considering their mechanism of action, potency, duration of efficacy, effect on the CNS, antiinflammatory effects, toxicity, metabolism, drug interactions, and price.*

pain control. They educate their clients about realistic expectations as well as the benefits, deficiencies, and toxicoses of different pain therapies. They also begin analgesics before the onset of pain and then continually change therapy to meet the pet's needs throughout the course of the disease and its therapy.

Nonopioids

Nonopioids, including NSAIDs (e.g., carprofen, etodolac, deracoxib, ketoprofen, piroxicam, meloxicam), provide mild to moderate antiinflammatory and analgesic effects. The older, nonspecific NSAIDs, such as aspirin, ibuprofen, ketoprofen, and piroxicam, may be associated with a greater risk for side effects because they inhibit two cyclooxygenase (COX) enzymes, COX-1 and COX-2. Inhibition of COX-1 can result in serious side effects such as gastrointestinal distress and perforation. However, these drugs are relatively simple to obtain, and their nonselective COX inhibition exerts central analgesic and peripheral antiinflammatory effects that make them useful in treating pain associated with intrathoracic and intraabdominal masses and bony metastases.

The newer NSAIDs, such as carprofen, etodolac, and deracoxib, primarily inhibit the COX-2 enzyme and are often associated with fewer side effects. Regardless, liver and renal function should be evaluated periodically in all animals receiving these drugs. Drugs such as misoprostol are concurrently prescribed by some clinicians to reduce the risk for toxicity to the gastrointestinal tract. Acetaminophen, which is believed to block the newly identified COX-3 enzyme, is related to NSAIDs but is not antiinflammatory; however, it is effective for treating discomfort without the side effects usually associated with NSAIDs. Newer drugs may inhibit only the COX-3 enzyme, resulting in fewer adverse effects.

α_2-Agonists

α_2-Agonists (e.g., clonidine, romifidine, medetomidine, xylazine) provide good to excellent analgesia with moderate to significant sedation and depression. Their short duration of action and tendency to reduce cardiac output and tissue oxygenation may make them an unwise choice for some frail or infirm patients. When combined with an opioid, they can enhance the analgesic effects of the opioid.

Opioids

Opioids (e.g., sustained-release morphine, fentanyl, oxymorphone, codeine) can result in excellent analgesia with low to moderate behavioral changes, such as depression. These drugs are the most predictable, effective analgesics for use in cancer patients. They can be administered orally, subcutaneously, intramuscularly, intravenously, or transdermally, but the efficacy of oral therapy has yet to be clearly documented. As the severity of discomfort increases, the dosage of the opiates can be increased. Toxicities can include bradycardia, diarrhea, vomiting, constipation, and sedation, although careful dosing can mitigate any problems.

Oral Morphine

Oral morphine is most commonly used for long-term cancer pain management. Morphine is a natural opioid agonist. On rare occasions, it may produce depression and seda-

> **KEY POINT**
>
> *Oral morphine, a common natural opioid agonist, is used for long-term cancer pain management. It may rarely produce depression and sedation or an initial excitement manifested by panting, salivation, nausea, vomiting, urination, defecation, and hypotension.*

tion or an initial excitement manifested by panting, salivation, nausea, vomiting, urination, defecation, and hypotension when administered to dogs. These reactions arise from activation of the chemoreceptor trigger zone, vagal stimulation, and histamine release.

Oxymorphone

Oxymorphone is a semisynthetic opioid agonist with analgesic properties that are approximately 10 times more potent than those of morphine; its adverse effects on the res-

Table 29-3 **Selected Analgesics**

Drug	Dosing Regimen
Opioid Agonists	
Fentanyl	2–5 µg/kg IV bolus before CRI
Postoperative	2–5 µg/kg/hr CRI for the duration of infusion
Operative	10–45 µg/kg/hr CRI for the duration of infusion
Patch	2–3 mg/kg/hr topical application; replace q3–5d
Hydromorphone	0.05–0.2 mg/kg IV, SC, or IM q2–6h
Meperidine	3–5 mg/kg SC or IM q1–2h
Methadone	1–1.5 mg/kg IV, SC, or IM once
Morphine	0.5–2 mg/kg PO, IM, or SC q2–4h
Morphine, sustained-release	2–5 mg/kg PO q1–4h
Oxymorphone	0.05–0.4 mg/kg IV, SC, or IM q2–4h
Remifentanil	4–10 µg/kg IV bolus before CRI q2–6h
Postoperative	4–10 µg/kg/hr CRI for the duration of infusion
Operative	20–60 µg/kg/hr CRI for the duration of infusion
Sufentanyl	5 µg/kg IV bolus before CRI q2–6h
Postoperative	0.1 µg/kg/hr CRI for the duration of infusion
Opioid Agonist–Antagonists	
Buprenorphine	0.005–0.02 mg/kg IV, IM, or SC q8–12h
Butorphanol	0.1–0.4 mg/kg IV, IM, or SC q1–4h or 0.5–2 mg/kg PO q6–8h
Nalbuphine	0.5–1 mg/kg IV, IM, or SC q4h
Pentazocine	1–3 mg/kg IV, IM, or SC q2–4h
NSAIDs	
Carprofen	2.2 mg/kg PO q12h
Deracoxib	1–2 mg/kg PO q24h
Etodolac	10–15 mg/kg PO q12h
Ketoprofen	1–2 mg/kg IV, IM, or SC q24h or 1 mg/kg PO q24h
Meloxicam	0.1–0.2 mg/kg IV, IM, or SC q24h; 0.1 mg/kg PO q24h
Piroxicam	0.3 mg/kg PO q24–48h
Tolfenamic acid	4 mg/kg PO or SC q24h for 3 days on, 4 days off
α_2-Agonists	
Medetomidine	5–10 µg/kg IM or SC once or 1–4 µg/kg IV once
Romifidine	10–20 µg/kg IM or SC once
Xylazine	0.2–0.5 mg/kg PO q12h

(Table continues)

Table 29-3 (continued)

Drug	Dosing Regimen
Local Anesthetics	
Bupivacaine	2 mg/4.5 kg as local nerve blocks q2–4h; intrapleural administration as needed
Lidocaine	1.5 mg/kg intrapleurally before bupivacaine q1–1.5h
Mepivacaine	1 mg/kg SC q1.5–2.5h
Ropivacaine	1 mg/kg SC q1.5–2.5h
Other Drugs	
Acetaminophen (paracetamol)	5–10 mg/kg PO q12h
Amantidine	3–5 mg/kg PO q24h
Amitriptyline	1–4 mg/kg PO q24h
Glucosamine, chondroitin	13–15 mg/kg PO q24h
Ketamine	0.5–1 µg/kg IM q30min or 1 µg/kg/min CRI for the duration of infusion and postinfusion
Pamidronate	1 mg/kg slow IV as needed q3–6wk with diuresis
Tramadol	2–4 mg/kg PO q6–8h

piratory, cardiovascular, and gastrointestinal systems are less pronounced. Oxymorphone is indicated for moderate to severe visceral or somatic pain. Lower doses are used for IV administration. When used alone, however, oxymorphone may result in excitement or hyperalgesia.[2,3,5] Diazepam given concurrently with oxymorphone may help reduce these side effects.

> **KEY POINT**
> *A transdermal analgesic patch system provides constant pain relief throughout the dosing period and obviates the need for constant reevaluation of schedules and dosing.*

Fentanyl

Fentanyl is an effective analgesic that can be given IM, SC, or IV as a preanesthetic. It can be administered via an IV bolus, CRI, or transdermal patch. Fentanyl can cause respiratory depression, bradycardia, and somnolence at higher dosages. It can also prolong return to normal body temperature during recovery from anesthesia. Fentanyl-impregnated transdermal patches (25, 75, and 100 µg/hr) reliably release a controlled amount of fentanyl over a 72-hour period (Figure 29-1). The patches maintain adequate blood levels of fentanyl for 72 hours, but therapeutic levels are not attained for 12 to 24 hours; thus, patches may be most effective when used in conjunction with other analgesics or in addition to fentanyl CRI during surgery or other painful procedures.

Opioid Antagonists

Opioid antagonists (e.g., butorphanol) are generally not as effective as opioids. Butorphanol is a synthetic opioid agonist–antagonist that has five times the analgesic potency of morphine, but its duration of analgesia is short (approximately 1 to 4 hours). Adverse effects such as nausea and vomiting are rare, but the drug can induce sedation. Higher dosages are needed for somatic pain, and analgesia lasts only about 2 to 4 hours. IV butorphanol

> **KEY POINT**
> *Butorphanol will reduce or eliminate the analgesic potential of opiates such as fentanyl.*

may result in transient hypotension or bradycardia.[2,3,5] Because butorphanol possesses antagonist properties, it reverses the effects of narcotics. Therefore, butorphanol must not be given within 12 hours of any pre- or intraoperatively administered narcotics. Buprenorphine HCl, an agonist–antagonist, can reverse opioid-induced respiratory depression while maintaining analgesia.

Ketamine

Ketamine is an *N*-methyl-D-aspartate (NMDA) receptor antagonist that is important in the wind-up phenomenon, in which pain makes certain nerve receptors more sensitive to subsequent impulses, which will be perceived as a greater degree of discomfort than before. When the drug is administered at microdosages during and up to 24 hours after a painful procedure, the need for additional analgesics is reduced and pain control maximized with few, if any, behavioral or cardiovascular effects. Typically, a bolus of 0.5 mg/kg IV is administered, followed by a CRI of 2 µg/kg/min for the first 24 hours after surgery. For simplicity, if an infusion pump is not available, 60 mg of ketamine (0.6 ml) can be mixed in a 1-L bag of crystalloids. When the fluid is administered at a drip rate of 10 ml/kg/hr, the

> **KEY POINT**
> *Ketamine, an NMDA-receptor antagonist that is important in the wind-up phenomenon, is commonly used in microdosages to reduce discomfort and pain and the subsequent need for other analgesics.*

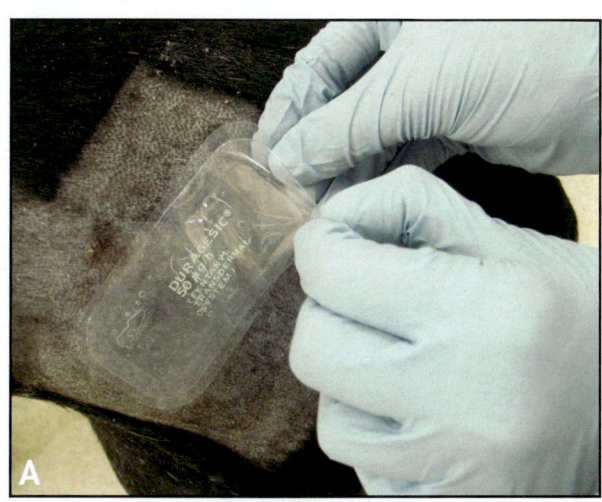 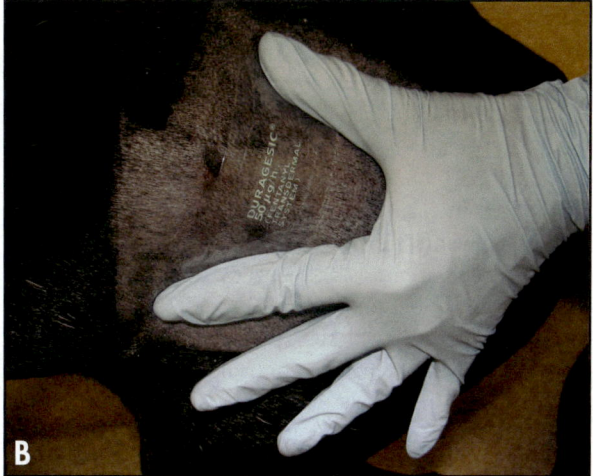

Figure 29-1. *Use of the fentanyl patch. The backing of the transdermal fentanyl patch is removed (**A**), and the patch is placed on a flat, hairless area of skin where it is unlikely to be removed by the dog (**B**). Latex rubber gloves should be worn when these patches are handled. The patches are capable of delivering the analgesic over a 72-hour period.*

ketamine is delivered at 10 µg/kg/min. To decrease the dosage to 2 µg/kg/min, the fluid rate should be reduced to 2 ml/kg/hr.

Tranquilizers

Tranquilizers (e.g., acepromazine, diazepam, midazolam) do not provide analgesia, but their use in the management of canine cancer patients can be profound because fear, apprehension, and anxiety may magnify the response to pain. To avoid excitation, diazepam and midazolam should only be administered with an opioid in alert patients.

Tricyclic Antidepressants

Tricyclic antidepressants (e.g., amitriptyline, imipramine) have antihistamine effects. They block the reuptake of serotonin and norepinephrine to the CNS. They are used at very low dosages to induce analgesic effects and enhance the analgesic effects of opiates.

Radiation

Palliative radiation is commonly used to reduce discomfort associated with some tumors, especially those involving the skeletal system. When combined with low-dosage chemotherapy (doxorubicin or cisplatin), the enhanced effect may be prolonged. Generally, one-third of the treated patients have good to excellent results, one-third have transient adequate responses, and one-third have no noticeable improvement in pain control.

Strontium-89, when administered intravenously, is taken up in places of active bone turnover. This uptake results in the local release of high quantities of radiation, with enhanced comfort in approximately 50% of cases.

Bisphosphonates

Bisphosphonates are being used more commonly in veterinary medicine to treat primary or metastatic bone disease. Pamidronate and alendronate given every 3 to 6 weeks have been associated with enhanced comfort and reossification of lytic sites associated with osteosarcoma, mammary cancer, prostate cancer, and other malignant processes.

Acupuncture

Acupuncture is used to treat many kinds of pain due to cancer or cancer therapy (e.g., surgery, radiation therapy). It is often used in concert with pharmacologic agents to reduce their dosage and enhance overall wellness. The effect of acupuncture appears to be mediated through opioids. Stimulation of acupuncture points induces the release of endogenous opioids. Opioid antagonists block acupuncture analgesia. Acupuncture analgesia is transferable with cerebrospinal fluid transfer. In human subjects, acupuncture analgesia appears to be most effective against the emotional aspects of pain.[6] Acupuncture can also be helpful in reducing nausea associated with chemotherapy, anesthesia, and the administration of certain antibiotics.

> *Bisphosphonates such as pamidronate and alendronate are given every 3 to 6 weeks to enhance comfort and to reossify lytic bone sites associated with osteosarcoma and bone metastases from mammary cancer, prostatic carcinoma, and multiple myeloma.*

Local Anesthesia: Nerve Blocks

Local anesthetic agents (e.g., lidocaine, bupivacaine) can be injected to block sensory or motor nerve fibers. Lidocaine HCl (2%) administered near an incision provides regional analgesia for about 1 hour. Bupivacaine HCl (0.75%) can be given to provide 6 to 10 hours of regional analgesia for periincisional pain. Lidocaine can be administered at or near intercostal nerves proximal to a thoracotomy incision to reduce postsurgical pain. This agent is also frequently administered into the pleural cavity before bupivacaine administration to decrease discomfort associated with thoracotomy. Lidocaine or bupivacaine can be used as a maxillary or mandibular nerve block for oral surgery or in the brachial plexus nerve roots before sectioning during forelimb amputation. Lidocaine can also be administered as a CRI to enhance the analgesic effect of other drugs while causing depression and anesthesia.

The specific nerve blocks commonly used to treat the cancer patient are the intercostal, infraorbital, and mandibular nerve blocks.

Intercostal Nerve Block

The intercostal nerve block (Figure 29-2) can be used to prevent or treat discomfort in the chest and cranial abdomen, including the area of the pancreas[1]:

- Attach a 22-gauge butterfly catheter to extension tubing. Advance the needle through the surgically prepared skin in each intercostal space from three ribs in front of to three ribs behind the area in question (Figure 29-2A; green dots). The optimal intercostal area is just caudal to the rib, where the nerves are located (Figure 29-2B).
- Perform aspiration to ensure there is no introduction of lidocaine or bupivacaine IV.
- Administer lidocaine (<1.5 mg/kg). The lidocaine can cause short-term discomfort upon injection because of its acidic pH. Some practitioners add injectable bicarbonate to the lidocaine (volume:volume ratio of bicarbonate:lidocaine = 25%:75%) to enhance comfort. After the lidocaine is injected, bupivacaine (<1.5 mg/kg) is injected. If injected first, bupivacaine can result in discomfort that may last for at least 15 minutes due to the slow onset of local anesthetic effects. Some practitioners combine the lidocaine and bupivacaine in one syringe. These drugs can also be administered through a chest tube to enhance comfort in the recovery period after a thoracotomy.
- This block can be repeated every 3 to 6 hours.

Infraorbital Block

Infraorbital nerve blocks (Figure 29-3) are used for analgesia to the rostral maxilla and nearby lip, nose, nasal cavity, and skin ventral to the infraorbital foramen. The infraorbital

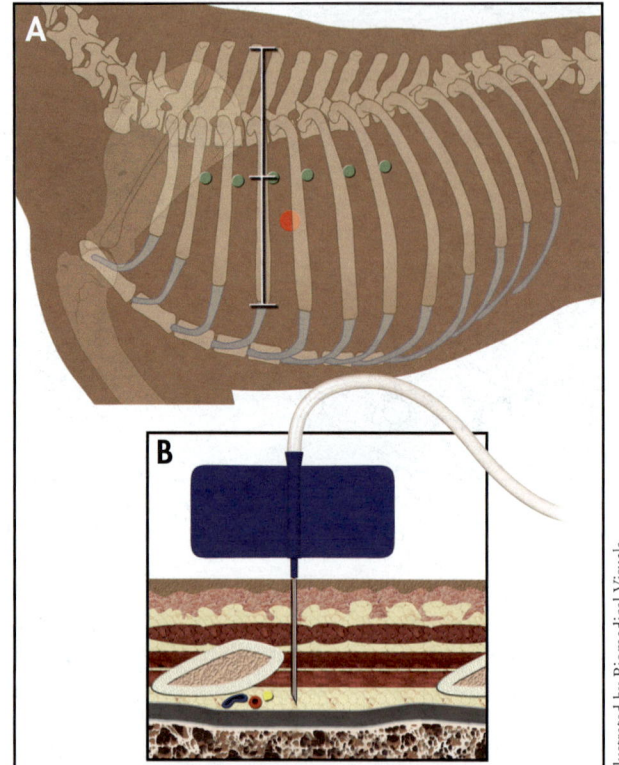

Figure 29-2. *An intercostal nerve block is very helpful in providing analgesia during thoracotomies and chest wall resections. See text for details on how to perform this block.*

foramen is palpated rostrally and distally to the medial canthus of either eye. A 25-gauge, 2.5-cm needle is inserted through the surgically prepared skin and into the foramen. The attached syringe is aspirated for blood, and a small (<1 ml) amount of lidocaine with or without bupivacaine is injected, ideally before any biopsy or surgical procedures.

Mandibular Nerve Block

The mandibular nerve block (Figure 29-4) is used to provide analgesia of the skin and mucosa at or near the incisor, canine, premolar, and molar teeth on the side to be injected. This is ideal for surgery to any of this tissue, including mandibulectomy and regional biopsies or tooth extractions.

- Clip and prepare the skin overlying the site to be blocked (medial to the mandible) as if for surgery. Insert a gloved hand into the mouth, and palpate the mucosa over the caudal and medial aspect of the mandible under the cheek mucosa for the mandibular nerve, which can feel like a submucosal thickening or "fibrous band."
- Direct the needle and attached syringe through the skin on the ventromedial aspect of the caudal mandible as indicated by the gloved hand. Use the inserted finger over the nerve to guide the needle placement within the tissue

next to the nerve. Aspirate the syringe for blood; if none is seen, inject the local anesthetic at a quantity that should not exceed 1 ml.

ROUTES OF ADMINISTRATION[1-5]

The efficacy of a drug or drug combination can be enhanced by using the optimal route of administration. As a general rule, oral analgesics can be effective for mild to moderate discomfort. However, when the degree of discomfort increases, efficacy can be increased by administering the same or related drugs IM, SC, or IV. The efficacy can be improved even further by giving the same drug epidurally. A brief discussion of the routes of administration follows:

- **Oral administration** is the easiest and cheapest route and can be performed on an outpatient basis, but it is associated with the lowest level of compliance or efficacy. NSAIDs are most often administered via this route; however, orally administered codeine, morphine, and sustained-release morphine are also effective for mild to moderate pain.
- **IV, IM, and SC administration** of drugs is associated with the most predictable efficacy. The IV CRI technique is optimal. However, this route cannot easily be used in an outpatient setting.
- **Epidural or subarachnoid drug therapy** can result in good to excellent long-term analgesia. Sterile, preservative-free drugs that have been used in this manner include opiates, NSAIDs, ketamine, α_2-agonists, and local anesthetic agents. However, this therapy cannot be performed on an outpatient basis.
- **Transdermal administration** of fentanyl and clonidine, or topical treatment with drugs such as lidocaine and eutectic mixture of local anesthetics (EMLA) cream, can result in good long-term pain management but is subject to many variables, such as rate of absorption and body condition. Transdermal pain management can be performed as outpatient therapy.
- **Transmucosal therapy** with drugs such as codeine, morphine, and buprenorphine may be very helpful in controlling mild discomfort.
- **Local nerve blocks** deliver local anesthetics precisely and directly to the anatomic site of choice with reduced toxicity.

> **KEY POINT**
> *Oral administration of analgesics is the easiest and cheapest route of administration and can be performed on an outpatient basis but is probably associated with the lowest level of compliance or efficacy.*

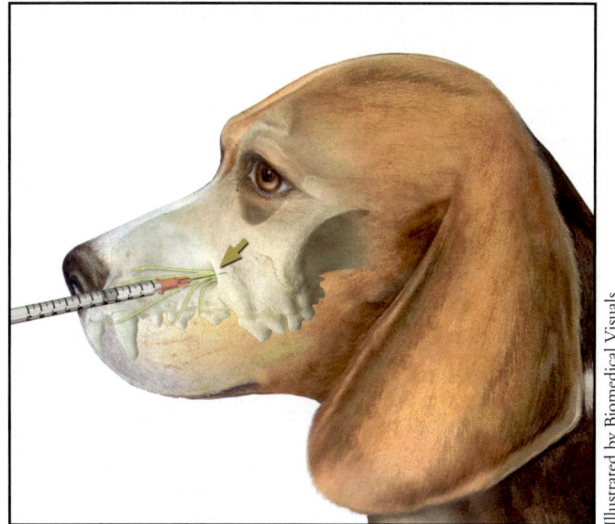

Figure 29-3. *An infraorbital block is an excellent method to provide good-quality analgesia to the rostral maxilla and nearby lip, nose, nasal cavity, and skin ventral to the infraorbital foramen (yellow arrow). See text for details on how to perform this block.*

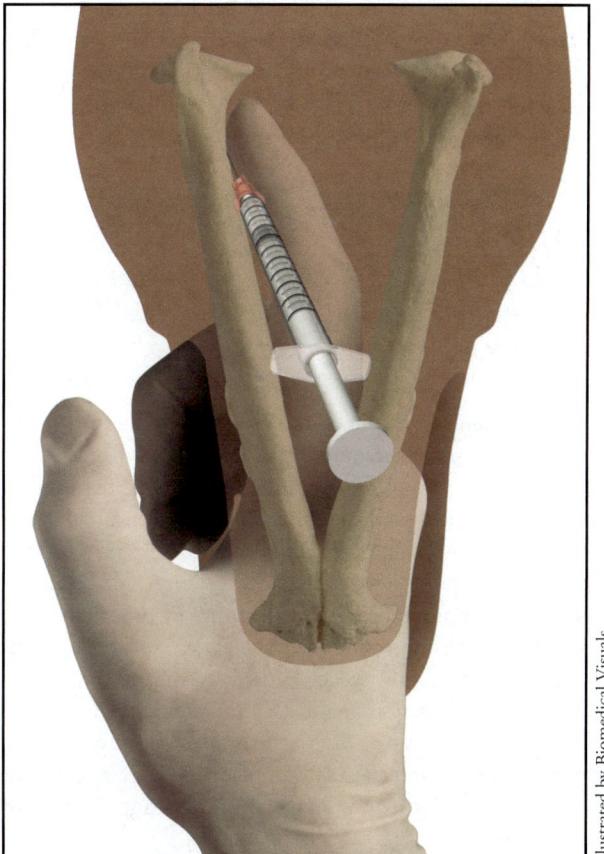

Figure 29-4. *Mandibular nerve blocks are very helpful in providing analgesia to the skin and mucosa at or near the incisor, canine, premolar, and molar teeth on the side to be injected. See text for details on how to perform this block.*

Preventing and Treating Pain and Discomfort[1]

The best way to manage pain is to prevent it. When prevention is not possible, discomfort and pain must be treated appropriately and the treatment adjusted continually as the disease or therapy progresses. Combinations of drugs are most effective and are less likely to result in side effects. Adequate pain therapy can only be achieved by ensuring that the entire team is highly knowledgeable about pain and all the approaches that can be employed to manage discomfort. This includes the client, who is most intimately aware of the patient's quality of life and behavior patterns. The client's perception of the animal's quality of life should be trusted and believed above all.

Pain may be best prevented and treated by dividing it into the categories of acute and chronic pain. In most species, severity is far more important than duration of pain with regard to the "memory" of pain: The severity of discomfort at any point in time will be repeated to the same degree when the same stimulus is applied subsequently. It is important to realize that pain is also increased through the *wind-up phenomenon*, defined as the enhanced perception of pain that occurs after the patient has experienced constant pain. This constant pain results in enhanced sensitivity to subsequent discomfort. Preventive analgesia helps avoid both the memory of pain and the wind-up phenomenon.

> **KEY POINT**
> *The best way to manage pain is to prevent it. When prevention is not possible, discomfort and pain must be treated appropriately and the treatment adjusted continually as the disease or treatment progresses.*

Acute pain can be due to the cancer itself, the treatment, or a diagnostic procedure. If discomfort is likely to be inflicted, then a preemptive, immediate, and poststimulus plan must be designed and implemented. To ensure that the plan is effective, the practitioner must determine whether the pain to be inflicted is likely to be mild, moderate, or severe and appropriately select the drugs or procedures that are likely to be effective to meet the patient's possible needs.

Chronic pain can also be caused by the cancer (e.g., a metastatic bone lesion in a dog with mammary adenocarcinoma) or, possibly, by a diagnostic or therapeutic procedure, such as chronic infection and implant, plate or screw loosening from limb-sparing surgery. Unrelenting pain from either cause can last for weeks or months.

MILD PAIN[1-3,5]

The treatment of mild pain must begin with eliminating the underlying cause and providing general compassionate care, including a comfortable environment, appropriate bedding, and effective bandaging, if indicated. Dogs respond well to comforting, petting, and talking. This is often followed with administration of an oral NSAID (e.g., carprofen, deracoxib, etodolac, aspirin, piroxicam, meloxicam, ketoprofen) and, if indicated, local nerve blocks, acupuncture, or both. Nonopioids may be used provided that renal and hepatic functions are normal and there is no evidence of gastric inflammation. If NSAIDs are ineffective, an agent from one of the other categories of analgesics should be selected based on the patient's response.

> **KEY POINT**
> *The treatment of mild pain must begin with eliminating the underlying cause and providing general compassionate care, including a comfortable environment, appropriate bedding, and effective bandaging, if indicated.*

Therapy for mild pain can include the use of a local lidocaine or bupivacaine nerve block to reduce the local acute discomfort from a needle-core biopsy. An oral NSAID can be given before and after the procedure to manage the relatively minor pain in the hours or few days that follow. If apprehension is an issue, a tranquilizer such as acepromazine can be used at the time of the procedure.

MODERATE PAIN[1-3,5]

Moderate pain can be treated by eliminating the cause while providing compassionate care, local analgesia, acupuncture when possible, and nonopioids, including NSAIDs (e.g., carprofen, etodolac, deracoxib, piroxicam, meloxicam, ketoprofen), in judicious combination with opiates. As with all analgesics, the parenteral, continuous administration of these drugs usually results in a more optimal effect than oral therapy. CRI of fentanyl or microdose ketamine is an excellent example. Transdermal delivery of drugs such as fentanyl can provide a background of analgesia via a continuous-release delivery system; however, this alone is rarely adequate to prevent perioperative or procedural discomfort. When these therapies are not adequate, an α_2-adrenergic agonist, opioid agonist–antagonist, anxiolytic, or tricyclic antidepressant can be considered.

When an acutely painful procedure is being considered, drugs for cancer patients are often divided into pre-, peri-, and postoperative analgesics.[1,3] Preoperative analgesics often include an opiate such as morphine with or without acepromazine to calm the patient and to relieve anxiety. Atropine or glycopyrrolate is often administered to prevent

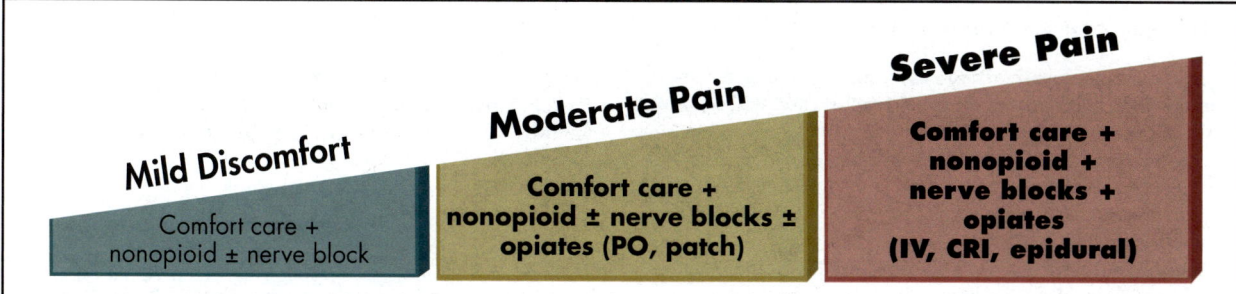

Figure 29-5. *General approach to the management of pain in dogs with cancer.*

bradycardia associated with the opiate. Nerve blocks are employed when possible. Perioperative therapy is often accomplished by adding fentanyl as a continuous IV infusion. This can decrease the need for additional analgesia and may be combined with microdose ketamine to prevent the wind-up phenomenon. Pain management in the immediate postoperative period is optimal when local nerve blocks are used in combination with fentanyl and microdose ketamine. Later, acepromazine, diazepam, or midazolam can be used to reduce dysphoria. See the box on this page for examples of pre-, peri-, and postoperative analgesia to treat moderate pain.

> **KEY POINT**
>
> *Moderate pain can be treated by eliminating the cause while providing compassionate care, local analgesia, acupuncture (when possible), and nonopioids, including NSAIDs (e.g., carprofen, etodolac, deracoxib, piroxicam, meloxicam, ketoprofen), in judicious combination with opiates.*

SEVERE PAIN[1,2,6]

Therapy for moderate to severe pain can be emotionally and physically difficult for the entire veterinary health care team and the family. Everyone should be aware of the difficulty associated with emotional and physical stress and be supported to prevent compassion fatigue (see Chapter 8).

Therapy for severe pain is as outlined for moderate pain (see above); however, the dosages of certain drugs, notably the opiates, are continually adjusted to a balance between maximum efficacy and minimal toxicity. The efficacy of drugs can be maximized by switching to more effective routes of administration such as epidural morphine and CRI of fentanyl. When drugs are combined, efficacy is often enhanced and reduction of dosages of individual drugs may be possible; however, the patient must be monitored for additive toxicity. Palliative procedures such as the

---

Treatment of Moderate Pain Associated with Invasive Procedures

Indication: Simple, minimally painful, short-term procedure (e.g., needle-core biopsy of tumor, small incisional biopsy)
- **Preemptive analgesia:** Oxymorphine (0.05–0.1 mg/kg SC), acepromazine (0.02–0.04 mg/kg SC), and atropine (0.04 mg/kg SC)
- **Anesthesia (as indicated):** Propofol or thiopental induction followed by inhalant anesthesia
- **Postoperative analgesia:** Ketoprofen 2.2 mg/kg SC

Indication: Simple, moderately painful, short-term procedure (e.g., nasal biopsy or bone biopsy in a dog with normal organ and cardiovascular function)
- **Preemptive analgesia:** Oxymorphine (0.05–0.1 mg/kg SC) and atropine (0.02–0.04 mg/kg SC)
- **Anesthesia (as indicated):** Propofol or thiopental induction followed by inhalant anesthesia; xylazine 0.1 mg/kg IV administered just before biopsy to enhance analgesia
- **Postoperative analgesia:** Ketoprofen 2.2 mg/kg SC

Indication: Relatively short, simple procedure (e.g., thoracoscopy, laparoscopy, abdominal exploratory, skin biopsy)
- **Preemptive analgesia:** Morphine (1 mg/kg SC), acepromazine (0.02 mg/kg SC), and atropine (0.04 mg/kg SC) with oral NSAID pre- and postoperatively (ensure adequate hydration and renal function)
- **Anesthesia (as indicated):** Propofol or thiopental induction followed by inhalant anesthesia
- **Postoperative analgesia (one of the following):**
  — Carprofen 4 mg/kg SC
  — Ketoprofen 2 mg/kg SC
  — Morphine 0.5–1 mg/kg SC as needed q4–6h
  — Nalbuphine 1 mg/kg SC as needed q4–6h
- **Home analgesia (one of the following):**
  — Morphine 0.5 mg/kg PO tid or qid
  — Transdermal fentanyl (2–3 mg/kg/hr); may be administered with or without one of the following: ketoprofen 1 mg/kg PO, piroxicam 0.3 mg/kg PO q24–48h, meloxicam 0.1 mg/kg PO q24h, carprofen 2.2 mg/kg PO q12h, etodolac 10–15 mg/kg PO q12h

> **Treatment of Severe Pain Associated with Invasive Procedures**
>
> **Indication:** Procedure thought to cause moderate to severe discomfort (e.g., maxillectomy, hemipelvectomy, chest wall resection)
> - **Preemptive analgesia:** Morphine (1 mg/kg SC) and acepromazine (0.02 mg/kg SC) with nerve block, if appropriate, to the local area of concern; ketamine microdose CRI at 10 µg/kg/min after an IV bolus of ketamine (0.5 mg/kg) can reduce the need for analgesics postoperatively
> - **Anesthesia (as indicated):** Propofol or thiopental induction followed by inhalant anesthesia
> - **Postoperative analgesia:** Fentanyl bolus (2 mg/kg IV) followed by fentanyl infusion 3–5 µg/kg/hr IV CRI by syringe pump or IV pump; bupivacaine nerve block and acupuncture
> - **Home analgesia (one of the following):**
>   — Morphine 0.5 mg/kg PO tid or qid
>   — Transdermal fentanyl (2–3 mg/kg/hr); may be administered with or without one of the following: ketoprofen 1 mg/kg PO, piroxicam 0.3 mg/kg PO q24–48h, meloxicam 0.1 mg/kg PO q24h, deracoxib 3–4 mg/day PO for 7 days then 1–2 mg/kg long-term, carprofen 2.2 mg/kg PO q12h, etodolac 10–15 mg/kg PO q12h
>
> **Indication:** Procedure thought to cause severe discomfort (e.g., mandibulectomy, laminectomy in combination with hemipelvectomy)
> - **Preemptive analgesia:** Hydromorphone (2 mg/kg SC) and atropine (0.04 mg/kg SC) with nerve block, if appropriate, to local area (e.g., infraorbital block for maxillectomy)
> - **Anesthesia (as indicated):** Propofol or thiopental induction followed by inhalant anesthesia
> - **Postoperative analgesia:** Fentanyl bolus (0.2 mg/kg SC) followed by fentanyl infusion 3–5 µg/kg/hr IV CRI by syringe pump or IV pump; bupivacaine nerve block
> - **Home analgesia (one of the following):**
>   — Morphine 0.5 mg/kg PO tid or qid
>   — Transdermal fentanyl (2–3 mg/kg/hr); may be administered with or without one of the following: ketoprofen 1 mg/kg PO, piroxicam 0.3 mg/kg PO q24–48h, meloxicam 0.1 mg/kg PO q24h, carprofen 2.2 mg/kg PO q12h, deracoxib 3–4 mg/day PO for 7 days then 1–2 mg/kg long term, etodolac 10–15 mg/kg PO q12h
>
> **Indication:** Procedure thought to cause severe discomfort (e.g., rear-limb amputation, hemipelvectomy)
> - **Preemptive analgesia:** Morphine (1 mg/kg SC) and atropine (0.04 mg/kg SC) with bupivacaine epidural
> - **Anesthesia (as indicated):** Propofol or thiopental induction followed by inhalant anesthesia
> - **Postoperative analgesia:** Fentanyl bolus (0.2 mg/kg SC) followed by fentanyl infusion 3–5 µg/kg/hr IV CRI by syringe pump or IV pump; bupivacaine nerve block
> - **Home analgesia:** Sustained-release morphine (0.5 mg/kg PO tid); may be administered with or without one of the following: ketoprofen 1 mg/kg PO, piroxicam 0.3 mg/kg PO q24–48h, meloxicam 0.1 mg/kg PO q24h, carprofen 2.2 mg/kg PO q12h, deracoxib 3–4 mg/day PO for 7 days then 1–2 mg/kg long term, etodolac 10–15 mg/kg PO q12h

KEY POINT

Therapy for moderate to severe pain can be difficult emotionally and physically for the entire veterinary health care team and the family and is as outlined for moderate pain. The dosages of certain drugs, notably the opiates, are continually adjusted to a balance between maximum efficacy and minimal toxicity.

use of radiation therapy at sites of bone pain can be profoundly beneficial, as can the IV infusion of bisphosphonates. When the degree of discomfort increases, dosages can be escalated for opiates with no ceiling effect (e.g., morphine); changing the route of analgesic administration (e.g., switching from SC to IV administration or to epidural therapy) may also be effective. As with moderate discomfort, sustained-release fentanyl patches, which are applied to the skin and slowly release the analgesic over 72 hours, may be helpful. See the box on this page for examples of pre-, peri-, and postoperative analgesia to treat severe pain.

Summary

Pain therapy is one of the most important aspects of cancer therapy, not only for the patient and the client but also for the entire veterinary health care team. Well-thought-out therapeutic approaches are key to the anticipation and prevention of pain (Figure 29-5). It is the responsibility of the veterinary health care team to stay up-to-date on the many current and emerging pain therapies and to gain experience in the optimal management of canine cancer patients.

REFERENCES

1. Gaynor JS, Muir WS (eds): *Handbook of Veterinary Pain Management.* St. Louis, Mosby, 2002 pp 13–447.
2. Lascelles BD: Relief of chronic cancer pain, in Dobson JM, Lascelles BD (eds): *BSAVA Manual of Canine and Feline Oncology,* ed 2. Gloucester, England. British Small Animal Veterinary Association, 2003, pp 137–151.
3. Tranquilli WK, Grimm KA, Lamont LA (eds): *Pain Management for the Small Animal Practitioner.* Jackson, WY, Teton NewMedia, 2000, pp 13–69.
4. Hendrix PK, Hansen B: Acute pain management, in Bonagura JD (ed): *Current Veterinary Therapy XIII: Small Animal Practice.* Philadelphia, WB Saunders, 2000, pp 57–61.
5. Hellyer PW, Gaynor JS: Acute postsurgical pain in dogs and cats. *Compend Contin Educ Pract Vet* 20:140–153, 1998.
6. Filshie J, Redman D: Acupuncture and malignant pain problems. *Eur J Surg Oncol* 11(4):389–394, 1985.

PREVENTION AND TREATMENT OF NAUSEA AND VOMITING

Gregory K. Ogilvie and Antony S. Moore

CLINICAL BRIEFING

Emetic potential	• Nausea and vomiting associated with the administration of chemotherapy are much less common in dogs than in humans. — Cisplatin is an exception. — Small dogs are at greater risk for vomiting than larger dogs when given cisplatin. • Emesis primarily originates from the CTZ and the emetic center. • Acute vomiting occurs shortly after the administration of chemotherapy. • Delayed vomiting may occur days to weeks after treatment.
Prevention	• When possible, anticipate nausea and vomiting by pretreating with antiemetics, especially in patients with a history of nausea and those receiving highly emetogenic chemotherapy. • In general, metoclopramide or a serotonin antagonist should be dispensed to each client for home care. • It may be good practice to have clients not feed patients before they are to receive chemotherapy.
Self-limiting vomiting	• Therapy: Treat with metoclopramide or oral serotonin antagonist. • Correct underlying cause. • Do not feed by mouth until vomiting ceases for 12 to 24 hours. • Initiate small amounts of water, then a bland, low-fat diet. • Monitor hydration and electrolytes.
Life-threatening vomiting	• Therapy: Follow the same protocol as for self-limiting vomiting, except administer IV fluids (maintenance needs + hydration deficits + losses) and correct electrolyte and pH abnormalities (e.g., serum potassium). — In addition, give antiemetics (e.g., metoclopramide) parenterally. — Concurrently administer serotonin antagonists such as ondansetron or dolasetron.

Nausea and vomiting are unacceptable consequences of cancer and cancer therapy.[1–5] They are common in humans: Combination chemotherapy induces vomiting in 75% of human cancer patients.[1] These problems are much less common in dogs. Risk factors for vomiting include administration of highly emetogenic chemotherapy, smaller patient size, repetitive administration of chemotherapy, and presence of underlying pathology in the gastrointestinal (GI) tract, such as dietary allergies.[2–5] Vomiting can lead to life-threatening problems, such as dehydration and metabolic imbalance, and wound dehiscence may occur after increased abdominal pressure. In addition, owners whose pets experience nausea and vomiting often get the impression that their pet is experiencing unnecessary toxicities, which may result in abandonment of life-saving treatment and subsequent euthanasia. Management of nausea and vomiting is important to improve the patient's quality of life, which subsequently can enhance response to therapy and increase survival time.

> **KEY POINT**
> *Nausea and vomiting are unacceptable consequences of cancer and cancer therapy.*

Chemotherapeutic Agents by Probability of Inducing Nausea or Vomiting[a]

Very Low	Low	Moderate	High	Very High
Chlorambucil	Mitoxantrone	Carboplatin	Dacarbazine	Cisplatin
Doxorubicin (liposomal)	Gemcitabine	Cyclophosphamide	Nitrogen mustard	Streptozocin
L-Asparaginase	Paclitaxel	Doxorubicin		
Vinblastine		Methotrexate		
Vinorelbine		Daunorubicin		
Steroids		Ifosfamide		
Bleomycin				

[a]To prevent emesis in patients taking drugs with very low to low emetic potential, administer metoclopramide as needed; for drugs with moderate emetic potential, administer metoclopramide preventively; and for drugs with high to very high emetic potential, administer a serotonin antagonist ± metoclopramide or butorphanol ± steroids preventively.

Mechanism of Vomiting

Tumor-induced vomiting may be caused by the presence of a tumor that physically obstructs the intestinal tract. Surgical resection of the tumor is the only solution to this clinical problem.

Chemotherapy may induce nausea and vomiting shortly after administration or as late as 5 to 10 days after administration. Chemotherapeutic agents differ in their emetic potential and in the length of time after administration that they cause emesis.[1-8] Unlike humans, animals rarely exhibit any evidence of nausea and vomiting at or shortly after the time drugs are administered, with the exception of dogs that receive cisplatin chemotherapy.[4,5]

The emetic potential of all chemotherapeutic drugs depends on the sensitivity of each patient as well as the route of administration and the dosage. Cisplatin may induce vomiting within 1 to 6 hours, whereas cyclophosphamide may induce vomiting within 4 to 12 hours. Doxorubicin may induce vomiting in a few patients 4 to 6 hours after treatment. All of these chemotherapeutic agents can induce vomiting 3 to 5 days after treatment because of damage to the GI tract. Drugs associated with low, moderate, and relatively high probabilities of vomiting are listed in the box on this page.

> **KEY POINT**
> *Acute nausea and vomiting are mediated by activation of serotonin type 3 receptors in the GI tract; therefore, serotonin receptor antagonists, such as ondansetron and dolasetron, are often effective.*

The mechanism of chemotherapy-induced vomiting is complex (Figure 30-1). The emetic center in the medulla coordinates vomiting and receives input from at least four sources: the chemoreceptor trigger zone (CTZ), peripheral receptors, the cerebral cortex, and the vestibular apparatus. The vestibular apparatus probably does not influence cancer- or chemotherapy-associated vomiting. The CTZ, located in the fourth ventricle of the medulla, is activated solely by chemical stimuli and plays an important role in chemotherapy-induced nausea and vomiting. Acute nausea and vomiting is mediated by the activation of serotonin (5-hydroxytryptamine) type 3 (5-HT-3) receptors in the GI tract.[1] Peripheral receptors can be triggered either directly by chemotherapeutic agents or indirectly by substances released by the agents' effects on other sites; these impulses arrive at the emetic center via the vagus nerve and other autonomic nerve afferents. Input from higher cognitive centers, a common source of vomiting in humans, is rarely identified in animals. The mechanism of delayed vomiting days to weeks after therapy is unknown. Pharmacologic intervention through any or all of these pathways is important in eliminating vomiting in patients with cancer.

> **KEY POINT**
> *Special attention should be focused on pretreating smaller patients, especially those that have vomited after a previous dosage of cisplatin, by administering drugs such as butorphanol.*

General Concepts of Emesis Therapy

Most chemotherapeutic agents are unlikely to induce vomiting in animals shortly after administration.[2-5] The exception is cisplatin, which is associated with brief, self-limiting vomiting within a few hours after treatment.[4,5] Moore and colleagues[5] demonstrated that butorphanol (0.4 mg/kg IM) at the end of cisplatin infusion was effective in reducing the incidence of cisplatin chemotherapy–induced vomiting from 90% to less than 20%. Another study[4] demonstrated that when vomiting occurred, it was almost always in smaller dogs. If an animal

> **KEY POINT**
> *When butorphanol was administered intramuscularly at the end of cisplatin infusion, the incidence of cisplatin chemotherapy–induced vomiting decreased from 90% to less than 20%.[5]*

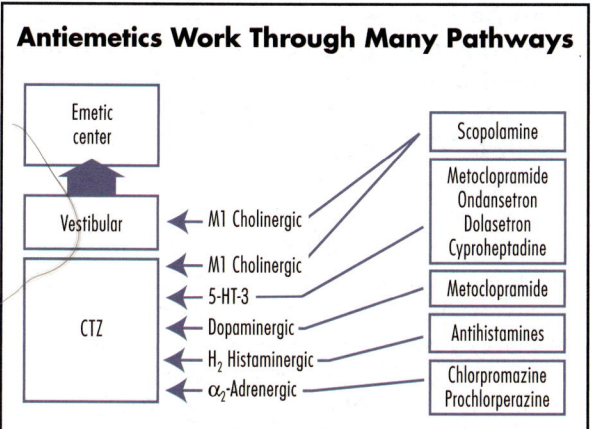

Figure 30-1. Vomiting results from a complex array of central and peripheral components that are common targets of therapy with antiemetics. The chemoreceptor trigger zone, vestibular system, and emetic center can all cause vomiting. Similarly, the vestibular system influences the emetic center. The drugs listed on the right work at the level of the brain noted on the left via the impulse pathways noted in the middle. Pharmacologic intervention through any or all of the impulse pathways is important in eliminating vomiting in the cancer patient.

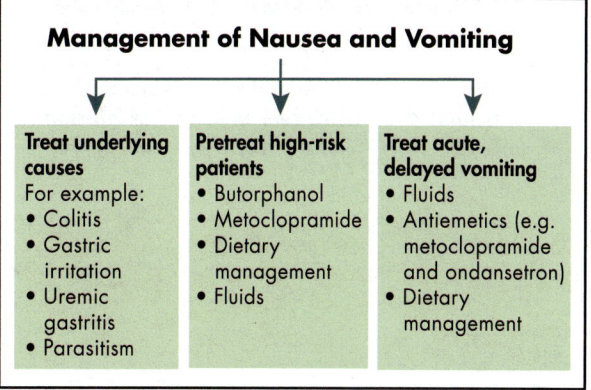

Figure 30-2. General scheme for the treatment of nausea and vomiting in veterinary cancer patients. Impulses are transmitted by both vagal and sympathetic afferents to the emetic center of the medulla. Appropriate motor reactions are then initiated to cause vomiting. The act of vomiting is initiated by motor impulses through several cranial nerves to the upper GI tract and through the spinal nerves to the diaphragm and abdominal muscles.[2]

vomited after the first dose of cisplatin, that animal was much more likely than other patients to vomit subsequently, implying that individual animals may be more susceptible to the emetic effects of chemotherapy. A general guide to the management of nausea and vomiting is presented in Figure 30-2.

Self-Limiting Vomiting[1-3]

An underlying cause of acute, potentially self-limiting vomiting should be identified and corrected whenever possible. Vomiting should be treated as soon as it is identified as follows:

- Give nothing by mouth until vomiting ceases for at least 12 hours.
- Administer metoclopramide or one of the serotonin antagonists to improve quality of life and to speed recovery. Ideally, the antiemetic should initially be administered parenterally. Some serotonin antagonists are available in a rapidly dissolving transmucosal oral delivery system, which is another good route of administration.
- Subsequently, very small amounts of water (e.g., ice cubes) followed by a bland diet can be offered every 2 to 4 hours.
- Once the animal is able to eat without vomiting, it can be slowly returned to a normal diet. During this transition period, the food should be soft in consistency, low in fat, and high in carbohydrates. Fat is a complex nutrient that is difficult to digest, can delay gastric emptying, and may induce diarrhea.

- Dogs with minimal dehydration can receive fluids subcutaneously; however, IV therapy is preferred for significantly dehydrated patients. Many dogs improve dramatically shortly after the administration of IV fluids.
- Potassium supplementation of IV fluids should be provided if hypokalemia is identified (Table 30-1).

Life-Threatening Vomiting[1-3,5]

Clients are often frightened that cancer and cancer therapy will degrade and destroy the quality of life of their pet. Therefore, life-threatening vomiting is not only a serious medical issue but also an emotional "emergency" for clients. The cause of life-threatening vomiting should be identified and corrected as soon as possible. Specific treatment recommendations include the following:

- Fluid therapy should be administered to all patients, especially those that are severely dehydrated (8% to 12% of normal hydration).
- Deficits in fluid and electrolytes secondary to dehydration should be replaced during the first 24 hours. In addition, approximately 66 ml/kg/day of maintenance fluids should be administered. Continued losses, such as from vomiting and diarrhea, should be estimated and replaced.
- Potassium chloride should be supplemented in the fluids, especially if hypokalemia is identified. Potassium should not be administered at a rate greater than 0.5 mEq/kg/hr because this may cause cardiac arrest and death.
- The patient should be monitored for fluid overload using the following parameters: body weight, capillary refill time, skin turgor, chest auscultation, packed cell volume, total solids, and central venous pressure. If vomiting is not

Table 30-1 Intravenous Potassium Supplementation to Correct Hypokalemia

Serum Potassium (mEq/L)	KCl Added to Each Liter of Fluid (mEq)	Maximum Rate of Infusion (ml/kg/hr)[a]
<2	80	6
2.1–2.5	60	8
2.6–3.0	40	12
3.1–3.5	28	16

[a]Above this rate, the risk of life-threatening complications increases.
KCl = potassium chloride.

Selected Antiemetics for Use in Dogs

Recommended
- Butorphanol: 0.4 mg/kg IM q8h
- Dolasetron: 0.1–0.3 mg/kg IV, PO 15 min before chemotherapy then daily to bid
- Metoclopramide: 1–2 mg/kg CRI IV over 24 hr
- Ondansetron: 0.1–0.5 mg/kg IV, PO 15 min before chemotherapy then daily to bid

Less Effective
- Chlorpromazine: 0.5 mg/kg IM, SC, rectal suppository q6–8h
- Dimenhydrinate: 8 mg/kg PO q8h
- Diphenhydramine: 2.0–4.0 mg/kg PO q8h
- Domperidone: 0.1–0.3 mg/kg IM, IV bid
- Prochlorperazine: 0.1–0.5 mg/kg IM, SC q6–8h or 1.0 mg/kg rectally q8h
- Prochlorperazine–isopropamide: 0.5–0.8 mg/kg IM, SC q12h
- Trimethobenzamide: 3 mg/kg IM q8h
- Yohimbine: 0.25–0.5 mg/kg SC, IM bid

Investigational
- Dexamethasone: 1–3 mg IV
- Haloperidol: 110 µg/kg q4d
- Pimozide: 100 µg/kg q6d

likely to subside in a short period, antiemetics such as metoclopramide (constant-rate infusion [CRI]) and a serotonin antagonist (e.g., ondansetron or dolasetron, especially the oral disintegrating tablets or the IV formulation) should be employed; they can be combined for greater efficacy. If vomiting is caused by chemotherapeutic agents, pretreatment with antiemetics is indicated for all future administrations.

Antiemetic Agents

The box on this page lists selected antiemetic agents and their recommended dosages for use in dogs.

METOCLOPRAMIDE[1-3,7]

Metoclopramide is one of the most commonly administered antiemetics in veterinary medicine. Its antiemetic effect is both central and peripheral. Centrally, metoclopramide is a dopamine antagonist that blocks the CTZ and prevents emesis. Peripherally, it increases the tone of the caudal esophageal sphincter and increases gastric antral contractions by relaxing the pylorus and duodenum, thereby reducing the rate of stomach emptying. Metoclopramide can be given to dogs at a dosage of 0.2 to 0.5 mg/kg IM or SC q8h or 1 to 2 mg/kg as a CRI by IV pump over a 24-hour period. This drug should not be given if there is an intestinal obstruction.

> **KEY POINT**
> *In veterinary medicine, metoclopramide is one of the most commonly administered antiemetics because it has both central and peripheral effects.*

Metoclopramide is dispensed at many veterinary health care centers with instructions to administer it before or immediately after chemotherapeutic agents to enhance and improve quality of life. The drug is relatively safe, inexpensive, and readily available. If nausea and vomiting occur, use of this drug alone or in combination with a serotonin antagonist, such as dolasetron or ondansetron, is recommended. Adverse effects are rare but can include extrapyramidal effects resulting in odd behavior when very high dosages are used.

> **KEY POINT**
> *Metoclopramide should not be administered if a GI obstruction is identified or suspected.*

SEROTONIN ANTAGONISTS[1-3,6]

Drugs that inhibit the 5-HT-3 receptor (e.g., ondansetron, dolasetron) constitute a newer and effective class of antiemetics to prevent and treat nausea. These drugs come in oral and IV formulations. The oral formulations are standard tablets and a formulation that dissolves and is absorbed transmucosally. Serotonin antagonists are most effective when used in combination with other drugs, such as metoclopramide. Ondansetron and dolasetron are two of the most commonly used antiemetics available. They are equipotent at recommended dosages; however, once the serotonin receptors are fully occupied, increasing the dosage does not enhance efficacy. Serotonin antagonists are effective in reducing vomiting from all chemotherapy agents, including cisplatin. They appear to be less toxic than other antiemetics, including metoclopramide. These drugs are expensive, but their cost is expected to decline in the future. In addition, early use of these drugs may reduce the need for hospitalization and length of hospital stay, thereby reducing costs. (For dosage recommendations, see the box on page 228.)

Cyproheptadine has some antiserotonin effects, but its efficacy in preventing severe vomiting is poor. It may be a better appetite stimulant.

NARCOTIC ANALGESICS[1-3]

Butorphanol (0.4 mg/kg IM) is a controlled drug that has been shown to reduce the prevalence of vomiting in response to the administration of cisplatin. The drug also has analgesic properties. For best results, butorphanol should be administered intramuscularly at the end of the cisplatin infusion. This drug has little effect in preventing streptozocin-induced vomiting.

> **KEY POINT**
> *Butorphanol (0.4 mg/kg IM) is a controlled drug that has been shown to reduce the prevalence of vomiting in response to the administration of cisplatin. It also has analgesic properties.*

PHENOTHIAZINES[1-3]

Phenothiazines (e.g., chlorpromazine, prochlorperazine) block the CTZ and are commonly used as antiemetics for mild chemotherapy-induced nausea. In human medicine, phenothiazines generally are not effective for reducing efferent GI irritation. These drugs can induce vasodilation and therefore should not be used in dehydrated patients or in those with poor cardiac output. In addition, phenothiazines can induce mild depression and make patient monitoring difficult. All phenothiazines can cause seizures in predisposed animals. For these reasons, the authors do not recommend their use as first-line therapy. Chlorpromazine can be administered at 0.5 mg/kg IM or SC q6–8h; prochlorperazine can be dosed at 0.1 to 0.5 mg/kg IM or SC q6–8h. A suppository form (Compazine, GlaxoSmithKline) is available for use in selected patients.

ANTIHISTAMINES[1-3]

Antihistamines (e.g., diphenhydramine, dimenhydrinate, trimethobenzamide) are another class of antiemetics. They block input from the vestibular system and work against motion-induced vomiting. Diphenhydramine can be administered at 2 to 4 mg/kg PO q8h; it can cause mild sedation.

DOPAMINE ANTAGONISTS AND DIPHENYLBUTYLPIPERIDINE[1-3]

Haloperidol is another dopamine antagonist that blocks the CTZ and can prevent vomiting for up to 4 days in dogs at a dose of 110 µg/kg. Pimozide, a long-acting diphenylbutylpiperidine, can protect dogs from drug-induced vomiting for up to 6 days when given at a dose of 100 µg/kg. Clinical experience with these two drugs in dogs is minimal.

CORTICOSTEROIDS[1-3]

Dexamethasone has been shown to have antiemetic activity. Its mechanism is unknown. Side effects are few except in patients with diabetes or gastric ulcers. Relatively small (1–3 mg) IV doses of dexamethasone are effective in humans; an appropriate dosage in dogs is not known at this time. In human cancer patients, combinations of dexamethasone with serotonin antagonists are very effective; therefore, these combinations are being explored in veterinary oncology.

CANNABINOIDS[1-3]

Many veterinarians are asked about the antiemetic effects of cannabinoids. Dranabinol is the only orally available formulation available at this time; however, its use and efficacy in dogs are unknown. In human patients, dranabinol is effective for moderate to mild vomiting, but much more effective and less toxic agents exist. The mechanism of cannabinoids is not clearly understood, but it appears to mediate their effects centrally. Until more definitive information is known, cannabinoids are not recommended for routine use in dogs.

NEUROKININ-1 RECEPTOR ANTAGONISTS[1-3]

Neurokinin-1 (NK-1) receptor antagonists are the newest antiemetics in human and veterinary medicine. The NK-1 receptor mediates the centrally mediated vomiting reflex, and its antagonists have been shown to be very effective in preventing and treating nausea and vomiting. Experience with use of these drugs in dogs is limited at this time.

REFERENCES

1. Hainsworth JD: Nausea and vomiting, in Abeloff MD, Armitage JO, Niedelhuber JE, et al (eds): *Clinical Oncology*, ed 2. Philadelphia, Elsevier, 2004, pp 759–773.
2. Tams TR: Vomiting, regurgitation and dysphagia, in Ettinger SJ (ed): *Textbook of Veterinary Internal Medicine: Diseases of the Dog and Cat*, ed 3. Philadelphia, WB Saunders, 1989, pp 27–32.
3. Leib MS: Acute vomiting: A diagnostic approach and systematic management, in Kirk RW, Bonagura JD (eds): *Current Veterinary Therapy XI*. Philadelphia, WB Saunders, 1992, pp 583–587.
4. Ogilvie GK, Moore AS, Curtis CR: Cisplatin-induced emesis in the dog with malignant neoplasia: 115 cases (1984–1987). *JAVMA* 195:1399–1403, 1989.
5. Moore AS, Rand WM, Berg J, L'Heureux DA: A randomized evaluation of butorphanol and cyproheptadine for prevention of cisplatin-induced vomiting in the dog. *JAVMA* 205:441–443, 1994.
6. Ogilvie GK: Dolasetron: A new option for nausea and vomiting. *JAAHA* 36(6):481–483, 2000.
7. Kosecki SM: Pharmacy profile: Metoclopramide. *Compend Contin Educ Pract Vet* 25(11):826–828, 2003.
8. Poirier VJ, Hershey AE, Burgess KE, et al: Efficacy and toxicity of paclitaxel (Taxol) for the treatment of canine malignant tumors. *J Vet Intern Med* 18(2):219–222, 2004.

NUTRITIONAL SUPPORT

Gregory K. Ogilvie and Antony S. Moore

CLINICAL BRIEFING

Cancer prevention and therapy	• Maintain lean body weight throughout life. Consider antioxidants and n-3 LC-PUFAs to assist in cancer prevention. • Cancer patients are best nourished via enteral routes. • Consider diets that are low in simple carbohydrates and moderate in fats and highly bioavailable proteins for prevention and therapy. • LC-PUFAs of the n-3 series may prevent cancer by delaying tumor growth. • Adequate fiber is essential for general health. • Energy requirements must be determined on an individual basis and may not be higher in a cancer patient than in a normal animal, even during recovery from surgery.

Enteral feeding	• Oral feeding
	  — Best enteral route.
	  — Enhance intake by providing highly palatable, warmed foods.
	  — Consider appetite stimulants, such as benzodiazepine derivatives and megesterol acetate.
	  — Consider assisted feeding long before weight loss approaches 10%.
	• Esophagostomy tube feeding
	  — Excellent for short- and long-term feeding as well as oral medication in all patients except those that have esophageal motility problems or are vomiting.
	  — Feed blenderized foods to meet nutritional needs.
	• Gastrostomy tube feeding
	  — Excellent for long-term feeding and oral medication in patients that are not vomiting and have functional GI tracts.
	  — Use blenderized foods to meet nutritional needs.
	• Jejunostomy tube feeding
	  — Excellent choice to bypass the upper GI tract in vomiting patients.
	  — Use liquid nutrient solutions.
	  — The use of a pump or frequent small feedings by syringe is required.
	  — Ideal if vomiting precludes feeding via the upper GI tract.

Parenteral feeding	• Excellent choice whenever enteral feeding is not possible. • An infusion pump, specially designed nutrients, absolute dedication to aseptic technique, and a separate indwelling catheter are needed.

Using specifically formulated diets or dietary supplements to prevent and to treat cancer is in its infancy; however, enough information exists to begin making some recommendations to prevent and treat cancer in humans and dogs.[1-5] Many clients are actively seeking specific dietary changes to reduce their own risk of developing cancer. It is natural for them to want to do the same for their pets. It has been estimated that 30% to 40% of all human cancers can be prevented by lifestyle and dietary measures alone.[5] The same may be true in veterinary medicine. In human medicine, several nutritional factors have been found to increase the risk and rate of developing cancer, including[3-5]:

- Obesity
- Consumption of nutrient-sparse foods, such as concentrated sugars and refined flour products

- Low fiber intake
- Inadequate consumption of polyunsaturated fatty acids (PUFAs) of the n-3 series (n-3 PUFAs) and an increased consumption of PUFAs of the n-6 series (n-6 PUFAs)

Many of these factors have already been implicated in augmenting cancer development and progression in dogs and other animals.[1,2,6–21] This chapter is presented to assist the clinician in making decisions about what to feed dogs to prevent or treat cancer.

Cancer, Metabolism, and Clinical Nutrition

Cancer cachexia is a complex paraneoplastic syndrome that results in profound metabolic changes that occur before weight loss is identified[1,2,6–20] (see Chapter 45 for more information on cancer cachexia as a paraneoplastic syndrome). Many veterinarians believe that this condition only exists at the end stages of progressive involuntary weight loss that occurs even in the face of adequate nutritional intake. The fact is that the metabolic alterations that lead to the end stages of cancer cachexia occur early in the course of the disease, with serious clinical consequences. The importance of this syndrome cannot be overstated. Humans with cancer cachexia have a decreased quality of life, decreased response to treatment, and shortened survival time compared with patients who have similar diseases but do not exhibit clinical or biochemical signs associated with this condition.

> **KEY POINT**
>
> *Cancer cachexia is a misnamed, complex paraneoplastic syndrome that results in profound metabolic changes that occur before weight loss is ever identified.*

The ideal way of treating cancer cachexia is to eliminate the underlying neoplastic condition. Unfortunately, this is not possible for many veterinary patients. Therefore, dietary therapy has been examined as a way to reverse or eliminate cancer cachexia. Although investigators have demonstrated concern about the possibility of increasing tumor growth by enhancing the nutritional status of the host, several studies have failed to show this correlation. The benefits that have been shown with dietary support include weight gain and increased response to and tolerance of radiation, surgery, and chemotherapy. Other factors that have been shown to improve with nutritional support include thymic weight, immune system responsiveness, and immunoglobulin and complement levels, as well as the phagocytic ability of white blood cells.[1–5] Understanding the alterations in carbohydrate, protein, and lipid metabolism in pets with cancer is essential to knowing what to feed the cancer patient.

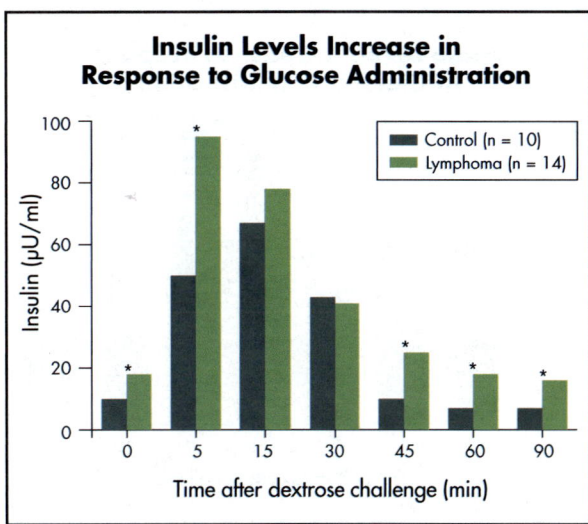

Figure 31-1. *Serum insulin concentrations in dogs with and without lymphoma before and after IV administration of 500 mg/kg dextrose. Asterisks (*) indicate values from dogs with lymphoma that differ significantly (P <0.001) from control dogs at the same time. (From Vail DM, Ogilvie GK, Wheeler SL, et al: Alterations in carbohydrate metabolism in canine lymphoma.* J Vet Intern Med *4:8–14, 1990; with permission)*

CARBOHYDRATES AND CANCER

Evidence is mounting that simple carbohydrates may be contraindicated for the nutritional management of cancer in dogs. For example, cancer cells display high rates of aerobic glycolysis, a phenomenon known as the *Warburg effect*.[21,22] This effect is characterized by the production of large quantities of lactate and pyruvate, the end products of glycolysis, even in the presence of oxygen. It has been found in vivo in human and veterinary cancer patients. Data demonstrating that insulin and lactate levels of dogs with cancer increase above levels in control dogs in response to glucose and a diet-tolerance test[8–11] (Figures 31-1 and 31-2) have been used to suggest that the metabolic alterations in carbohydrate metabolism worsen with the parenteral and enteral administration of simple carbohydrates.

> **KEY POINT**
>
> *The Warburg effect is characterized by the production of large quantities of lactate and pyruvate, the end products of glycolysis, by cancer cells even in the presence of oxygen and has been found in vivo in human and veterinary cancer patients.*

Research has documented that dogs with lymphoma and a wide variety of malignant diseases have significant alterations in carbohydrate metabolism[1,2,6–20]:

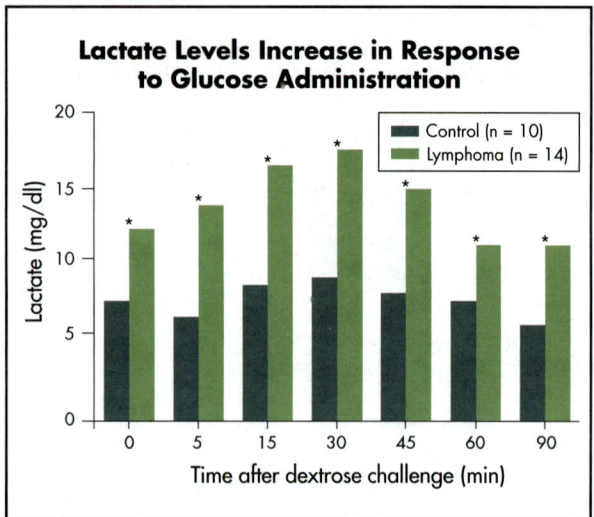

Figure 31-2. Serum lactate concentrations in dogs with and without lymphoma before and after IV administration of 500 mg/kg dextrose. Asterisks (*) indicate values from dogs with lymphoma that differ significantly (P <0.001) from control dogs at the same time. (From Vail DM, Ogilvie GK, Wheeler SL, et al: Alterations in carbohydrate metabolism in canine lymphoma. J Vet Intern Med 4:8–14, 1990; with permission)

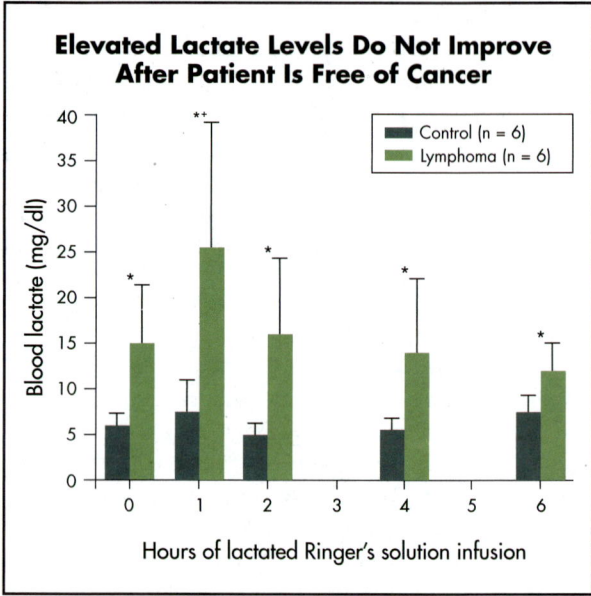

Figure 31-3. Blood lactate concentrations in dogs with and without lymphoma before and during IV infusion of lactated Ringer's solution. Asterisks (*) indicate values from dogs with lymphoma that differ significantly (P <0.05) from controls at the same time. Plus sign (+) indicates values that differ significantly (P <0.05) from preinfusion baseline values within the same test group. (From Vail DM, Ogilvie GK, Fettman MJ, et al: Exacerbation of hyperlactatemia by infusion of lactated Ringer's solution in dogs with lymphoma. J Vet Intern Med 4:228–232, 1990; with permission)

- Dogs with a wide variety of malignant conditions have elevated resting insulin and lactate levels compared with control animals[8–11,15] (Figures 31-1 and 31-2). It is unknown if the elevated insulin levels are a response to cancer or if they precede and possibly contribute to the development of cancer via stimulation of insulin-like growth-factor (IGF) pathways.
- Elevated lactate and glucose levels do not improve after dogs with cancer are rendered free of disease with chemotherapy and surgery[8] (Figure 31-3). This suggests that the malignancy causes a fundamental change in metabolism that persists after all clinical evidence of cancer is eliminated.
- Elevated lactate levels can result in inefficient Cori cycle activity to convert lactate back to glucose; this results in a net energy loss by the patient.[8–11,15]
- The administration of lactate-containing parenteral fluids such as lactated Ringer's solution has been shown to increase lactate levels in dogs with lymphoma, suggesting that these types of fluids may place an additional energy burden on the host.[9]
- Before the development of severe malnutrition, human patients with colon, gastric, sarcoma, endometrial, prostate, or localized head, neck, or lung cancer have many of the metabolic abnormalities of type 2 (non–insulin-dependent) diabetes mellitus.[21,22] These metabolic abnormalities include glucose intolerance; an increase in hepatic glucose production, glucose recycling, and insulin resistance; and an increase in anaerobic glycolysis causing increased lactate production. These are essentially the same findings as in dogs with cancer.[1,2,6–20]

The metabolic abnormalities noted above are only important if they affect the patient clinically. Studies done in human patients suggest that alterations in carbohydrate metabolism influence cancer prevention and outcome once cancer is diagnosed.[23–25] For example, one study evaluated the hypothesis that glucose, insulin, and IGFs contribute to breast cancer development in 10,786 women.[23] It was concluded in this research that higher levels of glucose, insulin, and IGF-1 were associated with a higher risk of developing breast cancer and a poorer survival after diagnosis. A second study involving 603 breast cancer patients was conducted to test the hypothesis that excess insulin and related factors are directly related to mortality after a diagnosis of breast cancer.[24] It was concluded in that study that high levels of insulin were associated with poorer survival for postmenopausal women.

Dietary Recommendations: It seems reasonable to limit the amount of simple carbohydrates in dogs with cancer. Similarly, because simple carbohydrates can cause elevated insulin levels, and because hyperinsulinemia has been associated with the development of cancer in some species, a diet lower in carbohydrates may be indicated throughout life, even in healthy dogs. Raghavan et al[26] showed that after adjustment for age, weight, neuter status, and coat color, there was an inverse association between consumption of vegetables at least three times per week and risk of developing transitional cell carcinoma in healthy Scottish terriers. Green leafy vegetables do not have a high glycemic index. A lower-carbohydrate diet may also help maintain a lean body mass and reduce the risks of dental disease and obesity, which may, in turn, enhance wellness by reducing the risk of cancer and metabolic diseases such as diabetes mellitus. As a general rule, inexpensive, extruded dry, and semimoist commercially available dog foods have the highest carbohydrate content.

> **KEY POINT**
> *Cancer patients have alterations in carbohydrate metabolism and should be fed diets that have limited amount of simple carbohydrates.*

PROTEINS AND CANCER

Dogs with cancer have alterations in protein metabolism that are very similar to those observed in humans and laboratory animals with cancer.[1] For example, there is a significant decrease in a wide variety of amino acids, suggesting that a high-quality, highly bioavailable protein source that would be beneficial to the animal would also encourage tumor growth.

Amino acids of particular importance to patients with cancer are glutamine, cysteine, and arginine. Glutamine supplementation may enhance the therapeutic index of chemotherapy and radiation by enhancing the efficacy of these treatments while reducing adverse effects such as mucositis, diarrhea, neuropathy, and cardiotoxicity.[27,28] Glutamine is conditionally essential for the health and function of the bowel. At least some of this amino acid is destroyed in the process of making many types of dried and canned pet food.

> **KEY POINT**
> *Optimally, the cancer patient should be fed a moderate quantity of highly bioavailable protein sources that contain adequate amounts of cysteine, glutamine, and arginine.*

Cysteine is critically important to replenish the glutathione antioxidant system.[29,30] This system is the principal protective mechanism of the cell and is a crucial factor in the development of the immune response. Cysteine supplementation has been shown to have anticancer activity via the glutathione pathway, the induction of p53 protein in cancer cells, and the inhibition of neoangiogenesis.[29,30]

Arginine is a conditionally essential amino acid that is necessary during periods of growth and recovery after injury. Arginine promotes wound healing, has several immunomodulatory effects such as stimulating T- and natural-killer cell activity, and influences proinflammatory cytokine levels.[31] L-Arginine is the sole precursor for the multifunctional messenger molecule nitric oxide, which appears to influence tumor initiation, promotion, and progression; tumor-cell adhesion; apoptosis angiogenesis; differentiation; chemosensitivity; radiosensitivity; and tumor-induced immunosuppression.[31] The administration of arginine to human and veterinary cancer patients has resulted in positive outcomes.

Dietary Recommendations: Optimally, the cancer patient should be fed a moderate quantity of highly bioavailable protein sources that contain adequate amounts of cysteine, glutamine, and arginine. Periodically evaluating the patient to ensure maintenance of body weight without the development of hypoalbuminemia is critical. Less expensive, commercially available dog foods, especially those that are extruded dry or semimoist, are less likely to have highly bioavailable proteins.

LIPIDS AND CANCER

Serum lipid profiles were conducted in dogs with lymphoma before and after the animals were put into remission with chemotherapy. These profiles were compared with those of normal dogs before and after they were given the same anticancer drug, with the following results[11]:

- The dogs with cancer had significantly lower levels of high-density lipoproteins. The total triglyceride levels and very low density triglycerides of untreated dogs with lymphoma were significantly higher than those of untreated control dogs.[11]
- After a total of five doses of doxorubicin chemotherapy, the total cholesterol level increased in dogs with lymphoma but decreased in treated control dogs.[11]
- All other parameters remained unchanged after doxorubicin therapy, suggesting that lipid abnormalities do not improve significantly, even after clinical remission is obtained.[11]

Abnormalities in lipid metabolism have been linked to a number of clinical problems, including immunosuppression, which correlates with decreased survival in affected humans.[1–5] The clinical impact of abnormalities in lipid metabolism may be lessened with dietary therapy. In contrast to carbohydrates and proteins, some tumor cells have difficulty using lipids as a fuel source, but host tissues continue to oxidize lipids for energy. This has led to the hypothesis that diets relatively high in fat may be beneficial for animals with cancer compared with diets that are high in simple carbohydrates, assuming that the protein content, caloric density, and palatability remain constant. One study suggested that a high-carbohydrate, low-fat diet induced elevated lactate and insulin levels compared with a diet relatively high in fat and low in carbohydrates.[2,12] It also suggested that a high-fat diet may result in a higher probability of going into remission with chemotherapy as well as a longer survival time. The kind of fat in the diet, rather than the amount, may be the important factor. For example, n-3 PUFAs have been shown experimentally to have many beneficial properties.[2,12,16]

Emerging Role of PUFAs

For the past decade, investigators have searched for dietary lipids associated with a delay in cancer relapse. The use of long-chain polyunsaturated fatty acids (LC-PUFAs) such as docosahexaenoic acid (DHA) and eicosapentaenoic acid (EPA) as adjuvant therapies to enhance the effect of chemotherapy and radiation therapy shows promise. LC-PUFAs have been shown to enhance disease-free interval, survival, and quality of life after surgery by reducing the rate of cancer development or incidence. This concept, known as *cancer prevention by delay* or *clinical cancer chemoprevention*, is an important mechanism behind the successes of several therapeutic agents, including tamoxifen, retinoids, interferon-α, and NSAIDs.[32]

> **KEY POINT**
> *LC-PUFAs, such as DHA and EPA, have been shown to enhance disease-free interval, survival, and quality of life after surgery or chemotherapy by reducing the rate of cancer development or incidence. This concept is known as* **cancer prevention by delay.**

Cancer prevention by delay is a valuable clinical tool until more effective cancer therapeutics can be developed. Unfortunately, while use of the most effective cancer therapies (i.e., surgery, radiation, and chemotherapy) is effective for improving the disease-free interval of many patients up to a point, it has not increased the cancer cure rate or survival time dramatically in the past 10 years. Therefore, it seems logical to add on relatively nontoxic therapies that can extend the disease-free interval, even if the absolute cure rate is not increased. Tamoxifen, retinoids, and NSAIDs are all recognized to improve disease-free interval without necessarily improving the absolute cure rate. Tamoxifen has been shown to significantly diminish the risk for human breast cancer; retinoids and interferon-α to reduce the risk of developing head and neck cancer in dogs, cats, and humans; and NSAIDs to delay or reduce the development of colorectal cancer in humans and transitional cell and squamous cell carcinomas in dogs.

Dietary lipids such as DHA and EPA appear to influence the growth of many types of cancer, including breast and prostate cancer.[33-36] A group of investigators in France used adipose tissue sampled during surgery as a biomarker of past dietary intake of PUFAs in a cohort of women treated for localized presentations of breast cancer.[37] They found elevated n-3 PUFAs, especially DHA, to be associated with a higher metastasis-free survival, suggesting that these PUFAs could potentially delay metastasis by decreasing tumor growth or development. Using a case-control approach comparing the fatty acid composition of adipose breast tissue obtained at the time of surgical removal of either malignant or benign breast tumors, they also found α-linoleic acid and DHA to be positively associated with a decreased risk of having breast cancer.[38]

The French investigators also explored the role of n-3 PUFAs in mammary tumor growth using the experimental system of *N*-methyl nitrosourea (NMU)–induced mammary tumors in rats. Because PUFAs are substrates for lipid peroxidation processes, the investigators studied the effects of n-3 PUFAs on tumor growth in interaction with anti- or prooxidant compounds. They found that dietary n-3 PUFAs in the form of DHA-containing fish oil inhibited tumor development. This inhibition was most evident in the absence of the antioxidant vitamin E. Inhibition of tumor growth was even greater when n-3 PUFAs were given in the presence of prooxidants.[39] Such effects were not found when the lipid diet was low in PUFAs. These data suggest that oxidized n-3 PUFAs have an inhibiting effect on tumor growth and emphasize the importance of the interaction of anti- and prooxidant compounds with n-3 PUFAs.

There is a growing body of data suggesting that the presence of n-3 PUFAs such as DHA and EPA affects several steps of tumor formation. N-3 PUFAs:

- Inhibit tumor vessel formation (angiogenesis)
- Inhibit cell proliferation in several epithelial cell lines
- Enhance the rate of tumor cell death
- Induce lipid peroxidation, which enhances the efficacy of radiation- and chemotherapy-induced cancer cell death; this effect is diminished or reduced dramatically with vitamin E
- Suppress the expression of cyclooxygenase-2 in tumors, thereby decreasing cancer cell proliferation
- Suppress nuclear factor κB activation and BCL-2 expression, thus allowing apoptosis of cancer cells

Dietary lipids have been shown to modify the sensitivity of tumors to reactive oxygen species–generating anticancer drugs. For example, when dogs with lymphoma were treated with doxorubicin chemotherapy and a diet supplemented with n-3 PUFAs in the form of fish oils, there was a direct correlation between the level of DHA in the blood and improved disease-free interval.[18] Another study, using the same randomized design, was used to assess the efficacy of n-3 PUFAs in combination with doxorubicin chemotherapy to improve the disease-free interval in dogs with hemangiosarcoma, a highly metastatic, rapidly fatal malignancy. There was a statistically significant positive correlation between the level of n-3 PUFAs in the serum and the disease-free interval.[40] A similar approach was used in rats bearing autochthonous, NMU-induced mammary tumors. It was found that dietary supplementation with fish oil or DHA increased the sensitivity of mammary tumors to anthracyclines compared with dietary supplementation with saturated fatty acids.[40]

Because DHA is the most polyunsaturated of the PUFAs, lipoperoxidation is a likely molecular mechanism implicated in the enhancement of the response of cancer cells to cytotoxic drugs. Addition of vitamin E to the diet provided to rats with mammary tumors abolished the enhancing effect of DHA on tumor sensitivity to anthracyclines.[40] In all studies done to date, there has been no clinically significant toxicity other than transient gastrointestinal (GI) distress linked to the dietary change.[17,18] Therefore, based on the safety and efficacy profile of n-3 PUFAs, it seems reasonable to further define the efficacy of n-3 PUFAs, especially DHA, for the treatment of spontaneously occurring cancer in dogs, with the intent to provide evidence for their use in randomized human clinical trials.

DHA and EPA also augment the efficacy of chemotherapy and radiation therapy, potentially enhancing the efficacy of traditional cancer therapies. Radiation therapy is currently the most effective treatment for many localized malignancies. Research is under way to identify methods to maximize its efficacy while minimizing the adverse effects associated with it. Among the agents being evaluated to minimize the damage to normal tissue are n-3 LC-PUFAs, which are readily incorporated into cell membranes and ameliorate inflammation and carbohydrate dyshomeostasis. In one study,[41] 12 dogs with histologically confirmed malignant carcinomas of the nasal cavity were randomized to receive isocaloric amounts of a diet supplemented with menhaden fish oil, including DHA (experimental diet), or an otherwise identical diet supplemented with corn oil (control diet). Megavoltage radiation was delivered to all dogs. The data in this study suggest that feeding a diet supplemented with fish oil and arginine is associated with decreased concentrations of inflammatory mediators of radiation damage in skin and mucosa and with improved performance scores in dogs with malignant nasal tumors.[41]

The ability of PUFAs to sensitize tumors to radiation has been investigated. Vartak et al[42,43] studied the in vitro response of a chemically induced rat malignant astrocytoma cell line to radiation after the cell culture medium was supplemented with γ-linoleic acid or n-3 LC-PUFAs. They found that n-3 PUFAs enhanced radiation-induced cell cytotoxicity. In a separate study, Colas et al[44] documented enhanced radiosensitivity of rat autochthonous mammary tumors after administration of dietary DHA.

Whether use of dietary n-3 PUFAs can enhance sensitivity of tumor tissue in the absence of a similar increase in the radiosensitivity of nontumor tissue remains a critical issue. Several studies, reviewed below, have suggested that PUFAs do not sensitize normal tissue to radiation. For example, because ionizing radiation generates reactive oxygen species, a study was initiated to determine whether dietary DHA might sensitize mammary tumors to irradiation, using a model in which mammary tumors were induced by NMU in Sprague-Dawley rats.[44] The study showed that dietary DHA sensitized mammary tumors to radiation. The addition of vitamin E inhibited the beneficial effect of DHA, suggesting that this effect might be mediated by oxidative damage to the peroxidizable lipids.[44]

Dietary Recommendations: N-3 LC-PUFAs may be beneficial for preventing and treating cancer in dogs. Therefore, n-3 PUFAs, such as DHA, should be used as dietary supplements. The addition of antioxidants such as vitamins A, E, or C is important to keep the PUFAs from oxidizing; however, excessive amounts may reduce or eliminate the beneficial effects of PUFAs.

> *N-3 PUFAs appear to be important in reducing toxicity induced by radiation and chemotherapy while increasing the efficacy of these therapies.*

NUTRITIONAL AND WATER NEEDS AND CANCER

Our knowledge of the nutrient and water needs of dogs is primarily based on work done years ago or extrapolated from research in rodents or humans. Most data concerning energy and water requirements in dogs may be overestimated.[45,46] It has been determined that the resting energy expenditure, which is an estimate of the nutrient and water needs of normal dogs, is lower than previously published data implied.[46] In addition, one study showed that dogs with lymphoma and dogs that have undergone surgery for various problems have resting energy requirements that are lower than those of normal animals.[45] This is in stark contrast to publications suggesting that cancer and surgery result in dramatic increases in the nutrient and water requirements of animals. This is of critical value for practicing veterinarians who are attempting to meet the nutrient and fluid needs of normal and ill veterinary patients. It also may be of great importance for pet owners.

Dietary Recommendations: The caloric needs of each cancer patient should be monitored carefully by evaluating body weight and serum albumin levels. Many dogs with cancer do not have dramatically elevated caloric needs compared with normal patients. Similarly, because the fluid needs of dogs are directly related to the number of kilocalories consumed on a basis of 1 ml of water to 1 kcal, the fluid needs of the cancer patient may be more conservative than once anticipated.

> **KEY POINT**
>
> *Dogs with cancer, especially those that have been recently anesthetized, may not have an increase in caloric needs, as is often stated in the older literature. Each patient should be periodically assessed to determine individual caloric and water needs.*

VITAMINS, MINERALS, AND ENZYMES AND CANCER

Vitamins

Retinoids, β-carotene, and vitamins C, D, and E may influence the growth and metastasis of cancer cells via a variety of mechanisms. These vitamins increase and decrease in popularity based on the results of select studies and the lay press. However, the weight of the literature suggests that many of these vitamins may be of value for some cancer patients.

Retinoids (Vitamin A)

Retinoids are not used as a mainstay of cancer therapy; however, there is a growing body of knowledge about the anticancer effect of vitamin A in humans and animals.[47–50] In humans, 13-*cis* retinoic acid prevents secondary tumors in patients treated for squamous cell carcinoma of the head and neck[47–50] and can reverse the effects of cervical human papillomavirus infection. Retinoic acid, when used in the adjuvant treatment of retinoblastoma (a childhood cancer), leads to translocation of bound receptor–vitamin complexes to the nucleus, which results in the regulation of the neuroblastoma gene.[48] Melanoma in mice has been successfully treated with retinoids.[49]

The efficacy of retinoids is not confined to rodents and humans. A study was completed to evaluate the synthetic retinoids isotretinoin and etretinate in treating dogs with intracutaneous cornifying epithelioma, other benign skin neoplasias, and cutaneous lymphoma.[50] This study showed reduction in the size of some tumors and elimination of others.

Vitamin C

Vitamin C has been studied continuously over the past several decades as an antioxidant and an agent that can effectively treat conditions such as colds, cardiovascular disease, and cancer. There have been some data suggesting that vitamin C may be of value for the prevention and treatment of certain types of cancers.[51,52] Water-soluble vitamin C has been widely reported to inhibit nitrosation reactions and prevent chemical induction of cancers of the esophagus and stomach.[52] Processed foods high in nitrates and nitrites, such as bacon and sausage, are often supplemented with vitamin C to reduce the carcinogenic capability of the resultant nitrosamines.

Vitamin E

Lipid-soluble vitamin E, or α-tocopherol, can inhibit nitrosation reactions, but vitamin E also has a broad capacity to inhibit mammary tumor and colon carcinogenesis in rodents.[52–54] In addition to its chemopreventive properties, vitamin E possesses antiproliferative activity that may convey potential therapeutic efficacy against certain malignancies.[52–54] As mentioned above, antioxidants may inhibit the effect of n-3 PUFAs, making it difficult to know how to administer these vitamins.

The effects of vitamins are not always positive. A meta-analysis of the dose-response relationship between vitamin E supplementation and total mortality was conducted using data from 135,967 human participants in 19 randomized, controlled clinical trials.[55] A dose-response analysis showed a statistically significant relationship between vitamin E dosage and all-cause mortality, with increased risk with dosages greater than 150 IU/day. The study concluded that high-dosage (≥400 IU/day) vitamin E supplements may increase all-cause mortality and should be avoided. Another study documented that higher dosages of β-carotene caused a poorer outcome in humans who smoked and had lung cancer.[56] Thus, vitamins have a complex role in the treatment and prevention of cancer, and more must be known about the impact of their dosage and form before they can be used effectively in the treatment of cancer.

Dietary Recommendations: Moderate quantities of vitamins are recommended for the cancer patient; however, megadosages of vitamins are not encouraged at this time.

Minerals

Minerals that have been suggested as having chemopreventive or anticancer effects and that are of value as nutrients include selenium, copper, zinc, magnesium, calcium, chromium, lead, iron, potassium, sodium, arsenic, iodine, and germanium. Zinc, chromium, and iron have been shown to be reduced in dogs with spontaneously occurring cancer.[19] Selenium is one of the most heavily studied minerals associated with the development of cancer.[57–60] Low serum selenium levels have been seen in human patients with prostate and GI cancer.[57] In rodents, dietary supplementation of selenium has been shown to inhibit colon, mammary gland, and stomach carcinogenesis.[57–60] Additional studies are essential to determine whether alteration of selenium levels would be of value for the treatment of veterinary or human cancer patients. Selenium may be toxic at high levels and thus should not be supplemented without first seeking advice from a veterinary nutritionist.

Dietary Recommendations: Care should be taken to ensure that the diet contains adequate levels of minerals for all life stages. Specific care should be taken to ensure that zinc, chromium, and iron are adequate in the diet. Selenium should be supplemented cautiously and without inducing selenium toxicity.

Therapeutic Enzymes

Enzymes have therapeutic potential but limited approval in the United States. L-Asparaginase is probably the most valuable therapy for the treatment of lymphoma and leukemia in animals and humans.[61] Oral enzyme preparations are used for the treatment of chronic pancreatic insufficiency and disaccharidase deficiency. Several enzyme preparations, including Wobenzym (Mucos Pharma, Czech Republic) and Musal, are available in Europe for oral adjuvant treatment of cancer and other diseases. Although manufacturers of these preparations note the efficacy of therapeutic enzymes in the treatment of cancer patients, the mechanism by which enzymes act is not precisely known. One hypothesis is that these enzymes eliminate pathogenic immune complexes. Therefore, enzymes may be of value as adjuvant treatment of cancer.

Information suggests that soybean-derived Bowman-Birk inhibitor (BBI) can inhibit or suppress carcinogenesis in vivo and in vitro.[62–66] Extracts of BBI have been shown to inhibit carcinogenesis in several animal model systems, including colon- and liver-induced carcinogenesis in mice, anthracene-induced cheek pouch carcinogenesis in hamsters, lung tumorigenesis in mice, and esophageal carcinogenesis in rats.[62–66] BBI concentration has been shown to inhibit metastasis and weight loss associated with radiation-induced thymic lymphoma in mice.[63] Irradiated rodents treated with dietary BBI concentration have fewer deaths, lower average grade of lymphoma, and larger fat stores than controls. Therefore, this protease inhibitor may be important as an adjunct to cancer chemotherapy protocols and in the prevention of secondary cancers.

Nutritional Prevention and Therapy of Cancer

The following general recommendations for cancer prevention and therapy are based on the information provided in this chapter. These recommendations should be revised as new knowledge is gained.

PREVENTION

Dogs generally eat the same diet for long periods of time; therefore, that diet should be designed to prevent the development of cancer. Until a special cancer prevention diet is developed, existing data can be employed to potentially reduce the risk of cancer in dogs eating commercially available food. Avoidance of obesity seems to be a basic preventive measure. As noted earlier, Raghavan et al[26] showed that after adjustment for age, weight, neuter status, and coat color, there was an inverse association between consumption of vegetables at least three times per week and risk of developing transitional cell carcinoma in healthy Scottish terriers. In addition, a lifetime study of restricted daily food intake was done in 48 Labrador retriever dogs from seven litters.[67,68] The dogs were paired; in each pair, the restricted-fed dog received 25% less food than the control-fed dog. The median life span of the restricted-fed dogs was significantly longer. While the prevalence of cancer between the groups was similar, dogs that received the restricted diet lived an average of 2 years longer before dying from cancer.

EPA and DHA have consistently been shown to inhibit the proliferation of breast and prostate cancer cell lines in vitro and to reduce the risk for and progression of these tumors in many species.[69,70] Adding these LC-PUFAs to the diet may be useful in preventing some types of cancer.

The following are basic dietary recommendations to prevent cancer in dogs:

- Restrict daily intake to maintain a low body weight throughout life.
- Minimize simple carbohydrates in the diet to reduce insulin levels and obesity; this may reduce the risk of developing a number of diseases.
- Feed a balanced diet specifically for dogs, with possible consideration of the use of n-3 PUFAs.

THERAPY

The ideal anticancer diet in dogs that already have cancer is unknown. However, as noted above, it may be logical to use a diet that contains 30% to 50% of nonprotein calories as fat, particularly n-3 PUFAs; a highly bioavailable protein source that has adequate amounts of glutamine, cysteine, and arginine; and a relatively low percentage of carbohydrates.[1–4] This type of diet may slow tumor growth and

> **KEY POINT**
>
> *Although the ideal "cancer diet" is not known, a diet composed of relatively low amounts of simple carbohydrates, moderate amounts of fats (especially n-3 PUFAs), and adequate amounts of highly bioavailable proteins may be beneficial.*

decrease glucose intolerance and fat loss. Glucose-containing fluids may result in increased lactate production, which may cause an energy drain on the host.

Enteral Nutrition

As a general rule, mature dogs with functional GI tracts and a history of inadequate nutritional intake for 5 to 7 days or a loss of at least 10% of their body weight over a 1- to 2-week period are candidates for enteral nutritional therapy. All methods to encourage food consumption should be attempted (Figure 31-4). These include warming the food to just below body temperature; providing a selection of palatable, aromatic foods; and providing comfortable, stress-free surroundings. When these simple procedures fail, such chemical stimulants as benzodiazepine derivatives (e.g., diazepam, oxazepam) and antiserotonin agents (cyproheptadine and pizotifen) can be used. Propofol at 1 mg/kg IV can also enhance the appetite in many hospitalized cancer patients. Megestrol acetate (2.5 mg PO daily for 4 days, then every 2–3 days thereafter) and diazepam (0.05–0.5 mg/kg IV) are effective for enhancing appetite. Dogs may have improved appetite when metoclopramide, ondansetron, or dolasetron is given orally to decrease nausea associated with chemotherapy or surgery. When all these measures fail, enteral nutritional support designed to deliver nutrients to the GI tract by various methods should be considered because it is practical, cost effective, physiologic, and safe.[1-4]

> **KEY POINT**
>
> *Enteral feeding should be used whenever possible—if the gut works, use it!*

Calculating Contents and Volumes

Calculation of the nutritional requirements for enteral feeding is essentially the same as for parenteral feeding,[1,2] which is relatively straightforward.[1-4] Parenteral feeding is discussed separately below. Although recent research suggests that animals with cancer do not have increased nutritional requirements, the following method is still in use:

- The basal energy requirement (BER, in kcal/day) is calculated by multiplying the animal's weight in $kg^{0.75}$ by 70.

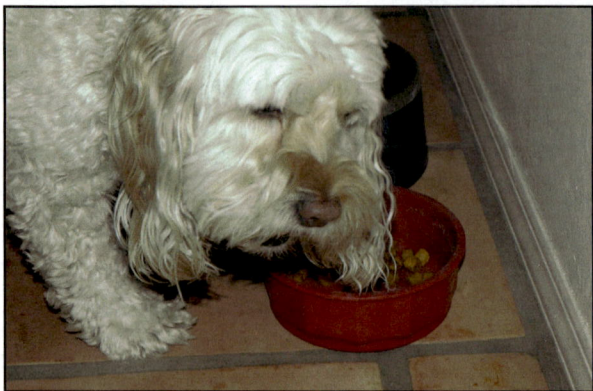

Figure 31-4. *All methods to encourage food consumption, including feeding a variety of highly palatable aromatic foods, warming the food to just below body temperature, and administering chemical stimulants, should be tried before starting enteral support. The optimum pharmacologic agent for use in the veterinary cancer patient is unknown; however, megestrol acetate has been shown to result in substantial weight gain in humans with cancer.*

This value is then multiplied by different factors to derive the maintenance energy requirement (MER) or illness energy requirement (IER).

- The standard guidelines state that to calculate the MER for normal dogs that are at rest in a cage, the BER is multiplied by a factor of 1.25. For dogs that have undergone recent surgery or that are recovering from trauma, the IER equals the BER multiplied by 1.2 to 1.6. To calculate the IER for dogs that are septic or have major burns, the BER is multiplied by 1.5 to 2.0.

- The IER (kcal/day as nonprotein calories) has not been determined for dogs with cancer but is reported to be high, even in animals without sepsis, burns, trauma, or surgery. The work of Ogilvie and colleagues[9,10] suggests that the energy requirement of dogs with cancer may not exceed that of normal dogs. Until this is confirmed, it may be better to overestimate, rather than underestimate, nutrient requirements of the cancer patient.

> **KEY POINT**
>
> *The energy needs of dogs with cancer may not be higher than the needs of normal dogs. Similarly, recent research has shown that energy needs may not increase after major or minor surgery.*

Some cancer patients have a very high energy expenditure that may exceed that seen in animals with infections, sepsis, or burns. Other research suggests that the energy needs of most cancer patients do *not* exceed those of a healthy animal. Dogs with renal or hepatic insufficiency should not be given high protein loads (>3 g/100 kcal in dogs). Because most high-quality pet foods can be put through a blender to form a gruel that can be passed through a large feeding tube, the IER of the animal is divided by the caloric density of the canned pet food to determine the amount of food to feed. The same calculation can be done with human enteral feeding products; the volume fed may need to be increased if the enteral feeding product is diluted to ensure it is approximately isoosmolar before administration.

Suggested Diets: There is one commercially prepared cancer diet, Hill's Prescription Diet Canine n/d (Topeka, KS). The recipe for a homemade alternative is provided in the box on this page.

Routes of Enteral Feeding

Esophagostomy Tubes: Recently, esophagostomy tube feeding has gained great popularity because the tube can be placed easily without special equipment, can be removed at any time, and requires no waiting time before feeding begins (Figure 31-5).[1-3,5] Tube sizes of 14 to 20 Fr are used in dogs. Esophagostomy tubes can be placed percutaneously with the use of a curved Rochester-Carmalt forceps or hemostat. Complications include local cellulitis and, occasionally, a dissecting abscess of the cervical tissues; these complications are rare and heal shortly after the tube is removed and the local reaction treated appropriately.

Gastrostomy Tubes: Gastrostomy tubes are used frequently in veterinary practice for animals that need nutritional support for more than 7 days.[1,2] These tubes can be placed surgically or with endoscopic guidance. A 5-ml balloon-tipped urethral catheter (e.g., Foley catheter, Bardex, Murray Hill, NJ) can be placed surgically, as can a mushroom-tipped Pezzer proportionate head urologic catheter (Bard Urological Catheter, Bard Urological Division, Covington, GA). For smaller dogs, an 18- to 24-Fr catheter is used; larger dogs require a 26- to 30-Fr tube. Low-profile gastrostomy tubes are also available. The procedure is as follows:

1. Before placing the tube, clip and prepare the left paracostal area just below the paravertebral epaxial musculature for surgery. Make a 2- to 3-cm incision just caudal to the last rib through the skin and subcutaneous tissue to allow blunt dissection through the musculature into the abdominal cavity.

2. Inflate the stomach through a tube placed down the esophagus to allow easy location of the stomach through the opening in the abdominal wall. Place stay sutures to temporarily fix the stomach against the abdominal wall; these stay sutures are used later to help close the muscular wall.

3. Place two concentric purse-string sutures of 2-0 nonabsorbable nylon suture deep in the stomach wall; the first purse-string suture is deeper than the second to allow a two-layered closure.

4. Place the feeding tube into the lumen of the stomach through a stab incision in the middle of the purse-string sutures. The tip of the catheter is usually clipped off to allow easy introduction of food through the tube and into the stomach.

5. If a balloon-tipped catheter is used, inflate the balloon with water after the tube is in place. The Pezzer catheter has an expanded head that flattens and then returns to its normal shape when a stylet is extended and then removed in the catheter lumen during placement through the stab incision into the stomach.

Homemade Canine Cancer Food

The following recipe will make 3 days' worth of food for a 25- to 30-lb dog.

Ingredients	Amount
Lean ground beef, fat drained	454 g (1 lb)
Rice, cooked	227 g (1⅓ cups)
Liver, beef	138 g (⅓ lb)
Vegetable oil	63 g (4½ Tbsp)
Fish oil	9 g (nine 1,000-mg fish oil capsules)[a]
Calcium carbonate	3.3 g[b]
Dicalcium phosphate[c]	2.9 g (¾ tsp)
Salt substitute (potassium chloride)	1.9 g (⅓ tsp)

Directions

Cook the rice with salt substitute added to the water. Cook the ground beef and drain the fat. Cook the liver and dice or finely chop into small pieces. Pulverize the calcium carbonate and vitamin/mineral tablets. Mix the vegetable oil, fish oil (break open capsules), and supplements with the rice; add the cooked ground beef and liver. Mix well, cover, and refrigerate. Feed approximately one-third of this mixture each day to a 25- to 30-lb dog. Palatability will be increased if the daily portion is heated to approximately body temperature. (Caution: When using a microwave to reheat, avoid "hot spots," which can burn the mouth.)

Nutrient Profile (% dry-matter basis)

Protein	35.3	Sodium	0.36
Fat	41.6	Potassium	0.68
Carbohydrate	17.8	Magnesium	0.05
Calcium	0.65	Energy	1,989 kcal/kg as fed
Phosphorus	0.54		

[a]Owners are encouraged to feed the highest dose of fish oil or, preferably, DHA oil tolerated by the dog.
[b]Calcium carbonate is available as oyster shell calcium tablets or Tums tablets (0.5 g in regular Tums, 0.75 g in Tums Extra, and 1.0 g in Tums Ultra; GlaxoSmithKline).
[c]Bone meal can be used in place of dicalcium phosphate.

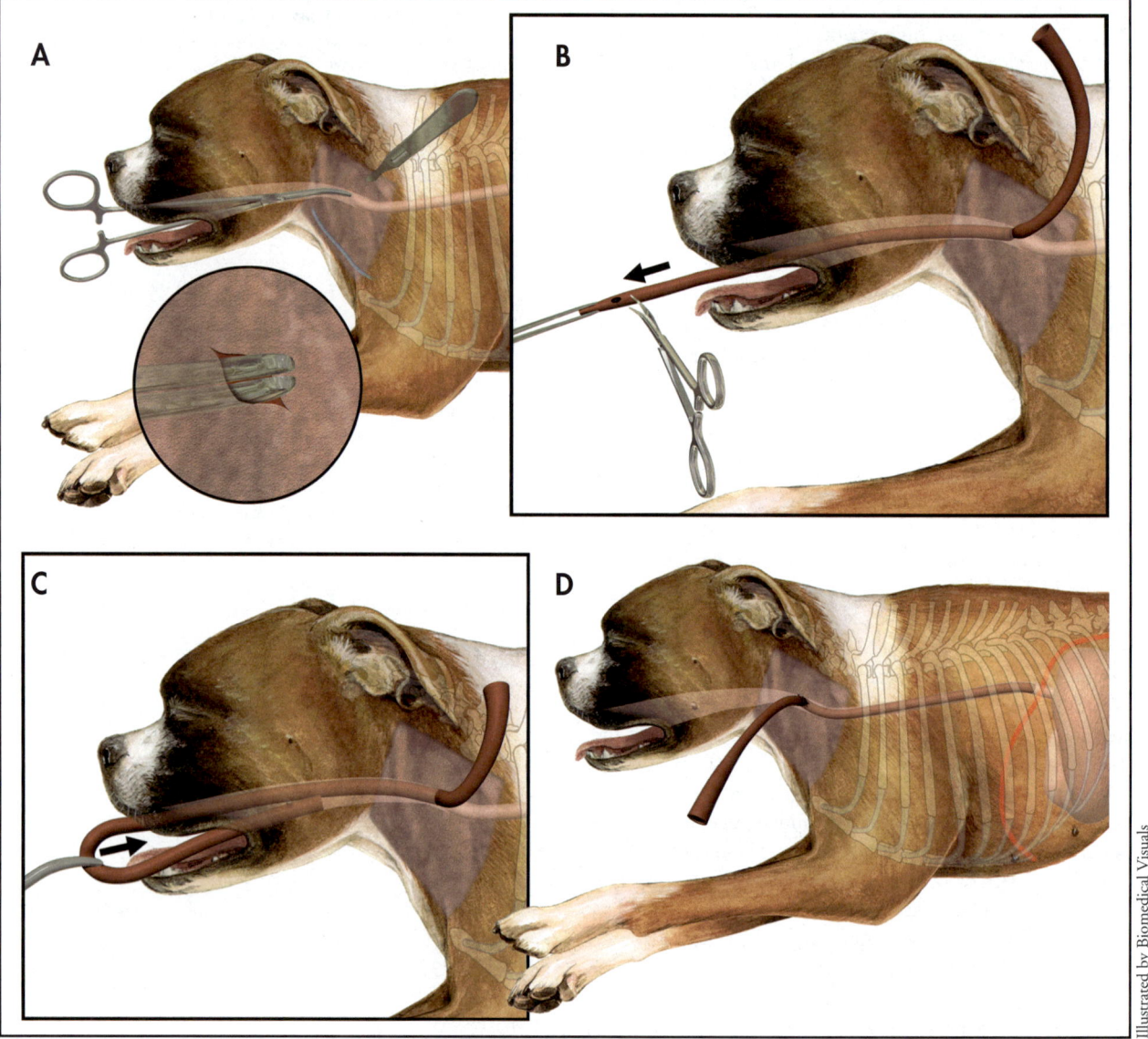

Figure 31-5. *Esophageal tube placement. Place the dog under anesthesia and clip and prepare the left lateral cervical skin for surgery. Place the esophagostomy tube in the midcervical region between the lateral spinous processes dorsally and the jugular vein and carotid artery ventrally. Then place a curved hemostat down the mouth into the esophagus with the curved portion of the instrument pointing laterally, halfway between the angle of the jaw and the thoracic inlet (**A**). Direct the hemostat laterally so that it "tents" the esophagus and overlying skin by pushing the tip laterally against the left lateral esophageal wall. Make a small incision (0.25–0.5 cm) over the tip of the hemostat. The key is to make a tiny incision through the esophagus just big enough to see the tip of the instrument (**B**). Push the instrument through the surgically created hole in the tissue. Open the jaws of the carmault or hemostat and grasp the tip of the red rubber feeding tube with the instrument, pulling it partially through the skin out the mouth (**C**). Push the tube aborally down the esophagus with the hemostat to the level of the ninth rib in dogs (**D**). To prevent any vomiting or reflux esophagitis, do not allow the tip of the tube to go into the stomach. Suture the esophagostomy tube into place and place a light wrap over the tube.*

6. With the tube in place, tie the purse-string sutures to cause the stomach to invert in the region adjacent to the tube. Then use the free ends of the sutures to close the lateral abdominal musculature and subcutaneous tissue.

7. Close the skin before securing the tube to the abdominal skin by sutures. To prevent the animal from removing the tube, an abdominal wrap and an Elizabethan collar are recommended.

Feeding can begin soon after the animal has recovered from anesthesia. The tube should be checked daily to ensure proper placement and should be flushed with warm water after each feeding to maintain patency. After 7 to 10 days,

NUTRITIONAL SUPPORT **241**

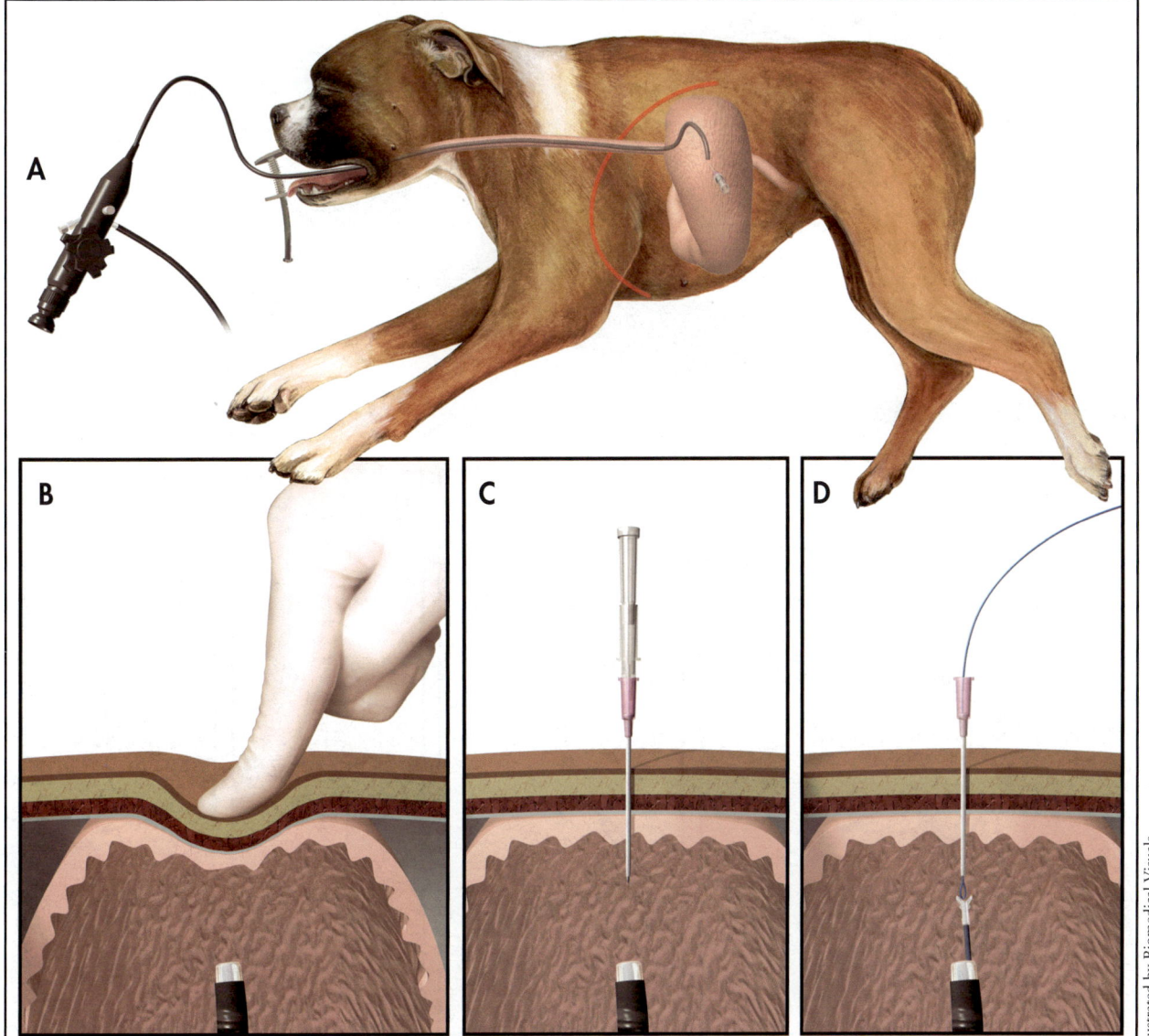

Figure 31-6. *Gastrostomy tube placement. An endoscope is used to insufflate the stomach so that a catheter can be placed through the skin and into the stomach to facilitate the passage of nylon suture into the stomach (**A**). The area caudal to the last left rib is depressed and located by endoscopy (**B**). A catheter is placed to allow the introduction of a piece of suture (**C**). The endoscope is used to grasp the suture, which is then pulled through the esophagus and out of the mouth (**D**). (Figure continues)*

an adhesion will form, allowing the tube to be removed or replaced as needed. The fistula generally heals within 1 week after the tube is permanently removed.

The percutaneous placement of a gastrostomy tube by endoscopic guidance is quick, safe, and effective.[1,2] In this procedure (Figure 31-6), a specialized 20-Fr tube (e.g., Dubhoff PEG, Biosearch, Summerville, NJ, or Bard Urological Catheter, Bard Urological Division, Covington, GA) is used.

1. Clip and surgically prepare an area of skin as described above. Distend the stomach with air from an endoscope placed into the stomach.

2. When the stomach is distended to the point that it is in apposition with the body wall, use a finger to depress an area just caudal to the last left rib below the transverse processes of the lumbar vertebrae. This area of depression is located by the person viewing the stomach lining by endoscopy.

3. Place a polyvinyl chloride (PVC) over-the-needle IV catheter through the skin and into the stomach in the

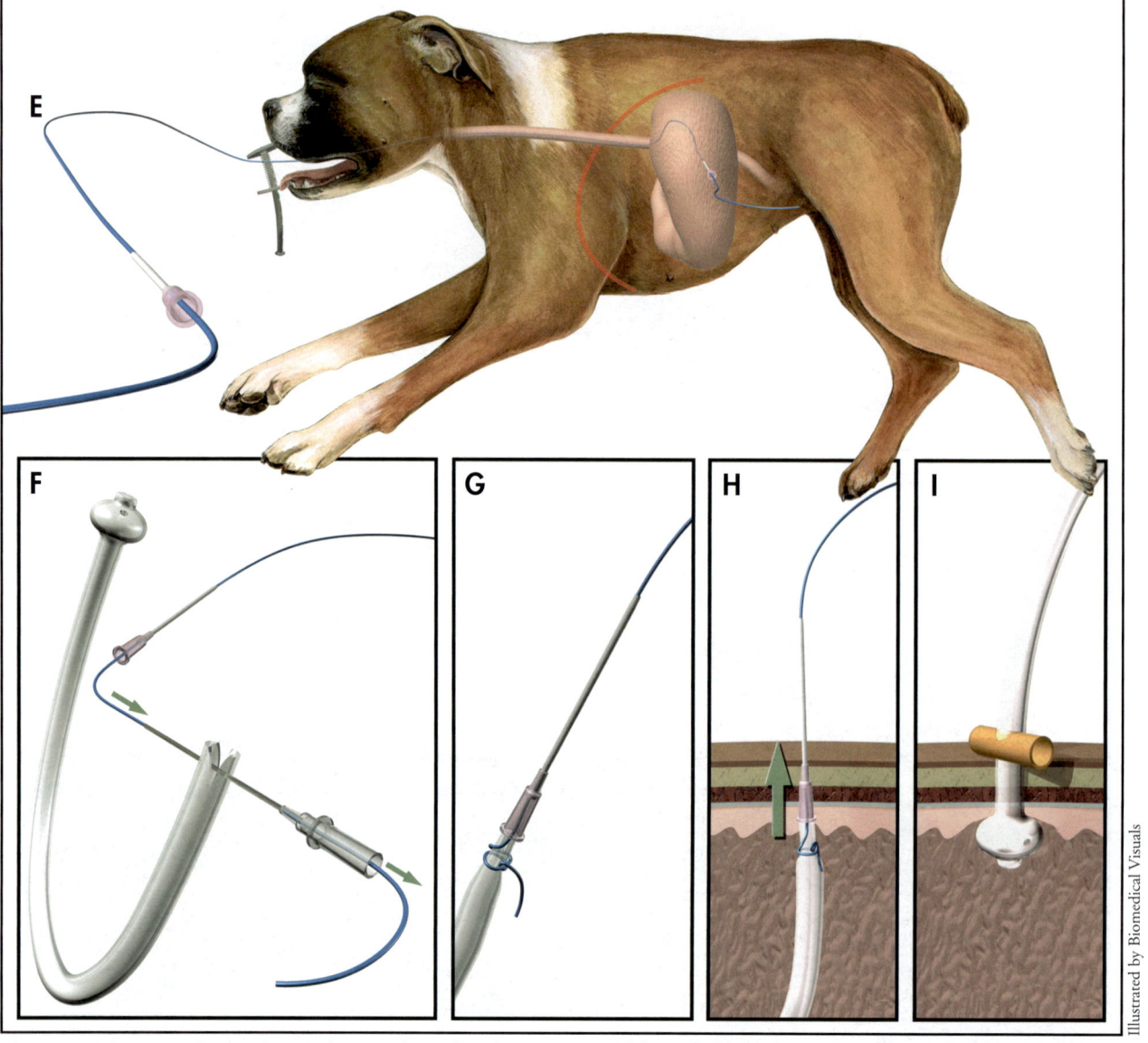

Figure 31-6 (continued). *A catheter is then passed over the nylon coming out of the animal's mouth (**E**). The Pezzer-tip gastrostomy tube is prepared (**F**) by cutting a "V" out of both sides of the open end of the tube. A needle is used to pass the nylon suture coming out of the mouth through the end of the tube, where a knot is securely fastened (**G**). The tube is then stretched and forced into the end of the catheter. The catheter–tube combination is pulled with the nylon suture down the esophagus, into the stomach, and through the abdominal wall (**H**), where a "bumper" is placed down the tube and against the body wall (**I**).*

area previously located by the endoscopist. Remove the stylet to allow the introduction of the first portion of a 5-ft piece of 8-lb test-weight nylon filament or suture.

4. Use a biopsy snare passed through the endoscope to grab the piece of nylon. Withdraw the endoscope and the attached nylon from the esophagus and oral cavity so that the piece of nylon extends through the body wall and out the mouth of the animal.

5. Trim the end of the gastrostomy tube opposite the mushroom tip so that it has a pointed end that will fit inside another PVC catheter after the stylet is removed and discarded. Place this second PVC IV catheter over the nylon suture so that the narrow end points toward the stomach. Suture the free end of the nylon emerging from the animal's mouth to the end of the tube and tie it securely.

6. Firmly but slowly, pull the end of the suture located outside the abdominal wall to advance the catheter–tube combination until the pointed end of the IV catheter passes down the esophagus and emerges from the abdominal wall.

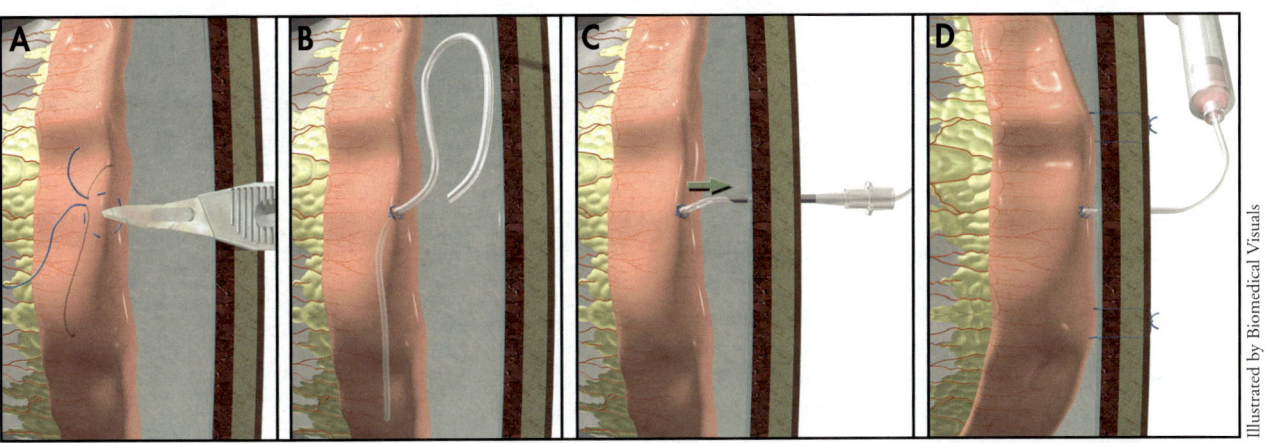

Figure: 31-7. A jejunostomy tube is surgically placed through a stab incision (**A**) in the antimesenteric side of the jejunum (**B**). The other end of the tube is then placed through the abdominal wall (**C**), whereupon the jejunum is securely sutured to the abdominal wall (**D**). Jejunostomy tubes are ideal for supporting cancer patients with alterations in the upper GI tract.

7. Grasp and pull the tube until the mushroom tip is adjacent to the stomach wall as viewed by endoscopy.

8. To prevent slippage, pierce the middle of a 3- to 4-inch piece of tubing completely through both sides and pass it over the feeding tube so that it is adjacent to the body wall. Glue or suture this bumper or retainer securely in place. Cap the tube and bandage it in place.

Complications with this method include peritonitis, diarrhea, and cramping.

An Elizabethan collar is almost always required to prevent the animal from removing the tube. To remove the tube once it has been in place for 7 to 10 days, the tube just below the bumper is severed to allow the mushroom tip to fall into the stomach. This piece may need to be removed by endoscopy in all but very large dogs.

Needle–Catheter Jejunostomy Tubes: Needle–catheter jejunostomy tubes should be considered for dogs with functional lower intestinal tracts that will not tolerate nasogastric or gastrostomy tube feeding.[1-4] This method is especially valuable in cancer patients that have had surgery of the upper GI tract. The procedure is as follows (Figure 31-7):

1. Locate the distal duodenum or proximal jejunum and isolate it by surgery. Place a purse-string suture of 3-0 nonabsorbable suture in the antimesenteric border of the isolated piece of bowel.

2. Place a 12-gauge needle from the serosa located at the center of the area encircled by the purse-string suture, subserosally 2 to 3 cm through the wall of the intestine, into the lumen of the loop of bowel. Alternatively, make a stab incision into the same location of the bowel using a No. 11 surgical blade.

3. Pass a 5-Fr nasogastric infant feeding tube through the hypodermic needle or the stab incision to an area down the bowel, 20 to 30 cm from the enterostomy site.

4. If a needle was used, remove it.

5. Tighten the purse-string suture and secure it around the tube.

6. Pass the free end of the feeding tube from the serosal surface of the abdominal wall out of the skin through a second hypodermic needle.

7. Secure the loop of bowel with the enterostomy site to the abdominal wall with four sutures. Cut these sutures after the tube is removed in 7 to 10 days, when feeding is complete.

As with gastrostomy tubes, complications with this method include peritonitis, diarrhea, and cramping.

Enteral Feeding Methods

The type of nutrients to be delivered depends largely on the enteral tube that is used and on the status of the patient.[1-4] Blended canned pet foods may be adequate for feeding by gastrostomy tube, and human enteral feeding products are easily administered through nasogastric and jejunostomy tubes. Feeding usually is not started until 24 hours after the tube is placed. Once feeding is started, the amount of nutrients is gradually increased over several days and is administered frequently in small portions, which allows the animal to adapt to this method of feeding. Continuous feeding may reduce the risk of vomiting caused by overloading the GI tract. Regardless, the tube should be aspirated three to four times a day to ensure there is not excessive residual volume in the GI tract. The tube should be flushed periodically with warm water to prevent clogging.

Parenteral Nutrition

Parenteral nutrition should be considered for animals with cancer whenever enteral feeding is not feasible. Parenteral feeding does require some specialized equipment, such as pumps, but the procedure can safely be carried out in private practice.

In veterinary medicine, parenteral nutrients are generally administered through a dedicated single-lumen polyurethane catheter or a more expensive multilumen catheter.[1,2] The catheter must be kept sterile to reduce the incidence of catheter-induced sepsis. One method of keeping the catheter port clean is to place a sealable plastic bag over the end. Most veterinary centers that administer parenteral nutrients use IV pumps to ensure a constant rate of infusion. The rate of infusion is simplified if lipid is used to provide a percentage of nonprotein calories because dextrose-containing fluids need to be gradually increased over several days.

With proper technique and patient care, problems associated with the administration of parenteral nutrition are relatively uncommon. Complications can result from destruction or occlusion of the catheter or tubing and pump failure; however, the most serious complication is catheter- or solution-related sepsis, which can be avoided by using aseptic technique. Other complications include metabolic and electrolyte abnormalities, including lactic acidosis. Mildly elevated blood urea nitrogen levels and hyperglycemia with glucosuria occasionally occur in dogs receiving parenteral nutrient therapy. Hypokalemia is perhaps the most common electrolyte disturbance related to parenteral feeding, but it is easily corrected with additional supplementation.

REFERENCES

1. Roudebush P, Davenport DJ, Novotny BJ: The use of nutraceuticals in cancer therapy. *Vet Clin North Am Small Anim Pract* 34(1):249–269, 2004.
2. Junien C, Gallou C: Cancer nutrigenomics. *World Rev Nutr Diet* 93:210–269, 2004.
3. Norman HA, Go VL, Butrum RR: Review of the International Research Conference on Food, Nutrition, and Cancer, 2004. *J Nutr* 134(12 Suppl):3391S–3393S, 2004.
4. Go VL, Wong DA, Wang Y, et al: Diet and cancer prevention: Evidence-based medicine to genomic medicine. *J Nutr* 134(12 Suppl):3513S–3516S, 2004.
5. Donaldson MS: Nutrition and cancer: A review of the evidence for an anti-cancer diet. *Nutr J* 3(1):19, 2004.
6. Vail DM, Ogilvie GK, Wheeler SL: Metabolic alterations in patients with cancer cachexia. *Compend Contin Educ Pract Vet* 12:381–395, 1990.
7. Ogilvie GK: Metabolic alterations and nutritional therapy for the veterinary cancer patient. *Compend Contin Educ Pract Vet* 15:925–937, 1993.
8. Ogilvie GK, Vail DM, Wheeler SL, et al: Effect of chemotherapy and remission on carbohydrate metabolism in dogs with lymphoma. *Cancer* 69(1):233–238, 1992.
9. Vail DM, Ogilvie GK, Fettman MJ, et al: Exacerbation of hyperlactatemia by infusion of lactated Ringer's solution in dogs with lymphoma. *J Vet Intern Med* 4:228–332, 1990.
10. Vail DM, Ogilvie GK, Wheeler SL et al: Alterations in carbohydrate metabolism in canine lymphoma. *J Vet Intern Med* 4:8–14, 1990.
11. Mazzaferro EM, Hackett TB, Stein TP et al: Metabolic alterations in dogs with osteosarcoma. *Am J Vet Res* 62(8):1234–1239, 2001.
12. Ogilvie GK, Ford RD, Vail DM: Alterations in lipoprotein profiles in dogs with lymphoma. *J Vet Intern Med* 8:62–66, 1994.
13. Ogilvie GK: Recent discoveries: Nutrition and cancer: Are eicosanoids the answer? *Vet Clin Nutr* 78:78–81, 1996.
14. McNiel EA, Ogilvie GK, Fettman MJ, Salman MD: Platelet hyperfunction in dogs with malignancies. *J Vet Intern Med* 11:178–182, 1997.
15. Ogilvie GK: Energy metabolism in diseased and critically ill dogs: New horizons. *Vet Clin Nutr* 4(4):138–142, 1997.
16. Lagutchik MS, Ogilvie GK, Hackett TM, Wingfield WE: Increased lactate concentrations in ill and injured dogs. *J Vet Emerg Crit Care* 8(2):117–127, 1998.
17. Hansen RA, Ogilvie GK, Davenport DJ, et al: Duration of effects of dietary fish oil supplementation on serum eicosapentanoic acid and doxocahexaenoic acid concentration in dogs. *Am J Vet Res* 59:864–868, 1998.
18. McNiel EA, Ogilvie GK, Mallinckrodt C, et al: Platelet function in dogs treated for lymphoma and hemangiosarcoma and supplemented with dietary n-3 fatty acids. *J Vet Intern Med* 13:574–580, 1999.
19. Ogilvie GK, Fettman MJ, Mallinckrodt CH, et al: Effect of fish oil, arginine, and doxorubicin chemotherapy on remission and survival time for dogs with lymphoma: A double-blind, randomized placebo-controlled study. *Cancer* 88(8):1916–1928, 2000.
20. Kazmierski KJ, Ogilvie GK, Fettman MJ, et al: Serum zinc, chromium, and iron concentrations in dogs with lymphoma and osteosarcoma. *J Vet Intern Med* 15(6):585–588, 2001.
21. Lu H, Forbes RA, Verma A: Hypoxia-inducible factor 1 activation by aerobic glycolysis implicates the Warburg effect in carcinogenesis. *J Biol Chem* 277(26):2311–2315, 2002.
22. Garber K: Energy boost: The Warburg effect returns in a new theory of cancer. *J Natl Cancer Inst* 96(24):1805–1806, 2004.
23. Muti P, Quattrin T, Grant BJ, et al: Fasting glucose is a risk factor for breast cancer: A prospective study. *Cancer Epidemiol Biomarkers Prev* 11(11):1361–1368, 2002.
24. Borugian MJ, Sheps SB, Kim-Sing C, et al: Insulin, macronutrient intake, and physical activity: Are potential indicators of insulin resistance associated with mortality from breast cancer? *Cancer Epidemiol Biomarkers Prev* 13(7):1163–1172, 2004.
25. Tayek JA: A review of cancer cachexia and abnormal glucose metabolism in humans with cancer. *J Am Coll Nutr* 11(4):445–456, 1992.
26. Raghavan M, Knapp DW, Bonney PL, et al: Evaluation of the effect of dietary vegetable consumption on reducing risk of transitional cell carcinoma of the urinary bladder in Scottish Terriers. *JAVMA* 227(1):94–100, 2005.
27. Mazzaferro E, Hackett T, Wingfield W, et al: Role of glutamine in health and disease. *Compend Contin Educ Pract Vet* 22(12):1094–1102, 2000.
28. Savarese DM, Savy G, Vahdat L, et al: Prevention of chemotherapy and radiation toxicity with glutamine. *Cancer Treat Rev* 29(6):501–513, 2003.
29. Fettman MJ, Valerius KD, Ogilvie GK, et al: Effects of dietary cysteine on blood sulfur amino acid, glutathione, and malondialdehyde concentrations in cats. *Am J Vet Res* 60(3):328–333, 1999.
30. Bounous G, Molson JH: The antioxidant system. *Anticancer Res* 23(2B):1411–1415, 2003.
31. Lind DS: Arginine and cancer. *J Nutr* 134(10 suppl):2837S–2841S, 2004.
32. Lippman SM, Hong WK: The biology behind cancer prevention by delay. *Clinical Cancer Research* 8:305–313, 2002.
33. Franceschi S, Favero A, La Vecchia C, et al: Influence of food groups and food diversity on breast cancer risk in Italy. *Int J Cancer* 63:785–789, 1995.
34. Fay MP, Freedman LS, Clifford CK, et al: Effect of different types and amounts of fat on the development of mammary tumors in rodents: A review. *Cancer Res* 57:3979–3988, 1977.
35. Thompson LU, Rickard SE, Orcheson LJ, et al: Flaxseed and its lignan and oil components reduce mammary tumor growth at a late stage of carcinogenesis. *Carcinogenesis* 17:1373–1376, 1996.
36. Braga C, La Vecchia C, Negri E, et al: Intake of selected foods and nutrients and breast cancer risk: An age- and menopause-specific analysis. *Nutr Cancer* 28:258–263, 1997.
37. Bougnoux P, Koscielny S, Chajes V, et al: Alpha-linolenic acid content of adipose breast tissue: A host determinant of the risk of early metastasis in breast cancer. *Br J Cancer* 70:330–334, 1994.
38. Maillard V, Bougnoux P, Ferrari P, et al: N-3 and n-6 fatty acids in breast adipose tissue and relative risk of breast cancer in a case-control study in Tours, France. *Int J Cancer* 98:78–83, 2002.
39. Denis F, Bougnoux P, de Poncheville L, et al: In vivo quantitation of tumour vascularisation assessed by Doppler sonography in rat mammary tumours. *Ultrasound Med Biol* 28(4):431–437, 2002.
40. Richardson KL, Lana SE, Fettman MJ, et al: Effect of fish oil and doxorubicin chemotherapy on remission and survival time in dogs with hemangiosarcoma: A double-blind, randomized, placebo-controlled study. *J Vet Intern Med,* in press.
41. Hansen RA, Slana SE, Anderson C, et al: Effect of fish oil on acute effects of radiation injury in dogs with nasal tumors: A double blind, randomized, placebo controlled study. *J Vet Intern Med,* in press.

42. Vartak S, Robbins ME, Spector AA: Polyunsaturated fatty acids increase the sensitivity of 36B10 rat astrocytoma cells to radiation-induced cell kill. *Lipids* 32(3):283–292, 1997.
43. Vartak S, McCaw R, Davis CS, et al: Gamma-linolenic acid (GLA) is cytotoxic to 36B10 malignant rat astrocytoma cells but not to 'normal' rat astrocytes. *Br J Cancer* 77(10):1612–1620, 1998.
44. Colas S, Paon L, Denis F, et al: Enhanced radiosensitivity of rat autochthonous mammary tumors by dietary docosahexaenoic acid. *Int J Cancer* 109(3):449–454, 2004.
45. Ogilvie GK, Walters LM, Fettman MJ, et al: Energy expenditure in dogs with lymphoma fed two specialized diets. *Cancer* 71:3146–3152, 1993.
46. Walters LM, Ogilvie GK, Fettman MJ, et al: Repeatability of energy expenditure measurements in normal dogs by indirect calorimetry. *Am J Vet Res* 54:1881–1885, 1993.
47. Clarke N, Germain P, Altucci L, Gronemeyer H: Retinoids: Potential in cancer prevention and therapy. *Expert Rev Mol Med* 6(25):1–23, 2004.
48. Brtko J, Thalhamer J: Renaissance of the biologically active vitamin A derivatives: Established and novel directed therapies for cancer and chemoprevention. *Curr Pharm Des* 9(25):2067–2077, 2003.
49. Niles RM, Loewy BP: Induction of protein kinase C in mouse melanoma cells by retinoic acid. *Cancer Res* 49:4483–4492, 1989.
50. White SD, Rosychuk RA, Scott KV, et al: Use of isotretinoin and etretinate for the treatment of benign cutaneous neoplasia and cutaneous lymphoma in dogs. *JAVMA* 202:387–391, 1993.
51. Block KI, Mead MN: Vitamin C in alternative cancer treatment: Historical background. *Integr Cancer Ther* 2(2):147–154, 2003.
52. Branda RF: Effects of folic acid deficiency on tumor cell biology, in Jacobs MM (ed): *Vitamins and Minerals in the Prevention and Treatment of Cancer.* Boca Raton, FL, CRC Press, 1991, pp 167–185.
53. Kline K, Sanders BG: Modulation of immune suppression and enhanced tumorigenesis in retrovirus tumor challenged chickens treated with vitamin E. *In Vivo* 3:161–185, 1989.
54. Kline K, Cochran GS, Sanders BG: Growth inhibitory effects of vitamin E succinate on retrovirus-transformed tumor cells in vitro. *Nutr Cancer* 14:27–35, 1990.
55. Miller ER 3rd, Pastor-Barriuso R, Dalal D, et al: Meta-analysis: High-dosage vitamin E supplementation may increase all-cause mortality. *Ann Intern Med* 142(1):37–46, 2005.
56. Paolini M, Abdel-Rahman SZ, Cantelli-Forti G, Legator MS: Chemoprevention or antichemoprevention? A salutary warning from the beta-carotene experience. *J Natl Cancer Inst* 93(14):1110–1101, 2001.
57. Shamberger RJ, Rukovena E, Longfield AK, et al: Antioxidants and cancer. I. Selenium in the blood of normals and cancer patients. *J Natl Cancer Inst* 50:863–870, 1973.
58. Ip C: Factors influencing the anticarcinogenic efficacy of selenium in dimethylbenzanthracene-induced mammary tumorigenesis in rats. *Cancer Res* 41:2638–2644, 1981.
59. Jacobs MM, Jansson B, Griffin AC: Inhibitory effects of selenium on 1,2-dimethylhydrazine and methylazoxymethanol acetate induction of colon tumors. *Cancer Lett* 2:133–2144, 1977.
60. Jacobs MM, Griffin AC: Effects of selenium on chemical carcinogenesis: Comparative effects on antioxidants. *Biol Trace Elem Res* 1:2–21, 1979.
61. Asselin BL, Ryan D, Frantz CN, et al: In vitro and in vivo killing of acute lymphoblastic leukemia cells by L-asparaginase. *Cancer Res* 49:4363–4369, 1989.
62. Weed H, McGandy RB, Kennedy AR: Protection against dimethylhydrazine induced adenomatous tumors of the mouse colon by the dietary addition of an extract of soybeans containing the Bowman-Birk protease inhibitor. *Carcinogenesis* 6:1239–1241, 1985.
63. Messadi DV, Billings P, Shklar G, Kennedy AR: Inhibition of oral carcinogenesis by a protease inhibitor. *J Natl Cancer Inst* 76:447–452, 1986.
64. St. Clair W, Billings P, Carew J, et al: Suppression of DMH-induced carcinogenesis in mice by dietary addition of the Bowman-Birk protease inhibitor. *Cancer Res* 50:580–586, 1990.
65. Kennedy AR: Effects of protease inhibitors and vitamin E in the prevention of cancer, in Prasad KN, Meyskens FL (eds): *Nutrients and Cancer Prevention.* Totowa, NJ, Humana Press, 1990, pp 79–98.
66. Witschi H, Kennedy AR: Modulation of lung tumor development in mice with the soybean-derived Bowman-Birk protease inhibitor. *Carcinogenesis* 10:2275–2277, 1989.
67. Kealy RD, Lawler DF, Ballam JM, et al: Influence of diet restriction on life span and age-related changes in Labrador retrievers. *JAVMA* 220:1315–1320, 2002.
68. Lawler DF, Evans RH, Larson BT, et al: Influence of lifetime food restriction on causes, time, and predictors of death in dogs. *JAVMA* 226(2):225–231, 2005.
69. Terry PD, Rohan TE, Wolk A: Intakes of fish and marine fatty acids and the risks of cancers of the breast and prostate and of other hormone-related cancers: A review of the epidemiologic evidence. *Am J Epidemiol* 141(4):352–359, 1995.
70. Sonnenschein EG, Glickman LT, Goldschmidt MH, McKee LJ: Body conformation, diet, and risk of breast cancer in pet dogs: A case-control study. *Am J Epidemiol* 133(7):694–703, 1991.

TRANSFUSION SUPPORT

Gregory K. Ogilvie and Antony S. Moore

CLINICAL BRIEFING

Blood donor characteristics	• The most common blood types are DEA 1.1, 1.2, 3, 4, 5, and 7. • Dogs with DEA 1.1 and 1.2 are group A positive; all others are group A negative. • Group–A negative donors are compatible with group A–negative and group A–positive recipients; major cross-match recommended after the first transfusion.
Indications	• Clinically significant acute blood loss, hemolytic anemia, nonregenerative anemia, thrombocytopenia, DIC, and hypoproteinemia.
Complications	• Clinical signs from incompatible blood: Hemolysis, hyperthermia, tachycardia, tachypnea, vomiting, collapse, urticaria and angioneurotic edema, and central nervous system alterations; treatment is to discontinue transfusion.
Rate of administration	• In an emergency situation, blood can be given rapidly (22 ml/kg/hr); otherwise, blood should be administered at a rate of 0.5 ml/kg/hr. • One unit of cryoprecipitate can be administered for every 5–10 kg and administered over 2 hours. • FFP can be given at 10 ml/kg administered over 2 hours.

Cancer patients, especially those presented for emergencies, frequently require blood component or transfusion therapy.[1-4] This type of treatment is essential for blood loss from the primary tumor, disseminated intravascular coagulation (DIC), clinical syndromes associated with the hypocoagulable state of malignancy, and other hematologic abnormalities.[1-3] In general, transfusions and administration of specific blood components should be given only when specifically indicated.

Serology

Blood typing for dogs is different than typing in human or feline medicine. Canine blood types have been defined based on the antigens on the cell surface of red blood cells (RBCs); however, only six blood types are currently identified in routine practice: dog erythrocyte antigens (DEAs) 1.1, 1.2, 3, 4, 5, and 7. A brief description of canine blood types follows[4-7]:

- **DEA 1:** The DEA 1 blood group has multiple alleles. These alleles define four DEA types: 1.1, 1.2, 1.3, and a negative or null type. The most clinically important canine antigens are DEA 1.1 and DEA 1.2; 40% of the canine population is DEA 1.1 positive, and 20% is 1.2 positive. Dogs positive for either of these antigens are considered group A positive; all other dogs are considered group A negative. Clinically significant antibodies against group A antigens do not exist naturally but can develop after exposure to group A–positive blood. DEA 1.1 is the most antigenic type, causing hemolytic transfusion reactions within 12 hours. Reactions to DEA 1.2 occur within 12 to 24 hours. A patient that has received an A-positive blood transfusion should be assumed to have developed antibodies and is at high risk for a transfusion reaction. The 1.3 antigen has not been extensively evaluated.

> **KEY POINT**
> *All canine blood donors should be group A negative unless the donor and recipient are both group A positive.*

- **DEA 3:** Once thought to be rare, DEA 3–positive RBCs may exist in up to 25% of greyhounds. DEA 3 alloantibody may occur naturally in up to 20% of all dogs. Delayed transfusion reactions can occur in these patients.
- **DEA 4:** DEA 4–positive dogs make up 98% of the canine population; therefore, dogs that are positive for DEA 4 and negative for other blood group antigens are considered universal donors. Alloantibodies to DEA 4 do not exist naturally, and antibodies that develop after transfusion are rarely a clinical problem.

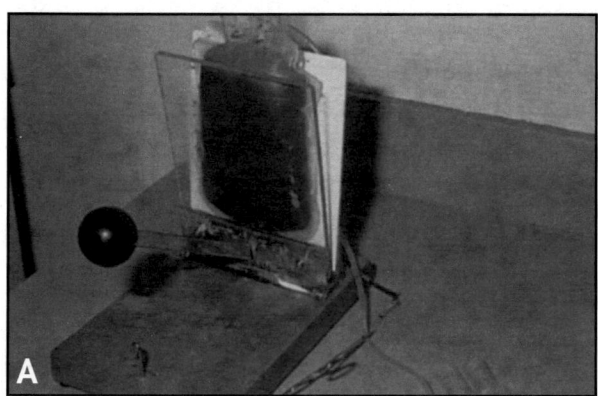 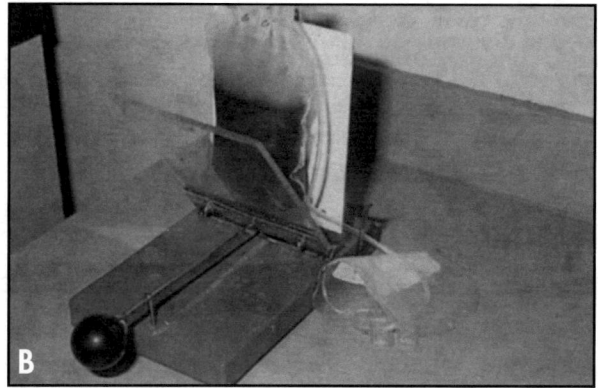

Figure 32-1. *Fresh whole blood is placed into a device (**A**) that squeezes the blood from the bottom of the bag (**B**), allowing the plasma to be decanted through a tube already in place into a separate bag. The process results in PRBCs and plasma that can be used for specific clinical settings. This procedure is also used to harvest platelet-rich plasma, which is located at, or just above, the interface between the RBCs and the plasma from a unit of blood that has been centrifuged.*

- **DEA 5:** This blood type is rare; however, up to 30% of greyhounds may be DEA 5 positive. Alloantibodies may exist in 10% of DEA 5–negative dogs, and delayed transfusion reaction can occur.
- **DEAs 6 and 8:** These antigens have been described, but their transfusion significance has not been evaluated.
- **DEA 7:** Antibodies to DEA 7 occur naturally in 50% of dogs. Antibody binding is weak; therefore, sensitized DEA 7–negative dogs show a delayed transfusion reaction when transfused with DEA 7–positive cells.

Dogs that have received previous transfusions should be cross-matched using only a major cross-match (e.g., testing the donor RBCs against the recipient's plasma), which allows determination of incompatibility in a cost-effective manner (Table 32-1). Donor plasma should not have antibodies to the recipient's RBCs unless the donor has been previously transfused.

> **KEY POINT**
>
> *Dogs that have received previous transfusions should be cross-matched using only a major cross-match (e.g., testing the donor RBCs against the recipient's plasma); this allows determination of incompatibility in a cost-effective manner.*

Blood is commercially available; however, larger practices often have their own blood donors. Although any large breed can make a good donor, greyhounds are more likely than Labrador retrievers to be only DEA 4 positive and have a quiet personality, high packed cell volume (PCV), and large body size, which makes them a popular choice. Sedation is rarely required during blood collection. Large dogs can safely donate 450 ml every 3 weeks for 2 years. The jugular or femoral vein is used, and the site is clipped and prepped as for surgery.

Plastic bags that hold 450 ml of whole blood and maintain a closed system are commercially available. Anticoagulants such as heparin or sodium citrate are used when the whole blood is to be used within 8 hours. Preservatives are used for blood products that are to be stored or shipped. Citrate phosphate dextrose adenine-1 (CPDA-1) is the most commonly used preservative. It has a shelf life of 20 days for dogs. Acid citrate dextrose A and B are also sometimes used and have a shelf life of 3 weeks. Additive nutrient solutions for processed packed red blood cells (PRBCs) (Nutricel (MEDSEP, Covina, CA) and Adsol (Baxter Healthcare, Round Lake, IL) increase the storage half-life of PRBCs up to 5 weeks.

Component Therapy

Blood components should be administered to dogs when clinically indicated. Blood component therapy can enhance the value of every unit of harvested blood.[1–4,8–11]

Whole blood or PRBCs[1–4, 8–11] may be administered immediately or stored for up to 21 days (Figures 32-1 and 32-2). PRBCs are obtained when whole blood is centrifuged and plasma is removed. The hematocrit is approximately 70% to 80%. When PRBCs are administered at 10 to 15 ml/kg, the PCV will increase by 10%. Packed cells are ideal for treatment of immune-mediated hemolytic anemia. It has been determined that human recombinant erythropoietin is a valuable adjuvant in canine blood banking for autotransfusion.[12] Erythropoietin enhances RBC vitality and stability. The safety of administering blood was exemplified in a study in which a total of 658 units of RBCs, including 474 units of PRBCs and 184 units of whole blood, were administered to 307 dogs.[13] Reasons for transfusion included hemorrhage, hemolysis, and ineffective erythropoiesis. The mean pre-

248 MANAGING THE CANINE CANCER PATIENT

Table 32-1 **Canine Transfusions**[1-4]

Blood Groups		Clinical Results
Recipient	Donor	
A+	A+	Compatible: no problems
A–	A–	Compatible: no problems
A–	A+	Compatible unless antibodies to DEA 1.1 or 1.2 (i.e., previously transfused)
A+	A–	Compatible: no problems

transfusion PCV of dogs with hemolysis was significantly lower than the mean pretransfusion PCV of dogs with hemorrhage or ineffective erythropoiesis. Overall, 67% of dogs were discharged from the hospital. Possible adverse events were observed during or shortly after RBC transfusion in 10 dogs (3.3%); all reactions were mild and self-limiting, and none was hemolytic.

Fresh frozen plasma (FFP)[8-11] is harvested and frozen within 6 hours of collection. FFP maintains adequate levels of clotting factors for up to 1 year. Frozen plasma stored for more than 1 year may have a diminished amount of clotting factors V, VII, and VIII and von Willebrand's factor (vWF). FFP is used to treat warfarin toxicity, DIC, vWF deficiency, hemophilia A, and sepsis. In one study, whole blood was collected from dogs to evaluate the effects of various storage conditions on one-stage prothrombin time (OSPT), activated partial thromboplastin time (APTT), and fibrinogen concentration of canine plasma collected for transfusion.[8] The investigators showed that storage for up to 30 days at 2°C versus -30°C did not have any significant effect on hemostatic parameters of canine plasma obtained for transfusion.

Cryoprecipitate[8-11] is made by ultrafreezing plasma for 24 hours, thawing in a refrigerator for 24 hours, and then removing the cryoprecipitate-free plasma. Cryoprecipitate concentrates factors VIII and XIII, fibrinogen, vWF, and fibronectin.

Cryoprecipitate-free plasma[8-11] is plasma left after the freezing/precipitation process for the making of cryoprecipitate. Cryoprecipitate-free plasma contains vitamin K–dependent proteins, with a slight decrease in factor IX and diminished factor VIII, factor XIII, fibrinogen, vWf, and fibronectin.

Oxyglobin[8-11] is a blood-substitute polymer. At the time of this writing, it is no longer commercially available; however, others of its type are likely to become available. Its IV half-life is 30 to 40 hours at the 30 ml/kg dose. More than 90% is eliminated within 5 to 7 days.

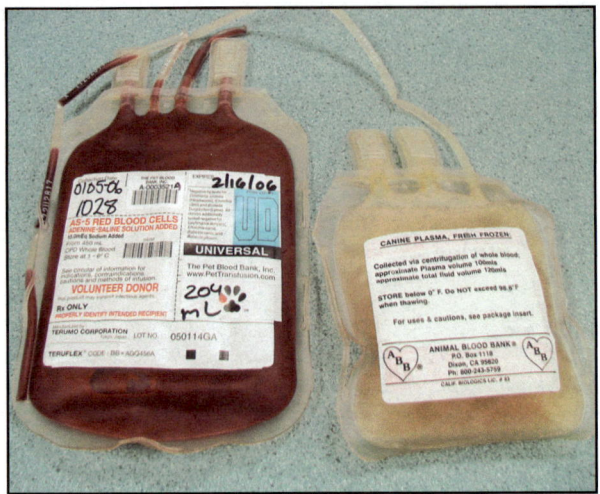

Figure 32-2. *The self-contained interconnected system allows separation of blood components without outside contamination. One unit (450 ml) of whole blood is equivalent to 270 ml of PRBCs. Whole blood or PRBCs may be administered immediately or stored for up to 21 days. Alternatively, FFP can be stored and used effectively for 1 year or longer.*

Indications for Transfusion Therapy[1-4]
HEMORRHAGE

Although there is a theoretical advantage to transfusing fresh whole blood, PRBCs can be administered with excellent results in cases of hemorrhage. Canine RBCs stored for more than 2 weeks can have a depletion of 2,3-diphosphoglycerate, which may decrease RBC oxygen-carrying capacity. When blood loss is chronic, transfusion should be performed to keep the hematocrit level above 15%. In acute and chronic blood loss, the patient's response to transfusion should be just as important a determinant as the hematocrit level or amount to be transfused. Dogs with acute blood loss are less tolerant of low hematocrit values, whereas those that have a gradual reduction in RBC numbers are able to adapt to extremely low RBC numbers.

HEMOLYTIC ANEMIA

Dogs with immune-mediated hemolytic anemia may require the administration of RBCs, even if it results in lysis of some of the transfused blood. Primary therapy with glucocorticoids, azathioprine, and cyclosporine is often essential to treat the underlying disease. The blood group of dogs with hemolytic anemia frequently cannot be determined adequately because of the presence of antibodies. Frequent evaluation of PCV is essential.

NONREGENERATIVE ANEMIA

Nonregenerative anemia can be relatively mild and often requires no transfusion. In some cases, however, nonregenerative anemia can be severe enough to require either fresh whole blood, when platelets are needed, or PRBCs. In addition, recombinant erythropoietin may be of value; however, antibodies directed to erythropoietin, which may cross-react with the animal's own erythropoietin, are a possible complication.

THROMBOCYTOPENIA

Platelet counts greater than 30,000/µl to 40,000/µl are rarely associated with bleeding disorders. A very gradual reduction in platelet counts can result in patients that appear healthy but have only 2,000 to 3,000 platelets/µl, especially when the platelets are relatively "young," as in immune-mediated thrombocytopenia. Recently released platelets have much greater function than older ones. Platelet transfusion is recommended only for dogs that exhibit clinical signs. Platelet-rich plasma may be considered in these patients; however, the circulating half-life of platelets may be only minutes, especially when immune-mediated conditions exist. One unit per 20 kg of platelet-rich plasma or fresh whole blood should be administered every hour until an adequate platelet count is reached. During this time, vincristine (0.5 mg/m² IV as a single dose or every 1–3 weeks) can be administered to induce premature release of platelets from the bone marrow. The platelet count usually increases 3 to 5 days after vincristine administration. This is especially valuable in immune-mediated thrombocytopenia because vincristine not only directly increases platelet numbers but also is taken up by platelets, where it is cytotoxic to phagocytic cells.

> **KEY POINT**
> *Platelet counts greater than 30,000/µl to 40,000/µl are rarely associated with bleeding disorders.*

DISSEMINATED INTRAVASCULAR COAGULATION

DIC can result in severe bleeding and consumption of clotting factors and platelets. In affected patients, approximately 1 U/10 kg of FFP can be given and repeated as needed to maintain prothrombin and partial thromboplastin time at 1 to 1.5 times the normal bleeding time. Heparin use is controversial; however, if given in conjunction with plasma, it may be of benefit. In patients in which all cell lines (RBCs and platelets) are decreased, fresh whole blood can be used (also see the Oncologic Emergencies section, Chapter 37).

HYPOPROTEINEMIA

Plasma transfusions can be valuable in patients that have decreased albumin levels. Increases in plasma proteins can be slower than expected after protein administration because only 40% of the body albumin is in the intravascular space, whereas 60% resides within the interstitial space. Thus, administration of FFP must increase albumin not only within the circulating space but also within interstitial spaces, which may require multiple units and repeated plasma administration. The administration of FFP from various donors can result in development of antibodies. Although their circulating half-life can be short, colloidal solutions, such as dextrans or hetastarch, may be more useful in these patients. Approximately 6 U of plasma are needed to raise the albumin of a 32-kg dog from 1.8 to 3 g/dL.

Amount to Transfuse[1-4]

Whole blood and PRBCs: Animals with significant acute blood loss should first be treated for shock with crystalloid solutions. Hypertonic saline is useful in selected patients. PRBCs can be given with crystalloid fluids, or whole blood may be used. As a general rule, 1 U of PRBCs is administered per 20 kg of body weight, with close adjustments to maintain the hematocrit values above 15%. Dogs that require whole blood for either acute or chronic anemia should be transfused using the general guideline below:

General Rule: Amount to Transfuse

Note: 2.2 ml of whole blood/kg or 1 ml/kg of PRBCs raises PCV 1% (transfused whole blood has a PCV of 40%).

$$\frac{ml}{donor} = [(2.2 \times wt_{kg}) \times (40)] \times \frac{(PCV_{desired} - PCV_{recipient})}{PCV_{donor}}$$

General Rule: Rate of Transfusion

0.5 ml/kg/h or faster (22 ml/kg/day) with close patient monitoring.

FFP: 10 ml/kg; repeat if necessary.

Cryoprecipitate and cryoprecipitate-free plasma: One unit to be given for every 5 to 10 kg of body weight and administered over 2 hours.

Oxyglobin: The labeled dose is 10 to 30 ml/kg; however, 7 to 10 ml/kg is the recommended starting dose for most patients.

> **KEY POINT**
> *In an emergency situation, blood can be given rapidly (22 ml/kg/hr); otherwise, blood should be administered at a rate of 0.5 L/kg/hr.*

Complications of Transfusions[1-4, 14]

Hemolysis is probably the most serious adverse effect of transfusion; however, it is relatively rare. Signs of an acute hemolytic reaction include elevated temperature, increased heart and respiration rates, and tremors, followed by vomiting and collapse. When this occurs, transfusion should be stopped and the patient's plasma should be checked for hemoglobinemia. Crystalloid fluids should be initiated and urine output monitored and preserved. Delayed hemolysis may occur in some patients.

> **KEY POINT**
> *Transfusion reactions are seen in less than 5% of canine patients.*

Fever that develops during transfusion can indicate either bacterial contamination of the blood or association with leukocyte antigens that elevate endogenous pyrogens. This elevation in body temperature is more common in cats than in dogs. Allergic reactions may manifest as urticaria and angioneurotic edema. If these occur, the transfusion should be discontinued and glucocorticoids should be administered. When large volumes of blood are administered, volume overload can occur; therefore, the patient's circulating volume should be monitored (e.g., central venous pressure, body weight) and treated appropriately (e.g., fluid restrictions, furosemide).

Citrate toxicity is a possible complication associated with stored whole blood and can cause an acute decrease in serum ionized calcium, especially in dogs with liver disease. Hypocalcemia results in muscle tremors, facial twitches, and seizures. IV calcium gluconate and cessation of transfusion is the treatment of choice. Rarely, blood ammonia levels can rise and cause associated clinical signs, such as mental dullness or seizures, particularly in animals with compromised liver function. This usually occurs in patients that receive blood that has been stored for a prolonged period and is usually associated with PRBCs. Treatment for this condition is the same as for hepatoencephalopathy, including a specialized diet such as Hill's Prescription Diet Canine l/d (Hill's Pet Nutrition, Topeka, KS); lactulose; antibiotics; non–lactate-containing fluids; Denosyl (Nutramax, Edgewood, MD); and, if indicated, ursodiol.

> **KEY POINT**
> *Hemolysis is probably the most serious adverse effect of transfusion, but it is relatively rare.*

REFERENCES

1. Stone MS, Cotter SM: Practical guidelines for transfusion therapy, in Kirk RW, Bonagura JD (eds): *Current Veterinary Therapy XI*. Philadelphia, WB Saunders, 1992, pp 479–485.
2. Giger U: The feline AB blood group system and incompatibility reactions, in Kirk RW, Bonagura JD (eds): *Current Veterinary Therapy XI*. Philadelphia, WB Saunders, 1992, pp 470–474.
3. Lanevschi A, Wardrop KJ: Principles of transfusion medicine in small animals. *Can Vet J* 42(6):447–454, 2001.
4. Feldman BF, Kristensen AT: Modern veterinary blood banking practices and their applications in companion animal practice. *Vet Clin North Am Small Anim Pract* 25(6):1231–1243, 1995.
5. Feldman BF: In-house canine and feline blood typing. *JAAHA* 35(6):455–456, 1999.
6. Hale AS: Canine blood groups and their importance in veterinary transfusion medicine. *Vet Clin North Am Small Anim Pract* 25(6):1323–1332, 1995.
7. Reine NJ: Infection and blood transfusion: A guide to donor screening. *Clin Tech Small Anim Pract* 19(2):68–74, 2004.
8. Iazbik C, Couto CG, Gray TL, Kociba G: Effect of storage conditions on hemostatic parameters of canine plasma obtained for transfusion. *Am J Vet Res* 62(5):734–735, 2001.
9. de Gopegui RR, Feldman BF: Use of blood and blood components in canine and feline patients with hemostatic disorders. *Vet Clin North Am Small Anim Pract* 25(6):1387–1402, 1995.
10. Rudloff E: The role of blood component therapy in the management of canine and feline patients with cancer. *Vet Clin North Am Small Anim Pract* 25(6):1403–1416, 1995.
11. Stokol T, Parry B: Efficacy of fresh-frozen plasma and cryoprecipitate in dogs with von Willebrand's disease or hemophilia A. *J Vet Intern Med* 12(2):84–92, 1998.
12. Suzuki K: Use of recombinant human erythropoietin as adjuvant therapy for blood banking for autotransfusion in dogs. *Vet J* 155(3):239–244, 1998.
13. Callan MB, Oakley DA, Shofer FS, Giger U: Canine red blood cell transfusion practice. *JAAHA* 32(4):303–311, 1996.
14. Harrell KA, Kristensen AT: Canine transfusion reactions and their management. *Vet Clin North Am Small Anim Pract* 25(6):1333–1364, 1995.

HEMATOPOIETIC GROWTH FACTOR SUPPORT

33

Gregory K. Ogilvie and Antony S. Moore

CLINICAL BRIEFING

Hematopoietic cytokines	• Glycoproteins such as G-CSF, GM-CSF, IL-3, and stem cell factor that all have profound effects on specific cell lines within the bone marrow and within other tissues of the body, including some tumors.
Recombinant erythropoietin	
Indications	• Anemia caused by inadequate production of red blood cells from normal bone marrow.
	• Especially effective when endogenous production of erythropcietin is low.
	• Patients with anemia caused by chronic renal failure, anemia of chronic malignant disease, chemotherapy, or radiation therapy.
Complications	• Erythrocytosis is a rare complication.
	• Antibodies can develop to recombinant human erythropoietin, rendering this therapy ineffective.
Recombinant granulocyte colony-stimulating factor	
Indications	• Neutropenia caused by inadequate production from the bone marrow.
	• rcG-CSF is effective for treating most neutropenias.
	• Response is directly proportional to the number of granulocyte precursors present and inversely proportional to the amount of endogenous G-CSF production.
	• rcG-CSF is effective for long-term therapy in dogs and cats.
Contraindications	• Neutrophilia can occur but is rarely a clinical problem.
	• Antibodies can develop to rhG-CSF, rendering this therapy ineffective.
Recombinant granulocyte–macrophage colony-stimulating factor	
Indications	• Neutropenia caused by inadequate production from the bone marrow.
	• rcGM-CSF is effective for treating neutropenia from most causes.
	• Response is directly proportional to the number of granulocyte precursors present and inversely proportional to the amount of endogenous GM-CSF production.
	• rcGM-CSF is effective for long-term therapy in dogs.
Contraindications	• Neutrophilia and monocytosis can occur but are rarely clinical problems.
	• Antibodies can develop to rhGM-CSF, rendering this therapy ineffective.

The use of hematopoietic growth factors has become an integral part of human cancer therapy. The limited availability of commercially available recombinant canine hematopoietic growth factors has limited the long-term use of these treatments in veterinary oncology. In the long-term, they have the potential to improve animal health.[1,2] The most clinically useful growth factors are erythropoietin, granulocyte colony-stimulating factor (G-CSF), and granulocyte–macrophage colony-stimulating factor (GM-CSF). Studies have been conducted in dogs using interleukin (IL)-3 and a fusion protein called PIXY321.

Erythropoietin

Recombinant human erythropoietin is commercially available and is similar to canine erythropoietin. The human and recombinant canine growth factors have been used clinically and experimentally in dogs with chronic renal failure with beneficial results.[2-4] For example, the efficacy and safety of recombinant canine erythropoietin therapy were evaluated in 19 dogs with chronic renal failure and significant anemia.[3] Recombinant canine erythropoietin stimulated erythrocyte production in dogs with nonregenerative anemia secondary to chronic renal failure without causing the profound erythroid hypoplasia that can occur in recombinant human erythropoietin–treated dogs. Although this study did not involve dogs with cancer, it did illustrate the value of using erythropoietin in dogs with renal disease.

> **KEY POINT**
> *The administration of erythropoietin is most effective in anemic patients that have low erythropoietin levels and normal bone marrow.*

Clinically, recombinant erythropoietin does improve quality of life in human cancer patients who have anemia of chronic disease due to their malignancies or associated chemotherapy and radiation therapy.[2] The response to therapy is directly related to the number of erythrocyte progenitor cells in the marrow and inversely related to the amount of endogenous erythropoietin in the patient. One area that is being explored is the use of recombinant erythropoietin as adjuvant therapy in banking blood used in autotransfusion.

Potential secondary effects of recombinant human erythropoietin include systemic hypertension, iron deficiency, hyperkalemia, polycythemia, and the development of antibodies to the recombinant protein in approximately 30% of patients weeks to months after treatment is initiated.[2-4] Antibody development does not appear to be a problem if recombinant canine erythropoietin is used. Indeed, investigators have shown that recombinant canine erythropoietin stimu-

> **KEY POINT**
> *Long-term use of recombinant human hematopoietic growth factors may result in antibody formation that can cross-react with the patient's own factors ("autoantibodies").*

lates erythrocyte production in clinically normal dogs during a 24-week period without causing the erythroid hypoplasia that is seen in recombinant human erythropoietin–treated dogs.[4] This reinforces the importance of using species-specific hematopoetic growth factors whenever possible.

Human or preferably recombinant canine erythropoietin can be administered to dogs at a dosage of 75 to 100 U/kg/day SC for 5 to 7 days, followed by the same dosage given two to three times a week until the hematocrit approaches the desired level. Erythropoietin can be administered weekly thereafter. Hematocrit levels should be monitored; if a decrease in the number of red blood cells occurs, steps should be taken to determine the cause. If the decrease is due to antibody formation to the erythropoietin, the therapy should be discontinued. Optimally, the hematocrit can increase by 1% per day; therefore, this type of therapy is not appropriate in cases of life-threatening anemia.

Granulocyte Colony-Stimulating Factor

Recombinant human G-CSF (rhG-CSF) and recombinant canine G-CSF (rcG-CSF) have been shown to induce their effect primarily on committed granulocytic precursors to increase neutrophil phagocytosis, superoxide generation, and antibody-dependent cellular cytotoxicity.[5] These proteins can be used whenever there is an inadequate number of neutrophils and in impending acute situations such as bone marrow toxicity and bacterial sepsis.[5-14] Both recombinant proteins have been produced in large quantities through recombinant technology using *Escherichia coli* bacteria. rcG-CSF is preferred over the human growth factor because it does not induce the formation of antibodies against the foreign or endogenous protein.

G-CSF is commonly used in human medicine to treat neutropenia and sepsis. In veterinary medicine, G-CSF has been used to treat neutropenia caused by chemotherapy and infections from conditions such as parvoviral enteritis.[15,16] There is no question that G-CSF reduces the duration and severity of chemotherapy-induced neutropenia; however, results vary concerning the value of this protein to enhance quality and quantity of life in puppies with parvoviral enteritis.[14,15]

Research has been conducted to evaluate the effect of dosage on the response of bone marrow to stimulation by G-CSF. One study showed a dosage-dependent increase in neutrophil and monocyte counts when rcG-CSF was given subcutaneously to normal dogs at dosages ranging from 3 to 25 µg/kg/day.[11] Another study evaluated the changes in neutrophil counts when rcG-CSF was administered at a dosage of 5 µg/kg/day to a group of healthy dogs.[11] At that dosage, mean neutrophil counts increased significantly to 26,330/µl within 24 hours after the first injection of rcG-CSF. The neutrophils reached a maximum of 72,125/µl by day 19. The neutrophil counts remained in this range until cytokine therapy was discontinued. Blood counts returned to normal within 5 days after discontinuing treatment. Re-initiation of rcG-CSF treatment resulted in a more rapid, dramatic increase in neutrophil numbers. Long-term (>30 days) use of rhG-CSF in dogs has been shown to induce significant decreases in neutrophil counts, presumably caused by antibody formation to the foreign rhG-CSF.[12] Therefore, rhG-CSF should only be used on a short-term

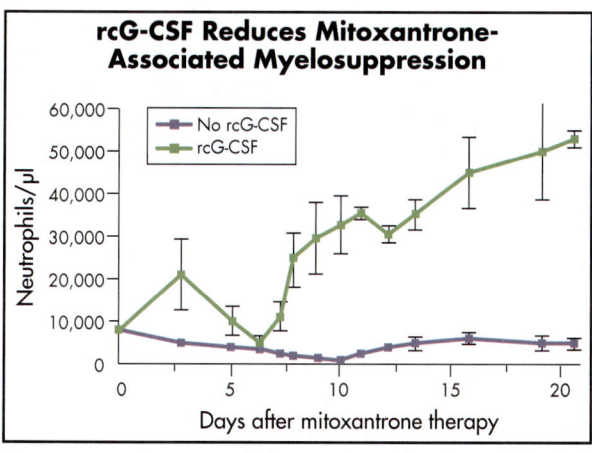

Figure 33-1. Mean neutrophil counts (±SD) from two groups of five normal dogs that received mitoxantrone (5 mg/m² IV) on day 0. Administration of rcG-CSF began on day 1 and ended on day 20. (From Ogilvie GK, Obradovich JA, Cooper MF: The use of recombinant colony-stimulating factor to decrease myelosuppression associated with the administration of mitoxantrone in the dog. J Vet Intern Med 6:44–47, 1992; with permission)

basis in dogs. Long-term treatment with rcG-CSF does not induce antibody formation in dogs.

> **KEY POINT**
> *One of the most promising areas of clinical application of G-CSF is in the prevention and treatment of chemotherapy- and radiation-induced cytopenias.*

One of the most promising areas of clinical application of G-CSF is in the prevention and treatment of chemotherapy- and radiation-induced cytopenia. It was shown that rcG-CSF is effective in significantly reducing the myelosuppression associated with mitoxantrone chemotherapy in dogs (Figure 33-1).[13] The dose-limiting toxicity associated with mitoxantrone therapy in dogs is myelosuppression. In that study, 10 healthy dogs were given IV mitoxantrone at a dose of 5 mg/m² body surface area.[13] rcG-CSF was administered to five of these dogs at 5 μg/kg/day SC for 20 days starting 24 hours after the chemotherapy was administered. The median neutrophil counts dropped below normal (<3,000/μl) for 2 days in dogs that received rcG-CSF and dropped for 5 days in dogs that only received mitoxantrone. Four of five dogs that were not treated with rcG-CSF, but none of the dogs receiving rcG-CSF developed serious neutropenia (<1,500/μl). Neutrophil counts were significantly higher in the dogs treated with rcG-CSF at all times evaluated except before administration of cytokine and mitoxantrone and on day 6 of therapy. Therefore, rcG-CSF seems to be safe and effective for preventing chemotherapy-induced myelosuppression in dogs.

G-CSF may be administered subcutaneously at 5 μg/kg/day to neutropenic dogs that are at risk of declining because of infection or sepsis. When the option exists, rcG-CSF should be chosen over rhG-CSF. As shown in the study above, G-CSF is more likely to be effective as a prophylactic measure rather than in the setting of emergency treatment of severe neutropenia. Using G-CSF when the neutrophil counts are already at the nadir does little to improve the already high levels of endogenous G-CSF and hence is unlikely to cause improvement in neutrophil numbers. An example in which G-CSF would be important is after an inadvertent overdose of a myelosuppressive chemotherapy agent; in this situation, starting G-CSF within 24 hours could make the difference between survival and death from sepsis.

Granulocyte–Macrophage Colony-Stimulating Factor

GM-CSF is a glycoprotein that is produced by a number of different tissues in the body, including T lymphocytes, monocytes, endothelial cells, and fibroblasts. As its name implies, GM-CSF stimulates the production of granulocytes and macrophages and acts in concert with erythropoietin and IL-3 to stimulate erythroid precursors.[16] This cytokine also acts along with IL-3 to regulate thrombopoiesis. This stimulator of multilineage and committed progenitors also increases the function of mature granulocytes, monocytes, macrophages, and eosinophils. More specifically, the cell-killing activity of neutrophils is enhanced by inhibiting migration of these cells, increasing chemotaxis, adhesion, phagocytosis, and superoxide generation; therefore, GM-CSF increases tumoricidal cytotoxicity.

> **KEY POINT**
> *G-CSF may be administered subcutaneously at 5 μg/kg/day to neutropenic dogs that are at risk of declining due to infection or sepsis.*

The use of GM-CSF in clinical medicine has the potential to be at least as profound and widespread as that of G-CSF. Recently, canine GM-CSF was shown to be effective for increasing granulocyte counts in dogs. We have used rhGM-CSF in dogs with chemotherapy-induced myelosuppression with variable results. One reason that GM-CSF may not have had as profound an effect as G-CSF in dogs is because of variable sequence homology between the recombinant products and the native GM-CSF of dogs. This has been shown in various species; for example, there is only a 57% sequence homology between human and murine GM-CSF and up to 75% homology between human and murine G-CSF.

In an attempt to overcome this problem, the use of nonspecific inducers of hematopoietic growth factors has been explored. For example, Imuvert (Cell Technologies, Inc, Boulder, CO), a biologic response modifier composed of ribosomes and other subcomponents of *Serratia marcescens*, is known to induce a variety of cytokines, including IL-1, IL-2, and GM-CSF.[17] Imuvert decreased the duration and severity of doxorubicin-induced myelosuppression in Imuvert-treated dogs compared with controls.[17] The mechanism of action of this biologic response modifier in dogs is unknown; endogenous G-CSF as determined by enzyme-linked immunosorbent assay (ELISA) methodology did not increase in response to administration of Imuvert.

Like G-CSF, GM-CSF has been shown to decrease the duration and severity of chemotherapy- and radiation-induced neutropenia in humans and laboratory animals. Because GM-CSF affects several cell lines, a variety of disease states can be treated with this growth factor. Diseases linked with leukopenia-associated AIDS, bone marrow failure states (e.g., myelodysplasia), aplastic anemia, and chronic and acute bacterial infections have been shown to be substantially improved with GM-CSF therapy. GM-CSF may be superior to G-CSF for rapid recovery from bone marrow transplantation. GM-CSF can stimulate some leukemic cells and therefore may be of value for forcing cells into the cell cycle, thus making them more susceptible to cell cycle–specific drugs. Some hypothesize that GM-CSF, like G-CSF, may force leukemic cells to differentiate and die. Finally, GM-CSF has been used experimentally to enhance the efficacy of liposome-encapsulated muramyl tripeptide for the successful treatment of canine malignant melanoma.[18]

G-CSF, but not GM-CSF, is currently being used to support clinical patients except in the experimental setting. The increased availability of rcGM-CSF may increase the use of this protein.

Interleukin-3, Stem Cell Factor, and PIXY321

IL-3, GM-CSF, G-CSF, and stem cell factor are members of a group of glycoproteins called *hematopoietic cytokines*.[19] These cytokines regulate the growth and differentiation of hematopoietic progenitor cells and functionally activate mature neutrophils or macrophages, a clinically useful function in cases of myelosuppression and sepsis.

Like GM-CSF, IL-3 affects multipotential marrow progenitors; however, IL-3 seems to have activity at an earlier stage than does GM-CSF. Humans with myelodysplasia and aplastic anemia treated with IL-3 showed dramatic increases in granulocytes, platelets, and red blood cells. Unlike G-CSF and GM-CSF therapy, responses to IL-3 do not occur until the fourth week after the start of treatment. Some investigators have shown that IL-3 can be used to decrease chemotherapy-induced myelosuppression in human patients. Sequential administration of IL-3 and GM-CSF has been shown to cause a marked increase in white blood cells, including myeloid lineages and platelets; the effect was clearly additive. We have used recombinant human IL-3 in dogs without significant changes in any cell line.

Stem cell factor may be a key treatment to enhance production and function of the bone marrow; however, some studies have shown that stem cell factor—like the other hematopoietic cytokines—can also stimulate the proliferation of nonhematopoietic cells. The receptors for these cytokines have been detected in cancer cell lines, and stimulation of these receptors induced proliferation of tumor cells.

One study demonstrated that recombinant human IL-3, GM-CSF, and a fusion protein of these cytokines, called PIXY321, did not significantly increase platelets, neutrophils, monocytes, or red blood cells in normal dogs.[20] This was unfortunate because these multilineage growth factors have the potential to treat a wide variety of bone marrow disorders in veterinary medicine.

Additional research is necessary before these cytokines are recommended for routine clinical use.

REFERENCES

1. Elmslie RE, Dow SW, Ogilvie GK: Interleukins: Biological properties and therapeutic potential. *J Vet Intern Med* 5:283–293, 1991.
2. Langston CE, Reine NJ, Kittrell D: The use of erythropoietin. *Vet Clin North Am Small Anim Pract* 33(6):1245–1260, 2003.
3. Randolph JF, Stokol T, Scarlett JM, MacLeod JN: Comparison of biological activity and safety of recombinant canine erythropoietin with that of recombinant human erythropoietin in clinically normal dogs. *Am J Vet Res* 60(5):636–642, 1999.
4. Randolph JE, Scarlett JM, Stokol T, MacLeod JN: Clinical efficacy and safety of recombinant canine erythropoietin in dogs with anemia of chronic renal failure and dogs with recombinant human erythropoietin-induced red cell aplasia. *J Vet Intern Med* 18(1):81–91, 2004.
5. Thomasson B, Peterson L, Thompson J, et al: Direct comparison of steady-state marrow, primed marrow, and mobilized peripheral blood for transduction of hematopoietic stem cells in dogs. *Hum Gene Ther* 14(17):1683–1686, 2003.
6. Sevransky JE, Parent C, Cui X, et al: Granulocyte colony-stimulating factor has differing effects comparing intravascular versus extravascular models of sepsis. *J Trauma* 57(3):618–625, 2004.
7. Yanay O, Barry SC, Katen LJ, et al: Treatment of canine cyclic neutropenia by lentivirus-mediated G-CSF delivery. *Blood* 102(6):2046–2052, 2003.
8. Suttorp M, Hoffmann B, Sippell WG: Prevention of oestradiol-associated toxicosis in a dalmatian by early intervention with granulocyte colony-stimulating factor. *Vet Rec* 151(8):244–245, 2002.
9. Kraft W, Kuffer M: Treatment of severe neutropenias in dogs and cats with filgrastim. *Tierarztl Prax* 23(6):609–613, 1995.
10. Obradovich JE, Ogilvie GK: Evaluation of recombinant canine granulocyte colony-stimulating factor as an inducer of granulopoiesis. *J Vet Intern Med* 5:75–79, 1991.
11. Obradovich JE, Ogilvie GK, Cooper MF, et al: Effect of increasing dosages of canine recombinant granulocyte colony-stimulating factor on neutrophil counts in normal dogs. *Proc Vet Cancer Soc 10ᵗʰ Annu Conf* 5, 1990.
12. Lorthrup CD Jr, Warren DJ, Souza LM, et al: Correction of canine cyclic hematopoiesis with recombinant human granulocyte colony-stimulating factor. *Blood* 72:1324–1334, 1988.
13. Ogilvie GK, Obradovich JE, Cooper MF, et al: The use of recombinant canine granulocyte colony-stimulating factor to decrease myelosuppression associated with the administration of mitoxantrone in the dog. *J Vet Intern Med* 6:44–47, 1992.
14. Mischke R, Barth T, Wohlsein P, et al: Effect of recombinant human granulocyte colony-stimulating factor (rhG-CSF) on leukocyte count and survival rate of dogs with parvoviral enteritis. *Res Vet Sci* 70(3):221–225, 2001.
15. Rewerts JM, McCaw DL, Cohn LA, et al: Recombinant human granulocyte colony-stimulating factor for treatment of puppies with neutropenia secondary to canine parvovirus infection. *JAVMA* 213(7):991–992, 1998.

16. Shin IS, Nam MJ, Park SJ, et al: Cloning of canine GM-CSF and SCF genes. *J Vet Sci* 2(3):159–166, 2001.
17. Ogilvie GK, Elmslie RE, Pearson F: The use of a biological extract of *Serratia marcescens* to decrease myelosuppression associated with doxorubicin-induced myelosuppression in the dog. *Am J Vet Res* 53:1787–1790, 1992.
18. MacEwen EG, Kurzman ID, Vail DM, et al: Adjuvant therapy for melanoma in dogs: Results of randomized clinical trials using surgery, liposome-encapsulated muramyl tripeptide, and granulocyte macrophage colony-stimulating factor. *Clin Cancer Res* 5(12):4249–4258, 1999.
19. Mroczko B, Szmitkowski M: Hematopoietic cytokines as tumor markers. *Clin Chem Lab Med* 42(12):1347–1413, 2004.
20. Ciekot PE, Ogilvie GK, Fettman MJ, et al: Evaluation of GM-CSF, IL-3, and GM-CSF/IL-3 fusion protein (PIXY 321) as multilineage colony stimulating factors in the dog [abstract]. *Vet Cancer 11th Annu Conf* 41–43, 1991.

SECTION 4

DIAGNOSIS AND THERAPY: PARANEOPLASTIC SYNDROMES AND ONCOLOGIC EMERGENCIES

Chapter 34 Paraneoplastic Syndromes and 259
Oncologic Emergencies: Overview

Chapter 35 Chemotherapy- or Radiation-Induced 261
Congestive Heart Failure

Chapter 36 Metabolic Manifestations of Malignancy: 266
Hypercalcemia, Hypocalcemia,
Hypoglycemia, and Hyponatremia (SIADH)

Chapter 37 Hematologic Manifestations of Malignancy 277

Chapter 38 Hypergammaglobulinemia 292

Chapter 39 Extravasation of Chemotherapeutic Agents 295

Chapter 40 Chemotherapy-Induced Anaphylaxis 298
and Hypersensitivity

SECTION 4

DIAGNOSIS AND THERAPY: PARANEOPLASTIC SYNDROMES AND ONCOLOGIC EMERGENCIES

Chapter 41   Cancer Therapy–Induced Renal Failure 301

Chapter 42   Acute Tumor Lysis Syndrome 306

Chapter 43   Disseminated Intravascular Coagulation 309

Chapter 44   Cancer-Related Disorders of the Central 314
Nervous System

Chapter 45   Cancer Cachexia as a Manifestation of 320
Malignancy

Chapter 46   Fever, Hypertrophic Osteopathy, and 323
Hypercortisolism

PARANEOPLASTIC SYNDROMES AND ONCOLOGIC EMERGENCIES: OVERVIEW   34

Gregory K. Ogilvie and Antony S. Moore

CLINICAL BRIEFING

Paraneoplastic syndromes	• Clinical signs induced by indirect means that may actually be more debilitating than the consequences of the cancer itself.
Types of emergencies	• True life-threatening emergencies. • Medical problems that are perceived as being life-threatening by well-meaning, concerned clients. • Emergencies of convenience (i.e., the caregiver wants the dog to be evaluated immediately despite non–life-threatening problems).
Initial approach to emergencies	• Identify the primary complaint. • Evaluate vital signs, including airway and breathing ability; heart rate, rhythm, and character; body temperature; and mucous membrane color and capillary refill time. • Perform a complete physical examination. • Obtain a complete history, including prior cancer treatment.

Cancer is a word feared throughout the world, regardless of the species affected. A diagnosis of cancer sets in motion feelings of fear and urgency. These feelings spur clients to demand that the veterinary health care team respond rapidly to their concerns. This heightened level of emotion is first witnessed during the initial diagnosis of cancer and the decision-making process but is often most apparent in emergency situations. It is important to note that dogs may hide their clinical signs until quite late in the disease process and thus are often in a debilitated state by the time cancer therapy begins; therefore, speed and decisiveness are key ingredients of successful emergency care.

This section is a prelude to the following chapters on paraneoplastic syndromes and oncologic emergencies. These two subjects are distinctly different; however, they are often intertwined because paraneoplastic syndromes are commonly responsible for oncologic emergencies.[1]

Paraneoplastic Syndromes

Cancer is a documented common cause of sickness and debilitation in dogs. Cancer may induce clinical signs not only directly by altering the body's structure or function but also indirectly by means that may actually be more debilitating than the consequences of the primary tumor. These indirect effects are known as *paraneoplastic syndromes* and are of profound importance to practicing veterinarians because of their devastating effects on dogs with cancer. The most common paraneoplastic syndromes in canine medicine are thought to be caused by the production of polypeptide hormones, most of which have endocrine-like effects. Other paraneoplastic syndromes include hematologic and cutaneous manifestations, hypergammaglobulinemia, cachexia, fever, neurologic syndromes, and hypertrophic osteopathy.

Detection of hormones or hormone-like substances that are directly elaborated or indirectly induced by the tumor can be used as a marker for the presence of a tumor. The most obvious examples are the detection of parathormone or insulin-like substances. Clinical evidence of an endocrine-associated paraneoplastic syndrome can also be used as a tumor marker. Complete workups of each condition are essential to unravel the typically vague clinical signs and subtle findings on physical examination. Therapy should be directed primarily at eliminating the underlying malignancy,

> *Many paraneoplastic syndromes in canine medicine are thought to be caused by the production of polypeptide hormones, the most common of which cause endocrine-like effects such as hypercalcemia and hypoglycemia.*

although modulation of tumor-induced hormones or hormone-like substances is an attractive alternative. In many cases, specific treatment of the paraneoplastic syndrome itself may be essential for the dog's survival.

Oncologic Emergencies

It is essential that canine oncologic emergencies be handled with extreme medical care as well as understanding. When an emergency or urgent situation arises, the entire veterinary health care team should be prepared to provide timely, compassionate care to meet the medical and nonmedical needs of both the patient and the caregiver. In some cases, this may mean referring the patient to another facility.

There are three types of emergencies:

- True life-threatening emergencies
- Medical problems that are perceived as being life-threatening by well-meaning, concerned clients
- Emergencies of convenience, in which the client wants the dog to be evaluated immediately despite non–life-threatening problems to accommodate the client's personal needs or schedule

Regardless of the type of emergency, the health care team should:

- Determine the primary complaint
- Evaluate vital signs, including:
  —Airway and breathing ability
  —Heart rate, rhythm, and character
  —Body temperature
  —Mucous membrane color and capillary refill time
- Perform a complete physical examination
- Obtain a complete history, including prior cancer treatment

> **KEY POINT**
>
> *When a dog is presented in an emergency situation, the team should rapidly assess the patient. First, ensure that there is a patent airway, adequate breathing, and cardiac output. Second, obtain blood and urine samples. Third, place an IV catheter while the needs of the patient are met.*

When a dog is presented in an emergency situation, blood and urine samples should be collected and an IV catheter placed as soon as possible. Blood and urine can be submitted at any time to determine pretreatment parameters based on a complete blood count, biochemical profile, activated clotting time, and urinalysis. Essential information that is rapidly obtainable and vital for initial decision making—and that should be obtained on admission—includes urine specific gravity, packed cell volume, white blood cell count, and blood glucose level.

As soon as a diagnostic and therapeutic plan is initiated, the client should be made aware of every aspect of the patient's condition. Measured, realistic information should be provided as soon as assessments are made and the information is available. It is also important to provide a cost estimate for initial care as well as updates on ongoing supportive care. The team approach to care is vital during emergencies. The client is an integral member of the team and, once empowered with information, is placed in a decision-making role that allows optimal medical care of the patient. Ongoing communication allows an open dialogue among team members regarding financial limitations, philosophy for continuing critical care in the face of diminishing hope, and advanced strategies for crisis situations, such as cardiac or respiratory arrest.

Oncologic emergencies, although rare, are potential risks associated with cancer and cancer therapy. Planning for these uncommon and unwanted problems is essential for a positive outcome. It is important to recognize that the true "first step" in handling oncologic emergencies is actually prevention. This step occurs before the initiation of treatment and encompasses time spent educating the caregiver about the nature of the disease, effects of each medication to be administered, and early and often subtle signs that should be dealt with to prevent a

> **KEY POINT**
>
> *True oncologic emergencies are rare. On the other hand, emergencies of emotion are extraordinarily common.*

true emergency from happening. Similarly, instructions about what clients can do at home to support their dogs are helpful. Always remember that the client is perhaps the most important member of the veterinary health care team.

The next step includes educating and empowering the entire veterinary health care team to take an active role in supporting the patient and the client. The words *cancer* and *cancer therapy* often frighten professional veterinary health care team members as much as they do clients. Developing a treatment strategy or "cookbook" approach to emergency situations empowers the staff to intervene quickly and efficiently on behalf of the patient. Providing the health care team with information about how to respond to the emotional component of the emergency on behalf of the caregiver is also essential. All members of the health care team must recognize that it is this emotional component that magnifies the seriousness of almost any health problem.

REFERENCE

1. Wingfield WE: *Veterinary Emergency Medicine Secrets.* Philadelphia, Hanley and Belfus, 2001, pp 1–3.

CHEMOTHERAPY- OR RADIATION-INDUCED CONGESTIVE HEART FAILURE

35

Gregory K. Ogilvie and Antony S. Moore

CLINICAL BRIEFING

History	• Acute decompensation, anorexia, lethargy, dyspnea, collapse, and exercise intolerance.
Clinical signs	• Pale mucous membranes; decreased capillary refill time; evidence of decreased cardiac output, such as poor femoral and jugular pulses, pulmonary edema, hepatomegaly, splenomegaly, and ascites.
Diagnostics	• Document myocardial failure and secondary heart failure by evaluating central venous pressure; obtain chest and abdominal radiographs, ECG, fluid analysis (if indicated), echocardiography, tissue Doppler, and (if indicated) sestamibi or other nuclear medicine studies.
Therapy	• Eliminate the underlying cause. • Initiate enforced rest. • Enhance oxygenation and reduce effusion or edema with thoracentesis and diuretics. • Increase contractility with digoxin or dobutamine. • Reduce afterload with enalapril, captopril, or hydralazine. • Control arrhythmias.

Primary cardiac disease is a cause of morbidity and mortality in cancer patients. In addition, heart disease secondary to anthracycline or anthracycline-like drugs is an uncommon problem that can become life threatening. Doxorubicin is the anthracycline most commonly associated with the development of cardiac diseases such as arrhythmias and dilatative cardiomyopathy. Cardiomyopathy can occur in response to the administration of doxorubicin after any dose, but the risk of developing this cardiac condition increases significantly in dogs that receive a total cumulative dose exceeding 240 mg/m^2.[1,2] Other anthracyclines that have been shown to cause heart disease in humans include daunorubicin, epirubicin, and idarubicin.[1,2] Other drugs and treatments also have the potential to induce cardiac damage (Table 35-1).

Radiation can induce cardiomyopathy if the heart is in the radiation therapy field and sufficiently high doses are used.[3] Histologic and clinically significant pericardial effusion can develop approximately 3 months after a 3-week radiation treatment schedule is completed. Radiation can induce a thinning of the myocardium and development of significant amounts of fibrosis 1 year after treatment.

> **KEY POINT**
> *Radiation can induce cardiomyopathy if the heart is in the radiation therapy field and if sufficiently high doses are used.*

Radiation therapy and doxorubicin may synergistically cause cardiotoxic effects.

Predisposing Factors

Doxorubicin-induced cardiac disease may occur more frequently in breeds with a predisposition to develop cardiomyopathy (e.g., boxers, Dobermans, Newfoundlands), in those that have preexisting cardiac disease such as viral myocarditis

> **KEY POINT**
> *Doxorubicin is the most common cause of chemotherapy-induced cardiomyopathy in dogs. The condition can occur after any dose, but the risk increases significantly in dogs with preexisting cardiac disease and in those that have received a total cumulative dose of more than 240 mg/m^2.*

ONCOLOGIC EMERGENCIES

Table 35-1 Cancer Therapies and Reported Effect on the Cardiovascular System in Humans and Dogs

Cancer Therapy	Potential Cardiovascular Complication	Reported in Dogs?
5-Fluorouracil	CHF	No
Anthracyclines	Cardiomyopathy, CHF, dysrhythmias	Yes
Cyclophosphamide	CHF, hemorrhagic myocarditis, pericardial effusion	No
Ifosfamide	CHF	No
Mitoxantrone	Cardiomyopathy, CHF	No
Paclitaxel	Dysrhythmias, ECG changes	Possibly?
Radiation	CHF, pericarditis, pericardial effusion	Yes
Thalidomide	Embolic events	No

or endocarditis, and in those that cannot metabolize or eliminate the drug adequately after administration. Similarly, rapid infusion of the drug, which establishes very high serum concentrations, may increase the prevalence of cardiac disease. Therefore, slowing the rate of doxorubicin infusion may reduce the prevalence of acute and chronic heart disease.

KEY POINT

Endomyocardial biopsy is still the gold standard for diagnosing doxorubicin-induced myocardial damage; however, few centers routinely conduct this test.

Ideally, breeds at risk should be carefully screened for pre-existing heart disease before they are treated with therapies that are known to be cardiotoxic. Screening patients for heart disease with a physical examination, thoracic radiograph, and echocardiogram is ideal.

Diagnosis

The process of diagnosing heart disease should begin with a physical examination to monitor for problems such as arrhythmias, murmurs, weak pulses, poor capillary refill, jugular pulses, hepatomegaly, and splenomegaly. A thoracic radiograph, electrocardiogram (ECG), or radionuclide scan may also be helpful. Monitoring should intensify in dogs with compatible clinical signs that have received a total cumulative dose of doxorubicin equal to or exceeding 180 mg/m². Endomyocardial biopsy is still the gold standard; however, few centers routinely conduct this test. Serum level measurement of troponin C, T, or I is being evaluated as a noninvasive test to monitor for myocardial damage.[4]

In one study,[5] 32 of 175 dogs treated with doxorubicin developed clinically evident cardiac disease at cumulative doses of 180 mg/m². Electrocardiographic abnormalities, including arrhythmias (i.e., atrial premature complexes, atrial fibrillation, paroxysmal atrial and sinus tachycardia, ventricular arrhythmias, bundle branch blocks, and atrioventricular dissociation) and nonspecific alterations in R wave, ST segment, or QRS duration, were seen in 31 dogs. Seven dogs had overt congestive heart failure (CHF) that resulted in death within 90 days despite supportive therapy. In contrast, a recent study found that of 303 dogs with osteosarcoma receiving five doses of doxorubicin (cumulative dose: 150 mg/m²), 23 developed cardiomyopathy (7.6%).[6] Dobermans, Great Danes, Newfoundlands, and Great Pyrenees accounted for 11 of these dogs. We have observed that careful screening and limiting the cumulative dose may reduce the incidence of cardiac disease in dogs receiving doxorubicin. Arrhythmias may occur at the time of treatment or after treatment is complete. In humans with doxorubicin-induced cardiac disease, significant dysrhythmias often occur in the absence of other physical or historical abnormalities.[6]

In dogs with cardiomyopathy and fulminant CHF, clinical signs vary from anorexia, lethargy, and weakness to more common signs associated specifically with decreased cardiac output and ensuing CHF. Owners may complain that their pet has exercise intolerance; coughing spells late at night, which may develop into a persistent cough at all times of the day; abdominal distention; increased respiratory effort and rate; and general malaise.

The physical examination can reveal much useful information, including identification of a jugular pulse, rapid heart and respiratory rates, ascites, cool extremities, blue mucous membranes, delayed capillary refill time, pitting edema of the lower extremities, enlarged liver and spleen, and rapid, weak pulses. The lung fields may sound dull because of pleural effusion, or pulmonary edema may cause crackling lung sounds. Heart murmurs and abnormal rhythms are frequently auscultated; heart sounds from dogs with atrial fibrillation may sound like "jungle drums" (i.e., irregularly irregular) on auscultation. ECG may suggest heart chamber enlargement or be diagnostic for arrhythmias, which may be supraventricular or ventricular in origin.

Thoracic and abdominal radiographs are valuable in identifying evidence of cardiac disease, including pericardial or pleural effusion; enlargement of the heart, liver, spleen, and pulmonary veins; and pulmonary edema, which usually is first noted around the hilar region. Echocardiography is extremely valuable in confirming pericardial effusion and documenting chamber size, myocardial wall thickness, and dynamic parameters (e.g., ejection fraction, cardiac output, contractility). Blood pressure measurements may assist in documentation of hyper- or hypotension. An elevated central venous pressure aids in making a diagnosis of cardiac insufficiency. Finally, some more specific tests can clarify a diagnosis of drug or radiation therapy–induced cardiac disease. They include fluid analysis of thoracic or abdominal effusion (usually a modified transudate with reactive mesothelial cells and macrophages) and contrast radiography. Unfortunately, no evaluation method can be performed routinely in veterinary practice to predict whether cardiotoxicity will occur in dogs that receive anthracycline agents or radiation therapy. This precludes withdrawal of therapy before overt signs of cardiac insufficiency occur. In humans, nuclear imaging techniques may be able to predict the development of doxorubicin-induced cardiomyopathy before it becomes clinically evident.

Prevention

The hallmark of doxorubicin-induced heart disease is the development of dilated cardiomyopathy. Many methods to prevent the development of this condition have been explored. Vitamin E, thyroxine, coenzyme Q10, IP-6, and selenium treatments are ineffective in preventing cardiomyopathy. We have observed that in humans, weekly low-dose doxorubicin therapy or administration of the total dose over 24 to 72 hours reduces the prevalence of cardiomyopathy. The compound ICRF-187 (dexrazoxane) is more effective. This compound substantially reduces the occurrence of cardiomyopathy in dogs treated concurrently with doxorubicin. ICRF-187 is administered intravenously just before the administration of doxorubicin at 30 mg of ICRF-187 for every 1 mg of doxorubicin. The following precautions should be taken when administering doxorubicin:

- **Identify patients at risk.** Boxers, Dobermans, and other predisposed breeds should be screened or perhaps not treated at all.
- **Minimize the cumulative dose.** Cumulative dosing is the most important factor in doxorubicin cardiomyopathy. Limit to 180 to 240 mg/m^2.
- **Use a different dosing schedule.** The risk of cardiac toxicity is related to peak plasma level rather than the area under the curve of the drug. There is evidence that continuous infusion causes less risk of cardiomyopathy than does slow bolus infusion. In humans, the rate of cardiomyopathy development was 21% with a bolus infusion and only 6% with a 6-hour infusion.
- **Consider using liposomal encapsulation.** Use of this technology enables the compound to be taken up by the reticuloendothelial system; however, data from clinical trials in humans do not necessarily support a resultant reduction in doxorubicin toxicity.

Drugs Used to Treat Supraventricular and Ventricular Tachyarrhythmias Induced by Anthracycline Antibiotics or Radiation Therapy
Atenolol: 0.25–1 mg/kg PO q12–24h
Digoxin: 0.003–0.005 mg/kg PO q12h
Diltiazem: 0.5–1.5 mg/kg PO q8h
Lidocaine: 2–4 mg/kg IV bolus, 40–80 µg/kg/min CRI
Mexiletine: 4–10 mg/kg PO q8h
Procainamide: 20 mg/kg PO q8h
Procainamide hydrochloride: 6–8 mg/kg IV bolus, 20–40 µg/kg/min CRI
Propranolol: 0.04–0.06 mg/kg IV slowly or 0.2–1.0 mg/kg PO bid or tid, often in combination with digoxin for supraventricular arrhythmias
Quinidine: 5–20 mg/kg PO q8h
Sotalol: 0.5–2 mg/kg PO q12h

- **Minimize cardiac irradiation** if concurrent doxorubicin will be used.

Treatment

The development of cardiomyopathy may be associated with a profound decrease in contractility without substantial alterations in quality of life. Indeed, some indoor pets live a normal life despite significant reductions in contractility and ejection fraction. Other patients exhibit signs of heart failure. Once these alterations in cardiovascular performance are documented, doxorubicin administration should be discontinued indefinitely. The important lesson to be learned from these data is that the presence or absence of clinical signs—not the results of diagnostic tests—should dictate whether cardiac drug therapy should be initiated.

Treatment of cardiomyopathy begins with the indefinite discontinuation of the inciting cause (e.g., radiation therapy, doxorubicin). Diuretics, a low-salt diet, rest, oxygen therapy, positive inotropes, and vasodilators should be used as dictated by the clinical status of the patient. For example, furosemide may be used two to three times a day in a compensated animal, or every few hours, if necessary, in patients in respiratory distress from severe, fulminant pulmonary edema. Digoxin, a positive inotrope, can be given orally or parenterally in combination with a preload or afterload reducer. When digoxin is given orally, therapeutic levels generally are not achieved for a few days, which may be adequate for animals that are relatively stable. Factors such as dehydration and electrolyte disturbances may promote the development of digoxin toxicoses. Because digoxin toxicity is a serious problem that occurs frequently, IV loading doses should not be used unless absolutely necessary. Regardless of the method of digitalization, periodic

Table 35-2 Potential Therapeutic Approach for Dogs with Drug- or Radiation-Induced Dilatative Cardiomyopathy

General Principle	Specific Details, Drug Dosages, and Toxicities
Discontinue cardiotoxic agents	Discontinue all cardiotoxic drugs indefinitely; avoid additional radiation therapy to the heart.
Enforce complete rest	Avoid any stressful environment; consider cage rest.
Oxygenate	• Acquire and maintain a patent airway. • Provide supplemental oxygen if needed; to avoid pulmonary toxicity, 50% oxygen should not be used for more than 24 hr. • Perform thoracentesis to reduce pleural effusion. • Initiate diuretic therapy for pulmonary edema (see below).
Reduce pulmonary edema	• Administer furosemide (drug of choice; monitor for such complications as dehydration and hypokalemia): 2–4 mg/kg IV or IM q2–12h depending on the severity of edema; decrease to 1–4 mg/kg PO sid or tid for maintenance therapy. • Administer hydrochlorothiazide–spironolactone combination (use with furosemide or as maintenance therapy; monitor for dehydration and electrolyte abnormalities): 2–4 mg/kg PO bid.
Increase contractility	• Perform pericardiocentesis to improve contractility if pericardial effusion is present in significant amounts. • Administer digoxin (monitor blood levels to acquire and maintain therapeutic blood levels [1–2 ng/ml]; watch for anorexia, vomiting, diarrhea, and ECG abnormalities suggestive of digoxin toxicity): dogs <22 kg should receive 0.011 mg/kg PO bid; dogs >22 kg should receive 0.22 mg/m^2 PO bid. • Administer dobutamine (monitor for tachycardia and arrhythmias): 1–10 μg/kg/min CRI, usually in combination with a pre- or afterload reducer and furosemide in severe, fulminant CHF. • Administer milrinone (monitor for gastrointestinal toxicity and hypotension): 0.5–1.0 mg/kg IV or PO bid.
Redistribute blood volume	• Administer vasodilators: —2% Nitroglycerin ointment (watch for hypotension): ¼–¾ inch on skin or in ear qid. —Sodium nitroprusside (watch for hypotension; prolonged use may result in cyanide toxicity): 5–20 μg/kg/min CRI. • Administer morphine (to reduce apprehension and redistribute blood volume): 0.05–0.5 mg/kg IV, IM, or SC.
Reduce afterload	• Administer enalapril (do not use in conjunction with nitroprusside; monitor for hypotension): 0.25–0.5 mg/kg PO sid or bid. • Administer hydralazine (do not use in conjunction with nitroprusside; monitor for hypotension): 0.5–2.0 mg/kg PO bid.
Control arrhythmias	See box on page 263.
Monitor response to therapy	Monitor pulse, respiratory rate, ECG, body weight, central venous pressure, urine output, hydration, electrolytes, blood urea nitrogen, creatinine, blood gases, and quality of life; adjust therapy as indicated.

determination of serum digoxin concentration is essential for adjusting the drug dosage and thereby maintaining therapeutic levels.

In an acutely decompensated dying dog with cardiomyopathy, a constant-rate infusion (CRI) of dobutamine combined with IV furosemide and an IV (e.g., nitroprusside) or transdermal (e.g., 2% nitroglycerin) application of a preload or afterload reducer may be more logical than oral treatment. Dobutamine may increase cardiac output within minutes to hours, whereas improvement of cardiac output with oral digoxin therapy may take days. A more detailed treatment regimen for cardiomyopathy is outlined in Table 35-2.

Arrhythmias may occur during infusion of a chemotherapeutic agent. If arrhythmias persist, interfere with a dog's quality of life, or pose a serious threat to the dog's survival, therapy should be instituted (see box on page 263) and the underlying cause identified and eliminated.

In each case, the potential adverse effects of the antiarrhythmic agents must be evaluated and considered before therapy is initiated. Treatments and their indications are:

- **Digoxin:** Supraventricular premature complexes, supraventricular tachycardia, and atrial fibrillation
- **Lidocaine:** Premature ventricular contractions and ventricular tachycardia
- **Procainamide:** Premature ventricular contractions and ventricular tachycardia
- **Atenolol, sotalol, and propranolol:** Supraventricular premature complexes, tachyarrhythmias, atrial fibrillation, and ventricular premature complexes
- **Diltiazem:** Supraventricular premature complexes, tachyarrhythmias, and atrial fibrillation

REFERENCES

1. Keefe DL: Anthracycline-induced cardiomyopathy. *Semin Oncol* 28(4 suppl 12):2–7, 2001.
2. Speyer JL, Ewer MS, Freedberg RS: Cardiac effects of cancer therapy, in Abeloff MD, Armitage JO, Niederhuber JE, et al (eds): *Clinical Oncology,* ed 3. Philadelphia, Elsevier, 2004, pp 1251–1268.
3. McChesney SL, Gillette EL, Powers BE: Radiation-induced cardiomyopathy in the dog. *Radiation Res* 113:120–132, 1988.
4. DeFrancesco TC, Atkins CE, Keene BW, et al: Prospective clinical evaluation of serum cardiac troponin T in dogs admitted to a veterinary teaching hospital. *J Vet Intern Med* 16(5):553–557, 2002.
5. Mauldin GE, Fox PR, Patnaik AK, et al: Doxorubicin-induced cardiotoxicosis: Clinical features of 32 dogs. *J Vet Intern Med* 6:82–88, 1992.
6. Jakacki RI, Larsen RL, Barber G, et al: Comparison of cardiac function tests after anthracycline therapy in childhood. *Cancer* 72:2739–2745, 1993.

36 METABOLIC MANIFESTATIONS OF MALIGNANCY: HYPERCALCEMIA, HYPOCALCEMIA, HYPOGLYCEMIA, AND HYPONATREMIA (SIADH)

Gregory K. Ogilvie and Antony S. Moore

▶ HYPERCALCEMIA OF MALIGNANCY

CLINICAL BRIEFING

Diagnosis

History
- Lethargy, anorexia, increased water consumption, increased urination, and vomiting due to hypercalcemic nephropathy.

Clinical signs
- Polyuria, polydipsia, vomiting, constipation, bradycardia, skeletal muscle weakness, depression, stupor, coma, and seizures.

Diagnostics
- Laboratory evidence of hypercalcemia and secondary renal damage. The underlying cause of this electrolyte abnormality may be identified with a complete blood count (CBC), biochemical profile, urinalysis, ionized calcium, bone-marrow aspirate, radiographs, adrenocorticotropic hormone stimulation, and, if indicated, parathyroid hormone and PTHrP concentrations.

Treatment
- Treat the underlying cause.
- Therapy depends on the severity of clinical signs and laboratory findings. Consider saline diuresis and furosemide; give prednisone only after a diagnosis has been made.
- In refractory cases, consider salmon calcitonin, bisphosphonates, gallium nitrate, and mithramycin.

Cancer is the most common cause of hypercalcemia in dogs.[1-4] This condition, known as *hypercalcemia of malignancy*, can result in an oncologic emergency. The tumors most often associated with this paraneoplastic syndrome are lymphoma, anal sac adenocarcinoma, multiple myeloma, and mammary gland adenocarcinoma, but any neoplastic process has the potential to elevate serum calcium. In 20% to 40% of dogs with lymphoma and hypercalcemia, the anterior mediastinum is involved. For dogs, therefore, thoracic radiographs are indicated when persistent hypercalcemia is identified. Parathyroid adenomas have been identified as malignancy-associated causes of hypercalcemia of malignancy in dogs; however, hypercalcemia caused by these adenomas is not a true paraneoplastic syndrome.

The potential causes of hypercalcemia of malignancy include[1-5]:

- Direct resorption of bone by tumor cells
- Tumor-induced production of osteoclast-activating factors, such as interleukins, tumor necrosis factor, lymphotoxin, colony-stimulating factors, and interferon-α
- Tumor-induced production of 1,25-dihydroxyvitamin D
- Tumor-induced production of prostaglandins
- Tumor-induced production of transforming growth factors
- Tumor-induced production of parathyroid hormone–related peptide (PTHrP)

> **KEY POINT**
> *Cancer is the most common cause of hypercalcemia in dogs and a common cause of hypercalcemia-induced clinical signs that can result in an oncologic emergency.*

While all of these mechanisms likely play a role in hypercalcemia, production of PTHrP is the most commonly documented. Dogs with lymphoma and anal sac adenocarcinoma most commonly develop cancer-induced hypercalcemia from production of PTHrP.[5] The cDNA of PTHrP has been cloned and found to encode a 16,000-dalton protein in which eight of 13 amino acids are identical to parathyroid hormone.

> **KEY POINT**
> *Alterations in renal function cause the most common life-threatening clinical consequences of hypercalcemia of malignancy in the veterinary patient.*

Clinical Presentation

Alterations in renal function cause the most common clinical manifestations of hypercalcemia of malignancy arising from malignant disease in the veterinary patient.[1,4] Polyuria and nocturia in the early phases of the disease are succeeded by anorexia, nausea, fatigue, dehydration, azotemia, and coma secondary to hypercalcemia-induced renal failure. Decreased sensitivity of the distal convoluted tubules and collecting ducts to antidiuretic hormone (ADH) causes polyuria and secondary polydipsia. Vasoconstrictive properties of calcium decrease the renal blood flow and glomerular filtration rate, resulting in degenerative changes, necrosis, and calcification of the renal epithelium.[1–4] Other clinical signs (e.g., constipation, muscle weakness, cardiac arrhythmias, seizures) may arise as direct effects of the electrolyte abnormality.

Diagnosis

Clinical pathology must be combined with a good history and physical examination to identify or rule out the differentials noted in the box on this page.[1–4] Calcium values must be interpreted in relation to serum albumin and blood pH. A correction formula that takes the albumin into account is as follows:

$$\text{Adjusted calcium (mg/dl)} = (\text{Calcium [mg/dl]} - \text{albumin [g/dl]}) + 3.5$$

> **KEY POINT**
> *The most common cause of confirmed hypercalcemia in dogs is neoplasia (lymphoma and anal sac adenocarcinoma).*

Clinical signs associated with hypercalcemia are intensified when the electrolyte is in the free, ionized fraction, which is increased by acidosis.

Ultimately, it may be difficult to identify malignancy as the cause of hypercalcemia (Figure 36-1). Laboratory

---

Common Differentials Associated with Hypercalcemia in Dogs

Nonpathologic
- Young growing dogs
- Hyperproteinemia
- Laboratory error
- Hypoadrenocorticism
- Spurious (lipemia)
- Severe hypothermia
- Hemoconcentration

Pathologic
- Neoplasia (e.g., humoral hypercalcemia of malignancy)
  — Lymphoma (common)
  — Anal sac apocrine gland adenocarcinoma (common)
  — Carcinoma (uncommon): Lung, pancreas, skin, nasal cavity thyroid, mammary gland, adrenal medulla all reported
  — Thymoma (uncommon)
  — Hematologic malignancies (bone marrow osteolysis): Multiple myeloma, myeloproliferative disease (uncommon), leukemia (rare), metastatic cancer of bone (uncommon)
  — Primary hyperparathyroidism: adenoma (common), adenocarcinoma (uncommon)
- Chronic renal failure
- Increased complexed fraction (common; low ionized calcium)
- Tertiary hyperparathyroidism
- Hypervitaminosis D
  — Iatrogenic (oversupplementation of vitamin D_3)
  — Plants (calcitriol glycosides)
  — Rodenticide exposure (cholecalciferol)
- Granulomatous disease
  — Blastomycosis
  — Injection site granuloma
- Parathyroid hyperplasia (uncommon)
- Acute renal failure
- Skeletal lesions (nonmalignant, uncommon)
  — Bacterial or mycotic osteomyelitis
  — Hypertrophic osteodystrophy
  — Disuse osteoporosis
- Excessive intestinal phosphate binders (uncommon)
- Excessive calcium supplementation (calcium carbonate)
- Hypervitaminosis A (uncommon)
- Mammary hyperplasia, severe (PTHrP associated)
- Thiazide diuretics

268 MANAGING THE CANINE CANCER PATIENT

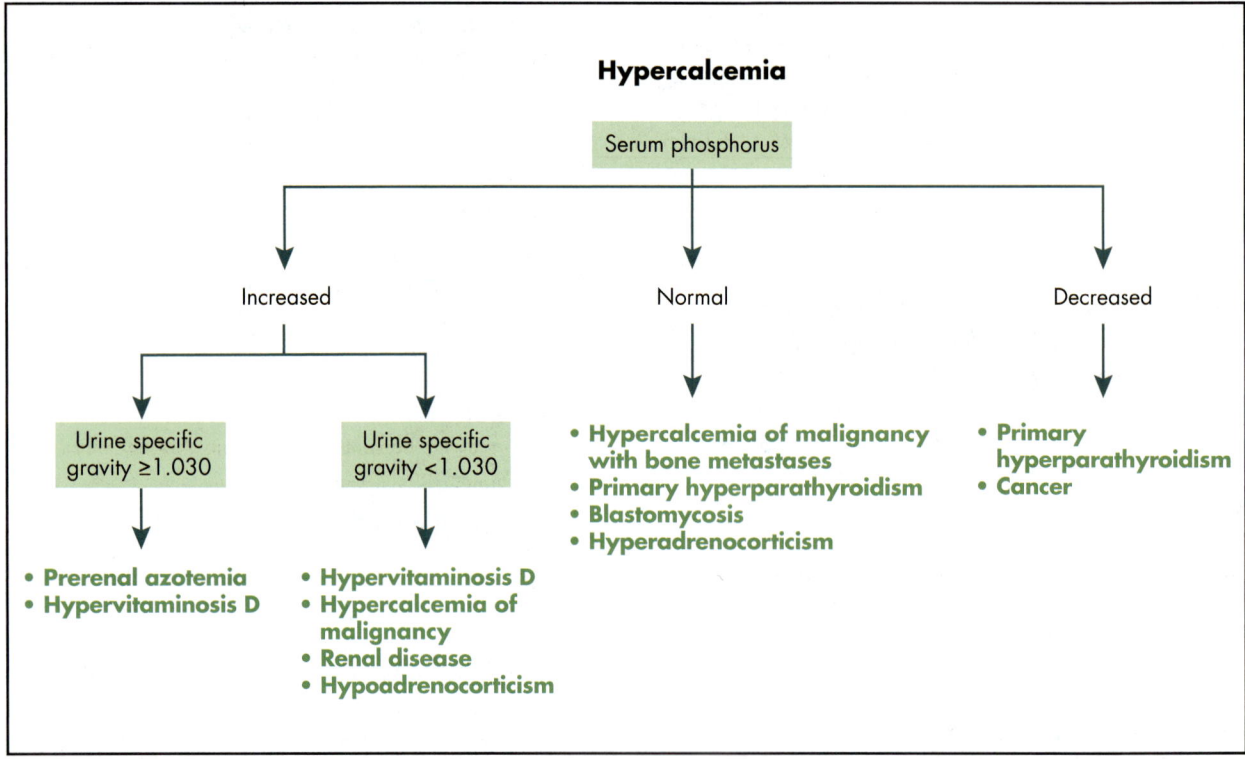

Figure 36-1. *The most common differentials and laboratory findings associated with hypercalcemia in relationship to serum phosphorus.*

findings that may accompany true hypercalcemia include elevated blood urea nitrogen, normophosphatemia or hypophosphatemia, hypercalciuria, hyperphosphaturia,

> **KEY POINT**
>
> *Laboratory findings that may accompany true hypercalcemia include elevated blood urea nitrogen, normophosphatemia or hypophosphatemia, hypercalciuria, hyperphosphaturia, hypernatriuria, and decreased glomerular filtration rate as determined by an exogenous or endogenous creatinine clearance study.*

hypernatriuria, and decreased glomerular filtration rate as determined by an exogenous or endogenous creatinine clearance study. Evaluating serum phosphorus levels in hypercalcemic dogs may be helpful in pursuing a diagnosis (Figure 36-2).

Treatment[1-4]

Eliminating the tumor is the first and most important therapy for hypercalcemia of malignancy. Clinical signs associated with hypercalcemia of malignancy can range from very mild to a full oncologic emergency. The approach to the treatment of this condition depends on the severity of the clinical signs (Table 36-1).

MILD HYPERCALCEMIA, MINIMAL CLINICAL SIGNS

- Restore and maintain hydration and ensure calciuresis, especially during anesthesia and surgery.
- Monitor calcium, phosphorus, and creatinine levels until the underlying cause can be identified and eliminated or until the hypercalcemia and subsequent clinical signs progress to a point requiring additional therapy.
- Avoid nephrotoxic drugs.

MODERATE HYPERCALCEMIA, MODERATE CLINICAL SIGNS

More aggressive management is indicated in these patients, including:

- Administer IV saline in volumes that exceed daily maintenance needs (>66 ml/kg/day) and result in urine output that exceeds 2 ml/kg/hr.
- Consider adding potassium chloride (KCl) to 0.9% sodium chloride (NaCl) to prevent potassium depletion (20–30 mEq KCl/L of 0.9% NaCl) (Table 36-2).

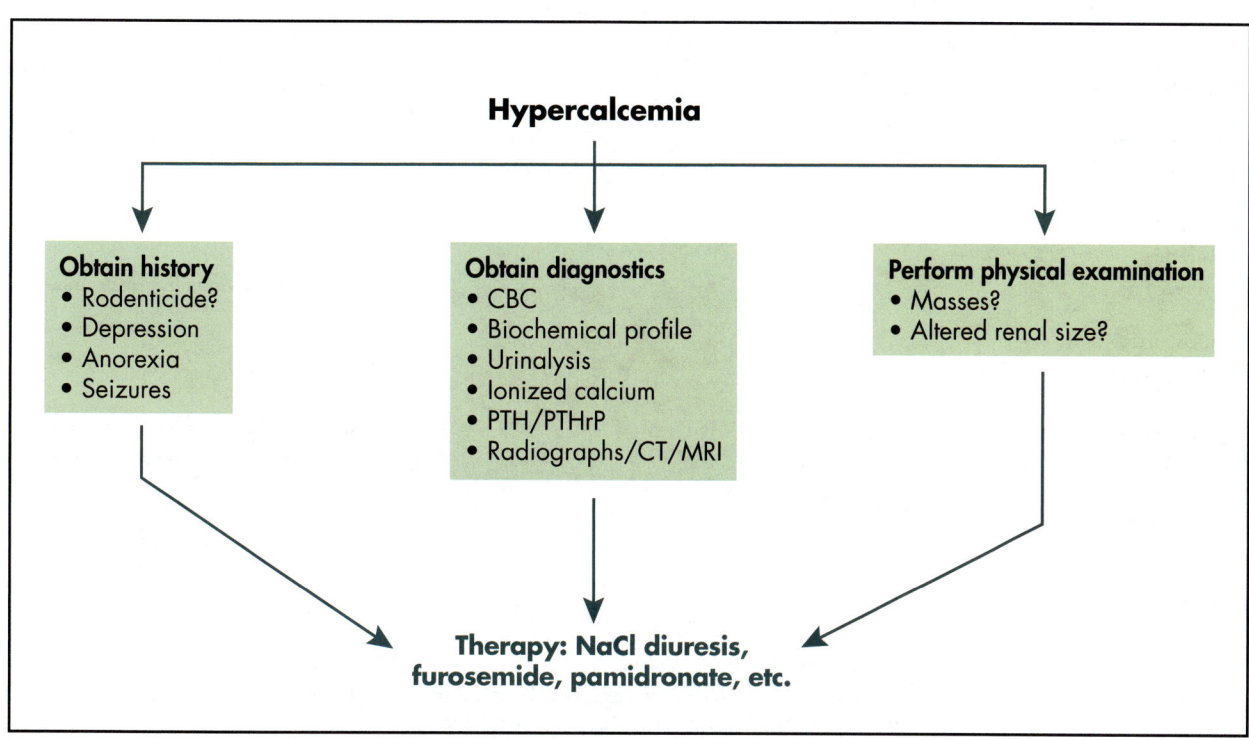

Figure 36-2. *Clinical approach for hypercalcemic dogs.* (PTH = *parathyroid hormone*)

- Repeatedly assess all electrolytes, blood urea nitrogen, and creatinine to reassess fluid rate, fluid choice, and potassium content of the fluid.

> **KEY POINT**
> *Glucocorticoids inhibit osteoclast-activating factor, prostaglandins, vitamin D, and the absorption of calcium across the intestinal tract; therefore, such drugs are effective in treating hypercalcemia of malignancy, including lymphoma and myeloma cells. Glucocorticoids should not be used until a histologic diagnosis of suspect tissue is made.*

- Monitor patient carefully for signs of overhydration and congestive heart failure. IV administration of 0.9% NaCl is effective in expanding the extracellular fluid volume, increasing glomerular filtration rate, decreasing renal tubular calcium reabsorption, and enhancing calcium and sodium excretion.
- In refractory cases, administer furosemide (2.2–8.8 mg/kg IV or PO bid), which is often administered concurrently with NaCl to well-hydrated hypercalcemic patients to prevent calcium reabsorption in the kidneys. This drug is also effective in treating many cases of anuria or oliguria.

Furosemide inhibits calcium resorption at the level of the ascending loop of Henle.

Prednisone (1.0–2.0 mg/kg PO bid) or any other glucocorticoid inhibits osteoclast-activating factor, prostaglandins, vitamin D, and the absorption of calcium across the intestinal tract; therefore, such drugs are effective in treating hypercalcemia of malignancy. However, glucocorticoids are cytotoxic to lymphoma and myeloma cells and, when administered, may obscure the extent of the tumor

> **KEY POINT**
> *Premature and inappropriate administration of symptomatic therapy, especially any glucocorticoid in any dosage or route of administration, may interfere with identification of the underlying cause of the electrolyte abnormality.*

and thus delay diagnosis of lymphoma and prevent definitive therapy. Therefore, glucocorticoids should not be used until a histologic diagnosis of suspect tissue is made. The diseases that cause hypercalcemia and appear to respond to steroid therapy include lymphoma and leukemia, multiple myeloma, thymoma, vitamin D toxicity, vitamin A toxicity, granulomatous disease, and hypoadrenocorticism.

Table 36-1 Treatment of Hypercalcemia[1-4]

Treatment	Dosage	Suggested Use
Volume expander IV saline (0.9%)	>66 ml/kg/day to achieve urinary output of 2 ml/kg/hr	Moderate to severe hypercalcemia Monitor serum potassium
Diuretic Furosemide	2–4 mg/kg PO, SC, IV bid to tid	Moderate to severe hypercalcemia
Glucocorticoids After diagnosis of underlying disease: Prednisone Dexamethasone	 1–2 mg/kg PO, SC, IV bid 0.1–0.22 mg/kg IV, SC bid	 Moderate to severe hypercalcemia Moderate to severe hypercalcemia
Bone resorption inhibitor Calcitonin	4–6 IU/kg SC bid to tid	Hypervitaminosis D toxicity
Bisphosphonates Etidronate disodium Clodronate Pamidronate	 5–15 mg/kg PO daily to bid 20–25 mg/kg in a 4-hr IV infusion 1–2 mg/kg in 150 ml 0.9% NaCl as a 2-hr IV infusion; can repeat in 1–3 wk. Package insert suggests giving during diuresis to reduce nephrotoxicity.	 Moderate to severe hypercalcemia Moderate to severe hypercalcemia Moderate to severe hypercalcemia
Chemotherapeutic drug Mithramycin	25 µg/kg IV in 5% glucose in water over 2-4 hr q2-4wk	Severe hypercalcemia

Table 36-2 IV Potassium Supplementation to Correct Hypokalemia

Serum Potassium (mEq/L)	KCl to Add to Each L of Fluids (mEq)	Maximum Rate of Infusion (ml/kg/hr)
<2.0	80	6
2.1–2.5	60	8
2.6–3.0	40	12
3.1–3.5	28	16

SEVERE HYPERCALCEMIA, SEVERE CLINICAL SIGNS

This is considered an oncologic emergency. Treatment is the same as for moderate hypercalcemia. In addition, the following drugs can be used (see also Table 36-1[1-4]):

- **Calcitonin:** A dosage of 4 to 8 MRC U/kg SC, given once, can cause a dramatic, rapid reduction in calcium levels, which may remain low for days.
- **Mithramycin:** This drug can be used at a dosage of 25 µg/kg IV once or twice weekly. At higher dosages, it has anticancer properties.
- **Bisphosphonates:** This class of agents is being explored for use in the therapy of hypercalcemia of malignancy. Etidronate disodium (5–15 mg/kg/day) is the most commonly used member of this class in human medicine. Clodronate (20–25 mg/kg in a 4-hr IV infusion) or pamidronate (1–2 mg/kg in 150 ml of 0.9% NaCl in a 2-hr IV infusion, to be repeated as needed every 1–6 weeks) can also be used with success. Studies of dogs with severe hypercalcemia and severe clinical signs suggest that pamidronate is effective in long-term control of chronic hypercalcemia.[2,3] Unlike phosphates, which bind calcium in the gastrointestinal tract, bisphosphonates bind to hydroxyapatite in bone and inhibit the dissolution of crystals.
- **Gallium nitrate:** This agent was recently approved in human medicine for the treatment of hypercalcemia. It appears to inhibit bone resorption by binding to and reducing the solubility of hydroxyapatite crystals.
- **Other agents to consider:** Calcium-channel blockers, somatostatin congeners, and calcium receptor agonists may be used.

HYPOCALCEMIA

CLINICAL BRIEFING

Diagnosis	
History	• Usually asymptomatic; occasional lethargy and anorexia.
Clinical signs	• Usually normal; occasional weakness, depression, and seizures.
Diagnostics	• Electrolyte abnormality can be identified with a biochemical profile, urinalysis, ionized calcium, and (if indicated) parathyroid hormone concentration.
Treatment	• Treat the underlying cause.
	• In severe cases, administer 10% calcium gluconate IV; oral calcium supplementation, with or without vitamin D, may be effective.

Hypocalcemia is an unusual complication in veterinary medicine. Hypocalcemia secondary to a malignancy and its treatment is much more common in human medicine.

Clinical Presentation

Hypocalcemia in dogs rarely causes clinical signs. In such cases, however, partial or generalized seizures are seen. In humans with bone metastases, hypocalcemia is more common than hypercalcemia.[1,4] Clinical signs are not usually seen in dogs until the total corrected serum calcium is less than 6.5 mg/dl or the ionized calcium is less than 0.7 mmol/L. Signs include seizures, fever, tense or painful abdomen, and rubbing of the face. In veterinary medicine, only a few possible causes of clinically significant hypocalcemia have been documented, including primary hypoparathyroidism, surgically induced iatrogenic hypoparathyroidism, eclampsia, ethylene glycol toxicity, and administration of phosphate-containing enemas, although this rarely occurs in dogs.[1,4] Another potential cause of hypocalcemia is magnesium deficiency, which can occur from prolonged intestinal drainage procedures, parenteral hyperalimentation without magnesium supplementation, cisplatin therapy, and severe liver disease.[1,4] Hypomagnesemia seems to impair the effect of parathyroid hormone on its target organs, resulting in hypocalcemia. Tumor lysis syndrome may be associated with hypocalcemia secondary to elevated phosphate levels. This is an oncologic emergency and should be addressed as such.

> **KEY POINT**
>
> *Clinical signs of hypocalcemia are not usually seen until the total corrected serum calcium is less than 6.5 mg/dl or the ionized calcium is less than 0.7 mmol/L. They include seizures, fever, tense or painful abdomen, and rubbing of the face.*

Treatment[1,4]

The underlying cause of hypocalcemia should be identified and treated as soon as possible. If clinical signs are present, calcium should be administered intravenously slowly with electrocardiographic monitoring (10% calcium gluconate given over 10–20 min, 1.0–1.5 ml/kg; maintenance therapy of 2 ml/kg over 6–8 hr), followed by oral calcium supplements (i.e., calcium lactate, 400–600 mg/kg/day in 3–4 divided doses/day). Oral vitamin D preparations are beneficial in increasing serum calcium concentrations. Several formulations are available with different times to onset of activity and durations of action. Short-acting formulations, such as calcitriol, should be used in dogs that may recover parathyroid activity (i.e., those with surgical trauma). Longer-acting preparations, such as dihydrotachysterol, can be initiated in dogs in which the underlying cause is not likely to be corrected. Oral calcium supplementation may be required in some dogs to maximize the effect of vitamin D therapy.

ALTERED GLUCOSE HOMEOSTASIS

CLINICAL BRIEFING

Diagnosis
- History
  - Weakness, confusion, seizures, and coma.
- Clinical signs
  - Same as for history. Clinical signs are often paroxysmal and subtle in the earlier phases of the disease and are followed by seizures, coma, and death.
- Diagnostics
  - CBC, biochemical profile, urinalysis, fasting blood glucose and insulin levels, radiography, abdominal ultrasonography, computed tomography, magnetic resonance imaging, exploratory surgery, and biopsy.

Treatment
- Treat the underlying cause.
- Give frequent feedings of a complex carbohydrate food.
- Administer glucose infusion, prednisone, and diazoxide ± hydrochlorothiazide.
- Propranolol may be of value in refractory cases.

Hypoglycemia

Hypoglycemia (blood glucose <70 mg/dl) can cause a wide variety of clinical signs ranging from generalized weakness to seizures and death.[1,6–12] Insulinoma is the malignancy most commonly associated with hypoglycemia in dogs,[6–12] but a wide variety of other non–islet cell tumors have also been shown to cause hypoglycemia in humans and dogs by inducing ectopic hormone production.[6–12] Non–islet cell tumors that have been reported to cause hypoglycemia include hepatocellular carcinoma, hepatoma, plasmacytoid tumor, lymphoma, leiomyosarcoma, oral melanoma, hemangiosarcoma, and salivary gland adenocarcinoma.[6–12]

> **KEY POINT**
> *Insulinoma is the malignancy most commonly associated with hypoglycemia (blood glucose <70 mg/dl) in dogs,[6–12] but a wide variety of other non–islet cell tumors have also been shown to cause hypoglycemia.*

Insulinomas produce excessive quantities of insulin that cause very low blood glucose levels. In contrast, hypoglycemia of extrapancreatic tumors in dogs has been associated with low to low-normal insulin levels.[6–11] Extrapancreatic tumors cause hypoglycemia by secreting an insulin-like substance, accelerating the utilization of glucose by the tumor, and causing failure of gluconeogenesis or glycogenolysis by the liver.[6–12] The most common nonmalignant causes of hypoglycemia are hyperinsulinism, hepatic dysfunction, adrenocortical insufficiency, hypopituitarism, extrapancreatic tumors, starvation, and sepsis. Laboratory error is perhaps the most common etiology of hypoglycemia.

> **KEY POINT**
> *Subtle neurologic signs such as weakness and facial twitching predominate in dogs with hypoglycemia because carbohydrate reserve is limited in neural tissue and brain function depends on an adequate quantity of glucose.*

CLINICAL SIGNS

Neurologic signs, including weakness, disorientation, behavioral changes, seizures, and coma, predominate in dogs with hypoglycemia secondary to a malignancy.[1,2,6–12] These clinical signs generally occur in dogs when the blood glucose concentration falls below 45 mg/dl. Death may also occur.

Catecholamines, growth hormone, glucocorticoids, and glucagon are released secondary to hypoglycemia and activate compensatory mechanisms to combat hypoglycemia by promoting glycogenolysis.

DIAGNOSIS

Currently, it is not possible to identify the cause of hypoglycemia in many extrapancreatic tumors. Insulin-producing tumors, such as insulinomas, may be diagnosed by identifying normal to elevated insulin levels in association with low blood glucose concentrations.[1,2,6–12] For accurate diagnosis, some patients require frequent evaluation of glucose and insulin concentrations during a 72-hour fast. Although controversial, the amended insulin:glucose ratio has been advocated as a method to help diagnose insulin-producing tumors in pets:

$$\text{Amended insulin:glucose ratio} = \frac{\text{Serum insulin (μU/ml)} \times 100}{\text{Serum glucose (mg/dl)} - 30}$$

Values above 30 are highly suggestive of an insulinoma or other insulin-producing tumor.

TREATMENT

Surgery is the only method of eliminating the underlying cause of malignancy-associated hypoglycemia. However, metastases are common with most malignant tumors associated with this condition. Therefore, surgery often is not curative. If an insulinoma is suspected, a partial pancreatectomy may be indicated. Complications include iatrogenic pancreatitis and diabetes mellitus. Medical management of the hypoglycemia is essential before, during, and after surgery because of the serious consequences of hypoglycemia and the high metastatic rate.[1,2,6–12] Dogs with severe cases of hypoglycemia should be treated with IV administration of 2.5% to 5% dextrose in parenteral fluids, such as 0.9% NaCl or Ringer's solution. Dogs that are convulsing should be given 0.5 g/kg dextrose intravenously slowly over 5 minutes.

Combined surgical and medical management of pancreatic tumors has been associated with remission periods of 1 year or more.[9,10] The following agents may be useful in the medical management of hypoglycemia:

- **Prednisone** (0.5–2.0 mg/kg PO divided bid) can induce hepatic gluconeogenesis and decrease peripheral utilization of glucose.
- **Diazoxide** (10–40 mg/kg PO divided bid), with or without hydrochlorothiazide (2-4 mg/kg PO daily), may be effective in elevating blood glucose levels by inhibiting pancreatic insulin secretion and glucose uptake by tissues, enhancing epinephrine-induced glycogenolysis, and increasing the rate of mobilization of free fatty acids. Diazoxide is expensive and difficult to obtain. Hydrochlorothiazide enhances the hyperglycemic effects of diazoxide.
- **Propranolol** (0.2–1.0 mg/kg PO tid) may be effective in increasing blood glucose levels by blocking insulin release through the blockade of β-adrenergic receptors at the level of the pancreatic β cell; inhibiting insulin release by membrane stabilization; and altering peripheral insulin receptor affinity.
- **Streptozotocin** (streptozocin), a nitrosourea chemotherapeutic agent that is specifically toxic to β cells and therefore specific for the treatment of insulinomas, is being evaluated by a number of oncologists. Streptozotocin can induce nephrotoxicity unless given with aggressive saline diuresis. The drug is also extremely emetogenic; pretreatment with butorphanol, metoclopramide, or ondansetron is required.
- **Glucagon** (5 ng/kg/min) can be used to increase gluconeogenesis. Glucagon can be used by reconstituting 1 mg of lyophilized glucagon with the diluent provided. This material can be added to 1 L of 0.9% NaCl. The resultant solution will have a 1-μg/ml concentration, which will allow for convenient administration rates. This treatment is most effective for the hypoglycemic crisis, but it may provide sustained benefits after infusion in some cases.

Survival times for dogs with insulinomas range widely in reported studies, based on the treatment selected (surgery alone, medical therapy alone, or both) and tumor stage. The stages are stage 1 (pancreatic nodule only), stage 2 (regional lymph node metastasis), and stage 3 (distant metastasis, usually the liver). In one study of 73 dogs,[6] dogs with stage 1 tumors had a median disease-free interval (no hypoglycemia) of 14 months; those with stage 1 or 2 tumors had similar median survival times of 12 to 18 months; and those with stage 3 tumors lived an average of 6 months. Five dogs lived between 24 and 36 months (two stage 1 tumors, three stage 2 tumors). Younger dogs generally had a poorer prognosis than older dogs.

Dogs with insulinomas managed surgically (with or without postoperative medical therapy) generally survive longer than those managed with medical therapy alone.[8,9–11] Debulking metastatic disease will increase survival times. In one study, the median survival with surgery was 381 days in 26 dogs compared with 70 days in 13 dogs treated with medical therapy alone.[8] In another study,[10] 31 dogs with resectable tumors or metastases had a median survival of 258 days. Dogs in that study that were hyperglycemic or normoglycemic after surgery had a median survival of 680 days; dogs that were hypoglycemic had a median survival of 90 days. In a third study, 18 dogs that were normoglycemic after surgery lived for more than 435 days. Eleven dogs that were hypoglycemic after surgery and were treated medically survived a median of 215 days (with one dog alive after 704 days).

▶ ALTERED SODIUM HOMEOSTASIS

CLINICAL BRIEFING

Diagnosis
History
Clinical signs
Diagnostics

- Anorexia, muscle stiffness, confusion or unresponsive state, and history of recent administration of a drug that may cause hyponatremia or SIADH.
- Anorexia, nausea, subtle neurologic signs, confusion, and coma.
- Biochemical profile to include serum sodium, urinalysis, fractional excretion of sodium, serum osmolality, and adrenal and thyroid function tests.

Treatment
- Treat the underlying cause.
- Use judicious water restriction.
- Administer demeclocycline and furosemide.
- Administer lithium carbonate, phenytoin, and hypertonic saline in refractory cases.

Syndrome of Inappropriate Secretion of Antidiuretic Hormone

Hyponatremia is the primary electrolyte defect associated with the syndrome of inappropriate secretion of

> **KEY POINT**
> *Hyponatremia is the primary electrolyte defect associated with SIADH.*

antidiuretic hormone (SIADH). However, before SIADH can be diagnosed, many other causes of hyponatremia must be ruled out (Table 36-3). While SIADH is one of the best characterized and most frequently encountered ectopic hormone syndromes in human medicine, it is underdiagnosed in veterinary medicine.[1,4] It is likely that SIADH will be identified more frequently in dogs as awareness of it grows.[1,4]

SIADH can be caused by increased expression of antidiuretic hormone (ADH) from the pituitary or as a true paraneoplastic syndrome secondary to ectopic production of ADH. In addition, several drugs can indirectly cause SIADH by potentiating the release of ADH.[1,4]

CLINICAL SIGNS[1,4]

Most dogs with SIADH are clinically normal. When sodium levels drop to 120 to 125 mEq/L, however, lethargy and mental dullness may be noted. When serum sodium levels drop below 115 mEq/L, more dramatic central nervous system problems can develop and may progress to convulsions and coma. When this occurs, the animal must be treated for a medical emergency.

DIAGNOSIS

The diagnosis of SIADH is based on the absence of hypovolemia and dehydration as well as on the following laboratory findings[1,4]:

- Hypoosmolality
- Hyponatremia of extracellular fluids
- Urine that is less than maximally dilute
- Absence of volume depletion
- Sustained renal excretion of sodium
- Normal renal, pituitary, and adrenal function

Spurious or artifactual hyponatremia can occur in dogs with marked increases in serum lipids or serum proteins. In addition, in dogs with marked hyperglycemia, water can be drawn into the circulatory system, diluting electrolytes and causing hyponatremia.

> **KEY POINT**
> *Drugs that can cause SIADH include chlorpropamide, vincristine, vinblastine, cyclophosphamide, opiates, histamine, thiazides, barbiturates, and isoproterenol.*

TREATMENT

The treatment of choice for patients with SIADH is to eliminate the underlying cause. The goal is to treat acute hyponatremia quickly and chronic hyponatremia slowly (<0.5 mEq/L/hr or 12 mEq/L/day). The change in serum sodium usually needed to alleviate the clinical signs of

Table 36-3 **Causes of Hyponatremia**

Associated with Hypovolemia	Associated with Euvolemia	Associated with Hypervolemia

• Excessive renal sodium loss
• Excessive external losses: diarrhea, vomiting, hemorrhage, third spacing, sweating
• Diuretics
• Renal tubular acidosis
• Hypoadrenocorticism (secondary to cranial radiation)
• Congestive heart failure
• Nephrotic syndrome
• Malignant ascites
• Cirrhosis, renal failure
	• Distal tubule diuretics
	• Loop diuretics
	• Hypothyroidism
	• SIADH
	• Cancer
	• Central nervous system lesions
	• Selected drugs
	  — Chlorpropamide
	  — Vincristine
	  — Vinblastine
	  — Cyclophosphamide
	  — Opiates
	  — Thiazide diuretics
	  — Barbiturates
	  — Isoproterenol
	  — Mannitol
	  — Morphine
	  — Other diuretics
	• Increased intrathoracic pressure of mediastinal tumor
		• Primary polydipsia
		• Excessive sodium depleted fluids
		• Tap water enemas

Adapted from Heideman RL, Heideman NH: Hyponatremia, in Abeloff MD, Armitage JO, Niederhuber JE, et al (eds): *Clinical Oncology*, ed 3. Philadelphia, Elsevier, 2004, page 978; with permission.

hyponatremia is small, usually 3 to 7 mEq/L. Once that change is seen, further correction of serum sodium should be slowed down. If clinical signs warrant treatment, the following measures may be helpful[1,4]:

- **Water restriction:** This is effective for mild cases in which the animal can be watched carefully for dehydration. The objective is to raise the serum sodium level while restricting water intake to approximately 66 ml/kg/day.

- **Demeclocycline:** This drug antagonizes the actions of ADH on the kidneys and thus causes reversible nephrogenic diabetes insipidus. In humans, nausea, vomiting, skin rashes, and hypersensitivity reactions are possible side effects. Demeclocycline is effective in treating patients with mild to moderate cases of SIADH. Other drugs, such as lithium carbonate and phenytoin, are not as effective as demeclocycline.

- **Hypertonic sodium chloride:** This IV solution is generally reserved for patients that have significant clinical signs related to hyponatremia. The following formula may help determine the approximate amount of sodium needed to correct hyponatremia[10]:

Sodium for replacement (mEq) =
(Desired serum sodium [mEq/L] − observed serum sodium [mEq/L]) × Body weight (kg) × 0.6

REFERENCES

1. Ogilvie GK: Metabolic emergencies and the cancer patient, in Wingfield WE (ed): *Veterinary Emergency Medicine Secrets*. Philadelphia, Hanley and Belfus, 2001, pp 247–251.
2. Hostutler RA, Chew DJ, Jaeger JQ, et al: Uses and effectiveness of pamidronate disodium for treatment of dogs and cats with hypercalcemia. *J Vet Intern Med* 19(1):29–33, 2005.
3. Milner RJ, Farese J, Henry CJ, et al: Bisphosphonates and cancer. *J Vet Intern Med* 18(5):597–604, 2004.
4. Feldman EC, Nelson RW: Hypercalcemia and primary hyperparathyroidism in dogs, in Bonagura JD (ed): *Kirk's Current Veterinary Therapy XIII*. Philadelphia, WB Saunders, 2000, pp 345–348.
5. Weir EC, Burtis WJ, Morris CA, et al: Isolation of a 16,000-dalton parathyroid hormone-like protein from two animal tumors causing humoral hypercalcemia of malignancy. *Endocrinology* 123(6):2744–2751, 1988.
6. Caywood DD, Klausner JS, O'Leary TP, et al: Pancreatic insulin-secreting neoplasms: Clinical, diagnostic, and prognostic features in 73 dogs. *JAAHA* 24:577–584, 1987.
7. Fischer JR, Smith SA, Harkin KR: Glucagon constant-rate infusion: A novel strategy for the management of hyperinsulinemic-hypoglycemic crisis in the dog. *JAAHA* 36(1):27–32, 2000.

8. Leifer CE, Peterson ME, Matus RE: Insulin-secreting tumor: Diagnosis and medical and surgical management in 55 dogs. *JAVMA* 188(1):60–64, 1986.
9. Steiner JM, Bruyette DS: Canine insulinoma. *Compend Contin Educ Pract Vet* 18:13–23, 1996.
10. Tobin RL, Nelson RW, Lucroy MD, et al: Outcome of surgical versus medical treatment of dogs with beta cell neoplasia: 39 cases (1990–1997). *JAVMA* 215(2):226–230, 1999.
11. Trifonidou MA, Kirpensteijn J, Robben JH: A retrospective evaluation of 51 dogs with insulinoma. *Vet Q* 20(suppl 1):S114–S115, 1998.
12. Moore AS, Nelson RW, Henry CJ, et al: Streptozotocin for treatment of pancreatic islet cell tumors in dogs: 17 cases (1989–1999). *JAVMA* 221(6):811–818, 2002.
13. Giger U, Gorman NT: Acute complications of cancer and cancer therapy, in Gorman NT (ed): *Oncology*. New York, Churchill Livingstone, 1986, pp 147–168.

HEMATOLOGIC MANIFESTATIONS OF MALIGNANCY

Gregory K. Ogilvie and Antony S. Moore

▶ ERYTHROCYTOSIS

CLINICAL BRIEFING	
Diagnosis	
History	• Patient may be asymptomatic; lethargy, anorexia, polyuria, and polydipsia may be noted by the owner.
Clinical signs	• Polyuria, polydipsia, and red mucous membranes.
Diagnostics	• Increased number of RBCs on CBC and hyperviscosity of the blood on visual inspection.
Definitions	
Paraneoplastic erythrocytosis	• Increased erythropoietin concentration, normal blood oxygenation, extramedullary hematopoiesis, and hyperplastic erythroid series on bone marrow examination.
Nonparaneoplastic erythrocytosis (including primary erythrocytosis)	• Normal blood oxygenation and erythropoietin levels, malignant erythron on bone marrow examination.
Secondary erythrocytosis caused by hypoxemia	• Elevated erythropoietin concentration, enlarged liver and spleen caused by extramedullary hematopoiesis and decreased arterial oxygen concentration.
Secondary erythrocytosis caused by renal disease	• Evidence of renal disease on CBC, biochemical profile, and urinalysis; normal arterial or venous oxygenation; and enlargement of spleen and liver caused by extramedullary hematopoiesis.
Treatment	• Treat the underlying cause and institute supportive care. • Repeated phlebotomy may be superior to other therapies. • Hydroxyurea in selected cases. Less proven therapies include radioactive phosphorus, chlorambucil, busulfan, pipobroman, and interferon-α.

An increase in the number of red blood cells (RBCs) (erythrocytosis) is relatively common in canine patients, but only a few cases can be classified as true paraneoplastic syndromes and are an indirect result of malignancy.[1-7] Erythrocytosis can also be caused by dehydration and secondary volume contraction, pulmonary and cardiac disorders, venoarterial shunts, Cushing's disease, chronic corticosteroid administration, and polycythemia vera. Erythrocytosis can produce significant clinical signs and a diagnostic dilemma.

Erythrocytosis secondary to elevated erythropoietin concentrations may be caused by four possible mechanisms[1-7]:

- Erythropoietin produced directly by the tumor
- Erythropoietin produced in response to either tumor-initiated hypoxia or vascular obstruction
- Erythropoietin produced by the kidney in response to a tumor-induced factor
- Tumor-induced change in metabolism of erythropoietin

Erythropoietin is normally produced by the kidney in dogs; thus, it is not surprising that renal tumors are associated with erythrocytosis.[1-4] Hepatic tumors and lymphoma have also been associated with erythrocytosis.[1-9]

Clinical Presentation

Many dogs with erythrocytosis are asymptomatic.[1-9] Others exhibit lethargy, anorexia, polydipsia, and polyuria. If the erythrocytosis is caused by generalized hypoxia, clinical signs referable to decreased oxygenation may predominate. In rare

Table 37-1 Examples of Alterations in Select Hemogram Parameters

Hematologic Parameter	Level	Cancer-Related Etiology	Non–Cancer-Related Etiology
WBC count	Increase	Leukemia, inflammatory or necrotic neoplastic process, paraneoplastic syndrome	Infection, (bacterial, mycotic, viral), inflammation (immune-mediated disease, tissue trauma), physiologic leukocytosis, metabolic (stress, endogenous or exogenous steroids), responsive anemia
	Decrease	Bone marrow infiltration by cancer	Decreased production, increased consumption, phenobarbital
RBCs	Increase	Polycythemia	Dehydration, splenic contraction, pulmonary and cardiac disorders, venoarterial shunts, Cushing's disease
	Decrease	Immune-mediated hemolytic anemia as a paraneoplastic syndrome, tumor hemorrhage, vascular neoplasia inducing hemolysis, cancer-induced coagulopathies and blood loss, cancer-induced anemia of chronic disease, estrogen-producing tumor, chemotherapy, myeloproliferative disease	Blood loss (trauma, ulcers, coagulopathies, parasites, hematuria), hemolytic anemia (microangiopathic due to dirofilariasis, vasculitis, DIC, RBC parasites, leptospirosis, *Escherichia coli*, oxidative injury caused by onions, kale, phenothiazines, methylene blue), nonresponsive anemias (renal failure, anemia of chronic disease, endocrine disease such as hypothyroidism and hyperestrogenism, idiopathic aplastic anemia, red cell aplasia, chloramphenicol, iron deficiency, lead poisoning, infections)
Hemoglobin, hematocrit	Increase	Polycythemia	Dehydration, splenic contraction
	Decrease	Bleeding tumor, bone marrow infiltration by tumor	Hemorrhage, decreased production
Neutrophils	Increase	Tumor inflammation, chronic granulocytic leukemia	Infection (bacterial, mycotic, protozoal), inflammation (immune mediated, tissue trauma or necrosis), responsive anemia, demargination associated with endogenous or exogenous steroids
	Decrease	Myelophthisis, chemotherapy	Myelofibrosis, drugs (chloramphenicol, trimethoprim–sulfamethoxazole, griseofulvin), idiopathic, cyclic neutropenia, immune mediated, hypersplenism, infection, endotoxemia, hypoadrenocorticism, margination
Lymphocytes	Increase	Lymphocytic leukemia	Physiologic leukocytosis, chronic antigenic stimulation
	Decrease	Chemotherapy	Stress, drugs (steroids), immunodeficiency, lymphangiectasia
Monocytes	Increase	Myelomonocytic or monocytic leukemia	Chronic inflammation, chronic infection, granulomatous disease, stress, glucocorticoids
Eosinophils	Increase	Mast cell tumor, paraneoplastic syndrome of solid tumors, eosinophilic leukemia	Allergic disease, enteritis, asthma, stomatitis, rhinitis, parasites, fungal infections, hypereosinophilic syndrome, hypoadrenocorticism, pregnancy
	Decrease	None	Stress, hyperadrenocorticism, exogenous steroids
Basophils	Increase	Mast cell tumors	Dirofilariasis
Platelets	Increase	Polycythemia vera	Essential thrombocytosis, rebound thrombocytosis
	Decrease	Paraneoplastic syndrome, myelophthisis	Infections, immune mediated, sequestration, hemorrhage, DIC, breed (King Charles spaniels and greyhounds)

Adapted from Dunfort RM: Abnormal laboratory findings, in Ettinger SJ, Feldman EC (eds): *Textbook of Veterinary Internal Medicine: Diseases of the Dog and Cat,* ed 6. 2005, Cover, with permission.

Table 37-2 **Results of Common Diagnostic Tests and Various Classifications of Erythrocytosis**

Classification	Erythropoietin Levels	Blood Oxygen	Bone Marrow	Renal Status	Extramedullary Hematopoiesis
(1°) Polycythemia vera	Normal to low	Normal	Malignant	Normal	No
(2°) Paraneoplastic syndrome	Increased	Normal	Hyperplastic	Normal	Yes
(2°) Tissue hypoxia	Increased	Low	Hyperplastic	Normal	Yes
(2°) Renal disease	Increased	Normal	Hyperplastic	Abnormal	Yes

cases, these signs may include cardiovascular decompensation, exercise intolerance, ascites, dyspnea, and cyanosis.

Diagnosis

The diagnosis of erythrocytosis is based on the results of a hemogram, a biochemical profile, blood gas analysis, erythropoietin levels, chest and abdominal radiography, a cardiovascular examination, renal imaging, and splenic aspiration (Tables 37-1 and 37-2).[1-3,7-9] Some keys to the classification of erythrocytosis include:

- Dogs with erythrocytosis of paraneoplastic origin have normal renal structure and function but show signs of extramedullary hematopoiesis and a hyperplastic erythroid series in the bone marrow.
- Dogs with secondary polycythemia have decreased arterial oxygen saturation or renal disease.[1-3,7-9]
- Dogs with polycythemia vera have normal to decreased erythropoietin concentrations. Polycythemia vera is a myeloproliferative disorder that results from clonal proliferation of RBC precursors. The diagnosis generally is made using histology and cytology of a bone marrow core biopsy specimen and aspirate after ruling out the presence of local or systemic hypoxia.

KEY POINT

Dogs with erythrocytosis of paraneoplastic origin have normal renal structure and function but show signs of extramedullary hematopoiesis and a hyperplastic erythroid series in the bone marrow.

Treatment

Patients usually require no treatment for erythrocytosis. Specific therapy for the underlying cause of the tissue hypoxia should be instituted in appropriate cases.[1-3,7-9] In emergency situations, patients with relative polycythemia should be treated with fluid therapy, whereas patients with absolute polycythemia should be treated by phlebotomy. Phlebotomy may assist in temporarily reducing the RBC load. This procedure is performed by withdrawing approximately 20 to 40 mL/kg of blood through a large-bore needle (e.g., 12-gauge) while simultaneously replacing the volume being removed with crystalloid fluids. With polycythemia vera, the chemotherapeutic agent hydroxyurea (30 mg/kg/day PO for 7 days, then 15 mg/kg/day) can be used to induce reversible bone marrow suppression and reduce RBC production[1,2,7] (see Chapter 48). Alternative chemotherapeutic agents are chlorambucil, busulfan, and pipobroman. Radioactive phosphorus and interferon-α can also be employed, but periodic phlebotomies may be as effective as any other therapy. If a solid tumor is responsible for the condition, surgery or radiation may be an effective treatment.

KEY POINT

The treatment of choice for a tumor that produces erythropoietin or induces regional or systemic hypoxia is surgical removal. Phlebotomy and hydroxyurea can also be used.

ANEMIA

CLINICAL BRIEFING

Diagnosis

History
- Lethargy, weakness, and exercise intolerance.

Clinical signs
- Pale mucous membranes, lethargy, and weakness.

Diagnostics
- CBC, biochemical profile, bone marrow aspirate and biopsy, serum iron, total iron-binding capacity, slide agglutination test, antinuclear antibody, and Coombs' test (if indicated).

Treatment
- Treat the underlying cause.
- Consider iron supplementation, erythropoietin, and immune modulation after specific diagnosis is identified.
- Transfusion after cross-match.

Anemia occurs frequently in veterinary cancer patients and may result from increased blood loss, decreased RBC production (e.g., abnormal bone marrow function), or increased RBC destruction (e.g., immune-mediated diseases).[1–6] More specific causes of malignancy-associated anemia include anemia of chronic disease, bone marrow invasion by tumor cells, marrow suppression by chemotherapy, hypersplenism, megaloblastic anemia, vitamin and iron deficiency, microangiopathic hemolytic anemia, and pure red cell aplasia.[1–6] Anemia of any cause arising as an indirect effect of the tumor is a paraneoplastic syndrome. In most patients, a clear cause of anemia is not found and a diagnosis of "anemia of chronic disease" is made.

> **KEY POINT**
>
> *Anemia occurs frequently in veterinary cancer patients and may result from malignancy-associated anemia of chronic disease, bone marrow invasion by tumor cells, marrow suppression by chemotherapy, hypersplenism, immune-mediated disease, megaloblastic anemia, vitamin and iron deficiency, microangiopathic hemolytic anemia, and pure red cell aplasia.*

Blood loss anemia is seen in many types of cancer. It can be a direct effect of the cancer or an indirect result of coagulopathies linked with hemangiosarcomas, thyroid carcinomas, and inflammatory mammary carcinomas. Histamine released from mast cell tumors may activate parietal cells in the stomach, increasing production of hydrochloric acid and inducing gastric or duodenal ulceration and consequent blood loss. If anemia is secondary to blood loss, the cause may be obvious (as with bleeding superficial tumors) or inconspicuous (as with bladder or gastrointestinal tumors).

Microangiopathic hemolytic anemia is commonly seen in dogs with splenic hemangiosarcoma and occurs secondary to hemolysis because of damage to arteriolar endothelium or fibrin deposition within the artery.[1–6] Disseminated intravascular coagulation (DIC) is an important cause of this type of anemia. Although hemangiosarcoma is the most common cause of DIC, a variety of other neoplastic diseases, such as thyroid carcinoma and inflammatory mammary adenocarcinoma, may result in anemia caused by DIC.

In dogs, immune-mediated hemolytic anemia (premature destruction of RBCs by immune mechanisms) is sometimes triggered by tumors (e.g., lymphoma).[1,2,5] Antibodies can be directed against the RBCs or against a hapten (e.g., virus, drug) that is associated with the RBCs.

Chemotherapy-induced nonregenerative anemia is common in dogs. The condition is frequently associated with chronic drug therapy. Although chemotherapeutic agents often decrease the number of white blood cells (WBCs) and platelets, anemia associated with administration of chemotherapeutic agents generally is mild and is not associated with clinical signs. Hydroxyurea may cause anemia as its primary hematologic toxicity.

Less common causes of cancer-induced anemia include leukoerythroblastic anemia, hematopoietic dysplasia, hypersplenism, erythrophagocytosis, megaloblastic anemia, and red cell aplasia.[1,2]

Clinical Presentation

Many of the mechanisms previously described work alone or in concert to decrease the population of RBCs.[1–3,5,6] Although clinical signs relating to the anemia may be overshadowed by aspects of the underlying neoplastic condition, the anemia can nevertheless impair the quality of life of the animal. Most patients remain asymptomatic if anemia develops gradually or if the number of RBCs is only slightly decreased. As the anemia progresses, lethargy and exercise intolerance may arise. Mucous membranes may be pale.

Diagnosis

The anemia must first be classified as regenerative or nonregenerative. If the anemia is regenerative and serum proteins are decreased, blood loss may be considered.[1,2,5] If serum proteins are increased, differentials of RBC destruction by immune-mediated diseases (e.g., immune-mediated hemolytic anemia), physical trauma (e.g., DIC, parasites), or toxins must be considered. If the anemia is nonregenerative, a bone marrow aspiration or biopsy should be performed to evaluate for erythroid hypoplasia (causes include anemia of chronic disease, endocrine deficiencies, renal disease, and lead toxicity), aplastic anemia (causes include estrogen toxicity and phenylbutazone), myeloproliferative disorders, and iron deficiency (Table 37-1).

Anemia of chronic disease in cancer patients is associated with a shortened erythrocyte life span, depressed bone marrow response, and disordered iron metabolism and storage.[1,2,5,6] Clinically, anemia of chronic disease is recognized as normocytic and normochromic, with normal bone marrow cellularity and reticuloendothelial iron sequestration. Blood loss anemia is recognized clinically when the RBCs are microcytic and hypochromic because of decreased hemoglobin synthesis.[1,2,5,6] Poikilocytosis, microleptocytosis, inadequate reticulocytosis, increased total iron-binding capacity, decreased serum-iron concentrations, and elevated platelet counts may also be seen with blood loss. Hemolysis and schistocytosis are the hallmarks of microangiopathic hemolytic anemia. The diagnosis of immune-mediated hemolytic anemia is based on finding antibody or complement on the surface of the patient's RBCs by a Coombs' test or slide agglutination test and spherocytosis, paired with nonregenerative anemia. Histologically, chemotherapy-induced changes include bone marrow hypoplasia of the erythroid or other cell lines that subsequently causes inadequate reticulocytes and decreased RBC mass with normal erythrocytic indexes.[1,2,5,6]

Treatment

As with all paraneoplastic syndromes, the best treatment is eliminating the underlying cancer.[1,2,5,6] Symptomatic treatment is usually needed only if the anemia produces clinical signs or if the animal is to undergo surgery. If acute correction of the condition is warranted, it is common to administer RBCs after a cross-match. Preparations of RBCs are listed in Table 37-3.

The following general guidelines for transfusion should be followed. More detailed recommendations can be found in Chapter 32.

Table 37-3 **Blood Products for Red Cell Replacement**

Product	Storage Conditions	Shelf Life	Dosage Guidelines
Fresh whole blood	Room temperature	<8 hr	12–20 ml/kg
Whole blood	Refrigeration	20–35 days	12–20 ml/kg
Packed RBCs	Refrigeration	20–35 days	5–10 ml/kg

General rule: Amount to transfuse

$$\frac{ml}{donor} = [(2.2 \times wt_{kg}) \times (40)] \times \frac{(PCV_{desired} - PCV_{recipient})}{PCV_{donor}}$$

- **Note:** 2.2 ml of whole blood/kg or 1 ml/kg of packed RBCs raises the packed cell volume (PCV) 1% (transfused whole blood has a PCV of 40%).

General rule: Rate of transfusion

0.5 ml/kg/hr or faster (22 ml/kg/day) with close patient monitoring

Transfusion-associated graft-versus-host disease is a risk for all patients, not just bone marrow transplant recipients. Some advanced centers therefore recommend irradiating blood with 2.5 Gy before transfusion. Transfusion is of great help for many patients; however, it also carries the risk of transmitting infectious diseases. Peripheral progenitor cells are the latest development in hematologic supportive care associated with chemotherapy, but more work is needed before they are used to treat anemia on a routine basis in veterinary medicine.

Canine recombinant erythropoietin will soon be available; however, until it is, human recombinant erythropoietin (75–100 U/kg/day SC for 3–5 days, then three times a week; decrease to once or twice weekly when the desired hematocrit level is reached) is being used more commonly for a variety of anemias.[2] Because recombinant erythropoietin is somewhat species specific, patients may develop antibodies to the recombinant protein, which may cross with the patient's own erythropoietin. Recombinant erythropoietin is most effective when endogenous erythropoietin levels are low and when adequate erythrocyte precursors are present in the bone marrow and other structures. If anemia is attributable to blood loss, the source of bleeding should be identified and eliminated. Medical management of immune-mediated hemolytic anemia can include prednisone (2 mg/kg PO daily); in addition, azathioprine (2 mg/kg PO daily for 4 days, then 0.5–1.0 mg/kg PO every other day) may be indicated if resolution of the underlying neoplastic condition is delayed.[1-3] Cyclosporine (5 mg/kg PO bid; dose adjusted by monitoring blood levels) is sometimes effective. Contrary to early reports, cyclophosphamide is probably of limited value in treating immune-mediated hemolytic anemia and associated conditions in dogs.[1,2]

THROMBOCYTOPENIA

CLINICAL BRIEFING

Diagnosis	
History	• Localized or systemic hemorrhage without due cause.
Clinical signs	• Evidence of bleeding, petechial and ecchymotic hemorrhages, hematuria, and hemarthrosis.
Diagnostics	• MDB[a] with platelet count and bone marrow aspirate; consider coagulation screening tests (APTT, OSPT, fibrinogen, and fibrin degradation products).
Therapy	• Treat the underlying cause; treat nonmedical needs of the patient. • Minimize activity and enforce rest. • Limit heparinized saline flushing of catheter; discontinue aspirin or other nonsteroidal medications. • Correct secondary conditions (e.g., treat DIC and drug-induced myelosuppression). • Consider low-dose vincristine therapy to cause premature release of platelets, transfusion with platelet-rich plasma, and epsilon aminocaproic acid. • Withhold additional chemotherapeutics until stabilized (except corticosteroids); consider dose reduction with next dosage of same drug.

[a]Minimum database (MDB) includes CBC, biochemical profile, urinalysis, and thoracic radiographs (three views).

Mechanisms associated with diminished platelet numbers in dogs with cancer include reduced platelet production from bone marrow, sequestration of platelets in capillaries, increased platelet consumption (e.g., as in DIC), increased platelet destruction, and reduction of hematopoietic growth factors. Consumption of platelets is considered the primary hemostatic abnormality in tumor-bearing dogs.[1-4,10,11]

> **KEY POINT**
>
> *Mechanisms associated with diminished platelet numbers in dogs with cancer include reduced platelet production from bone marrow, sequestration of platelets in capillaries, increased platelet consumption, increased platelet destruction, and reduction of hematopoietic growth factors.*

Diminished platelet numbers and elevated plasma-fibrinogen concentrations are common in dogs with extensive tumors involving spleen or marrow.[1,2,10,11] DIC, a common cause of platelet consumption, occurs in 39% of dogs with tumors that involve these structures.[11] In these dogs, eliminating the neoplastic condition and administering IV fluids and heparin may be of therapeutic value. Immune-mediated thrombocytopenia also significantly decreases platelet numbers in some dogs with cancer.[1,2,10,11]

Clinical Presentation

Dogs with thrombocytopenia may be clinically normal, or they may bleed for no reason into any part of the body. For example, these dogs may bleed excessively from a simple venipuncture and may have petechial or ecchymotic hemorrhages on physical examination.

Diagnosis

A complete blood count (CBC), platelet count, clotting profile, and bone marrow evaluation are essential to diagnose and evaluate the cause of thrombocytopenia in dogs[1,2] (Figure 37-1). Combined with a complete history and physical examination, this information helps determine whether thrombocytopenia results from decreased platelet production (e.g., tumor-induced myelophthisis, chemotherapy-induced marrow suppression), increased platelet consumption (e.g., DIC secondary to any malignancy, including hemangiosarcoma), or increased platelet loss (Table 37-1). If DIC is suspected, clotting times (activated clotting time, one-step prothrombin time [OSPT], activated partial thromboplastin time [APTT]) may be prolonged and fibrinogen levels elevated. Thrombocytopenia attributable to an immune mechanism is diagnosed when antibodies against bone marrow megakaryocytes are detected. Thrombocytopenia as a true paraneoplastic syndrome is diagnosed by eliminating all other causes and determining whether the animal responds to removal of an apparently unrelated tumor.

> **KEY POINT**
> *Vincristine and platelet transfusions can be administered to treat life-threatening thrombocytopenia.*

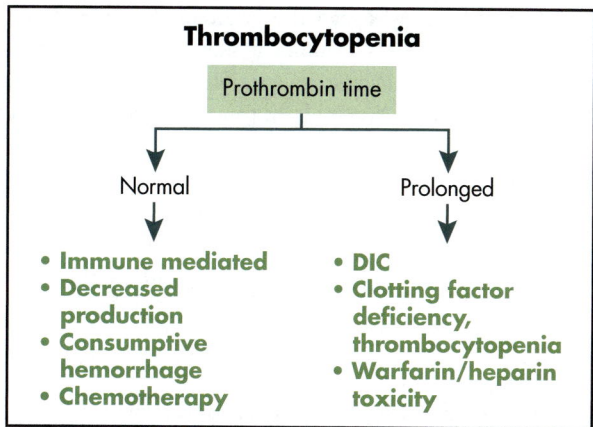

Figure 37-1. *Diagnostic differentials and laboratory findings associated with thrombocytopenia.*

Treatment

Activity should be restricted in dogs with thrombocytopenia to reduce the risk of painful or life-threatening hemorrhage. The primary treatment for the paraneoplastic syndrome is removal of the tumor.[1,2,10,11] Malignancy-associated, immune-mediated thrombocytopenia has been resolved successfully in dogs by treatment with immunosuppressive drugs such as prednisone (2 mg/kg PO daily) and azathioprine (2 mg/kg daily for 4 days, followed by 0.5–1.0 mg/kg PO every other day).[1–4] Cyclosporine may be helpful in refractory cases. In any case of thrombocytopenia secondary to a malignancy, vincristine (0.5–0.75 mg/m² IV) can be used to increase the number of platelets temporarily; response is directly proportional to the number of megakaryocytes and the rate of platelet removal from the body. Platelet counts increase 4 days after vincristine is given. In academic or large private practice settings, platelet transfusions can be administered to specific dogs that are, or have a high likelihood of, bleeding uncontrollably. The amount of random donor platelet transfusion generally is about 3 U/m² body surface area or 0.1 U/kg body weight. Each unit of platelets should be administered with 30 to 60 ml of plasma. When acute bleeding is not responsive to other treatments or procedures, epsilon aminocaproic acid (Amicar; Xanodyne Pharmaceuticals, Florence, KY) can be given IV or PO (250 mg/m² qid).

▶ LEUKOCYTOSIS

CLINICAL BRIEFING

Diagnosis	
History	• Patient usually asymptomatic; otherwise, lethargy and anorexia.
Clinical signs	• Bone marrow packing can result in shifting leg lameness due to bone pain; lethargy; and possibly splenomegaly, if the reticuloendothelial system is actively clearing abnormal cells.
Diagnostics	• CBC, bone marrow aspiration and biopsy, and special stains for abnormal cells; look for other cause with chest and abdominal radiography, biochemical profile, and urinalysis.
Treatment	• Treat the underlying cause. • Beware of and treat any underlying infection.

An increased WBC count attributable to increased production, decreased loss, or decreased destruction is common in veterinary cancer patients.[1,2,12–14] Any cell line can be involved.

When leukocytosis is a remote effect of underlying malignancy, the laboratory finding may be classified as a paraneoplastic syndrome. Paraneoplastic leukocytosis in dogs arises from a variety of malignancies, including lymphoma and hemangiosarcoma.[1,2,4,5,12–14] Although some cases of leukocytosis are caused by malignant clonal proliferation of a specific WBC line, they are not considered paraneoplastic syndromes.

Clinical Presentation

Dogs with paraneoplastic leukocytosis are often clinically normal (Table 37-1). Human patients occasionally describe bone pain due to the high proliferative rate in the bone marrow.

Diagnosis

The diagnosis is based on a CBC and bone marrow examination. Occasionally, special stains may be performed by the clinical pathology laboratory to determine whether the leukocytes are from a neoplastic clone.

> **KEY POINT**
>
> *The mechanism of malignancy-associated leukocytosis is not known but may involve the direct or indirect production of hematopoietic growth factors, such as granulocyte colony-stimulating factor, granulocyte–macrophage colony-stimulating factor, or interleukin-3. It may also be a result of tissue necrosis and granulocyte breakdown with positive feedback that increases neutrophil production.*

Treatment

The condition is not generally of clinical significance and requires no therapy.

▶ NEUTROPENIA AND SEPSIS

CLINICAL BRIEFING

Diagnosis

History	• Anorexia and general malaise, acute decompensation and collapse, usually 5–7 days after receiving myelosuppressive chemotherapy.
Clinical signs	• Depression, poor responsiveness, pyrexia, brick-red mucous membranes, tachycardia, rapid capillary refill (hyperdynamic shock) or pale mucous membranes, evidence of decreased cardiac output (hypodynamic shock), collapse.
Diagnostics	• CBC, biochemical profile, urinalysis, thoracic radiographs; cultures of blood, urine, stool, pulmonary airways, or other tissues as indicated; blood gas analysis and other diagnostics based on clinical signs.

Therapy

- Treat the underlying cause; support nonmedical needs of the patient.
- Restore tissue perfusion with fluids and stabilize cardiovascular system.
- Correct acid–base and electrolyte imbalances and hypoglycemia.
- Initiate parenteral bactericidal antibiotic therapy.
- Consider hematopoietic growth factor support, transfusions of fresh whole blood.
- Withhold additional chemotherapeutics until stabilized; consider dose reduction with next dosage of same drug.

Sepsis due to chemotherapy or cancer-related neutropenia is one of the more common emergencies in canine cancer medicine.[13–24] Bleeding due to thrombocytopenia is much less common. Both conditions are usually preventable by use of judicious monitoring and appropriate supportive care during cancer therapy. In addition, caregivers should be educated about the early clinical signs of neutropenia and thrombocytopenia induced by cancer treatment so that they can assist in early detection and seek immediate treatment.

In humans, sepsis is a common cause of death in cancer patients, exceeding all other causes combined.[14–21] As the

> **KEY POINT**
>
> *Sepsis due to chemotherapy or cancer-related neutropenia is one of the more common emergencies in canine cancer medicine.*

popularity of advanced medicine increases and the use of chemotherapy and radiation in private practice soars, this observation is likely to be repeated in canine cancer medicine. Because dogs may hide their clinical signs until late in the disease, the condition of sepsis may be advanced when first recognized and requires prompt intervention by the veterinary health care team.

Neutropenia secondary to malignancy or as a result of the myelosuppressive effects of chemotherapy or radiation therapy is a common predisposing factor for development of sepsis in dogs. Septic shock is the state of circulatory collapse that occurs secondary to overwhelming sepsis or endotoxemia. This syndrome is frequently fatal, with a mortality rate of 40% to 90%. The profound systemic effects of septic shock include:

- Vasoconstriction leading to multiorgan failure
- Cardiac dysfunction, in part from lactic acidosis
- Increased vascular permeability, leading to hyperviscosity and hypovolemia
- Liver dysfunction from splanchnic vascular pooling and tissue ischemia
- Acute renal failure
- Worsening neutropenia and thrombocytopenia
- Coagulopathies
- Severe gastrointestinal damage
- Decreased insulin release
- Initial hyperglycemia followed by hypoglycemia

The bacteria that most commonly cause morbidity and mortality in veterinary cancer patients arise from the dog's own flora.[21] The most important thing a clinician can do for the septic canine cancer patient is to quickly identify the source and type of bacterial infection and initiate therapy with broad-spectrum antibiotics as well as appropriate and aggressive supportive care. Factors such as prolonged hospitalization; the presence of urinary, venous, chest, endotracheal, and other tubes or catheters; and antibiotic administration may result in increased susceptibility to increasingly resistant strains of organisms. These factors should be avoided or minimized when possible. Minimizing the chance of exposure to, or the opportunity for development of, resistant strains of bacteria enhances the chance of rapid recovery in response to appropriate antibiotic therapy.

Predisposing Factors

The following are predisposing factors for neutropenia-associated sepsis in dogs with cancer[14–21]:

- **Defects in cellular immunity:** Cellular immune dysfunction, while extraordinarily difficult to diagnose in dogs, may

Table 37-4 **Myelosuppressive Effects of Chemotherapeutic Agents Used in Veterinary Medicine**

Highly Myelosuppressive	Moderately Myelosuppressive	Mildly Myelosuppressive
Doxorubicin	Melphalan	L-Asparaginase
Vinblastine	Chlorambucil	Vincristine
Cyclophosphamide	5-Fluorouracil	Bleomycin
Lomustine (CCNU)	Methotrexate	Corticosteroids

Table 37-5 **Myelosuppressive Drugs Associated with the Development of Pyrexia and Sepsis**

Delayed Myelosuppression (3–4 weeks)	Mid-range Myelosuppression (7–10 days)	Early Myelosuppression (<7 days)
Carmustine (BCNU)	Cyclophosphamide	Taxol
Lomustine (CCNU)	Doxorubicin	
Mitomycin C	Mitoxantrone	
Carboplatin ?		

be due to an underlying cause or the result of administration of antineoplastic agents or corticosteroids. These defects may result in various bacterial, mycobacterial, fungal, and viral infections. Humoral immune dysfunction is also associated with an increased prevalence of sepsis in human patients with cancer and may cause similar problems in animals. Agammaglobulinemic or hypogammaglobulinemic dogs may be considered susceptible to infections. Multiple myeloma and chronic lymphocytic leukemia are common neoplasms associated with humoral immune dysfunction in humans and are likely causes in dogs as well.

- **Myelosuppressive effects of chemotherapy:** The myelosuppressive effects of chemotherapeutic agents can be categorized as high, moderate, or mild (Table 37-4). These drugs cause a nadir (lowest level) in the WBC count at different times after administration (Table 37-5).
- **Splenectomy:** Splenectomized dogs are susceptible to overwhelming sepsis when infected with a strain of encapsulated bacteria against which they have not made antibodies.
- **Indwelling vascular or urinary catheters:** The longer a catheter is present, the higher the probability of infection, especially in neutropenic dogs (Figure 37-2).
- Frequent acquisition of **blood samples**.
- **Prolonged hospitalization:** The patient is continually exposed to bacterial strains that are resistant to the antibiotics most commonly used in that practice.

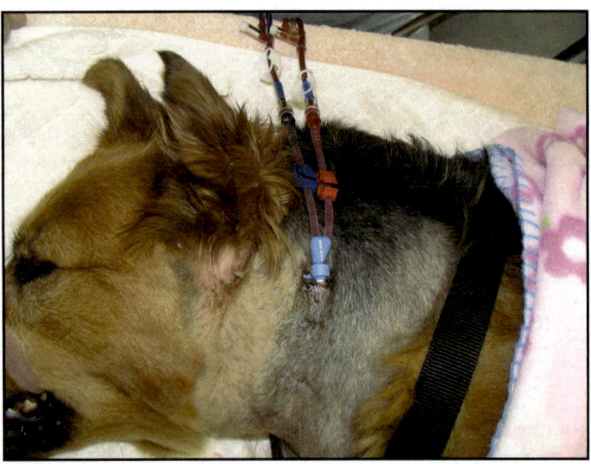

Figure 37-2. *Sepsis secondary to any indwelling catheter, especially one that has been in place for several days, is a serious problem in neutropenic animals. Strict aseptic technique should be adhered to when handling catheters, especially multilumen catheters.*

- **Malnutrition:** Malnutrition is a serious cause of debilitation and decreased resistance to bacterial infection, especially in dogs with neutropenia.
- **Neurologic dysfunction** or lack of ambulation from any cause.

When possible, these risk factors must be avoided or minimized and associated problems recognized and corrected early to reduce the probability of sepsis. The first approach for clinician and client is to understand the myelosuppressive effects of various drugs (Table 37-4). Clients and the veterinary health care team should be encouraged to be vigilant for the clinical signs associated with neutropenia and thrombocytopenia around the time of the nadir for the drug being used. With monitoring of CBCs at the appropriate times, especially early in the course of chemotherapy, the veterinarian will have a general idea of how low the WBC count is dropping. If the count is too low (<1,000/µl) or the patient becomes even mildly symptomatic, subsequent dose reduction of that drug should be considered.

> **KEY POINT**
>
> *The frequency and severity of infections are directly related to the severity and duration of neutropenia.*

Further steps can be taken to minimize the risk of sepsis in dogs with cancer. One logical step is to minimize the administration of immunosuppressive drugs, especially corticosteroids. When a splenectomized dog is treated for cancer, it should be watched carefully for complications, including sepsis. The risk of catheter-induced sepsis can be minimized by placing a new catheter in a new site every 2 to

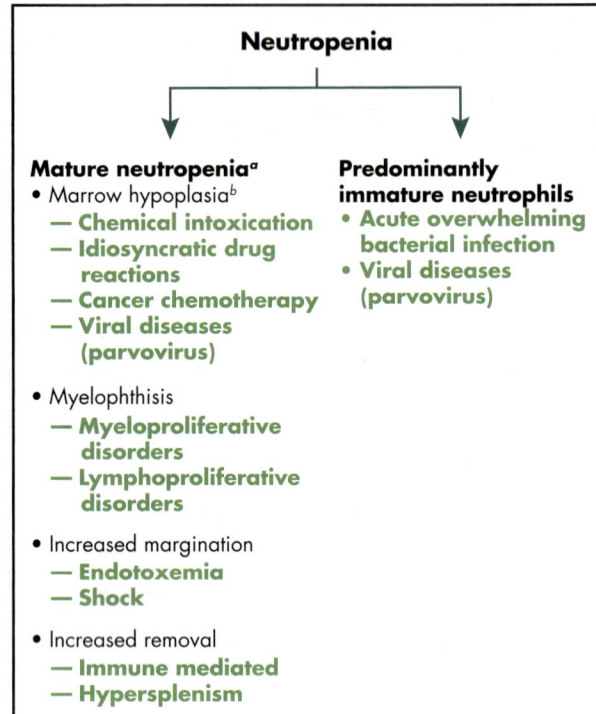

Figure 37-3. *Differential list for neutropenia in the canine cancer patient.* [a] *Bone marrow examination is recommended.* [b] *Marrow hypoplasia frequently involves more than one cell line.*

3 days. Strict aseptic procedures should be used, especially with dogs that are myelosuppressed. The use of semipermanent indwelling catheters in patients with cancer may be safe if strict aseptic procedures are followed by caregivers and health care professionals. Proper aseptic technique and changing of catheters are especially important in dogs with

> **KEY POINT**
>
> *The incidence of sepsis significantly increases when the neutrophil count drops to less than 1,000/µl.*

neurologic dysfunction because these dogs are at a much higher risk for sepsis. The duration of hospitalization should be kept short whenever possible to limit exposure to resistant bacteria.

Diagnosis

Dogs presented with septic shock secondary to neutropenia require immediate intervention and careful patient support. Diagnostic and therapeutic interventions must begin concurrently for the patient's benefit. The differential list for neutropenia is extensive (Figure 37-3).

The diagnosis of septic shock begins with the physical examination as a catheter is placed and blood samples are acquired for initial diagnostics. Mucous membrane color can be difficult to identify in dogs; however, in some dogs with septic shock, the mucous membranes may be brick red. In addition, tachycardia, short capillary refill time, gastrointestinal signs, altered mentation, and decreased blood pressure may be identified on physical examination in dogs in the hyperdynamic state of septic shock.[14–21] Thrombocytopenia and neutropenia are often identified during the course of septic shock. Hyperglycemia is an early finding that often is followed by hypoglycemia. Metabolic acidosis is commonly identified.

End-stage signs reflect a hypodynamic state and include hypothermia, mucous membrane pallor, marked mental depression, bloody diarrhea, and signs of multiorgan failure.[14–20]

Cultures of urine and blood should always be obtained, even though they may be negative and require a significant amount of time for results to be available. Appropriate broad-spectrum antibiotics and combinations must be available immediately for parenteral administration. When positive, the results of cultures will guide follow-up oral antibiotic selection.

Blood and urine taken at the time of initial presentation can be very helpful for supporting a diagnosis of septic shock. At a minimum, samples should be obtained for a CBC, biochemical profile, and urinalysis. These clinical pathologic findings are often combined with other tests.

The absence of circulating neutrophils affects many of the commonly used clinical, laboratory, and radiographic findings that may normally suggest localized or systemic infection. For example, neutropenia results in urine samples without pyuria, despite infection. Also, without a neutrophilic infiltrate, which is responsible for many of the radiographic changes associated with pneumonia, thoracic radiographs often appear "normal" even in the presence of significant pneumonia.

> **KEY POINT**
>
> *When laboratory and clinical data from a neutropenic dog are evaluated, the clinician must remember that many results may be surprisingly normal, even in the face of overt sepsis.*

Thus, any suspicious sites should be cultured.[21–24] At a minimum, cultures should include:

- **Blood cultures:** Two, and preferably four, sets of blood samples should be acquired for culture (aerobic and anaerobic). However, it is critical to be cognizant of the total volume of blood taken, including blood for hemograms, biochemical profiles, and other tests, because dogs with

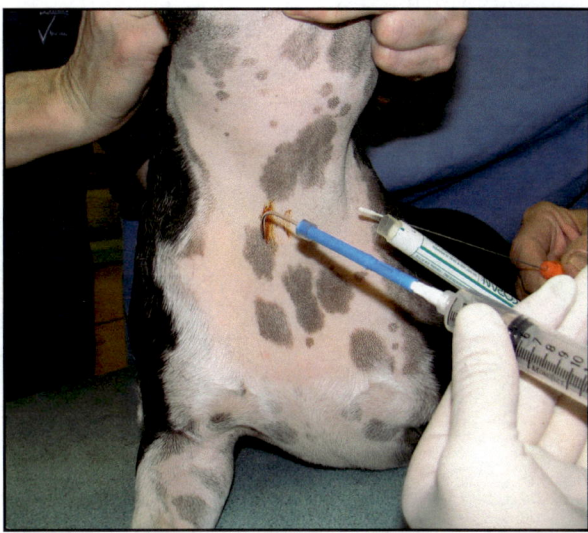

Figure 37-4. *Septic cancer patients with severe neutropenia may have bacterial pneumonia without any radiographic abnormalities, owing to the lack of inflammatory cells. Therefore, any septic, neutropenic animal that is coughing or that has abnormal lung auscultation should have a transtracheal wash for cytology and bacterial culture and sensitivity testing.*

cancer almost always have some degree of anemia of chronic disease. The timing of the sampling intervals is controversial; however, sampling every 20 to 30 minutes before initiation of antibiotic therapy may be adequate. At least 2 ml of blood should be injected into appropriate culture containers.

- **Catheter cultures:** If a central venous catheter is present, cultures of the port should be done. Ideally, culture bottles that contain an antibiotic-binding resin or other antibiotic-binding substance should be included with each culture for patients on antibiotics.

- **Urine culture:** A cystocentesis specimen for urine culture and analysis should be acquired in each case.

- **Cerebrospinal fluid (CSF) culture:** When neurologic signs are present, a CSF tap should be obtained and cultured appropriately. CSF should be sent for Gram staining, bacterial culture, cell count and differential, and glucose and protein determination. A cryptococcal antigen titer or India ink preparation should be performed in suspect cases. Acid-fast stains and culture are probably not indicated routinely.

- **Stool cultures:** For dogs with diarrhea, appropriate cultures should be done for clostridial bacteria, including appropriate assays for endotoxin.

- **Lung cultures:** Thoracic radiographs and a transendotracheal wash should be obtained, especially when the patient shows any sign of respiratory difficulty, such as increased respiratory effort or cough (Figure 37-4).

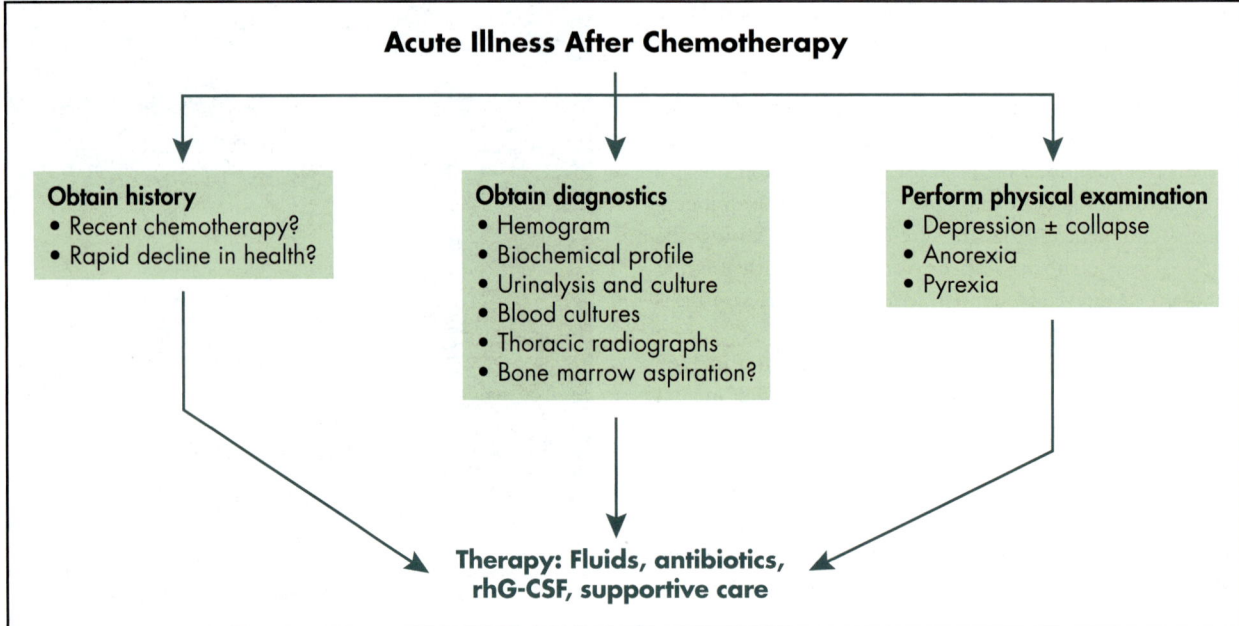

Figure 37-5. *Clinical approach to the septic, neutropenic dog.*

Other diagnostic studies that should be considered include[14–21]:

- CBC with differential, biochemical profile, and urinalysis
- Thoracic and abdominal radiographs to look for signs of infection
- Abdominal ultrasonography to look for pancreatitis, abscesses, abdominal effusion, and other signs of infection
- Echocardiography to identify the presence of valvular endocarditis
- Bronchoscopy with bronchoalveolar lavage if pulmonary disease is suspected
- Skin biopsy if deep cutaneous infection is identified
- Bone marrow aspiration or biopsy to determine the cause and severity of neutropenia
- Percutaneous or laparoscopic-guided liver biopsy or aspiration to evaluate for hepatic infection or abscessation
- Exploratory laparotomy in select cases when other, less invasive tests are not successful, yet there is clinical evidence of disease in the abdomen
- Blood gas analysis

KEY POINT

When possible, pyrexic, low-risk patients should be treated as outpatients with oral antibiotics to reduce the risk of nosocomial infections.

Treatment[21-24]

Treatment for septic shock should begin as soon as the condition is suspected. This is usually at the time the dog is initially presented for an acute, emergency condition. Treatment for the septic, neutropenic dog (Figures 37-4 and 37-5) is primarily directed at restoring adequate tissue perfusion, improving the alterations in metabolism, and controlling systemic infection.

RESTORING ADEQUATE TISSUE PERFUSION

Standard therapy includes crystalloid solutions and antibiotics. Although the use of hypertonic solutions for the treatment of shock is being investigated, balanced electrolyte solutions are cited in most canine textbooks as the first line of therapy. The infusion rate for critically ill dogs is initially 90 ml/kg IV for 1 hour, then 10 to 12 ml/kg/hr thereafter. The fluid rate should then be adjusted to meet the needs of the dog as determined by monitoring body weight, heart and respiratory rates, central venous pressure, ongoing losses (e.g., vomiting, diarrhea), and urine output. During the first hour of fluid administration, it is vitally important to monitor at 15-minute intervals for evidence of fluid overload and adjust appropriately.

IMPROVING ALTERATIONS IN METABOLISM

When choosing the type of fluid, some authorities prefer a non–lactate-containing fluid; lactate must be metabolized

Table 37-6 Approach to Febrile, Neutropenic Dogs[21-24]

Approach	Action
Identify the site of infection	• Perform complete physical examination. • Acquire CBC and platelet count, biochemical profile, and urinalysis. • Conduct four blood cultures, cystocentesis for culture and sensitivity, thoracic radiography, and transtracheal wash for culture and sensitivity. • If indicated, culture and sensitivity testing of CSF, catheters, joint fluid, and feces.
Initiate supportive care	• Establish indwelling IV catheter aseptically and initiate fluid therapy; for shock: 90 ml/kg for the first hour divided into quarter aliquots administered every 15 min, followed by 10–12 ml/kg/hr with very close monitoring to adjust fluid rate as needed. • Withhold any additional chemotherapeutic agents.
Initiate IV antibiotic	• Four-quadrant (gram-positive, gram-negative, aerobic, and anaerobic bacteria) antimicrobial therapy after cultures are obtained: Cefoxitin (22 mg/kg IV tid) or ampicillin (22 mg/kg IV tid) and enrofloxacin (5–10 mg/kg IV slowly daily). • If aminoglycosides not contraindicated (i.e., no evidence of dehydration, renal disease, low renal blood flow): Cefoxitin (22 mg/kg tid) and gentamicin (2–3 mg/kg tid over 30 min). • Monitor for nephrotoxicity (urinalysis, evaluate sediment for casts, monitor blood urea nitrogen/creatinine) if aminoglycosides, particularly gentamicin, administered; consider IV maintenance fluids. • Granulocyte-colony stimulating factor, if available (5 µg/kg/day SC).
Redefine antibiotic therapy based on culture and sensitivity results	Monitor fever and neutrophil count.
Discharge for home care	• Appropriate antibiotic therapy (e.g., trimethoprim–sulfamethoxazole 15 mg/kg PO bid). • Consider dose reduction with next chemotherapy (e.g., decrease by 25%).

Table 37-7 Antibiotics Used to Treat Sepsis[21-24]

Antibiotic	Potential Toxicoses
Gram-negative bacteria	
Gentamicin (2.2–4.4 mg/kg IV tid)	• Nephrotoxicity, especially when renal damage is present; ototoxicity; ensure adequate hydration and check frequently for renal damage during use
Cefazolin (22 mg/kg [10 mg/lb] IV q8h)	• Phlebitis, muscle pain after IV or IM administration; rare prevalence of nephrotoxicity
Cefoxitin (22 mg/kg IV tid)	• Phlebitis; discomfort with rapid IV injection; rare prevalence of nephrotoxicity
Gram-positive bacteria	
Sodium or potassium penicillin (22,000 U/kg IV qid)	• Allergy to penicillin can cause anaphylaxis, hives, fever, and pain; neurologic signs may occur with rapid infusion
Cefoxitin (22 mg/kg IV tid)	• Same as above
Enrofloxacin (10 mg/kg IV bid)	• Hives, fever, and pain
Anaerobic bacteria	
Metronidazole (15 mg/kg IV or IM tid)	• Anorexia, vomiting, and neurologic signs
Cefoxitin (22 mg/kg IV tid)	• Same as above

to bicarbonate by a functional liver that may be impaired during shock and sepsis. Normosol R and Plasmalyte are examples of non–lactate-containing fluids with acetate and gluconate as buffers. Dextrose should be included in fluids when systemic hypoglycemia is identified during constant patient monitoring.

CONTROLLING OR PREVENTING INFECTION

Asymptomatic dogs with fewer than 1,000 neutrophils/μl should be started prophylactically on antibiotics. Trimethoprim–sulfamethoxazole (7.5 mg/kg PO bid) is often recommended for prophylactic therapy in asymptomatic neutropenic patients. Neutropenic dogs in septic shock should be started on IV fluids and IV antibiotic therapy as soon as samples for bacterial cultures are acquired (Tables 37-6 and 37-7). Reevaluation of the initial antibiotic regimen is mandatory when the identity and sensitivity patterns of the bacteria become available. For gram-negative infections, two antibiotics that are effective against the isolated organism are often recommended.

Initial antibiotic therapy in dogs with sepsis commonly consists of broad-spectrum agents. Combinations of an aminoglycoside plus penicillin or a second-generation cephalosporin (e.g., cefoxitin, cefamandole, cefaclor, cefuroxime, cefonicid, ceforanide, cefotetan, cefmetazole) are often used. If the infection does not respond within 24 hours, the antibiotics should be changed. For gram-negative organisms, a different aminoglycoside, a fluoroquinolone, or aztreonam may be used. Extended-spectrum penicillins (e.g., ticarcillin, carbenicillin, azlocillin, piperacillin sodium, and mezlocillin), third-generation cephalosporins (e.g., cefotaxime, moxalactam, cefoperazone, ceftizoxime, ceftriaxone, ceftazidime, cefixime), or imipenem with cilastatin sodium have sufficiently broad spectrums to be used alone. Dogs treated with aminoglycosides, particularly gentamicin, should be monitored for nephrotoxicity via urinalysis (urine sediment should be examined for the presence of casts), blood urea nitrogen and creatinine concentrations, and good hydration.

Other treatments include:

- **Corticosteroids:** Steroids remain controversial in septic shock. Recommended doses for shock are hydrocortisone at 300 mg/kg, methylprednisolone or prednisone at 10 to 30 mg/kg, or dexamethasone at 4 to 8 mg/kg. Short-term use (i.e., <2 days of massive doses) does not result in as many adverse effects as long-term use.
- **Glucose:** If hypoglycemia is present, glucose at 0.25 g/kg IV bolus can be given, followed by infusions of 2.5% to 10% glucose solutions as needed to maintain normal blood glucose levels.
- **Bicarbonate:** Although very controversial, bicarbonate can be given if severe metabolic acidosis is present. The amount of bicarbonate to give can be calculated (i.e., base deficit × [0.3 × body weight in kg]) or estimated (mild, moderate, or severe acidosis is treated with 1, 3, or 5 mEq bicarbonate/kg IV, respectively). Bicarbonate should be given slowly IV (i.e., over 20 minutes or more).
- **Neutrophil-rich transfusions:** These transfusions have not been associated with beneficial responses in controlled trials. In addition, transfusion reactions and allosensitizations to specific antigens of the granulocytes may occur, and severe pulmonary reactions may be more prevalent.
- **Hematopoietic growth factors:** Canine recombinant granulocyte colony-stimulating factor (5 μg/kg/day SC) and canine recombinant granulocyte–macrophage colony-stimulating factor (10 μg/kg/day SC) have been associated with an increased rate of myeloid recovery in dogs with neutropenia. These hematopoietic growth factors increase cell numbers and enhance neutrophil function but are not widely available commercially. Human recombinant granulocyte colony-stimulating factor (rhG-CSF) and granulocyte–macrophage colony-stimulating factor are commercially available; however, long-term use may induce antibody formation to the protein. Of the two human recombinant proteins, rhG-CSF induces the most profound increase in neutrophil numbers before development of antibodies is noted (see Chapter 33).
- **Transfusions** of fresh, whole blood.
- **Other options:** Tumor necrosis factor antiserum, antibody to tumor necrosis factor, interleukin and interferon therapy, pooled immunoglobulin preparations, and monoclonal antibodies to neutralize endotoxin may be future treatments of choice.

REFERENCES

1. Ogilvie GK: Paraneoplastic syndromes, in Withrow SJ, MacEwen EG (eds): *Clinical Oncology.* Philadelphia, JB Lippincott, 1989, pp 29–40.
2. Ogilvie GK: Paraneoplastic syndromes, in Ettinger SJ, Feldman EC (eds): *Textbook of Veterinary Internal Medicine,* ed 4. Philadelphia, WB Saunders, 2000, pp 498–506.
3. Ogilvie GK: Anemia, thrombocytopenia, and hypoproteinemia, in Wingfield WE (ed): *Veterinary Emergency Medicine Secrets.* Philadelphia, Hanley and Belfus, 2001, pp 265–268.
4. Giger U, Gorman NT: Acute complications of cancer and cancer therapy, in Gorman NT (ed): *Oncology.* New York, Churchill Livingstone, 1986, pp 147–168.
5. Madewell BR, Feldman BF: Characterization of anemias associated with neoplasia in small dogs. *JAVMA* 176(5):419–425, 1980.
6. Comer KM: Anemia as a feature of primary gastrointestinal neoplasia. *Compend Contin Educ Pract Vet* 12(1):13–22, 1990.
7. Yamauchi A, Ohta T, Okada T, et al: Secondary erythrocytosis associated with schwannoma in a dog. *J Vet Med Sci* 66(12):1605–1608, 2004.
8. Bertazzolo W, Zuliani D, Pogliani E, et al: Diffuse bronchiolo-alveolar carcinoma in a dog. *J Small Anim Pract* 43(6):265–268, 2002.
9. Sato K, Hikasa Y, Morita T, et al: Secondary erythrocytosis associated with high plasma erythropoietin concentrations in a dog with cecal leiomyosarcoma. *JAVMA* 220(4):486–490, 2002.
10. Helfand SC, Couto CG, Madewell BR: Immune-mediated thrombocytopenia associated with solid tumors in dogs. *JAAHA* 21:787–794, 1985.

11. Hargis AM, Feldman BF: Evaluation of hemostatic defects secondary to vascular tumors in dogs: 11 cases (1983–1988). *JAVMA* 198(5):891–894, 1991.
12. Chinn DR, Myers RK, Matthews JA: Neutrophilic leukocytosis associated with metastatic fibrosarcoma in the dog. *JAVMA* 186(8):806–809, 1985.
13. Couto CG: Tumor-associated eosinophilia in the dog. *JAVMA* 184(7):837–838, 1984.
14. Ogilvie GK: Neutropenia, sepsis and thrombocytopenia, in Wingfield WE (ed): *Veterinary Emergency Medicine Secrets*. Philadelphia, Hanley and Belfus, 2001, pp 235–241.
15. Haskins SC: Shock, in Kirk RW (ed): *Current Veterinary Therapy VIII*. Philadelphia, WB Saunders, 1983, pp 2–27.
16. Kirk RW, Bistner SI: Shock, in *Handbook of Veterinary Procedures Emergency Treatment*, ed 4. Philadelphia, WB Saunders, 1985, pp 59–68.
17. Parker MM, Parrillo JE: Septic shock: Hemodynamics and pathogenesis. *JAMA* 250:2324–2230, 1983.
18. Hardie EM, Rawlings CA: Septic shock. *Compend Contin Educ Pract Vet* 5:369–373, 1983.
19. Wolfsheimer KJ: Fluid therapy in the critically ill patient. *Vet Clin North Am Small Anim Pract* 19(2):361–378, 1989.
20. Lazarus HM, Creger RJ, Gerson SL: Infectious emergencies in oncology patients. *Semin Oncol* 16(6):543–560, 1989.
21. Couto CG: Management of complications of cancer chemotherapy. *Vet Clin North Am Small Anim Pract* 4:1037–1053, 1990.
22. Woodlock TJ: Oncologic emergencies, in Rosenthal S, Carignan JR, Smith BD (eds): *Medical Care of the Cancer Patient*, ed 2. Philadelphia, WB Saunders, 1993, pp 236–246.
23. Hughes WT, Armstrong D, Bodey GP: Infectious Diseases Society of America: Guidelines for the use of antimicrobial agents in neutropenic patients with unexplained fever. *J Infect Dis* 161(3):381–390, 1990.
24. Quadri TL, Brown AE: Infectious complications in the critically ill patient with cancer. *Semin Oncology* 27(3):335–346, 2000.

HYPERGAMMAGLOBULINEMIA

Gregory K. Ogilvie and Antony S. Moore

38

CLINICAL BRIEFING

History	• Anorexia. • Lethargy. • Polyuria. • Polydipsia. • Spontaneous bleeding.
Clinical signs	• Bleeding from any site. • Petechial and ecchymotic hemorrhages. • Evidence of volume expansion. • Cardiovascular problems. • Blindness due to retinal hemorrhages. • Bone pain.
Diagnostics	• CBC. • Biochemical profile. • Urinalysis. • Immunoelectrophoresis demonstrating monoclonal gammopathy in blood and urine. • Bone marrow aspiration and cytology. • Retinal examination. • Coagulation profile (ACT, OSPT, APTT, fibrinogen, antithrombin III, platelet factor III, and FDPs). • Blood pressure. • Abdominal radiography and/or ultrasonography and bone marrow aspiration to help confirm or eliminate neoplastic etiology.
Therapy	• Eliminate underlying cause using surgery, chemotherapy (e.g., melphalan and prednisone), and radiation therapy. • Restore tissue perfusion with fluids, stabilize cardiovascular system, and reduce viscosity (if needed) with fluids, plasmapheresis, or plasma harvests from patient.

Hypergammaglobulinemia, also known as *M-component disorder* or *hyperviscosity syndrome,* is commonly associated with a variety of malignancies in dogs, particularly multiple myeloma.[1–8] About 75% of plasma cell tumors (i.e., plasma cell or multiple myeloma) exhibit hypergammaglobulinemia. Hypergammaglobulinemia results from excessive secretion of immunoglobulin (e.g., IgG, IgA, IgM, light-chain protein classes) by a monoclonal line of immunoglobulin-producing cells. Light chains, also known as Bence Jones proteins, may be present in the urine. Disorders associated with the production of large quantities of immunoglobulin include[1,2,5–9]:

• Acute inflammation
• Malignancy
• Trauma
• Necrosis
• Infarction
• Burns
• Chemical injury

Monoclonal gammopathies are associated with a malignant or potentially malignant clonal or biclonal process.

These processes include[1,2,5–9]:

- Multiple myeloma
- Waldenström's macroglobulinemia
- Solitary plasmacytoma
- Monoclonal gammopathy of undetermined significance
- Plasma cell leukemia
- Heavy chain disease
- Amyloidosis
- Rickettsial disease

The quantity of M protein, the results of bone marrow biopsy, and other characteristics can help differentiate multiple myeloma from other causes of monoclonal gammopathy. Paraneoplastic syndromes occur only with tumors that increase globulin concentration as an indirect, distant effect. In contrast, polyclonal gammopathies may be caused by any reactive or inflammatory process.

> **KEY POINT**
> *Hypergammaglobulinemia, also known as* **M-component disorder** *or* **hyperviscosity syndrome,** *is commonly associated with a variety of malignancies in dogs, particularly multiple myeloma.*

Clinical Presentation

Clinical signs associated with M-component disorders arise from increased viscosity associated with elevated globulins and from the tumor's direct effect on surrounding structures. Elevated proteins that interfere with normal platelet function can cause excessive bleeding from any site.[1,2,5–9] Hyperviscosity syndrome, which decreases blood fluidity, causes[1,2,5–9]:

- Polydipsia
- Central nervous system (CNS) signs, including confusion and seizures
- Retinopathies, including retinal hemorrhage
- Visual disturbances
- Secondary renal problems
- Congestive heart failure
- Hemarthrosis
- Epistaxis
- Hemothorax
- Hemoabdomen

Renal decompensation often follows renal amyloidosis or Bence Jones proteinuria; increased serum viscosity decreases renal perfusion, and concentrating ability is impaired. Neurologic signs arise when altered blood flow and diminished delivery of oxygen to neural tissue produce hypoxia in the CNS. Increased blood volume and viscosity place greater

> **KEY POINT**
> *Renal decompensation often follows renal amyloidosis or Bence Jones proteinuria; increased serum viscosity decreases renal perfusion, and concentrating ability is impaired.*

demands on the heart, which can produce decompensation of stable preexisting cardiac conditions or development of a hypertrophic cardiomyopathy-like state.

Diagnosis

The following baseline tests must be conducted to determine the underlying cause of each case of hypergammaglobulinemia[1–9]:

- Complete blood count (CBC), biochemical profile, and urinalysis
- Immunoelectrophoresis of serum and urine (± Bence Jones protein test of urine)
- Bone marrow aspiration and cytology
- Thoracic and abdominal radiography
- Survey skeletal radiography (± nuclear scintigraphy of the skeletal system)
- Retinal examination
- Coagulogram (activated partial thromboplastin time [APTT], one-stage prothrombin time [OSPT], activated clotting time [ACT], platelet count, fibrin degradation products [FDPs], and antithrombin III)
- Rickettsial titers, including titers for *Ehrlichia* and *Borrelia* spp.

Initial screening tests are conducted primarily to detect evidence of bone marrow involvement by tumor or *Ehrlichia* spp, monoclonal gammopathy, renal failure sec-

> **KEY POINT**
> *In the presence of a monoclonal gammopathy, initial screening tests are conducted primarily to detect evidence of bone marrow involvement by tumor or* **Ehrlichia** *spp, monoclonal gammopathy, renal failure secondary to hyperglobulinemia, coagulopathy distinct from increased globulins, lytic bone lesions suggestive of multiple myeloma, myelophthisis, or hypertension and bleeding.*

ondary to hyperglobulinemia, coagulopathy distinct from increased globulins, lytic bone lesions suggestive of multiple myeloma, myelophthisis, or hypertension and bleeding. Because it determines not only whether monoclonal gammopathy is present but also which class of immunoglobulins is involved, immunoelectrophoresis is generally preferred to serum protein electrophoresis. Multiple myeloma, which does not engender paraneoplastic syndrome, is described in Chapter 48; it is diagnosed by the presence of monoclonal gammopathy, Bence Jones or monoclonal proteinuria, the appearance of "punched-out" bone lesions on a nuclear bone scan, and more than 20% to 30% plasma cells in bone marrow. Clinical signs resolve when malignancy is controlled. If increased globulin concentrations are in response to *Ehrlichia* infection, titers should disclose the organism.

> **KEY POINT**
>
> *As an alternative to plasmapheresis, blood can be harvested from dogs with clinically significant hypergammaglobulinemia; the plasma can then be removed and the red blood cells resuspended in an equal volume of 0.9% NaCl for immediate reintroduction into the patient.*

Treatment[1,2,8]

The treatment of choice for multiple myeloma is melphalan (0.1 mg/kg PO daily for 10 days, then 0.5–1 mg/kg every other day) and prednisone (0.5–1 mg/kg PO daily for 21 days, then every other day thereafter). Plasmapheresis rapidly reduces protein levels and is useful in cases in which hyperviscosity requires symptomatic treatment.[1,2,8]

In one study,[8] each case of multiple myeloma was confirmed by observation of more than 5% plasma cells on examination of a bone marrow aspirate and detection of monoclonal gammopathy of immunoglobulin. Treatment with melphalan, cyclophosphamide, and prednisone was associated with long-term survival (median: 540 days). Negative prognostic factors included hypercalcemia and immunoglobulin light-chain proteinuria.

Other supportive care involves fluid therapy for dehydration. Because myeloma cells are believed to secrete a substance that suppresses macrophage and lymphocyte function, prophylactic administration of broad-spectrum antibiotics should be considered, particularly in the early phases of therapy.

REFERENCES

1. Ogilvie GK: Paraneoplastic syndromes, in Withrow SJ, MacEwen EG (eds): *Clinical Veterinary Oncology.* Philadelphia, JB Lippincott, 1989, pp 29–40.
2. Ogilvie GK: Paraneoplastic syndromes, in Ettinger SJ, Feldman EC (eds): *Textbook of Veterinary Internal Medicine,* ed 5. Philadelphia, WB Saunders, 2000, pp 498–506.
3. Griffin TW, Rosenthal PE, Costanza ME: Paraneoplastic and endocrine syndromes, in Cady B (ed): *Cancer Manual,* ed 7. Boston, American Cancer Society, 1986, pp 373–390.
4. Ogilvie GK: Metabolic emergencies and the cancer patient, in Wingfield WE (ed): *Veterinary Emergency Medicine Secrets.* Philadelphia, Hanley and Belfus, 2001, pp 247–251.
5. O'Connell TX, Horita TJ, Kasravi B: Understanding and interpreting serum protein electrophoresis. *Am Fam Physician* 71:105–112, 2005.
6. Ramaiah SK, Seguin MA, Carwile HF: Biclonal gammopathy associated with immunoglobulin A in a dog with multiple myeloma. *Vet Clin Pathol* 31:83–89, 2002.
7. Lautzenhiser SJ, Walker MC, Goring RL: Unusual IgM-secreting multiple myeloma in a dog. *JAVMA* 223:645–648, 2003.
8. Matus RE, Leifer CE, MacEwen EG, et al: Prognostic factors for multiple myeloma in the dog. *JAVMA* 188:1288–1292, 1986.
9. Lane IF, Roberts SM, Lappin MR: Ocular manifestations of vascular disease: Hypertension, hyperviscosity, and hyperlipidemia. *JAAHA* 29:28–36, 1993.

EXTRAVASATION OF CHEMOTHERAPEUTIC AGENTS

Gregory K. Ogilvie and Antony S. Moore

CLINICAL BRIEFING

Diagnosis

History
- Pain or discomfort during infusion or swelling at the injection site.

Clinical signs
- Initial swelling and discomfort followed by severe tissue necrosis and a nonhealing lesion 1 to 4 weeks after infusion.

Therapy
- Stop infusion, leave catheter in place, and aspirate as much fluid and drug as possible from the site.
- Administer antidote.
  - *For doxorubicin:* Apply cold compresses and infuse with saline; administer IV dexrazoxane; possibly use topical DMSO or infiltrate area with intralesional hydrocortisone.
  - *For vinca alkaloid:* Apply warm compresses and instill hyaluronidase; possibly use topical DMSO or infiltrate area with intralesional hydrocortisone.

Many chemotherapeutic agents induce significant tissue injury after extravasation. Some of these agents are severe irreversible vesicants; others induce irritation to tissue. The agents commonly used in canine oncology are listed in the box on this page. Every member of the veterinary health care team must be aware of the potential for drug extravasation and must do everything possible to prevent extravasations.

The best key to prevention is awareness and training of every member of the veterinary health care team. Atraumatic placement of "first-stick" catheters, appropriate use of butterfly catheters, and adequate patient restraint, along with careful monitoring during administration, will prevent

> **KEY POINT**
> *Atraumatic placement of "first-stick" catheters, appropriate use of butterfly catheters, and adequate patient restraint, along with careful monitoring during administration, will prevent extravasations and their devastating consequences.*

extravasations and their devastating consequences. Management of extravasations in human and canine medicine is anecdotal and extremely controversial. Despite this controversy, guidelines (Table 39-1) have been established for clinical use.

Predisposing Factors

Accurate and secure first-stick catheter placement is essential when administering drugs that can cause tissue damage if extravasated perivascularly. Generally, only small-gauge (22- to 23-gauge) indwelling IV catheters should be used when treatment volumes exceed 1 ml; 23- to 25-gauge butterfly needles can be used to administer smaller volumes of drugs such as vincristine. Everyone involved in patient care should note when and where blood samples are taken by venipuncture and where catheters have been placed previously to prevent administration of chemotherapeutic agents through veins that may leak because of previous procedures. Drawing blood samples from peripheral veins should be avoided if at all possible to preserve these veins for catheter access. Preferably, all blood samples should be taken from the jugular veins to reduce damage to the peripheral veins.

Potential Vesicants and Irritants Used in Canine Oncology[1-4]

Actinomycin D	Etoposide	Vinblastine
Daunorubicin	Mechlorethamine	Vincristine
Doxorubicin	Mithramycin	Vinorelbine
Epirubicin	Mitoxantrone	

Table 39-1 **General Treatment Guidelines for Extravasated Drugs**[1-4]

General Procedures	Details
Minimize amount of drug at site	• Do not remove the catheter or needle. • With a syringe, immediately withdraw as much drug as possible from the tissue, tubing, and catheter. • Administer antidote (see below) or sterile saline to neutralize or dilute the drug.
Extravasated Agent	*Antidote*
Doxorubicin, daunorubicin, epirubicin, idarubicin, or actinomycin D	• Apply topical cooling with ice or cold compresses and DMSO for 6–10 hr to inhibit vesicant cytotoxicity; do not apply heat. • Administer 10 mg of dexrazoxane IV for every 1 mg of doxorubicin over a 20- to 30-minute period. • Controversial: Infiltrate area with 1 mg/kg hydrocortisone. • Surgical debridement, plastic surgery, or limb amputation may be indicated in rare cases.
Vincristine, vinblastine, or etoposide	• Infiltrate area with 1 ml of hyaluronidase (150 U/ml) for every milliliter extravasated to enhance absorption and to disperse the drug. • Apply warm compresses to the site for several hours to enhance systemic absorption. — Controversial: — Apply topical DMSO. • Infiltrate area with 1 mg/kg hydrocortisone.
Mechlorethamine	Give local injection of sodium thiosulfate (sodium hyposulfite).

Only catheters that have been placed very recently (within 4 hours) should be used for administration of chemotherapeutic agents. Extreme care should be taken when administering drugs to all dogs; however, some patients have more fragile veins, including extremely debilitated patients, diabetic patients, some aged patients, and patients that have been receiving weekly or biweekly therapy for a significant period. The catheter should be checked for patency with a very large injection of saline (e.g., 12–15 ml) before and after administration of the drug. The catheter must also be closely monitored and checked for patency throughout drug infusion.

> **KEY POINT**
> *The catheter should be checked for patency with a very large injection of saline (e.g., 12–15 ml) before and after administration of the drug. The catheter must be closely monitored and checked for patency throughout drug infusion.*

Diagnosis

Usually, there is no doubt about whether extravasation has occurred. Some agents are very caustic if given perivascularly; dogs may vocalize or physically react to pain at the injection site. With small volumes, there may be no reaction from the patient, so lack of these signs does not rule out extravasation. Treatment for extravasation must begin immediately. Tissue necrosis generally becomes evident 1 to 10 days after injection and may progress for 3 to 4 weeks. The lesions occur early with vinca alkaloids and late with anthracycline antibiotics such as doxorubicin. Lesions may begin as mild erythema and progress to open, draining wounds. These wounds will not heal without extensive debridement and plastic surgery weeks to months after the perivascular slough begins, when all damage is evident.

Treatment[1-4]

Extensive training and awareness are the first steps to prevention. Everyone involved with the administration of chemotherapeutic agents should be aware of procedures for

> **KEY POINT**
> *The perivascular administration of doxorubicin should be immediately treated in part with cold compresses. The perivascular administration of vinca alkaloids should be immediately treated in part with warm compresses.*

treatment of extravasation (Figure 39-1). The procedures should be posted in a common area, and all materials needed to treat extravasations should be readily available and accessible. Because of their extensive use in canine practice, doxo-

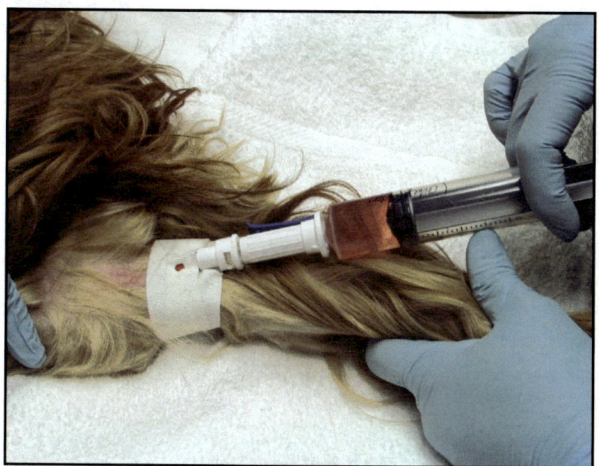

Figure 39-1. *When an extravasation occurs, do not remove the catheter or needle. With a syringe, immediately withdraw as much drug as possible from the tissue, tubing, and catheter and administer an appropriate antidote to neutralize or dilute the drug.*

rubicin and the vinca alkaloids are the most common causes of perivascular sloughs. Applying cold packs to a doxorubicin perivascular injection and warm packs to a vinca alkaloid perivascular injection may be helpful. Dexrazoxane and dimethyl sulfoxide (DMSO) may be of value for doxorubicin-induced perivascular injections. Regardless, no method effectively eliminates tissue necrosis. Sodium bicarbonate, corticosteroids, α-tocopherol, *N*-acetylcysteine, glutathione, lidocaine, diphenhydramine, cimetidine, propranolol, and isoproterenol are not known to be effective in the treatment of doxorubicin extravasations.[4]

Once tissue damage is identified, analgesics, an Elizabethan collar, and bandages with nonstick pads are essential to allow the area to heal without self-trauma. Bandages should be changed daily as long as the area is draining or has the potential for infection. If a bacterial infection is noted, culture and sensitivity testing and appropriate administration of antimicrobials are essential. Frequent cleansing and debridement may be necessary. Some cases require reconstructive surgical repair techniques. In the event of a doxorubicin extravasation, it may become necessary to amputate the limb.

REFERENCES

1. Ogilvie GK: Extravasation of chemotherapeutic agents, in Wingfield WE (ed): *Veterinary Emergency Medicine Secrets.* Philadelphia, Hanley and Belfus, 2001, pp 259–260.
2. Jordan K, Grothe W, Schmoll HJ: Extravasation of chemotherapeutic agents: Prevention and therapy. *Dtsch Med Wochenschr* 130:33–37, 2005.
3. Hubbard SM, Jenkins JF: Chemotherapy administration: Practical guidelines, in Chabner BA, Collins JM (eds): *Cancer Chemotherapy: Principles and Practice.* Philadelphia, JB Lippincott, 1990, pp 449–464.
4. Bertelli G: Prevention and management of extravasation of cytotoxic drugs. *Drug Saf* 12:245–255, 1995.

CHEMOTHERAPY-INDUCED ANAPHYLAXIS AND HYPERSENSITIVITY

Gregory K. Ogilvie and Antony S. Moore

CLINICAL BRIEFING

History	• Acute decompensation and collapse soon after the administration of any drug, including a chemotherapeutic agent.
Clinical signs	• Rapid onset of pale or cyanotic mucous membranes. • Decreased capillary refill time. • Evidence of decreased cardiac output. • Alterations in heart rate. • Cool extremities.
Diagnostics	• Eliminate other causes with complete blood count, biochemical profile, urinalysis, and cardiac evaluation.
Therapy	• Eliminate the underlying cause. • Ensure a patent airway and adequate cardiac output. • Establish vascular access. • Initiate fluid therapy. • Treat with dexamethasone $NaPO_4$ or hydrocortisone, diphenhydramine, and epinephrine (if indicated).

Although anaphylaxis or an anaphylaxis-like reaction can occur with any drug, these potentially life-threatening reactions usually happen soon after the administration of L-asparaginase. Hypersensitivity reactions can occur with any drug but are most common with doxorubicin,[1] paclitaxel,[2] and etoposide.[3]

> **KEY POINT**
>
> *Although anaphylaxis or an anaphylaxis-like reaction can occur with any drug, these potentially life-threatening reactions usually happen soon after the administration of drugs such as L-asparaginase. Hypersensitivity reactions can occur with any drug but are most common with doxorubicin,[1] paclitaxel,[2] and etoposide.[3]*

L-Asparaginase is well known for inducing anaphylaxis, hemorrhagic pancreatitis, diabetes mellitus, and coagulopathies in humans. In one study, 48% of dogs given L-asparaginase intraperitoneally developed adverse effects[4]; 30% of these dogs exhibited signs of anaphylaxis. These findings are similar to those in children given IV L-asparaginase.[5] The same study showed that administration of the drug intramuscularly completely eliminated signs associated with anaphylaxis but did not reduce remission rates (Figure 40-1). Although hemorrhagic pancreatitis, diabetes mellitus, and coagulopathies may be seen with use of L-asparaginase in humans, they have not been reported in any study in which this drug was administered to a large number of dogs.

L-Asparaginase–induced anaphylaxis and hypersensitivity are common because of enzyme immunogenicity. Anaphylaxis is usually caused by IgE-mediated mast cell degranulation; however, certain substances (e.g., bacterial and fungal cell walls) can trigger anaphylaxis by activating the alternate complement pathway. During the activation of this alternate pathway, C3a and C5a are formed. These are known potent anaphylatoxins capable of degranulating mast cells and basophils.[6] Although the exact mechanism of L-asparaginase–induced anaphylaxis in dogs is largely unexplored, induction of anaphylaxis in children with acute lymphoblastic leukemia is believed to result in part from com-

General Approach to Treatment of Animals with Drug-Induced Anaphylaxis

- **Examine the patient;** call for help.
- **Ensure that the patient has a good airway.** Provide oxygen via facemask or, if needed, intubation. If intubation is difficult to achieve because of upper airway or facial edema, epinephrine may rapidly reverse airway compromise; mask ventilation may be effective in the interim when intubation is not possible. Surgical airway intervention using standard tracheostomy is an option when intubation is not effective.
- **Provide mechanical ventilation** for the patient if necessary.
- **Support the patient's cardiovascular system:**
  — Initiate cardiac monitoring, establish a large-bore IV catheter, and initiate fluid therapy with isotonic crystalloid solution (70–90 ml/kg/hr) with patient reassessment every 15 minutes.
  — After the "shock dose" of fluid is administered, administer fluid as needed (e.g., 10 ml/kg/hr). Further intervention depends on severity of reaction and affected organ system(s).
  — Concurrently, initiate drug therapy: Dexamethasone NaPO$_4$ (2 mg/kg IV), diphenhydramine (2–4 mg/kg IM, watch for toxicoses), or epinephrine (0.1–0.3 ml of a 1:1,000 solution IV or IM for severe reactions). Hypotension in anaphylaxis is usually due to vasodilatation and capillary fluid leakage. Epinephrine is the primary pharmacologic treatment for these findings. H$_1$-blocking antihistamines may also have a role in reversing hypotension. Some authors also recommend H$_2$-blocking agents.
  — In cases of refractory hypotension, first administer large volumes of crystalloid and repeated doses of epinephrine or a continuous epinephrine infusion. If this is not effective, consider other pressors with α-adrenergic activity, such as norepinephrine or dopamine. Cases of effective use of military antishock trousers for refractory hypotension have been reported.
- **Treat any cutaneous effects.** These effects of anaphylaxis are uncomfortable but not life threatening. Patients often respond promptly to epinephrine and H$_1$ antihistamines. Some authors state that corticosteroids help prevent recurrence of signs (both cutaneous and systemic) that may occur 6 to 8 hours after successful treatment ("biphasic reaction"). H$_2$ blockers may have an added effect.

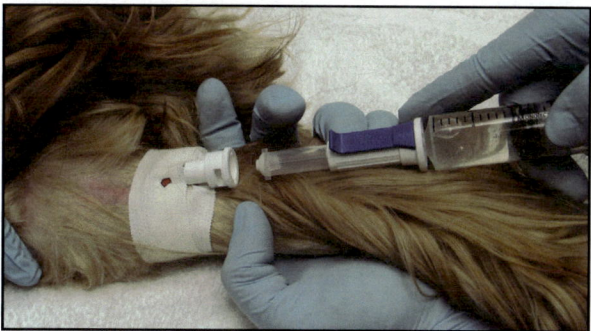

Figure 40-1. *The rapid intravenous administration of chemotherapeutic agents, especially L-asparaginase, can result in anaphylaxis. Whenever possible, administer L-asparaginase intramuscularly.*

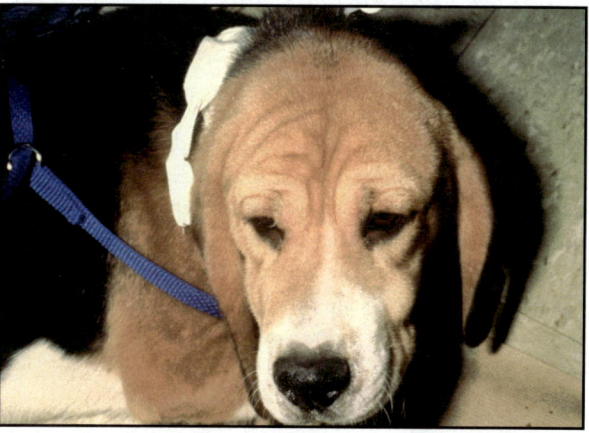

Figure 40-2. *The carriers in drugs such as etoposide and paclitaxel can induce a profound allergic reaction that can result in severe erythema, thickening of the skin, and pruritus, especially around the head and neck. This beagle was given etoposide, which resulted in an acute collapse and edema of the head and neck.*

plement activation induced by formation of immune complexes of L-asparaginase and specific antibodies.[7] Anaphylaxis usually occurs within seconds to minutes after administration of L-asparaginase; however, some dogs may have a delayed response that results in the same clinical signs hours after the drug is given.

The hypersensitivity reaction secondary to doxorubicin therapy is believed to be related, at least in part, to mast cell degranulation. Cremophor EL and polysorbate, the carriers used in formulations of taxol and etoposide, respectively, are responsible for the hypersensitivity reaction induced by these drugs (Figure 40-2). These two carriers are sometimes found in other medications marketed for use in human patients; for this and other reasons, off-label use of drugs should be undertaken with caution.

Predisposing Factors

One predisposing factor related to anaphylaxis secondary to L-asparaginase or other drug therapy is a history of exposure to the drug. Because L-asparaginase is a ubiquitous bacterial product in mammalian systems, anaphylaxis may occur after the first administration. In addition, anaphylactic and hypersensitivity reactions are worse in animals that have an existing condition such as atopy, which results in a buildup of mast cells and eosinophils before the drug treatment. As mentioned earlier, the route of administration of the drug may contribute to development of an anaphylactic or hypersensitivity reaction.

Diagnosis

The most common clinical signs associated with drug-induced anaphylaxis are acute collapse and cardiovascular failure, which lead to shock and death. The event usually occurs within minutes after parenteral injection of the offending drug, although some anaphylactic reactions that occurred hours to days after drug therapy have been reported. The patient is pale and weak and usually exhibits bradycardia or tachycardia and a rapid, thready pulse. Mucous membranes generally are pale to cyanotic. Peripheral extremities are often cool to the touch, and blood pressure is low.

> **KEY POINT**
> *The most common clinical signs associated with drug-induced anaphylaxis are acute collapse and cardiovascular failure, which lead to shock and death.*

Hypersensitivity reactions may result in profound pruritus during or after administration of the drug. Pruritus may result in head shaking, and there may be swelling of the ears, lips, or paws or near the vein or area being treated. The erythematous reaction usually lasts for the duration of treatment. Occasionally, the edematous and erythematous reactions last for hours after the treatment is finished.

Therapy[6,8,9]
PREVENTION

A prospective study[8] of 81 dogs with histologically confirmed, measurable malignant tumors was conducted to determine the prevalence of anaphylaxis associated with intramuscular administration of 232 doses of L-asparaginase (10,000 U/m^2). None of the dogs exhibited clinical signs associated with anaphylaxis. Therefore, to reduce the probability of anaphylaxis, L-asparaginase should be given intramuscularly rather than intravenously or intraperitoneally. In addition, because L-asparaginase is a potent inducer of anaphylaxis, administration of a test dose is advised.

Hypersensitivity reactions secondary to the administration of doxorubicin can be almost completely eliminated by slowly infusing the drug. One method includes diluting the drug into 150 to 500 mL of 0.9% NaCl and administering the solution over 20 to 40 minutes. Thousands of doses of doxorubicin have been administered by the authors, and less than 3% of patients show any signs of hypersensitivity reactions. Some advocate pretreatment with diphenhydramine and glucocorticoids before doxorubicin therapy to reduce the prevalence of hypersensitivity reactions. Because these drugs have their own adverse effects and cost factors, the benefits of premedication may be limited.

Reactions secondary to the carriers in paclitaxel and etoposide can be reduced by slowing the rate of infusion and by pretreating with dexamethasone (1–2 mg/kg IV), diphenhydramine (2–4 mg/kg IM), and cimetidine (2–4 mg/kg IV slowly) 1 hour before infusion of the chemotherapeutic agent. If a reaction is noted, the infusion can be discontinued temporarily until the animal is more comfortable.

Treatment

Anaphylaxis is a potentially fatal condition and should be treated immediately with supportive care, fluids, glucocorticoids, H$_1$-receptor antagonists, and epinephrine. Large-volume fluid resuscitation with isotonic crystalloid is often needed to support the circulation in patients with cardiovascular manifestations of anaphylaxis. The treatment outline is detailed in the box on page 299.

Hypersensitivity reactions can be treated by terminating drug therapy. Reactions usually subside within minutes. The patient can then be treated with H$_1$-receptor antagonists (see box) before reinitiating drug treatment at a much slower rate.

> **KEY POINT**
> *The risk of L-asparaginase–induced anaphylaxis can be reduced substantially by giving the drug intramuscularly rather than intravenously or intraperitoneally.*

REFERENCES

1. Ogilvie GK, Curtis C, Richardson RC, et al: Acute short term toxicity associated with the administration of doxorubicin to dogs with malignant tumors. *JAVMA* 195:1584–1587, 1989.
2. Ogilvie GK, Walters LM, Powers BE, et al: Organ toxicity of NBT taxol in the rat and dog: A preclinical study. *Proc 13th Annu Vet Canc Soc Conf*:90–91, 1993.
3. Ogilvie GK, Cockburn CA, Tranquilli WJ, Reschke RW: Hypotension and cutaneous reactions associated with etoposide administration in the dog. *Am J Vet Res* 49:1367–1370, 1988.
4. Teske E, Rutteman GR, van Heerde P, Misdorp W: Polyethylene glycol-L-asparaginase versus native L-asparaginase in canine non-Hodgkin's lymphoma. *Eur J Cancer* 26:891–895, 1990.
5. Nesbit M, Chard R, Evans A, et al: Evaluation of intramuscular versus intravenous administration of L-asparaginase in childhood leukemia. *Am J Pediatr Hematol Oncol* 1:9–13, 1979.
6. Degen MA: Acute hypersensitivity reactions, in Kirk RW (ed): *Current Veterinary Therapy X*. Philadelphia, WB Saunders, 1989, pp 537–542.
7. Fabry U, Korholz D, Jurgens H, et al: Anaphylaxis to L-asparaginase during treatment for acute lymphoblastic leukemia in children. Evidence of a complement-mediated mechanism. *Pediatr Res* 19:400–408, 1985.
8. Ogilvie GK, Atwater SW, Ciekot PA, et al: Prevalence of anaphylaxis associated with the intramuscular administration of L-asparaginase to 81 dogs with cancer: 1989–1991. *JAAHA* 4:3662–3665, 1994.
9. Ogilvie GK: Chemotherapy induced anaphylaxis, in Wingfield WE (ed): *Veterinary Emergency Medicine Secrets*. Philadelphia, Hanley and Belfus, 2001, pp 257–258.

CANCER THERAPY–INDUCED RENAL FAILURE

Gregory K. Ogilvie and Antony S. Moore

CLINICAL BRIEFING

History	• Acute decompensation, anorexia, and vomiting. • Damage to lower urinary tract can result in stranguria and hematuria.
Clinical signs	• Possible oliguria with increased body weight and central venous pressures with fluid therapy, uremic gastritis, and uremic breath. • Stranguria or hematuria may also be seen.
Diagnostics	• Ultrasonography, computed tomography, or magnetic resonance imaging of the urinary tract; CBC, biochemical profile, urinalysis, central venous pressures, and urine output quantification.
Therapy	• Treat or eliminate the underlying cause. • Correct dehydration. • Administer fluids to meet daily needs and external losses and induce a mild to moderate diuresis. • Correct acid–base and electrolyte abnormalities. • Treat oliguria with dobutamine, furosemide, and dextrose (if indicated).

Many cancer therapies, including radiation to the urinary tract, cisplatin, piroxicam, doxorubicin, and methotrexate, can induce renal failure (Table 41-1). Drugs such as ifosfamide, if administered without the thiol compound mesna, can cause sterile hemorrhagic cystitis and primary or secondary renal damage. Renal failure can also be caused by a malignant condition (e.g., transitional cell carcinoma, prostatic carcinoma) or the use of anesthetic agents, nephrotoxic antibiotics (e.g., gentamicin), or contrast agents.

Predisposing Factors

In veterinary medicine, the most common predisposing factors associated with the development of acute renal failure are cancer and nephrotoxic drugs, including chemotherapeutic agents. Therefore, when chemotherapeutic agents are used in veterinary patients, other nephrotoxic drugs, such as aminoglycosides, should be avoided. Other risk factors associated with the development of acute and chronic renal failure in dogs are decreased cardiac output, urinary tract infection, sepsis, preexisting renal disease, advanced age, dehydration, fever, liver disease, hypokalemia, and hypercalcemia. Several studies have shown that preexisting renal disease may be one of the most important predisposing factors for the development of cisplatin-induced acute renal failure.[1-13]

Dogs with transitional cell carcinoma of the bladder, urethra, or prostate commonly have urethral obstruction that may lead to hydroureter, hydronephrosis, and renal dysfunction. The concurrent septic cystitis seen in most patients with bladder tumors may induce secondary pyelonephritis. This can result in acute and chronic renal failure.

NEPHROTOXIC CHEMOTHERAPEUTIC AGENTS

The most nephrotoxic chemotherapeutic agent is cisplatin, a heavy-metal coordination compound that has antineoplastic activity.[1-7] The drug is not as commonly used today as it once was because of the increased availability and affordability of a less nephrotoxic compound, carboplatin. In dogs, 80% to 90% of cisplatin is eliminated in the urine within 48 hours. Nephrotoxicosis, characterized by reduced glomerular filtration rate (GFR) and tubular injury, is the major dose-limiting toxicosis. Renal toxicosis may range from brief increases in blood urea nitrogen and creatinine concentrations to irreversible renal failure. However, renal damage generally is not a clinical problem if adequate hydration is maintained.[6,7,10-12] A variety of administration protocols have been suggested to limit or eliminate cisplatin nephrotoxicosis in dogs.[1-7] Each

Table 41-1 **Anticancer Drugs Reported to Cause Damage to the Urinary Tract**

Drug	Potential Damage
• Cisplatin • Methotrexate • Mithramycin • Streptozocin • Ifosfamide	Commonly associated with renal disease
• Carboplatin • Ifosfamide • Doxorubicin • Bleomycin • Cyclophosphamide • Mitomycin • Nitrosoureas • Pamidronate (e.g., alendronate) • NSAIDs (e.g., piroxicam)	Less commonly associated with renal disease

protocol includes the use of IV 0.9% saline solution during the 4- to 24-hour diuresis period (see Prevention section, below).

Cisplatin is not the only drug to cause some degree of nephrotoxicosis. Doxorubicin, which can cause chronic renal failure in cats,[9] has also been noted to cause renal failure in dogs; however, this complication is rare. Methotrexate is eliminated primarily by the kidneys and has been associated with the development of nephrotoxicosis. Streptozocin, used to treat insulinomas, is a known nephrotoxin in dogs; however, an appropriate 0.9% saline diuresis, as is used for cisplatin, is effective in mitigating its toxicity. Piroxicam, the drug that is commonly used to treat transitional cell carcinoma, can also enhance the progression of renal disease, especially when it is used in combination with cisplatin.[13]

> **KEY POINT**
> *Preexisting disease of the urinary tract and concurrent use of nephrotoxic agents enhance the risk of developing renal disease due to the administration of chemotherapeutic agents.*

Diagnosis

Acute and chronic renal failure are results of decreased GFR with or without tubular damage. Therefore, the parameters used to diagnose these syndromes are related to damage of the glomeruli and tubules. Significant renal disease may exist long before clinical, hematologic, and biochemical abnormalities are identified because at least two-thirds of the kidney function must be abnormal before evidence of renal disease becomes overt.

Acute renal failure may occur with varying amounts of urine output, including oliguria or anuria. Regardless of the amount, the urine usually has a constant osmolality (isosthenuria) or is minimally concentrated with a high sodium content (>40 mEq/L). Glucose, protein, and renal epithelial cells may be noted in the urine. There is an acute increase in blood urea nitrogen, creatinine, and phosphorus concentrations. In oliguric or anuric renal failure, body weight, heart rate, and central venous pressure may increase if fluids are administered before urine flow is reestablished.

Therapy

The best treatment for acute or chronic renal failure is prevention. Substantial data show that cisplatin nephrotoxicity can be reduced and almost eliminated with adequate hydration. The incidence of chemotherapy-induced renal failure can be reduced by not treating dogs with preexisting renal disease with chemotherapeutic agents or by increasing the duration of time the chemotherapeutic drug is administered.

PREVENTION

Chemotherapy-induced nephrotoxicity is best prevented by identifying and treating patients with underlying renal disease before chemotherapy is initiated. Measuring creatinine clearance may be helpful in predicting preexisting renal disease. In human medicine, the creatinine clearance is used to guide dosage reduction for the drugs listed in Table 41-1. Few guidelines exist in veterinary medicine; however, the general concept of reducing the drug dosage to be administered and enhancing urine output is logical: In the event that chemotherapy must be given, concurrent administration of fluids is essential. Cisplatin nephrotoxicity may be reduced with the administration of amifostine (WR-2721).

Many diuresis protocols may prevent or delay the onset of cisplatin-induced nephrotoxicosis in dogs.[1,2] The 6- and 4-hour protocols are most commonly used.

Six-hour diuresis protocol: A study completed using normal dogs suggested that one dose of cisplatin could be administered safely at 70 mg/m^2 of body surface using a 6-hour diuresis protocol.[7] In that study, cisplatin was administered IV to six healthy dogs over a 20-minute period after 0.9% NaCl solution (saline) was administered IV for 4 hours at a rate of 18.3 ml/kg/hr. After cisplatin injection, saline diuresis was continued at the same rate for 2 hours. All dogs vomited within 8 hours after the drug was administered. Clinical status, weight gain, and food consumption remained normal throughout 27 days after the drug was administered. Nadirs in the daily neutrophil count were observed on days

Table 41-2 **Example of Fluid Therapy Needs for a 10-Kg Dog That Is 5% Dehydrated and Has Diarrhea**

Task	Calculation
Correct dehydration	• 5% (0.05) × 10 kg body weight = 0.5 kg of water needed to correct dehydration • 1,000 ml/kg of water × 0.5 kg = 500 ml of water needed to correct dehydration • 75% (0.75) × 500 ml = 375 ml of fluid should be administered to replace 75% dehydration
Meet daily needs	• 66 ml/kg (daily requirements) × 10 kg body weight = 660 ml needed on a daily basis • Increase this amount 1.5–3.0 times to induce a mild to moderate diuresis in renal failure patients, ensuring urine output exceeds 2 ml/kg/hr
Replace ongoing losses	• Estimated losses through diarrhea = 200 ml
Fluids needed (first 24 hr)	• 375 ml + 660 ml + 200 ml = 1,235 ml; increase fluid therapy judiciously to increase urine output, sustaining a mild to moderate diuresis

6 and 15. There were no significant gross or histologic abnormalities referable to cisplatin administration when the dogs were necropsied at the conclusion of the study.

To ensure that the 6-hour diuresis protocol was safe and effective in older, tumor-bearing dogs, cisplatin (70 mg/m^2 body surface area IV every 21 days) was given to 61 dogs with malignant neoplasia for a total of 185 doses in one (n = 9 dogs), two (n = 26 dogs), three (n = 4 dogs), four (n = 9 dogs), five (n = 2 dogs), or six (n = 11 dogs) treatments. The cisplatin was given over a 20-minute period after 0.9% NaCl solution was administered IV for 4 hours at a rate of 18.3 ml/kg/hr. After the cisplatin infusion, saline diuresis was continued at the same rate for 2 hours. Before each treatment with cisplatin, dogs were evaluated with at least a physical examination, complete blood count (CBC), blood urea nitrogen, and, in most cases, determination of serum creatinine and urine specific gravity. Four of the 61 dogs (6.6%) developed clinically evident renal disease after two (one dog), three (two dogs), and four (one dog) doses of cisplatin were administered. Three of the four dogs had disease of the urinary tract before beginning therapy. Survival time in dogs that developed renal disease (median: 145 days; range: 15–150 days) was similar to that of all of the dogs in this study (median: 154 days; range: 30–500 days); 13 dogs were still alive at the conclusion of the study. Three of the four dogs that developed renal disease were euthanatized because of tumor-related causes and chronic renal failure; the fourth dog died as a direct result of the nephrotoxicity. Therefore, the 6-hour saline diuresis protocol used to administer cisplatin in this study seems to be effective in preventing nephrotoxicity in tumor-bearing dogs without preexisting urinary tract disease.

Four-hour diuresis protocol: After the 6-hour diuresis protocol was determined to be safe and effective for administering cisplatin, a 4-hour diuresis protocol was designed.[10] In this study, cisplatin (70 mg/m^2 of body surface IV every 21 days) was given to 64 dogs that had malignant neoplasia for a total of 179 doses in one to four treatments. The cisplatin was given over a 20-minute period after 0.9% NaCl solution was administered IV for 3 hours at a rate of 25 ml/kg/hr. After cisplatin infusion, saline solution diuresis was continued at the same rate for 1 hour. Before each treatment with cisplatin, dogs were evaluated with at least a physical examination, CBC, and determination of serum phosphorus concentration and urine specific gravity. Exogenous creatinine clearance was evaluated in eight dogs. Five of the 64 dogs developed clinically evident renal disease after two and three doses of cisplatin were administered. Two of the five dogs had disease of the urinary tract before beginning treatment. Median survival time in dogs that developed renal disease was 114 days (range: 5–586 days). Thirty dogs were still alive at the conclusion of the study. Three of the five dogs that developed renal disease were alive at the conclusion of the study, the fourth dog died of the cancer, and the fifth dog died as a result of renal damage. The neutrophil counts decreased and creatinine concentrations increased before the third and fourth treatments compared with pretreatment values. It was concluded from this study that up to four doses of cisplatin can be safely administered using the 4-hour diuresis protocol with minimal nephrotoxicity. Because the 4-hour diuresis protocol was relatively safe, an additional study was initiated to determine whether a 1-hour diuresis protocol was safe. The 1-hour diuresis protocol was not very safe, so it is not recommended.

TREATMENT OF ACUTE RENAL FAILURE[12,13]

The initial goals for treating drug- and tumor-related acute renal failure in dogs are to discontinue all drugs that may be nephrotoxic, document prerenal or postrenal abnormalities, and initiate fluid therapy (Table 41-2). The primary objectives of fluid therapy are to:

• Collect urine for urinalysis and culture and sensitivity testing

Table 41-3 Support Measures for Patients in Renal Failure

General Principle	Specific Details
Stop nephrotoxins	Discontinue cisplatin, methotrexate, doxorubicin, aminoglycosides, NSAIDs; avoid anesthesia
Assess patient	• CBC, urinalysis, and biochemical profile • Urine culture and sensitivity • Specifically, determine: 　— Percentage of dehydration 　— Amount of ongoing losses (e.g., vomiting, diarrhea, blood loss) 　— Maintenance fluid requirements 　— Electrolyte and biochemical abnormalities 　— Cardiovascular performance 　— Urine output
Administer fluids	• Tailor therapy to needs of each patient: 　— Administer isotonic polyionic fluid initially. 　— Correct dehydration first over 6–8 hr to prevent further renal ischemia while watching carefully for pathologic oliguria and subsequent volume overload. 　— Meet maintenance requirements (approximately 66 ml/kg/day). 　— Meet ongoing losses (e.g., vomiting, diarrhea). 　— Induce a mild to moderate diuresis (>2 ml/kg/hr).
Monitor urine output	• Metabolism cage or indwelling catheter • For inadequate output (<0.5–2.0 ml/kg/hr): 　— Mannitol or dextrose 0.5–1.0 g/kg in a slow IV bolus 　— Furosemide 2–4 mg/kg IV q1–3h as needed 　— Dopamine 1–3 µg/kg/min IV (50 mg dopamine in 500 ml of 5% dextrose = 100 µg/ml solution)
Correct acid–base and electrolytes	Rule out hypercalcemia of malignancy; if identified, treat specifically.
Induce diuresis	Urine output: 2–5 ml/kg/hr; monitor body weight, heart and respiratory rate, and central venous pressure for signs of overhydration.
Consider peritoneal dialysis if not responsive	Temporary or chronic ambulatory peritoneal dialysis with specific dialysate solution may be helpful.
Initiate long-term plans	• Continue diuresis until blood urea nitrogen and creatinine normalize or until these values stop improving despite aggressive therapy and a clinically stable patient, then gradually taper fluids. • Control hyperphosphatemia, if indicated (e.g., aluminum hydroxide, 500 mg at each feeding). • Treat gastric hyperacidity, if indicated (cimetidine, 4 mg/kg IV or PO q6h).

- Correct deficits (such as dehydration) and excesses (such as volume overload) seen in oliguric renal failure
- Supply maintenance needs
- Supplement ongoing losses that occur with vomiting and diarrhea

Each patient must be assessed carefully, and a treatment plan must be tailored based on the hydration status, cardiovascular performance, and biochemical data. A general approach to patients in renal failure is shown in Table 41-3. Maintenance requirements vary from 44 to 110 ml/kg body weight; smaller animals generally require the larger amount because their metabolic rate per kilogram is higher than that of larger animals. A quick formula that can be used to

> **KEY POINT**
>
> *Maintenance requirements differ for each patient; however, a quick formula that can be used to approximate the fluid needs is 66 ml/kg/day plus an amount of fluid equal to external fluid losses, such as vomiting and diarrhea. Patients with renal failure require 1.5 to 3.0 times this amount to achieve diuresis.*

approximate the fluid needs for daily maintenance of an individual patient is 66 ml/kg/day plus an amount of fluid equal to external fluid losses, such as vomiting and diarrhea. In patients with renal failure, 1.5 to 3.0 times this amount of fluid is administered daily to achieve diuresis. The success of diuresis can be monitored by documenting adequate urine output (>2 ml/kg/hr).

Fluid therapy should meet daily needs, replace excessive losses, and correct dehydration. The percentage of dehydration should be determined; approximately 75% of the fluid needed to correct the dehydration should be administered during the first 24 hours. Fluid therapy should be altered to correct electrolyte and acid–base abnormalities. Potassium-containing fluids generally are not good choices for animals in acute renal failure because systemic hyperkalemia often occurs in these patients. Until more is known about the systemic effects of sepsis, lactate-containing fluids should be avoided because sepsis and cancer are associated with hyperlactatemia, which worsens with the administration of lactate-containing fluids.

> **KEY POINT**
>
> *The percentage of dehydration should be determined; approximately 75% of the fluid needed to correct the dehydration should be administered during the first 24 hours.*

If oliguric renal failure is present, a diligent and aggressive approach should be taken to increase urine output, starting with an effort to increase the GFR and renal blood flow. An osmotic diuresis can also be used. If urine output is less than 0.5 to 2.0 ml/kg/hr despite aggressive fluid therapy, furosemide should be administered every 1 to 3 hours. Furosemide increases the GFR and enhances diuresis in many patients. If furosemide is not effective, mannitol or 50% dextrose can be used as an osmotic diuretic to enhance urine production. The advantage of dextrose over mannitol is that it can be detected on a urine glucose test strip. If furosemide and osmotic diuretics are not effective, dopamine can be administered as a constant-rate infusion. Dopamine enhances renal blood flow and increases urine output secondarily.

Treatment of acute renal failure should be continued until the patient improves substantially and abnormal biochemical parameters have been corrected or are at least stable. The therapy should then be tapered off over several days, and a home treatment plan should be developed that includes avoiding nephrotoxic drugs; feeding a high-quality, low-quantity protein diet; maintaining a low-stress environment; and providing fresh, clean water ad libitum.

REFERENCES

1. Page R, Matus RE, Leifer CE, et al: Cisplatin, a new antineoplastic drug in veterinary medicine. *JAVMA* 186:288–290, 1985.
2. Mehlhaff CJ, Leifer CE, Patnaik AK, et al: Surgical treatment of pulmonary neoplasia in 15 dogs. *JAVMA* 20:799–803, 1984.
3. Himsel CA, Richardson RC, Craig JA: Cisplatin chemotherapy for metastatic squamous cell carcinoma in two dogs. *JAVMA* 89:1575–1578, 1986.
4. Shapiro W, Fossum TW, Kitchell BE, et al: Use of cisplatin for treatment of appendicular osteosarcoma in dogs. *JAVMA* 192:507–511, 1988.
5. LaRue SM, Withrow SJ, Powers BE, et al: Limb-sparing treatment for osteosarcoma in dogs. *JAVMA* 195:1734–1744, 1989.
6. Cvitkovic E, Spaulding J, Bethune V, et al: Improvement of *cis*-dichlorodiammineplatinum (NSC 119875): Therapeutic index in an animal model. *Cancer* 39:1357–1361, 1977.
7. Ogilvie GK, Krawiec DR, Gelberg HB, et al: Evaluation of a short-term saline diuresis protocol for the administration of cisplatin. *Am J Vet Res* 49:1076–1078, 1988.
8. Rassnick KM, Frimberger AE, Wood CA, et al: Evaluation of ifosfamide for treatment of various canine neoplasms. *J Vet Intern Med* 14(3):271–276, 2000.
9. Cotter SM, Kanki PJ, Simon M: Renal disease in five tumor-bearing cats treated with adriamycin. *JAAHA* 21:405–412, 1985.
10. Ogilvie GK, Straw RC, Jameson VJ, et al: Prevalence of nephrotoxicosis associated with a four-hour saline solution diuresis protocol for the administration of cisplatin to dogs with sarcomas: 64 cases (1989–1991). *JAVMA* 202:1845–1848, 1993.
11. Ogilvie GK, Fettman MJ, Jameson VJ, et al: Evaluation of a one-hour saline diuresis protocol for the administration of cisplatin to dogs. *Am J Vet Res* 53:1666–1669, 1992.
12. Couto CG: Management of complications of cancer chemotherapy. *Vet Clin North Am Small Anim Pract* 21:1037–1053, 1990.
13. Mohammed SI, Craig BA, Mutsaers AJ, et al: Effects of the cyclooxygenase inhibitor, piroxicam, in combination with chemotherapy on tumor response, apoptosis, and angiogenesis in a canine model of human invasive urinary bladder cancer. *Mol Cancer Ther* 2(2):183–188, 2003.

ACUTE TUMOR LYSIS SYNDROME

Gregory K. Ogilvie and Antony S. Moore

CLINICAL BRIEFING

History	• Uncommon condition. • Acute decompensation, anorexia, and collapse within days after chemotherapy for chemoresponsive tumor.
Clinical signs	• Pale mucous membranes. • Decreased capillary refill time. • Evidence of decreased cardiac output (hypodynamic shock) with or without arrhythmias. • Vomiting and diarrhea. • Evidence of lysis of tumor.
Diagnostics	• Complete blood count (CBC), biochemical profile, urinalysis, and thoracic radiography may reveal evidence of multiorgan failure, metabolic acidosis, azotemia, and, in a few cases, hypocalcemia, hyperkalemia, and hyperphosphatemia. • Hyperkalemia and hyperphosphatemia may have corrected if several hours have passed.
Therapy	• Prevention is essential with adequate hydration. • This condition is rare and should not be used as a reason to delay or reduce therapy unless azotemia is identified. • Restore tissue perfusion with fluids and stabilize the cardiovascular system. • Correct acid–base and electrolyte imbalances and azotemia. • Withhold additional chemotherapy pending patient recovery.

Acute tumor lysis syndrome (ATLS; Figure 42-1) is an underreported, rare condition of acute collapse that may lead to death soon after administration of a chemotherapeutic agent or radiation therapy for a chemotherapy- or radiation-sensitive tumor.[1-3] ATLS most often occurs shortly after the treatment of lymphoma and lymphoid leukemia and may occur after effective chemotherapy in dogs with rapidly growing, bulky, chemosensitive tumors.[4,5] Affected dogs present to the veterinary health

KEY POINT
Dogs with ATLS often present with a history of acute decompensation, sometimes to the point of imminent death (within hours of presentation).[1-3]

care team with a history of acute decompensation over a short period, sometimes to the point of imminent death. Rapid diagnosis and therapy are essential to reduce mortality.

Predisposing Factors

The actual pathophysiology of ATLS in dogs is unstudied and therefore unknown. In humans, and probably in dogs, rapid tumor lysis may cause an acute release of intracellular phosphate and potassium.[1-5] This release of electrolytes causes hypocalcemia, hyperkalemia, and hyperphosphatemia. In human patients with ATLS, hyperuricemia is also seen.[1-3] As noted earlier, ATLS is most common in lymphoma or leukemia patients; in human patients, this may be partly because the intracellular concentration of phosphorus in human lymphoma and leukemia cells is four to six times higher than in normal cells.[1] Unpublished clinical experience suggests that ATLS is most common in dogs with some degree of volume contraction and a large tumor mass that responds rapidly to cytolytic therapy. In addition, dogs that have sepsis or extensive neoplastic disease that infiltrates the parenchyma of organs are predisposed to ATLS. Canine patients at highest risk have volume contraction with stage IV or V lymphoma, are treated with chemotherapy or radiation therapy,

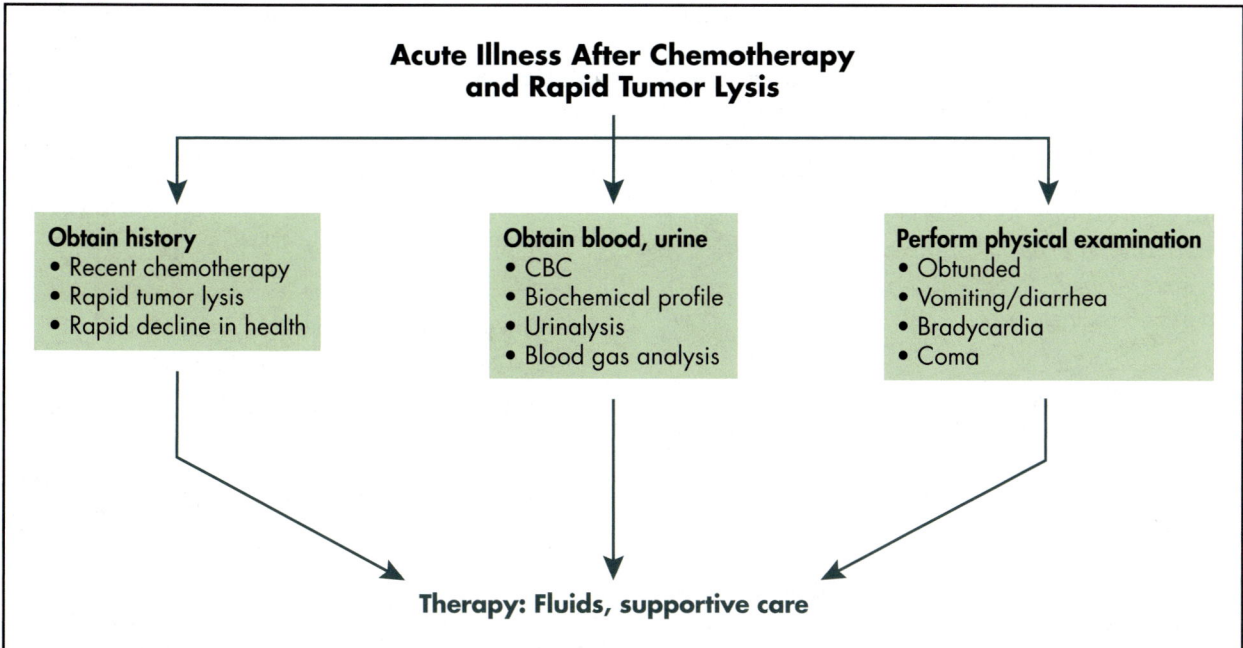

Figure 42-1. Clinical approach to ATLS.

Table 42-1 **Therapy for the Dog with ATLS**

Problem	Approach	
Acute decompensation (hours to days after therapy for a chemoresponsive tumor)	Evaluate the dog.	Determine whether the tumor has responded rapidly and dramatically. Perform complete physical examination to evaluate for systemic disease, cardiac output, and other parameters. Determine the presence or absence of neutropenia, sepsis, coagulopathies, and organ failure with CBC, biochemical profile, urinalysis, blood cultures, and other tests.
Initiate specific support	Treat for shock, provide daily fluid needs, correct dehydration, correct electrolyte abnormalities, and compensate for external fluid losses.	Consider non–lactate-containing fluids. In ATLS, 0.9% NaCl may be ideal until hyperkalemia and hyperphosphatemia are corrected. Fluids can be administered during acute shock or shock-like states at a rate of 40–60 ml/kg/hr for the first hour, followed by 10–12 ml/kg/hr with very close monitoring to adjust fluid rate as needed. If hypocalcemia secondary to hyperphosphatemia causes significant clinical signs (rare), exogenous parenteral calcium supplementation may be indicated.
Monitor dog	Monitor hydration, electrolytes, and renal and cardiovascular function.	Rate of fluid administration must be "fine-tuned" based on ongoing reevaluation of hydration, cardiovascular, renal, and electrolyte status.
Delay additional chemotherapy pending patient recovery	Monitor for patient recovery.	Resume chemotherapy after patient recovery.

and undergo very rapid remission; therefore, ATLS may be identified within 48 hours after the first treatment.

Diagnosis

Dogs with ATLS present with clinical signs similar to those seen in neutropenic, septic dogs and are often diagnosed after acute collapse and decompensation hours to days after the administration of chemotherapy.[4,5] To reduce morbidity and mortality, rapid diagnosis of and therapy for ATLS are essential. Dogs with ATLS may show cardiovascular collapse, pale mucous membranes, slow capillary refill time, vomiting, diarrhea, and ensuing shock. The hyperkalemia may result in bradycardia with diminished P-wave amplitude and spiked T waves on an electrocardiogram. Biochemical analysis of blood may confirm the presence of hypocalcemia, hyperkalemia, and hyperphosphatemia. However, if several hours

> **KEY POINT**
> *Rapid tumor lysis causes an acute release of intracellular phosphate and potassium, resulting in clinical signs associated with hypocalcemia, hyperkalemia, and hyperphosphatemia.*

have passed after decompensation, hyperkalemia and hyperphosphatemia may have corrected. Hyperuricemia has not been identified in dogs. In the presence of elevated serum phosphate levels, hypocalcemia develops as a result of calcium and phosphate precipitation. Without effective treatment, cardiovascular collapse, shock, or renal failure may occur; therefore, the blood urea nitrogen and creatinine concentrations should be monitored closely.

> **KEY POINT**
> *The metabolic disturbances associated with ATLS can lead to life-threatening complications, including arrhythmias and acute renal failure.*

Treatment

The best treatment is prevention. Because the kidneys are the main source of electrolyte excretion, metabolic abnormalities may be exacerbated in dogs with renal dysfunction. Identification and correction of any volume depletion or azotemia before initiation of therapy may reduce the risk of ATLS; chemotherapy should be delayed until metabolic disturbances, such as azotemia, are corrected.

If ATLS is identified, the patient should be treated with aggressive crystalloid fluid therapy (Table 42-1) and careful monitoring of electrolytes and renal parameters. The following general steps should be taken[1-5]:

- Establish central venous access.
- Obtain pretreatment blood and urine samples.
- Assess electrocardiogram continually.
- Start fluid therapy. Consider non–lactate-containing fluids and isotonic or hypotonic saline.
- Conduct serial laboratory evaluations to assess changes in electrolytes (serial lactate, Na^+, K^+, creatinine, blood urea nitrogen, phosphorus, Ca^+).
- Monitor urine output.
- Initiate hemodialysis if recovery is not rapid. Further chemotherapy should be withheld until the patient is clinically normal and all biochemical parameters have stabilized.

REFERENCES

1. Marcus SL, Einzig AI: Acute tumor lysis syndrome: Prevention and management, in Dutcher JP, Wiernik PH (eds): *Handbook of Hematologic and Oncologic Emergencies.* New York, Plenum Press, 1987, pp 9–15.
2. Woodlock TJ: Oncologic emergencies, in Rosenthal S, Carignan JR, Smith BD (eds): *Medical Care of the Cancer Patient,* ed 2. Philadelphia, WB Saunders, 1993, pp 236–246.
3. Couto CG: Management of complications of cancer chemotherapy. *Vet Clin North Am Small Anim Pract* 4:1037–1053, 1990.
4. Page RL: Acute tumor lysis syndrome. *Semin Vet Med Surg (Small Anim)* 1(1):58–60, 1986.
5. Piek CJ, Teske E: [Tumor lysis syndrome in a dog.] *Tijdschr Diergeneeskd* 121(3):64–66, 1996.

DISSEMINATED INTRAVASCULAR COAGULATION

Gregory K. Ogilvie and Antony S. Moore

CLINICAL BRIEFING

History	• Acute decompensation, anorexia, collapse, and inappropriate bleeding from any site.
Clinical signs	• Pale mucous membranes. • Decreased capillary refill time. • Evidence of decreased cardiac output due to blood loss or thrombosis. • Bleeding from any part of the body, including venipuncture sites. • Dyspnea from blood loss or pulmonary thrombosis.
Diagnostics	• Complete blood count, with platelet count, biochemical profile, urinalysis, blood gas analysis, and coagulation screening tests (PT, APTT, FDPs, ACT, fibrinogen, D-dimer, AT-III) may reveal evidence of blood loss, multiorgan failure, coagulopathies, or metabolic acidosis.
Therapy	• Treat the underlying cause. • Restore tissue perfusion with fluids. • Stabilize the cardiovascular system. • Correct acid–base and electrolyte imbalances. • Administer blood component therapy, including plasma for clotting factors. • Heparin therapy may be of value if thrombosis predominates. • Discontinue chemotherapy, including prednisone, pending patient recovery.

Disorders of hemostasis are an underreported and underrecognized cause of morbidity and mortality in canine and human cancer patients.[1-10] In one study,[3] the incidence of disseminated intravascular coagulation (DIC) in 208 dogs with a malignant tumor was 9.6%. In that same study, in 164 dogs with a malignant solid tumor, the incidence of DIC was 12.2%. The incidence of DIC in dogs with hemangiosarcoma, mammary gland carcinoma, or adenocarcinoma of the lung was significantly higher than that in dogs with other malignant tumors. These results suggest that special care should be taken to look for DIC in dogs with a malignant solid tumor.

The etiology of DIC is not as clearly defined in dogs as in humans. Until more is known, it may be helpful to characterize hemostatic disorders as follows[1-4]:

1. DIC
2. Malignancy-associated fibrinolysis
3. Platelet abnormalities
4. Clinical syndrome of the hypercoagulable state of malignancy
5. Chemotherapy-associated (e.g., L-asparaginase) thromboembolism

DIC, which has been associated with all the listed disorders, is a consumptive coagulopathy that often results in a life-threatening condition. It occurs with many malignancies when clotting factors are activated by tumor-induced procoagulants or when the tumor directly or indirectly stimulates platelet aggregation. The resultant formation of clots in the circulation consumes clotting factors and platelets, which leads to widespread bleeding. In addition, deposition of fibrin throughout the body may result in concurrent microangiopathic hemolytic anemia. To reduce morbidity and mortality, DIC must be identified and treated early.

Predisposing Factors

DIC occurs with a wide variety of malignant conditions, including hemangiosarcoma, lymphoma, and mammary adenocarcinoma. It may also be induced or exacerbated by concurrent infection, treatment with chemotherapeutic agents, or surgery. Renal failure and loss of low molecular

Table 43-1 **Clinical and Laboratory Parameters Used to Diagnose DIC**

Tests/Observations	Acute DIC	Chronic DIC
Clinical signs	Clinically evident coagulopathies	Few clinical signs evident
Onset and duration	Rapid onset and quick progression	Insidious and prolonged
PT, APTT, and ACT	Prolonged	Normal to slightly decreased
Platelets	Decreased	Often normal
FDPs	Very high	High
Fibrinogen	Decreased to normal	Normal
AT-III	Reduced	Normal
Prognosis	Grave	Good

weight coagulation factors through glomeruli may increase the risk of coagulation abnormalities. Thrombosis with or without DIC has been identified in dogs with hyperadrenocorticism and in dogs that have been treated with high doses of glucocorticoids. The syndrome of corticosteroid-induced thrombosis is more commonly recognized in dogs than in cats. Other predisposing factors include[1-4]:

- Extrinsic vascular compression or tumor invasion
- Tissue necrosis
- Production of procoagulants by the cancer
- Activation of platelets and increased accumulation of platelets around the cancer
- Inflammation induction of factor VIII, fibrinogen, and von Willebrand's factor
- Deficiencies in endogenous anticoagulants
- Presence of IV catheters
- Damage to endothelial cells by chemotherapeutic agents
- Doxorubicin-induced heart failure
- Immobility due to lethargy, anorexia, anemia

Diagnosis

Clinical signs that support a diagnosis of DIC include oozing from venipuncture sites, nosebleeds, oral bleeding, melena, ecchymoses and petechial hemorrhages anywhere on the body, and hematuria.[1-4,5-7] Widespread thrombosis can cause multiorgan failure that may result in a variety of clinical signs, such as acute renal failure and acute onset of respiratory distress.

Laboratory abnormalities associated with DIC vary depending on the organs involved and whether the DIC is acute or chronic (Table 43-1); the chronic form of DIC is rarely associated with clinical signs. In addition, alterations in red blood cell morphology, such as fragmentation, may result from microangiopathic events that occur in this syndrome.

There are many causes of the decreased platelet count and coagulation factor deficiencies seen with DIC (Figures 43-1 and 43-2).[1-4,5-7] Decreased platelet count can be caused by bone marrow failure, increased platelet consumption, or splenic pooling of platelets. Prolonged prothrombin time (PT) may result from lack of clotting factor I (fibrinogen), II (prothrombin), V, VII, or X. Increased activated partial thromboplastin time (APTT) may be caused by a deficiency in clotting factor I, II, V, VIII, IX, X, XI, or XII. Heparin and oral anticoagulant therapy also prolong the APTT. Low fibrinogen levels are associated with decreased production or increased consumption of fibrinogen.

A diagnosis of DIC is based on clinical findings and laboratory parameters (Table 43-1), including[1-4,5-7]:

- Decreased packed cell volume (<37%) that may be evident within a few hours
- Hypoproteinemia (<5.5 g/dL) with external blood loss
- Prolonged buccal mucosal bleeding time (>4 min), as seen in thrombopathies and von Willebrand's disease
- Reduced von Willebrand's factor (<65%), as seen in von Willebrand's disease
- Increased PT (>16 sec), as seen with extrinsic and common coagulopathies
- Increased APTT (>16 sec), as seen with intrinsic and common coagulopathies
- Thrombocytopenia (<8–15 platelets per high-power field or <150,000/μl)
- Prolonged activated coagulation time (ACT) (>110 sec), as seen with intrinsic and common coagulopathies
- Decreased antithrombin III (AT-III) concentrations (<90%), as seen with thrombosis

KEY POINT

Clinical signs that support a diagnosis of DIC include oozing from venipuncture sites, nosebleeds, oral bleeding, melena, ecchymoses and petechial hemorrhages anywhere on the body, and hematuria.

DISSEMINATED INTRAVASCULAR COAGULATION

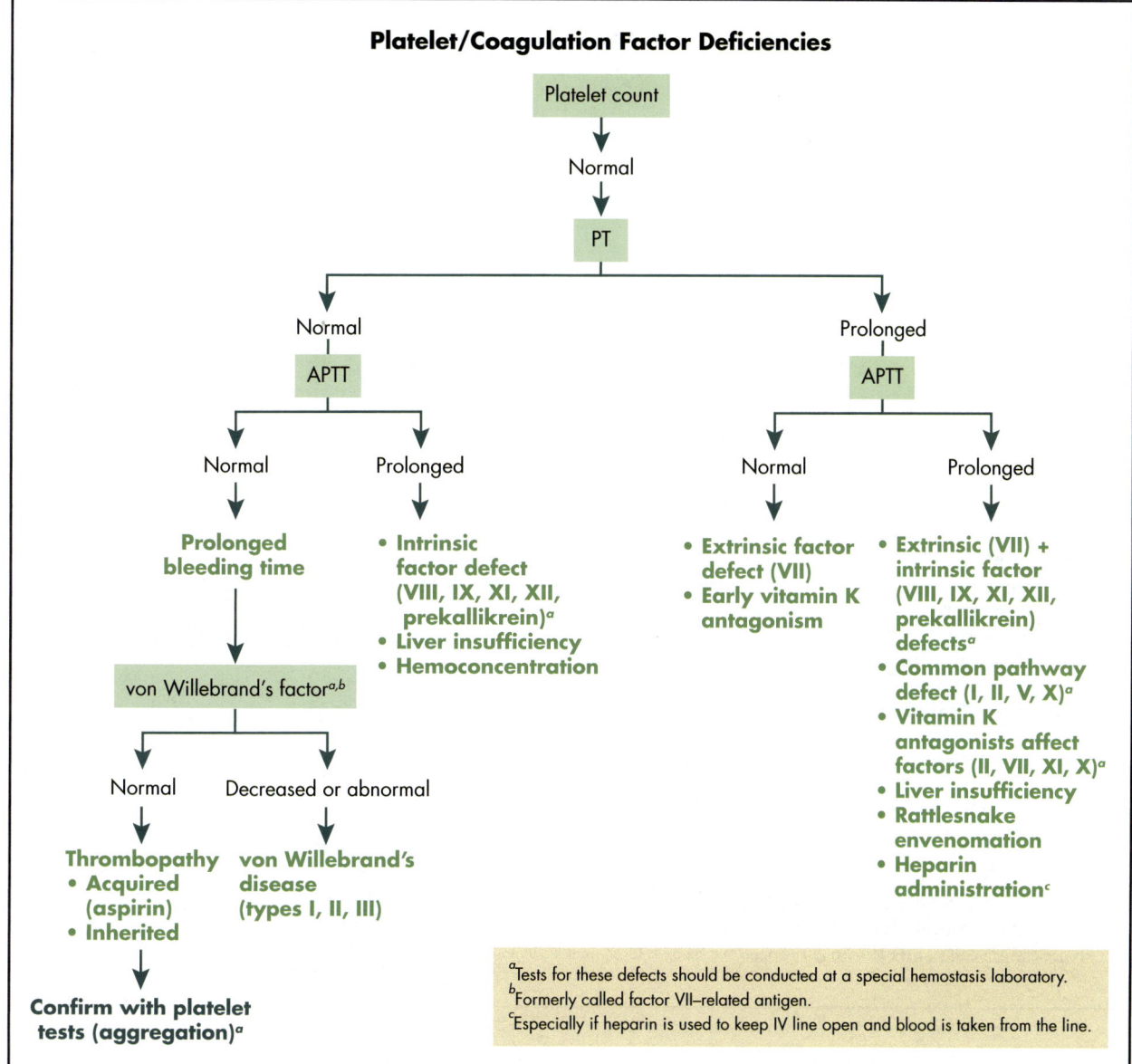

Figure 43-1. Suggested diagnostics and associated diagnoses for dogs with hemostatic disorders and normal platelet counts.

- Hypofibrinogenemia <100 mg/dl
- Increased fibrin degradation products (FDPs) (>1:5), as seen with fibrin degradation
- D-dimers >250 µg/dl, as seen with fibrin degradation

One of the consequences of DIC is deep venous thrombosis. Diagnosis of thromboses often relies on one or more of the following[1–4,5–7]:

- Contrast venography
- Sodium iodide I 125 fibrinogen scan
- Technetium Tc 99m apcitide scintigraphy
- Contrast ultrasonography
- Lung scintigraphy
- Duplex ultrasonography
- Magnetic resonance venography
- Helical computed tomography
- D-dimer levels, although these are less sensitive for cancer

Treatment[1–4]

Dogs with DIC often do not exhibit clinical signs until late in the course of the disease. Therefore, treatment must begin as soon as possible. Specific treatment for DIC is con-

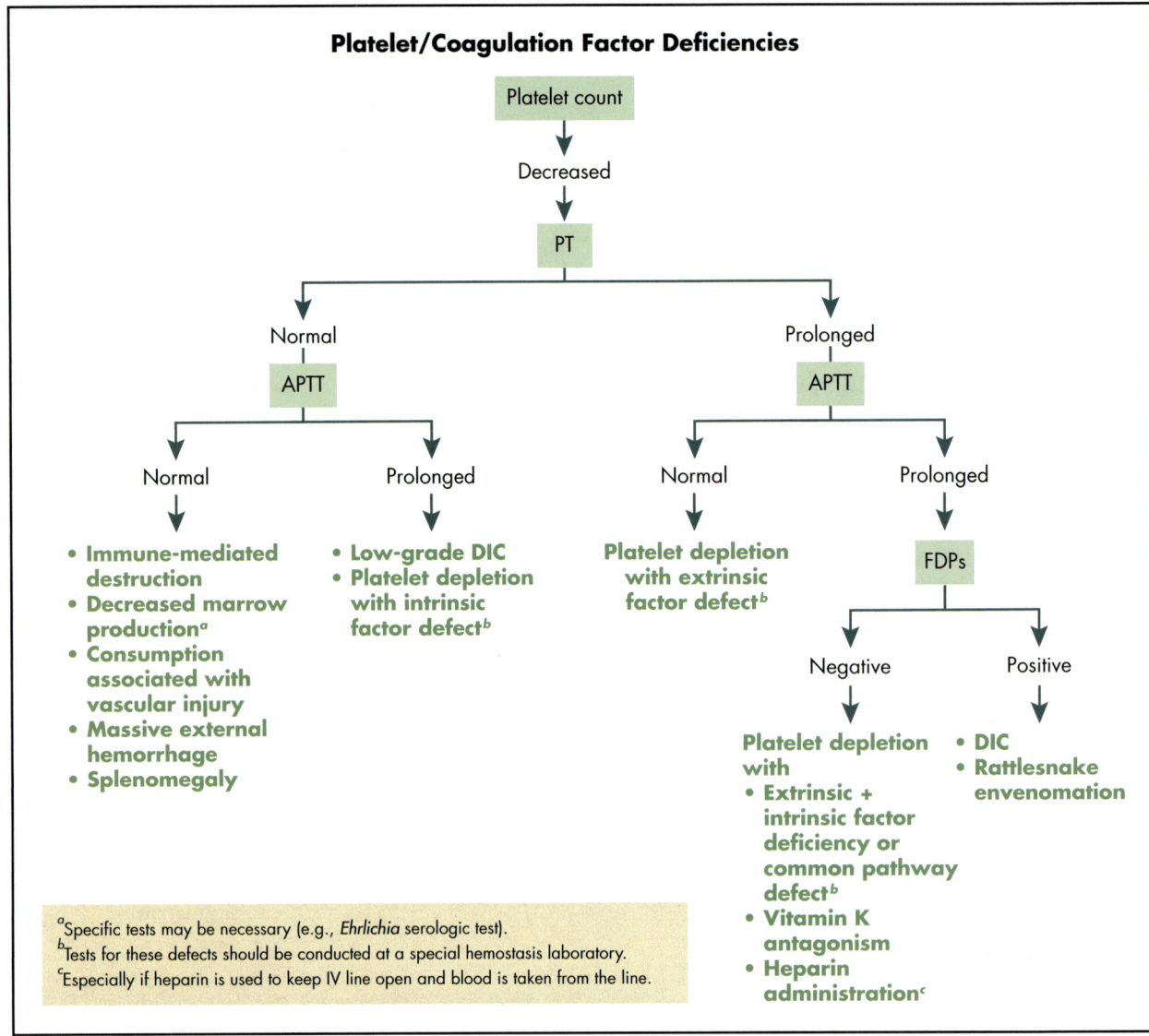

Figure 43-2. Suggested diagnostic plan for dogs with hemostatic disorders and low platelet counts.

troversial, but certain procedures are uniformly accepted despite the fact that few data document their efficacy. Treatment revolves around the following:

- **Elimination of the underlying cause:** The most important therapy for DIC is treatment of the underlying cause.
- **Fluids:** Fluid therapy is essential to correct volume contraction and to reduce the possibility of ensuing renal failure and acid–base abnormalities (Figure 43-2). Fluid administration, body weight, and urine output must be carefully monitored in all dogs. Increases in body weight, heart and respiratory rates, and central venous pressure may suggest volume overload. Volume overload is especially threatening in dogs that are anuric secondary to acute renal shutdown.

- **Transfusion support:** In dogs with severe bleeding diatheses, fresh blood or plasma with clotting factors and platelets may be useful in replacing components of the blood that are consumed.
- **Heparin therapy:** If thrombosis appears to be the most clinically evident problem, heparin therapy may reduce the formation of thrombi. The amount of heparin to be used is controversial. Methods include intermittent SC or IV administration and constant-rate infusion to prolong the APTT to 1.5 to 2 times its normal value. Mini-dose heparin therapy may be helpful in some cases. The following treatment protocols are used; however, data on efficacy are limited:

—Mini dose: 5 to 10 IU/kg SC q8h

- —Low dose: 50 to 100 IU/kg SC q8h
- —Intermediate dose: 300 to 500 IU/kg SC or IV q8h
- —High dose: 750 to 1,000 IU/kg SC or IV q8h
- **Discontinuation of therapy:** Chemotherapeutic agents, including prednisone, should be withheld until all evidence of DIC is eliminated and the patient has recovered completely. Dogs that receive glucocorticoid therapy are at major risk for thromboembolic events that can initiate or perpetuate DIC.

> **KEY POINT**
>
> *Treatment of the underlying cause and fluid therapy are two of the most effective and important treatments of DIC.*

Dogs with acute DIC have a poor prognosis; therefore, identification of patients at high risk and initiation of prophylactic treatment are of great value. Routine monitoring of ACT and platelet counts can identify dogs in the early phases of DIC.

REFERENCES

1. Ogilvie GK: Acute tumor lysis syndrome, in Wingfield WE. *Veterinary Emergency Medicine Secrets*. Hanley and Belfus, Philadelphia, 2001, pp 242–243.
2. Smith MR: Disorders of hemostasis and transfusion therapy, in Skeel RT (ed): *Handbook of Cancer Chemotherapy*, ed 3. Boston, Little, Brown & Co, 1991, pp 449–459.
3. Maruyama H, Miura T, Sakai M, et al: The incidence of disseminated intravascular coagulation in dogs with malignant tumor. *J Vet Med Sci* 66(5):573–575, 2004.
4. Woodlock TJ: Oncologic emergencies, in Rosenthal S, Carignan JR, Smith BD (eds): *Medical Care of the Cancer Patient*, ed 2. Philadelphia, WB Saunders, 1993, pp 236–246.
5. Hackner SG: Approach to the diagnosis of bleeding disorders. *Compend Contin Educ Pract Vet* 17:331–349, 1995.
6. Bateman SW, Mathews KA, Abrams-Ogg AC, et al: Diagnosis of disseminated intravascular coagulation in dogs admitted to an intensive care unit. *JAVMA* 215(6):798–804, 1999.
7. Nelson OL, Andreasen C: The utility of plasma D-dimer to identify thromboembolic disease in dogs. *J Vet Intern Med* 17(6):830–834, 2003.
8. Golden DL, Langston VC: Use of vincristine and vinblastine in dogs. *JAVMA* 193:1114–1117, 1988.
9. Slappendel RJ: Disseminated intravascular coagulation. *Vet Clin North Am Small Anim Pract* 18:169–184, 1988.
10. Couto CG: Disseminated intravascular coagulation in dogs. *Vet Med* 94:547–554, 1999.

CANCER-RELATED DISORDERS OF THE CENTRAL NERVOUS SYSTEM

Gregory K. Ogilvie and Antony S. Moore

Cancer- and cancer therapy–related disorders of the brain, spinal cord, and peripheral nerves are being recognized more and more often in veterinary medicine. Many causes of these disorders affect the central and peripheral nervous systems simultaneously, although they may be most often recognized as affecting the brain, spinal cord, or peripheral nerves. The ultimate therapeutic goals are to eliminate the underlying cause and to mitigate the clinical signs, which can range from very subtle weakness to overt seizures or paralysis.

▶ DISORDERS OF THE BRAIN

CLINICAL BRIEFING

Brain Herniation

History	• Acute or chronic neurologic decompensation.
Clinical signs	• Altered mentation. • Progressive drowsiness. • Altered pupil size and function. • Altered respiration. • Extensor rigidity. • Disconjugate eye movements. • Arrhythmias.
Diagnostics	• CT, MRI, CSF analysis, and EEG.
Treatment	• Control respiration. • Decrease intracranial pressure with mannitol, glucocorticoids, and surgical decompression in rare cases. • Treat the underlying cause.

Seizures

History	• Seizure preceded by an aura and followed by a postictal period.
Clinical signs	• Characterized as partial, simple partial, complex partial, generalized, or generalized nonconvulsive.
Diagnostics	• Metabolic and traumatic causes should be eliminated immediately and other causes evaluated after recovery via CBC, biochemical analysis, urinalysis, radiography, fasting blood glucose, CSF analysis, and brain imaging.

CANCER-RELATED DISORDERS OF THE CENTRAL NERVOUS SYSTEM

The most common brain disorders include those that cause subtle neurologic clinical signs secondary to a paraneoplastic syndrome; life-threatening emergencies due to meningitis; brain tumors; bleeding secondary to drug-induced thrombocytopenia; and chemotherapy-induced neurotoxicity.[1-5] The paraneoplastic syndromes most commonly recognized in veterinary medicine as affecting the central nervous system (CNS) include hypercalcemia of malignancy (e.g., secondary to anal sac adenocarcinoma or lymphoma), hypoglycemia (e.g., secondary to insulinoma or carcinoma of the liver), hyperviscosity syndrome caused by hyperglobulinemia (e.g., secondary to multiple myeloma), and erythrocytosis (e.g., polycythemia). Other, less defined paraneoplastic syndromes that cause disorders of the CNS are also suspected in dogs. Radiation can cause late effects within the brain, especially when larger dosages are given over a short period of time, resulting in mental dullness, depression, and, on occasion, seizures and death. Chemotherapy-induced seizures in dogs are reported with 5-fluorouracil. Other drugs that have been shown to cause clinical signs of CNS disorders in humans and possibly in dogs include:

- L-Asparaginase (may cause seizures by inducing cerebrovascular events)
- Cisplatin (may cause cortical blindness, reversible encephalopathy syndrome, and ototoxicity)
- Cytosine arabinoside (may cause leukoencephalopathy)
- Ifosfamide (may cause encephalopathy)
- Methotrexate (rarely associated with leukoencephalopathy)
- Thalidomide (causes a profound somnolence that can last for hours or days after each dose)

Brain herniation and seizures are relatively common, life-threatening emergencies.

Brain Herniation
PREDISPOSING FACTORS

Brain herniation can be caused by a wide variety of primary or secondary malignancies of the brain or by intracerebral hemorrhage and intradural hematoma, brain abscess, or acute hydrocephalus. Primary lung tumors, hemangiosarcoma, and malignant melanoma are examples of tumors that metastasize to the brain. Regardless of the cause, diagnosis must be made swiftly and therapy initiated without hesitation to prevent irreparable neurologic damage or death.

CLINICAL SIGNS

Brain herniation is characterized by any CNS abnormality, including progressive drowsiness, small reactive pupils, periodic respirations (Cheyne-Stokes), and, in the most severe cases, bilateral extensor rigidity.[2,4] As the herniation evolves, hyperventilation, disconjugate eye movements, pupillary fixation, and abnormal motor postures can be noted. The "brain–heart syndrome" may be evident if the brain stem is

> **KEY POINT**
>
> *In the "brain–heart syndrome," the clinician may be distracted by the occurrence of bizarre arrhythmias that are caused by compression of the cardiac control center and centers of the brain that regulate autonomic control of the heart.*

compressed. This syndrome is associated with potentially fatal arrhythmias caused by a CNS disturbance.

DIAGNOSIS

The diagnosis and decision to treat are based primarily on the presence of relatively rapidly developing abnormal neurologic signs. Because the decision to withhold therapy may result in death or severe, irreversible neurologic abnormalities, treatment should be initiated immediately or concurrently with diagnostic methods such as computed tomography (CT), magnetic resonance imaging (MRI), nuclear scans, and, if available, electroencephalography (EEG). A cerebrospinal fluid (CSF) tap at the cisterna magna may cause or exacerbate brain herniation; therefore, this procedure should not be used if increased intracranial pressure is suspected.

TREATMENT

The goals are to prevent further herniation and to treat existing herniation and the underlying cause.[2,4] Intubation and control of respiration may be required when hyperventilation produces cerebral vasoconstriction, decreased blood volume, and decreased intracranial pressure. Mannitol (1–2 g/kg IV qid slowly) can reduce brain water content, reduce brain volume, and decrease intracranial pressure rapidly. Steroids (e.g., dexamethasone NaPO$_4$ [2 mg/kg IV once, followed by 0.25 mg/kg IV qid]) can be administered acutely but may take hours to have full effect. Hydrocortisone (10–50 mg/kg IV) given at the time of brain trauma may be beneficial.[2,4] In rare cases, surgical decompression may help. Once treatment is under way, plain and contrast CT or other imaging techniques may help identify the cause of decompensation.

Seizures
PREDISPOSING FACTORS

A variety of metastatic and nonmetastatic conditions can cause seizures in veterinary cancer patients. Vascular disorders, such as intracerebral hemorrhage, subdural hematomas, and thrombosis of the CNS vessels, may be associated with

Table 44-1 Emergency Procedures for Status Epilepticus[1-5]

General Principle	Specific Details
Evaluate the patient	• Brief history and physical examination. • Place indwelling catheter. • Acquire blood samples; determine glucose and calcium levels while therapy is initiated.
Stop the seizures	• Administer diazepam IV (2.5–15.0 mg). • For hypoglycemia, administer 0.5 g of dextrose as a 25% solution given IV over 5 min; for hypocalcemia, administer 1.0–1.5 ml/kg of 10% calcium gluconate solution; if necessary, repeat diazepam bolus every 10 min for three doses. • If diazepam is inadequate for seizure control, administer phenobarbital IV (see Table 44-2). • Monitor acid–base status, ability to ventilate, body temperature, electrolyte balance, and hydration status, and treat appropriately.
Monitor during recovery	Phenobarbital may be administered (0.5 mg/kg IM tid) to reduce seizures; monitor blood levels. When seizures are controlled and the patient is able to swallow, oral phenobarbital therapy should be continued.
Initiate definitive diagnostics	CBC, biochemical profile, fasting blood glucose and insulin measurement, CSF tap, CT or MRI of the brain (if indicated), and EEG (if available).

Table 44-2 Anticonvulsants Used in an Acute Situation to Treat Seizures[2,4,5]

Anticonvulsant	Recommended Dosage	Half-Life	General Indications	Precautions
Phenobarbital	5–16 mg/kg/day, divided bid or tid	40 hr	Long-term seizure control; grand mal and partial seizures; effective in delaying progressive activity (kindling)	Monitor for sedation, ataxia, polydipsia, and polyuria (usually abate over time)
Primidone	15–80 mg/kg/day, divided bid	Metabolized to phenobarbital, then 40 hr	Not as effective as phenobarbital for emergency therapy Grand mal and partial seizures, status epilepticus; effective in delaying progressive activity (kindling)	Expensive Monitor for sedation, ataxia, polydipsia, polyuria, and personality trait changes (usually abate over time); hepatotoxicity
Diazepam	5–15 mg tid	2–4 hr	Grand mal seizures and status epilepticus	Monitor for sedation

seizures. Hypoglycemia secondary to insulinoma or hepatic tumor may induce CNS abnormalities.[1,2,4,5] Several chemotherapeutic agents (e.g., 5-fluorouracil, cisplatin, mitoxantrone, vincristine), radiation therapy, and radiosensitizers are reported to cause seizures.[3,4]

CLINICAL PRESENTATION

Seizures may appear clinically as partial (focal or local), simple partial (symmetric and rarely associated with loss of consciousness), complex partial (alterations in consciousness plus complex behavior), generalized (involuntary, uncontrolled motor activity), and generalized nonconvulsive (loss of consciousness with lack of spontaneous motor activity and transient collapse).[1,2] There is generally an aura or period of behavioral change before each type of seizure, followed by ictus or the actual clinical seizure, and finally a postictal period that lasts for approximately 30 minutes, during which the animal exhibits abnormal behavior that may include weakness and blindness. If malignancy is associated with the condition, the seizures tend to get progressively worse because of the enlarging intracranial mass or because of progressive worsening of hypoglycemia in insulin-producing tumors.

DIAGNOSIS

The diagnosis generally is evident from the historical or physical findings. In an emergency situation (often associated with a dog in status epilepticus), a definitive diagnosis is made after the patient is stabilized. Imaging techniques that include skull radiography, CT, nuclear imaging, or MRI of the brain are usually used. If a neoplasm is suspected, a complete staging scheme must be initiated as soon as the animal is stable. This should include a complete history, complete physical and neurologic examinations, complete blood count (CBC), biochemical profile, urinalysis, thoracic and abdominal radiography, fasting (>24 hr) blood glucose and insulin levels, a CSF tap if the animal is not at risk for brain herniation, and an EEG, if available.

TREATMENT

Caution should be used when handling a patient during a seizure. General procedures are noted in Table 44-1; Table 44-2 lists anticonvulsants used in acute situations. If a seizure is in progress, IV diazepam should be administered. Respiration should be monitored, and, when necessary, intubation and ventilation should be considered. In these patients, phenobarbital can be given via a loading dose, followed by a maintenance dose. Phenobarbital therapy also may be valuable when a single seizure is expected to continue or if clusters of seizures occur within a short period.

▶ DISORDERS OF THE SPINAL CORD

CLINICAL BRIEFING

Spinal Cord Compression

History	• Acute upper or lower neurologic decompensation.
Clinical signs	• Back pain. • Root signature. • Weakness. • Muscle atrophy. • Conscious proprioceptive deficits. • Altered spinal reflexes. • Upper or lower motor neuron damage.
Diagnostics	• Myelogram, CT, MRI, CSF analysis, spinal decompression, and biopsy.
Treatment	• Corticosteroids. • Spinal decompression. • Treat the underlying cause with chemotherapy, surgery, or radiation therapy.

Like brain disorders, disorders of the spinal cord range from almost undetectable conditions to life-threatening emergencies. Causes include meningitis, tumor of the spinal cord, radiation- or chemotherapy-induced neurotoxicity, and drug-induced thrombocytopenia.[1-5] Many of the paraneoplastic syndromes that are commonly recognized as having an effect on the brain, including hypercalcemia of malignancy, hypoglycemia, and hyperviscosity syndrome secondary to hyperglobulinemia, can also affect the spinal cord. Radiation can cause late effects within the spinal cord, especially when larger dosages are given over a short period of time, resulting in paresis or, occasionally, paralysis. Spinal cord compression is an important, relatively common, life-threatening emergency.

Spinal Cord Compression
PREDISPOSING FACTORS

Many malignancy-induced spinal cord compressions in veterinary cancer patients are extradural.[3,6] With the increased use of CT and MRI, the antemortem diagnosis of intradural and extradural lesions is increasing.

DIAGNOSIS

Clinical signs include back pain, a root signature, paresis, or paralysis.[6] Significant spinal cord compression may occur before clinical signs are evident because of slow progression of the tumor and compensation of the nervous tissue. In some cases, such as with neurofibrosarcomas, lower motor neuron signs (e.g., muscle atrophy, weakness, lack of spinal reflexes) may precede clinical signs that are referable to the spinal cord.

The importance of early diagnosis cannot be overemphasized. When spinal cord compression is identified, immediate action must be taken to ensure that the underlying cause is specifically diagnosed and treated. Diagnosis is based on clinical findings, including back pain; spinal tenderness; a root signature; abnormal findings on MRI, CT, or contrast myelogram; and bone scans via scintigraphy. In many animals with spinal cord compression, a diagnosis can be made by performing a surgical spinal cord decompression and biopsy.

TREATMENT[3,4,6]

The optimal treatment of epidural spinal cord compression caused by metastatic disease is debated in human medicine. Corticosteroids (i.e., prednisone, 2 mg/kg SC bid initially) and radiotherapy are the mainstays of therapy for most patients that have solid tumors of the spinal cord. Steroids reduce spinal cord edema and may be beneficial when administered before and during radiation treatment. Surgical intervention is indicated if tissue diagnosis is required, if the cause of the spinal cord compression is uncertain, if relapse occurs in the area of prior irradiation, if spinal instability is present, or if radiation therapy and steroid treatment fail.

▶ DISORDERS OF THE PERIPHERAL NERVES

CLINICAL BRIEFING

Paraneoplastic Neurologic Syndromes

History	• Abnormalities referable to peripheral nerves, muscle, and neuromuscular junctions.
Clinical signs	• Often subtle in the early phases. • May include peripheral nervous system lower motor dysfunction. • Behavioral abnormalities, neurologic dysfunction, and seizures possible with CNS involvement.
Diagnostics	• CBC, biochemical profile, and evaluation of thyroid and adrenal function. • Imaging (e.g., CT, MRI, myelogram), CSF analysis (if indicated), electrodiagnostics, biopsy of nervous tissue, and response tests (e.g., with edrophonium chloride [Tensilon; ICN Pharmaceuticals, Costa Mesa, CA]) to diagnose specific CNS disease.
Treatment	• Treat the underlying cause. • Treat symptomatically for specific disease with glucocorticoids, mannitol, or surgical decompression, as indicated.

Cancer and cancer therapy may disrupt the function of the peripheral nerves. The results range from subtle neurologic clinical signs secondary to a paraneoplastic syndrome to life-threatening emergencies. As with the brain and the spinal cord, chemotherapy-induced neurotoxicity or tumor-related disruption in neurotransmission may be the cause.[1-5] Paraneoplastic syndromes that can disrupt the entire peripheral nervous system include hypercalcemia of malignancy, hypoglycemia, thymoma-induced myasthenia gravis, and hyperviscosity syndrome secondary to hyperglobulinemia. Radiation can cause late effects within the peripheral nervous system, especially when larger dosages are given over a short period of time, resulting in paresis or, occasionally, paralysis.

Rarely, cisplatin, vincristine, cytosine arabinoside, paclitaxel, procainamide, or thalidomide causes peripheral neuropathy.

In human and veterinary patients, the remote effects of cancer on the nervous system induce a wide variety of clinical signs.[1-9] Cancer-induced neuropathies in dogs include peripheral neuropathy, trigeminal nerve paralysis, and Horner's syndrome.[6-11] Dogs also exhibit neurologic signs secondary to endocrine, fluid, and electrolyte disturbances attributable to neoplasia, such as hypercalcemia, hyperviscosity syndrome, and hepatoencephalopathy. The neurologic syndromes of myasthenia gravis secondary to thymoma (e.g., megaesophagus, acetyl cholinesterase–responsive neuropathy) are well described in the literature.[6-11]

Table 44-3 Neurologic Syndromes Caused by Paraneoplastic Syndromes of the CNS[6-11]

Site Involved	Syndrome
Brain	• Cerebellar degeneration • Optic neuritis • Progressive multifocal leukoencephalopathy
Spinal cord	• Subacute necrotic myelopathy • Subacute motor neuropathy
Peripheral nerves	• Sensory neuropathy • Peripheral neuropathy • Autonomic gastrointestinal neuropathy
Muscle and neuromuscular junction	• Dermatomyositis and polymyositis • Myasthenic syndrome (Eaton-Lambert syndrome) • Myasthenia gravis

> **KEY POINT**
>
> *In human and veterinary patients, the remote effects of cancer on the nervous system induce a wide variety of clinical signs, including peripheral neuropathy, trigeminal nerve paralysis, Horner's syndrome, hepatoencephalopathy, and myasthenia gravis.*

Paraneoplastic Neurologic Syndromes

CLINICAL SIGNS

Virtually any change in normal nervous system functions can be a manifestation of a neurologic paraneoplastic syndrome, including behavioral changes, peripheral and spinal cord neuropathies, and alterations in the function of the cerebrum, cerebellum, medulla, and neuromuscular junction in humans and dogs. Some of these aberrations are noted in Table 44-3.

DIAGNOSIS

The diagnosis of a neurologic paraneoplastic syndrome involves eliminating nonneoplastic causes using CBC, a biochemical profile, urinalysis, tests of the thyroid and adrenal axes, brain or spinal cord imaging (CT, MRI, and contrast radiography), biopsy of the affected nerves, CSF tap, and (if indicated) electrodiagnostics.

TREATMENT

Elimination of the neoplastic condition may result in resolution of neurologic syndromes. Immune-mediated conditions of the CNS or peripheral nervous system may require the use of immunosuppressive therapy, including glucocorticoids.

REFERENCES

1. Fenner WR: Seizures, narcolepsy and cataplexy, in Birchard SJ, Sherding RG (eds): *Saunders Manual of Small Animal Practice.* Philadelphia, WB Saunders, 1993, pp 1147–1156.
2. Fenner WR: Diseases of the brain, in Birchard SJ, Sherding RG (eds): *Saunders Manual of Small Animal Practice.* Philadelphia, WB Saunders, 1993, pp 1126–1146.
3. Couto CG: Management of complications of cancer chemotherapy. *Vet Clin North Am Small Animal Practice* 4: 1037–1053, 1990.
4. Woodlock TJ: Oncologic emergencies, in Rosenthal S, Carignan JR, Smith BD (eds): *Medical Care of the Cancer Patient,* ed 2. Philadelphia, WB Saunders, 1993, pp 236–246.
5. Bunch SE: Anticonvulsant drug therapy in companion animals, in Kirk RW (ed): *Current Veterinary Therapy IX, Small Animal Practice.* Philadelphia, WB Saunders, 1986, pp 836–844.
6. Luttgen PJ: Spinal cord disorders, in Birchard SJ, Sherding RG (eds): *Saunders Manual of Small Animal Practice.* Philadelphia, WB Saunders, 1993, pp 1157–1164.
7. Shahar R, Rosseau C, Steiss J: Peripheral polyneuropathy in a dog with functional islet B-cell tumor and widespread metastases. *JAVMA* 187:175–177, 1985.
8. Bergman PJ, Bruyette DS, Coyne BE et al: Canine clinical peripheral neuropathy associated with pancreatic cell carcinoma. *Prog Vet Neurol* 5:57–62, 1994.
9. Duncan ID: Peripheral neuropathy in the dog and cat. *Prog Vet Neurol* 2:111–121, 1990.
10. Braund KG, McGuire JA, Henderson RA: Peripheral neuropathy associated with malignant neoplasms in dogs. *Vet Pathol* 24:16–24, 1987.
11. Braund KG: Remote effects of cancer on the nervous system. *Semin Vet Med Surg (Small Anim)* 5:262–273, 1990.

CANCER CACHEXIA AS A MANIFESTATION OF MALIGNANCY

Gregory K. Ogilvie and Antony S. Moore

CLINICAL BRIEFING

History	• Decreased quality of life followed by weight loss in the face of adequate nutritional intake.
Clinical signs	• Anorexia, lethargy, increased toxicoses in response to radiation therapy, surgery, and chemotherapy. • Decreased response to therapy. • Weight loss despite adequate energy intake is a late result.
Diagnostics	• Hypoalbuminemia. • Elevated serum lactate and insulin concentrations; abnormal amino acid and lipid profiles.
Therapy	• Eliminate underlying cause by surgery, chemotherapy, and radiation therapy. • Feed complex carbohydrates and high-quality proteins; moderate amounts of fats, possibly enriched with omega-3 fatty acids. • Encourage oral feeding (when possible). • Use nasogastric, gastrostomy, or jejunostomy feeding (when necessary). • Parenteral support should be used if enteral feeding fails.

Cancer cachexia is a syndrome that affects many cancer patients. If not treated, it results in involuntary weight loss even when caloric intake is adequate.[1-4] As with all other paraneoplastic syndromes, this condition is a remote effect of cancer. Cancer cachexia has been shown to result in dramatic alterations in carbohydrate, lipid, and protein metabolism before clinical evidence of cachexia is detectable.[1-16] This syndrome is encountered by every practitioner who treats dogs with cancer but is often suspected only in patients with unexpected weight loss.

> **KEY POINT**
>
> *Dramatic alterations in carbohydrate, lipid, and protein metabolism are documented in cancer patients even before clinical evidence of cachexia is noted; these alterations fail to resolve after remission is achieved with surgery or chemotherapy.*

Dogs with cancer do not commonly have weight loss,[12] although many have dramatic alterations in metabolism regardless of the type, size, or stage of the cancer.[1-16] These effects impair quality of life, response to therapy, and overall survival. The actual cause of cancer cachexia is the subject of a great deal of research. A detailed description of this paraneoplastic syndrome and its treatment are provided in Chapter 31.

Mechanism

The mechanisms of cancer cachexia are complex and include[1-15]:

- Starvation and malnutrition
- Impaired oral intake
- Stomatitis, taste aversions, zinc deficiency
- Dehydration
- Nausea
- Constipation
- Bowel obstruction
- Pain
- Impaired gastrointestinal absorption
- Maldigestion
- Exocrine pancreatic insufficiency
- Diarrhea
- Development of ascites, pleural effusion
- Infections
- Heart, lung, kidney failure

- Prolonged deconditioning
- Growth hormone deficiency

In addition to these items, profound alterations in carbohydrate metabolism are seen in dogs and humans with cancer cachexia.[1-15] In dogs, elevated serum insulin and lactate concentrations associated with lymphoma and other malignancies rise higher still, compared with those in control dogs, in response to glucose-tolerance tests.[7] Increased lactate and insulin levels in dogs with cancer do not normalize even when complete remission is obtained after doxorubicin

> **KEY POINT**
> *The metabolic alterations associated with cancer cachexia begin long before any weight loss is seen and have negative and profound effects on the patient's quality of life.*

chemotherapy or surgery.[5] Dogs with lymphoma have even higher lactate and insulin levels on reevaluation after relapse and show signs of cachexia.[5] Additional studies suggest that dogs with lymphoma may have a postreceptor defect, indicating that dietary therapy may be effective in combating the problem. Hyperlactatemia becomes more pronounced on administration of lactate-containing parenteral fluids (e.g., lactated Ringer's solution) to dogs with lymphoma compared with control dogs.[6]

Dogs and humans with cancer show alterations in protein and lipid metabolism that remain after chemotherapy or surgery achieves remission.[4] Specifically, dogs with lymphoma have significant reductions in threonine, glutamine, glycine, valine, cystine, and arginine. In contrast, their isoleucine and phenylalanine levels are significantly increased.[1] Dogs and humans with cancer often have increased protein catabolism. Tumors produce proteolysis-inducing factor.

> **KEY POINT**
> *Dogs and humans with cancer show alterations in protein and lipid metabolism that remain after chemotherapy or surgery achieves remission, including significant reductions in threonine, glutamine, glycine, valine, cystine, and arginine.*

Dogs with untreated lymphoma have significantly higher free fatty acid, total triglyceride, and very low-density lipoprotein and triglyceride serum concentrations compared with untreated control dogs.[1-13] High-density lipoprotein cholesterol levels in dogs with lymphoma are significantly lower than those in control dogs. After doxorubicin treatment, dogs with lymphoma develop significantly elevated total cholesterol levels, as is noted in humans with cancer.

Indirect calorimetry has been used in clinical cancer patients to quantify nutritional and water requirements.[9-11] It demonstrates that energy expenditure and caloric needs in

> **KEY POINT**
> *Alterations in carbohydrate, protein, and lipid metabolism persist after the cancer is eliminated, suggesting that therapy is important before, during, and after the time of definitive cancer therapy.*

dogs with lymphoma and other malignancies are equal to or lower than those in normal dogs.[9,10] Furthermore, it demonstrates that major or minor surgery fails to significantly increase the energy expenditure of normal or cancer-bearing dogs. This is opposite to the common belief that animals and humans with cancer have elevated energy metabolism.

The above-mentioned alterations in carbohydrate, protein, and lipid metabolism are important to practitioners because they affect a diverse population of dogs with a wide variety of cancers.[1-15] Therapies to improve these changes must begin early and continue even after surgery or other treatment eliminates the malignancy.

Clinical Presentation

Dogs with cancer cachexia show few clinical signs of the paraneoplastic syndrome in the early stages. As the syndrome progresses, weight loss is noted despite a good appetite (Figure 45-1). Later, weight loss, anorexia, lethargy, and depression predominate. Anorexia, fatigue, chronic nausea or vomiting, decreased activity level, and weight loss are a few of the obvious clinical signs and clinical parameters associated with this condition.[1-13]

Diagnosis

The changes in metabolism noted above can be documented early in the course of malignant disease. Dogs in the early phase of cancer cachexia may only show exercise intol-

> **KEY POINT**
> *Dogs in the early phase of cancer cachexia may only show exercise intolerance, lethargy, and anorexia.*

erance, lethargy, and anorexia. Later in the course of the disease, there is overt wasting and loss of body condition despite adequate nutritional intake. Hypoalbuminemia is a notable finding in the later stages of the disease. The later stages are followed by death owing to failure of one or more organ systems.

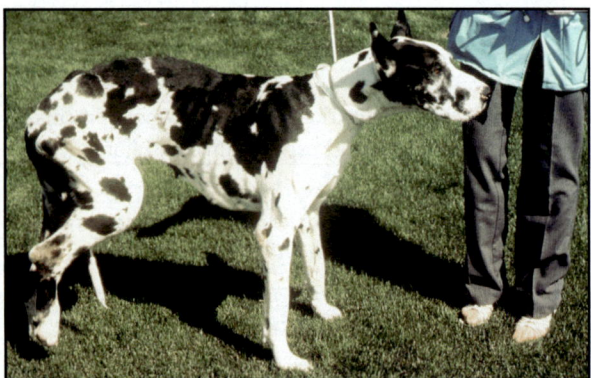

Figure 45-1. *A Great Dane with osteosarcoma and dramatic weight loss despite adequate nutritional intake, the hallmark for the very late stages of cancer cachexia. The metabolic alterations associated with this condition occur even before clinical signs are noted and continue after the animal is rendered free of the malignancy. Most dogs with the metabolic alterations associated with cancer cachexia do not exhibit weight loss.*

Treatment[1-15,17-19]

Detailed therapeutic strategies are found in Chapter 31. Some general principles are reviewed below.

- The patient should consume an adequate quantity of highly bioavailable nutrients presented in a palatable form.
- A diet composed of modest amounts of complex carbohydrates, minimal quantities of rapidly absorbed simple carbohydrates, relatively modest amounts of high-quality bioavailable proteins, and a modest amount of fats of the omega-3 (n-3) series may be ideal for supporting cancer patients without enhancing tumor growth.
  — Supplementing the diet with oils containing omega-3 or with purified omega-3 fatty acids has been shown to slow the growth of various types of cancers in animals.
  — The efficacy of cancer chemotherapeutic drugs such as doxorubicin, epirubicin, irinotecan, 5-fluorouracil, and tamoxifen and of radiation therapy has been improved when the diet included omega-3 fatty acids.
  — Omega-3 fatty acids induce beneficial effects in cancer patients, such as modulation of eicosanoid production and inflammation, angiogenesis, proliferation, and susceptibility for apoptosis.
  — Omega-3 fatty acids have been used to suppress cancer-associated cachexia and to improve the quality of life.
- Dogs should be fed enterally when possible. If appropriate, methods such as warming the food, increasing palatability, and using pharmacologic agents (e.g., megestrol acetate, benzodiazepine derivatives, cyproheptadine) to enhance appetite and stimulate oral feeding should be used before considering nasogastric, gastrostomy, or jejunostomy tube feeding.
- When enteral feeding is not feasible, parenteral feeding using minimal simple carbohydrates should be used.
- When possible, lactate- and glucose-containing fluids should be avoided because they may produce lactate and stimulate release of insulin. An exception is in cases of septic shock or during an insulin overdose, when glucose-containing fluids may be required specifically to treat hypoglycemia.
- Adequate calories should be provided; however, it may not be necessary to provide more nutrients than needed by disease-free dogs. The following formula is a general approximation of the amount of metabolizable food to feed (kcal/day): $2(30 \times \text{body weight [kg]}) + 70$. A more accurate formula is $70(\text{body weight in kg})^{0.75}$.
- Frequent, small, energy-dense meals should be provided.
- Metoclopramide should be given when possible to reduce nausea. Ondansetron may also be of value.
- The dog should be exercised regularly to maintain lean body mass and to keep the attitude positive.

REFERENCES

1. Ogilvie GK, Marks SL: Cancer, in Hand MS, Thatcher CD, Remillard RL, Roudebush P (eds): *Small Animal Clinical Nutrition*, ed 4. Topeka, KS, Mark Morris Institute, 2000, pp 887–906.
2. Ogilvie GK: Paraneoplastic syndromes, in Withrow SJ, MacEwen EG (eds): *Clinical Veterinary Oncology*. Philadelphia, JB Lippincott, 1989, pp 29–40.
3. Ogilvie GK: Paraneoplastic syndromes, in Ettinger SJ, Feldman EC (eds): *Textbook of Veterinary Internal Medicine*. Philadelphia, WB Saunders, 2000, pp 498–506.
4. Ogilvie GK: Alterations in metabolism and nutritional support for veterinary cancer patients: Recent advances. *Compend Contin Educ Pract Vet* 15:925–937, 1993.
5. Ogilvie GK, Vail DM, Wheeler SL, et al: Effects of chemotherapy and remission on carbohydrate metabolism in dogs with lymphoma. *Cancer* 69:233–238, 1992.
6. Vail DM, Ogilvie GK, Fettman MJ, Wheeler SL: Exacerbation of hyperlactatemia by infusion of LRS in dogs with lymphoma. *J Vet Intern Med* 4:228–232, 1990.
7. Vail DM, Ogilvie GK, Wheeler SL, et al: Alterations in carbohydrate metabolism in canine lymphoma. *J Vet Intern Med* 4:8–11, 1990.
8. Ogilvie, GK, Ford RD, Vail DM, et al: Alterations in lipoprotein profiles in dogs with lymphoma. *J Vet Intern Med* 8:62–66, 1994.
9. Ogilvie GK, Walters LM, Fettman MJ, et al: Energy expenditure in dogs with lymphoma fed two specialized diets. *Cancer* 71:3146–3152, 1993.
10. Walters LM, Ogilvie GK, Fettman MJ, et al: Repeatability of energy expenditure measurements in normal dogs by calorimetry. *Am J Vet Res* 54:1881–1885, 1993.
11. Ogilvie GK, Vail DM: Unique metabolic alterations associated with cancer cachexia in the dog, in Kirk RW (ed): *Current Veterinary Therapy XI*. Philadelphia, WB Saunders, 1992, pp 433–438.
12. Michel KE, Sorenmo K, Shofer FS: Evaluation of body condition and weight loss in dogs presented to a veterinary oncology service. *J Vet Intern Med* 18(5):692–695, 2004.
13. Krishnaswamy K: Effects of malnutrition on drug metabolism and toxicity in humans. *Nutritional Toxicology* 2:105–124, 1987.
15. Fields AL, Cheema-Dhadli S, Wolman SL, Halperin ML: Theoretical aspects of weight loss in patients with cancer. Possible importance of pyruvate dehydrogenase. *Cancer* 50(10):2183–2188, 1982.
16. Chlebowski RT, Heber D: Metabolic abnormalities in cancer patients: Carbohydrate metabolism. *Surg Clin North Am* 66:957–968, 1986.
17. Persson C, Glimelius B, Ronnelid J, Nygren P: Impact of fish oil and melatonin on cachexia in patients with advanced gastrointestinal cancer: A randomized pilot study. *Nutrition* 21(2):170–178, 2005.
18. Burns CP, Halabi S, Clamon G, et al: Phase II study of high-dose fish oil capsules for patients with cancer-related cachexia. *Cancer* 101(2):370–378, 2004.
19. Hardman WE: (n-3) Fatty acids and cancer therapy. *J Nutr* 134(suppl 12):3427–3430, 2004.

FEVER, HYPERTROPHIC OSTEOPATHY, AND HYPERCORTISOLISM

Gregory K. Ogilvie and Antony S. Moore

CLINICAL BRIEFING

Fever

History	• Lethargy and anorexia.
Clinical signs	• Lethargy, anorexia, increased body temperature, and weight loss (if condition is prolonged).
Diagnostics	• Confirm that elevated body temperature persists in a quiet patient. • Rule out infections and inflammatory or immune-mediated causes with a CBC, biochemical profile, urinalysis, echocardiogram, antinuclear antibody test, and cultures of blood, urine, and lung. • Determine the presence of disease of the hypothalamus with history, physical examination, brain imaging studies, and a CSF tap (if indicated).
Treatment	• Eliminate the underlying cause. • Therapy depends on the severity of clinical and laboratory parameters. • Consider fluids and steroidal and nonsteroidal antiinflammatory agents.

Hypertrophic Osteopathy

History	• Shifting leg lameness.
Clinical signs	• Swollen, warm extremities; may also involve the ribs and pelvis.
Diagnostics	• Radiography of affected bones to demonstrate unique periosteal reaction. • Search for underlying malignancy with thoracic radiography followed by abdominal radiography or ultrasonography, CBC, biochemical profile, and urinalysis.
Treatment	• Treat the underlying cause. • Antiinflammatory agents.

Ectopic Cushing's Syndrome

History	• Primary lung cancer in dogs.
Clinical signs	• Most patients are asymptomatic. • Some patients exhibit polyuria, polydipsia, weakness, lethargy, and weight loss.
Diagnostics	• Low- and high-dose dexamethasone suppression test, endogenous ACTH concentration, urine cortisol:creatinine ratio, CBC, biochemical profile, and urinalysis.
Treatment	• Treat the underlying cause. • Mitotane or ketoconazole.

Fever

Fever is a common complication of cancer.[1-3] In many cases, it is caused by infection, although noninfectious conditions, such as drug toxicity and adrenal insufficiency, have also been associated with fever.[2] Tumor-associated fever is usually defined as unexplained elevated body temperature that coincides with growth or elimination of a tumor. Tumor-induced fevers may result from the release of pyrogens from tumor cells, normal leukocytes, or other normal cells. These tumor-elaborated pyrogens may act on the hypothalamus, which governs thermoregulation, to upset temperature regulation of the body. Although the incidence of cancer-associated fever in dogs is unknown, in humans, up to 40% of fevers of unknown origin are found to be caused by cancer.[3]

> **KEY POINT**
>
> *Tumor-associated fever is usually defined as unexplained elevated body temperature that coincides with growth or elimination of a tumor. It may result from the release of pyrogens from tumor cells, normal leukocytes, or other normal cells.*

CLINICAL SIGNS

Clinical signs are directly related to the underlying malignant disease, elevated body temperature, and associated increase in energy expenditure. They include depression, anorexia, lethargy, and weight loss.

DIAGNOSIS

The diagnosis of fever as a paraneoplastic syndrome is essentially a diagnosis of exclusion and is supported by determining whether eliminating the underlying tumor resolves the elevated body temperature. All nontumor-related causes of increased body temperature are eliminated with the following procedures: complete blood count (CBC), biochemical profile, urinalysis, blood and urine cultures, thoracic radiography, echocardiography (to rule out bacterial endocarditis), and, if indicated, an antinuclear antibody test, a brain imaging study (computed tomography, magnetic resonance imaging, or both), a myelogram, and a cerebrospinal fluid (CSF) tap to evaluate hypothalamic function.

TREATMENT

Fever can be used as a tumor marker to document response to therapy.[1-3] Excessive fever that induces clinical signs and is directly related to malignant disease can be treated symptomatically with antipyretics or NSAIDs. Resolution of the underlying malignant condition usually eliminates the fever.

Hypertrophic Osteopathy

Hypertrophic osteopathy is a relatively common disease in dogs. It primarily occurs in the bones of the extremities and is often associated with primary and metastatic lung tumors.[2] Other neoplastic and nonneoplastic conditions have been associated with this disorder, including esophageal sarcoma, rhabdomyosarcoma of the urinary bladder, pneumonia, heartworm disease, congenital and acquired heart disease, and focal lung atelectasis.[2] Other factors include hyperestrogenism, deficient oxygenation, and increased blood flow.[2]

CLINICAL SIGNS

The disease produces an increase in peripheral blood flow and a periosteal proliferation along the shafts of long bones, often beginning with the digits and extending as far proximally as the femur and humerus. Initially, there is soft tissue proliferation. This is succeeded by osteophytes, which tend to radiate from the cortices at a 90° angle. This results in shifting leg lameness and swollen, warm extremities that seem to first involve long bones but can occasionally involve ribs and pelvis. The cause of this syndrome is unknown; however, successful treatment by vagotomy suggests a neurovascular mechanism that may involve a reflex emanating from the tumor and nearby pleura that is transmitted through afferent vagal fibers.[2]

> **KEY POINT**
>
> *Hypertrophic osteopathy results in an increase in peripheral blood flow and a periosteal proliferation along the shafts of long bones, often beginning with the digits and extending as far proximally as the femur and humerus. Initially, there is soft tissue proliferation. This is succeeded by osteophytes, which tend to radiate from the cortices at a 90° angle.*

DIAGNOSIS

Radiographs of affected limbs and the contralateral extremities often show increased soft tissue density and a unique osteophyte reaction that radiates outward at a 90° angle from the cortex of the bone (Figure 46-1). When hypertrophic osteopathy is identified, radiographs of the thorax (and of the abdomen, when indicated) should be done to identify the underlying cause. Although a biopsy is definitive, the classic history, physical examination, and radiographic changes are often enough to permit a definitive diagnosis of hypertrophic osteopathy.

TREATMENT

Prednisone offers temporary improvement of clinical signs and may reduce swelling.[1,2] Removal of the tumor can

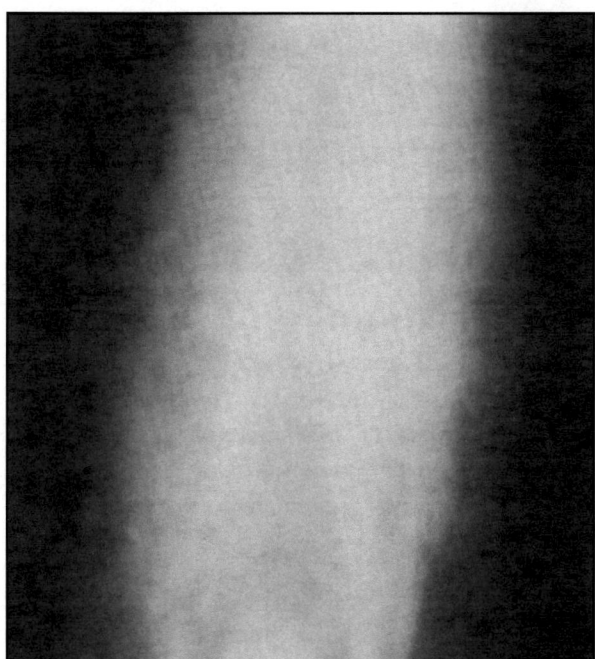

Figure 46-1. *Radiograph of a limb affected with hypertrophic osteopathy showing an increased soft tissue density and a unique osteophyte reaction that radiates outward at a 90° angle from the cortex of the bone.*

cause almost immediate resolution of clinical signs; regression of bony and soft tissue changes may take months or years. Other treatments, such as the use of analgesics, unilateral vagotomy on the side of the lung lesion, incision through the parietal pleura, subperiosteal rib resection, or bilateral cervical vagotomy, have been suggested.

Altered Corticosteroid Homeostasis

The ectopic production of adrenocorticotropic hormone (ACTH) or related polypeptides has been described in dogs with primary lung tumors as well as in a variety of human cancers, including small cell lung cancer, bronchial carcinoids, islet cell tumors of the pancreas, medullary cancer, and pheochromocytoma.[1-4] Ectopic Cushing's syndrome is caused by excessive steroid production from normal adrenal glands that are under the influence of ectopically produced ACTH or ACTH-like substances.

CLINICAL PRESENTATION

Most patients with this condition are asymptomatic. When clinical signs occur, they are similar to those of Cushing's disease.[1-3]

DIAGNOSIS

Ectopic production of ACTH produces a syndrome identified by pronounced hypokalemia, metabolic alkalosis, glucose intolerance, and mild hypertension. In humans, plasma cortisol concentrations are elevated and plasma ACTH levels are generally high. The tumors are rarely suppressible with dexamethasone.[1-4]

TREATMENT[1-4]

As in all paraneoplastic syndromes, elimination of the primary tumor is the treatment of choice. This is generally done while correcting any electrolyte or acid–base abnormalities. If sodium and water retention leads to clinical signs, thiazides or other diuretics may be indicated. If the underlying malignancy cannot be treated, the patient may need to be treated with mitotane (50 mg/kg/day PO for 5–10 days, then 25–50 mg/kg/week PO) or ketoconazole (15 mg/kg PO bid) using laboratory monitoring for Cushing's disease. In human cancer patients, aminoglutethimide, metyrapone, and mifepristone (RU 486) are viable alternative treatments.

REFERENCES

1. Ogilvie GK: Paraneoplastic syndromes, in Withrow SJ, MacEwen EG (eds): *Clinical Veterinary Oncology*. Philadelphia, JB Lippincott, 1989, pp 29–40.
2. Ogilvie GK: Paraneoplastic syndromes, in Ettinger SJ, Feldman EC (eds): *Textbook of Veterinary Internal Medicine*, ed 5. Philadelphia, WB Saunders, 2000, pp 498–506.
3. Griffin TW, Rosenthal PE, Costanza ME: Paraneoplastic and endocrine syndromes, in Cady B (ed): *Cancer Manual*, ed 7. Boston, American Cancer Society, 1986, pp 373–390.
4. Ogilvie GK, Weigel RM, Haschek WM, et al: Prognostic factors for tumor remission and survival in dogs after surgery for primary lung tumors: 76 cases (1975–1985). *JAVMA* 195:109–112, 1989.

SECTION 5

MANAGEMENT OF SPECIFIC DISEASES

Chapter 47   Lymphoma 329

Chapter 48   Bone Marrow Neoplasia 359

Chapter 49   Tumors of the Nervous System 379

Chapter 50   Tumors of the Eye and Ear 396

Chapter 51   Tumors of the Respiratory Tract 405

Chapter 52   Cardiac Tumors 420

Chapter 53   Tumors of the Gastrointestinal Tract 425

Chapter 54   Melanoma 457

Chapter 55   Tumors Affecting the Liver, Pancreas, ... 470
              and Spleen

SECTION 5

MANAGEMENT OF SPECIFIC DISEASES

Chapter 56   Tumors of Blood and Lymph Vessels 479

Chapter 57   Tumors of the Endocrine System 495

Chapter 58   Tumors of the Reproductive System 522

Chapter 59   Mammary Neoplasia. 537

Chapter 60   Tumors of the Urinary Tract 549

Chapter 61   Tumors of Bone 565

Chapter 62   Soft Tissue Sarcomas 590

Chapter 63   Tumors of the Body Cavities 603

Chapter 64   Tumors of the Skin and Surrounding Structures. . . 620

Chapter 65   Mast Cell Tumors 643

LYMPHOMA
Antony S. Moore and Gregory K. Ogilvie

CLINICAL BRIEFING

Clinical factors
- Generalized peripheral lymphadenopathy most commonly seen (clinical stage III).
- Diffuse large cell, immunoblastic, and small lymphocytic.
- B-cell immunophenotype more common than T cell.
- All breeds, middle aged; systemic disease.
- Associated with environmental factors.

Staging and diagnosis
- MDB (includes a CBC, biochemical profile, urinalysis, and thoracic radiography [three views]).
- Measure all lymph nodes and extranodal sites.
- Immunophenotype of biopsy.
- Possibly abdominal ultrasonography.
- Possibly bone marrow aspirate cytology.

Prognostic factors

Have a negative effect on prognosis:
- T-cell immunophenotype.
- Substage b (clinically ill).
- Higher stage.
- Hypercalcemia (may reflect T-cell immunophenotype; often associated with a mediastinal mass).
- Increasing grade of malignancy, proliferative indexes (AgNORs only).
- Presence of multidrug resistance protein.
- Pretreatment corticosteroids.
- Low serum albumin.

Have a positive effect on prognosis:
- B-cell immunophenotype.
- Low body weight (<15 kg).
- Complete response to therapy.
- Toxicity to chemotherapy.
- Low-grade lymphoma.
- Diet (n-3 fatty acids).
- Trisomy chromosome 13.

Treatment

Level		
Level 1	Single-agent prednisone.	50% in PR or CR for 2 to 3 months.
Level 2	COP.	70% in CR for median of 5 months.
	Doxorubicin.	60% to 75% in CR for median of 6 to 8 months.
Level 3	COP plus doxorubicin and L-asparaginase.	80% in CR for median of 12 months. • Can be given as a discontinuous protocol. • Include more alkylating agents if T cell. • Use supportive care if substage b.
Level 4	Level 3 plus —Radiation. —Autologous bone marrow.	CR for median of 16 months. CR for median of 12.5 months; 57% 1-year remission.

CR = complete remission (complete disappearance of all clinical evidence of lymphoma).
PR = partial remission (>50% reduction in clinical disease parameters, no new lesions, but less than CR).

The terms *lymphoma* and *lymphosarcoma* are interchangeable in veterinary medicine. Lymphoma is the most common hematopoietic tumor of dogs, and its natural history and progression are well described. Chemotherapy has been shown to be very effective in altering progression and prolonging quality of life in most animals.

Incidence, Signalment, and Etiology

Lymphoma accounts for approximately 90% of canine hematopoietic tumors and is the hematopoietic malignancy most responsive to chemotherapy in dogs. Its epidemiology is multifactorial, with both genetic and environmental influences playing a role. The incidence rate may be increasing, but this is difficult to assess accurately because not all cases are reported. A study in the 1960s found an incidence of 24 per 100,000[1] that increased to 30 per 100,000 in the same area over the next decade.[2] Another study in the Netherlands found an incidence of 33 per 100,000.[3] Data from insured dogs in the United Kingdom found an adjusted incidence rate of 114 per 100,000 dogs,[4] which is closer to Clancy et al's unpublished observations of 109 per 100,000 in Massachusetts.[5]

Lymphoma is uncommon in young dogs; affected dogs are typically middle aged. Neither gender nor neutering is a predisposing factor for developing lymphoma.

In two early studies of canine tumor epidemiology,[1,6] boxers had a risk of developing lymphoma that was approximately 10 times greater than that for all dogs combined. Boxers may be more likely to develop T cell–derived lymphoma.[7] In a group of 59 bullmastiffs, nine dogs developed lymphoma over a 3-year period; cases seemed to follow a familial distribution.[8] The predisposition of boxers, bulldogs, and bullmastiffs to lymphoma was confirmed in a British study, with estimated incidences of 178, 174, and 279 per 100,000 dogs, respectively.[9] Two studies suggested that golden retrievers were nearly three times more likely than other breeds to develop lymphoma.[10,11] Two studies also found that Rottweilers were between 2.5 and 6 times more likely to develop lymphoma than other breeds,[10,12] and one study found apparent familial trends in Rottweilers.[13]

Virus particles resembling a C-type retrovirus have been observed in cases of canine lymphoma and leukemia as well as in tissue cultures of canine lymphoma cells.[14,15] The purported retrovirus has also been found in normal dogs, however, and no etiologic involvement has been confirmed. In view of the lack of an early age–incidence peak for dogs with lymphoma and the lack of reports of "clustering" of unrelated cases, it seems unlikely that a viral etiology of the type seen for feline lymphoma is present in dogs.

One study found that the distribution of canine lymphoma was not random and that distinct clustering occurred in some counties in Michigan, which implies that environmental factors play a role in the epidemiology of lymphoma in dogs.[16] Dr. Moore has found similar clustering when geographic information systems technology was applied to dogs living in Massachusetts. An Italian study found that compared with the rest of the population, dogs living in an industrial area and dogs exposed to paints and solvents were at increased risk of developing lymphoma and developed lymphoma at a younger age.[17]

Evidence suggests that high exposure to some herbicides, notably 2,4-dichlorophenoxyacetic acid (2,4-D), is associated with an increased risk of non-Hodgkin's lymphoma in humans. A case-controlled study found that dogs with lymphoma were exposed to 2,4-D more frequently than were control dogs. In addition, the risk of a dog developing lymphoma increased twofold if the owner applied 2,4-D to the lawn four or more times per year.[18] A further study found that dogs exposed to a lawn treated with 2,4-D excreted metabolites in their urine.[19] These data remain controversial[20–22]; however, given the potential role of this chemical, dog owners may wish to be prudent in their use of herbicides.[22]

> **KEY POINT**
>
> *Genetic and environmental factors have been associated with an increased risk of lymphoma in dogs.*

Further evidence supporting environmental influences as a cause of lymphoma in dogs comes from a study of exposure to magnetic fields in the home. Dogs that lived in homes with a magnetic field derived from a "very high" current configuration wire code were nearly seven times more likely to develop lymphoma than the general canine population.[23]

Environmental causes of lymphoma may act through suppression of the immune system. One study found that dogs with immune-mediated thrombocytopenia were more likely to have lymphoma, but the cause and effect of the association could not be assessed.[24]

Clinical Presentation and History

The most common physical finding in dogs with lymphoma is peripheral lymphadenopathy, which is usually generalized but may be localized to a single lymph node or a region of the body. Involvement of other organs, such as spleen, liver, or bone marrow, is an indication of advanced disease. Involvement of other (extranodal) sites is rare in dogs.

Most canine patients with lymphoma present with generalized lymphadenopathy, often because their owners have noticed mandibular lymphadenopathy during petting or grooming (Figures 47-1 and 47-2). One study found that 63% of dogs presented for lymphadenopathy had lymphoma, and only 20% had inflammatory conditions.[25] Dogs with lymphoma have few, if any, clinical signs of illness, although owners may report reduced exercise tolerance, fatigability, and mild inappetence. This is in contrast to most systemic infections

LYMPHOMA

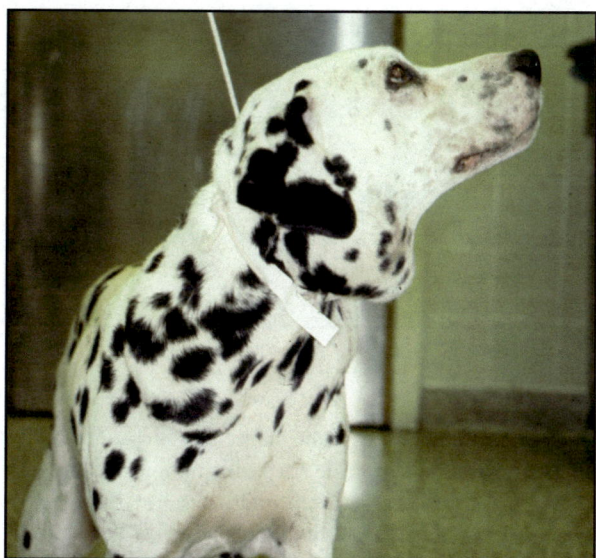

Figure 47-1. This 6-year-old dalmatian has extremely large peripheral lymph nodes. The dog had no organomegaly or evidence of bone marrow involvement and was clinically well. The lymphoma was therefore classified as clinical stage IIIa. Complete remission was achieved with combination chemotherapy.

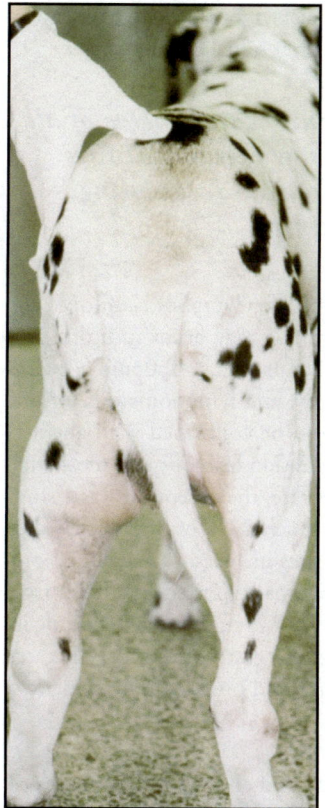

Figure 47-2. The same dog as in Figure 47-1. Note the lymphadenopathy causing distal edema of the left hindlimb.

Table 47-1 Clinical Stages of Canine Lymphoma (WHO)[26]

Clinical Stage[a]	Criteria
Stage I	Involvement limited to single node or lymphoid tissue in single organ (excluding the bone marrow)
Stage II	Regional involvement of many lymph nodes, with or without involvement of the tonsils
Stage III	Generalized lymph node involvement
Stage IV	Involvement of liver and/or spleen, with or without generalized lymph node involvement
Stage V	Involvement of blood, bone marrow, and/or other sites

[a]Stages are further classified to clinical substage a (no clinical signs) or b (with clinical signs). For example, stage IIIa describes a dog with generalized lymphadenopathy and no clinical signs.

(e.g., fungal, bacterial, rickettsial, viral, protozoal), which cause obvious signs of illness, as do immune-mediated diseases that cause lymphadenopathy. Lymphoma should always be suspected in a middle-aged, apparently healthy dog with lymphadenopathy.

If the disease is advanced and involves other organs, dogs may show weakness, depression, anorexia, vomiting, or diarrhea. Terminally ill dogs may be cachectic, dyspneic due to respiratory tract obstruction by lymph nodes, and pyrexic (dogs with lymphoma are immunocompromised and therefore are at high risk of developing severe infections, such as pneumonia) and have episodes of collapse.

Untreated lymphoma progresses rapidly (1–2 months) from presentation to terminal stages. However, chemotherapy can considerably improve the patient's duration and quality of life.

Staging and Diagnosis

When evaluating an animal for treatment of lymphoma, it is important to not only obtain a definitive diagnosis but also assess the general health of the patient by clinical examination and ancillary diagnostics.

Lymphoma is a systemic disease; therefore, it is important to determine the extent of organ involvement and to identify unrelated or secondary conditions that need to be treated or controlled before instituting appropriate therapy for lymphoma. Staging is a clinical process that enables the veterinarian to quantitate the extent of lymphoma involvement. Staging carries prognostic significance and enables the veterinarian and client to make informed and rational decisions as to the type of therapy best suited for the patient. In dogs, the most widely used staging scheme is the one developed by the World Health Organization (WHO; Table 47-1; Figure 47-3). In one study, the category of stage V was split so that dogs with extranodal lymphoma involving sites other than bone marrow and blood were labeled stage VI; this scheme has not been applied in other studies.[27]

CYTOLOGY

The diagnosis of lymphoma can be confirmed by cytologic or histologic demonstration of malignant lymphoid infiltration in organs that do not ordinarily contain such cells. Cytologic examination of lymph nodes may be suggestive of, or compatible with, a diagnosis of lymphoma but rarely provides a definitive diagnosis. In the presence of lym-

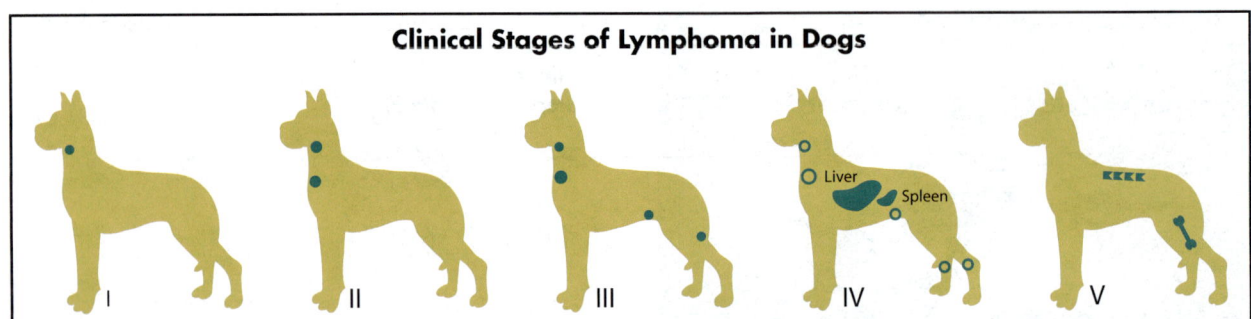

Figure 47-3. *A visual synopsis of the staging system for canine lymphoma outlined in Table 47-1.*

phadenopathy, a definitive diagnosis of lymphoma is based on histologic examination of a surgically resected lymph node. This is preferable to a needle or wedge biopsy because the entire node can be examined for key histopathologic evidence of malignancy, such as disruption of architecture and invasion of the capsule. The most accessible, most easily removed lymph node is the popliteal lymph node, which is the preferred biopsy site if it is enlarged.

Examination of nodal architecture enables the pathologist to assign a grade, which has been thought to be important for prognosis. However, the utility of immunophenotype, lack of repeatability for tumor grading, and subjective nature of morphologic classification have led to tumor grading being considered of less value for clinical prognosis in dogs with lymphoma. The one exception may be the finding of "low-grade" lymphoma.

Immunophenotyping should be requested on all biopsy specimens. Differentiation of phenotype is now widely available by immunostaining for CD3 (T cell) and CD79a (B cell) markers, which can be conducted on histopathology and acetone-fixed cytology specimens. The clinician should also inquire whether flow cytometry is available to quantitate multiple lymphocyte markers.

Occasionally, it may be difficult to differentiate a low-grade lymphoma from a reactive lymphoid disease. In this situation, the lymphocytes in the malignant disease would be expected to have a clonal population, but those in the reactive disease would not. This was shown to be true in one study.[28] Tests for clonality are available in some institutions in the United States.

PHYSICAL EXAMINATION

The clinical stage of a dog with lymphoma is often determined on physical examination. All lymph nodes should be palpated; accurate measurements should be recorded to help the clinician assess response to therapy. Each dog is clinically staged based on the results of physical examination, clinical laboratory testing (i.e., complete blood count [CBC], biochemical profile, urinalysis, and bone marrow cytology), and imaging procedures (i.e., radiography and ultrasonography). In each case, a biopsy of the affected lymphoid tissue is necessary to confirm the diagnosis and determine the cell type (histologic grading and immunophenotype). In addition, urine culture should be conducted to identify occult urinary tract infection. Abdominal ultrasonography is probably only warranted if organ involvement is suspected. Bone marrow aspiration is required to complete staging, but the finding of bone marrow involvement in a dog with no clinical or CBC changes suggesting marrow involvement is rare. Dogs with bone marrow involvement may be more likely to have myelosuppression at diagnosis and after initial chemotherapy.

> **KEY POINT**
>
> *Accurate pretreatment measurements of all affected lymph nodes or extranodal sites will assist the veterinarian in assessing response to chemotherapy.*

The eyes should be assessed for lymphoid infiltrate and secondary anterior uveitis, which may occur in up to 37% of dogs with multicentric lymphoma.[29] Abdominal palpation may reveal organomegaly, and lymphomatous infiltration of the spleen or liver can be confirmed with ancillary tests, such as fine-needle aspiration or biopsy. In most studies, extranodal lymphoma is rare; the exception was a study from Western Australia in which 27% of 85 affected dogs had unspecified extranodal sites involved.[30] The largest proportion of extranodal lymphomas reported in studies from the United States was 13%[27]; however, this may reflect deliberate exclusion of cutaneous and gastrointestinal (GI) cases, for which different treatments and prognoses are evident.

IMAGING STUDIES

Radiographs of the thorax and abdomen are valuable in determining the clinical stage of disease and prognosis. In one report, 75 of 100 dogs with lymphoma had abnormalities detected radiographically.[31] One study found that changes detected were often nonspecific.[32] A larger study

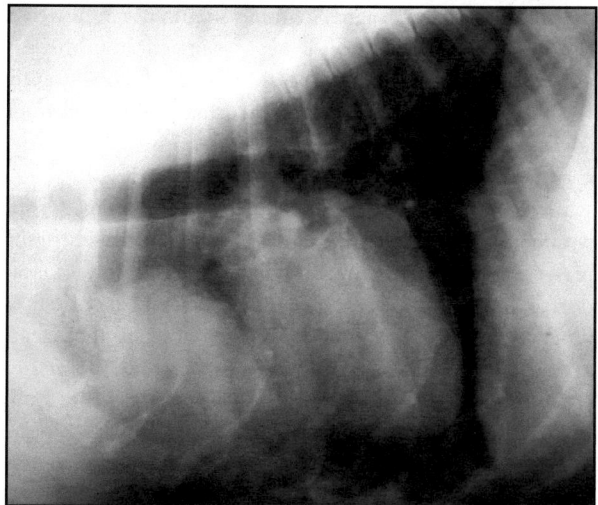

Figure 47-4. *A dog with anterior mediastinal lymphoma. This disease may be associated with pleural effusion and dyspnea or may cause dyspnea due to space-occupying pressure on the trachea. This anatomic form of lymphoma also may be associated with paraneoplastic hypercalcemia. The concurrent findings of hypercalcemia and anterior mediastinal lymphoma warrant a guarded prognosis. (Courtesy of Kenneth M. Rassnick, DVM, Cornell University College of Veterinary Medicine)*

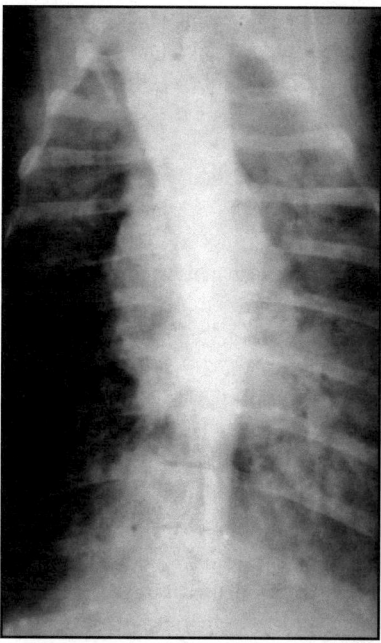

Figure 47-5. *Pulmonary lymphoma in a rottweiler. Note that the lung involvement has an infiltrative pattern rather than a nodular appearance.*

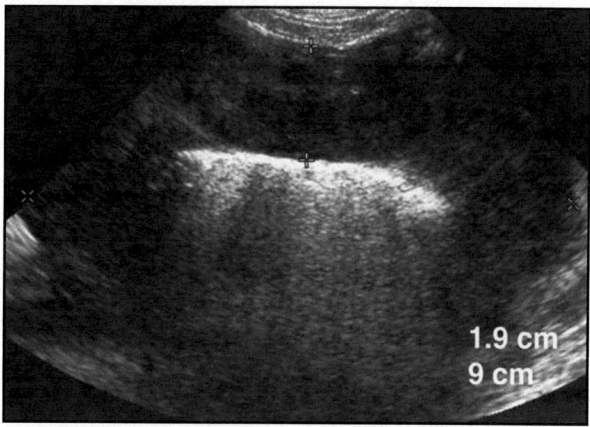

Figure 47-6. *A discrete large mass involving a long (>9 cm) bowel segment is noted. The marked wall thickening (0.9 cm) is associated with complete loss of layering. Regional lymphadenopathy (not present on this image) was also present. The large bright interface associated with dirty shadowing represents the lumen. (Courtesy of Dominique G. Pennick, DVM, Tufts Cummings School of Veterinary Medicine)*

found that dogs with cranial mediastinal lymphadenomegaly had shorter remissions and survival times regardless of immunophenotype.[33] Thoracic radiographs may allow appreciation of lymphadenopathy of mediastinal or tracheobronchial nodes. In addition, a mediastinal mass, pulmonary infiltration, or pleural effusion may be seen (Figures 47-4 and 47-5). Radiographs of the abdomen are principally used to identify hepatosplenomegaly or lymphadenopathy of the sublumbar nodes.

Technetium 99m methoxyisobutylisonitrile (sestamibi) has been used to image dogs with lymphoma.[34] This methodology is primarily useful in detecting lymphoma within extranodal sites rather than in lymph nodes or bone marrow. Sestamibi imaging has the potential to predict chemotherapeutic drug resistance; therefore, it has potential applications to predict response to treatment.

If biopsy of a mediastinal mass is being considered, particularly if pleural effusion is present, ultrasonography provides an accurate guide and a relatively safe means of obtaining a tissue or fluid sample. When involvement of abdominal viscera is suspected, ultrasonography allows evaluation of spleen and liver homogeneity and renal architecture and can be used to detect the presence of enlarged lymph nodes as well as GI involvement (Figure 47-6). Ultrasonography is relatively insensitive for the detection of hepatic involvement with lymphoma, presumably because the process is infiltrative and diffuse rather than nodular.[35]

COMPLETE BLOOD COUNT AND URINE TESTS

Anemia is common in animals with lymphoma, but it is usually low grade and characterized as normocytic normochromic anemia, which is compatible with anemia of chronic disease. Moderate to severe anemia may be present in animals that are experiencing blood loss from GI involvement and occasionally may result from immune-mediated destruction. Anemia rarely signals bone marrow infiltration, particularly if granulocyte and platelet counts are normal, because the life span of mature erythrocytes is relatively long (120 days) compared with that of platelets (5 to 6 days) or neutrophils (6 hours).

Thrombocytopenia, particularly in association with neutropenia, may indicate bone marrow infiltration by lymphoma, and bone marrow aspiration cytology should be conducted. Immune-mediated thrombocytopenia may occur in dogs with lymphoma. Thrombocytopenia may also be a sign of disseminated intravascular coagulation (DIC), a life-threatening complication. Intrinsic and extrinsic clotting pathways should be evaluated and appropriate therapy begun (see Chapter 43).

Lymphopenia (due to stress of disease) or normal lymphocyte counts may be found on the hemogram of animals with lymphoma. Lymphocytosis should prompt evaluation of lymphocyte morphology because circulating lymphoblasts imply bone marrow involvement and a higher clinical stage (stage V). In this situation, bone marrow aspiration should be performed. If the lymphocyte count is elevated and there is bone marrow infiltration but no other clinical findings, the disease is designated as lymphoid leukemia (see Chapter 48), and evaluation of lymphocyte morphology is critical for an accurate prognosis.

When cytopenia other than anemia occurs in an animal with lymphoma, neoplastic infiltration of the bone marrow must be suspected and should be confirmed by aspiration or biopsy (see Chapter 16). Lymphoma most often affects the marrow as a loose extension of malignant lymphocytes (75% of cases in one study[36]); focal (11%) or obliterating (14%) involvement is less common.[36] A single aspirate should be sufficient to diagnose infiltration in most dogs. However, in one study, bone marrow core biopsy was more effective in diagnosing marrow involvement; 55% of dogs with lymphoma had marrow involvement based on core biopsy compared with 34% diagnosed by aspiration cytology.[37] It is unclear whether more aggressive sampling has any prognostic significance. An earlier study showed that only 7% of dogs with lymphoma without circulating lymphoblasts had marrow involvement.[38] For dogs that do not have abnormal circulating cells and that have hematologic values within acceptable ranges, it may not be advantageous to perform a bone marrow aspirate. In one series of dogs, bone marrow positivity as a specific entity did not influence outcome.[39]

Myelosuppressive chemotherapeutic agents should not be used in animals with extensive neoplastic infiltration and cytopenia until the segmented neutrophil and platelet counts are in a noncritical range (>3,000 segmented neutrophils/μl; >50,000 platelets/μl).

Animals with lymphoma are often immunosuppressed and therefore susceptible to urinary tract infections, which may be subclinical. Bacterial cultures should be conducted if abnormalities in the urinalysis suggest infection; in this situation, antibiotics should be administered concurrently with chemotherapy. Animals with urinary tract infections are at high risk for sepsis when myelosuppressive chemotherapeutic drugs are used.

Biochemistry profiles are useful in staging animals with lymphoma. Elevated hepatic enzyme levels, particularly in the presence of cranial abdominal organomegaly, imply infiltration of the liver with lymphoma. If severe disturbances in liver function occur, the use of some chemotherapeutic agents should be reevaluated. Cyclophosphamide is metabolized to an active form in the liver; therefore, it may be ineffective if liver function is impaired. Doxorubicin is metabolized in the liver, so liver function impairment may lead to higher than expected serum concentrations and greater toxicity. Doxorubicin dosages should be reduced in dogs with poor liver function. Elevated blood urea nitrogen or serum creatinine levels may be associated with hypercalcemia in dogs. Primary renal involvement with lymphoma is rare in this species.

Hypercalcemia in association with lymphoma occurs in 10% to 15% of affected dogs as a result of tumor cell secretion of parathyroid hormone–related peptide.[40] It is most commonly associated with T-cell immunophenotype, and affected dogs often have a mediastinal mass. Polyuria, polydipsia, weakness, and anorexia may develop when serum calcium levels exceed 14 mg/dl. If serum calcium levels remain elevated, calcium nephropathy and resultant renal failure may ensue. Calcium levels may be reduced with bisphosphonates, saline diuresis (0.9% NaCl), or, if the patient is adequately hydrated, furosemide diuretic treatment. In addition, prednisone may be used to increase renal losses, decrease GI calcium absorption, and reduce osteoclast activity. A confirmed histologic diagnosis should be obtained before commencing prednisone therapy because complete clinical remission of lymphoma may occur, leaving the clinician uncertain as to the true cause of the hypercalcemia. The clinician should not delay obtaining a diagnosis while trying to reduce the calcium levels. Rapid diagnosis and initiation of chemotherapy will result in rapid normalization of serum calcium. A complete discussion of the treatment of hypercalcemia can be found in Chapter 36.

OTHER SYNDROMES

Other paraneoplastic syndromes are rare in dogs with lymphoma but include monoclonal gammopathy, which may be detected by serum electrophoresis. Most malignancy-associated monoclonal gammopathies in dogs are associated with multiple myeloma. Pemphigus has been associated with a thymic lymphoma,[41] as has nonspecific pruritus.[42] Renal lymphoma is rare in dogs but has been associated with excessive erythropoietin production and secondary erythrocyto-

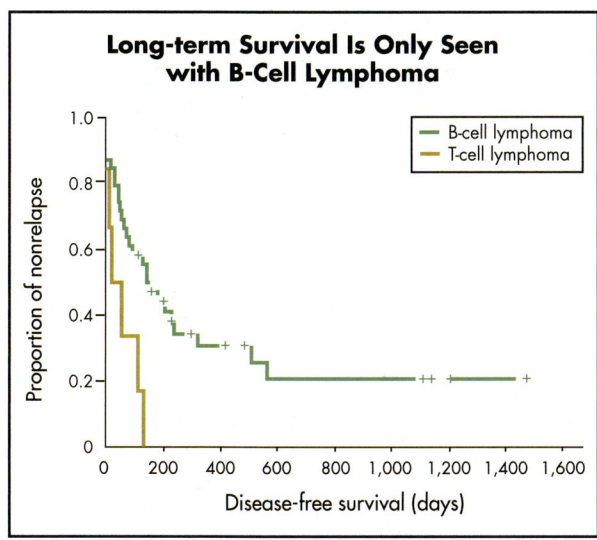

Figure 47-7. Overall remission duration for dogs treated for lymphoma. (From Dobson JM, Blackwood LB, McInnes EF, et al: Prognostic variables in canine multicentric lymphosarcoma. J Small Anim Pract 42:377–384, 2001; with permission)

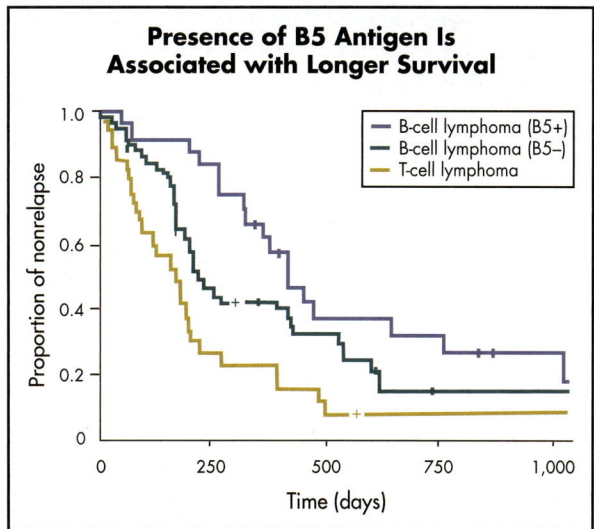

Figure 47-8. Overall survival for dogs treated for lymphoma. Dogs with B-cell lymphoma that were positive for B5 antigen lived longer than dogs with B-cell lymphoma that were negative for B5 antigen and dogs with T-cell lymphoma. (From Ruslander DA, Gebhard DH, Tompkins MB, et al: Immunophenotypic characterization of canine lymphoproliferative disorders. In Vivo 11:169–172, 1997; with permission)

sis.[43] Trigeminal neuropathy has been associated with lymphoma invasion of multiple nervous tissues.[44]

Prognostic Factors

General statistics for survival of canine lymphoma patients can be derived from reports of the efficacy of different chemotherapy protocols. Recent studies, reviewed below, have identified factors that can help provide a prognosis for the individual patient; lymphoma is one of the best-characterized canine tumors with regard to prognostic factors. Good clinical staging and ancillary laboratory testing provide important prognostic information.

In the future, histopathologic "subtyping" of lymphoma using specific antibodies and cell markers may provide prognostic information for individual patients. The features currently known to be important in predicting outcome for dogs with lymphoma patients are described below.

T-CELL VERSUS B-CELL PHENOTYPE

Differentiation of phenotype is now widely available by immunostaining for CD3 (T cell) and CD79a (B cell) markers, which can be conducted on histopathology and acetone-fixed cytopathology specimens.[45–48] Most canine lymphomas in all studies (74%–83%) have been B-cell type.[45,48–52] Only two studies have reported a high frequency of T-cell lymphoma: 38% in the Netherlands[53] and 48% in Mexico.[54] Some lymphoma cells fail to stain with either antibody. These so-called *null-cell tumors* account for less than 5% of cases in most studies, and no prognostic significance has so far been ascribed to them; they may reflect a failure of the staining rather than a true immunophenotype. The effect of phenotype on whether a dog achieves remission is variable. One study found no effect[49]; most others found that dogs with B-cell lymphoma were more likely to achieve a complete remission (CR) than dogs with T-cell lymphoma (81%–84% and 50%–67%, respectively).[51,52,55] Dogs with B-cell lymphoma have a much longer remission duration and survival than dogs with T cell–derived lymphoma.[33,49,51,56] Often, immunophenotype is a stronger predictor of remission duration than any other potential factor. Only dogs with B-cell lymphoma have long-term survival (Figure 47-7).[49]

In one study, the radiographic finding of mediastinal lymphadenomegaly and immunophenotype had a combined effect on survival duration.[33] Dogs with B-cell lym-

> *Immunophenotype is one of the strongest indicators of prognosis for a dog with lymphoma. Dogs with T cell–derived lymphoma have a worse prognosis. ("T is terrible, B is better.")*

phoma and no mediastinal lymphadenopathy had a median survival of 10.8 months compared with 6.4 months for dogs with B-cell lymphoma and enlarged mediastinal lymph nodes. Dogs with T-cell lymphoma and no mediastinal lymphadenopathy had a median survival of 6.4

Table 47-2 Percentage of Cells from 29 Lymph Node Aspirates Expressing Different Antigens on Flow Cytometry[57]

Antigen	Percentage of Cells
CD-1a	2.1–5.4
CD-1b	3.5–6.5
CD-1c	4.9–9.5
CD-3	45.7–63.4
CD-4	18.7–25.5
CD-8-α	7.3–10.7
CD-14	1.7–3.0
CD-18	40.0–57.3
CD-21	24.7–38.0
CD-45	19.1–40.4
CD-45RA	30.1–55.0
CD-90 (Thy-1)	22.9–39.7
TCR-αβ	22.9–35.8
TCR-γδ	2.0–4.0
MHC-II	41.7–59.0

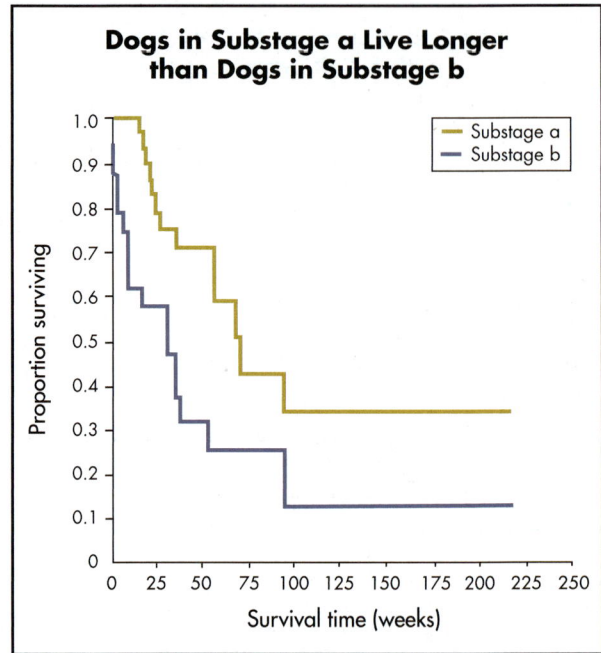

Figure 47-9. Survival curves for dogs with lymphoma treated with a five-drug protocol, separated according to clinical substage. Thirty-one dogs in substage a (no clinical signs) lived longer than 24 dogs in substage b (clinical signs of illness present). (From Keller ET, MacEwen EG, Rosenthal RC, et al: Evaluation of prognostic factors and sequential combination chemotherapy with doxorubicin for canine lymphoma. J Vet Intern Med 7:289–295, 1993; with permission)

months compared with 3.4 months for dogs with T-cell lymphoma and enlarged mediastinal lymph nodes.

Some studies have found that other antibodies may predict clinical outcome. Only dogs that expressed CD4 on lymphoma cells had hypercalcemia in one study.[51] In another study, a subtype of B-cell lymphoma was identified by staining for B5 antigen; these dogs survived longer (median: 13.8 months) than other dogs with B-cell lymphoma (median: 8 months) and dogs with T-cell lymphoma (median: 5.5 months; Figure 47-8).[51] Histologic classification in combination with immunophenotype may also allow identification of subtypes of lymphoma with differing prognoses.[56]

Most recently, fine-needle aspiration has been used to obtain cells for flow cytometry. This technique has the advantage of being able to measure percentages of cells with a range of antibodies directed against various surface antigens and other cell markers and is becoming commercially viable. The normal distribution of flow cytometry staining for normal canine lymph nodes was recently published.[57] It is presented in Table 47-2 as a reference for evaluation of dogs with lymphoma. Soon, flow cytometry may be able to identify subtypes of lymphoma immunophenotypes that have different prognoses and different sensitivities to treatment.

SUBSTAGE

While the stage of disease is not always of prognostic significance, the absence or presence of clinical illness (substage a and b, respectively) appears to reliably predict remission duration and survival; dogs in substage b have shorter remission and survival times (Figure 47-9).[52,58-63] Table 47-3 outlines some of the results from published studies. Although remission duration and survival times vary for dogs in substage a, presumably due to the different protocols used, the corresponding times for dogs in substage b are uniformly poor. Recent studies have further refined the substage category as detailed in the Stage of Disease section, below.

> **KEY POINT**
> *Dogs with advanced lymphoma, particularly if they are clinically ill, have a poor prognosis compared with healthy dogs with limited disease.*

As examples of clinical illness, fever[10] and dyspnea[10,11] have been noted as poor prognostic indicators, with affected dogs less likely to achieve a CR to induction chemotherapy.

Table 47-3 Effect of Substage or Anorexia on Remission and Survival in Dogs with Lymphoma

Number of Dogs	Remission Duration (months)		Survival (months)		Study
	Substage a	Substage b	Substage a	Substage b	
53	11	4	18	4.5	Garrett et al[59]
43	7	3	10.5	4.6	Jagielski et al[12]
121	7.1	3.4	8.4	4.4	Valerius et al[60]
55	10.2	3.5	15.9	6.5	Keller et al[27]
56 (anorexia)	12	5	—	—	Moore et al[10]
92 (anorexia)	—	—	13.4	5.3	Morrison-Collister et al[39]

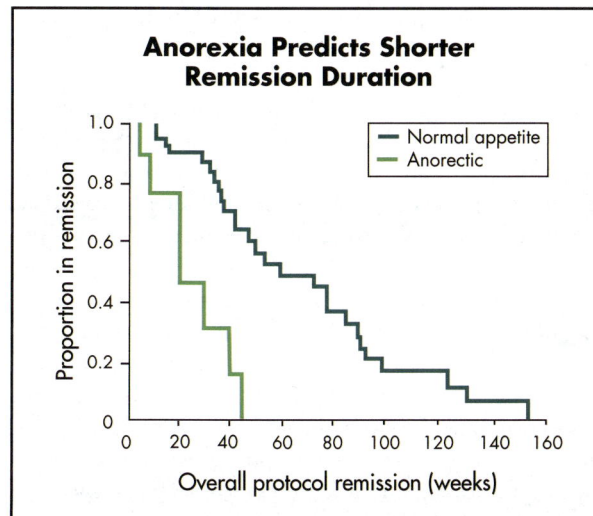

Figure 47-10. Lack of anorexia at presentation predicted remission duration for dogs that achieved CR. Ten dogs that were anorectic had a shorter remission (median, 5 months) than 46 dogs with a normal appetite (median, 12 months). (From Moore AS, Cotter SM, Rand WM, et al: Evaluation of a discontinuous treatment protocol (VELCAP-S) for canine lymphoma. J Vet Intern Med 15:348–354, 2001; with permission)

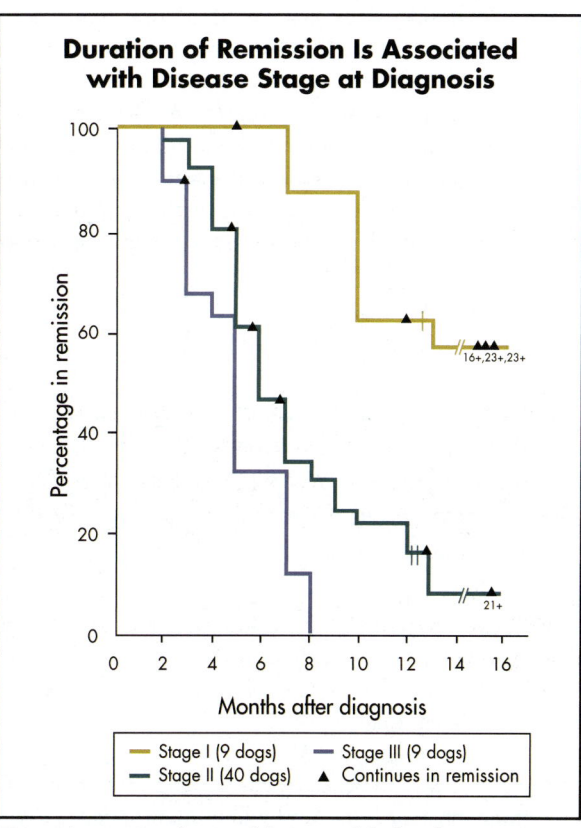

Figure 47-11. Populations of dogs treated for lymphoma using combination chemotherapy (COP) separated according to clinical stage. Dogs with localized disease at diagnosis (stage I) have longer remissions than dogs with more advanced disease. (From Cotter SM: Treatment of lymphoma and leukemia with cyclophosphamide, vincristine and prednisone: I. Treatment of dogs. JAAHA 19:159–165, 1983; with permission)

Anorexia has also been evaluated as a prognostic indicator. In one study, 35 of 40 dogs without anorexia (88%) achieved CR, while 30 of 52 dogs with anorexia achieved CR.[39] Of dogs that achieve CR, those that are anorectic at entry have shorter overall disease control and survival (Figure 47-10[10]).[39]

STAGE OF DISEASE

Although various studies have shown the prognostic importance of clinical staging, the details remain controversial. Some studies have suggested that dogs with less-extensive disease (i.e., stage I to III lymphoma) are more likely to achieve CR than are dogs in clinical stages IV and V.[64] In other studies, the percentage of dogs achieving remission did not correlate with stage of disease, but the duration of remission and survival were significantly longer in dogs with stage I to III lymphoma (Figure 47-11).[65–67] In yet other studies, dogs with stage IV lymphoma had longer remissions.[58]

Many studies do not report bone marrow aspirates on all patients. In one series of dogs that all had bone marrow aspirates performed, neither stage of disease nor bone marrow positivity as a specific entity influenced outcome.[39]

The differentiation between stage III, IV, and V lymphoma may depend on the aggressiveness of staging. Studies that report fine-needle cytology for all sites (e.g., spleen, liver) and perform multiple bone marrow aspirates may tend to stage patients "higher." It seems that dogs with stage I or II disease, while rarely seen, may have the best prognosis.[12]

HYPERCALCEMIA

Hypercalcemia is often associated with anterior mediastinal lymphoma; therefore, thoracic radiography should always be considered for dogs with confirmed hypercalcemia. A dog with lymphoma and hypercalcemia is, by convention, considered to be in clinical substage b. Early studies found that the average survival time for hypercalcemic dogs was shorter than that for normocalcemic dogs.[68] In a refinement of that finding, an anterior mediastinal mass (AMM) was found in 16 of 37 dogs (43%) with lymphoma and hypercalcemia. For dogs treated with chemotherapy, only the presence of an AMM was prognostic; dogs that did not have a mass had longer survival times (9.5 months) than dogs that did have an AMM (3 months).[69]

> **KEY POINT**
>
> *For hypercalcemic dogs, it is important to obtain a diagnosis and begin chemotherapy quickly rather than to delay while attempting to reduce serum calcium levels by other means.*

More recent studies[70,71] have found that hypercalcemic dogs (particularly those with an AMM) are more likely to have a lymphoma derived from T lymphocytes. It may be this factor, rather than hypercalcemia or the presence of an AMM, that is prognostic. Although the finding of hypercalcemia increases the chance that the dog could have a T-cell lymphoma, confirmation by immunohistochemistry is required (see also T-cell versus B-cell Phenotype section, above).

COMPLETE BLOOD COUNT FINDINGS

In two studies, of dogs that achieved a CR, those that were thrombocytopenic at entry had a shorter remission duration.[10,11] In contrast, longer survival was seen in dogs that were thrombocytopenic in another study.[59]

Dogs that were anemic had a shorter remission (6.2 months) than did dogs that had a normal hematocrit (11.4 months) at diagnosis in one study.[52]

BODY WEIGHT

Dogs that weigh less than 15 to 18 kg have been reported to have longer survival times than larger dogs.[11,59,66] It is possible that dosages based on body surface area (m^2) tend to deliver relatively higher doses to smaller animals.[72] Other studies have not confirmed this association between body weight and survival.[61]

RESPONSE TO THERAPY

Survival times of patients with canine lymphoma are often biased by the veterinarian's and the owner's levels of perseverance in treatment, and most dogs are euthanatized at the owner's request. Response to therapy and quality of life are, therefore, important criteria in prolonging survival. If a dog shows only a partial remission (PR), its survival time is significantly shorter than if it achieved a CR.[12,61,64] Response to therapy is linked to biologic characteristics of lymphoma.

HISTOLOGIC TYPE

Several histologic grading schemes, including the Rappaport system, have shown no correlation between histologic classification and prognosis. *Histiocytic lymphoma* is a little-used term in current pathologic description, and despite anecdotal reports of poor prognosis associated with this type of lymphoma, there is no statistical evidence for such an association.

Although the Rappaport system was not found to be of prognostic use, a system of histologic classification for canine lymphoma based on the National Cancer Institute's Working Formulation for classification of non-Hodgkin's lymphomas has shown some prognostic significance, as has the Kiel classification system.[53,67] Canine lymphoma is morphologically heterogeneous, almost always diffuse (versus nodular), and usually high grade. Most canine lymphomas seem to fit into three high-grade morphologic groups: diffuse large cell, immunoblastic, and small lymphocytic. It may be possible to grade lymphomas using cytology specimens.[45,73]

Counterintuitively, dogs with high-grade lymphoma are more likely to achieve CR than dogs with intermediate-grade lymphoma, possibly due to a higher proportion of "cycling" cells in the tumor.[67] In addition, remission and survival times are usually longer in dogs with high-grade lymphoma. In two studies, dogs with an immunoblastic cell type had higher CR rates and longer remission duration and survival times.[62–69,72–74] In some studies, however, no differences in remission duration or survival have been noted. There is no correlation between grade or morphologic classification and immunophenotype.[45,49,53]

The lack of repeatability between pathologists for tumor grading, combined with the subjective nature of morphologic classification, has led to tumor grading being considered of less value than immunophenotyping for clinical prognosis in dogs with lymphoma. The one exception may be the finding of "low-grade" lymphoma.

LOW-GRADE LYMPHOMA

Low-grade lymphoma is uncommon in dogs, accounting for approximately 5% to 10% of cases.[53,73] In the few reported cases, response rates have been lower than for high- or intermediate-grade lymphoma, but survival times are often long because of a more indolent clinical course. Some of these dogs have long survival times even when not treated. In one study, dogs with untreated low-grade lymphoma had a median survival time of 5 months compared with 1.3 months in dogs with untreated lymphoma that was not low grade.[70] Argyrophilic nucleolar organizer region (AgNOR) numbers (see Measurement of Tumor Proliferation section, below) may be able to distinguish dogs with low-grade lymphoma.

Most low-grade lymphomas appear to be B-cell derived, but immunophenotyping should be performed. In one study, 19% of T-cell lymphomas were low grade.[71] It is unknown whether dogs with low-grade T-cell lymphoma have a worse prognosis than dogs with low-grade B-cell lymphoma.

MEASUREMENT OF TUMOR PROLIFERATION

AgNORs are present in the nucleus, take up silver stain, and can be used as an indirect measure of cellular proliferation in histopathology or cytopathology specimens.[46] The average number of AgNORs per cell correlates well with tumor grade in histologic and cytologic specimens and, in some studies, appears to be an independent predictor of remission duration and survival, particularly when the mean AgNOR area is measured.[55,70,75] In other studies, AgNOR numbers had no influence on remission duration or survival.[49] AgNOR numbers may be able to distinguish dogs with low-grade lymphoma (see Low-Grade Lymphoma section, above).

Another method of measuring cellular proliferation, immunostaining for Ki67, was found to correlate well with tumor grade for lymphoma.[76] There was correlation between Ki67 and remission duration but not overall survival for 41 dogs in another study.[77] Immunohistochemical staining for Ki67 may be conducted on biopsy specimens.

A third method of measuring cellular proliferation, staining for proliferating cell nuclear antigen (PCNA), has failed to predict survival in dogs with lymphoma.[70,75]

Apoptotic index was predictive of remission duration but not overall survival in one study.[77] The ratio of Ki67 to apoptotic index was the most significant predictor of remission duration.

MULTIDRUG RESISTANCE

Multidrug resistance due to a transmembrane efflux pump protein (gp170) expressed by the *mdr* gene is able to reduce intracellular levels of vinca alkaloids, anthracyclines, and other "naturally" derived chemotherapeutics to non-toxic levels. Two studies have found that if gp170 is detected in pretreatment biopsies, the remission duration and survival times are shorter. Dogs with lymphoma that expressed gp170 lived a median of 7.4 months compared with 12 months if gp170 was not present.[78,79]

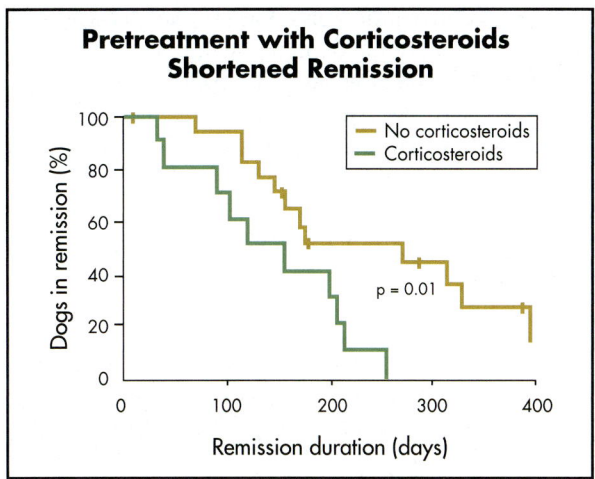

Figure 47-12. Remission duration in dogs with lymphoma treated with combination chemotherapy. Dogs that received corticosteroids before chemotherapy had shorter remission than dogs that did not receive corticosteroids before chemotherapy. (From Price GS, Page RL, Fischer BM, et al: Efficacy and toxicity of doxorubicin/cyclophosphamide maintenance therapy in dogs with multicentric lymphosarcoma. J Vet Intern Med 5:259–262, 1991; with permission)

CHROMOSOMAL ABNORMALITIES

Chromosomal aberrations are frequent in human cancer cells and often correlate with other clinical and histopathologic parameters. One study performed molecular cytogenetic analyses on samples from 25 dogs with lymphoma. Comparative genomic hybridization analysis demonstrated almost twice as many genomic gains as losses. In one study of dogs with lymphoma, gain of chromosome 13 was the most common aberration observed (12 of 25 dogs), followed by gain of chromosome 31 (eight dogs) and loss of chromosome 14 (five dogs).[80]

Although it may seem esoteric, another study showed that dogs with trisomy of chromosome 13 (25% of 61 dogs in that study) had longer remission and survival than did dogs with any other abnormality or parameter.[81] In the future, such testing could be a valuable tool to identify subgroups of dogs with lymphoma that have an excellent prognosis with treatment.

PRETREATMENT STEROID THERAPY

It has been postulated that administration of glucocorticoids before other chemotherapeutic agents may change clinical staging by causing incomplete remission, thereby masking more advanced disease, which is known to be a poor prognostic sign. It is also possible that glucocorticoid therapy may induce multidrug resistance in the malignant cells, as has been observed in human patients.

In two studies, dogs with lymphoma that received glucocorticoids before initiation of combination chemotherapy had significantly shorter remissions and survival times than dogs that did not receive glucocorticoids before treatment.[82,83] Duration of glucocorticoid treatment (>2 weeks versus <2 weeks) did not influence this finding (Figure 47-12).[83]

> **KEY POINT**
> *Glucocorticoids should not be given to dogs with lymphoma if future combination chemotherapy is planned.*

SPLENIC LYMPHOMA

Occasionally, the spleen will be the only site of lymphoma. The prognosis for diffuse involvement is worse than that for a single nodular lesion. One study showed that median survival for 13 dogs with diffuse splenic lymphoma was 1 month compared with 8 months for seven dogs with a solitary lymphoma nodule; only three of the 20 dogs received any chemotherapy.[84]

HYPOALBUMINEMIA

Hypoalbuminemia (albumin <2.8 g/dL) that was present before initiation of chemotherapy was a poor prognostic sign in one study[83]; hypoalbuminemic dogs had a mean remission time of 3.5 months compared with 7 months for dogs with normal serum albumin. The cause of the low serum albumin was not investigated, although no dogs had proteinuria. Other studies have not confirmed this prognostic association.

TREATMENT TOXICITY

Dogs that developed GI toxicity had shorter survival times in one study.[58] In another study, dogs that had a dose reduction in any chemotherapy because of toxicity had longer survival times: 65 dogs that had a dose reduction had a median survival of 13 months; 54% were alive 1 year after treatment. In contrast, 28 dogs that did not need a dose reduction had a median survival of 4 months, and only 14% were alive 1 year after treatment.[39] This is presumably because the dogs that experienced toxicity were being treated at or near their maximally tolerated dose of chemotherapy; it may be similar to the effect of weight, in which small dogs may have longer survival. This effect has been exploited by increasing dose intensity of chemotherapeutic drugs and providing supportive procedures to offset toxicity.

Only one study has examined which prognostic factors determine whether a dog develops toxicity.[39] Dogs with B-cell phenotype were significantly more likely to require a dose reduction of one or more drugs than dogs with T-cell phenotype, with the exception of doxorubicin, for which T-cell dogs were significantly more likely to require a dose reduction. Older dogs were significantly more likely to require a dose reduction of vincristine than younger dogs. Lighter dogs were significantly more likely to require cyclophosphamide dose reduction.

SEX

Some studies have found that female dogs, both sexually intact and spayed, had significantly longer remission and survival times than male dogs.[27,61] Regardless of disease, female dogs have a longer age-adjusted overall survival than their male counterparts.[2] This is particularly important in evaluating the reported prognostic value of sex on response to chemotherapy in dogs with lymphoma.

Treatment
DISCUSSION WITH THE CLIENT

Once a definitive diagnosis has been obtained and the patient has been staged accurately, the veterinarian should schedule a discussion with the owner regarding prognosis and treatment. This consultation should allow enough time to discuss the chances and length of remission and survival balanced against costs, time required for therapy, and side effects. The primary emphasis of all discussions should center on methods to enhance the patient's quality of life. One of the most important distinctions to make for the client is between remission and cure. Remission is the absence of clinical evidence of lymphoma, whereas cure really only becomes a reality when remission has been sustained for more than 2 years.

When toxicities are discussed, the owner should be given criteria by which to distinguish mild side effects from those that can be life threatening. Preventing toxicities is essential. The goal should be to have no toxicities related to drug therapy or lymphoma. This can be accomplished by educating the client in oral and written form about the potential toxicities and dispensing metoclopramide and, in some cases, tylosin (a macrolide antibiotic) to reduce nausea and diarrhea, respectively. When metoclopramide is inadequate to prevent nausea, serotonin antagonists such as ondansetron or dolasetron are excellent antinausea drugs, especially when combined with metoclopramide. Any dietary changes must be done slowly to reduce adverse dietary-induced GI problems. Emphasis should be placed on a diet that is relatively low in simple carbohydrates, has moderate amounts of proteins, and has enhanced quantities of polyunsaturated fatty acids of the n-3 series (see Chapter 31 for more information on nutritional support.) A copy of the protocol to be administered, with scheduled treatments, rechecks, and blood counts, will assist caregivers in remembering much of the information they receive at this time. Well-informed owners whose pets are receiving chemotherapy are reliable, cooperative, and appreciative of a veterinarian's efforts.

The major concern that caregivers voice during initial discussions about chemotherapy is their fear that the quality of their dog's life will be compromised by toxicity. Despite lymphoma being a very common disease that is widely treated, and despite numerous publications evaluating the toxicity of individual protocols, few data have been published regarding caregivers' assessments of quality of life during chemotherapy. One report detailed results of a small survey of 25 dog owners whose pets had lived a median of 8 months during treatment of lymphoma. Approximately half the clients reported no toxicity attributable to chemotherapy. Only one client would not pursue chemotherapy again with a pet and regretted the decision to treat.[85]

A common question from clients is whether to continue to vaccinate dogs that are undergoing chemotherapy. One concern is whether dogs that are immunosuppressed by lymphoma and chemotherapy are able to maintain a titer to distemper, parvovirus, and rabies. In one study, protective titers were found in all dogs before and during chemotherapy[86]; another preliminary study showed that dogs treated for lymphoma could mount an antibody response and had no decrease in CD4, CD8, or CD5 lymphocyte numbers.[87]

Whether to vaccinate during chemotherapy is less clear; many oncologists believe that vaccination could have the effect of altering growth patterns in lymphoma cells. This concern, combined with recent evidence that vaccination need not be done annually, leads us to recommend delaying vaccination during treatment for lymphoma.

TREATING LYMPHOMA IN PRACTICE

A survey of 382 small animal practitioners in the United Kingdom found that 87% treated more than half the cases of lymphoma that they diagnosed. Most used a protocol based on cyclophosphamide, vincristine, and prednisone (COP; see Combination Protocols with Maintenance Therapy section, below); the remainder used prednisolone alone. Only 2% used doxorubicin as first-line therapy for lymphoma, although 12% used it as a rescue agent, often in multidrug protocols.[88] There are no data from the United States.

> **KEY POINT**
>
> *If a dog with lymphoma is neutropenic, nonmyelosuppressive chemotherapeutic agents should be used, such as prednisone, vincristine, and L-asparaginase.*

Our recommendations are tiered and are found at the end of this section on treatment. In brief, palliative therapy would be corticosteroids; a low-cost, low-toxicity protocol would be COP or doxorubicin alone; treatment with potential curative intent would be five-drug protocols (COP plus doxorubicin and L-asparaginase), such as the "short" versions of VELCAP and Wisconsin protocols; and advanced therapy would be a five-drug protocol with consolidation using radiation therapy or autologous bone marrow transplantation. Details of each of these protocols are given below.

MONITORING REMISSION

Most monitoring of remission is done clinically (i.e., by physical examination and sometimes imaging such as radiography and ultrasonography). Two simple blood tests that normalize when remission is achieved and may detect early relapse have been evaluated in two small studies. In one study, serum $\alpha 1$-acid glycoprotein (AGP) was elevated before treatment in 12 dogs but reduced to normal levels when chemotherapy induced remission. Elevations in serum AGP levels preceded clinical relapse by 3 weeks.[89] Serum AGP levels were not evaluated prognostically. The second study monitored thymidine kinase (TK) activity, which reflects DNA synthesis. Serum TK may rise when replicating cells die and release the enzyme into the blood. In the second study, serum levels of TK had a normal upper limit of 7 U/L; 24 dogs with lymphoma that had a serum TK of >30 U/L had a median survival of 1 month compared with 9 months for 20 dogs with a serum TK <30 U/L.[90] Significantly, serum TK levels appeared to decrease during remission and to rise about 3 weeks before clinical relapse was recognized. Unfortunately, it is unclear whether the prognostic value of this test is independent of other established criteria.

MULTIDRUG RESISTANCE

Chemotherapeutic drugs act by many mechanisms. Resistance to individual drugs may be caused by cellular factors (e.g., altered target) or host factors (e.g., antibody formation to L-asparaginase). Cross-resistance between different classes of agents is a serious threat to successful treatment using combination chemotherapy. In particular, the *mdr* pump protein, gp170, is able to reduce intracellular levels of vinca alkaloids, anthracyclines, and other naturally derived chemotherapeutics to nontoxic levels. Because these drugs are often used in the treatment of lymphoma, it is wise to not overly rely on them in the "rescue" setting but rather to use them in combination in first-line therapy.

Studies have shown that levels of gp170 are low at the outset of chemotherapy for canine lymphoma but increase in approximately 75% of cases after chemotherapy is instituted.[78,79,91] In addition, pretreatment identification of multidrug resistance confers a worse prognosis for remission length and survival.[78,79] Interestingly, drugs classified as alkylating agents are not susceptible to resistance mechanisms. There is very little cross-resistance even between different alkylating agents. This may explain the success of the strategy of using alkylating agents as rescue therapy for animals with lym-

Table 47-4 **Stages of a Combination Treatment Protocol**

Treatment	Description	Toxicity	Response	Example
Induction	Intensely scheduled initial treatment	Higher risk	Greatest chance of response	First 12 weeks of VELCAP-SC; first 9 weeks of Wisconsin protocol
Consolidation	Unrelated, effective drugs after induction	Moderate risk	Further reduces surviving cancer cells	MOPP; lomustine in VELCAP-SC
Maintenance	Less-intense course; induction drugs	Lower risk	Slows time to relapse; may not affect cure	Decreased administration frequency
Rescue	Unrelated drugs used upon relapse after first 3 treatment phases	Moderate to higher risk	Lower chance of response	Alkylating agents often used for less cross-resistance

phoma. It is also possible that the use of alkylating agents in combination with drugs that are susceptible to gp170 during the early phases of treatment (induction) may slow the onset of resistance. Trials of agents that competitively "block" gp170 have not yet led to practical veterinary treatment strategies.

First-Line Therapy

In this chapter, *first-line therapy* pertains to drugs and protocols used to induce remission in animals that have received no previous therapy. *Rescue therapy*, discussed below, details drugs and protocols used to reinduce remission when lymphoma relapses during treatment with chemotherapy. Dogs with lymphoma that come out of remission during chemotherapy are generally more difficult to induce into a subsequent remission, and the duration of the subsequent remission is generally shorter than the previous remission.

Table 47-4 outlines the stages of a protocol used as chemotherapy treatment of a dog with lymphoma.

Combination chemotherapy has two major aims. The first is to slow the onset of drug resistance in tumor cells. As indicated above, the use of agents with different targets and mechanisms of action is most likely to provide long-term tumor control. In particular, the use of alkylating agents may slow the development of multidrug resistance (e.g., adding either cyclophosphamide or MOPP [see Combination Rescue Chemotherapy section, below]), to a chemotherapy protocol for lymphoma rather than using doxorubicin alone). The second aim of combination chemotherapy is to maximize tumor cell kill while minimizing toxicity and enhancing quality of life. Combinations that include myelosuppressive drugs and drugs that are minimally myelosuppressive (e.g., cyclophosphamide–vincristine, doxorubicin–cisplatin) may fulfill this aim. It is important that combinations be made of effective drugs; there is little utility in using a nontoxic combination when one drug has not been shown to be efficacious against the tumor type. Combinations, therefore, use drugs that have shown activity as single agents.

Some combinations may result in altered toxicity due to changes in the way a drug is metabolized or excreted. For example, L-asparaginase is thought to slow hepatic metabolism of drugs such as vincristine and doxorubicin, thereby increasing the risk of myelosuppression. Only combinations for which published efficacy and toxicity data are available should be used.

SINGLE-AGENT CHEMOTHERAPY

Vincristine, cyclophosphamide, and prednisone are the basis for most combination protocols to treat canine lymphoma, but surprisingly little information exists as to their efficacy as single agents. The results of studies using these and other drugs as single agents are summarized in Table 47-5.

Prednisone: Approximately 50% of dogs treated with prednisone have a PR or CR[92,101,102]; this response usually lasts between 14 and 240 days (average: 53 days).[65,92,101]

Cyclophosphamide: Cyclophosphamide is probably more effective than prednisone as a single agent. More CRs occur, with a median of 165 days.[92] The response rate appears to be dose related. In one early study, successful treatment with cyclophosphamide was hindered by high-dosage regimens (240 mg/m^2 PO for 5 consecutive days) that resulted in mortality due to bone marrow aplasia.[103] Lower doses given in combination with prednisone produced a response rate similar to that of prednisone alone.[65]

Vincristine: Vincristine was found in one study to be more efficacious and less toxic than vinblastine (which is myelosuppressive) in treating canine lymphoma[104]; however, no studies comparing vincristine with other single chemotherapeutic agents have been reported in detail.

Chlorambucil: This alkylating agent was not as successful as cyclophosphamide in causing remission, even when used in conjunction with prednisone.[92] The major clinical use of chlorambucil is as a substitute for cyclophosphamide if animals develop hemorrhagic cystitis.

L-Asparaginase: This agent has been used widely in the treatment of canine lymphoma because of its low rate of toxi-

Table 47-5 Canine Lymphoma Treatment with Single Agents

Drug	Number of Dogs in CR	Total Dogs Treated	Percentage in CR (%)	Remission Range (Months)	Study
Prednisone	26	57	46	0.5–7	Squire et al,[65] Brick et al[92]
Cyclophosphamide	17	30	57	2–3.5	Brick et al,[92] McClelland[93]
Chlorambucil	2	9	22	?–20	Brick et al[92]
Vincristine	—	—	—	<2	Theilen et al[63]
Vinblastine	5	8	63	1–6	Engstrom et al[94]
Methotrexate	1	3	33	—	Engstrom et al[94]
L-Asparaginase	26	134	19	—	MacEwen et al,[95] Teske et al[96]
Mitoxantrone	10	40	25	2–14	Moore et al[97]
Cytarabine	0	10	0	—	Ruslander et al[98]
Epirubicin	26	37	70	—	Hahn and Hahn[99]
9-Aminocamptothecin	1	10	10	—	Moore et al[100]

city. Although the CR rate is low when it is used as a single agent, most dogs show a PR with L-asparaginase; therefore, it is a useful addition to combination protocols.[95,96] L-Asparaginase and vincristine, when used in combination, cause severe myelosuppression (<1,000 segmented neutrophils/μl) in 18% of canine patients; this is presumably due to decreased hepatic clearance of the vincristine. If both drugs are to be used, some oncologists separate their administration by at least 24 hours.[61,105] A study that compared myelosuppression in dogs that received the two drugs together found no significant difference in the risk of neutropenia, regardless of whether the drugs were given at the same time or at an interval of 6, 18, or 24 hours.[106] Because individual dogs may be predisposed to myelosuppression, and because there are no predicting factors, it may be wise to administer prophylactic antibiotics when L-asparaginase and vincristine are combined in a protocol.

The most common toxicity of L-asparaginase is hypersensitivity (anaphylaxis). The covalent attachment of polyethylene glycol (PEG) conjugates to L-asparaginase produces a compound that is active, stable, and without significant immune response and has a greatly extended plasma half-life. Trials comparing "native" L-asparaginase with PEG-conjugated L-asparaginase in dogs demonstrated no differences in response rate, time to relapse, or overall survival between the two groups.[95,96] Adverse (allergic) reactions were uncommon in both groups; this was attributed to the intramuscular route of administration (compared with intraperitoneal or intravenous routes, which produce a 20% to 47% adverse reaction rate).[66,96,107,108] A recent study found a moderate reduction in time to response, duration of response, and survival when L-asparaginase was given subcutaneously compared with intramuscularly.[109] L-Asparaginase should be given intramuscularly to dogs.

The use of L-asparaginase in combination protocols is controversial. All published studies have shown better remission rates and remission duration and survival times if L-asparaginase is used, but with the exception of remission rates,[60] statistics have not upheld the differences to be significant. This has led some oncologists to suggest that the use of L-asparaginase is not warranted. Most protocols use L-asparaginase in the induction phase only; this may not be the best use of this drug. In two protocols that used L-asparaginase in the maintenance phase, 1- and 2-year survival rates were high (48%–53% and 23%–26%, respectively), but without randomized trials, statistical proof is lacking.[11,82] The drug was administered subcutaneously in these protocols, which has been shown to be inferior to intramuscular administration.

Our stance is that L-asparaginase should be used in combination protocols, but the use of multiple doses, preferably in the maintenance phase as well as during induction, is encouraged.

Doxorubicin: Doxorubicin is considered the most active single agent in the treatment of canine lymphoma, and protocols that contain doxorubicin are considered superior to those that do not. Doxorubicin was reported to be successful as a rescue agent (to reinduce clinical remission when the tumor was resistant to chemotherapy).[110] The response rates and durations in studies using doxorubicin as a single induction agent are found in Table 47-6. Overall, doxorubicin causes CR in about 70% of dogs treated, for a median of 165 days.

Table 47-6 Canine Lymphoma Treatment with Doxorubicin

Number of Dogs in CR	Total Dogs Treated	Percentage in CR (%)	Remission (Months) Median	Remission (Months) Range	Study
28	38	74	6	—	Vonderhaar et al[111]
7	11	64	4	0.7–7.2	Gray et al[112]
22	37	59	5	1.5–24	Postorino et al[113]
16	21	76	6.8	—	Carter et al[67]
18	38	47	1.2	—	Hahn et al[74]
31	42	74	4.8	4–7.2	Mutsaers et al[114]
84	121[a]	69	4.3	0–27.6	Valerius et al[60]

[a]43 also received L-asparaginase weekly for the first 3 weeks of induction.

Toxicities are relatively common in dogs treated with doxorubicin at a dose of 30 mg/m^2, but they are usually mild and well tolerated by dogs and their owners. Of 37 dogs with lymphoma treated with doxorubicin in one study, toxicities occurred in 21 dogs (five anaphylaxis, three cardiomyopathy, nine GI, and four hematologic) and were mild in most dogs. Large dogs apparently were at greater risk of developing cardiomyopathy, whereas smaller dogs were more likely to develop other toxicities.[113]

The standard dose of doxorubicin in dogs is 30 mg/m^2 every 3 weeks, but there is evidence that weekly administration of a lower dose decreases the prevalence of cardiotoxicity in humans. Nine dogs with lymphoma were treated with 15 weekly treatments of doxorubicin at a dose of 10 mg/m^2 in one study.[115] This protocol was found to be safe but was generally ineffective in achieving remission rates comparable with those provided by the standard protocol. Of nine dogs, two had a CR (for 14 and 231 days) and five had a PR. Median remission duration was 14 days. Mild toxicosis was seen in three dogs.

> **KEY POINT**
>
> *Doxorubicin is considered the most active single agent in the treatment of canine lymphoma.*

Mitoxantrone: When this drug was given as a single agent at a dose of 5 mg/m^2 IV to 40 dogs with untreated lymphoma, it induced a CR rate of 25% (10 dogs), with a median remission duration of 94 days (range: 49–440 days).[97] A dose of 6.0 mg/m^2 is more appropriate in dogs.[116]

Mitoxantrone was delivered as a 1-hour IV infusion at a dose of 5 to 6.5 mg/m^2 every 3 weeks to 30 dogs with lymphoma. Toxicities were similar to those described for mitoxantrone given as a bolus injection.[117]

Cytarabine (cytosine arabinoside, ara-C): Cytarabine used alone at various doses and schedules was not found to be a useful induction agent in one early study.[104] This was supported by a more recent trial in which 15 dogs with lymphoma received cytarabine (300 mg/m^2 continuous IV infusion for 2 consecutive days) as an induction agent.[98] No dog responded to this treatment, and there was evidence of myelosuppression (principally thrombocytopenia) in 10 of 15 dogs. Although the use of cytarabine has been recommended in combination protocols, its efficacy must be questioned, and although cytarabine may be more effective in combination with alkylating agents, such as cyclophosphamide, care should be used in such combination protocols.[98]

Epirubicin: This derivative of doxorubicin has equivalent antitumor activity to doxorubicin in the treatment of human cancer but puts patients at considerably less risk of cardiotoxicity. It is not currently available for the treatment of canine lymphoma. However, it has been compared with doxorubicin for efficacy in the treatment of canine lymphoma.[99] Dogs were given six treatments of 30 mg/m^2 IV doxorubicin or epirubicin at 3-week intervals. With doxorubicin, 74% of 38 dogs achieved CR, whereas with epirubicin, 70% of 37 dogs achieved CR. The median duration of remission was 180 and 143 days for doxorubicin and epirubicin, respectively.

Dactinomycin (actinomycin D): At a weekly dose of 0.75 mg/m^2 IV, dactinomycin caused remission in three of four dogs with lymphoma.[94] In a more recent study, dactinomycin (0.5–0.9 mg/m^2 IV every 3 weeks) was used to treat 12 dogs with lymphoma.[118] CR was seen in five dogs for a median duration of 63 days (range: 21–105 days). Three of the 12 dogs had not received previous treatment and had either a CR (84, 63 days) or a PR (42 days). Efficacy of dactinomycin as a single induction agent is still uncertain.

In a randomized trial, dogs received combination chemotherapy that included either doxorubicin (30 mg/m^2) or

COP Protocol

Vincristine is administered at 0.75 mg/m² IV. Cyclophosphamide[a] is given at 250 mg/m² PO or 200 mg/m² IV. The dose for prednisone is 1 mg/kg daily for 7 days, then PO every other day.

Week	Vincristine	Cyclophosphamide[a]	Prednisone
1	•	•	
2	•		
3	•		
4	•	•	
5			
6			
7	•	•	
10	•	•	
	⇓	⇓	↓

Repeat week 10 treatment every 3 weeks

[a]If hemorrhagic cystitis occurs, chlorambucil is substituted on the same schedule at 15 mg/m² PO daily for 4 consecutive days (or 6 to 8 mg/m² PO daily continuously).

Alternative COP Protocol

Vincristine is administered at 0.5 mg/m² IV. Cyclophosphamide[a] is given at 50 mg/m² PO daily for 4 consecutive days. The dose of prednisone is 10 mg/m² PO bid for 7 days, then 10 mg/m² daily.

Week	Vincristine	Cyclophosphamide[a]	Prednisone
1	•	•	
2	•	•	
3	•	•	
4	•	•	
5	•	•	
6	•	•	
7	•	•	
8	•	•	
	⇓	⇓	↓

The cycle is repeated to week 8, then repeated every 2 weeks to week 24, then every 3 weeks to week 48, and finally every 4 weeks.
[a]Chlorambucil 2 mg/m² PO is substituted on the same schedule from week 8.

dactinomycin (0.75 mg/m²).[119] While the remission rate was the same, dogs that received doxorubicin had a longer remission duration and survival, with no difference in toxicity. Dactinomycin is not an acceptable substitute for doxorubicin.

9-Aminocamptothecin (9-AC): The type-I topoisomerase inhibitor 9-aminocamptothecin was given as a 72-hour IV infusion to 10 dogs with untreated lymphoma at a dose of 3.35 to 3.69 mg/m² and caused objective responses in all dogs (one CR and nine PRs). The median remission was 3 months.[100]

Vinblastine: Vinblastine given at a weekly dose of 1.5 mg/m² IV resulted in objective responses in five of eight dogs. Remissions lasted 1 to 6 months.[94]

Methotrexate: At a weekly dose of 30 mg/m², methotrexate resulted in an objective response in one of three dogs.[94] GI toxicity is commonly encountered during treatment with methotrexate.

Mercaptopurine (6-mercaptopurine, 6-MP): This drug was not found to be a useful induction agent in the treatment of canine lymphoma.[104]

Carmustine (BCNU): This alkylating agent was given as a substitute for cyclophosphamide in the COP protocol (see Combination Protocols with Maintenance Therapy section, below) at a dosage of 50 mg/m² given in 150 ml of saline over 30 to 40 minutes every 6 weeks. Myelosuppression was the main side effect, with <1,000/μl segmented neutrophils seen following 37% of treatments; however, the combination appeared very effective, causing CR in six of seven dogs.[120]

COMBINATION PROTOCOLS WITH MAINTENANCE THERAPY

COP protocol: Much of the information regarding efficacy of treatment for canine lymphoma has come from studies using combinations of cyclophosphamide, vincristine (Oncovin, Eli Lilly), and prednisone. This combination, known colloquially as COP, forms the foundation for most currently used chemotherapy protocols.

COP is a relatively nontoxic protocol and is relatively inexpensive. Its efficacy has been evaluated in seven published reports with minor variations in dosage and schedule. A brief summary of these studies is included in Table 47-7, and the two most commonly used COP protocols are schematically represented in the boxes on this page. The two illustrated protocols appear equal in efficacy, and the choice between them is solely one of familiarity and comfort. Overall, COP chemotherapy causes complete remission in about 70% of dogs with lymphoma for a median of 4.3 months.

COP, L-asparaginase, and methotrexate: Methotrexate is not widely used as a single agent in treating canine lymphoma; however, it does have some role in combination with other drugs for maintenance of remission. In one study, 147 dogs with lymphoma were treated with vincristine, L-asparaginase, cyclophosphamide, and methotrexate.[61] CR was achieved in 77% of the dogs, and PR was seen in 17.7%. For dogs with CR, the median remission duration was 4.6 months and the median survival was 9.5 months. A similar protocol in which L-asparaginase was given more frequently during induction did not improve either remission duration or survival, although a higher proportion of dogs appeared to enter CR.[66]

COP and cytarabine (COAP): Cytarabine recently has been shown to be ineffective as a single induction agent[98]; however, reported synergy with alkylating agents has been the basis for including it with COP.[121] This synergy has not been marked in reported studies in which cytarabine at a dose of

Table 47-7 Canine Lymphoma Treatment with Cyclophosphamide, Vincristine, and Prednisone (COP)

Number of Dogs in CR	Total Dogs Treated	Percentage in CR (%)	Remission (Months)			Study
			Mean	Median	Range	
15	19	79	6	—	1–9.3	Squire et al[65]
13	20	65	3.5	3	1.5–21	Madewell[121]
58	77	75	—	6	—	Cotter[64]
20	30	67	—	—	—	Squire and Bush[104]
14	20	70	3.3	4.2	—	Carter et al[67]
36	67	54	—	1.5	—	Hahn et al[74]

100 mg/m² IV for the first 4 days of the first week was added to the COP protocol. CR occurred in 67% of dogs, which was essentially the same response rate seen for the protocol without cytarabine.[63] Response duration was evaluated in another study and was 6 months; median survival was 8 months.[12]

Vincristine, cyclophosphamide, prednisone, and doxorubicin (COPA): The exceptional efficacy of doxorubicin as an induction agent led to two studies using doxorubicin in combination with vincristine, cyclophosphamide, and prednisone.[122,123] In one study, doxorubicin was used for the maintenance of remission induced by COP.[122] Surprisingly, overall remission durations and survival did not differ greatly from those seen with the COP protocol; however, it is possible that the scheduling of doxorubicin in only the maintenance phase of the protocol influenced the outcome.

In two studies comparing COP, COAP or COP plus L-asparaginase, and COP plus doxorubicin, more dogs achieved remission and remission lasted longer if doxorubicin was administered.[58,123] Overall survival times did not differ.

In a recent preliminary report, the same four drugs were given sequentially (rather than in combinations) as the PVAC protocol, and the efficacy was markedly reduced.[124]

Vincristine, cyclophosphamide, prednisone, doxorubicin, and L-asparaginase combination protocols: A maintenance schedule of COP and doxorubicin[122] was given to 41 dogs that were induced into remission using weekly doses of a combination of vincristine, L-asparaginase, and prednisone (ACOPA-1).[105] CR was attained in 31 dogs (76%) for a median of 330 days; 48% were still in remission at 1 year. This group of dogs had longer remission times both overall and for dogs in clinical stage III than did dogs receiving COPA.[122] Toxicity of this protocol was most marked during the induction phase; five dogs (12%) died during this period.[105] Myelosuppression was marked during induction and was somewhat unexpected because the three induction drugs are not considered potent myelosuppressive agents. L-Asparaginase, however, decreases hepatic clearance of vincristine, leading to more pronounced myelosuppression. It is advisable to use prophylactic antibiotics when administering L-asparaginase and vincristine together (see L-Asparaginase section, above).

A similar protocol (ACOPA-2) used doxorubicin and prednisone for induction of remission and had a similar maintenance phase. ACOPA-2 was found to induce fewer dogs into remission than ACOPA-1 (44 dogs, 65%), and the dogs that achieved remission had a shorter median remission time (228 days; 34% still in remission at 1 year). ACOPA-2 had a lower rate of induction toxicity than did ACOPA-1.[125] These data imply that an aggressive induction is important for long-term remission.

A sequential chemotherapy protocol that used vincristine and cyclophosphamide in combination with L-asparaginase, doxorubicin, and prednisone for induction of remission and in combination with methotrexate for maintenance of remission was used in 55 dogs. CR was achieved in 46 dogs (84%) for a median of 252 days. Survival 1 year after starting chemotherapy was 52%. Toxicities that required dose reduction occurred in 40% of dogs.[27]

In a further study that used a protocol with these same five drugs, 75 dogs with high- and intermediate-grade lymphoma had an 80% CR rate and 12% PR rate with a median remission of 6 months; 17% were in remission at 1 year and 5% at 2 years.[126]

A five-drug combination chemotherapy regimen (VEL-CAP-L) was used in 98 dogs (see the VELCAP-L Protocol box on page 347). The CR rate was 69%, with a median remission duration of 12.7 months. Dogs that had advanced stage of disease, were in substage b, were older, or were dyspneic were less likely to achieve remission. Small dogs and dogs without pretreatment thrombocytopenia were likely to have longer remission duration. Toxicities were frequent but rarely fatal, and there were no predictive factors for a dog developing toxicity.[11] VELCAP-L is an effective treatment for dogs with stage I to III lymphoma, particularly in young, small animals.

SHORT-TERM COMBINATION PROTOCOLS (DISCONTINUOUS THERAPY)

Combination chemotherapy is a successful treatment strategy for canine lymphoma. Protocols using the five most active drugs (doxorubicin, vincristine, cyclophosphamide, L-asparaginase, and prednisone) with an extended maintenance phase provide high response rates and remission durations of 12 months or more. Despite differences in the details of these protocols, their overall effectiveness does not vary greatly, and it is unlikely that further minor manipulations in scheduling will provide major advances in response rate or duration.

Because palliation, rather than cure, is a major goal of chemotherapy in veterinary oncology, there has been recent interest in developing protocols that reduce the number of patient visits as well as cost and toxicity of treatment. The use of short-term chemotherapy given in pulse doses provides similar remission durations to long-term maintenance chemotherapy. Therefore, these short-term protocols are generally recommended over the longer-term variants.

In one such study, 82 dogs with lymphoma received a single 15-week course of chemotherapy and then no treatment until relapse.[10] This protocol, VELCAP-S, uses the first 12 weeks of the VELCAP-L protocol, after which corticosteroids are "weaned" to 15 weeks. At relapse, reinduction followed by maintenance chemotherapy (VELCAP-L) is used. In the study, 56 dogs (68%) achieved CR for a median first remission duration of 5 months. Of 48 dogs that relapsed, 30 repeated the induction cycle. First remission was short in 22 of these dogs, and they received maintenance chemotherapy after the induction cycle; the other eight dogs received two or three courses of induction chemotherapy. The second remission rate for all 30 dogs was 87% (26 dogs). Overall disease control in the 38 dogs that remained on protocol lasted 11 months, which was not significantly shorter than dogs treated with VELCAP-L. There was a correlation between first remission duration and the length of any subsequent remission. The incidence of toxicity was high, particularly after the combination of doxorubicin and vincristine; however, dose reductions because of toxicity did not significantly reduce remission duration. The authors concluded that discontinuous chemotherapy results in long-term disease control in a small number of patients and may therefore reduce patient visits. Delaying maintenance chemotherapy until after second remission is achieved does not significantly affect overall disease control.

A similar study that used a 25-week induction (Wisconsin protocol) had a high remission rate, and the median first remission length was longer than that with VELCAP-S (9 months).[59] The longer remission was probably due to the greater length of the protocol and to measurement of remission from first chemotherapy rather than from when remission was achieved, not to any inherent superiority of the protocol. As was seen with VELCAP-S, the second remission rate was also high. This protocol is described in the Wisconsin Protocol box on page 348.

Regardless of whether VELCAP-S or the Wisconsin protocol was used, most dogs relapsed between 3 and 4 months after stopping chemotherapy. A few dogs (10% to 15%) did not relapse. The advantage of discontinuous chemotherapy is most pronounced for these dogs. Dogs that are "cured" may be identified by using discontinuous therapy, and those that relapse have a chemotherapy "break" but reattain remission when chemotherapy is restarted. For the latter dogs, maintenance therapy after achieving a second remission is strongly recommended.

VELCAP-L Protocol[11]

An example of a protocol with a prolonged maintenance phase. The short-term version is described below.

Vincristine is administered at 0.75 mg/m² IV. Cyclophosphamide* is given at 250 mg/m² PO. The dose for L-asparaginase is 10,000 IU/m² IM (maximum treatment dose = 10,000 IU). Doxorubicin† is administered at 25 mg/m² IV. Prednisone is given at 40 mg/m² PO sid for 7 days, then every other day.

Week	Vincristine	Cyclophosphamide*	L-Asparaginase	Doxorubicin†
1	•			
2	•			•
3	•			
4				•
5				
6				
7	•	•	•	
8			•	
9			•	
12	•	•		
15	•	•		
18	•			•
21	•	•		
24		•	•	
25			•	
27	•			•

From week 28, repeat weeks 12 to 18 every 9 weeks until week 75, then stop.
*If hemorrhagic cystitis occurs, chlorambucil is substituted on the same schedule at 15 mg/m² PO daily for 4 consecutive days (or 6 to 8 mg/m² PO daily continuously).
†Echocardiograms are performed before each doxorubicin administration starting at sixth treatment.

The short-term VELCAP-S protocol uses the same first 12 weeks of the VELCAP-L protocol, and then treatment is ceased until relapse, at which time VELCAP-L is started.

Wisconsin Protocol[59]

Another example of a short-term protocol without a prolonged maintenance phase.

Vincristine is administered at 0.5 to 0.7 mg/m² IV. L-Asparaginase is given at 400 IU/kg IM. The dose of cyclophosphamide[a] is 200 mg/m² IV. Doxorubicin is administered at 30 mg/m² IV. The dose of prednisone is 2.0 mg/kg PO, week 1; 1.5 mg/kg PO, week 2; 1.0 mg/kg PO, week 3; and 0.5 mg/kg PO, week 4.

Week	Vincristine	L-Asparaginase	Cyclophosphamide[a]	Doxorubicin	Prednisone
1	•	•			•
2			•		•
3	•				•
4				•	•
5					
6	•				
7			•		
8	•				
9				•	
11	•				
13			•		
14	•				
17				•	
19	•				
21			•		
23	•				
25				•	

[a]Replace cyclophosphamide with chlorambucil 1.4 mg/kg PO from week 11 if dog is in CR.

Tufts VELCAP-SC Protocol[39]

Vincristine (0.75 mg/m² IV; 0.5 mg/m² IV on weeks 3 and 4), cyclophosphamide (200 mg/m² IV with furosemide 1–2 mg/kg IV), L-asparaginase (10,000 IU/m² IM; maximum treatment dose = 10,000 IU), doxorubicin (30 mg/m² IV), and prednisone (40 mg/m² PO sid for 14 days (1), then every other day for 7 days (2), then halved every week until stopped (3 and 4). Mechlorethamine (3.0 mg/m² IV) and procarbazine (50 mg/m² PO daily for 7 days). If mechlorethamine is not available, substitute dactinomycin at 0.5 mg/m² IV. The dose of CCNU is 90 mg/m² PO. CBCs are conducted at weeks 2, 4, 6, 8, 14, 18, and 21.

Week	Vincristine	L-Asparaginase	Cyclophosphamide[a] / Furosemide	Doxorubicin	Mechlorethamine / Procarbazine	CCNU	Prednisone
1		•					•1
2	•						•1
3				•			•2
4		•					•3
5	•		•				•4
6							
7				•			
8	•						
9	•		•				
11				•			
13	•				•		•
14	•				•		•
17						•	
20						•	

[a]Dogs that are considered to be in substage b should be hospitalized and treated supportively for the first 4 to 7 days of their treatment protocol. During this time, they should receive IV crystalloid fluids at a maintenance or higher rate as well as prophylactic cefazolin sodium and metoclopramide IV.

COMBINATION PROTOCOLS WITH ALKYLATING AGENT CONSOLIDATION

Combination chemotherapy with a long-term maintenance phase[11,125,126] and discontinuous chemotherapy[10] are the most commonly described protocols for treating dogs with lymphoma. Consolidation is a third treatment strategy used in regimens to treat human patients with lymphomas and leukemias. Consolidation therapy is administered to patients in CR after the induction phase. It may consist of treatment regimens similar to induction therapy, higher doses of active agents with hematologic support, radiation therapy, or the introduction of new drug combinations.

A protocol using a consolidation phase of alkylating agents was administered to 94 dogs with lymphoma (see the Tufts VELCAP-SC Protocol box on page 348).[39] Most dogs (57%) were stage V, 63% were in substage b, and 31% had T-cell lymphoma. The CR rate was 70%, which compares favorably with that of other protocols. The finding of pretreatment anorexia predicted remission. Of 40 dogs without anorexia, 35 (88%) achieved CR; of 52 dogs with anorexia, 30 (58%) achieved CR. Median duration of first CR was 168 days, and the CR rate at 1 and 2 years was 17.4% and 15.5%, respectively. Low platelet count had a significant negative effect on the length of the first CR. Median survival was 302 days. One- and 2-year survival rates were 44% and 13%, respectively. Anorexia and no dose reduction of any drug were independent negative variables. Of 93 dogs, 65 dogs (70%) required a dose reduction. Cyclophosphamide was the drug that most commonly required reduction (31 of 82 dogs; 38%). A dose reduction was significantly more likely in dogs with B-cell lymphoma than in those with T-cell lymphoma.

This protocol was compared with another series of dogs for which immunophenotype was known; the second series was treated at the same institution but received only a COPA-style protocol for 15 weeks. The results are in Table 47-8. It is clear that more intensive treatment, particularly treatment that includes consolidation, improves long-term prognosis for dogs with lymphoma. Furthermore, alkylating agents may have a greater effect on T-cell lymphoma than conventional "five-drug" combinations.

COMBINATION PROTOCOLS WITH RADIATION THERAPY

A clinical technique using half-body irradiation has been reported; half the body receives 7 Gy of megavoltage radiation, and the other half is irradiated 28 days later. This technique has toxicities that are difficult to justify. Acute radiation sickness was seen in eight normal dogs when they received caudal irradiation.[127] The second treatment, regardless of anatomy, was more likely to cause bone marrow toxicity, and platelets were more affected. Pneumonitis was common, and there was permanent bone marrow atrophy (cellularity less than 20%) 1 year after radiation, implying that combining this technique with chemotherapy would be risky. Similar toxicities were seen when 14 dogs with failed lymphoma were treated; five dogs had a CR or PR.[128] Acute radiation sickness was seen in 30% of dogs after cranial irradiation and in 80% of dogs after caudal irradiation. Four dogs died. Pneumonitis was seen in six dogs and was progressive until death in two.

Table 47-8 **Comparison of a Low-Intensity Protocol (PVAC) with a High-Intensity Protocol Including a Consolidation Phase (VELCAP-SC)**[39,124]

Protocol	VELCAP-SC	PVAC
Number of dogs	94	36
Stage V (%)	57	5
Substage a (%)	37	72
B cell (%)	51	73
CR rate (%)	70	42
First remission (wk)	24	22
Remission at 1 year (%)	44	20
Remission at 2 years (%)	13	10

In contrast, when half-body radiation therapy was given in two consecutive daily 4 Gy fractions (instead of a single dose), toxicities were mainly mild and self-limiting.[52] Dogs in remission from lymphoma after chemotherapy appeared to benefit from the addition of radiation as a consolidation phase. In this study, 52 dogs received a short (11-week) chemotherapy protocol followed by radiation therapy if they were in CR. Median first remission was 10 months; 31 dogs relapsed, and 20 went on to receive further chemotherapy. The second remission rate was 85%. The overall median remission (which included remission after first relapse) was 16 months.[52] Similar efficacy was seen in another preliminary report of a study in which the radiation therapy was given during chemotherapy.[129] These results appear to be substantially better than those achieved with chemotherapy alone, and this combination should be investigated further.

COMBINATION PROTOCOLS WITH INCREASED DOSE INTENSITY ± AUTOLOGOUS BONE MARROW SUPPORT

One study compared two discontinuous protocols (high dose and conventional dose) that differed in the dosages of doxorubicin and cyclophosphamide.[130] In the high-dose protocol, doxorubicin and cyclophosphamide were each increased by 25% to 37 mg/m^2 and 250 mg/m^2 IV, respectively. No additional supportive care was given. Remission rate, remission duration, and survival times did not differ between the high-dose and conventional-dose protocols, possibly because dogs treated with the higher dosages were more likely to die from toxicity than dogs treated with conventional dosages (death rate of 27% and 4%, respectively). This study indicates the need for supportive care when higher dosages are used.

High-dose chemotherapy with hematopoietic stem cell support or bone marrow transplantation (BMT) has become an important component of therapy for lymphoma and other malignancies in humans. Although combination chemotherapy results in a complete remission rate of 75% or greater in dogs, relapses frequently occur after a median of 10 to 12 months. It appears that autologous BMT allows dogs to receive intensified doses of myelosuppressive chemotherapy without increased toxicity and that this intensification improves remission duration and overall survival.

In a reported protocol based on VELCAP-S, dogs in CR at week 8 were treated with filgrastim (G-CSF) followed by bone marrow collection.[131] A high dose of cyclophosphamide was given with mesna followed by prophylactic antibiotics, and bone marrow was administered intravenously. Three dosage levels of cyclophosphamide were used: 300 mg/m^2 (three dogs), 400 mg/m^2 (12 dogs), and 500 mg/m^2 (13 dogs). Toxicity was acceptable, with only one dog requiring hospitalization after transplantation for complications that resolved in 24 hours. Remission duration was not significantly different for dogs receiving 300 mg/m^2 or 400 mg/m^2. For dogs receiving 500 mg/m^2, the median remission was 12.4 months, significantly longer than for dogs receiving 400 mg/m^2, with 6 of 13 dogs still in remission between 6 and 33 months after starting chemotherapy and 1-year survival of 57.1%. Using autologous bone marrow to support chemotherapy dose intensification allows dogs to receive 2.5 times the standard dose of cyclophosphamide without any increase in clinical toxicity. This dose intensification results in significant prolongation of remission.

CURRENT RECOMMENDATIONS

It is important that the client be given all the options and that the best option be used first. As a general rule, combination chemotherapy is superior to single-agent therapy. Each time an effective drug is added to the COP protocol, the remission duration increases; however, so do the cost and the potential for toxicity. It is also important that clients realize that a second or third remission is possible with appropriate therapy but that these subsequent remissions are more difficult to attain and that their duration is generally half the duration of the previous remission.

The treatment options below are tiered according to risk of toxicity, cost, and efficacy. First-level protocols provide a low risk of toxicity at low cost but have low efficacy; as the level rises, so do efficacy, cost, and risk of toxicity.

First level: For clients who cannot afford or will not accept a combination chemotherapy protocol because of the risks of toxicity, a protocol using prednisone alone (40 mg/m^2 PO daily for 7 days then every other day) or in combination with chlorambucil (6 to 8 mg/m^2 PO every other day) may provide palliation with few risks of side effects. A CBC should be collected every 2 to 3 weeks to make sure that myelosuppression is not occurring.

Second level: The COP protocol (either version) is a relatively inexpensive chemotherapy protocol with a low risk of toxicity. Dogs tolerate the treatments, and veterinarians find the protocol very manageable. CBCs should be taken 1 week after each dose of cyclophosphamide to ensure that myelosuppression (if it occurs) is not severe and that doses do not need to be adjusted.

Doxorubicin administered every 3 weeks for five to eight treatments at a dosage of 30 mg/m^2 (1 mg/kg for small dogs) is the most effective single chemotherapeutic agent. This treatment regimen results in a relatively high remission rate with relatively few serious life-threatening toxicities (<5%). With the advent of generic doxorubicin, the cost is reasonable for most clients. Because the drug is given every 3 weeks, this treatment approach is less time intensive than most chemotherapy protocols. A second remission seems more likely if doxorubicin is used as first-line therapy and COP is used after relapse than if COP is used first.[67] Overall remission time for the two-protocol treatment approach is similar to that of the COPA protocol.[122]

Third level: The most effective chemotherapy protocols use a five-drug combination of L-asparaginase, vincristine, cyclophosphamide, doxorubicin, and prednisone. Similar remission rates and survival times have been obtained for the protocols that include these drugs.[11,27,105,125] Although these protocols require more intense client–veterinarian communication and monitoring for toxicity, the overall level of satisfaction for owners, pets, and veterinarians is high. Most oncologists recommend discontinuous protocols such as VELCAP-S or the Wisconsin protocol; however, some clients will not restart chemotherapy when first remission is over.[10,59]

> **KEY POINT**
>
> *Combination chemotherapy using vincristine, cyclophosphamide, prednisone, doxorubicin, and L-asparaginase provides long remission times with good quality of life for dogs with lymphoma.*

For dogs with T-cell lymphoma, protocols that rely heavily on alkylating agents, such as Tufts VELCAP-SC, should be used.[39]

Fourth level: The addition of radiation therapy or, if available, autologous bone marrow support to allow chemotherapy dose intensification represents the best possible treatment option for a dog with lymphoma. The potential for long-term remission and possibly cure is much higher than with other protocols. Dogs with T-cell lymphoma may not benefit to the same extent as those dogs with B-cell lymphoma. Although risks of toxicity are higher, the addition of radiation or chemotherapy dose intensification has not negatively affected the quality of life for treated dogs (Figure 47-13).

Table 47-9 illustrates some parameters for a series of protocols used at Tufts University from 1977 to 2003. It illustrates the differences that more aggressive protocols can make in improving long-term remission and survival. There is insufficient information to truly compare populations of dogs (e.g., immunophenotype was only known for dogs treated after 1997), so some of the differences may be due to other factors. This is true for any protocol comparison. Clinicians should understand that there is probably no "best" protocol that uses only standard-dose chemotherapy. Each clinician should find a protocol that he or she is comfortable with and use it for all qualified patients.

SUPPORTIVE AND NUTRITIONAL TREATMENT OF CANINE LYMPHOMA

Table 47-9 also illustrates another interesting point. The induction death rate decreased markedly for the VELCAP-SC protocol compared with previous protocols, despite an increase in the percentage of dogs needing a dose reduction of at least one chemotherapy drug (toxicity) and despite a higher proportion of substage b dogs undergoing therapy. We attribute the difference in death rate to careful staging that required the owners' commitment to therapy as well as strict use of hospitalized induction for any animal that was in substage b.

We suggest that any dog that has signs compatible with substage b (particularly anorexia and other GI signs) be admitted for IV fluid therapy (maintenance × 1.5), broad-spectrum antibiotics (cefazolin sodium or enrofloxacin), and GI prophylaxis (metoclopramide and bland diet). This supportive care should be continued for at least 4 days after induction and preferably for a week. Dogs can be discharged to the owner as soon as they are self-supporting. Antibiotics and prophylactic metoclopramide are continued for the first 3 weeks of the protocol.

In addition, in one study, administration of trimethoprim–sulfadiazine (Tribrissen, Schering-Plough Animal Health) to dogs for 14 days, starting on the day of treatment with doxorubicin, markedly reduced the likelihood of GI toxicity (vomiting or diarrhea), hospitalization, and lower quality-of-life (Karnofsky) score. The effect was most marked in dogs with lymphoma and may be due to reduced bacterial translocation in damaged intestinal epithelial layers.[133]

Nutrition is an important part of supportive care for any dog with cancer, particularly dogs with a systemic disease like lymphoma. Lactate and insulin concentrations in untreated dogs with lymphoma are higher than in dogs without lym-

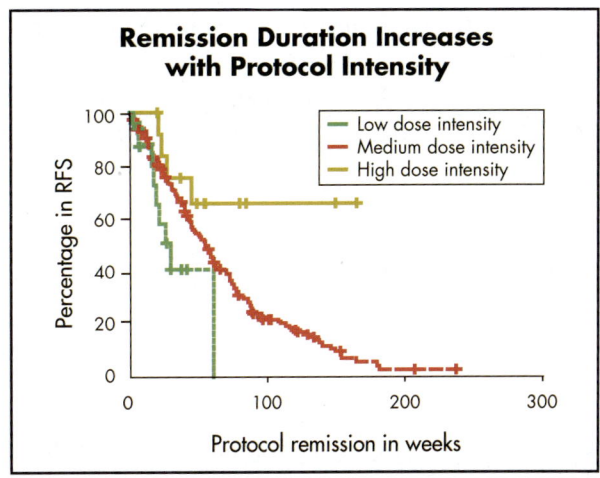

Figure 47-13. *A comparison of remission durations for dogs treated with a low-intensity protocol (PVAC), medium-intensity five-drug protocol (VELCAP-L, VELCAP-S and VELCAP-SC data combined; not different from one another) or high-intensity protocol with autologous bone marrow support (VELCAP-BM). The differences between each curve are significant.* RFS =*remission-free survival*

phoma and do not improve when dogs enter chemotherapy-induced remission.[134,135]

Nutrition may also play a role in prolonging remission and survival. Polyunsaturated n-3 fatty acids have been shown to inhibit the growth and metastasis of tumors. In one study, 32 dogs with lymphoma were randomized to receive a diet supplemented with polyunsaturated n-3 fatty acids (menhaden fish oil and arginine) or an otherwise identical diet supplemented with soybean oil.[136] Diets were fed from the start of doxorubicin chemotherapy and continued after remission was attained. Dogs fed the diet supplemented with n-3 fatty acids had higher serum levels of n-3 fatty acids (docosahexaenoic acid and eicosapentaenoic acid) and lower plasma lactate responses to carbohydrate testing. Increased serum levels of docosahexaenoic acid were associated with longer remission and survival times for dogs with stage III lymphoma. Nutrition therapy is described in detail in Chapter 31.

OTHER TREATMENT MODALITIES FOR CANINE LYMPHOMA

Chemoimmunotherapy: The potential use of chemoimmunotherapy appears promising. As further information is obtained using antibodies with different chemotherapeutic protocols, chemoimmunotherapy may prove to be an efficacious and well-tolerated treatment modality.

On the premise that immunotherapy is more effective after reduction of tumor burden, some dogs with lymphoma that achieved CR with chemotherapy have been treated with immunotherapy.

Table 47-9 Comparison of Protocols Used to Treat Canine Lymphoma at Tufts University from 1977–2003

Protocol	CR (%)	CR Duration (months)	1-Year Survival (%)	2-Year Survival (%)	Induction Death (%)	Toxicity (%)	Study
COP	75	6	19	—	6	19	Cotter[132]
COPA	84	7	22	—	6	29	Cotter and Goldstein[122]
ACOPA-1	76	11	48	—	12	37	Stone et al[105]
ACOPA-2	65	10	40	21	22	64	Myers et al[125]
VELCAP-L	69	13	53	25	19	55	Zemann et al[11]
VELCAP-S	68	11	36	12	27	48	Moore et al[10]
VELCAP-SC	70	12	44	13	4	70	Morrison-Collister et al[39]

Early studies used an autochthonous tumor vaccine, which is made from tumor cells that have been extracted and acetoacetylated. This vaccine is administered intramuscularly to dogs in CR with Freund's complete adjuvant at 2, 3, 4, 6, and 8 weeks after finishing chemotherapy. Results of early studies did not show any benefit to this therapeutic approach.[137]

Antibody 231: Monoclonal antibodies have been obtained from mice immunized with cultured canine lymphoma cells. One of these antibodies (CL/MAb 231, Synbiotics Corporation, San Diego, CA) bound to the cells of 73% of 15 lymphoma samples tested. In vitro studies showed enhanced antibody-dependent cell-mediated cytotoxicity against canine lymphoma cells when canine mononuclear cells were combined with these antibodies. A weekly cyclic chemotherapy protocol was followed by administration of CL/MAb 231 daily for 5 days to dogs in CR.

Although preliminary results showed a median survival time of 19 months, with 40% of dogs still alive, further evaluation of this antibody was apparently unsuccessful, and the product is no longer listed as available.[138]

Cyclooxygenase-2 inhibition: Piroxicam, a nonsteroidal inhibitor of cyclooxygenase-2 (COX-2), given at a dose of 0.3 mg/kg PO sid, may inhibit tumor angiogenesis. Addition of piroxicam to doxorubicin chemotherapy did not improve either remission rate or remission duration.[114]

Antiangiogenic drugs: Antiangiogenic therapy is a new area of interest in veterinary medicine. Angiogenesis is a complex process by which new blood vessels sprout from existing vessels and then dissolve surrounding matrix to extend further into tumors. New blood vessel growth is rarely needed in existing normal tissue (except in wound healing, pregnancy, and fetal growth), so inhibiting aspects of the angiogenic pathway should target tumors specifically. Without new blood vessels, tumors cannot expand beyond a size that allows passive diffusion of nutrients and oxygen to the tumor cells, and existing tumors may reduce in size.

Tumors also need to dissolve surrounding cellular matrix in order to allow angiogenesis and tumor invasion. Various drugs may target angiogenesis and matrix dissolution through various pathways. A large, multiinstitutional, randomized clinical trial found no survival benefit to oral administration of an inhibitor of metalloproteinases 2 and 9 (MMP-2 and MMP-9) in conjunction with doxorubicin chemotherapy, except in a small subset of dogs that were older than 7 years and had measurable MMP-9 plasma levels.[139]

Rescue Therapy

Durable first remissions in dogs with lymphoma are achievable with available schedules and protocols, and most efforts are directed toward reducing toxicity and cost of therapy. In contrast, success in achieving durable second remis-

> **KEY POINT**
> *For most dogs with lymphoma, if relapse occurs during treatment, second remissions are difficult to obtain and are short.*

sions is rare. Most "rescue" protocols result in remission rates of 30% or less, and the duration of these second remissions is generally short. More work is needed to develop efficacious rescue protocols.

SINGLE-AGENT RESCUE CHEMOTHERAPY

Mitoxantrone: Mitoxantrone was given as a single agent at a dose of 5 mg/m² IV to 34 dogs that had failed to respond to, or relapsed from, other chemotherapy. Nine dogs (26%) had a CR for a median of 4 months (range: 1.5–26 months).[97] Although the response rate was low, it is similar to that for mitoxantrone used for induction of remission as first-line therapy. Further evaluation of mitoxantrone as rescue therapy has shown that 6 mg/m^2 may be a more appropriate dosage than 5 mg/m^2; another study of 15 dogs with advanced stage (IV or V) lymphoma treated at 6 mg/m^2 reported a 47% CR rate for a median of 2.8 months.[140]

Dactinomycin: In one study, this drug was given to dogs that had failed previous chemotherapy, and a high response rate was seen.[118] In another study, however, 30 dogs that had relapsed on combination chemotherapy protocols were treated with dactinomycin at a dose of 0.5 to 0.9 mg/m^2 IV every 3 weeks.[141] None of the dogs in this group responded, despite a higher average dose rate than the previous study. The efficacy of dactinomycin as a rescue agent for dogs that have received doxorubicin appears poor, possibly as a result of tumor-cell cross-resistance to these two agents.

Etoposide (VP-16): Etoposide was given intravenously at a dosage of 100 mg/m^2 IV or 25 mg/m^2 IV for 4 days to 13 dogs that had failed to respond to, or had relapsed on, combination chemotherapy. Only one dog responded completely for 30 days (and partially for another 90 days). Eleven dogs showed cutaneous reactions; these reactions were severe in three dogs and were not alleviated by diphenhydramine or corticosteroids. Six dogs were sedated using ketamine and diazepam to minimize discomfort from toxic reactions,[142] which are believed to result from sensitivity to polysorbate 80, a drug-delivery vehicle used in etoposide.[143] Intravenously administered etoposide is not recommended for routine use in dogs. Oral etoposide has not been well evaluated for the treatment of lymphoma in dogs, but Dr. Moore's experience suggests that there is limited efficacy, probably due to variable absorption from the GI tract.

CCNU (lomustine): CCNU was used at a dose of 90 mg/m^2 PO every 3 weeks to treat 43 dogs with lymphoma that had relapsed or had failed to achieve CR with previous chemotherapy. Durable CR or PR was achieved in 11 dogs for a median of 3 months. The acute dose-limiting toxicity was neutropenia 7 days after administration, and cumulative thrombocytopenia occurred in dogs receiving continued CCNU treatment.[144] Hepatotoxicity and renal toxicity have also been seen in approximately 5% of dogs.[145] A dose interval of 4 to 6 weeks may be preferred for continued administration of this drug (i.e., more than 2 treatments). Patients should be monitored for thrombocytopenia and elevations in serum liver enzyme activities and creatinine. Remission was less frequent and much shorter when a lower dosage of 70 mg/m^2 was used.[146]

Ifosfamide: Ifosfamide (350–375 mg/m^2), in combination with saline diuresis and the thiol compound mesna, was used to treat 40 dogs with lymphoma. One dog had a PR for 3.7 months. The acute dose-limiting toxicity was neutropenia 7 days after administration of ifosfamide.[147] At current doses, ifosfamide appears ineffective as a rescue agent.

Vinblastine: Kenneth Rassnick, DVM, Cornell University, reports that vinblastine at a dose of 3.5 mg/m^2 has caused 3 PRs in 17 treated dogs.

COMBINATION RESCUE CHEMOTHERAPY

Dacarbazine and doxorubicin: Dacarbazine (DTIC) has not been evaluated for single-agent activity in the treatment of canine lymphoma. Synergy with doxorubicin has been observed in the treatment of human lymphoma patients; therefore, DTIC was given in combination with doxorubicin to nine dogs with lymphoma. Six dogs had failed to respond to doxorubicin; five of these dogs achieved CR with the combination therapy for a median of 87 days (range: 32–281 days). Another three previously untreated dogs that were treated with the combination achieved CR for 30, 89, and 106 days, respectively. The DTIC dosage was 133 to 167 mg/m^2 IV as a 5-day course every 3 weeks. The doxorubicin dose ranged from 36.5 to 40.0 mg/m^2 every 3 weeks.[112]

Doxorubicin and DTIC were given to 15 dogs with lymphoma resistant to a combination chemotherapy protocol that included doxorubicin. The doxorubicin dosage was 30 mg/m^2 every 3 weeks, and dacarbazine was given at 200 mg/m^2 IV for 5 days every 3 weeks. CR was achieved in five dogs.[148]

MOPP: The combination of mechlorethamine, vincristine, procarbazine, and prednisone (MOPP) has been relatively effective in the treatment of Hodgkin's disease in humans. As a rescue protocol, MOPP was given on a 28-day course to 17 dogs with relapsed lymphoma. Mechlorethamine (6 mg/m^2 IV) and vincristine (0.7 mg/m^2 IV) were given on day 1, and procarbazine (100 mg/m^2 PO) and prednisone (30 mg/m^2 PO) were given daily on days 1 through 14. This protocol was severely myelosuppressive; two-thirds of the dogs became leukopenic, and six died from this toxicity.[149] Severe myelosuppression necessitated dose reductions to 3 mg/m^2 of mechlorethamine and 50 mg/m^2 of procarbazine.

MOPP was used at these lower dosages to treat 117 dogs that had resistance to a median of six chemotherapeutic drugs following a first median remission of 7 months. A CR was seen in 36 dogs (31%) for a median of 2 months, and 40 (34%) had a PR for a median of 1.5 months. There were no predictors for response to MOPP. GI toxicity occurred in 28% of the dogs, and 13% required hospitalization. Five dogs developed septicemia, and two died as a result. MOPP was an effective treatment for dogs with resistant lymphoma and was well tolerated by most affected dogs.[150]

An additional finding in this study was that some dogs responded to MOPP, relapsed during the period between day 7 and 28, and subsequently responded again to another treatment with MOPP. Median response duration for dogs achieving this type of response was not significantly different from that of a sustained response.[150] Clinicians using the MOPP protocol for rescue of dogs with refractory lymphoma should not be discouraged, even if there is an apparent relapse in the 3-week rest period between courses.

DOPP: Mechlorethamine has recently become difficult, and in some places impossible, to obtain. In the experience of Rassnick and Moore, the substitution of dactinomycin (0.5 mg/m² IV) for mechlorethamine appears to result in similar efficacy.

BOPP: A study reported preliminary findings substituting carmustine (BCNU; 50 mg/m² IV) for mechlorethamine. In that study, 13 dogs were treated; five had a CR and four had a PR, but many were of short duration (median 9 days). The median increase in survival for treated dogs was 51 days.[151]

Cisplatin and cytarabine: Ten dogs with resistant lymphoma were treated with cisplatin (50 mg/m² IV every 3 weeks) and cytarabine (100 mg/m² every 7 days, IV on day 0 and SC on days 7 and 14). Although this protocol had little associated toxicity, only one dog had a CR, which lasted 2 months, and two dogs had PRs for 1 and 3.6 months.[152] Rassnick and Moore have further explored this combination and shown similar efficacy with increased dosages and altered scheduling.

Antiangiogenic drugs: A preliminary report of use of a thrombospondin-I peptide known to inhibit angiogenesis, in combination with lomustine chemotherapy, for the treatment of dogs with resistant lymphoma showed that while the remission rate did not differ from that of lomustine therapy alone, the median length of remission was nearly twice as long if the antiangiogenic therapy was used.[146]

Lymphoma of Extranodal Sites

The information above is applicable to lymphoma of all sites, but there are some prognostic and behavioral differences for lymphoma of extranodal sites. By convention, dogs with lymphoma involving these sites are considered to be in stage V. Cutaneous lymphoma is covered in more detail in Chapter 64. Pulmonary lymphomatoid granulomatosis is discussed in Chapter 51.

LYMPHOMA OF THE GASTROINTESTINAL TRACT

One author described GI lymphoma as being primary if the only additional sites involved were within the abdominal cavity and bone marrow; other dogs were described as having GI lymphoma with multicentric disease.[153] In that study, 15 of 20 dogs had primary GI lymphoma. Although an early study found males to be overrepresented, a larger study found no gender predilection.[153,154] In one series of 44 dogs, there were six boxers and six shar-peis.[154] Most dogs have involvement of the small intestine.

In one study, dogs were most commonly presented for depression, vomiting, anorexia, and diarrhea, with half of the dogs presented for noticeable weight loss. Multiple segments of bowel were affected in most dogs.[153] Perforation of bowel wall is possible in affected dogs.[153]

Anemia and hypoalbuminemia were seen in 30% of dogs,[153] which is in contrast to a series of dogs seen by Moore and Penninck in which 32 of 38 affected dogs (84%) were hypoalbuminemic (albumin <3.0 mg/dl).

Ultrasonography is the preferred method of evaluating, staging, and directing a biopsy in dogs with intestinal lymphoma (Figure 47-6). Ultrasonography is usually performed through the abdominal wall but can be performed endoscopically.[155]

Canine primary GI lymphoma was believed to be of B-cell origin based on the morphology and behavior of the neoplastic cells and evidence from the human medical field. However, canine primary GI lymphoma is more commonly of T-cell origin. Of 50 dogs in three reports, 39 (78%) had T-cell lymphoma, three (6%) had B-cell lymphoma, and eight (16%) had null-cell lymphoma.[154-156] Many of the dogs with T-cell lymphoma had epitheliotropic lymphoma (localized in the lamina propria and epithelium of the mucosa), which is also described in mycosis fungoides, a T-cell variant of cutaneous lymphoma.[154] This has implications for treatment.

Of eight dogs treated in one series, five that received corticosteroids alone or with vincristine and azathioprine responded either briefly or not at all; four were dead within 14 weeks of diagnosis. COP plus L-asparaginase and COAP were used in three dogs, but only one had prolonged survival and was alive 54 months later.[153]

Dr. Moore's experience is similar. Of 110 dogs treated with VELCAP-SC, those with GI involvement did statistically worse than those with multicentric lymphoma, even those with multicentric T-cell lymphoma. In another series, dogs that were treated with any chemotherapy lived longer than those treated with either surgery alone or with supportive care, but most dogs were dead within a year of diagnosis. One dog with a solitary intestinal mass of B-cell origin was alive more than 3 years after surgical resection, having received no chemotherapy.

LYMPHOMA OF THE NERVOUS SYSTEM

It is rare that lymphoma involves a single location in the central nervous system (CNS).[157] In two series of 18 dogs with lymphoma of the nervous system, spinal involvement was usually multifocal, and most dogs also had brain involvement.[158,159] Two dogs with peripheral nerves involved also had CNS disease.[158] Spinal lymphoma is usually extradural, but it can be intradural[158,159] and is usually associated with systemic disease. Most commonly, CNS involvement occurs in a dog that has been treated with chemotherapy for a long period, and it may be associated with relapse of systemic disease.[159]

Signs in these dogs may include seizures, but subtle changes in mentation and alertness are more common.

Occasionally, lymphoma cells will be detected in the cerebrospinal fluid (CSF) and counts may be high, but a negative result does not rule out lymphoma. Herniation is a potential complication of CSF collection.[160,161]

Immunophenotype has been reported for one dog with CNS lymphoma, and that dog had a T-cell lymphoma.[162]

Chemotherapy may cause complete remission of peripheral lymphoma, yet lymphoma may progress in the CNS.[158] This is presumably because the blood–brain barrier creates a "sanctuary site" from chemotherapy, although meningeal infiltration by lymphoma cells would be expected to disrupt this barrier. Chemotherapy alone has caused a remission in some dogs.[159] There is one report of cytarabine used as an intrathecal injection in four dogs, although the contribution to remission was difficult to assess because some dogs received concurrent radiation therapy and/or systemic chemotherapy.[159] Cytarabine will cross the blood–brain barrier, although a continuous infusion is required to obtain therapeutic levels. Prednisone also crosses the blood–brain barrier, as do the alkylating agents lomustine and carmustine.

Radiation should be directed at the entire craniospinal axis because multiple sites are usually involved. While there may be marked improvement in neurologic status, chemotherapy is warranted for systemic lymphoma. One dog with extradural lymphoma affecting the lumbar spine was treated with 24 Gy radiation and COP-L after decompressive surgery. Subjectively, there was decreased pain but no neurologic improvement 2 weeks after treatment.[163]

INTRAVASCULAR LYMPHOMA

Intravascular lymphoma (malignant angioendotheliomatosis, angiotrophic lymphoma) is a rare variant of lymphoma in dogs, characterized by thromboses, infarction, and hemorrhage. It has most commonly been reported in the brain and spinal cord. In a series of 17 dogs, eight had T-cell lymphoma, six had non-T, non-B cell (null-cell) lymphoma, and only one had B-cell lymphoma.[164] The disease may progress to involve other organs, but survival is often poor, and dogs are often euthanatized with only CNS involvement.[164,165]

Because of the vascular distribution of the lesions, there may be little visible effect on the structure of the CNS, and computed tomography (CT) may fail to detect a lesion. Magnetic resonance imaging is more sensitive and may detect multiple CNS infarctions.[166] CT-guided biopsy was used to diagnose this disease in one dog.[167]

Corticosteroids may result in improvement in neurologic status, but improvement is usually incomplete and short-lived.[165,166] The addition of vincristine and L-asparaginase did not improve response in one dog.[167]

MUSCULOSKELETAL LYMPHOMA

Lymphoma of bone has been reported as a primary site rarely and only as case reports. In one study, lymphoma accounted for less than 1% of bone tumors.[168]

Lymphoma of bone rarely involves one site.[169] Although a dog may present for lameness due to a single lesion, further radiography or scintigraphy usually reveals multiple sites of involvement. Other extranodal sites may also be involved, as in two dogs with skeletal muscle and cardiac involvement[170,171] and another dog with synovial and skin lymphoma.[172] One dog had most of the axial and appendicular skeleton involved (polyostotic),[173] as did two young dogs (<9 months of age).[174,175]

Reports of immunophenotype are rare, although one dog with a concurrent mediastinal mass and hypercalcemia presumably had a T-cell lymphoma.[176] One dog had a synovial and cutaneous T-cell lymphoma.[172]

Chemotherapy alone (COP) was unsuccessful in causing a remission in one dog.[170] In contrast, a more aggressive five-drug protocol caused long-term remission, including healing of pathologic fractures, in a dog with multiple lesions. The dog died with no lymphoma detected 41 months after diagnosis.[168]

Radiation therapy would appear to be a good adjunct to chemotherapy; however, there are few reports to gauge efficacy. A dog with a solitary lymphoma of the ulna and adjacent joint was treated with 45 Gy of radiation alone and had no evidence of disease 34 months later.[169]

It appears that lymphoma may be a solitary lesion in bone only rarely; careful and complete staging should be performed before localized therapy is undertaken. Most dogs will need chemotherapy and, from the limited data, it seems that multidrug protocols as described for multicentric lymphoma should be used.

PERICARDIAL AND CARDIAC LYMPHOMA

The heart is a rare location for lymphoma. In a series of 52 dogs with pericardial neoplasia, six had lymphoma,[177] and of 1,383 dogs in another series, 34 (2.5%) had lymphoma.[178] Myocardial lymphoma was seen in three related otter hounds in one study.[13]

In one report of a small series of dogs with pericardial lymphoma, only six were treated with chemotherapy, and the median remission time was 5.2 months.[179] Two dogs were long-term survivors for more than 1 year. One dog with myocardial lymphoma responded for more than a year to prednisolone alone.[13]

LOWER URINARY TRACT LYMPHOMA

In the two case reports of lymphoma primarily affecting the urinary tract, both dogs had a T-cell lymphoma, and neither was treated.[180,181]

NASAL LYMPHOMA

A case report of solitary, T cell–derived, nasal lymphoma described doxorubicin chemotherapy and radiation therapy causing a durable CR for more than 30 months.[182]

REFERENCES

1. Dorn CR, Taylor DO, Hibbard HH: Epizootiologic characteristics of canine and feline leukemia and lymphoma. *Am J Vet Res* 28:993–1001, 1967.
2. Schneider R: Comparison of age- and sex-specific incidence rate patterns of the leukemia complex in the cat and the dog. *J Natl Cancer Inst* 70:971–977, 1983.
3. Teske E: Canine malignant lymphoma: A review and comparison with human non-Hodgkin's lymphoma. *Vet Q* 16:209–219, 1994.
4. Dobson JM, Samuel S, Milstein H, et al: Canine neoplasia in the UK: Estimates of incidence rates from a population of insured dogs. *J Small Anim Pract* 43:240–246, 2002.
5. Clancy E, McConnell W, Patronek G, Moore A: Epidemiological study of canine lymphoma in New England. *Proc 19th Ann Conf Vet Cancer Soc* 71. 1999.
6. Priester WA: Canine lymphoma: Relative risk in the boxer breed. *J Natl Cancer Inst* 39:833–845, 1967.
7. Lurie D, Lucroy MD, Griffey SM, et al: T-cell-derived malignant lymphoma in the boxer breed. *Vet Comp Oncol* 2:171–175, 2004.
8. Onions DE: A prospective survey of familial canine lymphosarcoma. *J Natl Cancer Inst* 72:909–912, 1984.
9. Edwards DS, Henley WE, Harding EF, et al: Breed incidence of lymphoma in a UK population of insured dogs. *Vet Comp Oncol* 1:200–206, 2003.
10. Moore AS, Cotter SM, Rand WM, et al: Evaluation of a discontinuous treatment protocol (VELCAP-S) for canine lymphoma. *J Vet Intern Med* 15:348–354, 2001.
11. Zemann BI, Moore AS, Rand WM, et al: A combination chemotherapy protocol (VELCAP-L) for dogs with lymphoma. *J Vet Intern Med* 12:465–470, 1998.
12. Jagielski D, Lechowski R, Hoffmann-Jagielska M, Winiarczyk S: A retrospective study of the incidence and prognostic factors of multicentric lymphoma in dogs (1998-2000). *J Vet Med A Physiol Pathol Clin Med* 49:419–424, 2002.
13. Teske E, de Vos JP, Egberink HF, Vos JH: Clustering in canine malignant lymphoma. *Vet Q* 16:134–136, 1994.
14. Onions D: RNA-dependent DNA polymerase activity in canine lymphosarcoma. *Eur J Cancer* 16:345–350, 1980.
15. Tomley FM, Armstrong SJ, deSouza PN: Retrovirus particles associated with canine lymphosarcoma and leukemia. *Br J Cancer* 45:644, 1982.
16. O'Brien DJ, Kaneene JB, Getis A, et al: Spatial and temporal distribution of selected canine cancers in Michigan, USA, 1964-1994. *Prev Vet Med* 42:1–15, 1999.
17. Gavazza A, Presciuttini S, Barale R, et al: Association between canine malignant lymphoma, living in industrial areas, and use of chemicals by dog owners. *J Vet Intern Med* 15:190–195, 2001.
18. Hayes HM, Tarone RE, Cantor KP, et al: Case-control study of canine malignant lymphoma: Positive association with dog owners use of 2,4-dichlorophenoxyacetic acid herbicides. *J Natl Cancer Inst* 83:1226–1231, 1991.
19. Reynolds PM, Reif JS, Ramsdell HS, Tessari JD: Canine exposure to herbicide-treated lawns and urinary excretion of 2,4-dichlorophenoxyacetic acid. *Cancer Epidemiol Biomarkers Prev* 3:233–237, 1994.
20. Carlo GL, Cole P, Miller AB, et al: Review of a study reporting an association between 2,4-dichlorophenoxyacetic acid and canine malignant lymphoma: Report of an expert panel. *Regul Toxicol Pharmacol* 16:245–252, 1992.
21. Kaneene JB, Miller R: Re-analysis of 2,4-D use and the occurrence of canine malignant lymphoma. *Vet Human Toxicol* 41:164–170, 1999.
22. Hayes HM, Tarone RE, Cantor KP: On the association between canine malignant lymphoma and opportunity for exposure to 2,4-dichlorophenoxyacetic acid. *Environ Res* 70:119–125, 1995.
23. Reif JS, Lower KS, Ogilvie GK: Residential exposure to magnetic fields and risk of canine lymphoma. *Am J Epidemiol* 141:352–359, 1995.
24. Keller ET: Immune-mediated diseases as a risk factor for canine lymphoma. *Cancer* 70:2334–2337, 1992.
25. Day MJ, Whitbread TJ: Pathological diagnoses in dogs with lymph node enlargement. *Vet Rec* 136:72–73, 1995.
26. Owen LN: TNM classification of tumours in domestic animals. Geneva: World Health Organization. 1st. 1980.
27. Keller ET, MacEwen EG, Rosenthal RC, et al: Evaluation of prognostic factors and sequential combination chemotherapy with doxorubicin for canine lymphoma. *J Vet Intern Med* 7:289–295, 1993.
28. Burnett RC, Vernau W, Modiano JF, et al: Diagnosis of canine lymphoid neoplasia using clonal rearrangements of antigen receptor genes. *Vet Pathol* 40:32–41, 2003.
29. Krohne SG, Henderson NM, Richardson RC, Vestre WA: Prevalence of ocular involvement in dogs with multicentric lymphoma: Prospective evaluation of 94 cases. *Vet Comp Ophthalmology* 4:127–135, 1994.
30. Wyatt KM, Robertson ID: Canine lymphosarcoma: A West Australian perspective. *Aust Vet Pract* 28:63–66, 1998.
31. Ackerman N, Madewell BR: Thoracic and abdominal radiographic abnormalities in the multicentric form of lymphosarcoma in dogs. *JAVMA* 176:36–40, 1980.
32. Blackwood L, Sullivan M, Lawson H: Radiographic abnormalities in canine multicentric lymphoma: A review of 84 cases. *J Small Anim Pract* 38:62–69, 1997.
33. Starrak GS, Berry CR, Page RL, et al: Correlation between thoracic radiographic changes and remission/survival duration in 270 dogs with lymphosarcoma. *Vet Radiol Ultrasound* 38:411–418, 1997.
34. Steyn PF, Ogilvie G: 99m Tc-methoxy-isobutyl-isonitrile (sestamibi) imaging of malignant canine lymphoma. *Vet Radiol Ultrasound* 36:411–416, 1995.
35. Lamb CR, Hartzband LE, Tidwell AS, Pearson SH: Ultrasonographic findings in hepatic and splenic lymphosarcoma in dogs and cats. *Vet Radiol* 32:117–120, 1991.
36. Raskin RE, Krehbiel JD: Histopathology of canine bone marrow in malignant lymphoproliferative disorders. *Vet Pathol* 25:83–88, 1988.
37. Raskin RE, Krehbiel JD: Prevalence of leukemic blood and bone marrow in dogs with multicentric lymphoma. *JAVMA* 194:1427–1429, 1989.
38. Madewell BR: Hematological and bone marrow cytological abnormalities in 75 dogs with malignant lymphoma. *JAAHA* 22:235–240, 1986.
39. Morrison-Collister KE, Rassnick KM, Northrup NC, et al: A combination chemotherapy protocol with MOPP and CCNU consolidation (Tufts VELCAP-SC) for the treatment of canine lymphoma. *Vet Comp Oncol* 1:180–190, 2003.
40. Rosol TJ, Nagode LA, Couto CG, et al: Parathyroid hormone (PTH)-related protein, PTH, and 1,25-dihydroxyvitamin D in dogs with cancer-associated hypercalcemia. *Endocrinology* 131:1157–1164, 1992.
41. Lemmens P, De Bruin A, De Meulemeester J, et al: Paraneoplastic pemphigus in a dog. *Vet Dermatol* 9:127–134, 1998.
42. Anderson RK, Carpenter JL: Severe pruritus associated with lymphoma in a dog. *JAVMA* 207:455–456, 1995.
43. Nelson RW, Hager D, Zanjani ED: Renal lymphosarcoma with inappropriate erythropoietin production in a dog. *JAVMA* 182:1396–1397, 1983.
44. Mayhew PD, Bush WW, Glass EN: Trigeminal neuropathy in dogs: A retrospective study of 29 cases (1991-2000). *JAAHA* 38:262–270, 2002.
45. Fournel-Fleury C, Magnol JP, Bricaire P, et al: Cytohistological and immunological classification of canine malignant lymphomas: Comparison with human non-Hodgkin's lymphomas. *J Comp Pathol* 117:35–59, 1997.
46. Vail DM, Kravis LD, Kisseberth WC, et al: Application of rapid CD3 immunophenotype analysis and argyrophilic nucleolar organizer region (AgNOR) frequency to fine needle aspirate specimens from dogs with lymphoma. *Vet Clin Pathol* 26:66–69, 1997.
47. Fisher DJ, Naydan D, Werner LL, Moore PF: Immunophenotyping lymphomas in dogs: A comparison of results from fine needle aspirate and needle biopsy samples. *Vet Clin Pathol* 24:118–123, 1995.
48. Caniatti M, Roccabianca P, Scanziani E, et al: Canine lymphoma: Immunocytochemical analysis of fine-needle aspiration biopsy. *Vet Pathol* 33:204–212, 1996.
49. Dobson JM, Blackwood LB, McInnes EF, et al: Prognostic variables in canine multicentric lymphosarcoma. *J Small Anim Pract* 42:377–384, 2001.
50. Appelbaum FR, Sale GE, Storb R, et al: Phenotyping of canine lymphoma with monoclonal antibodies directed at cell surface antigens: Classification, morphology, clinical presentation and response to chemotherapy. *Hematol Oncol* 2:151–168, 1984.
51. Ruslander DA, Gebhard DH, Tompkins MB, et al: Immunophenotypic characterization of canine lymphoproliferative disorders. *In Vivo* 11:169–172, 1997.
52. Williams LE, Johnson JL, Hauck ML, et al: Chemotherapy followed by half-body radiation therapy for canine lymphoma. *J Vet Intern Med* 18:703–709, 2004.
53. Teske E, Wisman P, Moore PF, van Heerde P: Histologic classification and immunophenotyping of canine non-Hodgkin's lymphomas: Unexpected high frequency of T cell lymphomas with B cell morphology. *Exp Hematol* 22:1179–1187, 1994.
54. Alvarez-Berger FJ, Chavez-Gris G, Aburto-Fernandez E, Aristi-Urista G: Histopathologic and immunophenotypic study of lymphoma in Mexico. *Proc 23rd Annu Conf Vet Cancer Soc*: 28, 2003.
55. Kiupel M, Teske E, Bostock D: Prognostic factors for treated canine malignant lymphoma. *Vet Pathol* 36:292–300, 1999.
56. Ponce F, Magnol JP, Ledieu D, et al: Prognostic significance of morphological subtypes in canine malignant lymphomas during chemotherapy. *Vet J* 167:158–166, 2004.
57. Gibson D, Aubert I, Woods JP, et al: Flow cytometric immunophenotype of canine lymph node aspirates. *J Vet Intern Med* 18:710–717, 2004.
58. Baskin CR, Couto CG, Wittum TE: Factors influencing first remission and survival in 145 dogs with lymphoma: A retrospective study. *JAAHA* 36:404–409, 2000.
59. Garrett LD, Thamm DH, Chun R, et al: Evaluation of a 6-month chemotherapy protocol with no maintenance therapy for dogs with lymphoma. *J Vet Intern Med* 16:704–709, 2002.
60. Valerius KD, Ogilvie GK, Mallinckrodt CH, Getzy DM: Doxorubicin alone or in combination with asparaginase, followed by cyclophosphamide, vincristine,

and prednisone for treatment of multicentric lymphoma in dogs: 121 cases (1987-1995). *JAVMA* 210:512–516, 1997.
61. MacEwen EG, Hayes AA, Matus RE, Kurzman I: Evaluation of some prognostic factors for advanced multicentric lymphosarcoma in the dog: 147 cases (1978-1981). *JAVMA* 190:564–568, 1987.
62. Greenlee PG, Filippa DA, Quimby FW, et al: Lymphomas in dogs. A morphologic, immunologic, and clinical study. *Cancer* 66:480–490, 1990.
63. Theilen GH, Worley M, Benjamini E: Chemoimmunotherapy for canine lymphosarcoma. *JAVMA* 170:607–610, 1977.
64. Cotter SM: Treatment of lymphoma and leukemia with cyclophosphamide, vincristine and prednisone: I. Treatment of dogs. *JAAHA* 19:159–165, 1983.
65. Squire RA, Bush M, Melby EC, et al: Clinical and pathologic study of canine lymphoma: Clinical staging, cell classification, and therapy. *J Natl Cancer Inst* 51:565–574, 1973.
66. MacEwen EG, Brown NO, Patnaik AK, et al: Cyclic combination chemotherapy of canine lymphosarcoma. *JAVMA* 178:1178–1181, 1981.
67. Carter RF, Harris CK, Withrow SJ, et al: Chemotherapy of canine lymphoma with histopathological correlation: Doxorubicin alone compared to COP as first treatment regimen. *JAAHA* 23:587–596, 1987.
68. Weller RE, Theilen GH, Madewell BR: Chemotherapeutic responses in dogs with lymphosarcoma and hypercalcemia. *JAVMA* 181:891–893, 1982.
69. Rosenberg MP, Matus RE, Patnaik AK: Prognostic factors in dogs with lymphoma and associated hypercalcemia. *J Vet Intern Med* 5:268–271, 1991.
70. Kiupel M, Bostock D, Bergmann V: The prognostic significance of AgNOR counts and PCNA-positive cell counts in canine malignant lymphomas. *J Comp Pathol* 119:407–418, 1998.
71. Fournel-Fleury C, Ponce F, Felman P, et al: Canine T-cell lymphomas: A morphological, immunological, and clinical study of 46 new cases. *Vet Pathol* 39:92–109, 2002.
72. Price GS, Frazier DL: Use of body surface area (BSA)-based dosages to calculate chemotherapeutic drug dose in dogs: I. Potential problems with current BSA formulae. *J Vet Intern Med* 12:267–271, 1998.
73. Teske E, van Heerde P: Diagnostic value and reproducibility of fine-needle aspiration cytology in canine malignant lymphoma. *Vet Q* 18:112–115, 1996.
74. Hahn KA, Richardson RC, Teclaw RF, et al: Is maintenance chemotherapy appropriate for the management of canine malignant lymphoma? *J Vet Intern Med* 6:3–10, 1992.
75. Vail DM, Kisseberth WC, Obradovich JE, et al: Assessment of potential doubling time (Tpot), argyrophilic nucleolar organizer regions (AgNOR), and proliferating cell nuclear antigen (PCNA) as predictors of therapy response in canine non-Hodgkin's lymphoma. *Exp Hematol* 24:807–815, 1996.
76. Fournel-Fleury C, Magnol JP, Chabanne L, et al: Growth fractions in canine non-Hodgkin's lymphomas as determined *in situ* by the expression of the KI-67 antigen. *J Comp Pathol* 117:61–72, 1997.
77. Phillips BS, Kass PH, Naydan DK, et al: Apoptotic and proliferation indexes in canine lymphoma. *J Vet Diagn Invest* 12:111–117, 2000.
78. Lee JJ, Hughes CS, Fine RL, Page RL: P-glycoprotein expression in canine lymphoma: A relevant, intermediate model of multidrug resistance. *Cancer* 77:1892–1898, 1996.
79. Bergman PJ, Ogilvie GK, Powers BE: Monoclonal antibody C219 immunohistochemistry against P-glycoprotein: Sequential analysis and predictive ability in dogs with lymphoma. *J Vet Intern Med* 10:354–359, 1996.
80. Thomas R, Smith KC, Ostrander EA, et al: Chromosome aberrations in canine multicentric lymphomas detected with comparative genomic hybridisation and a panel of single locus probes. *Br J Cancer* 89:1530–1537, 2003.
81. Hahn KA, Richardson RC, Hahn EA, Chrisman CL: Diagnostic and prognostic importance of chromosomal aberrations identified in 61 dogs with lymphosarcoma. *Vet Pathol* 31:528–540, 1994.
82. Piek CJ, Rutteman GR, Teske E: Evaluation of the results of a L-asparaginase-based continuous chemotherapy protocol versus a short doxorubicin-based induction chemotherapy protocol in dogs with malignant lymphoma. *Vet Q* 21:44–49, 1999.
83. Price GS, Page RL, Fischer BM, et al: Efficacy and toxicity of doxorubicin/cyclophosphamide maintenance therapy in dogs with multicentric lymphosarcoma. *J Vet Intern Med* 5:259–262, 1991.
84. Spangler WL, Kass PH: Pathologic factors affecting postsplenectomy survival in dogs. *J Vet Intern Med* 11:166–171, 1997.
85. Mellanby RJ, Herrtage ME, Dobson JM: Owners' assessments of their dog's quality of life during palliative chemotherapy for lymphoma. *J Small Anim Pract* 44:100–103, 2003.
86. Henry CJ, McCaw DL, Brock KV, et al: Association between cancer chemotherapy and canine distemper virus, canine parvovirus, and rabies virus antibody titers in tumor-bearing dogs. *JAVMA* 219:1238–1241, 2001.
87. Walter CU, Lana SE, Laible IJ, et al: Effects of chemotherapy on adaptive immunity in cancer-bearing dogs: A prospective evaluation. *Proc 23rd Annu Conf Vet Cancer Soc*: 4, 2003.
88. Mellanby RJ, Herrtage ME, Dobson JM: Treatment of canine lymphoma by veterinarians in first opinion practice in England. *J Small Anim Pract* 43:198–202, 2002.
89. Hahn KA, Freeman KP, Barnhill MA, Stephen EL: Serum alpha 1-acid glycoprotein concentrations before and after relapse in dogs with lymphoma treated with doxorubicin. *JAVMA* 214:1023–1025, 1999.
90. von Euler H, Einarsson R, Olsson U, et al: Serum thymidine kinase activity in dogs with malignant lymphoma: A potent marker for prognosis and monitoring the disease. *J Vet Intern Med* 18:696–702, 2004.
91. Moore AS, Leveille CR, Reimann KA, et al: The expression of P-glycoprotein in canine lymphoma and its association with multidrug resistance. *Cancer Invest* 13:475–479, 1995.
92. Brick JO, Roenigk WJ, Wilson GP: Chemotherapy of malignant lymphoma in dogs and cats. *JAVMA* 153:47–52, 1968.
93. McClelland RB: Cyclophosphamide therapy in lymphoma of the dog. *Cornell Vet* 53:319–322, 1963.
94. Engstrom D, Shumay J, Jonas AM, Bertino JR: Dog lymphosarcoma as a model system for experimental chemotherapy. *Clin Res* 13:337, 1965.
95. MacEwen EG, Rosenthal GR, Fox LE, et al: Evaluation of L-asparaginase: Polyethylene glycol conjugate versus native L-asparaginase combined with chemotherapy. A randomized double-blind study in canine lymphoma. *J Vet Intern Med* 6:230–234, 1992.
96. Teske E, Rutteman CG, van Heerde P, Misdorp W: Polyethylene glycol-L-asparaginase versus native L-asparaginase in canine non-Hodgkins lymphoma. *Eur J Cancer* 26:891–895, 1990.
97. Moore AS, Ogilvie GK, Ruslander D, et al: Evaluation of mitoxantrone for the treatment of lymphoma in dogs. *JAVMA* 204:1903–1905, 1994.
98. Ruslander D, Moore AS, Gliatto JM, et al: Cytosine arabinoside as a single agent for the induction of remission in canine lymphoma. *J Vet Intern Med* 8:299–301, 1994.
99. Hahn KA, Hahn EA: Epirubicin (4'-epi-doxorubicin) chemotherapy, in Kirk RW, Bonagura JD (eds): *Current Veterinary Therapy XI*. Philadelphia, WB Saunders, 1992, pp 393–395.
100. Moore AS, Imondi AR, de Souza PL, Wood CA: Intravenous administration of 9-aminocamptothecin to dogs with lymphoma. *Vet Comp Oncol* 1:86–93, 2003.
101. Moldovenu G, Friedman M, Miller DG: Experience with the management of malignant lymphoma in dogs. *Sangre (Barc)* 17:253–262, 1964.
102. Bell R, Cotter S, Lillquist A, et al: Characterization of glucocorticoid receptors in animal lymphoblastic disease: Correlation with response to single-agent glucocorticoid treatment. *Blood* 63:380–383, 1984.
103. Moldovanu G, Friedman M, Miller DG: Treatment of canine malignant lymphoma with surgery and chemotherapy. *JAVMA* 148:153–156, 1966.
104. Squire RA, Bush M: The therapy of canine and feline lymphosarcoma. *Bibl Haematol* 39:189–197, 1973.
105. Stone MS, Goldstein MA, Cotter SM: Comparison of two protocols for induction of remission in dogs with lymphoma. *JAAHA* 27:315–321, 1991.
106. Northrup NC, Rassnick KM, Snyder LA, et al: Neutropenia associated with vincristine and L-asparaginase induction chemotherapy for canine lymphoma. *J Vet Intern Med* 16:570–575, 2002.
107. Bowles CA, Lucas D, Norton L, Graw RG Jr: Immunologic studies of canine lymphosarcoma: Mixed leukocyte reactivity following chemotherapy. *Clin Immunol Immunopathol* 9:211–217, 1978.
108. Ogilvie GK, Atwater SW, Ciekot PA, et al: Prevalence of anaphylaxis associated with the intramuscular administration of L-asparaginase to 81 dogs with cancer: 1989-1991. *JAAHA* 30:62–64, 1994.
109. Valerius KD, Ogilvie GK, Fettman MJ, et al: Comparison of the effects of asparaginase administered subcutaneously versus intramuscularly for treatment of multicentric lymphoma in dogs receiving doxorubicin. *JAVMA* 214:353–356, 1999.
110. Calvert CA, Leifer CE: Doxorubicin for treatment of canine lymphosarcoma after development of resistance to combination chemotherapy. *JAVMA* 179:1011–1012, 1981.
111. Vonderhaar M, Morrison WB, DeNicola D, et al: Comparison of duration of first remission using doxorubicin versus epirubicin as single agent therapy for canine multicentric malignant lymphoma. *Proc 11th Annu Conf Vet Cancer Soc*: 87, 1991.
112. Gray KN, Raulston GL, Gleiser CA, Jardine JH: Histologic classification as an indication of therapeutic response in malignant lymphoma of dogs. *JAVMA* 184:814–817, 1984.
113. Postorino NC, Susaneck SJ, Withrow SJ, et al: Single agent therapy with adriamycin for canine lymphosarcoma. *JAAHA* 25:221–225, 1989.
114. Mutsaers AJ, Glickman NW, DeNicola DB, et al: Evaluation of treatment with doxorubicin and piroxicam or doxorubicin alone for multicentric lymphoma in dogs. *JAVMA* 220:1813–1817, 2002.
115. Ogilvie GK, Vail DM, Klein MK, et al: Weekly administration of low-dose doxorubicin for treatment of malignant lymphoma in dogs. *JAVMA* 198:1762–1764, 1991.
116. Ogilvie GK, Moore AS, Chen C, et al: Toxicoses associated with the administration of mitoxantrone to dogs with malignant tumors: A dose escalation study. *JAVMA* 205:570–573, 1994.

117. Hauck ML, Price GS, Ogilvie GK, et al: Phase I evaluation of mitoxantrone alone and combined with whole body hyperthermia in dogs with lymphoma. *Int J Hyperthermia* 12:309–320, 1996.
118. Hammer AS, Couto CG, Ayl RD, Shank KA: Treatment of tumor-bearing dogs with actinomycin D. *J Vet Intern Med* 8:236–239, 1994.
119. Khanna C, Lund EM, Redic KA, et al: Randomized controlled trial of doxorubicin versus dactinomycin in a multiagent protocol for treatment of dogs with malignant lymphoma. *JAVMA* 213:985–990, 1998.
120. Ricci Lucas SR, Pereira Coelho BM, Marquezi ML, et al: Carmustine, vincristine, and prednisone in the treatment of canine lymphosarcoma. *JAAHA* 40:292–299, 2004.
121. Madewell BR: Chemotherapy for canine lymphosarcoma. *Am J Vet Res* 36:1525–1528, 1975.
122. Cotter SM, Goldstein MA: Comparison of two protocols for maintenance of remission in dogs with lymphoma. *JAAHA* 23:495–499, 1987.
123. Crow SE, Carter RF: Chemotherapy of canine lymphoma: CHOP vs. COP. *Proc 10th Annu Conf Vet Cancer Soc*: 11–12, 1990.
124. Calo A, Barber LG, Chretin J, et al: Evaluation of a short canine lymphoma protocol with low-dose intensity. *Proc 23rd Annu Conf Vet Cancer Soc*: 29, 2003.
125. Myers NC 3rd, Moore AS, Rand WM, et al: Evaluation of a multidrug chemotherapy protocol (ACOPA II) in dogs with lymphoma. *J Vet Intern Med* 11:333–339, 1997.
126. Boyce KL, Kitchell BE: Treatment of canine lymphoma with COPLA/LVP. *JAAHA* 36:395–403, 2000.
127. Laing EJ, Fitzpatrick PJ, Norris AM, et al: Half-body radiotherapy. Evaluation of the technique in normal dogs. *J Vet Intern Med* 3:96–101, 1989.
128. Laing EJ, Fitzpatrick PJ, Binnington AG, et al: Half-body radiotherapy in the treatment of canine lymphoma. *J Vet Intern Med* 3:102–108, 1989.
129. Gustafson NR, Lana SE, Mayer MN, LaRue SM: A preliminary assessment of whole-body radiotherapy interposed within a chemotherapy protocol for canine lymphoma. *Vet Comp Oncol* 2:125–131, 2004.
130. Chun R, Garrett LD, Vail DM: Evaluation of a high-dose chemotherapy protocol with no maintenance therapy for dogs with lymphoma. *J Vet Intern Med* 14:120–124, 2000.
131. Frimberger AE, Moore AS, Rassnick KM, et al: A combination chemotherapy protocol with dose intensification and autologous bone marrow transplant (VELCAP-HDC) for canine lymphoma. *J Vet Intern Med* 20:355–364, 2006.
132. Cotter SM: Treatment of lymphoma and leukemia with cyclophosphamide, vincristine, and prednisone: I. Treatment of dogs. *JAAHA* 19:159–165, 1983.
133. Chretin JD, Shaw NA, Hahn KA, et al: Prophylactic trimethoprim-sulfadiazine during chemotherapeutic induction: A double-blind placebo-controlled study. *Proc 20th Annu Conf Vet Cancer Soc*: 47. 2000.
134. Ogilvie GK, Vail DM, Wheeler SL, et al: Effects of chemotherapy and remission on carbohydrate metabolism in dogs with lymphoma. *Cancer* 69:233–238, 1992.
135. Ogilvie GK, Ford RB, Vail DM, et al: Alterations in lipoprotein profiles in dogs with lymphoma. *J Vet Intern Med* 8:62–66, 1994.
136. Ogilvie GK, Fettman MJ, Mallinckrodt CH, et al: Effect of fish oil, arginine, and doxorubicin chemotherapy on remission and survival time for dogs with lymphoma: A double-blind, randomized placebo-controlled study. *Cancer* 88:1916–1928, 2000.
137. Weller RE, Theilen GH, Madewell BR, et al: Chemoimmunotherapy for canine lymphosarcoma: A prospective evaluation of specific and nonspecific immunomodulation. *Am J Vet Res* 41:516-521, 1980.
138. Jeglum KA: Chemoimmunotherapy of canine lymphoma with adjuvant canine monoclonal antibody 231. *Vet Clin North Am Small Anim Pract* 26:73–85, 1996.
139. Ogilvie GK, Lana S, Bachand A, et al: Effect of BAY-129566 and chemotherapy on remission time in dogs with lymphoma: a double blind, randomized study. *Proc 22nd Ann Conf Vet Cancer Soc* 11, 2002.
140. Lucroy MD, Phillips BS, Kraegel SA, et al: Evaluation of single-agent mitoxantrone as chemotherapy for relapsing canine lymphoma. *J Vet Intern Med* 12:325–329, 1998.
141. Moore AS, Ogilvie GK, Vail DM: Actinomycin D for reinduction of remission in dogs with resistant lymphoma. *J Vet Intern Med* 8:343–344, 1994.
142. Hohenhaus AE, Matus RE: Etoposide (VP-16): Retrospective analysis of treatment in 13 dogs with lymphoma. *J Vet Intern Med* 4:239–241, 1990.
143. Ogilvie GK, Cockburn CA, Tranquilli WJ, et al: Hypotension and cutaneous reactions associated with intravenous administration of etoposide in the dog. *Am J Vet Res* 49:1367–1370, 1988.
144. Moore AS, London CA, Wood CA, et al: Lomustine (CCNU) for the treatment of resistant lymphoma in dogs. *J Vet Intern Med* 13:395–398, 1999.
145. Kristal O, Rassnick KM, Gliatto JM, et al: Hepatotoxicity associated with CCNU (lomustine) chemotherapy in dogs. *J Vet Intern Med* 18:75–80, 2004.
146. Rusk T, Cozzi E, Sharpee R, et al: A randomized placebo-controlled clinical trial of ABT-526 angiogenic inhibitor plus lomustine chemotherapy versus lomustine chemotherapy alone in dogs with relapsed lymphoma. *Proc 23rd Annu Conf Vet Cancer Soc*: 59, 2003.
147. Rassnick KM, Frimberger AE, Wood CA, et al: Evaluation of ifosfamide for treatment of various canine neoplasms. *J Vet Intern Med* 14:271–276, 2000.
148. Van Vechten M, Helfand SC, Jeglum KA: Treatment of relapsed canine lymphoma with doxorubicin and dacarbazine. *J Vet Intern Med* 4:187–191, 1990.
149. Rosenberg M, Matus R: The use of MOPP as rescue treatment for dogs with lymphoma. *Proc 11th Annu Conf Vet Cancer Soc*: 56, 1991.
150. Rassnick KM, Mauldin GE, Al-Sarraf R, et al: MOPP chemotherapy for treatment of resistant lymphoma in dogs: A retrospective study of 117 cases (1989-2000). *J Vet Intern Med* 16:576–580, 2002.
151. Mauldin GE, Mauldin GN: Efficacy of BOPP rescue for the treatment of relapsed canine lymphoma. *Proc 21st Annu Conf Vet Cancer Soc*: 82, 2001.
152. Ruslander D, Moore AS, Cotter SM: Cisplatin and ara-C as rescue treatment for dogs with lymphoma. *Proc 11th Annu Conf Vet Cancer Soc*: 61, 1991.
153. Couto CG, Rutgers HC, Sherding RG, Rojko J: Gastrointestinal lymphoma in 20 dogs: A retrospective study. *J Vet Intern Med* 3:73–78, 1989.
154. Coyle KA, Steinberg H: Characterization of lymphocytes in canine gastrointestinal lymphoma. *Vet Pathol* 41:141–146, 2004.
155. Miura T, Maruyama H, Sakai M, et al: Endoscopic findings on alimentary lymphoma in 7 dogs. *J Vet Med Sci* 66:577–580, 2004.
156. French RA, Seitz SE, Valli VE: Primary epitheliotropic alimentary T-cell lymphoma with hepatic involvement in a dog. *Vet Pathol* 33:349–352, 1996.
157. Dennis JS, Schmidt DA: Cutaneous and central nervous system lymphoma in a dog. *JAAHA* 23:31–34, 1987.
158. Rosin A: Neurologic diseases associated with lymphosarcoma in ten dogs. *JAVMA* 181:50–53, 1982.
159. Couto CG, Cullen J, Pedroia V, Turrel JM: Central nervous system lymphosarcoma in the dog. *JAVMA* 184:809–813, 1984.
160. Berg RJ, Wingfield W: Pericardial effusion in the dog: a review of 42 cases. *JAAHA* 20:721–730, 1984.
161. Lefbom BK, Parker GA: Ataxia associated with lymphosarcoma in a dog. *JAVMA* 207:922–923, 1995.
162. Long SN, Johnston PE, Anderson TJ: Primary T-cell lymphoma of the central nervous system in a dog. *JAVMA* 218:719–722, 2001.
163. Turner JL, Luttgen PJ, VanGundy TE, et al: Multicentric osseous lymphoma with spinal extradural involvement in a dog. *JAVMA* 200:196–198, 1992.
164. McDonough SP, Van Winkle TJ, Valentine BA, et al: Clinicopathological and immunophenotypical features of canine intravascular lymphoma (malignant angioendotheliomatosis). *J Comp Pathol* 126:277–288, 2002.
165. Cullen CL, Caswell JL, Grahn BH: Intravascular lymphoma presenting as bilateral panophthalmitis and retinal detachment in a dog. *JAAHA* 36:337–342, 2000.
166. Kent M, de laHunta A, Tidwell AS: MR imaging findings in a dog with intravascular lymphoma in the brain. *Vet Radiol Ultrasound* 42:504–510, 2001.
167. Bush WW, Throop JL, McManus PM, et al: Intravascular lymphoma involving the central and peripheral nervous systems in a dog. *JAAHA* 39:90–96, 2003.
168. Turnwald GH, Pechman RD, Shires PK, et al: Lymphosarcoma with osseous involvement in a dog. *JAAHA* 24:350–354, 1988.
169. Giger U, Evans SM, Hendrick MJ, Dudek SM: Orthovoltage radiotherapy of primary lymphoma of bone in a dog. *JAVMA* 195:627–630, 1989.
170. Ogilvie GK, Brunkow CS, Daniel GB, Haschek WM: Malignant lymphoma with cardiac and bone involvement in a dog. *JAVMA* 194:793–796, 1989.
171. Harkin KR, Kennedy GA, Moore WE, Schoning P: Skeletal muscle lymphoma in a bullmastiff. *JAAHA* 36:63–66, 2000.
172. Lahmers SM, Mealey KL, Martinez SA, et al: Synovial T-cell lymphoma of the stifle in a dog. *JAAHA* 38:165–168, 2002.
173. Berzon JL: Disseminated reticulum cell sarcoma in a dog: Case report and discussion. *JAAHA* 15:491–496, 1979.
174. Thomas HL, Pressler BM, Robertson ID: Radiographic diagnosis–polyostotic lymphoma in a 5 month old dog. *Vet Radiol Ultrasound* 42:521–523, 2001.
175. Langley-Hobbs SJ, Carmichael S, Lamb CR, et al: Polyostotic lymphoma in a young dog: A case report and literature review. *J Small Anim Pract* 38:412–416, 1997.
176. Barthez PY, Davis CR, Pool RR, et al: Multiple metaphyseal involvement of a thymic lymphoma associated with hypercalcemia in a puppy. *JAAHA* 31:82–85, 1995.
177. Girard C, Helie P, Odin M: Intrapericardial neoplasia in dogs. *J Vet Diagn Invest* 11:73–78, 1999.
178. Ware WA, Hopper DL: Cardiac tumors in dogs: 1982-1995. *J Vet Intern Med* 13:95–103, 1999.
179. MacGregor JM, Faria ML, Moore AS, et al: Cardiac lymphoma and pericardial effusion in dogs: 12 cases (1994–2004). *JAVMA* 227:1449–1453, 2005.
180. Forterre F, Kaiser S, Schmahl W, Brunnberg L: Rückenmarkstumoren beim Hund: 33 Fälle (retrospektive Studie). *Kleintierpraxis* 47:357–364, 2002.
181. Maiolino P, DeVico G: Primary epitheliotropic T-cell lymphoma of the urinary bladder in a dog. *Vet Pathol* 37:184–186, 2000.
182. Ueno H, Isomura H, Tanabe S, et al: Solitary nonepitheliotropic T-cell lymphoma in a dog. *J Vet Med Sci.* 66:437–439, 2004.

BONE MARROW NEOPLASIA
Antony S. Moore and Gregory K. Ogilvie

CLINICAL BRIEFING

Myelodysplasia

Clinical factors
- Clinical signs attributable to cytopenias (e.g., fever and neutropenia, petechiation and thrombocytopenia).
- Differentiated from leukemias by <30% blasts in dysplastic bone marrow.
- No age, gender, or breed predilection.
- May progress to acute leukemia.

Staging and diagnosis
- MDB (includes a CBC, biochemical profile, urinalysis, and thoracic radiography [three views])
- Bone marrow aspiration and biopsy.

Prognostic factors
- None identified.

Treatment

Initial
- Erythropoietin and corticosteroids may minimize clinical signs and cause remission in dogs with myelodysplastic syndrome with refractory anemia.
- Differentiating agents, cytarabine, and retinoids are under investigation.

Supportive
- Probably most important.
- Antibiotics and transfusions of blood and blood products.

Acute Myeloid Leukemia

Clinical factors
- Nonspecific, lethargy, and weight loss; clinical signs also result from cytopenias.
- Females, large breeds, all ages; median age: 6 years.
- Rapidly progressive, terminating in pancytopenia attributable to myelophthisis.

Staging and diagnosis
- MDB.
- Bone marrow aspiration.
- Immunostaining and histochemical staining for subtype.
- Multiple subtypes and subclassifications are recognized; myelomonocytic (M4) is most common.
- Dogs with any subtype have a poor prognosis.

Prognostic factors
- None identified.

Treatment

Initial
- Chemotherapy has not demonstrated efficacy in this disease.
- Aggressive chemotherapy often causes marrow ablation.

Supportive
- Antibiotics and transfusions of blood and blood products.

Acute Lymphoblastic Leukemia

Clinical factors
- Acute-onset lethargy, weight loss, and anorexia; splenomegaly common; mild lymphadenopathy.
- Clinical signs also result from cytopenias.
- No age or gender predilection; large-breed dogs.
- Rapidly progressive; pancytopenia caused by myelophthisis.

Staging and diagnosis
- MDB.
- Bone marrow aspiration.
- Immunostaining for CD3 and CD79a.
- Differentiate from stage V lymphoma with CD34 immunostaining.

Prognostic factors
- None identified.

Treatment

Initial
- Use nonmyelosuppressive chemotherapeutic agents, at least initially (e.g., vincristine, prednisone, L-asparaginase) until normal neutrophil counts are obtained, then use standard lymphoma protocols.
- Median survival is 120 days, with a 40% response rate to vincristine and prednisone.

Supportive
- Antibiotics and transfusions of blood and blood products.

Chronic Lymphocytic Leukemia

Clinical factors
- Nonspecific, often asymptomatic and found on routine blood work.
- Older dogs affected.
- Mature lymphocytosis; differentiate from reactive lymphocytosis and well-differentiated lymphoma.
- Slowly progressive.

Staging and diagnosis
- MDB.
- Bone marrow aspiration.
- Immunostaining for CD3 and CD79a.

Prognostic factors
- None identified.

Treatment

Observation
- Repeated monitoring by blood counts may be all that is required in asymptomatic animals.

Chemotherapy
- Prednisone and chlorambucil provide long-term remissions in symptomatic dogs.

Polycythemia (Primary Erythrocytosis)

Clinical factors
- Polyuria, polydipsia, bleeding, seizures, and hyperemic mucous membranes.
- Mature erythrocytosis; rule out relative and secondary polycythemia.
- Middle-aged dogs; no breed predilection.
- Elevated red cell mass without increase in erythropoietin.

Staging and diagnosis	• MDB. • Bone marrow aspiration. • Rule out causes of secondary erythrocytosis. • Serum erythropoietin level.
Prognostic factors	• None identified.
Treatment	
Phlebotomy	• Periodic removal eventually induces iron deficiency and microcytic cells that may assist in palliation.
Chemotherapy	• Hydroxyurea gives long-term control.
Multiple Myeloma	
Common clinical presentation	• Anemia and secondary infections caused by myelophthisis. • Lameness and pain from bone lytic lesions. • Polyuria and polydipsia from hypercalcemia, renal disease, and paraproteinuria. • Hemorrhage and retinal lesions caused by hyperviscosity. • Median age: 8 to 9 years; most cases occur in purebred dogs.
Staging and diagnosis	• MDB. • Bone marrow aspiration. • Radiography of ribs, spine, and any painful sites. • Serum protein electrophoresis and immunoelectrophoresis. • Urine Bence Jones protein test (or urine immunoelectrophoresis).
Prognostic factors	• Dogs with hypercalcemia have a worse prognosis. • Dogs with extensive bone lysis have a worse prognosis. • Dogs with light-chain (Bence Jones) proteinuria have a worse prognosis.
Treatment	
Initial	• Prednisone alone only palliative; median survival: 220 days. • Melphalan and prednisone causes CR in 40% and PR in 50% of dogs for median survival of 540 days. • Cyclophosphamide or chlorambucil may be effective.
Adjunctive	• Radiation therapy palliative for localized bone lesions.

It is more realistic to think of neoplastic disorders of the bone marrow elements as presenting a continuum of disease rather than as discrete pathophysiologic entities. The earliest stages in myeloproliferative disease reflect decreased or inappropriate bone marrow production; signs may reflect functional problems without overt evidence of neoplasia. When cytopenias and morphologic abnormalities are noted, they are termed *myelodysplasia* (MDS) or *preleukemia*. MDS may progress to a true neoplastic process or leukemia, which may be "aleukemic" when it involves only bone marrow, not peripheral blood. Leukemias may affect any of the cell lines in the marrow and are classified based on the type of cell from which they derive (Figure 48-1). Clinically, it is important to distinguish chronic leukemias and myeloproliferative diseases from acute leukemias and to distinguish acute lymphoblastic leukemia (ALL) from acute myeloid (nonlymphoid) leukemia (AML).

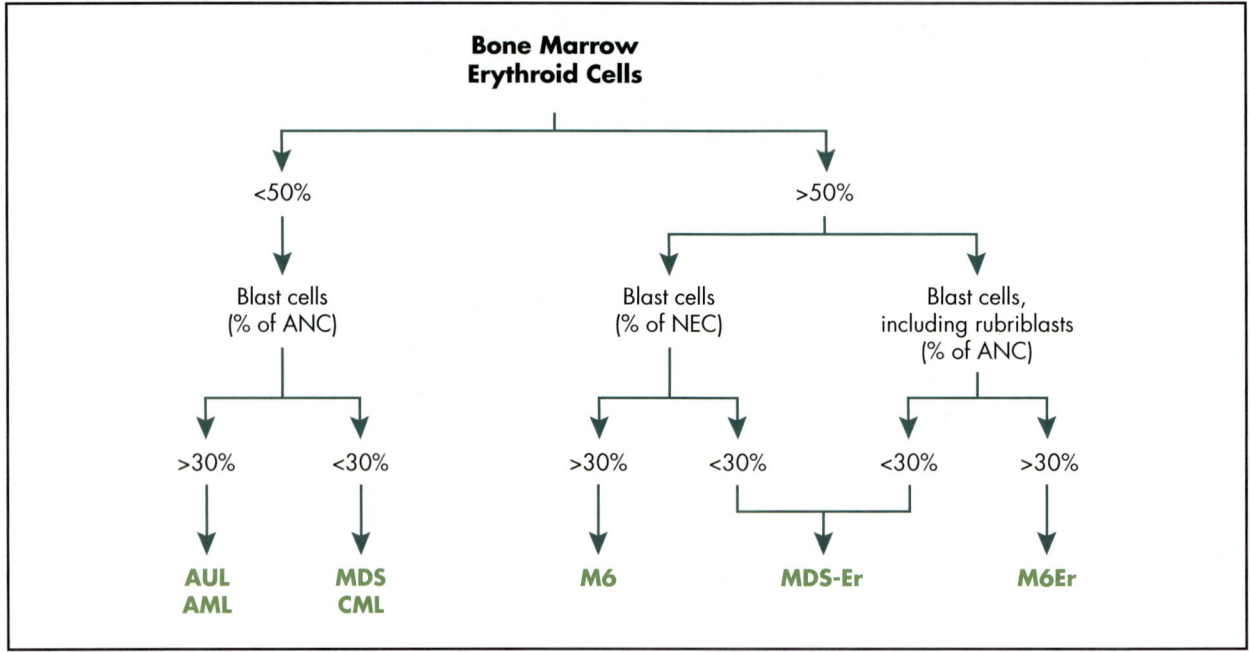

Figure 48-1. *A scheme to classify myelodysplastic syndromes and myeloid leukemias in dogs. Blast cells include myeloblasts, monoblasts, and megakaryoblasts. (AML = acute myeloid leukemias M1 to M5 and M7; ANC = all nucleated cells in bone marrow, excluding lymphocytes, plasma cells, macrophages, and mast cells; AUL = acute undifferentiated leukemia; CML = chronic myeloid leukemia, including chronic myelogenous, chronic myelomonocytic, and chronic monocytic leukemias; MDS-Er = myelodysplastic syndrome with erythroid predominance; M6 = erythroleukemia; M6Er = erythroleukemia with erythroid predominance; NEC = nonerythroid cells in bone marrow) (From Jain NC, Blue JT, Grindem CB, et al: Proposed criteria for classification of acute myeloid leukemia in dogs and cats.* Vet Clin Pathol *20:63–82, 1991; with permission)*

Myelodysplasia (Preleukemia)
INCIDENCE, SIGNALMENT, AND ETIOLOGY

MDS is rarely recognized in dogs, but its true prevalence may be underestimated because it is difficult to diagnose. It is often described retrospectively after development of acute leukemia. Theoretically, defects in stem cells impair hematopoiesis, which produces a wide variety of abnormalities, including disordered granulopoiesis accompanied by abnormal cellular morphology or maturation arrest. The progeny of these stem cells have dysplastic features and an accelerated rate of apoptosis.[1] There is no apparent breed, gender, or age predilection to canine MDS. Most affected dogs are between 4 and 11 years of age.[2] MDS is usually defined as peripheral cytopenia with normocellular to hypercellular bone marrow that manifests abnormalities in nuclear and cytoplasmic maturation (dysgranulopoiesis, dyserythropoiesis, dysthrombopoiesis, or a combination of the three in >10% of the affected cell line) but is composed of less than 30% blast cells.[1] In leukemia, more than 30% of nucleated bone marrow cells are blast cells.[3] Dogs with radiation-induced nonlymphoid leukemia have a preleukemic transition stage that is similar to MDS.[4]

MDS has been classified as primary (refractory anemia or MDS) or secondary (caused by lymphoma, multiple myeloma, drug therapy, immune-mediated hematologic disease, polycythemia vera, or overwhelming infection). In one series of 34 dogs with MDS, 13 were characterized as having primary MDS.[1] Primary MDS is further divided into MDS with refractory anemia (MDS-RA), MDS with refractory cytopenias (MDS-RC), and MDS with excess myeloblasts (MDS-EB).[5] A dog with naturally occurring MDS-EB had progression to AML over a 4-month period.[6]

> **KEY POINT**
> *Myelodysplasia is characterized by bone marrow that contains abnormalities in cellular maturation but less than 30% blast cells.*

CLINICAL PRESENTATION AND HISTORY

MDS is characterized by cytopenias in blood and cytologic features of dysplasia in marrow.[1] Peripheral cytopenias may produce a number of clinical signs and physical findings. Fever is common and may reflect production of pyrogens in response to the disease or, more often, may arise from infections that the neutropenic animal is unable to overcome.[2,7,8] Anemia and thrombocytopenia may cause petechiation, pallor, and lethargy. Inappetence and other nonspecific signs of illness can be seen. Clinical examination may detect hepatomegaly and splenomegaly, which possibly arise from extramedullary hematopoiesis or from increased sequestration and destruction of abnormal cells.

Because it may be difficult to distinguish between primary and secondary MDS on the basis of blood and bone marrow changes, primary MDS is often a disease of exclusion. It is imperative to obtain a thorough history and to evaluate the patient for any other disease process or drug therapy that could result in secondary MDS.

Table 48-1 Hematologic Features of Primary and Secondary MDS in Dogs[1]

Variable	MDS-RA	MDS-EB	Secondary MDS
Blood			
Circulating cells	Anemia	Pancytopenia	Variable
Bone Marrow			
Myeloblasts (%)	<5	>5	<5%
Red cell blasts (%)	>5	>5	Variable
Granulocyte maturation ratio	<0.15:1	>0.15:1	Variable
Erythroid maturation ratio	>0.12:1	>0.12:1	Variable
Dysplastic cell line(s)	Erythroid	Erythroid, myeloid (>20%), megakaryocytic	Variable

STAGING AND DIAGNOSIS

Staging animals with MDS includes a complete blood count (CBC), biochemical profile, urinalysis, bone marrow cytology, core biopsy, and special stains of abnormal cells. The hemogram of MDS usually reveals cytopenias involving any or all of the hematopoietic cell lines. Some dogs with MDS have been reported to have pancytopenia with marked normoblastemia. The bone marrow of animals with MDS is usually normocellular to hypercellular and often contains an increased number of plasma cells and macrophages.[2]

Granulocytes may be immature or show abnormal morphology (e.g., hypersegmentation, giant forms). There may be an abnormal progression in the granulocyte maturation series with an increased percentage of progranulocytes, cells with abnormal nuclear to cytoplasmic maturation, skipped mitoses, giant granulocytes, or megaloblastic cells. Nucleated red blood cells are often present in numbers disproportionate to reticulocytes. Megakaryocytes may be numerous but are often dysplastic with small nuclei or cytoplasmic vacuolization.

Blast cells may be absent; if present, they may account for up to 30% of the marrow without fulfilling the criteria for leukemia. Progression to acute leukemia is often rapid and has been reported to occur in dogs within 5 to 10 weeks.[2,8,9]

Veterinary authors have separated primary MDS into MDS-RA and MDS-EB; however, MDS-RC has not been recognized.[1,5] MDS-RA was diagnosed in four dogs and was characterized in the blood by a nonregenerative anemia without leukopenia or thrombocytopenia and in the bone marrow by erythroid hyperplasia with prominent dysplastic features in more than 15% of the red cell series (binucleate cells, sideroblasts, or both), less than 5% myeloblasts, and a normal granulocyte maturation ratio. MDS-EB was diagnosed in nine dogs and was characterized in the blood by pancytopenia and in the bone marrow by dysplastic features in all cell lines (dysgranulopoeisis in all nine dogs, dyserythropoiesis in eight, and dysthrombopoiesis in seven), more than 5% myeloblasts, and a high granulocyte maturation ratio (Table 48-1).[1]

TREATMENT

In human medicine, treatment of MDS is controversial. Some authors recommend no therapy until development of acute leukemia. Treatment with so-called *differentiating agents* such as low-dose cytarabine (5–10 mg/m^2/day SC) has been of benefit for some human patients, but its use has rarely been reported in dogs. Other differentiating agents being explored include etretinate. Transfusions are considered supportive for anemic patients but must be given at frequent intervals to maintain a reasonable quality of life for the dog.[2,8]

A dog with MDS-RA was treated with blood transfusion, prednisone, and human recombinant erythropoietin. Response to erythropoietin was slow, taking more than 2 weeks for an increase in the packed cell volume (PCV). Therapy was only given for 2 months, and the dog was normal 30 months later.[10] Another dog with liver disease and MDS-RA was treated with supportive blood transfusions, prednisolone, and cytarabine ocfosfate 200 mg/m^2 PO sid. The anemia (but not the hepatopathy) resolved, and the dog was clinically normal more than 1 year later.[11] This dog was considered refractory to human recombinant erythropoietin; however, the drug was only given for 7 days, which may not have been long enough to see a peripheral response. The use of human erythropoietin in dogs may result in pure red cell aplasia caused by cross-reactivity between antibodies to the human product and native canine erythropoietin; a canine recombinant product has been developed but is not commercially available at the time of writing.[12] One author has suggested that dogs with MDS-RC and MDS-RA seem to have prolonged survival with erythropoietin treatment. Dogs with MDS-EB respond poorly to any treatment.[13]

Given the difficulties in differentiating primary and secondary MDS, it is possible that some patients with immune-

Table 48-2 Types of AML Diagnosed by the ALSG[3]

ASLG Classification	Acute Leukemia Type	Comments
AUL	Undifferentiated	—
M1	Myeloblastic	Myeloblastic leukemia without maturation (>90% blasts)
M2	Myeloblastic	Myeloblastic leukemia with maturation (<90% blasts)
M4	Myelomonocytic	Morphology similar to ALL
M5a M5b	Monocytic	a = without maturation (>80% blasts) b = with maturation (<80% blasts)
M6 M6Er	Erythroblastic (erythroid)	Er = >50% erythroid cells and <30 myeloid cells
M7	Megakaryoblastic	—

mediated disease and MDS respond to immunosuppressive therapy (as described for the two cases above). A careful history should be obtained in any dog with characteristics of MDS.

Supportive treatment with transfusions and broad-spectrum antibiotics for neutropenic animals should be considered for dogs with MDS. Aggressive chemotherapy is not warranted; however, differentiating agents may be worth considering on an investigational basis.

Acute Leukemias
ACUTE MYELOID (NONLYMPHOID) LEUKEMIA

Although the cell of derivation for an acute leukemia can often be suspected on the basis of conventionally stained blood or bone marrow cytologic preparations, special cytochemical stains are usually necessary to confirm the lineage of a particular leukemia. For veterinary clinicians, the primary application of these stains is to distinguish ALL from AML. The prognosis for AML is poor, and further delineation of the specific leukemia cell type is often clinically unnecessary but can be of academic interest.

Acute nonlymphoid leukemia may be a better term than AML, which also has been used to describe granulocytic leukemia and may exclude leukemias that are erythroid in derivation. However, we follow the findings of the Animal Leukemia Study Group (ALSG) in characterizing these diseases as AML (Figure 48-1 and Table 48-2). Subtypes proposed by this group include undifferentiated myeloid leukemia and M1 to M7 AML. There is considerable overlap between the older terms of acute myelogenous, acute myelomonocytic, and acute monocytic leukemia within the ALSG classifications.[3] Dogs with myelomonocytic (M4) leukemia may be misdiagnosed as having ALL when cytochemical staining is not used.[14]

Incidence, Signalment, and Etiology

There are some reports that AML is more common than ALL in dogs, and AML accounts for approximately 70% of leukemias described in three studies.[15–17] The most common subclassification is acute myelomonocytic leukemia (M4).[3,15,16,18] AML is more likely to affect female dogs than males.[16,18–21] There seems to be no breed predisposition, although large-breed dogs may be overrepresented.[18–20] The age of affected dogs ranges from 1 to 12 years, with a median age of 6 years[16,18]; the median age of seven dogs with AML-M7 was 2.5 years.[22–26] AML can be induced experimentally in dogs by chronic radiation exposure.[4]

Clinical Presentation and History

Nonspecific clinical signs such as lethargy, anorexia, and sudden weight loss are most commonly noticed by caregivers.[16,19–21] In one study, more than one-third of dogs had a shifting-limb lameness that was attributed to subendosteal infiltration by malignant cells or bone infarcts.[16] The duration of signs is rarely longer than 1 month and is often less than 2 weeks.[19]

On physical examination, the most frequent findings are splenomegaly, lymphadenopathy, and hepatomegaly.[16,18,20,21] Pale mucous membranes, sometimes with petechiation, are common.[16,20] Ocular changes are more frequently described in association with AML than with ALL. Ocular changes include retinal detachment, often with hemorrhage; hyphema; glaucoma; chorioretinitis; chemosis; and conjunctivitis. These changes occur in approximately 30% of dogs with AML.[16,18]

Staging and Diagnosis

Staging for animals with suspected leukemia includes a CBC, a biochemical profile, urinalysis, bone marrow cytology, a core biopsy, and special stains of abnormal cells. Dogs with acute leukemia have a predominance of blast cells in their blood and bone marrow, which makes this disease difficult to diagnose accurately using only morphologic criteria. Cytochemical stains are required to determine the cell of origin. Some authors believe that bone marrow blast cells stain with greater intensity than do cells in the peripheral circulation,[12] but others believe that cells in a buffy-coat preparation provide better morphology.[15] To improve specificity, dogs with leukemia should have cytochemical stains conducted on samples of bone marrow as well as peripheral blood. Cytochemical staining provided the basis for changing the diagnosis from ALL to AML or vice versa in seven of 22 cases of leukemia in one study[27] and in eight of 17 cases in another.[15] Techniques such as electron microscopy and cytogenetics are not readily available or reliable for distinguishing leukemic cells from normal cells.[17,28]

Most dogs with AML are truly leukemic (i.e., abnormal cells circulate rather than appear only in bone marrow), and mean or median leukocyte counts are between 85,000 and 95,000 cells/µl, with a range of 1,500 (aleukemic) to 191,000.[16,19] Affected dogs are often pancytopenic, although anemia and thrombocytopenia are more common than other hematologic abnormalities.[18] A leukoerythroblastic reaction (increases in nucleated red blood cells and immature granulocytes) may be seen because of crowding of the bone marrow and disruption of the marrow–blood barrier.[16] Some dogs with AML have circulating micromegakaryocytes, as do some dogs with MDS before the development of AML.[9,29]

Newer techniques using flow cytometry and immunohistochemical staining have enabled some investigators to establish the type of leukemia by analyzing peripheral blood, even in dogs that are not overtly leukemic.[30,31] Although this technique is limited because of access to appropriate machines, the next few years will undoubtedly see increasing clinical use of this technology. Immunostaining using cluster of differentiation (CD) markers may help to differentiate AML from ALL. AML cells stain with CD1c, CD11, CD4, CD14, or DM-5; ALL cells stain with CD3 (T cell), CD79a (B cell), or CD8.[32]

Treatment

Untreated dogs with AML have a life expectancy of less than 2 weeks, with death often resulting from infection, bleeding, or both; most dogs are euthanatized because of poor quality of life soon after diagnosis.[29,33,34] Consequently, there are few reports of treatment.

Subtypes of AML seem to matter little to the prognosis for veterinary patients. Of seven dogs with AML-M7 (megakaryoblastic leukemia) treated with supportive treatment, anemia, bleeding, and pulmonary infiltrates caused death in all dogs by 4 weeks after diagnosis.[22-26,35]

Chemotherapy for AML in dogs has been uniformly disappointing; death commonly occurs either from progressive disease or from marrow ablation by overzealous treatment.

In one series of 10 dogs with AML, treatment with vinblastine, prednisone, cyclophosphamide, and cytarabine produced an average survival of 3 weeks, with a range of 1 day to 6 weeks.[19] Similarly, in two other studies, treated dogs survived from 4 to 12 weeks[16] and from 1 to 42 days (median: 10 days).[17] Death occurred as a result of sepsis or from hemorrhage caused by thrombocytopenia.

Case reports have documented similar clinical courses with chemotherapy. M4 leukemia, lymphadenopathy, and hepatosplenomegaly was misdiagnosed as ALL in one dog that responded to combination chemotherapy using vincristine, cyclophosphamide, cytarabine, and prednisone.[14] This dog had improvement in hematologic parameters for approximately 2 weeks, then slowly declined until euthanasia 8 weeks after the start of treatment. A short-term response to vincristine, cyclophosphamide, and prednisone was seen in another dog with AML-M6 that died 3 weeks after treatment was started.[36]

Combination therapy using vincristine, busulfan (4 mg/m^2 PO sid), and prednisolone caused a dramatic response in a dog with AML, but the dog died with pulmonary leukemic infiltrates less than 1 month after treatment.[37]

The best reported results come from using antimetabolites, but in only one dog. Cytarabine (100 mg/m^2 IV q12h for 4 days), 6-thioguanine (40 mg/m^2 PO bid for 4 days), and prednisone (20 mg/m^2 PO bid reduced to 10 mg/m^2 bid every other day) were used to treat a dog with AML and central nervous system (CNS) infiltration. The dog responded but relapsed 120 days later. Reinduction of remission was successful for an additional 120 days, at which time the dog was euthanatized.[18] Two other dogs treated with the same regimen were euthanatized 10 days after starting treatment.

In human patients with AML, doxorubicin is a useful agent, as is another anthracycline, daunorubicin. In two veterinary reports that used doxorubicin (30 mg/m^2 IV) in combination with prednisone and cyclophosphamide[20] or with vincristine, thioguanine, and prednisone,[21] death occurred within 7 and 30 days, respectively. The dog treated with the latter regimen had less than 5% blasts in the bone marrow after treatment; however, normal marrow elements also were ablated. Dr. Cotter at Tufts University reports that six other dogs treated with doxorubicin and prednisone did not respond and had short survival. The use of related chemotherapeutic agents, such as daunorubicin and idarubicin, has not been evaluated in dogs with AML.

> *Chemotherapy for AML in dogs has not yet met with any success. The prognosis for these animals is very poor.*

The prognosis for dogs with AML is poor because of lack of proven efficacy for chemotherapeutic agents at currently used dosages and lack of adequate support by specialized transfusions (e.g., granulocytes) and antimicrobial coverage. The use of colony-stimulating factors to support normal

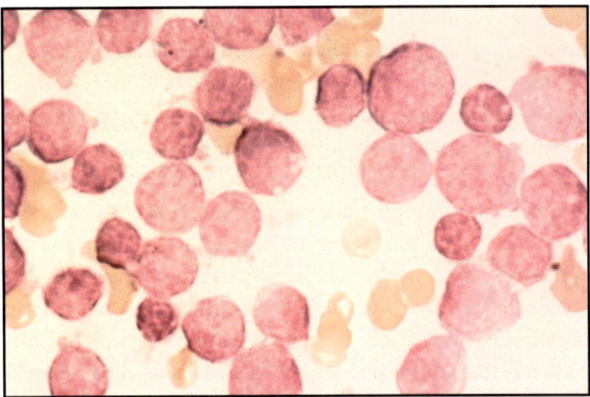

Figure 48-2. *This bone marrow aspirate from a dog with AML shows a predominant population of blast cells. It is necessary to conduct special cytochemical and immunohistochemical stains to determine whether this dog has ALL or which subtype of AML is present. (Courtesy of Susan M. Cotter, DVM, Tufts Cummings School of Veterinary Medicine)*

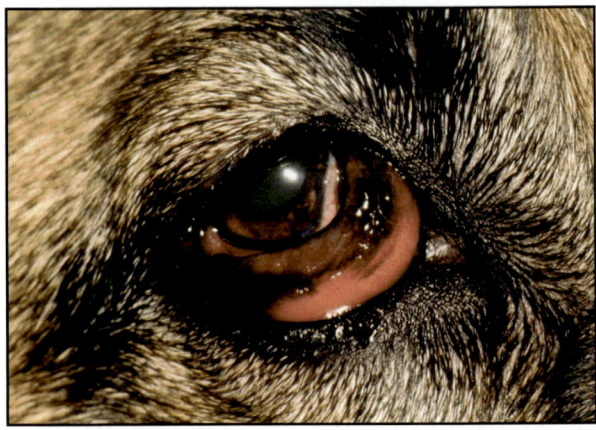

Figure 48-3. *ALL can cause infiltrates, as in this dog with nictitans lymphoblastic infiltration. In these dogs, it may be difficult to distinguish between ALL and stage V lymphoma. Immunostaining for CD34 is seen in ALL but not lymphoma.*

marrow elements is controversial because these factors may also stimulate the growth of malignant cells. Stimulated growth may, however, make tumor cells more susceptible to chemotherapy.

ACUTE LYMPHOBLASTIC LEUKEMIA
Incidence, Signalment, and Etiology

ALL is used to describe a lymphoid malignancy primarily involving bone marrow that is hypercellular and usually replaced by blasts (Figure 48-2). ALL affects dogs of all ages. German shepherds and other large-breed dogs may be overrepresented. There seems to be no strong gender predilection for ALL.[16,19,38]

Clinical Presentation and History

Clinical signs are usually acute with ALL and occur for 1 to 12 weeks before diagnosis; the median duration is 2 weeks. Nonspecific signs such as lethargy and anorexia are common; vomiting, diarrhea, abdominal pain, polyuria, polydipsia, and shifting lameness are occasionally seen.[16,19,38]

Affected dogs are usually thin. Between 50% and 60% have lymphadenopathy, which is often mild compared with the dramatic lymphadenopathy seen in dogs with lymphoma. Splenomegaly, hepatomegaly, and pale mucous membranes are the most common abnormalities detected on physical examination and occur in up to 70% of affected dogs. Infiltration of the CNS with lymphoblasts may occur, and dogs may present for incoordination and depression or acute paresis.[16] Additional infiltration of other organs may occur, making differential diagnosis between advanced lymphoma and ALL difficult (Figure 48-3).

This condition should be distinguished from stage V lymphoma, which primarily involves marked lymphadenopathy and may also cause splenomegaly and hepatomegaly. Dogs with lymphoma are frequently in good clinical condition. Whereas the prognosis for stage V lymphoma is guarded (see Chapter 47), the prognosis for ALL is poor.

Staging and Diagnosis

Staging animals with suspected ALL includes a CBC, a biochemical profile, urinalysis, bone marrow cytology, a core biopsy, and special stains of abnormal cells, specifically, markers for CD3, CD79a, or CD8. Staging dogs should also differentiate the disease from lymphoma with thoracic radiography, abdominal ultrasonography, and (if available) staining for CD34. Distinguishing between advanced (stage V) lymphoma and ALL can be clinically difficult, but dogs with leukemia have cells that stain with the progenitor cell marker CD34, and dogs with lymphoma do not.[32] Similar to dogs with lymphoma, dogs with ALL can be hypercalcemic.[39]

As with AML, dogs with ALL often have a predominance of primitive undifferentiated cells that are difficult to identify definitively. Cytochemical staining is important to distinguish ALL from AML. Both diseases are difficult to treat, but they may differ in their prognoses. More recently, immunostaining using CD markers has been used to differentiate ALL from AML. Dogs with ALL have cells that stain with CD3, CD79a, or CD8; AML cells stain with CD1c, CD11, CD4, CD14, or DM5.[32,40]

White blood cell counts are frequently high in dogs with ALL. Counts of greater than 100,000 cells/µl were reported in one study,[38] and counts were greater than 600,000/µl in another study.[16] Some dogs may be aleukemic or pancytopenic because of myelophthisis.[38] Thrombocytopenia and anemia are frequent in dogs with ALL.[16,38] Because white blood cell counts may rapidly normalize after treatment with corticosteroids, these drugs should be avoided until samples needed to reach a definitive diagnosis have been obtained.

A subtype of lymphoid leukemia has been described that consists of large granular lymphocytes (LGL). Although the cells are immunohistochemically distinct, it seems that the spectrum of diseases (reactive leukemia, chronic leukemia, and acute leukemia) is clinically indistinguishable from ALL not associated with LGL.[32,41]

Treatment

If thrombocytopenia and anemia are present, particularly if the dog is slow to respond to chemotherapy, supportive therapy with blood products, such as fresh whole blood and platelet-rich plasma, should be initiated. Hematopoietic growth factors may be useful to increase the number of neutrophils, but as mentioned earlier, it is theoretically possible that these factors can also enhance the growth of the tumor cells.

One of three dogs with ALL had a complete response for 8.5 years after receiving cyclophosphamide alone; the other two dogs failed to respond.[42] In a larger study, nine dogs that received either no treatment (n = 3) or single-agent treatment with prednisone (n = 3) or cyclophosphamide (n = 3) did not achieve remission.[38] All nine dogs died within 60 days. Median survival was 12 days. Another 21 dogs received vincristine (0.025 mg/kg/week IV) and prednisone (2.2 mg/kg PO sid). Four dogs (20%) achieved a complete remission (CR), and four dogs achieved a partial remission (PR). The median survival for these eight dogs was 120 days and ranged from 8 to 241 days. The median time to achieve a measurable response was 14 days, and the dogs that responded earlier lived longer.[38]

> **KEY POINT**
> *Dogs with ALL may be pancytopenic because of myelophthisis. Nonmyelosuppressive drugs, such as vincristine, L-asparaginase, or prednisone, should be used initially in these dogs.*

Dogs with ALL are often pancytopenic because of bone marrow crowding by tumor cells. This pancytopenia may be exacerbated by aggressive chemotherapy. Neither vincristine nor prednisone is strongly myelosuppressive, which is important in allowing normal marrow elements to repopulate while the dog enters remission. In addition, prednisone is one of the few drugs that crosses the blood–brain barrier, which is important in view of the risk of CNS involvement with ALL.[16] L-Asparaginase is another nonmyelosuppressive chemotherapeutic agent that has indirect action across the blood–brain barrier by reducing asparagine levels. Care should be taken when administering L-asparaginase at the same time as vincristine because the combination can be extremely myelosuppressive (see Chapter 47).

Prednisone (40 mg/m^2 PO sid for 3 weeks, then every other day) and vincristine (0.75 mg/m^2 IV q7d) followed 1 day later by L-asparaginase (10,000 IU/m^2 IM q7d) should be used until the neutrophil count is above 3,000 cells/µl. This induction chemotherapy reduces the tumor cell burden while maintaining normal marrow elements. More aggressive therapy with myelosuppressive agents, such as cyclophosphamide and doxorubicin, may be used to "consolidate" the remission when normal myeloid elements are restored. Even with this approach, prognosis is guarded for dogs with ALL because relapse is common when the chemotherapeutic regimen is eased into a maintenance phase.

Immunotherapy has been described only once for the treatment of ALL in a dog, and its use may more correctly be termed supportive care.[43] Five units of fresh heparinized canine plasma and two units of fresh whole blood were given over a period of 42 days, and the dog achieved a remission for 19 months. Relapse at that time did not respond to treatment. It is possible that remission was caused by a "graft versus leukemia" effect.

Chronic Leukemias and Myeloproliferative Disorders
CHRONIC LYMPHOCYTIC LEUKEMIA
Incidence, Signalment, and Etiology

Chronic lymphocytic leukemia (CLL) is an uncommon myeloproliferative disease characterized by an increased number of circulating lymphocytes with normal morphology; the bone marrow is often infiltrated with similar cells. Affected dogs are usually older (median age: 10 years).[32,44–49] There is no obvious gender or breed predisposition, with the exception of a subtype derived from large granular lymphocytes (LGL-CLL), which is most common in females.[32]

Clinical Presentation and History

Patients may be asymptomatic, in which case the diagnosis may be made only when a hemogram is evaluated for some other reason.[45,48] The most common client complaint is lethargy (>50% of affected dogs). Inappetence, sporadic vomiting, polyuria, polydipsia, and lymphadenopathy each occur in about 20% of cases. Other signs include lameness and diarrhea, both of which may be intermittent, and weight loss. Infiltration by abnormal lymphocytes produces such signs as buccal ulceration[47] and pruritic dermatitis.[49] On clinical examination, mild lymphadenopathy is noted in up to 80% of affected dogs.[45] Splenomegaly and hepatomegaly attributable to cellular infiltration or to extramedullary hematopoiesis are often found.[44,45,47] The duration of these signs is often long, and some dogs have had an elevated lymphocyte count for up to 2.5 years before definitive treatment.[44,49]

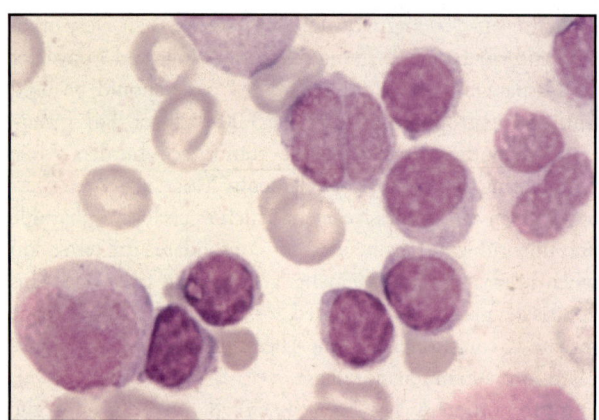

Figure 48-4. *CLL is characterized by a very high number of circulating lymphocytes that are morphologically normal. Lymphocyte counts in excess of 100,000/µl can occur with this disease; however, the prognosis with treatment is very good. (Courtesy of S. M. Cotter)*

CLL apparently occurs in three distinct stages: an asymptomatic period, which may last for months despite a high number of circulating lymphocytes; a symptomatic stage, when therapy is required; and a third stage, malignant transformation (blast crisis), which is rarely recognized in dogs.[45] Three dogs with CLL developed lymphoma after achieving stable remission between 460 and 730 days.[45] This may represent transformation of an otherwise well-differentiated disease to a more malignant stage.

Staging and Diagnosis

Staging animals with suspected CLL includes a CBC, a biochemical profile, urinalysis, bone marrow cytology (possibly with a core biopsy), and special lymphocyte stains (specifically, markers for CD3 and CD79a or CD8). Hematologic evaluation reveals a lymphocytosis composed of well-differentiated cells (Figure 48-4). Occasionally, "reactive" forms are noted. Lymphocytosis varies widely, with lymphocyte counts from 6,000 to more than 1,600,000 cells/µl in two studies.[32,45] Dogs with unexplained or persistent lymphocytosis should have a bone marrow aspirate evaluated cytologically to disclose infiltration by small lymphocytes and confirm the diagnosis of CLL. Infiltration explains other hematologic abnormalities, such as nonregenerative anemia and thrombocytopenia, which are usually mild, with a hematocrit level above 20% and a platelet count above 100,000/µl.[44,45] Unlike in acute leukemias, severe cytopenias are rare because marrow is rarely replaced.

Early studies assumed that CLL in dogs was usually derived from B lymphocytes because of the finding of a monoclonal gammopathy in nearly 70% of 22 dogs in one study.[45] However, a small study found that most cells in dogs with CLL were T-cell derived and CD8 positive.[40] This finding mirrored the results in a series of 73 dogs with CLL, in which lymphocytes from 52 dogs (73%) were found to be of T-cell derivation, and many were LGL, which are mostly cytotoxic T cells.[32] Some investigators have found that LGL mainly derive from the splenic red pulp and have suggested that CLL in dogs may often arise from the spleen rather than the bone marrow.[41] The major clinical differences between LGL-CLL and other types of CLL are that neutropenia is less common and abnormal cell counts are high, with a median of 54,000/µl.[32]

Protein electrophoresis and immunoelectrophoresis should be conducted, particularly if the globulin concentration is increased. Abnormal immunoglobulins may interfere with normal immune function as well as with coagulation and circulation (see Multiple Myeloma section, below). Hypercalcemia may be identified on a minimum database (MDB), even in dogs with a B cell–derived CLL, but resolves with therapy.[50]

Rarely, it may be necessary to decide whether a dog has CLL or ALL (e.g., when cells are reactive on cytology). Whereas dogs with ALL have cells that stain with the progenitor cell marker CD34, dogs with CLL do not.[32]

Treatment

Dogs with lymphoma derived from T lymphocytes are thought to have a worse prognosis. However, dogs with CLL, despite 70% of lymphocytes being derived from T cells, appear to have an excellent chance of responding, and remissions are often long lasting.

> **KEY POINT**
> *Clinical improvement is usually evident soon after treatment for CLL is started, but lymphocyte counts may not decrease appreciably until the dog has been treated for up to 3 months.*

Although patients with CLL are very responsive to treatment, for asymptomatic dogs, the clinician should consider a trial period of observation during which serial hematologic evaluations are performed every 3 months. One dog observed in this manner showed no clinical deterioration for 23 months.[48]

The presence or development of clinical signs should lead to prompt chemotherapy. Chlorambucil and prednisone are the most active agents in dogs as well as in humans. In a study of 20 dogs treated for 1 to 3 weeks with vincristine (0.75 mg/m² IV q7d) followed by chlorambucil (6 mg/m² PO daily for 1 week, then 3 mg/m² PO daily) and prednisone (30 mg/m² PO daily decreasing over 3 weeks), 14 achieved long-term remission for an average survival of 452 days (median: 348 days; range: 30–1,000 days).[45] Three dogs died or were lost to follow-up, and three dogs failed to respond. Some dogs took up to 3 months to achieve a remission.[45,46] The contribution of vincristine to this protocol is uncertain because similar results have been achieved with chlorambucil and prednisone alone; in other studies, chlorambucil and prednisone, even on intermittent schedules, have caused remissions of 10 months to 3 years.[44,46,49] Responses to melphalan and prednisone were also seen in dogs with CLL[51]; alkylating agents other than chlorambucil may be useful in refractory patients. Fludarabine is a useful agent in human patients with refractory CLL, but its use has not been reported in dogs.

In human patients with CLL, treatment may be administered in "pulses." With this therapy, the dog would be treated until the lymphocyte counts have normalized and for 6 weeks afterward; then therapy would be discontinued and the patient monitored by monthly blood counts until the lymphocyte counts began to rise again. This therapy has the appeal of allowing a period "off" chemotherapy, but results have not been published in the veterinary literature.

CLL in humans is often treated with combination chemotherapy protocols, such as cyclophosphamide, doxorubicin, and prednisone (CAP) or cyclophosphamide, vincristine, prednisone, and doxorubicin (CHOP), with good results. More recently, fludarabine has been shown to have efficacy similar to that of combination chemotherapy in humans.[52] No data exist on these approaches in dogs; however, CHOP is preferred by some over chlorambucil and prednisone because it may shorten the time to remission and lengthen the duration of remission.

CHRONIC MYELOID LEUKEMIA
Incidence, Signalment, and Etiology

Chronic myeloid leukemia (CML) is extremely rare in dogs, and a lack of defined diagnostic criteria makes it difficult to diagnose except by elimination of other diseases, such as systemic infections, immune-mediated disease, and other inflammatory diseases. The finding of granulocyte series overproduction in the absence of other causes is the best diagnostic criterion. Chromosomal abnormalities that are seen in human chronic granulocyte leukemia and used to confirm the diagnosis of CML in humans have not been identified in dogs.

The median age of affected dogs is 7 to 8 years.[20,53–55] There is no obvious gender or breed predilection.

Clinical Presentation and History

Affected dogs have nonspecific signs such as lethargy, weight loss, and inappetence for months before diagnosis of CML.[54,55] Some dogs may be asymptomatic.[53] Enhanced neutrophil activity, including phagocytosis, superoxide generation, and secretion of elastase and lysozyme, may cause degranulation in the circulation and thus contribute to clinical signs such as intermittent fever.[54] Although neutrophil function may increase, some dogs show signs of immune compromise.[20] Hepatosplenomegaly is common and is due to organ infiltration by abnormal cells or to extramedullary hematopoiesis.[53,55]

Staging and Diagnosis

Staging animals with suspected CML includes a CBC, a biochemical profile, urinalysis, and bone marrow cytology, possibly with a core biopsy. Leukocyte counts with CML range from 16,000[20] to 169,000 cells/µl; the median in one study was 98,000 cells/µl.[53] Anemia and thrombocytopenia are common, and nucleated red blood cells are a consistent finding.[20] Sometimes a more distinct lineage is obvious, as seen in two dogs with chronic basophil leukemia[56,57] and another four with eosinophilic differentiation.[55,58,59]

On bone marrow aspiration cytology, the myeloid:erythroid (M:E) ratio ranges from 3:1 to 24:1,[53] making accurate interpretation difficult. Because the circulating leukocyte pattern also varies, the definitive diagnosis is one of exclusion. The primary differential diagnosis for CML is leukemoid reaction to another tumor; however, in leukemoid responses, anemia and thrombocytopenia are not characteristic findings.[54]

Treatment

Hydroxyurea was used to treat 10 dogs with CML at a dose of 50 mg/kg PO daily for 14 days. If the dog was in remission, the treatment interval was lengthened to 2 days and then to 3 days. All 10 dogs attained CR within 1 month. Two untreated dogs died 80 and 703 days after diagnosis. Seven of 10 dogs that responded to hydroxyurea and did not develop a blast transformation ("blast crisis") survived in remission for 14 to 24 months.[20,53,56,60,61] One dog required transfusions every 2 months to treat persistent anemia that may have been compounded by hydroxyurea therapy. This dog developed multisystemic and meningeal neoplastic infiltrates 21 months after treatment was initiated.[20] Acute leukemia (blast crisis) was the cause of death in three of these 10 dogs and in another two dogs that were untreated from 2 to 24 months after diagnosis.[20,53,62] Hypereosinophilic syndrome was diagnosed in one dog based on high circulating counts and increased numbers of morphologically normal eosinophil precursors in marrow. The dog responded well to twice-daily treatment with hydroxyurea and prednisolone. Clinical signs of episodic vomiting, diarrhea, abdominal discomfort, and coughing were well controlled 16 months later.[59]

Busulfan at 2 to 8 mg/day per dog has been recommended for treatment of canine patients with CML, although details and response rates were not provided.[7]

Gastrointestinal (GI) absorption of busulfan is erratic and unpredictable in dogs,[63] and other therapies may be necessary in dogs that fail to respond. Of three dogs with CML that failed to respond to busulfan and were subsequently treated with cyclophosphamide, one responded to cyclophosphamide for 22 months, and the other two failed to respond.[42] Busulfan at 0.1 mg/kg PO daily was used to treat another dog with chronic basophilic leukemia. When no response was achieved with this therapy, hydroxyurea at a high dosage (50 mg/kg PO bid) was substituted. The dog subsequently achieved CR within 5 weeks and was still in remission 62 weeks after diagnosis despite receiving no treatment for the final 32 weeks.[57]

Hydroxyurea at 50 mg/kg PO daily seems to be the treatment of choice for dogs with CML. The PCV of dogs receiving hydroxyurea should be monitored every 1 to 3 months, and doses should be individualized through a compounding pharmacy. Anemia is the most common side effect, and stopping hydroxyurea until the PCV is again in normal range is recommended. Anecdotally, dogs may rarely have paronychia and sloughing of the toenails as a side effect of chronic hydroxyurea therapy.

ESSENTIAL THROMBOCYTHEMIA
Incidence, Signalment, and Etiology

Essential thrombocythemia, also called *primary thrombocytosis*, is rarely reported in dogs. When it occurs, it affects older dogs. There is no apparent gender or breed predilection. Strict definitions are used in the human literature for the diagnosis of essential thrombocythemia; however, it is unclear in the veterinary literature whether some dogs have had a reactive thrombocytosis or thrombocytosis as a part of CML (see Chronic Myeloid Leukemia section, above).

Clinical Presentation and History

Essential thrombocythemia is often a diagnosis of exclusion. Reactive thrombocytosis may be a sequel to splenectomy or a response to iron-deficiency anemia, may be associated with myelofibrosis or acute and chronic inflammatory conditions, and is sometimes seen accompanying primary erythrocytosis (polycythemia vera). In humans, thrombocytosis can accompany cancers such as breast and lung carcinoma and Hodgkin's disease. Affected dogs are reported to have nonspecific signs such as listlessness and weight loss that may be related to a concurrent anemia.[64]

Some of the reported canine cases were possibly reactive; two dogs developed pancreatitis within 1 month of diagnosis.[65,66] Another dog had polycythemia and myelofibrosis; it was unclear whether the myelofibrosis developed secondary to radiophosphorus treatment or was primary.[67,68] One dog developed CML 18 months after initial diagnosis.[60]

Staging and Diagnosis

Staging animals with suspected essential thrombocythemia includes a CBC, a biochemical profile, urinalysis, and bone marrow cytology, possibly with a core biopsy. In addition to thrombocytosis, basophilia may be seen, and bone marrow may contain abnormally shaped megakaryocytes. After causes of secondary thrombocytosis are ruled out, the diagnosis of essential thrombocythemia may be confirmed by serum thrombopoietin assay. Thrombopoietin levels should be low or normal in dogs with essential thrombocythemia. Serum thrombopoietin measurement was normal in one affected dog.[69] In most other reported cases, the diagnosis was by exclusion, although the thoroughness of that exclusion varied.

Treatment

There have been few reports of successful treatment. In one series that included a literature review, three dogs were treated with radiophosphorus (^{32}P).[67] One dog was given ^{32}P after failure to respond to melphalan. The dog also failed to respond to ^{32}P and then developed CML, which was controlled for 14 months with hydroxyurea.[60,67] The other dogs either failed to respond to ^{32}P or responded but had polycythemia vera (probably not essential thrombocythemia).[67,68]

In two other dogs, treatment with vincristine given once initially and hydroxyurea (500 mg/m^2 PO sid) caused no real response.[64] After 3 weeks, the dosage of hydroxyurea was increased in both dogs to 2,000 mg/m^2 PO sid. After 6 weeks of treatment, both dogs died with pancytopenia thought to be an effect of high-dose hydroxyurea. Another dog failed to respond to hydroxyurea but was alive and well and receiving no treatment 17 months after initial diagnosis.[69] Two dogs were not treated.[66]

POLYCYTHEMIA (PRIMARY ERYTHROCYTOSIS)

Polycythemia is characterized by an increase in the PCV, hemoglobin concentration, and red blood cell count. When this increase follows changes in plasma volume, such as occur with dehydration, it is termed *relative polycythemia*. *Absolute polycythemia*, which is the increased production of red blood cells, may be primary (polycythemia vera, primary erythrocytosis) or secondary to an increase in serum erythropoietin. Secondary polycythemia may be caused by systemic hypoxia arising from cardiopulmonary disease, hemoglobinopathies, and high altitude. It may also be the result of erythropoietin secretion by tumors, particularly renal tumors (see Chapter 37). In dogs, renal carcinomas and renal lymphoma have been reported to result in increased serum erythropoietin levels. Some breeds of dogs, such as greyhounds, have a higher normal range of PCV.

Polycythemia vera results from a clonal proliferation of the erythroid series and does not require erythropoietin for continued stimulus. In humans, this disorder usually includes thrombocytosis and hepatosplenomegaly and progresses to myelofibrosis or acute leukemia. This combination is rare in dogs.[68] We therefore use the term *primary erythrocytosis*.

Incidence, Signalment, and Etiology

Primary erythrocytosis is rarely reported in dogs. When it occurs, it affects middle-aged dogs.[67,70–72] There is no apparent gender or breed predilection.

Clinical Presentation and History

Affected dogs are reported to have hyperemic (brick-red) mucous membranes.[67,71–73] They may also have polyuria and polydipsia, lethargy, inappetence, or restlessness. Other clinical signs include bleeding, which has been reported as hematochezia, hematemesis, and hematuria, and neurologic disturbances, such as seizures, posterior weakness, ataxia, and blindness.[70,72] Increased blood viscosity leading to dilation and weakening of peripheral vessels may cause bleeding. Dogs with primary erythrocytosis have dilated retinal vessels,[67] and one dog had bilateral anterior uveitis and active chorioretinitis.[73] Seizures and other neurologic manifestations are presumably also caused by increased blood viscosity. Signs have been reported to occur from 1 week to 12 months before diagnosis, with an average of 6 weeks.[67] Mild splenomegaly is occasionally noted.[70,72]

Staging and Diagnosis

The PCV of dogs reported to have primary erythrocytosis ranges from 65% to 85%; the median in two studies was 73% to 78%.[70,74] Staging animals with suspected primary erythrocytosis includes a CBC, a biochemical profile, urinalysis, and possibly bone marrow cytology. Possible causes of secondary polycythemia must be ruled out. Thoracic radiography may detect changes consistent with chronic pulmonary disease or cardiac changes, and echocardiography can detect underlying cardiac disease. Arterial blood gas measurement is the best method to rule out systemic hypoxia, although it is usually not available in general practice. Renal architecture may be examined by abdominal ultrasonography.

After causes of secondary polycythemia are ruled out, the diagnosis of primary erythrocytosis may be confirmed by serum erythropoietin assay. Erythropoietin levels should be low or normal in dogs with primary erythrocytosis. In one study, the serum erythropoietin concentration ranged from 7 to 37 mU/ml in 25 normal dogs (median: 20 mU/ml), from 13 to 103 mU/ml in seven dogs with secondary polycythemias (median: 31 mU/ml), and from 10 to 57 mU/ml in eight dogs with primary erythrocytosis (median: 17 mU/ml).[74] All 15 affected dogs had a serum erythropoietin concentration in the normal range, but the median was significantly lower in the dogs with primary erythrocytosis. In some dogs with primary erythrocytosis, serum erythropoietin has been undetectable.[67,71]

Treatment

Phlebotomy may be successfully used to manage dogs with primary erythrocytosis and should be performed as the initial therapy in all dogs. The procedure usually followed is

> **KEY POINT**
> *Phlebotomy to remove 20 ml/kg body weight of blood reduces the dog's PCV by approximately 15%.*

to remove 20 ml/kg body weight of blood, which reduces the PCV by approximately 15%. This volume is replaced with crystalloid solutions.

Repeated phlebotomy maintains the PCV in the high-normal range. Iron supplementation is not required because iron deficiency will produce erythrocyte microcytosis and assist in controlling the red cell mass. The PCV should be checked every 3 to 4 weeks, and phlebotomy should be performed when appropriate. Phlebotomy every 2 to 4 weeks successfully maintained a high normal PCV in two dogs for more than 1 year.[72,75] Although repeated procedures may decrease patient tolerance, phlebotomy is safe. Apheresis to remove red cells was performed in one dog before hydroxyurea treatment.[74]

Chemotherapy with hydroxyurea is probably the treatment of choice for dogs with primary erythrocytosis.[67,72] Initial phlebotomy to reduce the PCV should be followed by a loading dose of hydroxyurea 30 mg/kg/day PO for 7 days, then 15 mg/kg/day PO for maintenance. Three dogs treated in this way achieved a normal PCV in 2 to 6 weeks.[72] Two dogs relapsed on treatment at 2 years and at 8 months after initial treatment, respectively; both were successfully reinduced with a 7-day loading dose. Chemotherapy with alkylating agents has been shown to be effective for primary erythrocytosis in dogs; however, uracil mustard[76] and busulfan have no advantage over hydroxyurea.

Other treatments have been attempted in dogs with primary erythrocytosis. ^{32}P accumulates in bone, resulting in bone marrow irradiation and myelosuppression. It is difficult to assess the response of dogs to this therapy because doses have varied from 1.5 mCi (total dose) to 3.25 mCi/m^2 and were sometimes combined with phlebotomy and busulfan (2 mg PO daily).[67,70] GI absorption of busulfan is erratic and unpredictable in dogs,[63] and one of the treated dogs died because of busulfan toxicity.[70] Of four dogs treated with ^{32}P alone, one achieved a CR for 2 years and another had a

PR for a number of months. In the dogs that failed or relapsed, repeated phlebotomy or chemotherapy with hydroxyurea controlled the disease. ^{32}P treatment is not widely available. It probably has an adjunctive role in the treatment of canine primary erythrocytosis, but it is difficult to draw conclusions on the basis of the available literature.

Initially, the PCV of dogs receiving hydroxyurea should be monitored every month. As the PCV stabilizes, monitoring can take place every 3 months. Doses should be individualized through a compounding pharmacy. Anemia is the most common side effect, and stopping hydroxyurea until the PCV is again in normal range is recommended in these cases. Anecdotally, dogs may rarely have paronychia and sloughing of the toenails as a side effect of chronic hydroxyurea therapy.

Multiple Myeloma

The diagnosis of multiple myeloma may be made in a dog when two or more of the following criteria are detected:

- Monoclonal gammopathy
- Lytic bone lesions
- Bence Jones (light-chain) proteinuria
- Neoplastic plasma cells or plasmacytosis in bone marrow

By strict definition, whereas *multiple myeloma* is the term used when monoclonal IgG, IgA, or light chains are produced, *Waldenström's macroglobulinemia* is associated with IgM overproduction. Monoclonal gammopathies may be seen with other neoplasms (e.g., lymphoma) or with infectious diseases (e.g., ehrlichiosis), in which plasmacytosis may also be found on bone marrow aspiration. Rarely, a dog may have multiple myeloma and no monoclonal gammopathy in serum or urine electrophoresis (nonsecretory multiple myeloma).

Solitary plasma cell tumors of the skin are benign tumors (see Chapter 64) that are rarely associated with multiple myeloma.[77,78]

INCIDENCE, SIGNALMENT, AND ETIOLOGY

Most published data regarding multiple myeloma in dogs are case reports. There are, however, two large reviews: one series of 60 dogs[79] and one retrospective study of 20 dogs.[80] The median age of dogs with multiple myeloma is between 8 and 9 years; ages range from 18 months to 16 years.[80,81] There is no apparent gender predilection. German shepherds were found to be at higher risk in one study, accounting for more than 20% of affected dogs.[79] Most reported cases have occurred in purebred dogs.

CLINICAL PRESENTATION AND HISTORY

The pathophysiology of multiple myeloma is complex and affects multiple systems. Clinical signs vary and are usually noticed by caregivers for 1 month or more before the dog is presented to the veterinarian. Tumor proliferation in the bone marrow causes myelophthisis when plasmacytosis becomes severe. Peripheral blood counts may reflect this occurrence, and affected dogs are often anemic and thrombocytopenic; some are neutropenic. In one group of dogs, nearly 70% were anemic, 25% were leukopenic, and 30% were thrombocytopenic.[79] Neutropenic patients are at increased risk for developing infections, particularly if normal immunoglobulin levels are also suppressed. Dogs may present with signs referable to secondary infections, such as cystitis.[82,83]

Bone involvement may manifest as multiple lytic lesions that primarily affect the axial skeleton, or affected dogs may appear diffusely osteoporotic. These changes result from osteoclast activation, which may also cause hypercalcemia. Pathologic fractures may cause lameness if the appendicular skeleton is involved. When the axial skeleton is involved, dogs may have pain from fractured ribs or may become paretic or acutely paralyzed from vertebral body collapse. Weakness was a presenting sign in more than 60% of 60 dogs, with lameness or paresis in 50% of dogs.[79] Lameness, paresis, and pain were the reasons for presentation in 18 of 42 other reported cases.[80,82,84-90]

Most reported cases of canine multiple myeloma involve overproduction of IgA or IgG. In one survey, IgA and IgG were each found in 30 of 60 dogs.[79] Of 16 other reported cases of multiple myeloma, IgA was found in 11 dogs[83,88-94] and IgG in 5 dogs.[82,83,90] Macroglobulinemia is less commonly reported.[84]

Normal immunoglobulin production is often suppressed; thus, it is possible for a dog with multiple myeloma and an abnormal monoclonal immunoglobulin level to still have a normal total globulin level. Serum protein electrophoresis or immunoelectrophoresis is necessary to confirm a diagnosis in these dogs. Abnormal immunoglobulin may be produced as incomplete fragments, which are usually light chains of myeloma protein. Occasionally, they may be heavy chains.[93] These abnormal proteins are excreted in the urine (Bence Jones proteins), but they are undetectable on routine urinalysis.

Abnormal immunoglobulin, particularly IgM or IgA (which, as dimers, may form high-molecular-weight polymers in circulation), may produce hyperviscosity of the blood when high protein levels are reached.[95] Hyperviscosity is recognized clinically as bleeding caused by paraprotein coating of platelets and as "sludging" of blood in vessels. Bleeding is often compounded by thrombocytopenia caused by bone marrow infiltration by plasma cells. Hyperviscosity may cause CNS signs such as dementia, confusion, and seizures, as well as funduscopic changes and retinal detachment causing blindness (Figure 48-5).[96] In one study,

19 of 60 dogs had evidence of hyperviscosity; 14 of these dogs had an elevation in IgA, and five had IgG paraproteinemia.[79] There were signs of bleeding in 37% of 60 dogs,[79] and bleeding (i.e., petechiation, epistaxis, and hematuria) was a presenting sign in another seven of 22 reported cases.[80,82,90,91,94,97,98] Signs referable to the CNS were less common and were seen in 12% of 60 dogs.[79]

Paraprotein light chains (Bence Jones proteins) and hypercalcemia may contribute to renal dysfunction; these changes may be exacerbated by renal infiltration with neoplastic plasma cells. Light-chain nephropathy, renal tubular damage from hypercalcemia, and glomerulosclerosis may all contribute to irreversible azotemia; however, azotemia may be prerenal in dogs with hypercalcemia and thus is often reversible when chemotherapy succeeds. Polydipsia and polyuria were reasons for presentation in 15 of 60 dogs.[79] In the same study, azotemia was documented in 20 dogs, and hypercalcemia was noted in 10 dogs. Bence Jones proteinuria was found in 24 of 60 dogs with multiple myeloma in the same study and in 11 of 19 other dogs reported.[80,83,88–92,94,98]

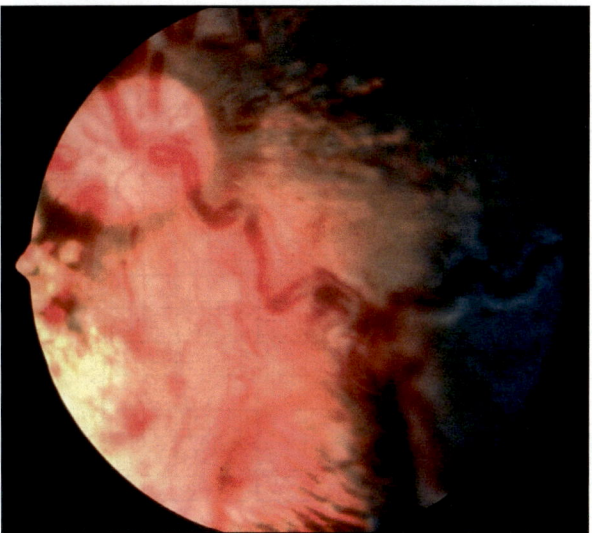

Figure 48-5. *A complete ocular examination may reveal tortuous vessels and hemorrhage in a dog that has multiple myeloma complicated by hyperviscosity.*

STAGING AND DIAGNOSIS

Complete staging of a dog with suspected multiple myeloma involves collection of an MDB, spinal and rib (rather than lung-field) radiography, electrophoresis and immunoelectrophoresis of serum and urine, and bone marrow aspiration.

> **KEY POINT**
>
> *Normal serum immunoglobulin levels are often suppressed when a monoclonal gammopathy is present; therefore, a dog with multiple myeloma may still have a normal total globulin level.*

In dogs with a monoclonal or biclonal gammopathy and plasmacytosis of the bone marrow but no bone lesions or light chains in the urine, the primary differential diagnoses are ehrlichiosis and leishmaniasis in areas where these diseases occur.[99] Serum titers and polymerase chain reaction (PCR) assays for *Ehrlichia* and *Leishmania* spp should be conducted. Other tumors that have been associated with a monoclonal gammopathy include lymphoma and CLL.

A CBC should be obtained to identify patients at increased risk for infection arising from neutropenia or bleeding from thrombocytopenia. A biochemistry profile may identify an increase in total protein levels that is primarily serum globulins. In addition, dogs with azotemia should be evaluated for renal dysfunction and hypercalcemia. Urinalysis can provide information about the patient's renal function, particularly if azotemia is present; however, although proteinuria may be an indication of glomerular damage, it is not an indication of Bence Jones proteinuria. Urine-protein detection strips detect albumin; special heat-precipitation methods are needed to detect Bence Jones protein. Urine immunoelectrophoresis may be a more sensitive method than heat precipitation to document Bence Jones protein[94] and to detect heavy chains in the urine.[93] Immunoelectrophoresis of the urine may also detect abnormal light- or heavy-chain paraproteins.

Serum protein electrophoresis and immunoelectrophoresis should be performed in dogs that have characteristics of multiple myeloma, even in the presence of a normal globulin level (nonsecretory multiple myeloma[100]). Suppression of normal circulating immunoglobulin levels may cause overall normal serum globulin in a dog that has a monoclonal gammopathy (Figure 48-6). A monoclonal gammopathy may be further characterized by immunoelectrophoresis, which quantitates IgA, IgG, and IgM. Occasionally, a dog with multiple myeloma may have a biclonal gammopathy with IgG, IgA, or both.[95,98,101,102]

Bone lesions from multiple myeloma are almost purely lytic, with very little new bone production; therefore, radionuclide bone scans may not be effective for imaging myeloma-induced bone lesions.[85,100] Plain radiograph skeletal surveys are the most sensitive method for detecting such abnormalities, although the increasing use of magnetic resonance imaging means that this modality may have a role in the diagnosis of bony lesions.[103] For dogs with large lytic bone lesions, samples may be obtained for histopathology by fluoroscopically guided biopsy; aspiration can secure samples for cytology (Figure 48-7).

Bone marrow aspiration should be conducted from any of the routinely used sites (see Chapter 16). Some investigators consider a finding of more than 30% plasma cells on bone marrow cytology to be diagnostic of multiple myeloma, but

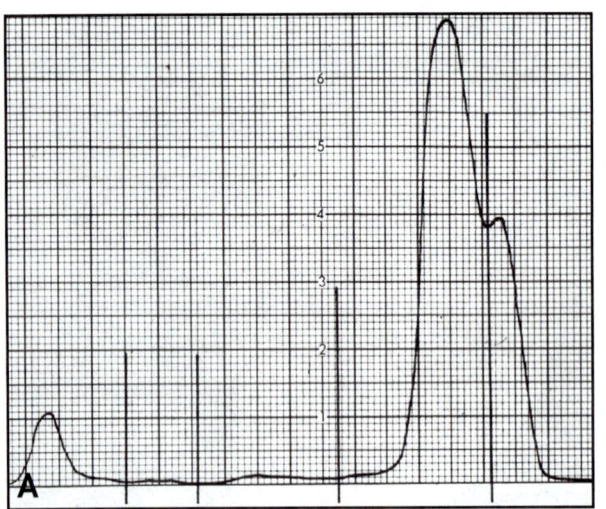 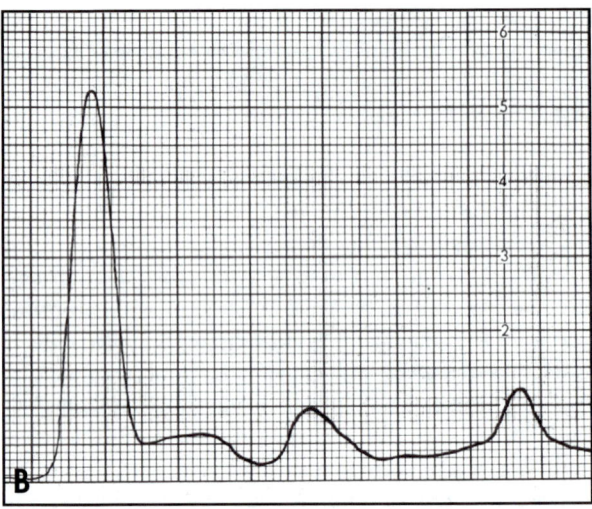

Figure 48-6. (A) *Electrophoretogram of a 6-year-old dog showing a monoclonal gammopathy. The total serum protein for this dog was 12.0 mg/dl. The dog was hypoalbuminemic at presentation.* (B) *Electrophoretogram of the same dog 3 months after starting treatment with melphalan and prednisone. Note the decrease in the gammopathy. The total serum protein is now 6.2 mg/dl, and the albumin level is normal.*

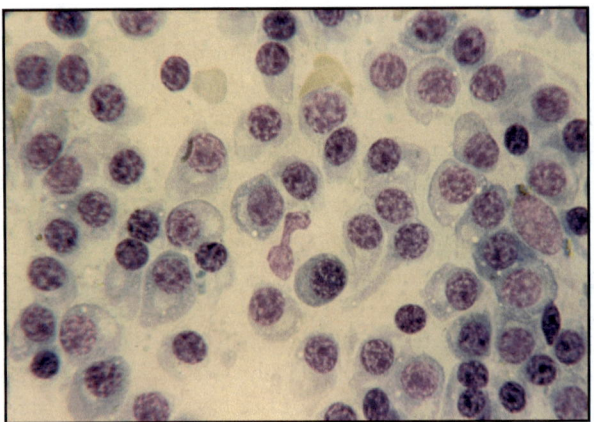

Figure 48-7. *Bone marrow aspirate from a dog with multiple myeloma showing a predominant population of plasma cells.*

most believe that a level between 5% and 20% supports such a diagnosis.[79]

There is a solitary case report of a dog with multiple myeloma, hypercalcemia, bone lesions, and a paraneoplastic polyneuropathy causing quadriplegia. The polyneuropathy resolved with treatment of the myeloma, and the dog was walking normally within 1 month.[104]

In dogs that are not treated or that fail to respond to treatment, neoplastic plasma cells are frequently found as discrete masses (sometimes large) in several organs.[80,91] Sites of involvement include the lymph nodes, pharynx, esophagus, GI tract, liver, pancreas, skin, muscle, and lung.

In a series of 38 dogs with multiple myeloma that died from their disease, six dogs with spinal cord paralysis were euthanatized at the time of diagnosis. Pancytopenia was the reason for later euthanasia of three dogs, and 11 dogs died from hemorrhage or infection. Progressive renal failure was the cause of death in 13 dogs; another five dogs failed to respond to chemotherapy.[79]

PROGNOSTIC FACTORS

There has only been one study of sufficient magnitude to identify prognostic factors in dogs with multiple myeloma.[79] In this study of 60 patients, dogs that were hypercalcemic, had extensive bone lysis, or had evidence of myeloma light chains in the urine (Bence Jones proteinuria) all had significantly shortened survival times (Figure 48-8). Gender, class of immunoglobulin (IgA or IgG), presence of hyperviscosity, and azotemia did not affect survival (Figure 48-9). Of the 49 dogs that were treated, chemotherapy with a combination of alkylating agents and prednisone enabled significantly longer survival than treatment with prednisone alone (see Treatment section below).

> **KEY POINT**
>
> *Dogs with multiple myeloma that are hypercalcemic, have extensive bony lysis, or have light-chain proteinuria do not survive as long as dogs without these findings.*

TREATMENT
Chemotherapy

Chemotherapy is the treatment of choice for canine multiple myeloma. The primary goal of chemotherapy is control of the disease. It is probably not possible to cure multiple myeloma in dogs, and it may not be possible to completely

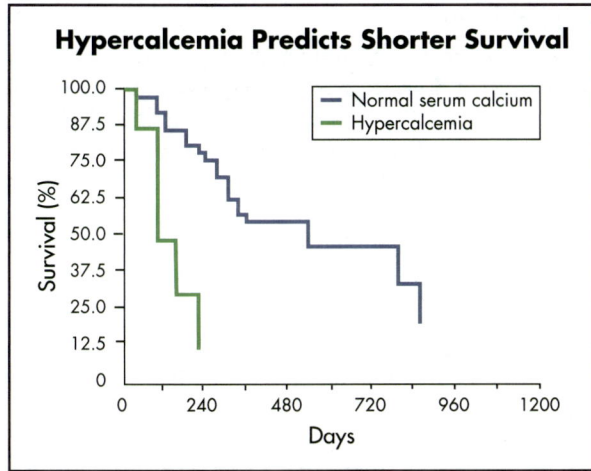

Figure 48-8. Survival data for dogs with multiple myeloma that were treated with melphalan and prednisone. Serum calcium was normal (<11.5 g/dl) in 31 dogs and elevated in six dogs. The difference in survival was significant. (From Matus RE, Leifer CE, MacEwen EG, Hurvitz AI: Prognostic factors for multiple myeloma in the dog. JAVMA 188: 1288–1292, 1986; with permission)

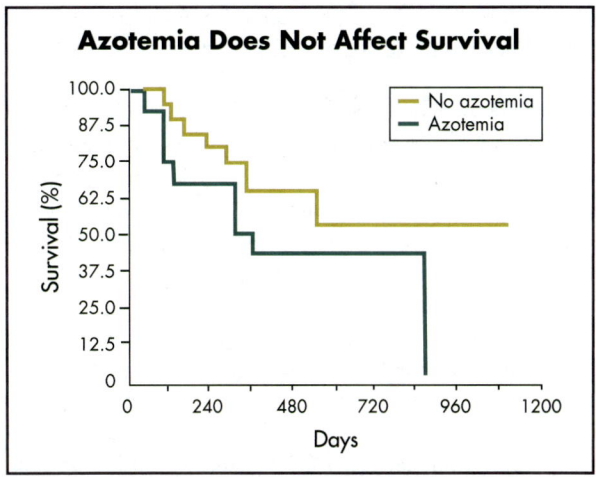

Figure 48-9. Survival data for dogs with multiple myeloma that were treated with melphalan and prednisone. The difference in survival between dogs with azotemia (n = 13) and those without (n = 24) was not significant. (From Matus RE, Leifer CE, MacEwen EG, Hurvitz AI: Prognostic factors for multiple myeloma in the dog. JAVMA 188:1288–1292, 1986; with permission)

resolve the abnormal globulin levels with chemotherapy. However, symptomatic relief is almost always achieved, even in dogs that achieve less than a CR. There is probably an undefined threshold that needs to be achieved for long-term control to be realized. Most clinicians believe that a reduction in the abnormal globulin of more than 50% is a reasonable goal.

Most reported dogs are treated with chemotherapy or euthanatized at diagnosis. Three dogs that received no treatment for their disease[80,83,90] and one dog that failed to respond to treatment[81] all died within 40 days of initial presentation.

In a series of 12 dogs treated with prednisone (0.5 mg/kg PO sid) for palliation, median survival was 220 days.[79] In the same study, another 37 dogs received melphalan (0.1 mg/kg PO sid for 10 days, then 0.05 mg/kg PO sid) and prednisone (0.5 mg/kg PO sid for 10 days, then 0.5 mg/kg PO every other day). Of these 37 dogs, 21 also received a single initial dose of cyclophosphamide (7 mg/kg IV). Only three of the 37 dogs (8%) failed to respond to treatment. CR was attained in 16 dogs (43%), and PR occurred in 18 (49%). Median survival for all 37 dogs was 540 days, which was significantly longer than for dogs treated with prednisone alone. The addition of cyclophosphamide did not influence survival times; however, complete response to therapy was associated with longer survival.[79]

Other dogs have been treated with combinations of melphalan and prednisone with or without cyclophosphamide[85,89,98] or vincristine.[85,98] Survival times of 9, 14, 18, and 22 months were reported in four dogs[88,89,105]; these times do not differ greatly from survival times of dogs treated with melphalan and prednisone alone.

When resistance to melphalan and prednisone arises, most dogs are euthanatized. In one report, a second PR was obtained with cyclophosphamide administered for 2 months in a dog resistant to the former combination.[85] In another report, a dog that relapsed after a 5-month remission, which had been achieved with prednisone and melphalan, responded for another 7 months to chlorambucil (4 mg/m² PO for 5 days q3wk).[83] In Dr. Moore's experience, one dog obtained a second remission of 18 months with combined cyclophosphamide (50 mg/m² PO every other day) and chlorambucil (6 mg/m² PO every other day) chemotherapy when the dog became resistant to melphalan and prednisone after 26 months of treatment. Doxorubicin is also an active agent for achieving second remission, and in one report, liposome-encapsulated doxorubicin was successful in achieving a CR in a dog that was resistant to a number of chemotherapeutic agents.[106] Thus, second remissions may be possible with appropriate therapy.

> **Combination chemotherapy using melphalan and prednisone often results in longer survival for dogs with multiple myeloma.**

A clinical distinction has been made between multiple myeloma (secreting IgA and IgG) and macroglobulinemia (IgM); chlorambucil has been recommended for treatment of macroglobulinemia.[107] Dogs with macroglobulinemia may still respond to treatment with melphalan and prednisone.[84] If macroglobulinemia is diagnosed, treatment with prednisone and melphalan should be instituted, and if less than a 50% response is seen after 6 weeks, chlorambucil should be substituted for the melphalan.

Supportive Therapy

As already mentioned, dogs with multiple myeloma are at high risk for infection caused by myelosuppression secondary to myelophthisis and effects on humoral immunity caused by monoclonal gammopathy. Dogs with fever or other evidence of infection require immediate broad-spectrum antibiotic therapy.

Dogs with renal dysfunction, particularly those with hypercalcemia, should be supported with aggressive fluid therapy to maintain hydration and to enhance renal perfusion. Dogs with hypercalcemia should also be treated with furosemide while receiving 0.9% sodium chloride diuresis. Chemotherapy should be started in these patients as soon as diagnosis is confirmed. Care should be taken when administering melphalan to dogs with renal dysfunction. Melphalan-induced myelosuppression is more severe in dogs with renal dysfunction when delivered intravenously, probably because of decreased clearance of the drug and a resultant longer half-life.[108] Absorption is more varied with oral administration; therefore, careful monitoring of blood counts when melphalan is administered, rather than an empiric dose reduction, is recommended.

Exercise should be restricted for dogs with severe bone lysis, particularly of the vertebrae. If the lesions in these dogs are large and localized, the lesions may resolve with radiation therapy.[85] Pathologic fractures have been treated with radiation therapy (18 Gy[106] to 36 Gy[85]) either alone or with internal fixation. A combination of polymethyl methacrylate and internal fixation was successful in one dog.[109] Healing seems to be progressive over months and therefore depends on control of the systemic disease. Some dogs develop other bone lesions if the myeloma does not enter remission[110] or if they relapse.[103] Dogs with bony lysis have a worse prognosis,[79] and most dogs are euthanatized with progressive and uncontrollable pain, lameness, or spinal lesions.

In dogs with hyperviscosity, chemotherapy usually causes improvement within weeks of initiation. In critical situations, plasmapheresis can reduce plasma protein levels.[111] In the absence of equipment to perform plasmapheresis, blood can be harvested in anticoagulant, the serum harvested, and the red blood cells returned to the patient after being resuspended in saline. Although this does not dramatically reduce globulin levels, clinical signs associated with the hyperviscosity syndrome may be reduced.

Four dogs with multiple myeloma presented for blindness caused by retinal detachment and hemorrhages; any secondary uveitis was controlled with topical corticosteroids. Three of the four dogs regained vision after the retina reattached after 2 to 6 months of chemotherapy.[96]

Future Therapy

Newer methods of treating multiple myeloma may come from targeted drugs currently under investigation; antiangiogenic drugs such as thalidomide have caused responses in human patients. The novel multitargeted indolinone-receptor tyrosine-kinase inhibitor SU11654 causes both antitumor and antiangiogenic activity. An objective response was seen in a dog with multiple myeloma treated in a preliminary trial of this compound.[112]

REFERENCES

1. Weiss DJ, Aird B: Cytologic evaluation of primary and secondary myelodysplastic syndromes in the dog. *Vet Clin Pathol* 30:67–75, 2001.
2. Weiss DJ, Raskin R, Zerbe C: Myelodysplastic syndrome in two dogs. *JAVMA* 187:1038–1040, 1985.
3. Jain NC, Blue JT, Grindem CB, et al: Proposed criteria for classification of acute myeloid leukemia in dogs and cats. *Vet Clin Pathol* 20:63–82, 1991.
4. Seed TM, Kaspar LV: Acquired radioresistance of hematopoietic progenitors (granulocyte/monocyte colony-forming units) during chronic radiation leukemogenesis. *Cancer Res* 52:1469–1476, 1992.
5. Raskin RE: Myelopoiesis and myeloproliferative disorders. *Vet Clin North Am Small Anim Pract* 26:1023–1042, 1996.
6. McManus PM, Hess RS: Myelodysplastic changes in a dog with subsequent acute myeloid leukemia. *Vet Clin Pathol* 27:112–115, 1998.
7. Gorman NT, Evans RJ: Myeloproliferative disease in the dog and cat: Clinical presentations, diagnosis and treatment. *Vet Rec* 121:490–496, 1987.
8. Couto CG, Kallet AJ: Preleukemic syndrome in a dog. *JAVMA* 184:1389–1392, 1984.
9. Tolle DV, Cullen SM, Seed TM, Fritz TE: Circulating micromegakaryocytes preceding leukemia in three dogs exposed to 2.5 R/day gamma radiation. *Vet Pathol* 20:111–114, 1983.
10. Boone LI, Knauer KW, Rapp SW, et al: Use of human recombinant erythropoietin and prednisone for treatment of myelodysplastic syndrome with erythroid predominance in a dog. *JAVMA* 213:999–1001, 1998.
11. Ide K, Momoi Y, Minegishi M, et al: A severe hepatic disorder with myelodysplastic syndrome, treated with cytarabine ocfosfate, in a dog. *Aust Vet J* 81:47–49, 2003.
12. MacLeod JN, Tetreault JW, Lorschy KA, Gu DN: Expression and bioactivity of recombinant canine erythropoietin. *Am J Vet Res* 59:1144–1148, 1998.
13. Weiss DJ: New insights into the physiology and treatment of acquired myelodysplastic syndromes and aplastic pancytopenia. *Vet Clin North Am Small Anim Pract* 33:1317–1334, 2003.
14. Graves TK, Swenson CL, Scott MA: A potentially misleading presentation and course of acute myelomonocytic leukemia in a dog. *JAAHA* 33: 37–41, 1997.
15. Grindem CB, Stevens JB, Perman V: Cytochemical reactions in cells from leukemic dogs. *Vet Pathol* 23:103–109, 1986.
16. Couto CG: Clinicopathologic aspects of acute leukemias in the dog. *JAVMA* 186:681–685, 1985.
17. Grindem CB: Cytogenetic analysis of leukaemic cells in the dog: A report of 10 cases and a review of the literature. *J Comp Pathol* 96:623–635, 1986.
18. Jain NC, Madewell BR, Weller RE, Geissler MC: Clinical-pathological findings and cytochemical characterization of myelomonocytic leukaemia in 5 dogs. *J Comp Pathol* 91:17–31, 1981.
19. Grindem CB, Stevens JB, Perman V: Morphological classification and clinical and pathological characteristics of spontaneous leukemia in 17 dogs. *JAAHA* 21:219–226, 1985.
20. Grindem CB, Steven JB, Brost DR, Johnson DD: Chronic myelogenous leukaemia with meningeal infiltration in a dog. *Compar Haematol Int* 2:170–174, 1992.
21. Rohrig KE: Acute myelomonocytic leukemia in a dog. *JAVMA* 182:137–141, 1983.
22. Colbatzky F, Hermanns W: Acute megakaryoblastic leukemia in one cat and two dogs. *Vet Pathol* 30:186–194, 1993.
23. Messick J, Carothers M, Wellman M: Identification and characterization of megakaryoblasts in acute megakaryoblatic leukemia in a dog. *Vet Pathol* 27: 212–214, 1990.
24. Bolon B, Buergelt CD, Harvey JW, et al: Megakaryoblastic leukemia in a dog. *Vet Clin Pathol* 18:69–72, 2003.

25. Cain GR, Feldman BF, Kawakami TG, Jain NC: Platelet dysplasia associated with megakaryoblastic leukemia in a dog. JAVMA 188:529–530, 1986.
26. Miyamoto T, Hachimura H, Amimoto A: A case of megakaryoblastic leukemia in a dog. J Vet Med Sci 58:177–179, 1996.
27. Facklam NR, Kociba GJ: Cytochemical characterization of leukemic cells from 20 dogs. Vet Pathol 22:363–369, 1985.
28. Grindem CB: Ultrastructural morphology of leukemic cells from 14 dogs. Vet Pathol 22:456–462, 1985.
29. Canfield PJ, Watson ADJ, Begg AP, Dill-Macky E: Myeloproliferative disorder in four dogs involving derangements of erythropoiesis, myelopoiesis and megakaryopoiesis. J Small Anim Pract 27:7–16, 1986.
30. Weiss DJ: Evaluation of proliferative disorders in canine bone marrow by use of flow cytometric scatter plots and monoclonal antibodies. Vet Pathol 38:512–518, 2001.
31. Fernandes PJ, Modiano JF, Wojcieszyn J, et al: Use of the cell-Dyn 3500 to predict leukemic cell lineage in peripheral blood of dogs and cats. Vet Clin Pathol 31:167–182, 2002.
32. Vernau W, Moore PF: An immunophenotypic study of canine leukemias and preliminary assessment of clonality by polymerase chain reaction. Vet Immunol Immunopathol 69:145–164, 1999.
33. Cooper BJ, Watson AD: Myeloid neoplasia in a dog. Aust Vet J 51:150–154, 1975.
34. Alroy J: Basophilic leukemia in a dog. Vet Pathol 9:90–95, 1972.
35. Holscher MA, Collins RD, Cousar JB, et al: Megakaryocytic leukemia in a cat. Feline Pract 13:8–12, 1983.
36. Capelli JL: Érythroleucémie chez un chien. J Pratique Medicale & Chirurgicale de l'Animal de Compagnie 26:337–340, 1991.
37. Mori T, Kadosawa T, Okada Y, et al: Acute respiratory failure caused by leukaemic infiltration of the lung of a dog. J Small Anim Pract 42:349–351, 2001.
38. Matus RE, Leifer CE, MacEwen EG: Acute lymphoblastic leukemia in the dog: A review of 30 cases. JAVMA 183:859–862, 1983.
39. Henry CJ, Lanevschi A, Marks SL, et al: Acute lymphoblastic leukemia, hypercalcemia, and pseudohyperkalemia in a dog. JAVMA 208:237–239, 1996.
40. Ruslander DA, Gebhard DH, Tompkins MB, et al: Immunophenotypic characterization of canine lymphoproliferative disorders. In Vivo 11:169–172, 1997.
41. McDonough SP, Moore PF: Clinical, hematologic, and immunophenotypic characterization of canine large granular lymphocytosis. Vet Pathol 37:637–646, 2000.
42. Moldovanu G: Continuing long-term remission after cyclophosphamide (NSC-26271) therapy for canine leukemia. Cancer Chemother Rep 53:223–227, 1969.
43. MacEwen EG, Patnaik AK, Hayes AA, et al: Temporary plasma-induced remission of lymphoblastic leukemia in a dog. Am J Vet Res 42:1450–1452, 1981.
44. Hodgkins EM, Zinkl JG, Madewell BR: Chronic lymphocytic leukemia in the dog. JAVMA 177:704–707, 1980.
45. Leifer CE, Matus RE: Chronic lymphocytic leukemia in the dog: 22 cases (1978–1984). JAVMA 189:214–217, 1986.
46. Kristensen AT, Klausner JS, Weiss DJ, et al: Spurious hyperphosphatemia in a dog with chronic lymphocytic leukemia and an IgM monoclonal gammopathy. Vet Clin Pathol 20:45–48, 1998.
47. Olivry T, Atlee BA: Leucemie lymphoide chronique avec ulcerations buccales chez un chien. J Pratique Medicale & Chirurgicale de l'Animal de Compagnie 27:177–181, 1992.
48. Harvey JW, Terrell TG, Hyde DM, Jackson RI: Well-differentiated lymphocytic leukemia in a dog: Long-term survival without therapy. Vet Pathol 18:37–47, 1981.
49. Couto GC, Sousa C: Chronic lymphocytic leukemia with cutaneous involvement in a dog. JAAHA 22:374–379, 1986.
50. Kleiter M, Hirt R, Kirtz G, Day MJ: Hypercalcaemia associated with chronic lymphocytic leukaemia in a giant schnauzer. Aust Vet J 79:335–338, 2001.
51. Fujino Y, Sawamura S, Kurakawa N, et al: Treatment of chronic lymphocytic leukaemia in three dogs with melphalan and prednisolone. J Small Anim Pract 45:298–303, 2004.
52. Leporrier M, Chevret S, Cazin B et al: Randomized comparison of fludarabine, CAP, and ChOP in 938 previously untreated stage B and C chronic lymphocytic leukemia patients. Blood 98:2319–2325, 2001.
53. Leifer CE, Matus RE, Patnaik AK, MacEwen EG: Chronic myelogenous leukemia in the dog. JAVMA 183:686–689, 1983.
54. Thomsen MK, Jensen AL, Skak-Nielsen T, Kristensen F: Enhanced granulocyte function in a case of chronic granulocytic leukemia in a dog. Vet Immunol Immunopathol 28:143–156, 1991.
55. Ndikuwera J, Smith DA, Obwolo MJ, Masvingwe C: Chronic granulocytic leukaemia/eosinophilic leukemia in a dog? J Small Anim Pract 33:553–557, 1992.
56. Mears EA, Raskin RE, Legendre AM: Basophilic leukemia in a dog. J Vet Intern Med 11:92–94, 1997.
57. MacEwen EG, Drazner FH, McClelland AJ, Wilkins RJ: Treatment of basophilic leukemia in a dog. JAVMA 166:376–380, 1975.
58. Jensen AL, Nielsen OL: Eosinophilic leukaemoid reaction in a dog. J Small Animal Pract 33:337–340, 1992.
59. Perkins M, Watson A: Successful treatment of hypereosinophilic syndrome in a dog. Aust Vet J 79:686–689, 2001.
60. Degen MA, Feldman BF, Turrel JM, et al: Thrombocytosis associated with a myeloproliferative disorder in a dog. JAVMA 194:1457–1459, 1989.
61. Fine DM, Tvedten HW: Chronic granulocytic leukemia in a dog. JAVMA 214:1809–1812, 1791, 1999.
62. Tarrant JM, Stokol T, Blue JT, et al: Diagnosis of chronic myelogenous leukemia in a dog using morphologic, cytochemical, and flow cytometric techniques. Vet Clin Pathol 30:19–24, 2001.
63. Ehninger G, Schuler U, Renner U, et al: Use of a water-soluble busulfan formulation—Pharmacokinetic studies in a canine model. Blood 85:3247–3249, 1995.
64. Favier RP, van Leeuwen M, Teske E: Essential thrombocythaemia in two dogs. Tijdschr Diergeneeskd 129:360–364, 2004.
65. Hopper PE, Mandell CP, Turrel JM, et al: Probable essential thrombocythemia in a dog. J Vet Intern Med 3:79–85, 1989.
66. Dunn JK, Heath MF, Jefferies AR, et al: Diagnostic and hematologic features of probable essential thrombocythemia in two dogs. Vet Clin Pathol 28:131–138, 1999.
67. Smith M, Turrel JM: Radiophosphorus (32P) treatment of bone marrow disorders in dogs: 11 cases (1970–1987). JAVMA 194:98–102, 1989.
68. Kammermann-Luscher B: Polycythaemia vera beim hund. Schweiz Arch Tierheilk 117:557–568, 1975.
69. Bass MC, Schultze AE: Essential thrombocythemia in a dog: Case report and literature review. JAAHA 34:197–203, 1998.
70. McGrath CJ: Polycythemia vera in dogs. JAVMA 164:1117–1122, 1974.
71. Quesnel AD, Kruth SA: Polycythemia vera and glomerulonephritis in a dog. Can Vet J 33:671–672, 1992.
72. Peterson ME, Randolph JF: Diagnosis of canine primary polycythemia and management with hydroxyurea. JAVMA 180:415–418, 1982.
73. Gray HE, Weigand CM, Cottrill NB, et al: Polycythemia vera in a dog presenting with uveitis. JAAHA 39:355–360, 2003.
74. Cook SM, Lothrop CD Jr: Serum erythropoietin concentrations measured by radioimmunoassay in normal, polycythemic, and anemic dogs and cats. J Vet Intern Med 8:18–25, 1994.
75. Meyer HP, Slappendel RJ, Greydanus-van der Putten SW: Polycythaemia vera in a dog treated by repeated phlebotomies. Vet Q 15:108–111, 1993.
76. Carb AV: Polycythemia vera in a dog. JAVMA 154:289–297, 1969.
77. Lester SJ, Mesfin GM: A solitary plasmacytoma in a dog with progression to a disseminated myeloma. Can Vet J 21:284–286, 1980.
78. Walton GS, Gopinath C: Multiple myeloma in a dog with some unusual features. J Small Anim Pract 13:703–708, 1972.
79. Matus RE, Leifer CE, MacEwen EG, Hurvitz AI: Prognostic factors for multiple myeloma in the dog. JAVMA 188:1288–1292, 1986.
80. Osborne CA, Perman V, Sautter JH, et al: Multiple myeloma in the dog. JAVMA 153:1300–1319, 1968.
81. Stone RW: The unexpected diagnosis of multiple myeloma in a Shiba Inu incidental to warfarin intoxication. Canine Pract 18:26–28, 1993.
82. Orr CM, Higginson J, Baker JR, Jones DR: Plasma cell myeloma with IgG paraproteinemia in a bitch. J Small Anim Pract 22:31–37, 1981.
83. Pechereau D, Lanore D, Martel PH: Le mylome multiple: Mise au point a partir de neuf cas. Pract Med Chirurgicale 26:369–378, 1991.
84. Lautzenhiser SJ, Walker MC, Goring RL: Unusual IgM-secreting multiple myeloma in a dog. JAVMA 223:645–648, 636, 2003.
85. MacEwen EG, Patnaik AK, Huruitz AI, et al: Non-secretory multiple myeloma in two dogs. JAVMA 184:1283–1286, 1984.
86. Oduye OO, Losos GJ: Multiple myeloma in a dog. J Small Anim Pract 13:257–263, 1972.
87. Breuer W, Colbatzky F, Platz S, Hermanns W: Immunoglobulin-producing tumours in dogs and cats. J Comp Pathol 109:203–216, 1993.
88. Maeda H, Ozaki K, Abe T, et al: Bone lesions of multiple myeloma in three dogs. Zentralbl Veterinarmed A 40:384–392, 1993.
89. Cayzer J, Jones BR: IgA multiple myeloma in a dog. N Z Vet J 39:139–144, 1991.
90. Finnie JW, Wilks CR: Two cases of multiple myeloma in the dog. J Small Anim Pract 23:19–27, 1982.
91. Day MJ, Penhale WJ, McKenna RP, et al: Two cases of IgA multiple myeloma

in the dog. *J Small Anim Pract* 28:147–156, 1987.

92. Zinkl JG, LeCouteur RA, Davis DC, Saunders GK: "Flaming" plasma cells in a dog with IgA multiple myeloma. *Vet Clin Pathol* 12:15–19, 1998.

93. Hoenig M: Multiple myeloma associated with the heavy chains of immunoglobulin A in a dog. *JAVMA* 190:1191–1192, 1987.

94. Kirschner SE, Niyo Y, Hill BL, Betts DM: Blindness in a dog with IgA-forming myeloma. *JAVMA* 193:349–350, 1988.

95. Kato H, Momoi Y, Omori K, et al: Gammopathy with two M-components in a dog with IgA-type multiple myeloma. *Vet Immunol Immunopathol* 49:161–168, 1995.

96. Hendrix DV, Gelatt KN, Smith PJ, et al: Ophthalmic disease as the presenting complaint in five dogs with multiple myeloma. *JAAHA* 34:121–128, 1998.

97. Doppa T, Simpson K: What is your diagnosis? Multiple myeloma. *J Small Anim Pract* 38:327, 357, 1997.

98. Jacobs RM, Couto CG, Wellmann ML: Biclonal gammopathy in a dog with myeloma and cutaneous lymphoma. *Vet Pathol* 23:211–213, 1986.

99. Giraudel JM, Pages JP, Guelfi JF: Monoclonal gammopathies in the dog: A retrospective study of 18 cases (1986–1999) and literature review. *JAAHA* 38:135–147, 2002.

100. Marks SL, Moore PF, Taylor DW, Munn RJ: Nonsecretory multiple myeloma in a dog: Immunohistologic and ultrastructural observations. *J Vet Intern Med* 9:50–54, 1995.

101. Ramaiah SK, Seguin MA, Carwile HF, Raskin RE: Biclonal gammopathy associated with immunoglobulin A in a dog with multiple myeloma. *Vet Clin Pathol* 31:83–89, 2002.

102. Peterson EN, Meininger AC: Immunoglobulin A and immunoglobulin G biclonal gammopathy in a dog with multiple myeloma. *JAAHA* 33:45–47, 1997.

103. Reitemeyer S, Kohn B, Leibold W, et al: Multiples myelom bei einem deutschen schäferhund. *Kleintierpraxis* 44:43–55, 1999.

104. Villiers E, Dobson J: Multiple myeloma with associated polyneuropathy in a German shepherd dog. *J Small Anim Pract* 39:249–251, 1998.

105. MacEwen EG, Patnaik AK, Johnson GF, et al: Extramedullary plasmacytoma of the gastrointestinal tract in two dogs. *JAVMA* 184:1396–1398, 1984.

106. Kisseberth WC, MacEwen EG, Helfand SC, et al: Response to liposome-encapsulated doxorubicin (TLC D-99) in a dog with myeloma. *J Vet Intern Med* 9:425–428, 1995.

107. MacEwen EG, Hurvitz AI: Diagnosis and management of monoclonal gammopathies. *Vet Clin North Am* 7:119–132, 1977.

108. Alberts DS, Chen HG, Benz D, Mason NL: Effect of renal dysfunction in dogs on the disposition and marrow toxicity of melphalan. *Br J Cancer* 43:330–334, 1981.

109. Banks T, Langova V, Straw R: Repair of three pathologic fractures in a dog with multiple myeloma. *Austr Vet Pract* 33:102, 2003.

110. Cowgill ES, Neel JA, Ruslander D: Light-chain myeloma in a dog. *J Vet Intern Med* 18:119–121, 2004.

111. Matus RE, Leifer CE, Gordon BR: Plasmapheresis and chemotherapy of hyperviscosity syndrome associated with monoclonal gammopathy in the dog. *JAVMA* 183:215–218, 1983.

112. London CA, Hannah AL, Zadovoskaya R, et al: Phase I dose-escalating study of SU11654, a small molecule receptor tyrosine kinase inhibitor, in dogs with spontaneous malignancies. *Clin Cancer Res* 9:2755–2768, 2003.

TUMORS OF THE NERVOUS SYSTEM
Antony S. Moore and Gregory K. Ogilvie

49

Tumors of the nervous system are rare in dogs. Brain tumors are diagnosed more commonly than spinal cord tumors. Tumors of the nervous system rarely metastasize; their effects are the result of slow expansion and displacement or destruction of surrounding nervous tissue. Therefore, signs may be mild and overlooked by owners until the advent of more serious neurologic disturbances, such as seizures or paresis.

▶ TUMORS OF THE BRAIN

CLINICAL BRIEFING

Clinical factors	• Seizures and temperament changes. • Meningioma most common tumor. • Brachycephalic breeds predisposed. • Older dogs (10 years of age and older). • Slight male predilection. • Meningiomas locally invasive, rare metastases. • Gliomas may be more aggressive.
Staging and diagnosis	• Minimum database (MDB; includes a CBC, biochemical profile, urinalysis, and thoracic radiography [3 views]). • CT or MRI of the brain. • Consider proliferation markers if meningioma biopsied.
Prognostic factors	• Worse prognosis with severe neurologic dysfunction, abnormal CSF, or multiple tumors.
Treatment	
Initial	• Surgery (± radiation therapy) may be beneficial for meningiomas.
Adjunctive	• Radiation therapy is treatment of choice for gliomas. • Useful alone or as an adjunct to surgery for meningiomas • Chemotherapy is theoretically hindered by blood–brain barrier. • Possible role for carmustine (BCNU) and lomustine (CCNU).
Palliative	• Corticosteroids and anticonvulsants.
Supportive	• As for palliative, plus pain relief after surgery; nutritional support as needed.

Incidence, Signalment, and Etiology

Although most canine brain tumors are meningiomas, tumors of neuroectodermal origin (e.g., astrocytomas, gliomas, ependymomas, choroid plexus papillomas) have been described (Table 49-1). Most brain tumors in dogs occur in the cerebrum rather than in the brain stem or cerebellum. The cerebrum is the most accessible area for surgery. Most studies of canine brain tumors do not separate data by histologic type, so much of the information refers to a conglomerate of tumor types. Overall, affected dogs are older (mean age: 9–10 years; range: 1–17 years). There is a slightly higher incidence in males than females (1.5:1).[1,2] In studies, mixed-breed dogs were the most commonly affected and boxers were the purebreds most often affected.[1-3] The term *glioma* encompasses a range of tumors, including astrocytomas and oligodendrogliomas. Astrocytomas arise most fre-

Table 49-1 **Primary Tumors Involving the Cerebrum in Dogs**

Tumor	N/44 Dogs[1] (%)	N/39 Dogs[2] (%)
Meningioma	27 (48)	13 (33)
Astrocytoma	7 (12)	7 (18)
Neuroblastoma	Not reported	5 (13)
Ependymoma	Not reported	1 (3)
Nasal tumor (by extension)	4 (7)	13 (33)
Choroid plexus	6 (11)	Not reported

quently in the rostral and middle fossa of older, brachycephalic-breed dogs. Gliomas, often astrocytomas, appear more frequently than other tumors in young dogs and may be low grade.[4,5]

Gliomatosis cerebri is a rare variant of glioma in which neoplastic glial cells diffusely infiltrate the neural axis. The features were described in six dogs; four had an acute history (2 weeks or less), but two had neurologic abnormalities for 6 months before presentation.[6] Magnetic resonance imaging (MRI) or computed tomography (CT) was conducted in five dogs and was normal or showed only mild diffuse abnormalities in three dogs. Clinically, the major differential diagnosis is lymphoma.

Glioblastoma multiforme is an aggressive (undifferentiated) variant of astrocytoma that is rare in dogs.[7,8] MRI may not accurately demonstrate microscopic extension into surrounding normal tissues, underestimating the extension of the tumor.[9] This should be compensated for if radiation therapy is contemplated.

Clinical Presentation and History

An early study found that temperament changes and locomotor deficiencies were the most common clinical signs associated with cerebral tumors.[3] Three other studies reported that seizures were the most common sign in dogs with brain tumors, occurring in 94 of 171 dogs.[2,10,11] Dogs with tumors in the supratentorial region (frontal, olfactory and parietal lobes) were more likely to have seizures,[2,11] whereas head tilt and ataxia were more common in dogs with lesions in the infratentorial region.[11] Of 43 dogs, 31 had a normal neurologic examination on presentation despite a history of seizures, but 25 of these 31 dogs later developed persistent deficits, usually within 3 months. Lack of persistent neurologic deficits at presentation was ascribed to initial involvement of the rostral cerebrum, which contains neither motor nor sensory areas. Progression of the tumor to involve other structures could produce persistent deficits.[2] In a series of 194 dogs with seizures, an underlying neoplastic lesion in the central nervous system (CNS) was identified in 7.7% (granulomatous meningoencephalitis in 4.1%), making this diagnosis less common than idiopathic epilepsy or encephalitis.[12]

Other common clinical signs were circling (seen in 23% of 97 dogs), ataxia (21%), head tilt (13%), lethargy (11%), pacing (10%), behavior changes (7%), blindness (6%), aggression (5%), and wandering (5%).[11] Pain (hyperesthesia) is rare.[13]

Visual deficits are recognized as an uncommon presenting sign in dogs with cerebral neoplasia and may signal neoplasia with involvement of the optic chiasm.[3,14] However, this manifestation is rare even for pituitary macroadenomas and adenocarcinomas.[14,15] Blindness may occur without other neurologic signs and may persist even after tumor excision. Meningiomas are associated with slow progression of clinical signs.[1] Meningiomas of the orbit arise from the cells of the arachnoid cap of the optic nerve and are described in more detail in Chapter 50.

Nasal tumors occasionally cause neurologic signs such as seizures because of extension through the cribriform plate. These tumors may occur with no sign of nasal disease.[2,16]

Staging and Diagnosis

If a brain tumor is suspected, metabolic causes of signs should be eliminated by routine blood work and urinalysis. Thoracic radiography and CT or MRI of the brain should be performed. CT and MRI techniques are reviewed in several publications.[17]

Radiography of the cranium rarely reveals changes, although meningiomas are sometimes associated with hyperostosis or skull lysis. Cerebrospinal fluid (CSF) is rarely abnormal in dogs with brain tumors; when abnormalities occur, they often indicate only nonspecific inflammation or necrosis. Similarly, electroencephalographic (EEG) changes are rarely specific.[18]

CT scans can be used to localize tumors and delineate tissue margins within structures. The scans locate the tumor precisely, increasing the accuracy of surgery and radiation therapy and thereby reducing injury to surrounding normal tissue. CT scans can sometimes indicate probable tumor type. Delineation between tumor and normal tissue during CT scanning is enhanced with an IV contrast material that pools within the imperfect microvasculature of the tumor. Uniformly contrast-enhanced, well-marginated, broad-based, peripherally located lesions are commonly meningiomas (Figure 49-1). Tumors associated with hemorrhage are more likely to be high-grade astrocytomas or glioblastomas[17] (Figure 49-2). Although much has been made of "ring enhancement" on CT images, this finding has been shown to be nonspecific.[19] CT may also be used to monitor patients postoperatively for early relapse or response to radiation therapy.[20]

MRI is becoming more common in veterinary practice and provides better resolution of intracranial structures than CT scanning (Figure 49-3).[21] Like CT, MRI may allow a presumptive diagnosis of brain tumor type and determination of whether the margins are well defined (as they are in most meningiomas). Dural thickening adjacent to the tumor (dural "tail") indicates extension into the dura mater and is diagnostic of a meningioma.[22] Cysts may be identified on MRI in many dogs with meningioma. In general, meningiomas enhance with contrast and are extraaxial; gliomas are usually intraaxial and have significant surrounding edema and irregular enhancement with contrast. Pituitary tumors are differentiated by location, and choroid plexus carcinomas are usually associated with ventricles with marked contrast enhancement. In one study, prediction of tumor type based on MRI was correct in 24 of 25 dogs; the exception was an intraaxial cystic meningioma.[23] Because meningiomas can occur at the sella, paranasal, and intraventricular sites, they are most likely to be confused with other tumors based on location. Differentiation of intraaxial tumors such as oligodendrogliomas and astrocytomas is not possible with MRI; however, these are rare in dogs.[24] In one study, MRI was able to image and allowed provisional diagnosis of tumors in all dogs with central vestibular disease.[25]

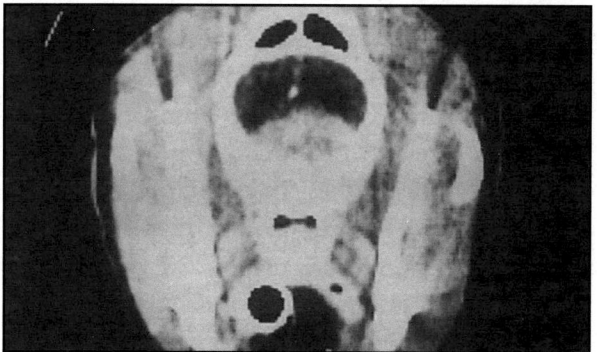

Figure 49-1. *CT scans usually reveal meningiomas as peripherally located, broad-based lesions. A CT scan can assist in planning surgery and radiation therapy. (Courtesy of Amy S. Tidwell, DVM, Tufts Cummings School of Veterinary Medicine)*

KEY POINT

CT or MRI is usually required to localize brain tumors and to delineate the extent of tissue involvement.

The use of CT to position the biopsy needle accurately has allowed preoperative biopsy and diagnosis of brain lesions to become more common in veterinary medicine. In a series of 22 brain biopsies directed by CT, the diagnostic yield was 89% for brain tumors, with 100% accuracy for meningiomas.[26] While most dogs (90%) had no complications, brain herniation and intracranial bleeding were sometimes seen (<5%) and were often fatal. Another study evaluated the accuracy of stereotactic CT-guided brain biopsy in 23 dogs.[27] Biopsy of the lesion was achieved in all but one dog. Complications included death from bleeding in two dogs with brain stem tumors. Minor neurologic deficits were seen in four other dogs. A diagnosis was reached in 70% of dogs after cytology and in more than 90% after histology. Fine-needle aspiration cytology was accurate in diagnosing a mass as neoplastic in another small study, but only 50% of diagnoses of histologic type correlated with biopsy; in contrast, needle-core biopsy obtained an accurate diagnosis in 90% of cases.[28]

Immunohistochemical staining for intermediate filaments may help distinguish different tumor types (Table 49-2).[29] Meningiomas have been histopathologically subclassified as meningothelial, transitional, fibroblastic, psammomatous, angiomatous, granular cell, papillary, and anaplastic (malignant); the clinical relevance of these subclassifications is still uncertain in dogs.[30] Meningothelial and transitional are the two most common variants seen in dogs. Papillary and anaplastic meningiomas are considered more biologically aggressive.[31]

Cystic meningiomas have been diagnosed more frequently since the use of CT and, particularly, MRI became routine.[32-35] Cysts can form in any of the histologic subtypes, and therapy is no different than that used for noncystic meningiomas.

Immunohistochemical staining may allow identification of estrogen and progesterone receptors in meningiomas. Estrogen receptors are rare, but progesterone receptors were seen in 100% of the tumors in one study,[36] in nearly 90% in another study,[37] and in 70% of meningiomas in a third study.[38] The percentage of positive cells appeared to decrease with increased staining for Ki67, a marker of cellular proliferation.[36] Another marker of cellular proliferation, proliferating cell nuclear antigen (PCNA), has been correlated with prognosis in dogs with meningiomas.[38]

Rarely, a primary brain tumor will metastasize outside the cranial vault. Pulmonary metastases of meningiomas were described in four dogs.[39,40] In addition, metastatic disease to the brain from other primary sites, such as primary lung tumors and hemangiosarcomas, may occur. For this reason, complete staging should include thoracic radiography.

Prognostic Factors

Dogs with mild or moderate neurologic impairment at presentation have a more favorable prognosis than dogs with severe initial neurologic signs.[1] Dogs with multiple tumors or intracranial metastasis have a shorter survival than dogs with a solitary tumor, and dogs with normal CSF fluid analysis have longer survival times.[1] Dogs with meningiomas live longer than dogs with other types of brain tumors.[1]

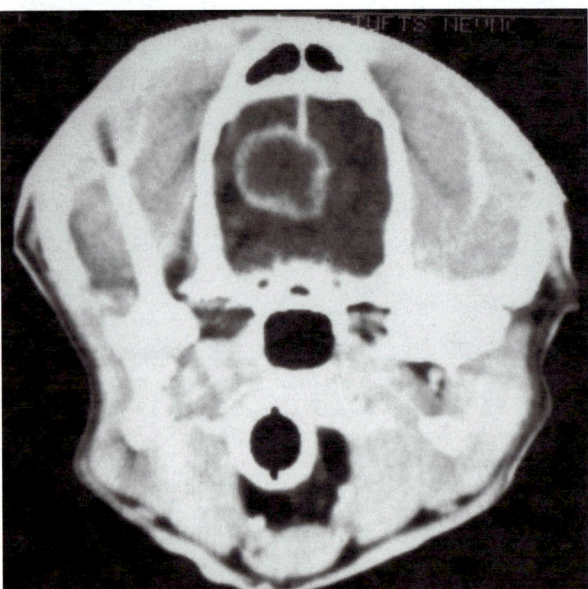

Figure 49-2. *A ring-enhancing astrocytoma of the cerebrum is demonstrated by CT scan. Ring enhancement is not specific for tumor type, but the location (away from periphery) is consistent with a parenchymal tumor rather than a meningioma. CT scanning allows accurate planning of megavoltage radiation therapy. (Courtesy of A. S. Tidwell)*

In a series of 20 dogs with meningiomas, the only prognostic factor was PCNA level. Tumor-free survival 1 and 2 years after surgery and radiation was 63% and 42%, respectively, for dogs with a high PCNA level and 91% at both time points for dogs with a low PCNA level.[38] Tumors with a high PCNA level were more than nine times as likely to recur.

Treatment

PALLIATIVE TREATMENT

Many neurologic signs and impairments seen in dogs with brain tumors arise from peritumoral edema that puts pressure on normal tissue. Neurologic status and, therefore, quality of life can be improved with corticosteroids (e.g., prednisone 1 mg/kg PO sid or every other day) and anticonvulsants (e.g., phenobarbital). Supportive measures do not improve survival times.[1] The median survival for eight dogs treated symptomatically was less than 2 months.[41]

SURGERY ALONE

Definitive therapy consists of surgery, which is usually reserved for superficial tumors (e.g., meningiomas). Perioperative mortality from bleeding and edema may follow excision of large tumors. Careful selection of anesthesia during surgery can help prevent increases in intracranial pressure that could cause brain herniation and death. Administering mannitol and corticosteroids, elevating the animal's head, and hyperventilating the patient help to control intracranial pressure.

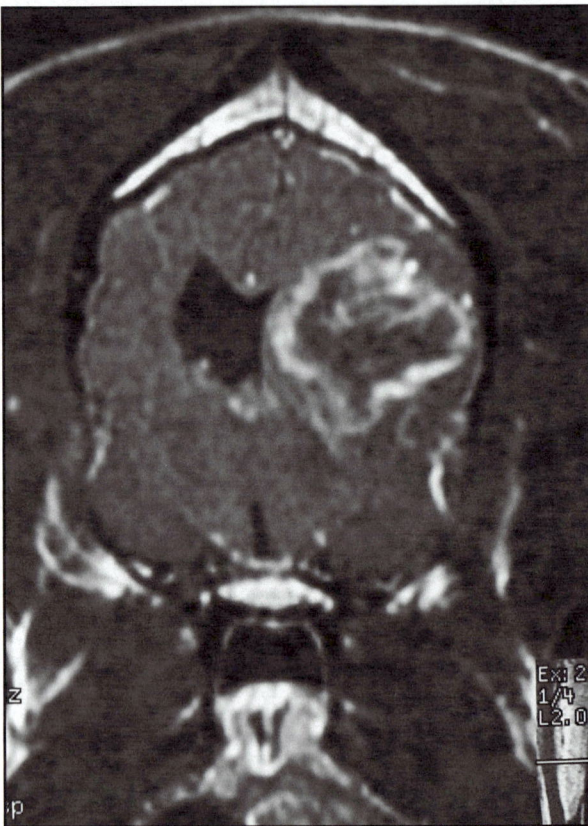

Figure 49-3. *A transverse T1-weighted postcontrast MRI image of the brain of a dog evaluated for generalized seizures. There is a hypointense intraaxial mass with peripheral enhancement (ring enhancing) at the level of the diencephalon (thalamus). There is also deviation of the midline and complete attenuation of the lateral ventricle. At necropsy, the mass appeared to be arising from the internal capsule. Histopathologic diagnosis was oligodendroglioma. (Courtesy of Marc Kent, DVM, University of Georgia College of Veterinary Medicine)*

Surgical access to the brain stem and cerebellar area is difficult, mainly hindered by the transverse sinus that overlies the area. Acute, permanent unilateral occlusion was safely performed in seven dogs with brain tumors (mostly meningiomas); however, no tumors could be resected due to adhesions to surrounding structures.[42] Tumors in this area are probably better treated by radiation therapy.

Surgery is at least moderately successful for treatment of meningiomas; however, incomplete excisions are common because these tumors have poorly defined borders. Complete excision of a meningioma may be associated with long survival.[37] Even with incomplete excision, survival is prolonged because regrowth of meningiomas is usually slow. Surgical excision may be complicated by bleeding and increases in intracranial pressure, leading to brain stem signs and death.[37] Careful attention to postsurgical management is crucial to survival of these patients. In one study, two of 31 dogs treated for meningioma died in the first week after surgery.[10] Of the surviving dogs, 14 were treated with surgery alone and had a median survival time of 7 months (range: 0.5–22 months).[10] Surgical resection of a granular cell neoplasm (presumably of meningeal origin) from the left rostral frontal lobe was successful in another dog, and the dog was clinically normal 4 months later.[43]

Most other reports of tumors are of histologic, rather than clinical, interest, and few treatment details are provided.

Table 49-2 **Intermediate Filament Staining in Brain Tumors**

Tumor Type	GFAP	Vimentin	Pancytokeratin	NSE	S-100
Meningioma	–	+	+/–		
Astrocytoma	+	+	–		Not useful
Oligodendroglioma		No pattern			
Choroid plexus papilloma		–		+	+

GFAP = glial fibrillary acidic protein; NSE = neuron-specific enolase

RADIATION THERAPY ALONE

Radiation therapy, which is used for more deep-seated tumors alone or as an adjunct to surgery, is important in treating brain tumors and prolonging survival in dogs. Unfortunately, most studies report only survival times because repeated CT or MRI is needed to document tumor response; similarly, most studies do not have histologic confirmation of tumor type and rely on imaging for a tentative diagnosis. Because of the depth of these tumors and protection by overlying bony structures, megavoltage (rather than orthovoltage) teletherapy is recommended. Megavoltage radiation also allows "splitting" of doses by using multiple fields for treatment, thereby reducing damage to normal surrounding brain tissues.

> **KEY POINT**
> *Postoperative radiation therapy is an effective modality in the treatment of brain tumors and may be more effective than surgery alone for some tumors such as meningiomas.*

In one retrospective study, dogs receiving cobalt-60 (^{60}Co) megavoltage, with or without other treatment modalities, lived longer than dogs undergoing surgery or supportive care only,[1] echoing the results of an earlier, smaller study.[41] In another study of 29 dogs, the overall median survival was 8 months; 75% of dogs had tumor recurrence or progression.[44]

Despite the theoretical disadvantages of orthovoltage radiation in treating deep-seated tumors, 14 dogs treated with orthovoltage alone for brain tumors had a median survival of 489 days; seven of 10 dogs had improved clinical signs.[45]

One of the main problems with radiation therapy to the brain is that surrounding normal brain tissue may be damaged, causing late effects that may result in clinical signs similar to those of the tumor. This limits the dose of radiation, and the tumor may be inadequately treated as the therapist tries to reduce the radiation field size surrounding the tumor. A CT scanner fitted with a collimator may allow more accurate delivery of radiation to the tumor alone. Preliminary results in dogs were encouraging.[46] A linear accelerator mounted on a rotating gantry that is centered on the brain tumor provides accurate results (radiosurgery), allowing a single large dose (10–15 Gy) of radiation to be delivered. In a preliminary report, control of tumors for more than 1 year was seen in three dogs, despite the relatively low total dose of radiation.[47] Another preliminary report indicated that radiosurgery may be most effective in treating pituitary macroadenomas.[48] A third method of increasing the radiation dose to a brain tumor while limiting exposure of surrounding normal tissue is the delivery of a boronated compound that localizes within the tumor before neutron beam radiation. Preclinical studies have been conducted in dogs, but none has reported a therapeutic outcome.[49]

Dogs treated with radiation for meningiomas seem to have longer survival times than dogs treated with radiation for other types of brain tumors. Median survival for 16 dogs with meningiomas treated with radiation alone was 7.7 months. For 10 dogs with gliomas treated solely by radiation, median survival was 5.8 months.[50] Another study found that, regardless of tumor type, dogs receiving radiation had a median survival of approximately 5 months, whereas dogs with meningiomas that were irradiated had a median survival that approached 9 months.[1] In another series of 18 dogs with meningiomas receiving 45 Gy of radiation alone, five dogs survived 10 months or longer after treatment.[46] Cystic meningiomas should be treated in the same way as other meningiomas; the outcome for affected dogs appears to be similarly encouraging.[33–35]

COMBINED SURGERY AND RADIATION

A series of 20 dogs with meningioma were treated with megavoltage radiation therapy to a total dose of 48 Gy after an incomplete surgical resection, and the median tumor-free survival was 30 months.[38] One year after treatment, 79% were tumor free; 2 years after treatment, 68% were tumor free. Dogs with a high PCNA fraction had shorter tumor-free survival and were more likely to have a recurrence (see Prognostic Factors section, above). Long-term side effects

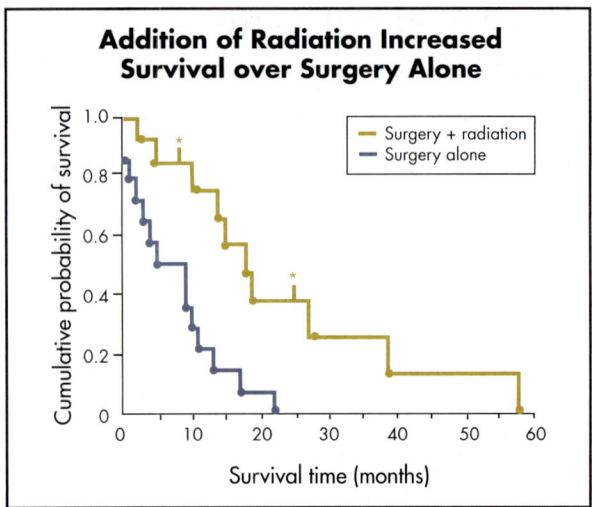

Figure 49-4. *Survival duration for 14 dogs with meningioma treated by surgery alone that survived a median of 7 months and 12 dogs with meningioma treated with surgery and radiation therapy that survived a median of 16.5 months. (From Axlund TW, McGlasson ML, Smith AN: Surgery alone or in combination with radiation therapy for treatment of intracranial meningiomas in dogs: 31 cases (1989-2002).* JAVMA 221:1597–1600, 2002; with permission)

were common and included keratoconjunctivitis sicca in three dogs, cataracts in one dog, possible brain necrosis in two dogs, and a second brain tumor in one dog, all occurring more than 12 months after treatment. Smaller doses per fraction may reduce the risk of late side effects.

Dogs treated with surgery and radiation (40–49.5 Gy) for meningiomas lived longer (median: 20 months; range: 3–58 months) than those treated with surgery alone (median: 7 months; range: 0.5–22 months) (Figure 49-4).[10]

There are only anecdotal reports of tumors other than meningiomas treated with surgery and radiation therapy; one dog with an astrocytoma lived 6 months after treatment.[51]

OTHER LOCAL THERAPIES

Laser therapy caused localized tumor reduction and resolution of clinical signs for 7 months in a boxer with an invasive meningioma.[52]

CHEMOTHERAPY

Chemotherapy is theoretically inconsequential in the treatment of brain tumors because of poor penetration of most drugs across the blood–brain barrier. Experimental chemical disruption of the blood–brain barrier in dogs has been achieved using mannitol, but the technique has not been clinically applied.[53,54] In reality, many large tumors disrupt the barrier and allow penetration of chemotherapeutic agents. The lipid-soluble nitrosourea compounds carmustine (BCNU) and lomustine (CCNU) enter the CSF in animals to achieve concentrations of 15% to 30% of concurrent plasma levels. CCNU is completely absorbed orally and is well tolerated by this route. BCNU is administered intravenously. Both compounds have been evaluated clinically for treatment of brain tumors in dogs.

CCNU (60–80 mg/m^2 q6–8wk) was administered orally to eight dogs with brain tumors. Of the three dogs with measurable disease, one had complete remission, one had stable disease, and one had progression of the disease. Histopathology was not available for these three dogs.[55] In another report, 51 dogs with brain tumors were treated with CCNU (80–100 mg/m^2 PO q4–6wk), and their median survival was 6 months; dogs that had surgery before CCNU lived longer (see Combined Surgery and Chemotherapy section, below).[56]

BCNU was administered intravenously to 15 dogs with brain tumors at a dose of 50 mg/m^2 every 6 weeks.[57] Neutropenia occurred with a nadir at 7 to 9 days after treatment and continued for 15 days. One dog developed histologic evidence of pulmonary fibrosis without clinical signs after eight treatments with BCNU. Six of the 15 dogs had gliomas, as did another dog in a different study[58]; all had partial remissions. The median survival of dogs with glioma was 218 days; responders had a median survival of 288 days,[57] which is comparable with that of radiation therapy. Another report documented responses in three dogs with astrocytoma or oligodendroglioma.[59] Both BCNU and CCNU should be further evaluated for treatment of canine gliomas.

COMBINED SURGERY AND CHEMOTHERAPY

In a preliminary report, CCNU (60–80 mg/m^2 q6–8wk) was administered orally to five dogs after surgery to remove the tumor. For these five dogs, median survival was 3 months (range: 1–21 months), with two dogs still alive at last report.[55] Fourteen dogs that were treated after surgery with CCNU at a higher dosage of 80 to 100 mg/m^2 every 4 to 6 weeks had a median survival of 16.7 months, which is similar to that achieved with surgery and radiation therapy.[56]

HORMONAL THERAPY

The finding of progesterone receptors in meningiomas has led some investigators to speculate that antiprogesterone agents may be useful in the treatment of meningiomas in dogs. Preliminary results using mifepristone in humans for palliation of unresectable meningioma have been encouraging; however, such trials have not been reported in dogs. One dog with an unresectable meningioma was treated with gestrinone at 1.25 mg PO twice a week but failed to respond after 6 weeks. This dog was the only one (of eight total) that did not have progesterone receptors on immunostaining, and the outcome may reflect a hormonal response.[37]

IMMUNOTHERAPY

A preliminary report of intercisternal administration of interleukin-2–stimulated lymphocytes after surgery in five dogs recorded marked regression of gliomas in four dogs for some months, but two dogs developed necrotic inflammatory lesions.[60]

Choroid Plexus Tumors

INCIDENCE, SIGNALMENT, AND ETIOLOGY

Choroid plexus tumors arise adjacent to the ventricles of the brain. Most reported tumors are well-differentiated papillomas.[23,24,61] Choroid plexus tumors may exist as a spectrum of malignancy, rather than in benign and malignant forms; one study classified tumors as papillomas (no mitoses, resembles normal choroid) and atypical papillomas (moderate cellular atypia, moderate mitotic rate, and focal necrosis with infiltration of surrounding brain). The atypical form occurred in a slightly older age group of dogs; only one of five dogs was less than 6 years of age compared with five of 11 with papillomas.[61] Choroid plexus tumors occur most commonly in male dogs (13 of 18 cases).[61–63] Choroid plexus carcinomas have also been reported in dogs with a median age of 6.5 years (range: 2.5–10 years).[64,65] Whether the diagnosis is papilloma or carcinoma, the lateral, third, and fourth ventricles are each affected with equal frequency, although occasionally multiple papillomas may be present; one dog had three tumors involving three different ventricles.[23]

Surprisingly, hydrocephalus is relatively uncommon with choroid plexus tumors.

STAGING AND DIAGNOSIS

Papillomas are solitary and enhance uniformly on MRI.[23,24] Evidence of spread within the ventricular system, presumably through the CSF, was seen in 25% of papillomas and 60% of atypical papillomas in one study; in addition, 25% of papillomas showed brain infiltration, while all of the atypical papillomas invaded surrounding brain.[61] Another dog had widespread cystic carcinomatosis affecting the parenchyma of the whole brain.[65] There is not, therefore, complete correlation between histologic appearance and biologic behavior. Despite involvement of the ventricular system, CSF samples do not contain malignant cells. Extracranial metastases have not been reported.

TREATMENT

The common finding of microscopic evidence of spread means that surgical excision is unlikely to be curative, and radiation therapy would need to take into account this potential distribution throughout the leptomeninges and subarachnoid space, leading to large fields that encompass the whole brain.[61,64] There have been no reports of definitive treatment for this uncommon tumor.

Palliative therapy has been reported in one dog; a ventriculoperitoneal shunt was successful in relieving clinical signs associated with a third ventricle papilloma in this dog.[63] The shunt blocked after 3 weeks, and the signs returned.

Pituitary Macroadenomas and Adenocarcinomas

INCIDENCE, SIGNALMENT, AND ETIOLOGY

Although most pituitary adrenocorticotropic hormone (ACTH)-secreting tumors are microadenomas, macroadenomas (diameter >1 cm) occasionally are reported. In 320 dogs with pituitary-dependent hyperadrenocorticism (PDH), 40 (12.5%) had a large tumor of the pituitary, and all showed neurologic dysfunction.[66] Small-breed dogs commonly develop PDH.[15] Adenomas are more common than adenocarcinomas.[67] Tumors may occur in any area of the pituitary, and carcinomas may invade the thalamus and hypothalamus, causing hemorrhage and death.[68] Most affected dogs develop neurologic signs after being treated with mitotane (o,p'-DDD) for PDH.[68] Any dog with hyperadrenocorticism that develops neurologic signs after treatment with mitotane should be evaluated for the presence of a pituitary mass. Neurologic signs not explained by PDH or mitotane can occur in these dogs as soon as 1 month after treatment but may not appear until 30 months or more after mitotane therapy was commenced.[69] These tumors affect older dogs (average age: 10–12 years). There is no sex predilection.[68]

CLINICAL PRESENTATION AND HISTORY

Clinical signs of hyperadrenocorticism include polydipsia and polyuria, truncal alopecia, and abdominal enlargement (i.e., pot-bellied appearance). The most common neurologic signs in dogs with pituitary macroadenoma are dullness or listlessness (90%), disorientation (75%), nystagmus, behavior changes, pacing, and difficulty lying down. Ataxia, head pressing, circling, and seizures also may occur.[66,68–70] Symmetric tetraparesis was common in one group of dogs.[68] Despite the proximity of these tumors to the optic chiasm, blindness is uncommon,[14,15] even with invasive tumors.[71] The absolute size of a pituitary tumor may be less important than other relative factors, such as calvarium size and tumor location and growth rate. Hence, small dogs may show neurologic signs with quite small (<1 cm) tumors.[15]

Dogs that develop neurologic signs while being treated with mitotane for PDH should be evaluated for a large pituitary tumor (Figure 49-5). Mitotane is cytotoxic to the adrenal cortex but will not affect growth of a pituitary tumor.[66,68] Inadequate serum cortisol suppression during a high-dose

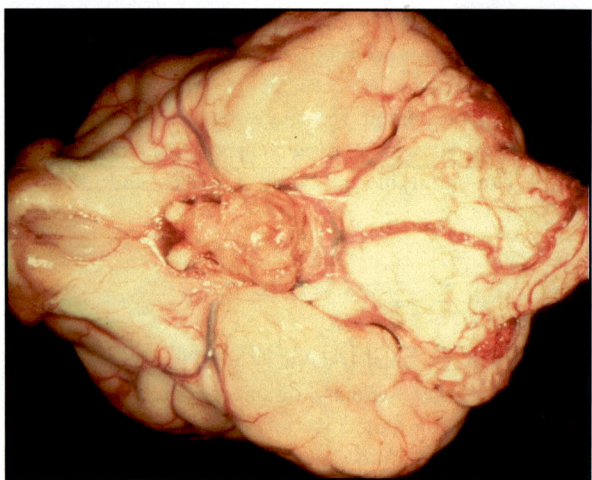

Figure 49-5. *A large pituitary tumor in a 13-year-old boxer that developed neurologic signs several months after treatment for PDH. (Courtesy of Gordon H. Theilen, DVM, University of California, Davis)*

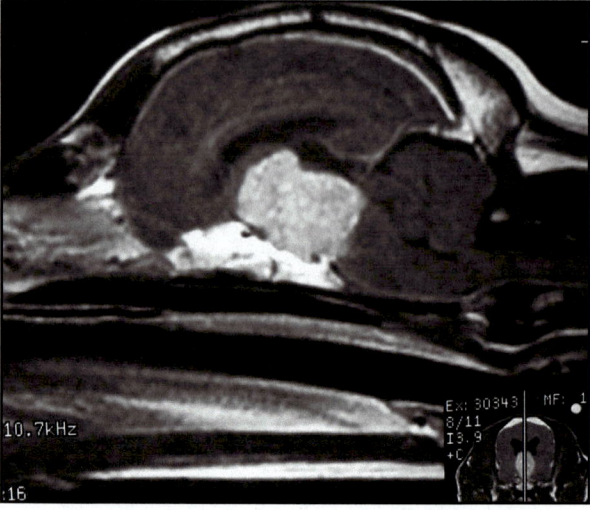

Figure 49-7. *A sagittal post-contrast T1-weighted MRI image of the brain of a cairn terrier that presented for polydipsia and generalized seizures. Hyperadrenocorticism was diagnosed with an ACTH-stimulation test. There is a well-delineated, strongly and homogenously enhancing mass arising from the sella turcica and compressing the diencephalon (thalamus). (Courtesy of M. Kent)*

ble of producing very high levels of ACTH and are not easily suppressed by exogenous corticosteroid administration. In one study, dogs that had large pituitary tumors and eventually developed neurologic signs had higher average plasma ACTH levels at presentation than dogs with small tumors, although endocrine testing alone was unlikely to distinguish between dogs with large pituitary tumors and those with small or microscopic tumors.[15]

> **KEY POINT**
>
> *Dogs that develop neurologic signs while being treated for hyperadrenocorticism should be evaluated by CT or MRI for a large pituitary tumor.*

STAGING AND DIAGNOSIS

In any dog suspected of having a pituitary tumor, staging should include endogenous ACTH levels, low- and high-dose dexamethasone suppression tests, thoracic radiography, and CT or MRI imaging of the brain (Figures 49-6 and 49-7). A presumptive diagnosis of pituitary macroadenoma or adenocarcinoma may be made by detection of a mass in the sella turcica that exceeds the dorsal limits of the sella.[69] Evidence of compression of surrounding structures as well as displacement and dilation of the third and lateral ventricles is common. In one study of 28 dogs with PDH imaged by CT, 11 dogs had neurologic signs and a median pituitary adenoma height of 1.5 cm compared with 0.6 cm in dogs

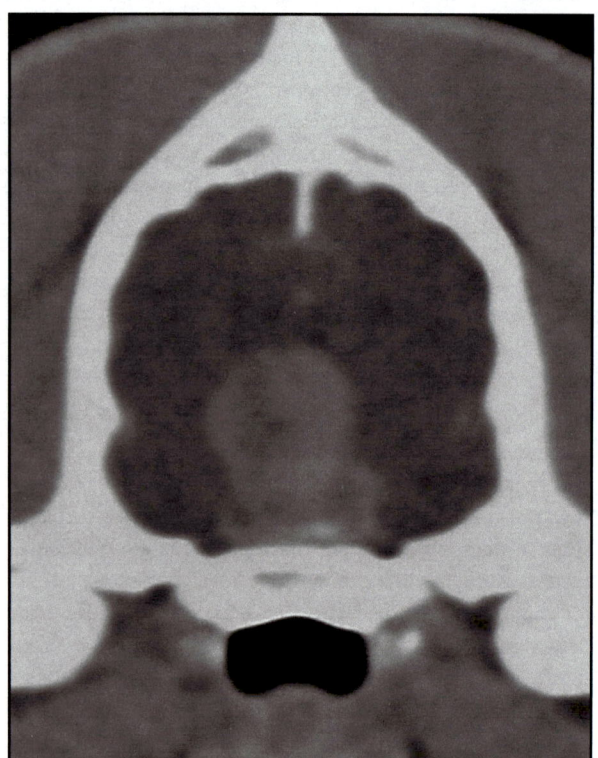

Figure 49-6. *CT scan of a large pituitary tumor. Severity of neurologic signs is related to tumor height relative to calvarium size. (Courtesy of Nicole Northrup, DVM, University of Georgia College of Veterinary Medicine)*

dexamethasone suppression test may indicate an adrenal tumor. In an animal with PDH, inadequate suppression may indicate the potential for subsequent development of a large or invasive pituitary tumor.[68] Large pituitary tumors are capa-

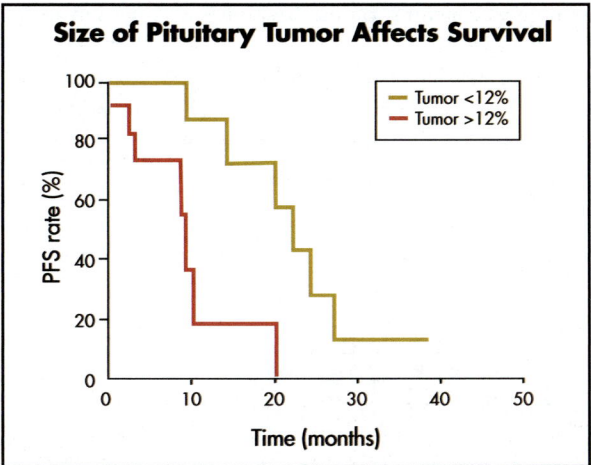

Figure 49-8. Progression-free survival (PFS) duration for dogs with a pituitary tumor smaller than 12% of calvarium was significantly longer than that for dogs with a pituitary tumor larger than 12% of calvarium. (From Theon AP, Feldman EC: Megavoltage irradiation of pituitary macrotumors in dogs with neurologic signs. JAVMA 213:225–231, 1998; with permission)

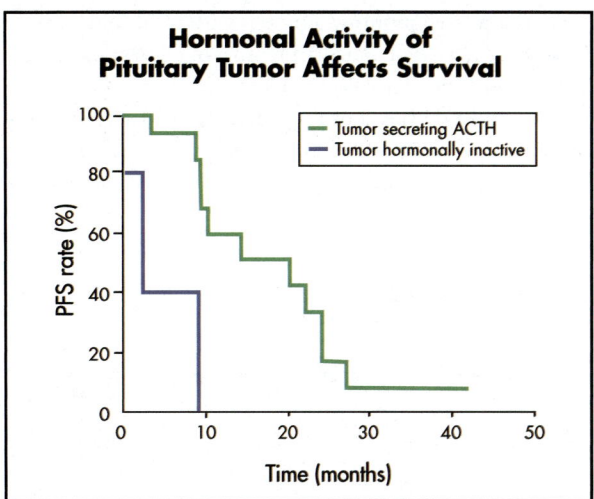

Figure 49-9. Progression-free survival duration for 19 dogs with pituitary tumors that were hormonally inactive was significantly shorter than for 19 dogs with pituitary tumors secreting ACTH. (From Theon AP, Feldman EC: Megavoltage irradiation of pituitary macrotumors in dogs with neurologic signs. JAVMA 213:225–231, 1998; with permission)

without neurologic signs; only two dogs with a tumor smaller than 1 cm had neurologic signs.[72] In another study, the relative size of the pituitary tumor (tumor to calvarium) was correlated with severity of neurologic signs.[73]

Periodic MRI may predict which dogs with a small pituitary tumor and PDH will develop a macroadenoma and neurologic signs. In one study, a year after initial diagnosis, four of eight dogs with visible pituitary tumors had increases in height of the mass; of these four dogs, two developed neurologic signs within a year of the MRI.[74] Neurologic signs developed in 10 of 20 dogs many months after central diabetes insipidus was diagnosed; most of these dogs had a pituitary tumor on CT scan or at necropsy.[75]

CSF analysis is not useful in diagnosing this type of tumor. Definitive diagnosis by biopsy is rare unless surgical resection is performed. Occasionally, pituitary adenocarcinoma may metastasize intracerebrally.[76]

PROGNOSTIC FACTORS

Dogs with mild or moderate neurologic impairment at presentation have a more favorable prognosis than dogs with severe initial neurologic signs when treated with radiation therapy.[67,73] The relative size of the pituitary tumor (tumor to calvarium) was correlated with progression-free survival (Figure 49-8).[73] Dogs with tumors that are not hormonally active have a poor prognosis (Figure 49-9).[73]

TREATMENT

Without treatment for a pituitary macroadenoma, survival is short. In a series of seven dogs treated supportively, five dogs survived less than 2 months.[67]

Hypophysectomy has been reported for the treatment of PDH caused by small adenomas.[77] One dog with a pituitary macroadenoma treated with hypophysectomy was still alive 8 months after surgery.[66] This surgery is technically difficult, particularly if the tumor is large; most studies concur that tumors larger than 1 cm can only be debulked for palliation.[77]

Radiation therapy is the preferred treatment for large pituitary tumors. For dogs with macroadenoma of the pituitary confirmed on CT or MRI, megavoltage radiation to the tumor and 1 cm of adjacent normal tissue resolves neurologic signs within 6 months of therapy in most reported cases; tumor shrinkage often continued for more than 1 year.[78] Resolution of signs of hyperadrenocorticism is more variable. ACTH levels decreased to normal over a period of months in some dogs, but other dogs required concurrent mitotane therapy.[73,78]

In two preliminary studies, dogs with large pituitary tumors treated with 38 to 40 Gy had a median survival of more than 24 months.[78,79] In another study, 10 dogs were treated to a total dose of 54 Gy, and their median survival was 2.5 months; five dogs that had minimal neurologic signs were more likely to have a long response (median: 21 months).[67] In a further study, radiation to 48 Gy was used to treat 24 dogs with pituitary macroadenomas and neurologic signs. Three dogs did not complete treatment due to progression of neurologic signs. The relative size of the tumor (compared with calvarium) predicted the remission of neurologic signs after therapy; smaller size correlated with a higher likelihood of complete resolution. Severity of neurologic signs also predicted survival. Overall median remission was 13 months, but dogs with mild to moderate neurologic signs had a median remission of 20 months (25 months for mild signs alone). Dogs with tumors not associated with PDH (i.e., hormone inactive) had a poorer survival, but plasma cortisol levels within the PDH group were not predictive of survival.[73] Tumor size itself was not a prognostic factor for tumor response or survival in any of these studies.

The major side effects of radiation are acute, with otitis and skin changes predominating. Late effects do not appear to be a problem; however, pituitary tumor necrosis may lead to worsening of neurologic signs.[67,73]

▶ TUMORS OF THE SPINE

CLINICAL BRIEFING

Clinical factors	• Pain; slow onset of ataxia and paresis. • Extradural tumors most common; vertebral body affected. • Large-breed dogs, young to middle aged. • Locally invasive.
Staging and diagnosis	• MDB. • Plain radiography of the spine may show vertebral lysis. • Myelogram may be helpful in localizing lesion. • CT or MRI of the spine.
Prognostic factors	• None identified.
Treatment	
Initial	• Surgery is the treatment of choice for extradural and intradural–extramedullary tumors. • Intramedullary tumors are not amenable to surgical excision.
Adjunctive	• Radiation therapy may be a useful adjunct to incomplete surgery. • Chemotherapy not described.
Palliative	• Corticosteroids.
Supportive	• As for palliative, plus pain relief after surgery; nutritional support as needed.

Tumors of the spine are classified not only by histology but also by their anatomic position within the spinal canal. *Intramedullary tumors* are located within the parenchyma of the spinal cord; *intradural–extramedullary tumors* are outside the spinal cord but inside the dura; and *extradural tumors* are those arising from outside the dura, usually involving the vertebral bone and often causing signs because of compression.

Incidence, Signalment, and Etiology

Most canine spinal tumors (up to 50%) are extradural, and most of these are primary or secondary bone tumors, such as osteosarcoma and multiple myeloma (Figure 49-10). Other tumors, such as fibrosarcoma, chondrosarcoma, hemangiosarcoma, and liposarcoma, are less common. These tumors rarely invade through the dura. Lymphoma is usually extradural but can be intradural[80,81] and is usually associated with systemic disease.

Intradural–extramedullary spinal neoplasms account for 35% of canine spinal tumors and are most likely to be neurofibrosarcomas (nerve sheath tumors) arising from the nerve roots or meningiomas; both tumor types are most common in the cervical spinal cord. In three series totaling 73 dogs with intradural or intramedullary tumors, the most common diagnosis was nerve sheath tumor (35 dogs); meningiomas and fibrosarcomas/myxosarcomas were the next most common (12 and 13 dogs, respectively). Other tumor types included primary nephroblastoma, glioma, and astrocytoma.[82–84]

Intramedullary tumors are rare in dogs. They are most commonly gliomas/astrocytomas but are occasionally metastatic lesions or part of a systemic disease, particularly lymphoma or hemangiosarcoma.[85]

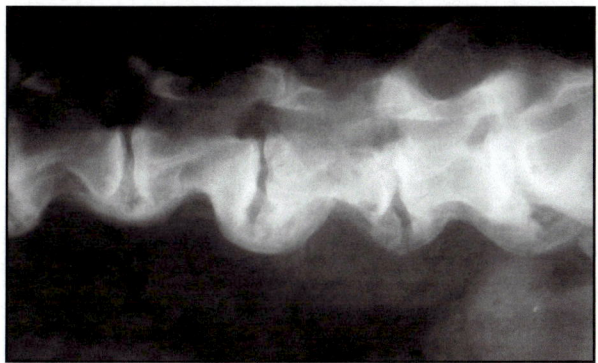

Figure 49-10. *An osteosarcoma of the sixth lumbar vertebra causing extradural compression of the associated spinal cord. Surgical decompression may relieve clinical signs, but definitive surgery requires vertebral removal and is unlikely to achieve complete resection. (Courtesy of John Berg, DVM, Tufts Cummings School of Veterinary Medicine)*

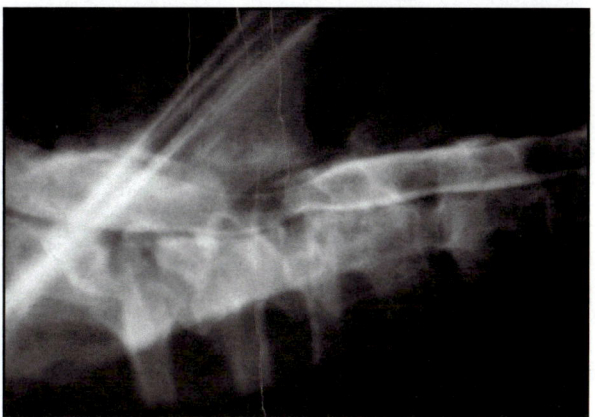

Figure 49-11. *An extradural tumor at the level of T1 is outlined by myelography showing an obvious compressive lesion. (Courtesy of J. Berg)*

Spinal tumors are more common in large-breed dogs (67%–90% of dogs with spinal tumors).[86] There is no gender predisposition overall, although meningiomas may be more common in male dogs.[87] The average age of affected dogs is 5 to 7 years, although dogs with nephroblastoma are considerably younger.[82,86] In two studies, more than 25% of dogs with spinal tumors were 3 years of age or younger.[82,86] Intramedullary tumors are more common in young animals.

Clinical Presentation and History

In animals with extradural spinal tumors, the first sign is pain that results from the destruction of bone and compression of nerve roots. Most extradural tumors occur at the thoracolumbar junction.

In tumors arising within the spinal canal, regardless of histogenesis, pain and paresis are the most common signs. Pain was the reason owners sought veterinary advice for 23 of 33 dogs with spinal canal tumors in one study. The pain was characterized as acute or chronic in equal numbers of patients in that study.[82] Paresis, alone or with pain, was the reason for presentation in 20 of 33 dogs with spinal canal tumors; six dogs were paralyzed.[82] Ataxia and paresis usually develop slowly with extradural and intradural–extramedullary spinal tumors, although rapid progression may occur and produce acute onset of paresis or paralysis. Most intradural–extramedullary tumors occur in the cervicothoracic spine. Nerve sheath tumors usually arise from dorsal nerve roots. The initial pain develops into paresis as the tumors slowly grow within the spinal canal and through the intervertebral foramen along peripheral nerves. Meningiomas cause similar signs; however, these tumors may invade the dura.

Signs of intramedullary tumors usually progress rapidly (<2 weeks), whereas signs of other spinal tumors have an average duration of 1 to 2 months.[86]

Meningiomas are most common in the cervical spine.[82,83,87,88] Most meningiomas are solitary and localized, but a meningioma and a meningeal sarcoma extending from the cervical to the thoracolumbar spine in one dog and the length of the entire lumbosacral spine in another have been described.[89,90]

Nerve sheath tumors occur in either the cervical or lumbar spine but rarely in the thoracic spine.[82,83] Nerve sheath tumors can be multifocal.[82,86] Whether this represents metastasis or synchronous primaries is not clear, but complete spinal evaluation is recommended in a patient with this diagnosis.

Staging and Diagnosis

An MDB is recommended for all dogs with a diagnosis of spinal tumor. Dogs with lymphoma should also be staged as outlined in Chapter 47. Additional imaging of a suspected spinal tumor is recommended to accurately plan biopsy and treatment.

Any imaging of the spine should be conducted under anesthesia. Plain radiography rarely demonstrates a lesion unless there is marked bony destruction.[83,91] Histopathology is needed for definitive diagnosis, but myelography can often distinguish between extradural, intradural–extramedullary, and intramedullary tumors. Decisions regarding the possible success of treatment can often be made using myelographic information alone. Extradural tumors compress the dura and cord, obstructing the flow of dye in the column (Figure 49-11), whereas intramedullary tumors cause diverging myelographic lines on both lateral and dorsoventral views. For intradural–extramedullary tumors, the mass may be outlined by contrast media, creating a "golf-tee" appearance[82,92] (Figure 49-12).

CT scanning and MRI have largely supplanted the use of myelography in veterinary practice. CT allows better evaluation of bony changes associated with extradural lesions

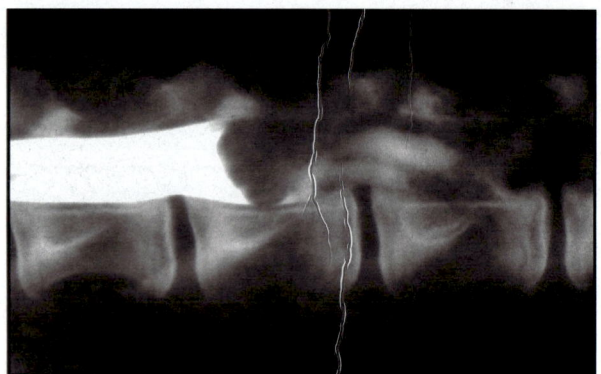

Figure 49-12. *An intradural–extramedullary neurofibrosarcoma is outlined by myelography to show a classic "golf-tee" appearance. (Courtesy of Karl Kraus, DVM, Tufts Cummings School of Veterinary Medicine)*

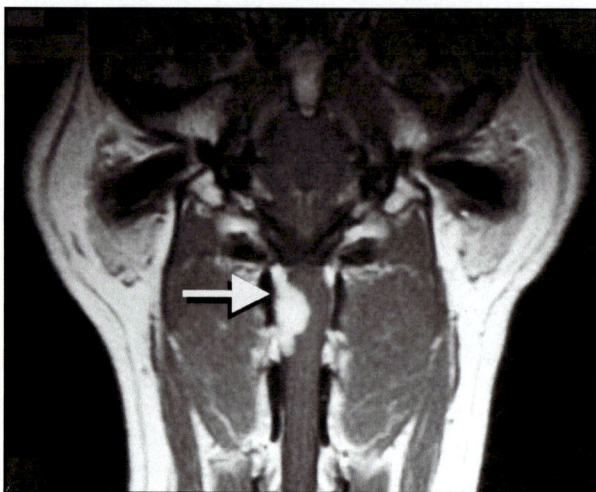

Figure 49-13. *A dorsal T1-weighted postcontrast MRI image of a caudal fossa and cranial cervical vertebral column. There is a well-delineated, strongly enhancing extraaxial mass* (arrow) *within the vertebral canal within the atlas. The mass was a meningioma. (Courtesy of M. Kent)*

than does radiography but does not show much advantage for intramedullary lesions.[91] MRI is probably the imaging modality of choice for spinal cord tumors. The resolution obtained with MRI, particularly for intramedullary tumors, is superior to that of any other imaging technique (Figure 49-13).[84,93] MRI allows differentiation of an intramedullary tumor from an extramedullary one, which can be difficult on myelography.[94] This is of major importance to therapy, as an extramedullary tumor may be amenable to surgery, whereas an intramedullary one is less likely to be resectable.

> **KEY POINT**
>
> *CT and MRI are useful imaging modalities that have largely replaced myelography in distinguishing extradural, intradural–extramedullary, and intramedullary spinal tumors.*

Electromyography was more helpful in precisely localizing a lesion than was neurologic examination in one early study[95]; however, MRI has largely supplanted this as a method of staging and diagnosis.

CSF analysis is not usually helpful in specifically diagnosing spinal tumors; with the exception of some spinal lymphomas, spinal tumors rarely exfoliate.[80,81]

Treatment

EXTRADURAL

Surgery is the treatment of choice for most extradural tumors. The exceptions are extradural lymphoma, which may respond to chemotherapy or radiation therapy; and multiple myeloma of the vertebrae, for which chemotherapy with prednisone and alkylating agents is the treatment of choice (see Chapter 48). In dogs with extensive bony lysis of a vertebra, removal of the vertebra may be the only option; however, vertebral removal does not often result in complete resection. Removal of extradural tumors is usually confined to tumors that have not yet damaged the vertebra structurally (Figures 49-14 and 49-15). Two dogs with surgically treated osteosarcomas had reported survival times of 3 weeks and 10 months.[96]

Incomplete resection of a lumbar extradural ganglioneuroma resolved all clinical signs for 8 months in a 10-year-old dog. At recurrence, a second surgery again resolved all clinical signs.[97] Recurrence 7 months after surgery was seen in a dog with a thoracolumbar liposarcoma.[98]

Radiation therapy, as described in Chapter 62, may be warranted in these dogs; however, the risk of spinal damage with high doses of radiation could limit efficacy (see Intradural–Extramedullary section, below).

INTRADURAL–EXTRAMEDULLARY

Intradural–extramedullary tumors that have not invaded the spinal cord may be amenable to surgical excision. Treatment of meningiomas is reported most frequently, but most reports describe few cases. Although meningiomas are benign and surgical resection can be curative, ventral location or location at an intumescence is associated with poor surgical outcome. Spinal cord invasion is seen in about 25% of spinal meningiomas; invasive tumors often are not operable. Even in the absence of cord invasion, surgery is complicated by the friable nature of these tumors and by numerous adhesions to surrounding structures. Neurologic improvement was seen in six of nine dogs that underwent surgery for spinal meningioma.[87] Five of the nine dogs lived more than 6 months, and one dog was free of disease 3 years

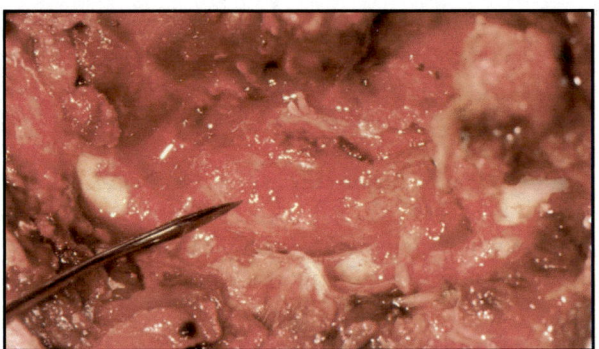

Figure 49-14. *The tumor seen in Figure 49-11 after surgical exposure through laminectomy* (arrowed by probe). *(Courtesy of J. Berg)*

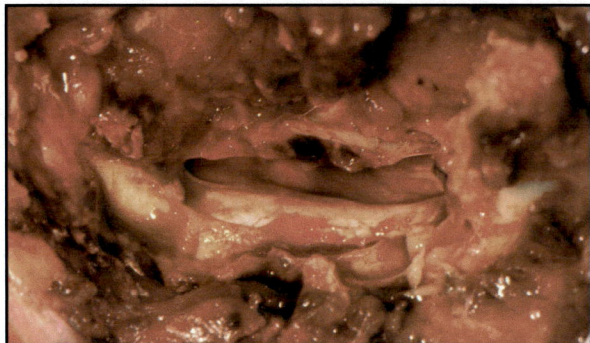

Figure 49-15. *The tumor seen in Figures 49-11 and 49-14 after surgical removal. (Courtesy of J. Berg)*

after surgery. Two additional dogs with meningiomas survived more than 46 months after surgery.[96] Tumor recurred 1.5 years after surgery in two of three dogs with meningiomas of the atlantooccipital region; one of these was treated surgically for a second time and was free of signs 8 months later.[88]

Six dogs with intradural–extramedullary tumors (three meningiomas and three neurofibrosarcomas) were treated surgically and survived a median of 12 months; the longest survivor was a dog with meningioma.[82] Median survival after surgery was 7 months in seven dogs with nerve sheath tumors.[96] The tumor recurred in most of these dogs despite apparent complete excision in three dogs. Another dog had no clinical evidence of tumor recurrence 8 months after resection of a cervical nerve sheath tumor.[99]

Spinal myxosarcoma is a recently described entity that is poorly understood. Three dogs with spinal myxosarcoma survived between 11 and 36 months after surgery.[96]

Radiation therapy may delay recurrence of an incompletely excised extradural or intradural–extramedullary tumor. However, there are few results published, and often prognosis is assumed based on data derived from treatment of brain tumors with the same histology.

One dog with intradural–extramedullary meningioma was treated by surgery and had a local recurrence 15 months later. Treatment with megavoltage (^{60}Co) radiation therapy alone provided a second remission of 19 months.[100] Tumor control for a median of 15 months was seen in six dogs with spinal meningiomas treated with postoperative radiation therapy of 33 to 48 Gy. Recurrence was seen in four dogs between 12 and 25 months after treatment.[101]

A dog with a nerve sheath tumor received 35 Gy of postoperative radiation therapy and had no recurrence 25 months later.[101] Radiation therapy alone in another dog controlled the tumor for 15 months, but this was similar to results gained with surgery alone.[96]

Higher doses of radiation may be more effective, but as the dose increases above 50 Gy, so does the risk of delayed spinal cord damage. Small doses per fraction (2.5 Gy or less) should be used if higher total doses are anticipated.

INTRAMEDULLARY

Intramedullary tumors usually cannot be resected surgically. Radiation therapy, either alone or postoperatively, provides the best chance of controlling these tumors. Surgical excision of an ependymoma was followed by radiation therapy in two dogs. One received 48 Gy and had no recurrence 70 months later[101]; the second dog received 35 Gy and was euthanatized 3 months later for persistent fecal incontinence.[102] A dog with a glioma in the atlantooccipital region was treated with surgery and radiation therapy. Signs of respiratory acidosis caused by spinal cord compression resolved, but the dog died suddenly 5 months later.[103]

Difficulties in penetrating the CSF may limit the efficacy of chemotherapy in treating spinal tumors. Intrathecal chemotherapy with cytarabine was used in three dogs with spinal lymphoma in conjunction with craniospinal irradiation to a total dose of 30 Gy. Responses were dramatic but short lived (6, 14, and 84 days) and were probably due to radiation rather than to chemotherapy.[81] CCNU is a lipophilic chemotherapeutic agent that has efficacy in the treatment of brain tumors in dogs, and responses have been seen in meningiomas. One dog with a spinal meningioma received CCNU postoperatively and developed a recurrence 15 months later. The contribution of chemotherapy to tumor control in this dog is difficult to assess.[88]

Corticosteroids (e.g., prednisone, 1 mg/kg PO bid) have been palliative for some intramedullary tumors[85] and for compressive extradural tumors,[104] but this presumably is a result of indirect antiinflammatory effects on edema rather than of direct effects on the tumor.

Spinal Nephroblastoma
INCIDENCE, SIGNALMENT, AND ETIOLOGY

Spinal nephroblastoma has been described under many names. It is usually found in very young dogs and has been called *intradural–extramedullary tumor of young dogs*; most cases have been described to arise in the thoracolumbar spine. Other terms for this tumor include medulloepithelioma, spinal cord blastoma, and neuroepithelioma.[105] One study demonstrated immunohistochemical staining for the Wilm's gene product in a dog with a neuroepithelioma, defining it as a spinal nephroblastoma.

Affected dogs are between 6 months and 3 years of age with no obvious gender predilection. Large breeds, possibly German shepherds and golden retrievers, are overrepresented.[106]

CLINICAL PRESENTATION AND HISTORY

Signs consistent with a thoracolumbar myelopathy are seen in affected dogs, and an intradural–extramedullary location is suggestive of this tumor type.

STAGING AND DIAGNOSIS

Staging as described for other dogs with spinal tumors is recommended, including MRI of the whole spinal cord.[94] Abdominal ultrasonography is also recommended. These are young dogs, and intercurrent disease is not expected; however, a report of a dog with spinal, renal, and bone marrow nephroblastoma means that staging should be complete in an affected dog.[107] One dog had two separate nephroblastoma lesions in the spinal canal.[108] While it is uncertain whether this represented metastasis or synchronous primaries, the whole spinal cord should be examined in affected animals.

CSF contained tumor cells in one dog,[109] although this appears to be rare.[105]

Immunohistochemistry to stain the Wilm's tumor gene product can be used to confirm the diagnosis.[110]

TREATMENT

Surgery has been described but is often impossible because of adhesions to the adjoining spinal cord.[111] Surgical excision has been reported in five dogs. Complete excision appears to be curative, with reported control over 2 years in two of four dogs.[102,112–114] One of these four dogs had a recurrence 12 months after the first surgery; a second surgery caused a 5-month additional remission.[114] Incomplete excision is associated with rapid return of signs within 2 to 6 months.[106,115,116] One dog treated with an incomplete surgery and 44 Gy of radiation therapy was apparently cured but developed a radiation-induced osteosarcoma at the radiation site 5 years later.[105]

▶ TUMORS OF PERIPHERAL NERVES

CLINICAL BRIEFING

Clinical factors	• Slowly progressive lameness. • Neurofibrosarcoma most common.[a] • Large-breed dogs, middle aged (average age is 7 years). • Local disease, rare metastasis.
Staging and diagnosis	• MDB. • Myelogram may be helpful in localizing lesion that is invading nerve root. • MRI of the spine and nerve roots.
Prognostic factors	• None identified.
Treatment	
Initial	• Surgical resection of tumor for small masses. • Amputation and resection for large masses or if severe neurologic deficits are present.
Adjunctive	• Radiation therapy used for incompletely excised tumors. • Chemotherapy not reported, as for soft tissue sarcomas.
Palliative	• Corticosteroids.
Supportive	• As for palliative, plus pain relief after surgery; nutritional support as needed.

[a]More detail is provided in Chapter 62.

Neurofibrosarcoma is the most common tumor of peripheral nerve tissue in the dog. It is sometimes termed schwannoma, neurilemmoma, perineural fibroblastoma, or nerve-sheath tumor. This neoplasm arises from the fibrous nerve sheath and most commonly occurs in the brachial plexus. Neurofibrosarcomas are classified as soft tissue sarcomas and are discussed in depth in Chapter 62. They are prone to regrowth and are invasive but rarely metastasize. As for all soft tissue sarcomas, the clinical behavior is similar regardless of whether the diagnosis is neurofibroma or neurofibrosarcoma. Neurofibrosarcomas also occur in the cervical and thoracolumbar region as intradural–extramedullary tumors (see Tumors of the Canine Spine section, above).

Peripheral Neuroblastoma

INCIDENCE, SIGNALMENT, AND ETIOLOGY

Peripheral neuroblastoma, also called *ganglioneuroblastoma* or *ganglioneuroma*, has been reported in a small number of dogs. Neuroblastoma is a primitive neuroectodermal tumor that occurs in the CNS and peripheral nervous system. Most are described in dogs younger than 4 years of age, although older dogs may be affected. There is no obvious breed or gender predilection. Large-breed dogs are most often affected.

CLINICAL PRESENTATION AND HISTORY

Neuroblastomas have been described in the adrenal medulla and retroperitoneum, olfactory bulb, mediastinum, and cranial cervical ganglia.[117–119] Metastases, including intracranial sites, have been described for approximately 50% of these tumors.

STAGING AND DIAGNOSIS

After an MDB is conducted, staging will depend on the site(s) affected. CT scanning or MRI may be necessary to accurately image these tumors.

TREATMENT

There are no reports of treatment of this rare tumor. Radiation therapy may be palliative for localized tumors that cannot be surgically resected. A similar tumor in cats (esthesioneuroblastoma) appears to be sensitive to radiation therapy.

REFERENCES

1. Heidner GL, Kornegay JN, Page RL, et al: Analysis of survival in a retrospective study of 86 dogs with brain tumors. *J Vet Intern Med* 5:219–226, 1991.
2. Foster ES, Carrillo JM, Patnaik AK: Clinical signs of tumors affecting the rostral cerebrum in 43 dogs. *J Vet Intern Med* 2:71–74, 1988.
3. Palmer AC, Malinowski W, Barnett KC: Clinical signs including papilloedema associated with brain tumours in twenty-one dogs. *J Small Anim Pract* 15:359–386, 1974.
4. Kube SA, Bruyette DS, Hanson SM: Astrocytomas in young dogs. *JAAHA* 39:288–293, 2003.
5. Uchida K, Nakayama H, Endo Y, et al: Ganglioglioma in the thalamus of a puppy. *J Vet Med Sci* 65:113–115, 2003.
6. Porter B, de Lahunta A, Summers B: Gliomatosis cerebri in six dogs. *Vet Pathol* 40:97–102, 2003.
7. Lipsitz D, Higgins RJ, Kortz GD, et al: Glioblastoma multiforme: Clinical findings, magnetic resonance imaging, and pathology in five dogs. *Vet Pathol* 40:659–669, 2003.
8. Uchida K, Kuroski K, Priosoeryanto BP, et al: Giant cell glioblastoma in the frontal cortex of a dog. *Vet Pathol* 32:197–199, 1995.
9. Kraft SL, Gavin PR, Leathers CW, et al: Diffuse cerebral and leptomeningeal astrocytoma in dogs: MR features. *J Comput Assist Tomogr* 14:555–560, 1990
10. Axlund TW, McGlasson ML, Smith AN: Surgery alone or in combination with radiation therapy for treatment of intracranial meningiomas in dogs: 31 cases (1989-2002). *JAVMA* 221:1597–1600, 2002.
11. Bagley RS, Gavin PR, Moore MP, et al: Clinical signs associated with brain tumors in dogs: 97 cases (1992-1997). *JAVMA* 215:818–819, 1999.
12. Bateman SW, Parent JM: Clinical findings, treatment, and outcome of dogs with status epilepticus or cluster seizures: 156 cases (1990-1995). *JAVMA* 215:1463–1468, 1999.
13. Holland CT, Charles JA, Smith SH, Cortaville PE: Hemihyperaesthesia and hyperresponsiveness resembling central pain syndrome in a dog with a forebrain oligodendroglioma. *Aust Vet J* 78:676–680, 2000.
14. Davidson MG, Nasisse MP, Breitschwerdt EB, et al: Acute blindness associated with intracranial tumors in dogs and cats: Eight cases (1984-1989). *JAVMA* 199:755–758, 1991.
15. Kipperman BS, Feldman EC, Dybdal NO, Nelson RW: Pituitary tumor size, neurologic signs, and relation to endocrine test results in dogs with pituitary-dependent hyperadrenocorticism: 43 cases (1980-1990). *JAVMA* 201:762–767, 1992.
16. Smith MO, Turrel JM, Bailey CS, Cain GR: Neurologic abnormalities as the predominant signs of neoplasia of the nasal cavity in dogs and cats: Seven cases (1973-1986). *JAVMA* 195:242–245, 1989.
17. Kornegay JN: Imaging brain neoplasms. Computed tomography and magnetic resonance imaging. *Vet Med Report* 2:372–390, 1990.
18. Steiss JE, Cox NR, Knecht CD: Electroencephalographic and histopathologic correlations in eight dogs with intracranial mass lesions. *Am J Vet Res* 51:1286–1291, 1990.
19. Wolf M, Pedroia V, Higgins RJ, et al: Intracranial ring enhancing lesions in dogs: A correlative CT scanning and neuropathologic study. *Vet Radiol Ultrasound* 36:16–20, 1995.
20. Bergman R, Jones J, Lanz O, et al: Post-operative computed tomography in two dogs with cerebral meningioma. *Vet Radiol Ultrasound* 41:425–432, 2000.
21. Kraft SL, Gavin PR: Intracranial neoplasia. *Clin Techn Small Anim Pract* 14:112–123, 1999.
22. Hathcock JT: Low field magnetic resonance imaging characteristics of cranial vault meningiomas in 13 dogs. *Vet Radiol Ultrasound* 37:257–263, 1996
23. Thomas WB, Wheeler SJ, Kramer R, Kornegay JN: Magnetic resonance imaging features of primary brain tumors in dogs. *Vet Radiol Ultrasound* 37:20–27, 1996.
24. Kraft SL, Gavin PR, DeHaan C, et al: Retrospective review of 50 canine intracranial tumors evaluated by magnetic resonance imaging. *J Vet Intern Med* 11:218–225, 1997.
25. Garosi LS, Dennis R, Penderis J, et al: Results of magnetic resonance imaging in dogs with vestibular disorders: 85 cases (1996-1999). *JAVMA* 218:385–391, 2001.
26. Koblik PD, LeCouteur RA, Higgins RJ, et al: CT-guided brain biopsy using a modified Pelorus Mark III stereotactic system: Experience with 50 dogs. *Vet Radiol Ultrasound* 40:434–440, 1999.
27. Moissonnier P, Blot S, Devauchelle P, et al: Stereotactic CT-guided brain biopsy in the dog. *J Small Anim Pract* 43:115–123, 2002.
28. Platt SR, Alleman AR, Lanz OI, Chrisman CL: Comparison of fine-needle aspiration and surgical-tissue biopsy in the diagnosis of canine brain tumors. *Vet Surg* 31:65–69, 2002.
29. Ribas JL: Application of immunohistochemistry in canine neuro-oncology. *Schweiz Arch Tierheilk* 132:463–464, 1990.
30. Barnhart KF, Wojcieszyn J, Storts RW: Immunohistochemical staining patterns of canine meningiomas and correlation with published immunophenotypes. *Vet Pathol* 39:311–321, 2002.
31. Kaldrymidou E, Polizopoulou ZS, Papaioannou N, et al: Papillary meningioma in the dog: A clinicopathological study of two cases. *J Comp Pathol* 124:227–230, 2001.
32. Schulman FY, Carpenter JL, Ribas JL, Brum DE: Cystic papillary meningioma in the sella turcica of a dog. *JAVMA* 200:67–69, 1992.

33. Kitagawa M, Kanayama K, Sakai T: Cystic meningioma in a dog. *J Small Anim Pract* 43:272–274, 2002.
34. Bagley RS, Kornegay JN, Lane SB, et al: Cystic meningiomas in 2 dogs. *J Vet Intern Med* 10:72–75, 1996.
35. Bagley RS, Silver GM, Gavin PR: Cerebellar cystic meningioma in a dog. *JAAHA* 36:413–415, 2000.
36. Mandara MT, Ricci G, Rinaldi L, et al: Immunohistochemical identification and image analysis quantification of oestrogen and progesterone receptors in canine and feline meningioma. *J Comp Pathol* 127:214–218, 2002.
37. Adamo PF, Cantile C, Steinberg H: Evaluation of progesterone and estrogen receptor expression in 15 meningiomas of dogs and cats. *Am J Vet Res* 64:1310–1318, 2003.
38. Théon AP, LeCouteur RA, Carr EA, Griffey SM: Influence of tumor cell proliferation and sex-hormone receptors on effectiveness of radiation therapy for dogs with incompletely resected meningiomas. *JAVMA* 216:701–707, 2000.
39. Schulman FY, Ribas JL, Carpenter JL, et al: Intracranial meningioma with pulmonary metastasis in three dogs. *Vet Pathol* 29:196–202, 1992.
40. Schmidt P, Geyer C, Hafner A, et al: Malignes meningeommit lungenmetastasen bei einem Boxer. [Malignant meningioma with lung metastases in a Boxer] *Tierarztl Prax* 19:315–319, 1991.
41. Turrel JM, Fike JR, LeCouteur RA, et al: Radiotherapy of brain tumors in dogs. *JAVMA* 184:82–86, 1984.
42. Bagley RS, Harrington ML, Pluhar GE, et al: Acute, unilateral transverse sinus occlusion during craniectomy in seven dogs with space-occupying intracranial disease. *Vet Surg* 26:195–201, 1997.
43. Higgins RJ, LeCouteur RA, Vernau KM, et al: Granular cell tumor of the canine central nervous system: Two cases. *Vet Pathol* 38:620–627, 2001.
44. Spugnini EP, Thrall DE, Price GS, et al: Primary irradiation of canine intracranial masses. *Vet Radiol Ultrasound* 41:377–380, 2000.
45. Evans SM, Dayrell-Hart B, Powlis W, et al: Radiation therapy of canine brain masses. *J Vet Intern Med* 7:216–219, 1993.
46. Iwamoto KS, Norman A, Freshwater DB, et al: Diagnosis and treatment of spontaneous canine brain tumors with a CT scanner. *Radiother Oncol* 26:76–78, 1993.
47. Lester NV, Hopkins AL, Bova FJ, et al: Radiosurgery using a stereotactic headframe system for irradiation of brain tumors in dogs. *JAVMA* 219:1562–1567, 1550, 2001.
48. Fidel J, Kippenes-Skogmo H, Gavin PR, et al: Radiosurgery for selected canine and feline brain tumors: A retrospective analysis. *Proc 23rd Annu Conf Vet Cancer Soc*: 48, 2003.
49. Kraft SL, Gavin PR, DeHaan CE, et al: Borocaptate sodium: A potential boron delivery compound for boron neutron capture therapy evaluated in dogs with spontaneous intracranial tumors. *Proc Natl Acad Sci USA* 89:11973–11977, 1992.
50. Turrel JM, Higgins RJ, Child G: Prognostic factors associated with irradiation of canine brain tumors. *Proc 6th Annu Conf Vet Cancer Soc*: 1986.
51. Nakaichi M, Taura Y, Nakama S, et al: Primary brain tumors in two dogs treated by surgical resection in combination with postoperative radiation therapy. *J Vet Med Sci* 58:773–775, 1996.
52. Feder BM, Fry TR, Kostolich M, et al: Nd: YAG laser cytoreduction of an invasive intracranial meningioma in a dog. *Progress Vet Neurol* 4:3–9, 1993.
53. Neuwelt EA, Maravilla KR, Frenkel EP, et al: Osmotic blood-brain barrier disruption. Computerized tomographic monitoring of chemotherapeutic agent delivery. *J Clin Invest* 64:684–688, 1979.
54. Culver B, Inzana K, Jones J, et al: Technique of, and complications attributable to, repeated hyperosmotic blood-brain barrier disruption in dogs. *Am J Vet Res* 59:1503–1510, 1998.
55. Fulton LM, Steinberg HS: Preliminary study of lomustine in the treatment of intracranial masses in dogs following localization by imaging techniques. *Semin Vet Med Surg (Small Anim)* 5:241–245, 1990.
56. McDonnell JJ, Potthoff AD, Frimberger AE, Moore AS: Lomustine for treatment of canine intracranial masses. *Proc 23rd Annu Conf Vet Cancer Soc*:84, 2003.
57. Hamilton TA, Cook JR, Scott-Moncreif C, et al: Carmustine chemotherapy for canine brain tumors. *Proc 11th Annu Conf Vet Cancer Soc*:43–44, 1991.
58. Dimski DS, Cook JR Jr: Carmustine-induced partial remission of an astrocytoma in a dog. *JAAHA* 26:179–182, 1990.
59. Cook JR Jr: Chemotherapy for brain tumors. *Vet Med Report* 2:391–396, 1990.
60. Ingram M, Jacques DB, Freshwater DB, et al: Adoptive immunotherapy of brain tumors in dogs. *Vet Med Report* 2:398–402, 1990.
61. Ribas JL, Mena H, Braund KG, et al: A histologic and immunocytochemical study of choroid plexus tumors of the dog. *Vet Pathol* 26:55–64, 1989.
62. Leschnik M, Kolm S, Konar M, et al: Vegetative dysfunktionen bein einem hund mit einem plexus chorioideus papillom: Klinische, diagnostische und pathomorphologische befunde. *Kleintierpraxis* 47:35–42, 2002.
63. Flegel T, Podell M, March PA: Ventrikel-peritoneum drainage für die behandlung eines sekundären hydrozephalus bei einem Brittany spaniel. *Kleintierpraxis* 47:95–102, 2002.
64. Cantile C, Campani D, Menicagli M, Arispici M: Pathological and immunohistochemical studies of choroid plexus carcinoma of the dog. *J Comp Pathol* 126:183–193, 2002.
65. Lipsitz D, Levitski RE, Chauvet AE: Magnetic resonance imaging of a choroid plexus carcinoma and meningeal carcinomatosis in a dog. *Vet Radiol Ultrasound* 40:246–250, 1999.
66. Nelson RW, Ihle SL, Feldman EC: Pituitary macroadenomas and macroadenocarcinomas in dogs treated with mitotane for pituitary-dependent hyperadrenocorticism: 13 cases (1981-1986). *JAVMA* 194:1612–1617, 1989.
67. Mauldin GN, Burk RL: The use of diagnostic computerized tomography and radiation therapy in canine and feline hyperadrenocorticism. *Probl Vet Med* 2:557–564, 1990.
68. Sarfaty D, Carrillo JM, Peterson ME: Neurologic, endocrinologic, and pathologic findings associated with large pituitary tumors in dogs: Eight cases (1976-1984). *JAVMA* 193:854–856, 1988.
69. Duesberg CA, Feldman EC, Nelson RW, et al: Magnetic resonance imaging for diagnosis of pituitary macrotumors in dogs. *JAVMA* 206:657–662, 1995.
70. Feldman EC, Nelson RW: *Canine and Feline Endocrinology and Reproduction*, ed 3. Philadelphia, WB Saunders, 2003.
71. Puente S: Pituitary carcinoma in an Airedale terrier. *Can Vet J* 44:240–242, 2003.
72. Reusch C, Stankeova S, Geissbühler U, et al: Zusammenhang zwischen computertomographisch ermittelter hypophysengröße und dem auftreten neurologischer symptome bei hunden mit cushing syndrom. *Kleintierpraxis* 46:133–139, 2001.
73. Theon AP, Feldman EC, Megavoltage irradiation of pituitary macrotumors in dogs with neurologic signs. *JAVMA* 213:225–231, 1998.
74. Bertoy EH, Feldman EC, Nelson RW, et al: One-year follow-up evaluation of magnetic resonance imaging of the brain in dogs with pituitary-dependent hyperadrenocorticism. *JAVMA* 208:1268–1273, 1996.
75. Harb MF, Nelson RW, Feldman EC et al: Central diabetes insipidus in dogs: 20 cases (1986-1995). *JAVMA* 209:1884–1888, 1996.
76. Boujon CE, Ritz U, Rossi GL, Bestetti GE: A clinico-pathological study of canine Cushings disease caused by a pituitary carcinoma. *J Comp Pathol* 105:353–365, 1991.
77. Meij B: Hypophysectomy in dogs: A review. *Vet Q* 21:134–141, 1999.
78. Dow SW, LeCouteur RA, Rosychuk AW, et al: Response of dogs with functional pituitary macroadenomas and macrocarcinomas to radiation. *J Small Anim Pract* 31:287–294, 1990.
79. Kaser-Hotz B, Stankeova S, Fidel J, et al: Strahlentherapeutische behandlkung von hypophysären makrotumoren bei vier hunden. *Kleintierpraxis* 46:197–206, 2001.
80. Rosin A: Neurologic diseases associated with lymphosarcoma in ten dogs. *JAVMA* 181:50–53, 1982.
81. Couto CG, Cullen J, Pedroia V, Turrel JM: Central nervous system lymphosarcoma in the dog. *JAVMA* 184:809–813, 1984.
82. Forterre F, Kaiser S, Schmahl W, Brunnberg L: Rückenmarkstumoren beim Hund: 33 Fälle (retrospektive studie). *Kleintierpraxis* 47:357–364, 2002.
83. Wright JA, Bell DA, Clayton-Jones DG: The clinical and radiological features associated with spinal tumours in thirty dogs. *J Small Anim Pract* 20:461–472, 1979.
84. Kippenes H, Gavin PR, Bagley RS, et al: Magnetic resonance imaging features of tumors of the spine and spinal cord in dogs. *Vet Radiol Ultrasound* 40:627–633, 1999.
85. Waters DJ, Hayden DW: Intramedullary spinal cord metastasis in the dog. *J Vet Intern Med* 4:207–215, 1990.
86. Luttgen PJ, Braund KG, Brawner WR Jr, Vandevelde M: A retrospective study of twenty-nine spinal tumours in the dog and cat. *J Small Anim Pract* 21:213–226, 1980.
87. Fingeroth JM, Prata RG, Patnaik AK: Spinal meningiomas in dogs: 13 cases (1972-1987). *JAVMA* 191:720–726, 1987.
88. Van Winkle TJ, Steinberg HS, DeCarlo AJ, et al: Myxoid meningiomas of the rostral cervical spinal cord and caudal fossa in four dogs. *Vet Pathol* 31:468–471, 1994.
89. Yeomans SM: Short paper—Extensive spinal meningioma in a young dog. *J Comp Pathol* 122:303–306, 2000.
90. Hopkins AL, Garner M, Ackerman N, et al: Spinal meningeal sarcoma in a rottweiler puppy. *J Small Anim Pract* 36:183–186, 1995.

91. Drost WT, Love NE, Berry CR: Comparison of radiography, myelography and computed tomography for the evaluation of canine vertebral and spinal cord tumors in sixteen dogs. *Vet Radiol Ultrasound* 37:28–33, 1996.
92. Luttgen PJ: Spinal neoplasia: Diagnosis and treatment. *Semin Vet Med Surg (Small Anim)* 5:246–252, 1990.
93. Levitski RE, Lipsitz D, Chauvet AE: Magnetic resonance imaging of the cervical spine in 27 dogs. *Vet Radiol Ultrasound* 40:332–341, 1999.
94. McConnell JF, Garosi LS, Dennis R, Smith KC: Imaging of a spinal nephroblastoma in a dog. *Vet Radiol Ultrasound* 44:537–541, 2003.
95. Rendano VT, de Lahunta A, King JM: Extracranial neoplasia with facial nerve paralysis in two cats. *JAAHA* 16:921–925, 1980.
96. Levy MS, Kapatkin AS, Patnaik AK, et al: Spinal tumors in 37 dogs: Clinical outcome and long-term survival (1987-1994). *JAAHA* 33:307–312, 1997.
97. Schueler RO, Roush JK, Oyster RA: Spinal ganglioneuroma in a dog. *JAVMA* 203:539–541, 1993.
98. Lewis DD, Kim DY, Paulsen DB, Kerwin SC: Extradural spinal liposarcoma in a dog. *JAVMA* 199:1606–1607, 1991.
99. Sullivan SA, Coates J, Chambers J: What is your neurologic diagnosis? Intradural-extramedullary malignant sarcoma at C1-2 vertebrae in a dog. *JAVMA* 207:563–565, 1995.
100. Bell FW, Feeney DA, O'Brien TJ, et al: External beam radiation therapy for recurrent intraspinal meningioma in a dog. *JAAHA* 28:318–322, 1992.
101. Siegel S, Kornegay JN, Thrall DE: Postoperative irradiation of spinal cord tumors in 9 dogs. *Vet Radiol Ultrasound* 37:150–153, 1996.
102. Jeffery ND, Phillips SM: Surgical treatment of intramedullary spinal cord neoplasia in two dogs. *J Small Anim Pract* 36:553–557, 1995.
103. Hara Y, Nezu Y, Harada Y, et al: Secondary chronic respiratory acidosis in a dog following the cervical cord compression by an intradural glioma. *J Vet Med Sci* 64:863–866, 2002.
104. Reif U, Lowrie CT, Fitzgerald SD: Extradural spinal angiolipoma associated with bone lysis in a dog. *JAAHA* 34:373–376, 1998.
105. Dickinson PJ, McEntee MC, Lipsitz D, et al: Radiation induced vertebral osteosarcoma following treatment of an intradural extramedullary spinal cord tumor in a dog. *Vet Radiol Ultrasound* 42:463–470, 2001.
106. Summers BA, deLahunta A, McEntee M, Kuhajda FP: A novel intradural extramedullary spinal cord tumor in young dogs. *Acta Neuropathol (Berl)* 75:402–410, 1988.
107. Gasser AM, Bush WW, Smith S, Walton R: Extradural spinal, bone marrow, and renal nephroblastoma. *JAAHA* 39: 80–85, 2003.
108. Terrell SP, Platt SR, Chrisman CL, et al: Possible intraspinal metastasis of a canine spinal cord nephroblastoma. *Vet Pathol* 37:94–97, 2000.
109. Vaughan-Scott T, Goldin J, Nesbit JW: Spinal nephroblastoma in an Irish wolfhound. *J S Afr Vet Assoc* 70:25–28, 1999.
110. Pearson GR, Gregory SP, Charles AK: Immunohistochemical demonstration of Wilms tumour gene product WT1 in a canine "neuroepithelioma" providing evidence for its classification as an extrarenal nephroblastoma. *J Comp Pathol* 116:321–327, 1997.
111. Malik R, Allan GS, Osuna DJ, et al: Diagnostic challenge. Intradural extramedullary tumour (nephroblastoma?) at T13-L1. *Aust Vet Pract* 20:90–92, 1990.
112. Ferretti A, Scanziani E, Colombo S: Surgical treatment of a spinal cord tumor resembling nephroblastoma in a young dog. *Prog Vet Neurol* 4:3, 84–87, 1993.
113. Macri NP, Van Alstine W, Coolman RA: Canine spinal nephroblastoma. *JAAHA* 33:302–306, 1997.
114. Sale CS, Skerritt GC, Smith KC: Spinal nephroblastoma in a crossbreed dog. *J Small Anim Pract* 45:267–271, 2004.
115. Moissonnier P, Abbott DP: Canine neuroepithelioma: Case report and literature review. *JAAHA* 29:5, 397–401, 1993.
116. Neel J, Dean GA: A mass in the spinal column of a dog. *Vet Clin Pathol* 29:87–89, 2000.
117. Schulz KS, Steele KE, Saunders GK, et al: Thoracic ganglioneuroblastoma in a dog. *Vet Pathol* 31:716–718, 1994.
118. Suzuki M, Uchida K, Taniguchi K, et al: Peripheral neuroblastoma in a young Labrador retriever. *J Vet Med Sci* 65:271–274, 2003.
119. Forrest LJ, Galbreath EJ, Dubielzig RR, MacEwen EG: Peripheral neuroblastoma in a dog. *Vet Radiol Ultrasound* 38:457–460, 1997.

TUMORS OF THE EYE AND EAR

Antony S. Moore and Gregory K. Ogilvie

50

CLINICAL BRIEFING

Tumors of the Eye

Clinical factors
- Glaucoma, uveitis, hyphema, or visible mass.
- Melanoma is most common ocular tumor, followed by epithelial tumors of the ciliary body.
- Melanomas and epithelial tumors both have low potential for metastasis.
- Older dogs are affected.

Staging and diagnosis
- MDB (includes a complete blood count, biochemical profile, urinalysis, and thoracic radiography [three views]).
- Ocular examination.
- Ultrasonography, CT, or MRI.
- Biopsy (may require surgery).

Prognostic factors
- None identified.

Treatment

Initial
- Enucleation is usually curative, even after failure of local excision.
- Other treatment modalities usually not required.

Supportive
- Pain medications after surgery.

Retrobulbar Tumors

Clinical factors
- Exophthalmos, nictitans protrusion, and deviation of globe.
- Multiple types; osteosarcoma, fibrosarcoma, mast cell tumor, and lymphoma are most common.
- Most tumors are locally aggressive; metastatic rate varies with tumor type.

Staging and diagnosis
- MDB.
- Ocular examination.
- Ultrasonography, CT, or MRI.
- Biopsy (may require surgery).

Prognostic factors
- Bony lysis on radiography may be a poor prognostic sign.

Treatment

Initial
- Orbital exenteration may be curative for small tumors.

Adjunctive
- Radiation therapy may be useful as an adjunct to surgery for some tumor types but is still under investigation.
- Chemotherapy may be useful for lymphoma; can also be an adjunct to local modalities for treatment of osteosarcoma and osteochondrosarcoma.

Supportive
- Pain medications after surgery.

Tumors of the Ear Canal	
Clinical factors	• Suppurative to pyogranulomatous otitis; either secondary to tumor, or tumor develops secondary to chronic preexisting otitis. • Multiple types; adenomas and adenocarcinomas (particularly ceruminous gland) are most common. • Usually older animals; cocker spaniels are predisposed.
Staging and diagnosis	• MDB. • Aural examination. • CT or MRI to evaluate middle ear and bulla. • Biopsy (may require surgery). • Malignant tumors are locally aggressive; metastasis rare, primarily via the lymphatics to parotid and mandibular lymph nodes.
Prognostic factors	• None identified.
Treatment	
Initial	• Local excision may be curative for small and benign tumors. • Total ear canal ablation with lateral bulla osteotomy required for malignant tumors.
Adjunctive	• Radiation therapy for incompletely excised tumors. • Chemotherapy anecdotal and rarely needed. • Doxorubicin and platinum drugs may be useful for metastatic ceruminous adenocarcinomas.
Supportive	• Symptomatic treatment for otitis. • Pain medications after surgery.

Tumors of the Eye
INCIDENCE, SIGNALMENT, AND ETIOLOGY

Melanoma accounts for more than half of ocular tumors in dogs. Melanoma of the eye is reviewed in detail in Chapter 54. Ciliary body adenomas and ciliary adenocarcinomas are the next most common ocular tumor types.[1] Less frequently diagnosed tumors are medulloepitheliomas, sarcomas, and hemangiomas. Retinal tumors are rare.[2,3]

Benign tumors accounted for nearly 90% of palpebral tumors in a study of 255 eyelid tumors in 200 dogs.[4] After melanomas, sebaceous gland adenomas and papillomas were the most common palpebral tumors. Beagles, Siberian huskies, and English setters had a higher risk of tumor development, and older dogs (average age: 10 years) were most commonly affected. The malignant tumor types seen were melanoma, adenocarcinoma, basal cell carcinoma, mast cell tumor, squamous cell carcinoma, hemangiosarcoma, and myoblastoma. Benign hemangiomas or angiokeratomas occur on the conjunctiva,[5] nictitans,[6,7] and ciliary body.[5,8] Hemangiosarcomas of the conjunctiva may be more common in English setters[6,8,9] (see also Chapter 56). There is no age or gender predilection for ocular tumors of any type.

Papilloma of the bulbar conjunctiva has been described as a manifestation of the canine papillomavirus.[10]

The lacrimal gland may develop adenoma or adenocarcinomas, but such tumors are rare,[11,12] as are tumors of the apocrine sweat glands of the eye.[13] Meibomian gland adenomas occur most frequently in older neutered dogs, and Saint Bernards, Gordon setters, malamutes, and Samoyeds are predisposed.[14] Meibomian carcinomas are very rare. Mast cell tumors may occur in the conjunctiva.[15]

Metastases from carcinomas and occasionally sarcomas may involve the eye but are usually accompanied by widespread involvement of other organs.[16] Lymphoma was the most common secondary or metastatic tumor in one study.[1]

CLINICAL PRESENTATION AND HISTORY

Some ocular tumors are detected as an incidental finding; others are noticed as a mass by the owner. Conjunctival masses may lead to chronic irritation and persistent "red eye." Duration of signs in one report was 4 to 6 months.[17]

Papillomas of the bulbar conjunctiva may appear as pigmented lesions with a frond-like appearance.[10] If the tumor extends into the retrobulbar space, exophthalmos may be the presenting sign.[13]

STAGING AND DIAGNOSIS

Epithelial tumors of the ciliary body, whether adenomas or adenocarcinomas, metastasize infrequently to the lungs.[18] Similarly, squamous cell carcinoma of the cornea or corneoscleral limbus does not seem to metastasize.[19,20] Carcinomas may, however, progress to invade the orbit.[21] Radiographs are not very sensitive for detecting minor or early invasion of an ocular tumor into the surrounding orbital bone.[21] For tumors that may be invasive, or for retrobulbar tumors, further imaging using magnetic resonance imaging (MRI) or computed tomography (CT) will describe tumor margins before surgery or radiation therapy (see Retrobulbar Tumors section, below).[22]

> **KEY POINT**
>
> *CT scan or MRI is suggested for evaluation of the eye and orbit before surgery or radiation therapy for a tumor of the globe.*

TREATMENT

Surgery is the treatment of choice for almost all ocular tumors. Local excision is an option, particularly for tumors of the limbus. Partial iridectomy and lamellar keratectomy also can achieve local removal. Although recurrence is possible after local excision, enucleation after recurrence is usually curative for intraocular lesions and for epithelial tumors of the eye, including ciliary body adenomas and adenocarcinomas.[18]

In a study of 255 eyelid tumors, both surgery and cryosurgery were used to treat tumors, of which 90% were benign.[4] Tumor recurrence rates were not significantly different between dogs treated with cryosurgery (15.1%) and those treated surgically (10.5%). However, tumors recurred more quickly after cryosurgery than after surgery alone (7 months and 28 months, respectively).[4] In other studies, an adenocarcinoma of the nictitans did not recur within 1 year after excision,[23] and papillomas did not recur after excision.[10] Local excision of hemangiomas and hemangiosarcomas of the nictitans or conjunctiva appears curative in most cases,[5-7] although one dog had a recurrence 28 months after surgery.[6] Enucleation is curative when recurrence is seen.

A retinal neuroepithelial tumor, presumed to be a retinoblastoma, was removed by enucleation, and the dog had no evidence of disease 10 months later.[2]

For owners who think that removal of the globe will have a negative effect on their pet's appearance, a silicone prosthesis may improve cosmetics. However, in one study, recurrence of the tumor was not prevented, and enucleation of the globe and prosthesis was required in two of five dogs with a neoplasm (including one dog with a ciliary body adenoma).[24]

Cryosurgery may reduce the chance of local recurrence after excision, but overzealous freezing can cause ocular damage. Local excision of squamous cell carcinoma followed by nitrous oxide cryosurgery gave long-term control in two dogs for 1 year or longer.[19,20] One of these two dogs had recurrence of squamous cell carcinoma years after the first treatment; the tumor recurred 9 months after a second treatment but did not metastasize.[20] The overall cosmetic appearance was thought to be better with cryosurgery than with surgery alone in one study[4]; otherwise, efficacy is similar, and it is difficult to see the advantage of cryosurgery after surgery compared with surgery alone.

Other methods of local treatment have been reported, including complete to minor regression of some ciliary body tumors after neodymium:yttrium–aluminum–garnet (YAG) laser treatment.[25] The best responses to laser therapy were in tumors that were confined to the ciliary body.

Surgery and postoperative chemotherapy with weekly 5-fluorouracil for 6 weeks was the treatment in five dogs with adenocarcinoma of the ciliary body and iris. There was no evidence of regrowth or metastases in any dog between 1 and 2.5 years after therapy.[17] Because of good reported tumor control after surgery alone, the contribution of chemotherapy to this outcome is difficult to assess.

Retrobulbar Tumors
INCIDENCE, SIGNALMENT, AND ETIOLOGY

Many tumor types occur in the retrobulbar (orbital) space. In two surveys, 64 of 67 tumors were malignant.[26,27] In order of prevalence, the most common tumors were osteosarcoma, fibrosarcoma, mast cell tumor, and lymphoma. The benign tumors were meningioma and leiomyoma.[26] Most tumors were primary; however, other tumors (e.g., nasal tumors, tumors affecting the vertical portion of the mandible, osteochondromas) occasionally invade the retrobulbar space.[28,29] Most affected dogs were older (average age: 8 years), but some, including those with lymphoma, were young.[26,27] There was no gender or breed predilection.

Tumors of the optic nerve that may invade the retrobulbar space include gliomas,[30] ganglioneuroblastomas,[31] and meningiomas.[32-37] Meningiomas of the orbit arise from the arachnoid cap cells within the optic nerve sheath. Meningiomas were described in 22 dogs between the ages of 3 and 17 years (median: 8 years) and were more common in males. Poodles, Samoyeds, and German shepherds (or their crosses) accounted for eight of 22 cases.[32]

CLINICAL PRESENTATION AND HISTORY

Dogs with tumors of the retrobulbar space usually present with exophthalmos, deviation of the eye, and nictitans pro-

TUMORS OF THE EYE AND EAR

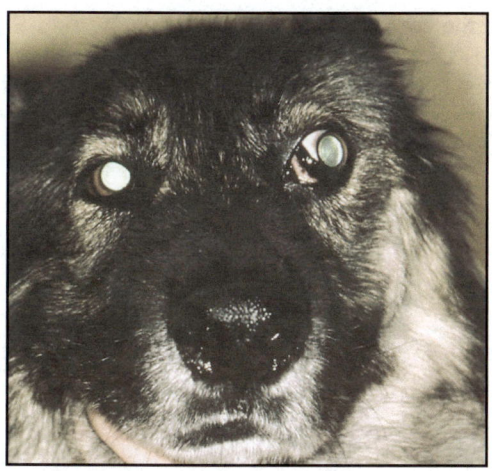

Figure 50-1. This dog has a retrobulbar osteochondrosarcoma that is displacing the left eye laterally and rostrally. Although ultrasonography may provide guidance for a biopsy, a CT scan would be needed to define the bony limits of the tumor.

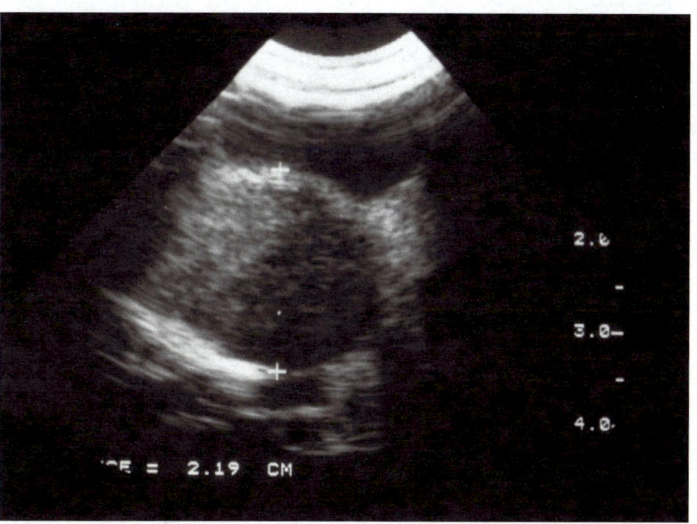

Figure 50-2. Ultrasonography of a retrobulbar mass. The globe is closest to the transducer and is compressed concavely by a 2-cm mass. (Courtesy of Dominique G. Penninck, DVM, Tufts Cummings School of Veterinary Medicine)

trusion (Figure 50-1). On physical examination, it is difficult to retropulse the globe; however, animals show pain on palpation less commonly than dogs with retrobulbar infections or abscesses. In one study, more than 30% of dogs with a retrobulbar tumor had signs that were compatible with a retrobulbar inflammatory process, probably as a result of necrosis.[26] Ocular examination may reveal loss of direct and consensual pupillary light reflexes, and the eye may be blind. Exophthalmos, orbital swelling, or a prolapsed globe was observed in 22 dogs with meningiomas of the orbit, and a fundic examination was abnormal in one-third of dogs.[32] Of 15 dogs in which vision was evaluated, 12 were blind in the affected eye.

STAGING AND DIAGNOSIS

Any retrobulbar mass should be imaged by ultrasonography, MRI, or CT to determine the site of origin and to guide a biopsy. Staging should also include thoracic radiography. Most retrobulbar tumors are aggressively invasive, and these tumors can metastasize. The primary differential diagnosis in these patients is an orbital abscess or cellulitis.

Radiography is rarely helpful in delineating either the nature of the mass or the origin or extent of orbital involvement[27] unless the tumor is mineralized[28] or extends to involve the nasal cavity and paranasal sinuses, causing bony lysis.[21] In one study, more than 60% of tumors showed radiographic evidence of bony lysis.[26] Radiographs were also not very sensitive for detecting minor or early invasion from an ocular tumor into the surrounding orbital bone in one study[21] and were not helpful in identifying a mass in dogs with meningiomas of the orbit in another.[32] Ultrasonography is more helpful in delineating the extent of retrobulbar disease, but it is not able to provide a definitive diagnosis and may even overlook large masses.[21,38,39] In one study, only 60% of masses were detected by ultrasonography.[26] Another study found that dogs with tumors (19 of 26) were more likely to show a mass effect on the medial aspect of the orbit than dogs with an abscess (four of 10), and most dogs that showed orbital bone lesions had a tumor (10 of 26 compared with one of 10 dogs with an abscess).[38] It may be difficult to distinguish neoplastic from inflammatory changes; however, ultrasonographic guidance may improve the success rate in obtaining biopsy samples or needle aspirates for cytology and microbiology (Figure 50-2). If the exophthalmos is mild and space for biopsy is limited, then CT provides more accurate guidance than ultrasonography.[40] CT and MRI are superior tools for evaluating the extent of ocular disease.

It is best to assume that all retrobulbar tumors are invasive and to use MRI or CT to determine invasiveness and describe tumor margins before surgery or radiation therapy.[21,22,40] The combination of high spatial and contrast resolution, cross-sectional format, and ability to demonstrate tissues beyond bony margins gives MRI significant advantages over radiography and ultrasonography. MRI correctly diagnosed whether the retrobulbar lesion was neoplastic or inflammatory in 19 of 22 dogs in one study[21]; however, biopsy is recommended for definitive diagnosis.

Ultrasonographic guidance can be very useful for obtaining retrobulbar biopsy specimens or aspirates.

In one study, the yield of positive diagnoses for samples collected by fine-needle aspiration was 97%.[41] In contrast, another study found the positive yield to be approximately 50%, regardless of whether the aspiration was guided by ultrasonography.[26] Similarly, biopsies obtained by needle or trephine were diagnostic in only about half of cases, and ultrasonography did not improve the yield. Ultrasonography is very operator dependent. When results of fine-needle aspiration and needle biopsy were combined in one study, a diagnosis was reached in less than 80% of cases.[26] In contrast, surgical biopsy was diagnostic in all cases; these samples were usually obtained at the time of definitive treatment.

Retrobulbar meningioma is rare in dogs. It may be imaged by ultrasonography,[33] CT, or MRI.[34] Many orbital meningiomas contain areas of bony metaplasia.[32] The tumor grows primarily by extension along the optic nerve, and in the largest reported series of 22 meningiomas of the orbit, no metastases were reported.[32] Although metastasis is rare, the risk appears to increase if definitive treatment is delayed.[33,34]

Table 50-1 **Types of Tumors in the Ear Canals of 81 Dogs**[42]

Benign	Number of Dogs	Malignant	Number of Dogs
Polyp	8	Ceruminous adenocarcinoma	23
Papilloma	6	Undifferentiated carcinoma	9
Sebaceous adenoma	5	Squamous cell carcinoma	8
Basal cell tumor	5	Round cell tumor	3
Ceruminous adenoma	4	Sarcoma	2
Histiocytoma	2	Melanoma	2
Plasmacytoma	1	Hemangiosarcoma	1
Fibromas	1		
Melanoma	1		
Total	*33*		*48*

> **KEY POINT**
> *A combination of fine-needle aspiration and needle biopsy gave a definitive result in less than 80% of cases. Surgical biopsy at the time of definitive treatment may be required for a diagnosis.*

PROGNOSTIC FACTORS

Dogs with evidence of bony lysis on radiography lived an average of 5 months after diagnosis compared with more than 18 months if no lysis was seen.[26] The authors of this report commented that bony lysis may have been a disincentive to treatment and therefore may not be an independent predictor of survival.

TREATMENT

Orbital exenteration is the treatment of choice for all retrobulbar tumors. However, it is rarely curative because of the infiltrative and destructive nature of these tumors. Even benign tumors may recur after surgery.[27]

If treatment is possible, then survival is improved. In one study, whereas only two of 18 dogs that were not treated were alive 6 months after diagnosis, 12 of 14 dogs that were treated were alive 6 months after diagnosis.[26] Treatment included exenteration, zygomatic arch resection (osteosarcoma), rhinotomy and radiation therapy (nasal tumor), and chemotherapy, either alone or with surgery.

A dog with a retrobulbar mast cell tumor was treated by exenteration and radiation therapy and was alive with no evidence of recurrence 4 years later.[27] Radiation therapy may be a useful adjunct to surgery for other tumor types, such as osteochondrosarcoma, but there are few reports of this approach.[29]

Early resection by orbital exenteration may be curative for orbital meningioma.[26,33] Although this tumor grows slowly, it is aggressive; therefore, delays in therapy may lead to incomplete excision. Extension along the optic nerve may make surgical excision impossible; however, it is uncommon for the tumor to invade the globe or cause bony lysis.[26] Recurrence and metastasis are rare and occur long after surgery.[34] In one survey of orbital tumors, the only dog with a meningioma was alive 12 months after

> **KEY POINT**
> *Orbital meningioma is best treated early because extension along the optic nerve and late metastases have been reported.*

presentation.[26] In a larger series of 17 dogs with orbital meningioma and known outcome, six dogs had recurrence a median of 2 years after surgery, and in two of these, the vision of the contralateral eye was lost. The remaining 11 dogs were free of disease at a median of 1 year after surgery, with four dogs free of disease more than 2 years after surgery.[32]

Table 50-2 **Clinical Signs Associated with Tumors in the Ear Canals of 81 Dogs**[42]

Clinical Sign	Benign (% of dogs)	Malignant (% of dogs)
Mass	63	72
Discharge	50	82
Odor	25	34
Pruritus	25	26
Pain	19	26
Neurologic signs (facial nerve paralysis, head tilt, circling)	0	13
Clinical appearance of tumors in the ear canals of 81 dogs		
Raised	55	42
Pedunculated	52	0
Irregular	30	0
Ulcerated	18	29
Broad based	0	23
Location of tumors in the ear canals of 81 dogs		
Vertical canal	52	29
Horizontal canal	36	35
Canal and bulla	0	23
Bulla	3	4

Tumors of the Ear

Ceruminous gland tumors are the most common ear canal tumor and are discussed separately below. The following is a general description of tumors found in the ear canal.

INCIDENCE, SIGNALMENT, AND ETIOLOGY

In a study of 81 dogs with ear canal tumors, 48 tumors (60%) were malignant and 33 (40%) were benign.[42] Cocker spaniels were overrepresented in both groups (see also Ceruminous Gland Tumors section, below). There was no difference between the groups with respect to age or gender. Of the dogs with malignant tumors, 17 (35%) had a history of otitis externa that had been present for more than 6 months.[42]

The types of tumors in this study are listed in Table 50-1 and are mostly (with the exception of ceruminous gland tumors) common cutaneous tumors.

CLINICAL PRESENTATION AND HISTORY

Dogs with malignant tumors were more likely to have an aural discharge, and if a dog had associated neurologic signs, then the diagnosis was invariably a malignant tumor, probably reflecting the increased tendency for invasion.[42] More than two-thirds of malignant tumors invaded the surrounding epithelium (10%), subcutaneous tissue (25%), or cartilage (31%), but none of the benign tumors invaded surrounding tissue. Malignant tumors were also more likely to involve both the ear canal and the bulla than were benign tumors (Table 50-2).

> **KEY POINT**
> *Neurologic signs in a dog with an aural tumor greatly increase the likelihood that the tumor is malignant.*

Regardless of whether a tumor was malignant or benign, the average duration of clinical signs was 3 to 4 months, but duration in individual cases ranged up to 4 and even 8 years.[42]

STAGING AND DIAGNOSIS

Most tumors of the ear canal are associated with otitis, either as a direct cause or secondary to the invasive or obstructive nature of the lesion causing increased production and decreased efflux of secretions. In addition to a minimum database (MDB), appropriate staging includes thorough examination of the ear canal under anesthesia and radiographic studies of the bullae. Radiographic evidence of invasion of the bulla has been seen for 30% to 80% of malignant tumors, depending on the study. CT scanning may be a more effective method of imaging the bullae. For invasive tumors, either a CT scan or an MRI study helps to define tumor borders and to assess the likelihood of surgery being successful. In one study, 25% of dogs with peripheral vestibular disease had a middle ear tumor imaged on MRI.[43] Advanced imaging also allows radiation therapy planning. Metastasis appears to be uncommon, and the regional lymph node was involved in only one of 48 dogs with a malignant ear canal tumor (including ceruminous gland carcinomas).[42]

TREATMENT

The surgical approach of choice is total ear canal ablation with lateral bulla osteotomy. Complications of surgery include facial nerve injury, inner ear injury, hemorrhage, and wound dehiscence in less than 30% of dogs. Careful dissection and familiarity with the procedure appear to lower complication rates.[44,45]

In one study of 81 dogs, 32 of the 33 dogs (97%) with a benign tumor and 32 of the 48 dogs (67%) with a malignant tumor were treated surgically.[42] Dogs with tumors that were confined to the vertical and horizontal canals had a median survival of 30 months. If the tumor was invasive,

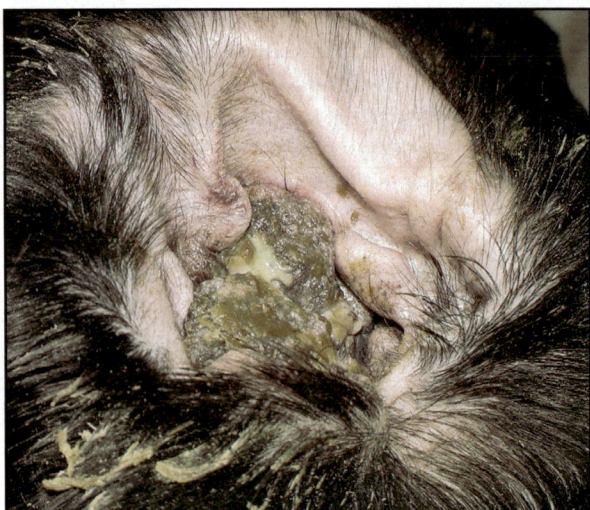

Figure 50-3. *A ceruminous gland carcinoma in the external ear canal of a dog. Note the severe accompanying otitis. (Courtesy of N. Northrup)*

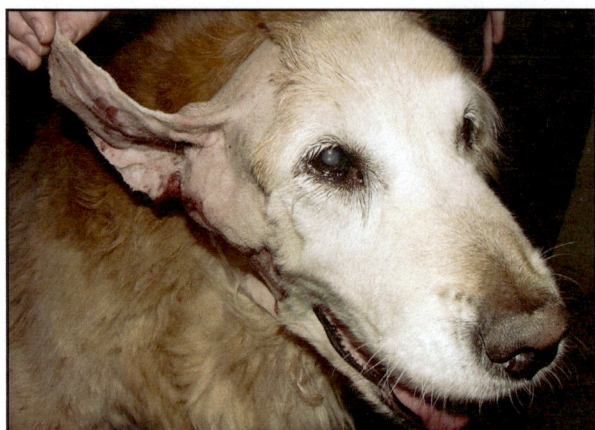

Figure 50-4. *An advanced ceruminous gland carcinoma that has extended out of the vertical canal of the ear and is invading surrounding skin and other structures. Staging dogs with a suspected ceruminous gland tumor should include a CT scan of the skull to evaluate the ear canal and bullae. (Courtesy of Nicole Northrup, DVM, University of Georgia College of Veterinary Medicine)*

median survival was 5 months. Benign tumors had a good prognosis after surgery in another study, and two of three sebaceous adenocarcinomas had no recurrence 8 and 12 months after aggressive surgery.[46]

Ceruminous Gland Tumors
INCIDENCE, SIGNALMENT, AND ETIOLOGY

The sweat glands of the skin in dogs are mainly apocrine glands; eccrine glands are found only on the footpads. Apocrine glands are found in many different parts of the body, and their tumors are named accordingly. In the ear, for example, they are called ceruminous gland tumors. In a survey of ear canal tumors, ceruminous adenocarcinoma was the most common malignancy in dogs.[42] Other apocrine tumors include mammary gland tumors, anal sac tumors, and tumors of the glands at the anal mucocutaneous junction. Adenomas of the ceruminous glands are more common than adenocarcinomas.[47]

Ceruminous gland tumors most often affect older dogs, with an average age of 10 years for dogs with adenomas or adenocarcinomas. Diagnosis of either of these tumors is unlikely in dogs younger than 4 years.[47] Adenomas and, to a lesser degree, adenocarcinomas appear be most common in males. Toy poodles are at increased risk (12 times the rest of the population) for adenomas, and several studies have noted that cocker spaniels have a predilection for adenomas and adenocarcinomas.[42,48] The only other breed at increased risk for adenocarcinomas is the German shepherd (three times).[47]

In a separate study, cocker spaniels were more likely to need total ear canal ablation than dogs of any other breed, accounting for 60% of ablations but only 4% of the hospital population.[49] In addition, cocker spaniels were more likely to develop a proliferative ceruminous gland response pattern (hyperplasia and ceruminous gland ectasia) than any other breed (73% of cocker spaniels compared with 28% of all other breeds). This pattern undoubtedly plays a role in carcinogenesis, and early aggressive treatment of otitis externa is probably warranted in cocker spaniels.

CLINICAL PRESENTATION AND HISTORY

Adenomas are small, elevated, well-demarcated nodules. They often have an ulcerated surface as a result of trauma and are generally firm but may have cystic areas. Malignant tumors of ceruminous gland origin are often indistinguishable from adenomas, but some ceruminous gland carcinomas present as firm, poorly circumscribed masses diffusely infiltrating the skin and producing an ulcerated, moist, and sometimes hemorrhagic skin surface that is frequently misdiagnosed as acute dermatitis (Figure 50-3). One study found that invasion of cartilage was common in malignant tumors of the ear canal[42] (Figure 50-4); in contrast, another study found cartilage invasion to be rare.[48]

Suppurative to pyogranulomatous inflammation is very common with both adenomas and adenocarcinomas, although whether this is a secondary change or reflects chronic otitis with recent neoplastic transformation is difficult to determine.[48]

STAGING AND DIAGNOSIS

Ceruminous gland carcinomas may metastasize, although metastasis appears to be uncommon, and the regional lymph node was involved in only one of 48 dogs with a malignant ear canal tumor.[42] Hematogenous spread to the lungs is rare.[50] An MDB (consisting of a complete blood count, bio-

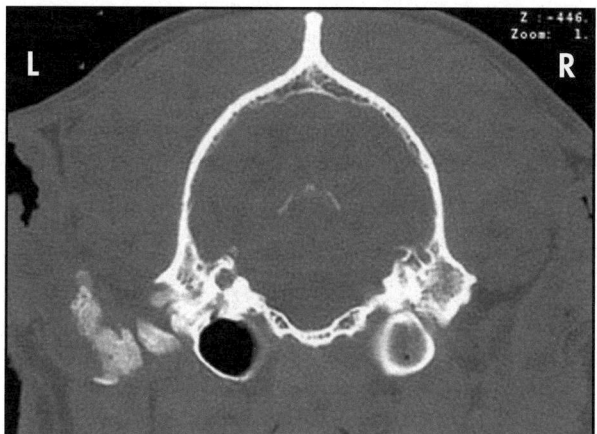

Figure 50-5. *A CT scan of a dog with a left ear canal mass. The left and right external ear canals are filled with a fluid density. The left external ear canal is mineralized. The right tympanic bulla appears thick and slightly irregular. The right tympanic cavity is filled with fluid and gas bubbles. The left external ear canal contained a ceruminous gland carcinoma; the right-sided changes were a result of chronic otitis media/externa and chronic right bulla osteitis. (Courtesy of Kenneth M. Rassnick, DVM, Cornell University College of Veterinary Medicine)*

chemistry panel, urinalysis, and thoracic radiography [three views]) should be obtained. In addition, appropriate staging includes thorough examination of the ear canal under anesthesia and either radiographic or, preferably, CT studies of the bullae. In one study, radiographs showed invasion of the bulla for nearly 80% of malignant tumors.[42] For invasive tumors, either a CT scan or an MRI study will help the veterinarian define tumor borders, assess the regional lymph nodes, and evaluate the likelihood of surgery being successful (Figure 50-5). Advanced imaging will also allow for radiation therapy planning.

> **KEY POINT**
> *CT scan or MRI should be used to evaluate the bullae before surgery for a ceruminous gland tumor.*

Because of the difficulty in clinically distinguishing between adenomas and adenocarcinomas, the veterinarian should consider either presurgical biopsy or a wide surgical excision as an initial therapeutic approach. Ceruminous gland adenocarcinoma may be bilateral.[50]

TREATMENT

Surgical removal of ceruminous gland adenomas is usually curative, but local recurrence after surgical removal is possible. Aggressive surgery is required for successful treatment of invasive ceruminous gland adenocarcinomas. The surgical approach of choice is total ear canal ablation with lateral bulla osteotomy. As with other tumors of the ear, complications of surgery include facial nerve injury, inner ear injury, hemorrhage, and wound dehiscence in less than 30% of dogs. Careful dissection and familiarity with the procedure appear to lower complication rates.[44,45]

Despite this aggressive surgical option, ceruminous gland adenocarcinomas are often incompletely excised or considered inoperable because they encroach on the middle ear.[45,46] In this situation, radiation therapy may improve local control and may significantly improve survival in dogs without metastases. Megavoltage radiation therapy (48 Gy in 12 fractions) was used to treat five dogs with ceruminous gland carcinoma. Some dogs had been treated surgically with incomplete margins; therefore, radiation was adjuvant. Two dogs had local recurrence that was more anaplastic than the original tumor; one of these was treated with further radiation and survived another 20 months. Three dogs were alive and free of disease between 2 and 5 years after treatment.[50] Surgical excision followed by radiation therapy for incompletely excised tumors is probably the treatment of choice for dogs with ceruminous adenocarcinomas.

Results of chemotherapy for metastatic tumors are anecdotal only. Based on information for mammary, anal sac, and perianal tumors (i.e., other apocrine gland tumors), doxorubicin and platinum derivatives may be useful agents in dogs.

REFERENCES

1. Peiffer RL Jr: Primary intraocular tumors in the dog. Part I. *Mod Vet Pract* 60:383–387, 1979.
2. Jensen OA, Kaarsholm S, Prause JU, Heegaard S: Neuroepithelial tumor of the retina in a dog. *Vet Ophthalmol* 6:57–60, 2003.
3. Syed NA, Nork TM, Poulsen GL, et al: Retinoblastoma in a dog. *Arch Ophthalmol* 115:758–763, 1997.
4. Roberts SM, Severin GA, Lavach JD: Prevalence and treatment of palpebral neoplasms in the dog: 200 cases (1975–1983). *JAVMA* 189:1355–1359, 1986.
5. Murphy CJ, Bellhorn RW, Buyukmihci NC: Bilateral conjunctival masses in two dogs. *JAVMA* 195:225–228, 1989.
6. George C, Summers BA: Angiokeratoma: a benign vascular tumour of the dog. *J Small Anim Pract* 31:390–392, 1990.
7. Peiffer RL Jr., Duncan J, Terrell T: Hemangioma of the nictating membrane in a dog. *JAVMA* 172:832–833, 1978.
8. Read RA: Ciliary body haemangioma in a dog with secondary glaucoma. *J Small Anim Pract* 34:405–408, 1993.
9. Muhgannam AJ, Hacker DV, Spangler WL: Conjunctival vascular tumours in six dogs. *Vet Comp Ophthal* 7:56–59, 1997.
10. Sansom J, Barnett KC, Blunden AS, et al: Canine conjunctival papilloma: A review of five cases. *J Small Anim Pract* 37:84–86, 1996.
11. Hirayama K, Kagawa Y, Tsuzuki K, et al: A pleomorphic adenoma of the lacrimal gland in a dog. *Vet Pathol* 37:353–356, 2000.
12. Morgan G: Ocular tumours in animals. *J Small Anim Pract* 10:563–570, 1969.
13. Hirai T, Mubarak M, Kimura T, et al: Apocrine gland tumor of the eyelid in a dog. *Vet Pathol* 34:232–234, 1997.
14. Goldschmidt MH, Shofer FS: Meibomian tumors, in Goldschmidt MH, Shofer FS (eds): *Skin Tumors of the Dog and Cat.* Tarrytown, NY, Pergamon Press, 1992, pp 75–79.
15. Johnson BW, Brightman AH, Whiteley HE: Conjunctival mast cell tumor in two dogs. *JAAHA* 24:439–442, 1988.
16. Barron CN, Saunders LZ, Jubb KV: Intraocular tumors in animals. III. Secondary intraocular tumors. *Am J Vet Res* 24:835–853, 1963.
17. Clere B: Surgery and chemotherapy for the treatment of adenocarcinoma of the

iris and ciliary body in five dogs. *Vet Comp Ophthal* 6:265–270, 1996.
18. Peiffer RL Jr, Gwin RM, Gelatt KN, et al: Ciliary body epithelial tumors in four dogs. *JAVMA* 172:578–583, 1978.
19. Latimer KS, Kaswan RL, Sundberg JP: Corneal squamous cell carcinoma in a dog. *JAVMA* 190:1430–1432, 1987.
20. Ward DA, Latimer KS, Askren RM: Squamous cell carcinoma of the corneoscleral limbus in a dog. *JAVMA* 200:1503–1506, 1992.
21. Dennis R: Use of magnetic resonance imaging for the investigation of orbital disease in small animals. *J Small Anim Pract* 41:145–155, 2000.
22. Morgan RV, Ring RD, Ward DA, Adams WH: Magnetic resonance imaging of ocular and orbital disease in 5 dogs and a cat. *Vet Radiol Ultrasound* 37:185–192, 1996.
23. Grahn B, Wolfer J: Diagnostic ophthalmology. *Can Vet J* 23:683, 1992.
24. McLaughlin SA, Ramsey DT, Lindley DM, et al: Intraocular silicone prosthesis implantation in eyes of dogs and a cat with intraocular neoplasia: Nine cases (1983–1994). *JAVMA* 207:1441–1443, 1995.
25. Nasisse MP, Davidson MG, Olivero DK, et al: Neodymium: YAG laser treatment of primary canine intraocular tumors. *Prog Vet Comp Ophthalmol* 3:152–157, 1993.
26. Hendrix DV, Gelatt KN: Diagnosis, treatment and outcome of orbital neoplasia in dogs: A retrospective study of 44 cases. *J Small Anim Pract* 41:105–108, 2000.
27. Kern TJ: Orbital neoplasia in 23 dogs. *JAVMA* 186:489–491, 1985.
28. Groff JM, Murphy CJ, Pool RR, et al: Orbital multilobular tumor of bone in dog. *J Small Anim Pract* 33:597–600, 1992.
29. Straw RC, LeCouteur RA, Powers BE, Withrow SJ: Multibular osteochondrosarcoma of the canine skull: 16 cases (1978–1988). *JAVMA* 195:1764–1769, 1989.
30. Spiess BM, Wilcock BP: Glioma of the optic nerve with intraocular and intracranial involvement in a dog. *J Comp Pathol* 97:79–84, 1987.
31. Brooks DE, Patton CS: An ocular ganglioneuroblastoma in a dog. *Prog Vet Comp Ophthalmol* 1:299–302, 1991.
32. Mauldin EA, Deehr AJ, Hertzke D, Dubielzig RR: Canine orbital meningiomas: A review of 22 cases. *Vet Ophthalmol* 3:11–16, 2000.
33. Paulsen ME, Severin GA, LeCouteur RA, Young S: Primary optic nerve meningioma in a dog. *JAAHA* 25:147–152, 1989.
34. Dugan SJ, Schwarz PD, Roberts SM, Ching SV: Primary optic nerve meningioma and pulmonary metastasis in a dog. *JAAHA* 29:11–16, 1993.
35. Barnett KC, Kelly DF, Singleton WB: Retrobulbar and chiasmal meningioma in a dog. *J Small Anim Pract* 8:391–394, 1967.
36. Geib LW: Ossifying meningioma with extracranial metastasis in a dog. *Pathol Vet* 3:247–254, 1966.
37. Langham RF, Bennett RR, Zydeck FA: Primary retrobulbar meningioma of the optic nerve of a dog. *JAVMA* 159:175–176, 1971.
38. Mason DR, Lamb CR, McLellan GJ: Ultrasonographic findings in 50 dogs with retrobulbar disease. *JAAHA* 37:557–562, 2001.
39. Morgan RV: Ultrasonography of retrobulbar diseases of the dog and cat. *JAAHA* 25:393–399, 1989.
40. Tidwell AS, Johnson KL: Computed tomography-guided percutaneous biopsy in the dog and cat: Description of technique and preliminary evaluation in 14 patients. *Vet Radiol Ultrasound* 35:445–446, 1994.
41. Boydell P: Fine needle aspiration biopsy in the diagnosis of exophthalmos. *J Small Anim Pract* 32:546, 1991.
42. London CA, Dubilzeig RR, Vail DM, et al: Evaluation of dogs and cats with tumors of the ear canal: 145 cases (1978–1992). *JAVMA* 208:1413–1418, 1996.
43. Garosi LS, Dennis R, Penderis J, et al: Results of magnetic resonance imaging in dogs with vestibular disorders: 85 cases (1996–1999). *JAVMA* 218:385–391, 2001.
44. Matthiesen DT, Scavelli TD: Total ear canal ablation and lateral bulla osteotomy in 38 dogs. *JAAHA* 26:257–267, 1990.
45. White RAS, Pomeroy CJ: Total ear canal ablation and lateral bulla osteotomy in the dog. *J Small Anim Pract* 31:547–553, 1990.
46. Little CJ, Pearson GR, Lane JG: Neoplasia involving the middle ear cavity of dogs. *Vet Rec* 124:54–57, 1989.
47. Goldschmidt MH, Shofer FS: Ceruminous gland tumors, in Goldschmidt MH, Shofer FS (eds): *Skin Tumors of the Dog and Cat*. Tarrytown, NY, Pergamon Press, 1992, pp 96–102.
48. Moisan PG, Watson GL: Ceruminous gland tumors in dogs and cats: A review of 124 cases. *JAAHA* 32:448–452, 1996.
49. Angus JC, Lichtensteiger C, Campbell KL, Schaeffer DJ: Breed variations in histopathologic features of chronic severe otitis externa in dogs: 80 cases (1995–2001). *JAVMA* 221:1000–1006, 2002.
50. Theon AP, Barthez PY, Madewell BR, Griffey SM: Radiation therapy of ceruminous gland carcinomas in dogs and cats. *JAVMA* 205:566–569, 1994.

TUMORS OF THE RESPIRATORY TRACT 51
Antony S. Moore and Gregory K. Ogilvie

CLINICAL BRIEFING

Nasal Tumors

Clinical factors
- Unilateral epistaxis, facial deformity, and epiphora.
- Most common tumor type is adenocarcinoma.
- Most common in older dogs; no breed or gender predisposition.

Risk factors
- Coal and kerosene heaters in the home for all dogs.
- Tobacco smoke exposure for long-nosed dogs.

Staging and diagnosis
- Tumor is locally invasive and rarely metastasizes to distant sites until late in the course of the disease.
- MDB (includes a CBC, biochemical profile, and urinalysis; thoracic radiography [three views]) and a clotting profile.
- Regional lymph node assessment (mandibular).
- Nasal radiographs or, preferably, CT scan.
- Closed biopsy preferred, but open may be necessary.

Prognostic factors
- Brain invasion by tumor is a poor prognostic sign.
- Bilateral tumors that cause any bony erosion have a worse prognosis.
- Remission of clinical signs after radiation therapy is a good prognostic sign.

Treatment

Initial
- Surgery contraindicated unless it is combined with radiation therapy.

Adjunctive
- Radiation therapy, with or without surgery, is the treatment of choice.
- Median survival rates vary from 8 to 23 months.
- Chemotherapy with platinum drugs may improve survival and local control.

Supportive
- Neurologic signs: corticosteroids and anticonvulsants.
- After radiation therapy: nutritional support, possibly feeding tube.
- Topical eye care, pain relief, and topical skin treatments.
- Antibiotics for secondary infections.
- Intracavitary or local nerve blocks, piroxicam, or opiates (or all three) for discomfort.

Lung Tumors

Clinical factors
- Chronic nonproductive cough, dyspnea, lethargy, lameness (hypertrophic osteopathy), and weight loss; some dogs are asymptomatic.
- Most common tumor type is adenocarcinoma.
- Older, large-breed dogs.

Risk factors
- Passive smoking may increase risk of developing primary lung tumor in brachycephalic breeds.

Staging and diagnosis	• MDB. • Metastasizes within lung and to regional lymph nodes. • CT or possibly ultrasonography to guide preoperative biopsy if excisional biopsy is not preferred.
Prognostic factors	• Normal regional lymph nodes are associated with longer survival than enlarged (11 versus 2 months). • Absence of clinical signs at diagnosis is a good prognostic factor. • Tumor staging predictive of survival after surgery.
Treatment Initial Adjunctive Supportive	 • Lung lobectomy is the treatment of choice. • Chemotherapy anecdotal, but vindesine, vinorelbine, and platinum drugs may have efficacy. • Pain relief postoperatively. • Nutritional support as needed.
Other Tumors Reviewed	• Tracheal and laryngeal tumors. • Canine lymphomatoid granulomatosis.

Nasal Tumors

INCIDENCE, SIGNALMENT, AND ETIOLOGY

Tumors involving the nasal cavity and nearby sinuses are uncommon in dogs, and the median age of affected animals is 10 years. Carcinomas, especially adenocarcinoma, represent at least 66% of all tumors in the canine nasal cavity.[1-3] Sarcomas (e.g., chondrosarcoma, osteosarcoma, fibrosarcoma, undifferentiated sarcoma) are less common and tend to occur in large-breed dogs.[2,4] Rare nasal carcinoids and transmissible venereal tumors arising from the nasal cavity have also been described (see Chapter 58).[5,6]

Male dogs were more likely to develop a nasal tumor in a study of more than 500 dogs.[7] Dolichocephalic breeds, particularly collies and Shetland sheepdogs, have been shown to be predisposed. Other predisposed breeds include Airedale terriers, basset hounds, Old English sheepdogs, Scottish terriers, and German shorthaired pointers.[7]

> **KEY POINT**
> *Dogs with nasal tumors often have unilateral epistaxis, epiphora, and facial deformity. Some clinical signs may resolve transiently with antibiotic therapy.*

Environmental factors may increase the risk of developing canine nasal tumors. Although an urban environment has been suggested as a risk factor, no association was found in one study.[8] Another study showed no increased risk overall for dogs exposed to environmental tobacco smoke in the home; however, dolichocephalic breeds were twice as likely as the general population to develop nasal cancer when exposed to tobacco smoke.[9] This predisposition is attributed to the greater filtering capacity of these dogs, exposing the nasal mucosa to a higher dose of tobacco-related carcinogens. In another study, exposure to indoor coal or kerosene heaters was the strongest risk factor for developing nasal cancer (4.2 times and 2.2 times the risk of the general population, respectively).[10] Again, nasal length was a modifier of this effect, with increased risk for dolichocephalic dogs. Environmental tobacco smoke exposure was not a risk factor in this study.

CLINICAL PRESENTATION AND HISTORY

Dogs with nasal tumors frequently have facial deformity, epiphora, and unilateral epistaxis. This epistaxis may become bilateral as the disease progresses. Less specific clinical signs include a purulent or mucoid nasal discharge, dyspnea, coughing, sneezing, ocular discharge, prolapse of the third eyelid, and neurologic signs. These clinical signs persist for months. Owners often report that antibiotic therapy alleviates clinical signs transiently, probably because of a decrease in secondary bacterial infections, which are often associated with nasal tumors. Many different diseases of the nasal and paranasal sinuses have identical clinical signs,[1-3] and diagnos-

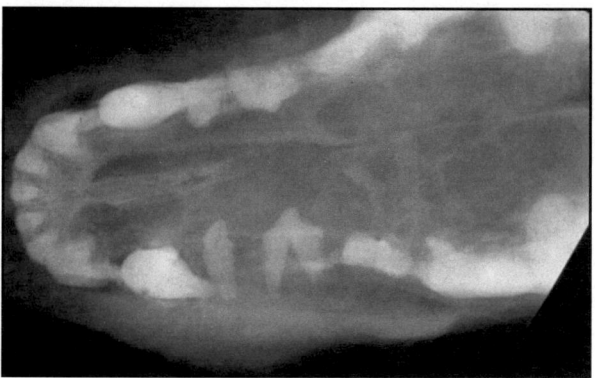

Figure 51-1. Open-mouth radiograph of a dog with a nasal cavity tumor of the right nasal passage. Note the bone destruction and soft tissue density of the tumor. Open-mouth radiographs are often ideal for delineating the location of the tumor in a private practice setting.

tic differentials that must be considered include bacterial, allergic, or fungal rhinitis; foreign bodies; nasal parasites; bleeding disorders; and trauma. *Aspergillus* spp are the most common cause of fungal rhinitis.

Neurologic signs (often increased aggression) may accompany extension of the tumor through the cribriform plate into the olfactory bulbs of the brain.[11]

STAGING AND DIAGNOSIS

Diagnosis of a nasal tumor begins with a good history and physical examination. A definitive diagnosis can be confirmed only by histology. Supportive data can be obtained with rhinoscopy, plain radiography, and computed tomography (CT) imaging. For fungal rhinitis, serology or mycotic cultures are indicated. Bacterial cultures are rarely of value. Before rhinoscopy, radiography, or biopsy procedures are considered, routine screening tests to eliminate the possibility of bleeding disorders are recommended. These tests include a complete blood count (CBC), biochemical profile, urinalysis, and clotting profile and blood pressure measurements (if indicated).

Nasal radiographs can help determine the extent and location of the disease, which is useful in directing biopsy procedures and planning treatment.[12] As a general rule, the most valuable views are the frontal sinus and ventrodorsal views. With the ventrodorsal open-mouth view, a high-resolution detail screen is placed as far caudal in the nasal cavity as possible. The open-mouth view shows the caudal nasal cavity and cribriform plate. Destruction and proliferation of bone and soft tissue densities within the nasal cavity suggest neoplasia.[1,3,12–15] Rhinitis is less likely to show involvement of the frontal sinus and to have lucent foci in the nasal cavity[15] (Figure 51-1).

The World Health Organization (WHO) staging scheme does not seem to predict survival after radiation therapy.[16–18] One study developed an alternative scoring system to indi-

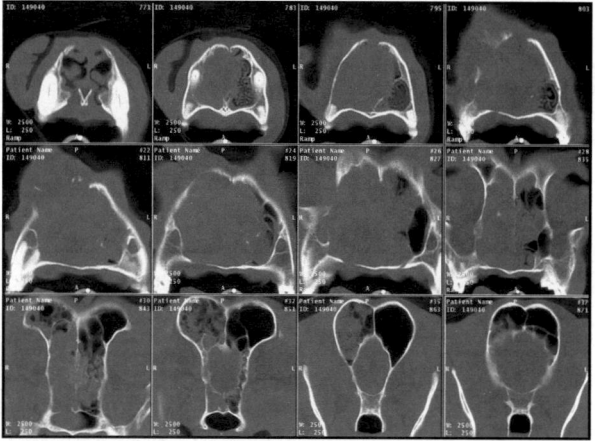

Figure 51-2. A series of CT images of a skull of a dog with a left-sided nasal chondrosarcoma that fills one entire side of the nasal cavity and then crosses to the right and erodes through the dorsal bony structures. Note the fluid in the frontal sinus, which may be tumor extension, although air bubbles make it unlikely. CT is an ideal imaging modality for determining the extent of disease in dogs with nasal tumors, particularly if radiation therapy is planned. (Courtesy of Kenneth M. Rassnick, DVM, Cornell University College of Veterinary Medicine)

cate nasal tumor severity based on radiographic changes; it was predictive of survival in 35 dogs in the study.[19] However, treatment may have influenced the outcome because dogs with worse scores were less likely to be treated. Another radiographic scoring system based on prognostic factors that seemed to correlate best with response to treatment was found to predict survival after radiation therapy.[17] In that system, dogs with stage I disease had a unilateral or bilateral neoplasm that was confined to the nasal passages (no frontal sinus involvement), and dogs with stage II disease had a bilateral nasal tumor that caused bony erosion.[17]

CT is more accurate than radiography in staging because it can differentiate unilateral from bilateral nasal cavity disease and can identify tumor extension into nearby structures, such as the hard palate, pterygopalatine fossa, cribriform plate, and cranial cavity (Figure 51-2). More accurate tumor staging improves prediction of treatment-related complications and planning of surgery and radiation therapy.[14,20] When brain involvement is suspected on the basis of history, physical examination, or radiographic findings, an iodinated contrast agent should be injected intravenously before CT is done. If the blood–brain barrier is broken, the agent will extend into the brain and surrounding tissue and will be visible on the scan as an area of increased radiodensity (contrast enhancement), which is a poor prognostic sign. Magnetic resonance imaging (MRI) may also be used to demonstrate potential invasion of the calvarium.[21]

Rhinoscopy and nasal flushing can help determine the extent of disease and support a diagnosis, but they are less effective than curettage or open biopsy. Rhinoscopy can be

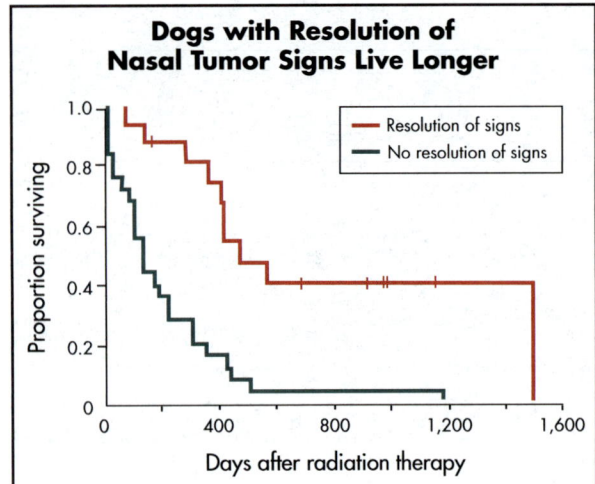

Figure 51-3. Survival curves for dogs with nasal tumors treated with radiation therapy with and without resolution of signs after treatment. Whereas 16 dogs that had complete resolution lived a median of 476 days, 25 dogs that had continued clinical signs lived a median of 133 days. (From Northrup NC, Etue SM, Ruslander DM, et al: Retrospective study of orthovoltage radiation therapy for nasal tumors in 42 dogs. J Vet Intern Med 15:183–189, 2001; with permission)

performed using a flexible rhinoscope or rigid cystoscope; either allows direct visualization of the nasal cavity and surrounding structures. When a flexible rhinoscope is used, the caudal nasopharynx should be examined for neoplastic tissue by extending the rhinoscope through the oral cavity and then retroflexing it over the soft palate. It should then be directed toward the nares to locate any tumor or other abnormality in the most caudal aspect of the nasopharyngeal area. Biopsy specimens can be taken concurrently through the rhinoscope. In one study, only 72% of animals with nasal neoplasia were diagnosed by rhinoscopic biopsy, implying that further biopsies should be obtained with a transnasal core biopsy procedure as insurance against a poor diagnostic sample.[22]

Nasal washings or flushes reportedly have mixed results. One investigator reported a 50% success rate by flushing the nasal cavity and examining the resultant fluid cytologically, but others believe that the yield is much lower with the flushing procedure.[1,3] Even when a "brushing" technique is used, the positive yield is less than 60%.[23]

The cornerstone of diagnosis of nasal tumors is obtaining adequate tissue for histopathology. In most cases, the tumor can be biopsied while the dog is anesthetized for radiography or rhinoscopy. The simplest, cheapest, and most accurate method of obtaining adequate tissue in a dog without resorting to surgery is transnostril core sampling (see Chapter 15). If nonsurgical approaches do not work, rhinotomy may be considered to obtain tissue for definitive diagnosis.

A trephine is used to gain entry into the nasal cavity or sinus, and a curette is used to sample tumor tissue. If cancer is diagnosed after rhinotomy, the entire biopsy tract must be considered contaminated with tumor and the size of the radiation field increased to include the incision site and nearby tissue. This may result in increased toxicity.

> **KEY POINT**
>
> *The simplest, cheapest, and most accurate method of obtaining adequate tissue for diagnosis in dogs without resorting to surgery is the transnostril core-sampling procedure.*

At the time of initial diagnosis of nasal tumors, approximately 6% of lymph node biopsy specimens and aspirates contain tumor cells; thus, biopsies should be performed in dogs with regional lymphadenopathy and considered even in dogs with normal-sized lymph nodes.[16] Metastasis to regional lymph nodes occurs in approximately 40% of cases during late stages of the disease.[2] Metastatic disease to the lungs is rare at the time of initial presentation (seen in approximately 5% of dogs with carcinomas),[16] and thoracic radiographs should be obtained as part of a minimum database (MDB). Metastasis to the brain and liver has also been reported.[2] Nonepithelial tumors have the lowest metastatic rate,[2,4] although metastases may occur widely.[24]

PROGNOSTIC FACTORS

In one study, dogs with facial deformity as measured by CT scan had shorter survival times than those without deformity.[18] Only 39% of all dogs in this study became free of clinical signs, but those that did lived longer than those with chronic nasal signs (Figure 51-3).[18] Dissolution of the cribriform plate by nasal squamous cell carcinoma (SCC) was associated with a poor prognosis in one study: Whereas dogs without dissolution survived a median of 16 months, dogs with cribriform destruction lived 2 months.[25]

The WHO staging scheme does not seem to predict survival after radiation therapy.[16–18] Using a modified staging scheme, one study found that dogs with stage II disease were 2.3 times more likely to relapse than dogs with stage I disease.[17] Similarly, the presence of either regional lymph node or pulmonary metastasis was associated with significantly shorter median survival time (3.5 months) compared with dogs without metastases (13 months).[16] It is possible that the WHO staging scheme should be altered to emphasize the finding of metastases.

In two studies, dogs with carcinomas had a poorer prognosis than dogs with sarcomas (predominantly chondrosarcoma).[17,26] Approximately 15% of dogs with chondrosarcomas had not relapsed 4 years after radiotherapy, but all dogs with carcinomas had relapsed by 3 years after therapy. Dogs with carcinomas were more than three times as likely to relapse as dogs with sarcomas.[17] Dogs with chondrosarcomas lived longer (median: 11 months) than dogs with other sarcomas (5.6 months) in another preliminary study.[27]

TREATMENT

Because nasal tumors metastasize rarely and late in the course of disease, therapy is directed at controlling localized disease.

Surgery

Surgical excision alone is not considered effective in treating nasal tumors in dogs because bone invasion occurs early in the pathogenesis of the disease and because the tumor is often located near the brain and eyes, which makes it impossible to obtain tumor-free surgical margins. Indeed, surgery alone is associated with acute and chronic morbidity without significant extension of life. Therefore, surgery is generally indicated only when combined with radiation therapy. In one study, dogs that received megavoltage radiation therapy had a significantly longer median survival time (14 months) than dogs treated by surgery alone (4 months) (Figure 51-4).[16]

Radiation Therapy

Radiation therapy with or without surgical debulking is the only treatment modality that increases survival time of dogs with nasal tumors.[3,16,26,28] Survival times for dogs with nasal carcinomas are modest, ranging from 8 to 16 months.[16–18,26,29] There is no difference between orthovoltage and megavoltage, and many dogs have residual nasal signs.

Surgical debulking is necessary before orthovoltage radiotherapy to reduce tumor volume and allow adequate delivery of radiation to the nasal cavity. Megavoltage radiotherapy is usually delivered without previous surgical debulking because the distribution of dose is less hindered by bone and tissue depth. In practical terms, megavoltage radiation without pretreatment surgical debulking and orthovoltage radiation after surgical debulking are approximately equipotent. However, the belief that surgical debulking should not be performed before megavoltage radiotherapy because the air-filled nasal cavity would result in inconsistent dosing has recently been shown to be untrue, and future studies in which debulking of tumors is performed before megavoltage radiation may demonstrate improved response rates.[30] To date, cytoreductive surgery has not significantly altered survival when megavoltage radiation is used.[17,31]

Early reports of the use of orthovoltage radiotherapy were encouraging. Orthovoltage radiotherapy dosages of 40 to 50 Gy delivered in 10 to 12 fractions were reported to result in a median survival of 16 to 23 months; 1- and 2-year survival

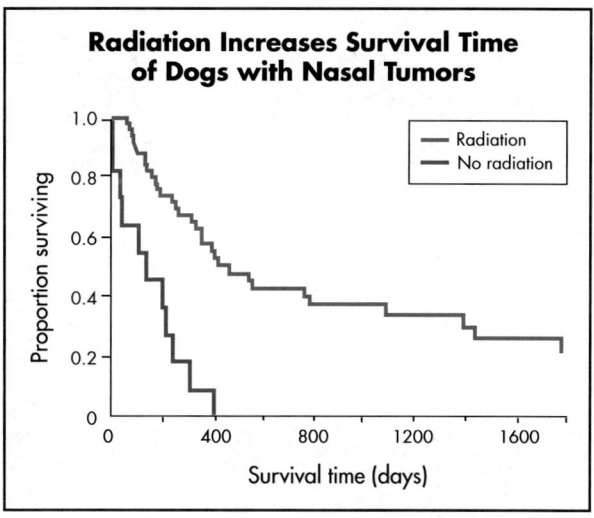

Figure 51-4. These survival curves demonstrate that whereas dogs with nasal tumors treated with radiation therapy lived a median of 424 days, dogs that did not receive radiation therapy lived a median of 126 days. (From Henry CJ, Brewer WG Jr, Tyler JW, et al: Survival in dogs with nasal adenocarcinoma: 64 cases (1981–1995). J Vet Intern Med 12:436–439, 1998; with permission)

rates were 57% and 43%, respectively.[26,28] For some time, it was believed that orthovoltage treatment was more effective than megavoltage. A more recent evaluation of orthovoltage, in a larger number of dogs, showed that median remissions are similar to those obtained with megavoltage therapy.[18] In this study, median survival was 7.4 months, and 1- and 2-year survival rates were 37% and 17%, respectively. Acute radiation toxicity that healed within 1 month of radiation therapy was seen in the skin and eyes but not in the oral mucosa. Only 39% of dogs achieved a disease-free period.

Early reported median survival of dogs with nasal tumors treated with megavoltage radiation alone was approximately 8 months.[31] More recent reports of larger numbers of dogs have found median survival times of between 12 and 14 months.[16,17] One- and 2-year survival rates in one report were 59% and 22%, respectively. Dogs received from 41.8 to 54.0 Gy on a Monday/Wednesday/Friday schedule over 4 weeks. The improvement in survival over that reported previously was attributed to the use of CT for tumor localization and treatment plans (Figure 51-5).

Radiation therapy always produces some acute adverse effects, including oral mucositis, rhinitis, moist desquamation, and alteration of pigment and hair color. These usually arise in the final third of the radiation course and are often severe but resolve over the 2 weeks after radiation therapy (Figures 51-6 and 51-7). Most dogs also have residual nasal signs such as sneezing and serous discharge as a result of tumor damage to turbinates and changes in mucosa caused by radiation therapy. Ocular effects are a significant factor in

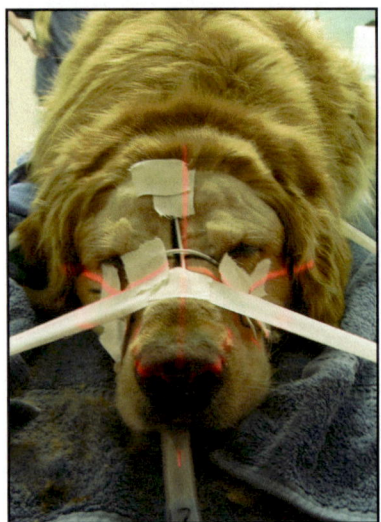

Figure 51-5. *The use of CT scans, positioning devices, and laser localization of landmarks has allowed repeatable radiation treatments and improved the efficacy of therapy.*

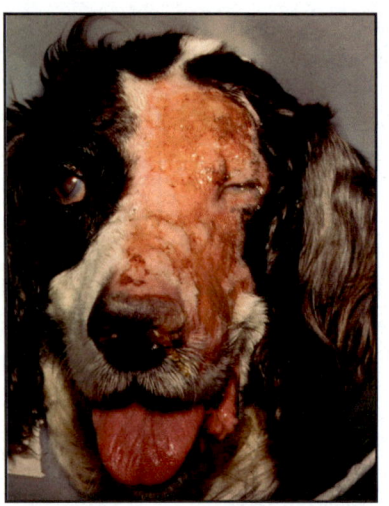

Figure 51-6. *This springer spaniel is pictured on the last day of a course of orthovoltage radiation therapy for a unilateral nasal carcinoma. Acute cutaneous reactions are often less severe after megavoltage treatment, but oral mucositis predominates.*

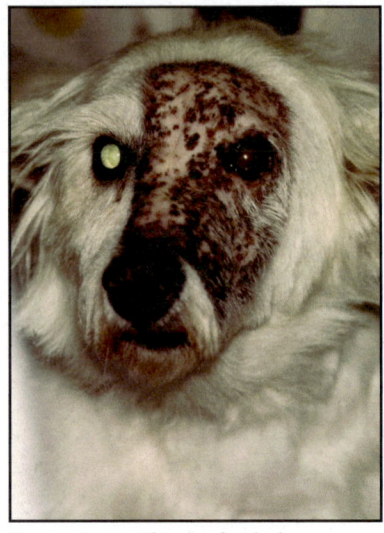

Figure 51-7. *This dog finished orthovoltage radiation therapy for a nasal carcinoma 3 months previously, healing is complete, and pigmentation of the site is progressing.*

the quality of life, but the eyes cannot be protected without shielding the underlying tumor tissue. Most ocular effects are acute and resolve after treatment; late effects of cataract formation and keratoconjunctivitis sicca may affect vision.[32]

Nasal tumors in dogs may have a short doubling time. Rapid proliferation of tumor cells creates a higher risk of tumor escape through accelerated repopulation during the intertreatment interval of alternate-day treatment. The delay between surgery and radiotherapy may also allow regrowth in tumors with a high proliferative fraction. Tumors with a high proliferative component are probably not treated adequately using a regular veterinary fractionation scheme. Shortening the time between radiation doses may hinder repopulation by tumor cells.

The poor response of nasal tumors to conventional radiation treatments has led to studies that attempted to improve control by dose-schedule manipulation. Two studies investigated an accelerated radiation course for nasal tumors in dogs. Radiation was delivered in daily fractions over 11 to 13 days or twice a day over 21 days.[33,34] Acute toxicities were common, including mucositis that was severe and protracted (up to 5 weeks); skin necrosis occurred in one dog. Few dogs lived more than 6 months, and late effects were seen in nearly all of them. Unilateral or bilateral blindness occurred 6 months after treatment. Osteonecrosis was seen in three dogs and seizures in one dog. Five dogs died because of acute or late tissue reactions. Theoretically, these protocols should have resulted in equivalent or better tumor control and a reduced risk of late effects. However, there was no reduction in recurrence rate compared with standard protocols; in fact, survival times were worse.[35] In addition, the high incidence of late effects and the high rate of acute side effects made these approaches unacceptable.

A retrospective study was undertaken in 56 dogs treated for nasal tumors with a hypofractionated schedule consisting of four doses of 9 Gy given once a week. Clinical signs improved in 53 of the 56 dogs by the end of the treatment schedule. Mild acute radiation side effects were observed in most dogs; late radiation side effects were rare. The median survival time after the final dose of radiation was 7 months. The 1- and 2-year survival rates were 45% and 15%, respectively, which is little different from those of more conventional dosing schemes.[29] A palliative course of three weekly 8-Gy treatments controlled chondrosarcoma in two dogs in another report.[36] Many oncologists believe that the "palliative" approach used in this study may provide the optimal balance between acute and late side effects and control of the disease.

Other sources of radiation, such as proton-beam therapy, may be available in some countries. The use of proton beams may reduce the risk of late side effects to underlying brain and allow increased doses of radiation to be delivered safely to the tumor.[37]

Some investigators think that SCC of the nasal cavity is a more aggressive tumor than the more commonly encountered adenocarcinoma. One study seemed to support that claim: Six dogs lived a median of 5 months after receiving radiation doses of 54 Gy and greater, even though none developed metastases.[38]

Other Local Therapies

Photodynamic therapy (PDT) was reported in a series of three dogs. Repeated treatments given as clinical signs returned provided palliation of signs for 6 months or more in two dogs with minimal side effects, despite apparent tumor progression at each treatment.[39] Access to PDT is limited because few facilities perform the procedure. PDT is not a substitute for radiation therapy.

> **KEY POINT**
> *Radiation therapy with or without surgery is the only treatment modality that increases survival time of dogs with nasal tumors.*

Systemic Therapies

Chemotherapy is not usually considered an effective treatment when used alone for canine nasal tumors, especially when compared with radiation therapy. Cisplatin may be effective in some cases. One report documented two complete remissions and one partial remission in 11 dogs treated with cisplatin. The duration of responses ranged from 3 to 13 months.[40] Five dogs treated with platinum drugs after relapsing from radiation therapy had no response.[18] Gemcitabine has been used as a radiation therapy "sensitizer" in the treatment of dogs with nasal carcinomas, but outcomes have not yet been reported.[41]

The findings that normal nasal tissue has no evidence of cyclooxygenase-2 (COX-2) expression and that 81% of malignant nasal tumors express COX-2 has led to speculation that nonsteroidal inhibitors of COX-2 may play a role in the treatment of nasal carcinoma.[42] In an early evaluation of piroxicam (an NSAID) in the treatment of canine cancer, only one dog with nasal carcinoma was treated, without response.[43] A preliminary report of 18 dogs treated with piroxicam alone resulted in clinical improvement in half the patients and a median survival time of 8 months.[44] In another preliminary report, eight dogs were treated with alternating carboplatin (300 mg/m^2) and doxorubicin (30 mg/m^2) every 3 weeks with concurrent piroxicam. Four dogs achieved a complete response, and two dogs had a partial response, with a median survival of 7 months (five dogs were still alive at last follow-up).[45]

Combined Radiation and Chemotherapy

A cisplatin-impregnated, slow-release polymer (OPLA-Pt) was implanted at a distant site on the body in 13 dogs treated with radiation therapy (50–56 Gy). The median survival of 19 months compared favorably with other reports indicating a potential benefit to combination therapy for nasal tumors.[46] Addition of a further 38 dogs confirmed these results.[47]

In another study of dogs treated with radiation therapy, some dogs also received chemotherapy consisting of either 5-fluorouracil and cyclophosphamide in combination (15 dogs) or mitoxantrone (seven dogs). However, neither chemotherapy group was associated with improvement in survival time compared with radiation therapy alone.[16]

Supportive Therapies

Dogs with neurologic signs attributable to extension of the tumor through the cribriform plate should be treated concurrently with corticosteroids and anticonvulsants if needed.[11]

Dogs undergoing aggressive megavoltage radiation therapy may experience significant oral mucosal side effects of mucositis and ulceration. These effects usually worsen during the third week of radiation therapy and resolve within 3 weeks after finishing the treatment course. During this time, pain and loss of appetite are major factors influencing the patient's quality of life. These dogs will benefit from antiinflammatory drugs, pain relief, and appetite stimulants. Consideration should be given to placing an esophagostomy tube before the side effects begin.

Ocular effects of radiation therapy are common. In one study of dogs that had one or both eyes in the radiation field, ocular side effects were categorized as mild in 17% of dogs and severe in 59% of dogs; only 24% had no ocular complications.[32] Complications included severe keratitis (40% of dogs), conjunctivitis (62%), and keratoconjunctivitis sicca (24%) caused by damage to the lacrimal gland. Most mild reactions resolved with supportive care only (control of bacterial infection, antiinflammatory drugs, and ocular surface protection). The caregiver should be instructed to use prophylactic eye lubricants until a Schirmer's tear test result is normal. Occasionally, keratoconjunctivitis sicca makes the need for eye lubrication permanent. Approximately 30% of dogs that have an eye included in the treatment field develop cataracts an average of 10 months after radiation therapy.[32]

Tumors of the Larynx
INCIDENCE, SIGNALMENT, AND ETIOLOGY

Tumors of the larynx are very rare in dogs, and there are few data concerning their prevalence. A review paper described 38 cases.[48] The most common tumors of the canine larynx are carcinomas (including SCC; 34%) and oncocytomas or rhabdomyomas (24%).[48,49] Benign laryngeal oncocytomas that occur in middle-aged and young dogs are most probably rhabdomyomas, based on special stains and ultrastructure.[50,51] Other reported laryngeal tumor types include mast cell tumor, chondrosarcoma, osteosarcoma, melanoma, lipoma, adenocarcinoma, fibrosarcoma, and papilloma.[48,52-55] Metastases are less common than primary tumors.[52]

CLINICAL PRESENTATION AND HISTORY

The two most common clinical signs associated with a laryngeal tumor are dyspnea and voice change, both occurring in more than half of affected dogs.[48] Laryngeal tumors may also cause coughing, respiratory stridor, and ptyalism, but rarely choking. These masses usually are not palpable.

STAGING AND DIAGNOSIS

Most tumors can be assessed by laryngeal examination, although the depth and extension of an invasive tumor can be hard to determine. Radiographs of the neck may show a laryngeal mass, but soft tissue discrimination to define borders is difficult.[56] Ultrasonography may direct preoperative biopsy and show distortion of the normal laryngeal structures.[57] CT or MRI is usually required to determine the extent of the tumor and is mandatory if surgical excision is contemplated.[58] Tissue for histopathology should be obtained with endoscopy or during open surgical biopsy.

Because of the chance of metastatic disease and the increased risk of concurrent problems, such as bronchopneumonia, thoracic radiographs should be taken as part of an MDB.

TREATMENT

Surgery is probably the treatment of choice for most laryngeal tumors, but the reported outcomes are mixed, even for benign tumors. Unilateral partial laryngectomy was described in one report, but improvement was reported in only one dog treated with repeated surgeries and chemotherapy for a laryngeal adenocarcinoma over a 16-month period.[59] Localized and benign laryngeal tumors, such as oncocytomas, may be removed by regional resection of the larynx. Local excision of malignant tumors is usually incomplete, and recurrence within months of surgery is common.[50,55] Attempted surgery may need to be abandoned if the margins have not been clearly defined before surgical approach.[60]

Most patients with a malignant laryngeal tumor require laryngectomy with permanent tracheostomy, but few clinical cases have been treated by this methodology. One dog with a laryngeal rhabdomyosarcoma was treated with a laryngectomy and tracheostomy and was alive with no evidence of disease 18 months later.[58] The authors ascribed their success to presurgical preparation in the form of placing and establishing feeding through a gastrostomy tube, a presurgical CT scan to delineate margins of the tumor, and a dedicated owner who was well informed about the care needed postoperatively. Despite the risks of aspiration pneumonia, this dog had not developed a complication. Complete laryngectomy was associated with considerable morbidity in two other dogs with a mast cell tumor and a rhabdomyosarcoma. Complications of stomal collapse, formation of a tracheoesophageal fistula, pharyngeal dehiscence, and ablation of the parathyroid glands were described.[61,62] Success probably depends on completing presurgical preparation as outlined above.

Tumors of the Trachea
INCIDENCE, SIGNALMENT, AND ETIOLOGY

Tumors of the trachea in dogs are even rarer than tumors of the larynx; a review paper described 23 cases.[48] There are few other data concerning the prevalence of tumors at this site. Benign tracheal osteocartilaginous tumors (osteochondromas) are the most common tumors and occur in dogs younger than 1 year of age. These tumors show active osteochondral ossification but are rarely malignant (chondrosarcoma).[48,55] Other reported tracheal tumors are leiomyoma, adenocarcinoma and other carcinoma, mast cell tumor, and plasmacytoma.[48,63]

CLINICAL PRESENTATION AND HISTORY

Tracheal tumors may cause coughing, dyspnea, respiratory stridor, and, in extreme cases, collapse and fainting after respiratory distress.[48] Tracheal masses are not usually palpable.

STAGING AND DIAGNOSIS

Tracheoscopy and radiography are usually required to determine the extent of the tumor. Because of the chance of metastatic disease and the increased risk of concurrent problems such as bronchopneumonia, thoracic radiography should be taken as part of an MDB. Radiographs of the neck may demonstrate a calcified mass if the tumor is an osteochondroma or chondroma. Other tumors may appear radiographically as discrete intraluminal masses.[48] Tissue should be obtained with tracheoscopy or during an open surgical biopsy. Pulmonary metastases have been reported in young dogs with tracheal chondrosarcomas.[48]

TREATMENT

Localized, relatively small tracheal tumors such as osteochondromas are treated effectively by removing the affected tracheal rings. Some suggest that up to four tracheal rings may be removed and the stoma closed by an end-to-end anastomosis without complications, but others suggest that the length can be much greater. One 28-kg dog had a 3-cm section of the trachea removed for a tracheal plasmacytoma and recovered uneventfully. There was no evidence of systemic disease or recurrence 3 months later.[63] Radiation therapy may be a useful adjunct to surgery because most tracheal tumors are benign.

> **KEY POINT**
>
> *Up to four tracheal rings can be removed with reasonable closure by an end-to-end anastomosis.*

Table 51-1 **Clinical Signs Associated with Primary Lung Tumors in Dogs**

Clinical Sign	Frequency (%)
Cough	52.0
Dyspnea	24.0
Lethargy	18.0
Weight loss	12.0
Tachypnea	5.0
Pyrexia	6.4
Lameness	3.8

Primary Lung Tumors

INCIDENCE, SIGNALMENT, AND ETIOLOGY

Primary lung tumors are uncommon in animals compared with humans but are more common in dogs than in other animal species.[64-66] In a lifetime study of normal beagles, 39 of 398 dogs (10%) developed a primary lung tumor.[65] The most common tumor type was carcinoma (35 dogs), with papillary adenocarcinoma in 20 dogs, bronchioalveolar carcinoma in nine dogs, adenosquamous carcinoma in five dogs, and SCC in one dog. In addition, adenomas developed in three dogs, and a fibroma was seen in one dog.[65] This distribution follows that of clinical studies.[64] Rare carcinoids have been reported.[67]

The average age of a dog with primary lung tumor is 10.9 years (range: 2–18 years), and the risk increases substantially after 13 years of age.[65,68] Male and female dogs are affected with equal frequency. Approximately 60% of dogs with primary lung tumors weigh between 20 and 30 kg.[64]

Many investigators suggest that carcinogens in the environment may directly influence the incidence of lung tumors in dogs. In one study, 75% of dogs with primary lung tumors lived in urban environments,[64] although two other studies found no association with urban living.[8,69] There is a weak association between exposure to secondhand smoke and the prevalence of primary lung tumors in dogs. The association is stronger in brachycephalic dogs than dolichocephalic dogs, presumably because of the increased filtration capacity of dolichocephalic dogs.[70]

CLINICAL PRESENTATION AND HISTORY

The primary complaint noted by owners of dogs with primary lung tumors is chronic, nonproductive cough.[68,71] These and other clinical signs of primary lung tumors are listed in Table 51-1. Some clinical signs are relatively nonspecific, and approximately 25% to 30% of dogs with primary lung tumors are asymptomatic at the time of diagnosis.[64,67,71]

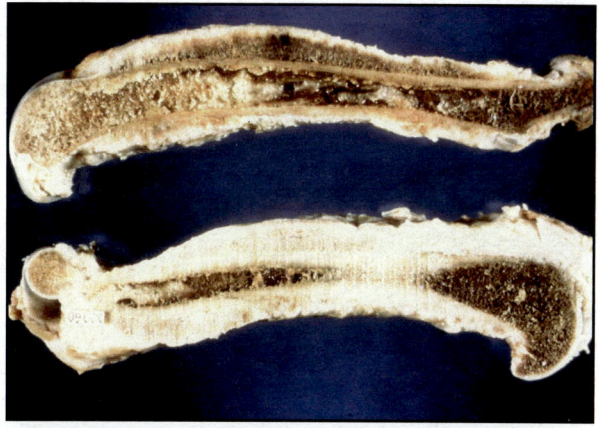

Figure 51-8. *This necropsy specimen clearly shows the periosteal proliferation associated with hypertrophic osteopathy. Clinical improvement is seen within 3 to 6 weeks after lung mass removal, but periosteal changes may not completely resolve.*

Rare clinical complications of a pulmonary tumor include compression of the anterior vena cava, which can cause edema of the head and neck (anterior vena cava syndrome). This finding usually signals a mediastinal mass. Invasion of pleura or regional pulmonary lymphatics by tumor cells can produce pleural effusion and cause severe dyspnea. Pleural effusion is seen in some cases of both primary and metastatic lung tumors. Although alveolar or bronchiole rupture may be caused by an invasive tumor, it is a rare cause of pneumothorax.[72] In a series of 38 dogs with pneumothorax, only three had a primary lung tumor, and one had a metastatic lung tumor.[73] Similarly, hemoptysis caused by neoplastic erosion of a pulmonary blood vessel is possible. However, of 36 dogs with hemoptysis, only three had a primary lung tumor; another three dogs had metastatic pulmonary disease.[74]

The most common paraneoplastic syndrome associated with primary and metastatic canine pulmonary neoplasia is hypertrophic osteopathy, occurring in nine of 277 (3%) cases in two studies[64,71] (Figure 51-8). Dogs with this condition often present with lameness in one or more limbs. Radiographs reveal a characteristic periosteal proliferation perpendicular to the long shaft of the bone. Surgical resection of the pulmonary mass often causes rapid resolution of the clinical signs (within 3 to 5 weeks), although resolution of radiographic changes may take much longer.[71,75] Lameness caused by metastatic spread of a lung tumor to the bones of the limbs is rare. Other paraneoplastic syndromes include hypercalcemia, polyneuropathy, polymyopathy, fever, and ectopic production of adrenocorticotropic hormone, which causes hyperadrenocorticism (seen in two of 210 dogs with primary lung tumors[64]). A dog with paraneoplastic polyneuropathy and tetraparesis was normal 4 years after a papillary adenoma was removed.[76] A paraneoplastic

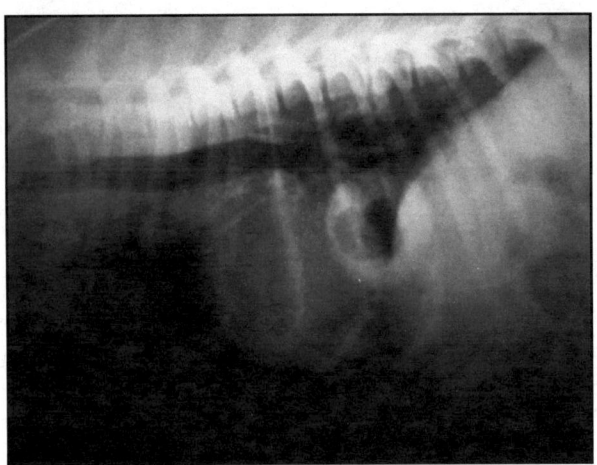

Figure 51-9. Thoracic radiograph of a canine primary lung tumor that appears as a cavitated mass. Most primary lung tumors appear radiographically as a well-circumscribed solitary mass within the lung fields.

leukocytosis (mainly neutrophils) was associated with production of filgrastim by a pulmonary papillary carcinoma and resolved within 1 month of tumor resection.[77]

STAGING AND DIAGNOSIS

Thoracic radiography is the most important preoperative diagnostic tool in the diagnosis of primary lung tumors.[64,71] Information gained from radiographic procedures directs subsequent diagnostic steps. Most dogs have a solitary, well-circumscribed pulmonary mass that may cause airway obstruction. Other common radiographic findings are pleural extension and regional lymph node enlargement. In one study, 54% of respiratory tumors were solitary, 37% were multiple, and 5% invaded neighboring tissues.[64] Cavitation of pulmonary tissue secondary to primary lung tumors occasionally occurs. Abscess formation can also cause a cavitary lesion (Figure 51-9).

> **KEY POINT**
>
> *Hypertrophic osteopathy is the most common paraneoplastic syndrome associated with primary lung tumor in dogs. Affected dogs are often lame.*

Because primary lung tumors tend to metastasize to other lung areas and regional lymph nodes, special attention should be directed to obtaining and evaluating high-quality thoracic radiographs. If lameness is noted, radiographs of the affected area should be evaluated for hypertrophic osteopathy. A CBC, biochemical profile, and urinalysis are required to identify paraneoplastic syndromes or organ dysfunctions secondary to the neoplastic disease. Lymph node biopsy specimens are valuable in identifying the extent of primary disease and any metastasis. Dogs with larger primary tumors are more likely to have lymph node involvement.[68]

A pulmonary mass that is not close to large, vascular structures can be aspirated safely; however, the risk of disseminating the tumor cells within the thoracic cavity must be recognized.[64] During transthoracic aspiration, a 3- to 5-ml syringe with a 22-gauge needle is directed into the mass while negative pressure is applied with the syringe. A quick "in-and-out" aspiration is done. There must be no negative pressure in the syringe when the needle is withdrawn from the mass and skin. This procedure has minimal risk. Possible complications include pneumothorax and hemoptysis. Ultrasonographic or CT guidance improves the accuracy of this procedure. A histologic scoring system devised for primary lung tumors has prognostic significance (Table 51-2).

An assessment of the metastatic potential for different malignant pulmonary carcinomas can be gleaned from a study of beagles that developed lung tumors and were followed with serial radiography but not treated. In that study, 67% of the dogs with bronchioalveolar carcinoma, 60% of the dogs with adenosquamous carcinoma, and 25% of the dogs with adenocarcinomas developed metastases.[65] Systemic metastases are less common than metastases to the rest of the lungs or to lymph nodes, but they can be widespread (as is seen more commonly in cats).[78]

Pleural effusion may obscure details of thoracic structures on radiographs; however, it may enhance the diagnostic potential of ultrasonography. Therefore, ultrasonography should be considered when fluid is present. If radiography is to be used, thoracic fluid should be drained to allow better visualization of intrathoracic structures. Most pleural effusions associated with malignancies are exudates (total protein >3.0 g/dl; specific gravity >1.015). Some tumors do not exfoliate into the pleural fluid; therefore, lack of tumor cells in an exudative pleural effusion should not exclude a diagnosis of primary lung neoplasia.

Ultrasonography is not better than radiography at detecting pulmonary lesions. Reflection of the ultrasound beam prevents evaluation of lesions surrounded by aerated lung. However, ultrasonography can be useful in guiding a biopsy of lung lesions that are not obscured by gas; in one study, more than 90% of ultrasound-guided biopsies were diagnostic.[79]

Helical CT scanning may be helpful in distinguishing small, potentially metastatic nodules from alveolar disease in lung lobes away from the primary tumor. It may also be helpful in delineating tumor margins, particularly around the hilus. CT may also be used to assess the size of tracheobronchial lymph nodes[80] as well as to guide a biopsy or fine-needle aspiration of the pulmonary mass and the hilar lymph nodes preoperatively.[81,82] Excessive movement of the thorax makes MRI less successful than CT in imaging lung tissue.

Table 51-2 **Histologic Grading of Primary Pulmonary Tumors**[71]

Score[a]	Parameter						
	Differentiation	Nuclear pleomorphism	Mitotic index	Nucleolar size	Tumor necrosis (%)	Fibrosis	Demarcation
0					None	None	
1	Well	Mild	1–10	Small	1–20	0.5 (1%–20%)	Well
2	Moderate	Moderate	11–20	Medium	21–50	1.0 (21%–50%)	Moderate
3	Poor	Severe	21–30	Large	>50	1.5 (>50%)	Invasive
4			31+				

[a]Total cumulative score: grade 1: <8.5; grade 2: 9–14; grade 3: >14.5.

Although bronchoscopy may be used to visualize the airways, most dogs with lung tumors have compressive lesions that can be visualized only indirectly.[68] Tumors are often peripherally located and therefore inaccessible by bronchoscopy. If cells or fluid are needed for cytology and bacterial culture, a transtracheal aspirate can be obtained from most conscious animals. Carcinomas are more likely than sarcomas to exfoliate into the pulmonary airways.

Pulmonary lymph node enlargement can be a sign of diseases other than a metastatic lung tumor. In the midwestern United States, fungal diseases must always be considered in dogs with pulmonary lymph node enlargement.

PROGNOSTIC FACTORS

Enlarged lymph nodes were identified in 25% of dogs with primary lung tumors before surgery in one study, and this number increased after surgical exploration of the area allowed more accurate detection.[68] In two studies, dogs with lymph nodes that were normal at the time of surgery had a significantly longer disease-free interval than dogs with enlarged nodes (11 months versus 2 months; 15 months versus 1 month; Figure 51-10). The type of tumor did not influence survival times or the disease-free interval.[68,71] If the dog had clinical signs at the time the tumor was detected,

> **KEY POINT**
>
> *Enlarged regional lymph nodes and tumor grade are the most important prognostic factors influencing disease-free interval and survival.*

the prognosis was worse than if there were no clinical signs (8 months versus 18 months; Figure 51-11).[71]

The histologic grade (as described above) was important: 26 dogs with grade 1 tumors had a median survival time of 26 months, 32 dogs with grade 2 tumors had a median survival of 8 months, and nine dogs with grade 3 tumors had a median survival of 5 days (Figure 51-12).[71]

TREATMENT

In a study of 24 beagles with lung carcinomas that were followed with serial radiography but only treated palliatively, the median survival was 10 months (range: 5 days to 42 months).[65] Diagnosis was made after routine thoracic radiography; patients were not presented for clinical signs associated with the tumor.

Surgery is the treatment of choice for dogs with primary lung tumors. For best results, the animal must be in relatively good health and have localized disease. Secondary infection of devitalized tissue may be possible in a dog with a large, rapidly growing lung tumor; prophylactic antibiotics after collection of samples for bacteriologic culture are suggested.[83]

A partial or complete lobectomy is the best choice. Automatic stapling devices reduce surgery time and patient morbidity (Figures 51-13 and 51-14). The average survival after lung lobectomy was 13 months in an early study.[84] In two further studies,[68,71] 143 dogs with a primary lung tumor had a therapeutic lobectomy. Complete removal of the tumor was possible in 110 dogs. These dogs had a median survival time of 11 months compared with 1 to 2 months for the 33 dogs in which excision was incomplete. The presence of clinical signs before surgery, tumor grade, and lymph node involvement all affected the prognosis. These results, together with the finding that dogs with larger primary tumors are more likely to have lymph node involvement, emphasize the importance of performing early surgical intervention rather than adopting a "wait and see" approach.

Most of the information in the literature refers to epithelial tumors; relatively little is found regarding mesenchymal

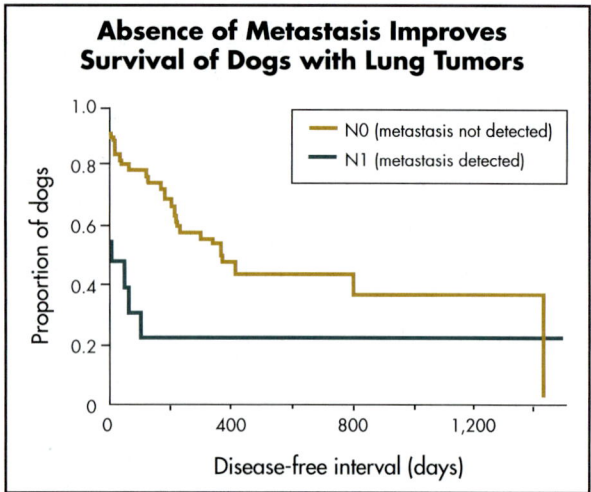

Figure 51-10. *Survival curves for dogs with lung tumors treated with surgery. Dogs that had metastasis to lymph nodes lived a median of 26 days; dogs that had no metastasis lived a median of 452 days. (From McNiel EA, Ogilvie GK, Powers BE, et al: Evaluation of prognostic factors for dogs with primary lung tumors: 67 cases (1985–1992). JAVMA 211:1422–1427, 1997; with permission)*

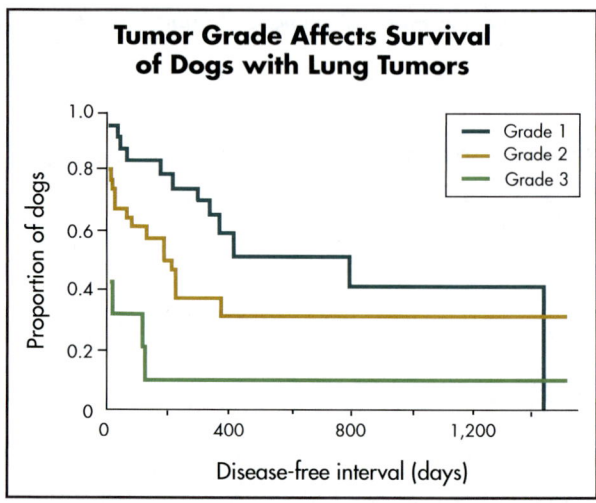

Figure 51-12. *Survival curves for dogs with lung tumors treated with surgery. Dogs that had grade 1 tumors lived a median of 790 days; dogs that had grade 2 tumors lived a median of 251 days. Dogs that had grade 3 tumors lived a median of 5 days (From McNiel EA, Ogilvie GK, Powers BE, et al: Evaluation of prognostic factors for dogs with primary lung tumors: 67 cases (1985-1992). JAVMA 211:1422–1427, 1997; with permission)*

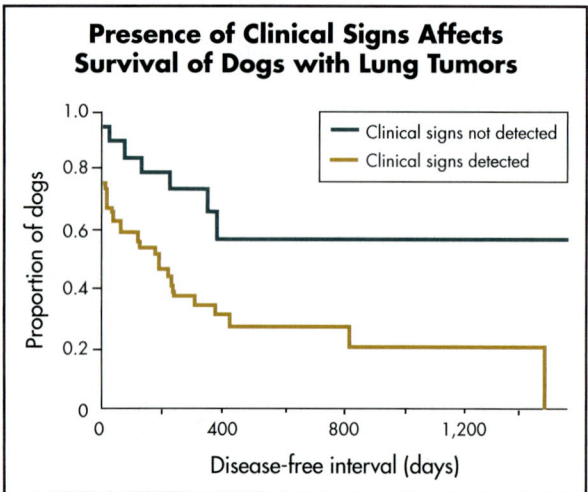

Figure 51-11. *Survival curves for dogs with lung tumors treated with surgery. Dogs that had clinical signs before surgery lived a median of 240 days compared with 545 days for asymptomatic dogs. (From McNiel EA, Ogilvie GK, Powers BE, et al: Evaluation of prognostic factors for dogs with primary lung tumors: 67 cases (1985–1992). JAVMA 211:1422–1427, 1997; with permission)*

lung tumors. In one case report, a primary pulmonary chondrosarcoma was removed by lobectomy. The dog developed oral metastases 6 months after surgery and widespread pulmonary metastases 12 months after surgery.[85]

Although no reports document the efficacy of radiation therapy in the treatment of primary lung tumors in dogs, it is likely that such treatment would significantly extend the survival time of dogs with incompletely excised lung tumors. A linear accelerator or cobalt-radiation therapy unit is required to treat these tumors; however, radiation pneumonitis may be dose limiting if a large area of the lung needs to be treated. In an experimental study, no clinical signs of pneumonitis occurred if less than one-third of the lung volume was irradiated.[86] In another study, intraoperative electron-beam radiation therapy was delivered to the hilar region, but the mediastinal vascular, bronchial, and esophageal structures are sensitive to doses greater than 20 Gy, and nearly 30% of dogs treated died from complications.[87]

PDT has not been reported in the clinical setting, but experimentally induced pulmonary SCC in dogs regressed when treated by this modality.[88]

There are few reports of chemotherapy for primary lung tumors in dogs. Early reports suggested efficacy for vindesine alone and in combination with cisplatin, but most dogs were treated after surgery, so the contribution of chemotherapy to survival is difficult to assess. Partial responses were seen in two dogs treated with the combination.[84] Recent preliminary experience with vinorelbine, a drug related to vindesine, has shown partial responses in two of seven dogs (29%) with metastatic bronchoalveolar carcinoma. Additional use as an adjuvant to surgery in three dogs with lymph node metastases or incomplete excision showed a possible improvement in survival for one dog.[89] It appears that vinorelbine may be the drug of choice for dogs with this disease, possibly in combination with platinum derivatives.

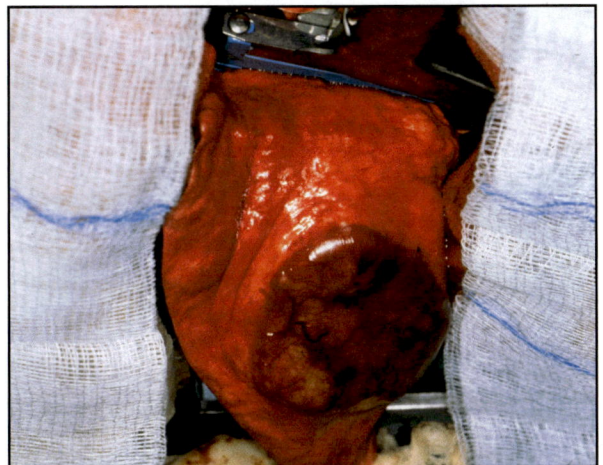

Figure 51-13. Bronchoalveolar adenocarcinoma of the right caudal lung lobe exposed at surgery. (Courtesy of John Berg, DVM, Tufts Cummings School of Veterinary Medicine)

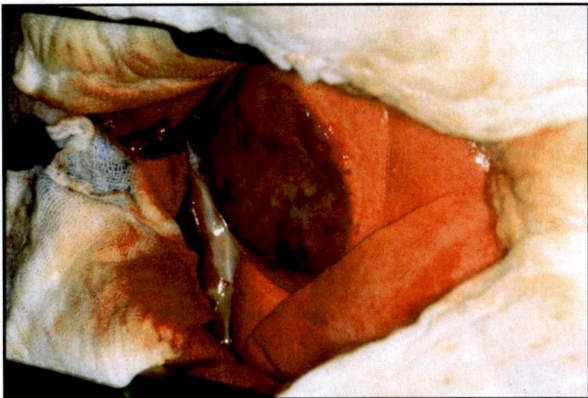

Figure 51-14. The primary lung tumor in Figure 51-13 is quickly and efficiently removed by using an automatic stapling device. Alternatively, the base of the lung can be clamped off and the tumor resected; the lung remnant is then sutured. Regional lymph nodes should be examined and biopsied during surgery, if possible. (Courtesy of J. Berg)

Canine Lymphomatoid Granulomatosis

INCIDENCE, SIGNALMENT, AND ETIOLOGY

Canine lymphomatoid granulomatosis, also known as *pulmonary lymphomatoid granulomatosis*, is a rare neoplastic disease that affects young to middle-aged dogs.[90–92] It appears to be a variant of lymphoma. This disease resembles other malignant pulmonary diseases clinically, but it has a more favorable prognosis than most.

CLINICAL PRESENTATION AND HISTORY

Canine lymphomatoid granulomatosis produces diffuse or well-defined pulmonary masses that can induce significant pulmonary dysfunction. The most common clinical signs are abnormal lung sounds, coughing, dyspnea, anorexia, fever, weight loss, and lymphadenopathy.

STAGING AND DIAGNOSIS

Radiographic changes associated with lymphomatoid granulomatosis include lobar consolidation, poorly defined pulmonary masses, hilar lymphadenopathy, and pleural effusion.[90–92] Transthoracic fine-needle aspirates may reveal a sterile eosinophilic and neutrophilic inflammatory reaction. The most common laboratory abnormalities include basophilia, eosinophilia, and leukocytosis.[91–93] Most dogs test negative for heartworm disease, although a similar syndrome of eosinophilic granulomatosis has been reported in dogs with heartworm.[94] Tissues obtained at the time of thoracotomy or percutaneous biopsy are required for definitive diagnosis.

This disease is considered by some to be a variant of, or a preneoplastic condition for, lymphoma, and responses to treatment of lymphoma have been seen. Some dogs have developed lymphadenopathy and lymphoma after a diagnosis of lymphomatoid granulomatosis.[91,92] Immunohistochemistry has shown that despite morphologic similarities to disseminated histiocytic sarcoma, there is no staining for lysozyme, indicating that the tumor cells are not of histiocytic origin.[95] Another study found that this disorder appears to be a form of atypical T-cell lymphoma.[96]

Involvement of other organs, such as the heart, liver, spleen, pancreas, and kidney, has been noted.[90,92,93]

TREATMENT

Chemotherapy is the treatment of choice for lymphomatoid granulomatosis. Five dogs were given cyclophosphamide, vincristine, and prednisone; three had clinical and radiographic resolution of their disease for 7, 12, and 32 months.[91] In another report, various combinations of cyclophosphamide, vincristine, cytarabine, and prednisone were used to treat six dogs. The response to therapy was favorable in two of these dogs. Survival times ranged from 6 days to 4 years; median survival was 3 months.[92] Another report documented a complete response for 22 months in a dog with this disease.[97] This low rate of response is consistent with responses in T-cell lymphoma of other sites in dogs (see Chapter 47).

REFERENCES

1. Madewell BR, Priester WA, Gillette EL, Snyder SP: Neoplasms of the nasal passages and paranasal sinuses in domesticated animals as reported by 13 veterinary colleges. *Am J Vet Res* 37:851–856, 1976.
2. Patnaik AK: Canine sinonasal neoplasms: Clinicopathological study of 285 cases. *JAAHA* 25:103–114, 1989
3. Norris AM: Intranasal neoplasms in the dog. *JAAHA* 15: 231–236, 1979.
4. Patnaik AK, Lieberman PH, Erlandson RA, Liu SK: Canine sinonasal skeletal eoplasms: Chondrosarcomas and osteosarcomas. *Vet Pathol* 21:475–482, 1984.
5. Patnaik AK, Ludwig LL, Erlandson RA: Neuroendocrine carcinoma of the nasopharynx in a dog. *Vet Pathol* 39:496–500, 2002.
6. Ginel PJ, Molleda JM, Novales M, et al: Primary transmissible venereal tumour in the nasal cavity of a dog. *Vet Rec* 136:222–223, 1995.
7. Hayes HM Jr, Wilson GP, Fraumeni HF Jr: Carcinoma of the nasal cavity and

paranasal sinuses in dogs: descriptive epidemiology. *Cornell Vet* 72:168–179, 1982.
8. Reif JS, Cohen D: The environmental distribution of canine respiratory tract neoplasms. *Arch Environ Health* 22:136–140, 1971
9. Reif JS, Bruns C, Lower KS: Cancer of the nasal cavity and paranasal sinuses and exposure to environmental tobacco smoke in pet dogs. *Am J Epidemiol* 147:488–492, 1998.
10. Bukowski JA, Wartenberg D, Goldschmidt M: Environmental causes for sinonasal cancers in pet dogs, and their usefulness as sentinels of indoor cancer risk. *J Toxicol Environ Health A* 54:579–591, 1998.
11. Smith MO, Turrel JM, Bailey CS, Cain GR: Neurological abnormalities as the predominant signs of neoplasia of the nasal cavity in dogs and cats: Seven cases (1973–1986). *JAVMA* 195:242–245, 1989.
12. Gibbs C, Lane JG, Denny HR: Radiological features of intra-nasal lesions in the dog: A review of 100 cases. *J Small Anim Pract* 20:515–535, 1979.
13. Harvey CE, Biery DN, Morello J, O'Brien JA: Chronic nasal disease in the dog: Its radiographic diagnosis. *Vet Radiol Ultrasound* 20:91–98, 1979.
14. Park RD, Beck ER, LeCouteur RA: Comparison of computed tomography and radiography for detecting changes induced by malignant nasal neoplasia in dogs. *JAVMA* 201:1720–1724, 1992.
15. Russo M, Lamb CR, Jakovljevic S: Distinguishing rhinitis and nasal neoplasia by radiography. *Vet Radiol Ultrasound* 41:118–124, 2000.
16. Henry CJ, Brewer WG Jr, Tyler JW, et al: Survival in dogs with nasal adenocarcinoma: 64 cases (1981–1995). *J Vet Intern Med* 12:436–439, 1998.
17. Theon AP, Madewell BR, Harb MF, Dungworth DL: Megavoltage irradiation of neoplasms of the nasal and paranasal cavities in 77 dogs. *JAVMA* 202:1469–1475, 1993
18. Northrup NC, Etue SM, Ruslander DM, et al: Retrospective study of orthovoltage radiation therapy for nasal tumors in 42 dogs. *J Vet Intern Med* 15:183–189, 2001.
19. Morris JS, Dunn KJ, Dobson JM, White RA: Radiological assessment of severity of canine nasal tumours and relationship with survival. *J Small Anim Pract* 37:1–6, 1996.
20. Thrall DE, Robertson ID, McLeod DA, et al: A comparison of radiographic and computed tomographic findings in 31 dogs with malignant nasal cavity tumors. *Vet Radiol* 30:59–66, 1989.
21. Voges AK, Ackerman N: MR evaluation of intra- and extracranial extension of nasal adenocarcinoma in a dog and cat. *Vet Radiol Ultrasound* 36:196–200, 1995.
22. Willard MD, Radlinsky MA: Endoscopic examination of the choanae in dogs and cats: 118 cases (1988–1998). *JAVMA* 215:1301–1305, 1999.
23. Clercx C, Wallon J, Gilbert S, et al: Imprint and brush cytology in the diagnosis of canine intranasal tumours. *J Small Anim Pract* 37:423–427, 1996.
24. Hahn KA, McGavin MD, Adams WH: Bilateral renal metastases of nasal chondrosarcoma in a dog. *Vet Pathol* 34:352–355, 1997.
25. Somae T, Minami T, Minami N, et al: Study on dissolution of cribriform plate in 13 dogs with squamous cell carcinoma in nasal cavity and therapeutic effects of radiation therapy. *Proc 22nd Annu Conf Vet Cancer Soc*:53, 2002.
26. Evans SM, Goldschmidt M, McKee LJ, Harvey CE: Prognostic factors and survival after radiotherapy for intranasal neoplasms in dogs: 70 cases (1974–1985). *JAVMA* 194:1460–1463, 1989.
27. Taylor K, Smith A, Brawner W, Higginbotham ML: Nasal sarcomas (1996–2004): A review of 20 dogs treated with megavoltage radiation therapy. *Proc 24th Annu Conf Vet Cancer Soc*:20, 2004.
28. Thrall DE, Harvey CE: Radiotherapy of malignant nasal tumors in 21 dogs. *JAVMA* 183:663–666, 1983.
29. Mellanby RJ, Stevenson RK, Herrtage ME, et al: Long-term outcome of 56 dogs with nasal tumours treated with four doses of radiation at intervals of seven days. *Vet Rec* 151:253–257, 2002.
30. Cohen M, Brawner WR, Henderson R, et al: Use of a soft tissue equivalent material inside the canine nasal cavity to maximize megavoltage dose distribution to the floor. *Proc 22nd Annu Conf Vet Cancer Soc*:18, 2002.
31. Adams WM, Withrow SJ, Walshaw R, et al: Radiotherapy of malignant nasal tumors in 67 dogs. *JAVMA* 191:311–315, 1987.
32. Roberts SM, Lavach JD, Severin GA, et al: Ophthalmic complications following megavoltage irradiation of the nasal and paranasal cavities in dogs. *JAVMA* 190:43–47, 1987.
33. Adams WM, Miller PE, Vail DM, et al: An accelerated technique for irradiation of malignant canine nasal and paranasal sinus tumors. *Vet Radiol Ultrasound* 39:475–481, 1998.
34. Thrall DE, McEntee MC, Novotney C, et al: A boost technique for irradiation of malignant canine nasal tumors. *Vet Radiol Ultrasound* 34:295–300, 1993.
35. LaDue TA, Dodge R, Page RL, et al: Factors influencing survival after radiotherapy of nasal tumors in 130 dogs. *Vet Radiol Ultrasound* 40:312–317, 1999.

36. Kleiter M, Kren G, Pangratz-Führer S, et al: Palliative röntgenbestrahlung nach turbinalienektomie bei zwei hunden mit nasalem chondrosarkom. *Tierarztl Prax* 30:355–360, 2002.
37. Kaser-Hotz B, Sumova A, Lomax A, et al: A comparison of normal tissue complication probability of brain for proton and photon therapy of canine nasal tumors. *Vet Radiol Ultrasound* 43:480–486, 2002.
38. Correa SS, Mauldin GN, Mauldin GE, Patnaik AK: Efficacy of cobalt-60 radiation therapy for the treatment of nasal cavity nonkeratinizing squamous cell carcinoma in the dog. *JAAHA* 39:86–89, 2003.
39. Lucroy MD, Long KR, Blaik MA, et al: Photodynamic therapy for the treatment of intranasal tumors in 3 dogs and 1 cat. *J Vet Intern Med* 17:727–729, 2003.
40. Hahn KA, Knapp DW, Richardson RC, Matlock CL: Clinical response of nasal adenocarcinoma to cisplatin chemotherapy in 11 dogs. *JAVMA* 200:355–357, 1992.
41. LaDue TA, Boshoven EW, Shaw N, Klein MK: Gemcitabine as a radiosensitizer for canine sinonasal carcinoma and feline oral squamous cell carcinoma. *Vet Radiol Ultrasound* 41:574, 2000.
42. Kleiter M, Malarkey DE, Ruslander DE, Thrall DE: Expression of cyclooxygenase-2 in canine epithelial nasal tumors. *Vet Radiol Ultrasound* 45:255–260, 2004.
43. Knapp DW, Richardson RC, Bottoms GD, et al: Phase I trial of piroxicam in 62 dogs bearing naturally occurring tumors. *Cancer Chemother Pharmacol* 29:214–218, 1992.
44. Husbands B, McNiel E, Larson V: Canine nasal carcinoma with piroxicam. *Proc 23rd Annu Conf Vet Cancer Soc*:47, 2003.
45. Langova V, Mutsaers AJ, Phillips B, Straw RC: Treatment of eight dogs with nasal tumours with alternating doses of doxorubicin and carboplatin in conjunction with oral piroxicam. *Aust Vet J* 82:676–680, 2004.
46. Lana SE, Dernell WS, LaRue SM, et al: Slow release cisplatin combined with radiation for the treatment of canine nasal tumors. *Vet Radiol Ultrasound* 38:474–478, 1997
47. Lana SE, Dernell WS, Lafferty MH, et al: Use of radiation and a slow-release cisplatin formulation for treatment of canine nasal tumors. *Vet Radiol Ultrasound* 45:577–581, 2004.
48. Carlisle CH, Biery DN, Thrall DE: Tracheal and laryngeal tumors in the dog and cat: Literature review and 13 additional patients. *Vet Radiol Ultrasound* 32:229–235, 1991.
49. Pass DA, Huxtable CR, Cooper BJ, et al: Canine laryngeal oncocytomas. *Vet Pathol* 17:672–677, 1980.
50. Liggett AD, Weiss R, Thomas KL: Canine laryngopharyngeal rhabdomyoma resembling an oncocytoma: Light microscopic, ultrastructural and comparative studies. *Vet Pathol* 22:526–532, 1985.
51. Meuten DJ, Calderwood Mays MB, Dillman RC, et al: Canine laryngeal rhabdomyoma. *Vet Pathol* 22:533–539, 1985.
52. Wheeldon EB, Suter PF, Jenkins T: Neoplasia of the larynx in the dog. *JAVMA* 180:642–647, 1982.
53. Saik JE, Toll SL, Diters RW, Goldschmidt MH: Canine and feline laryngeal neoplasia: A 10 year survey. *JAAHA* 22:359–365, 1986.
54. Bright RM, Gorman NT, Goring RL, Calderwood-Mays M: Laryngeal neoplasia in two dogs. *JAVMA* 184:738–740, 1984.
55. Flanders JA, Castleman W, Carberry CA, Tseng FS: Laryngeal chondrosarcoma in a dog. *JAVMA* 190:68–70, 1987.
56. Gibbs C: Radiographic examination of the pharynx, larynx and soft-tissue structures of the neck in dogs and cats. *Vet Annu* 26:227–241, 1986.
57. Rudorf H, Brown P: Ultrasonography of laryngeal masses in six cats and one dog. *Vet Radiol Ultrasound* 39:430–434, 1998.
58. Block G, Clarke K, Salisbury SK, DeNicola DB: Total laryngectomy and permanent tracheostomy for treatment of laryngeal rhabdomyosarcoma in a dog. *JAAHA* 31:510–513, 1995.
59. Harvey CE, O'Brien JA: Surgical treatments of miscellaneous laryngeal conditions in dogs and cats. *JAAHA* 18:557–562, 1982.
60. Clercx C, Desmecht D, Michiels L, et al: Laryngeal rhabdomyoma in a golden retriever. *Vet Rec* 143:196–198, 1998.
61. Henderson RA, Powers RD, Perry L: Development of hypoparathyroidism after excision of laryngeal rhabdomyosarcoma in a dog. *JAVMA* 198:639–643, 1991.
62. Crowe DT, Goodwin MA, Greene CE: Total laryngectomy for laryngeal mast cell tumor in a dog. *JAAHA* 22:809–816, 1986.
63. Chaffin K, Cross AR, Allen SW, et al: Extramedullary plasmacytoma in the trachea of a dog. *JAVMA* 212:1579–1581, 1998.
64. Ogilvie GK, Haschek WM, Withrow SJ, et al: Classification of primary lung tumors in dogs: 210 cases (1975–1985). *JAVMA* 195:106–108, 1989.
65. Hahn FF, Muggenburg BA, Griffith WC: Primary lung neoplasia in a beagle colony. *Vet Pathol* 33:633–638, 1996.

66. Dorn CR, Taylor DO, Schneider R, et al: Survey of animal neoplasms in Alameda and Contra Costa Counties, California. II. Cancer morbidity in dogs and cats from Alameda County. *J Natl Cancer Inst* 40:307–318, 1968.
67. Saegusa S, Yamamura H, Morita T, Hasegawa A: Pulmonary neuroendocrine carcinoma in a four-month-old dog. *J Comp Pathol* 111:439–443, 1994.
68. Ogilvie GK, Weigel RM, Haschek WM, et al: Prognostic factors for tumor remission and survival in dogs after surgery for primary lung tumor: 76 cases (1975–1985). *JAVMA* 195:109–112, 1989.
69. Nielsen SW, Horava A: Primary pulmonary tumors of the dog. A report of sixteen cases. *Am J Vet Res* 21:813–830, 1960.
70. Reif JS, Dunn K, Ogilivie GK, Harris CK: Passive smoking and canine lung cancer risk. *Am J Epidemiol* 135:234–239, 1992.
71. McNiel EA, Ogilvie GK, Powers BE, et al: Evaluation of prognostic factors for dogs with primary lung tumors: 67 cases (1985–1992). *JAVMA* 211:1422–1427, 1997.
72. Dallman MJ, Martin RA, Roth L: Pneumothorax as the primary problem in two cases of bronchioloalveolar carcinoma in the dog. *JAAHA* 24:710–714, 1988.
73. Puerto DA, Brockman DJ, Lindquist C, Drobatz K: Surgical and nonsurgical management of and selected risk factors for spontaneous pneumothorax in dogs: 64 cases (1986–1999). *JAVMA* 220:1670–1674, 2002.
74. Bailiff NL, Norris CR: Clinical signs, clinicopathological findings, etiology, and outcome associated with hemoptysis in dogs: 36 cases (1990–1999). *JAAHA* 38:125–133, 2002.
75. Madewell BR, Nyland TG, Weigel JE: Regression of hypertrophic osteopathy following pneumonectomy in a dog. *JAVMA* 172:818–821, 1978.
76. Mariani CL, Shelton SB, Alsup JC: Paraneoplastic polyneuropathy and subsequent recovery following tumor removal in a dog. *JAAHA* 35:302–305, 1999.
77. Sharkey LC, Rosol TJ, Grone A, et al: Production of granulocyte colony-stimulating factor and granulocyte-macrophage colony-stimulating factor by carcinomas in a dog and a cat with paraneoplastic leukocytosis. *J Vet Intern Med* 10:405–408, 1996.
78. Meinkoth JH, Rochat MC, Cowell RL: Metastatic carcinoma presenting as hindlimb lameness: Diagnosis by synovial fluid cytology. *JAAHA* 33:325–328, 1997.
79. Reichle JK, Wisner ER: Non-cardiac thoracic ultrasound in 75 feline and canine patients. *Vet Radiol Ultrasound* 41:154–162, 2000.
80. Paoloni MC, Dubielzig RR, O'Brien RT, et al: Use of CT imaging for lymph node assessment in dogs with primary lung tumors. *Proc 22nd Annu Conf Vet Cancer Soc*:37, 2002.
81. Tidwell AS, Johnson KL: Computed tomography-guided percutaneous biopsy in the dog and cat: Description of technique and preliminary evaluation in 14 patients. *Vet Radiol Ultrasound* 35:445–446, 1994.
82. Tidwell AS, Johnson KL: Computed tomography-guided percutaneous biopsy: Criteria for accurate needle tip identification. *Vet Radiol Ultrasound* 35:440–444, 1994.
83. Davies DR, Lucas J: *Actinomyces* infection in a dog with pulmonary carcinoma. *Aust Vet J* 81:132–135, 2003.
84. Mehlhaff CJ, Leifer CE, Patnaik AK, Schwarz PD: Surgical treatment of primary pulmonary neoplasia in 15 dogs. *JAAHA* 20:799–803, 1984.
85. Gressus JC, Debray B: Surgical treatment of a primary chondrosarcoma of the lung in a dog. *Pract Med Chirurgicale de L'animal Compagnie* 37:69–79, 2002.
86. Poulson JM, Vujaskovic Z, Gillette SM, et al: Volume and dose-response effects for severe symptomatic pneumonitis after fractionated irradiation of canine lung. *Int J Radiat Biol* 76:463–468, 2000.
87. de Boer WJ, Mehta DM, Timens W, Hoekstra HJ: The short and long term effects of intraoperative electron beam radiotherapy (IORT) on thoracic organs after pneumonectomy an experimental study in the canine model. *Int J Radiat Oncol Biol Phys* 45:501–506, 1999.
88. Hayata Y, Kato H, Konaka C, et al: Fiberoptic bronchoscopic photoradiation in experimentally induced canine lung cancer. *Cancer* 51:50–56, 1983.
89. Poirier VJ, Burgess KE, Adams WM, Vail DM: Toxicity, dosage, and efficacy of vinorelbine (Navelbine) in dogs with spontaneous neoplasia. *J Vet Intern Med* 18:536–539, 2004.
90. Baum B, Winkenwerder F, Nolte I, Hewicker-Trautwein M: Lymphomatoid granulomatosis in a borzoi. *Teirartzl Prax* 30:427–431, 2002.
91. Postorino NC, Wheeler SL, Park RD, et al: A syndrome resembling lymphomatoid granulomatosis in the dog. *J Vet Intern Med* 3:15–19, 1989.
92. Berry CR, Moore PF, Thomas WP, et al: Pulmonary lymphomatoid granulomatosis in seven dogs (1976–1987). *J Vet Intern Med* 4:157–166, 1990.
93. Fitzgerald SD, Wolf DC, Carlton WW: Eight cases of canine lymphomatoid granulomatosis. *Vet Pathol* 28:241–245, 1991.
94. Calvert CA, Mahaffey MB, Lappin MR, Farrell RL: Pulmonary and disseminated eosinophilic granulomatosis in dogs. *JAAHA* 24:311–320, 1988.
95. Moore PF: Utilization of cytoplasmic lysozyme immunoreactivity as a histiocytic marker in canine histiocytic disorders. *Vet Pathol* 23:757–762, 1986.
96. Smith KC, Day MJ, Shaw SC, et al: Canine lymphomatoid granulomatosis: An immunophenotypic analysis of three cases. *J Comp Pathol* 115:129–138, 1996.
97. McKay LW, Levy JK, Thompson MS: What is your diagnosis? Pulmonary lymphoma. *JAVMA* 224:1587–1588, 2004.

CARDIAC TUMORS
Antony S. Moore and Gregory K. Ogilvie

52

CLINICAL BRIEFING

Clinical factors	• Most common reasons for presentation are pericardial effusion and signs of cardiac failure. • Most common tumor type is hemangiosarcoma; next most common is chemodectoma. Other tumor types are rare.
Staging and diagnosis	• Minimal database (includes a complete blood count, biochemical profile, urinalysis, and thoracic radiography [three views]). • Cardiac ultrasonography and biopsy, which may require surgery.
Prognostic factors	• Pericardectomy improves survival for dogs with chemodectoma.
Treatment	
Initial	• Surgical removal of chemodectoma is difficult. • Carotid body tumors may be resected. • Surgery for hemangiosarcomas may provide short-term palliation; however, chemotherapy is recommended.
Adjunctive	• Chemotherapy (doxorubicin based) only reported for hemangiosarcoma.
Supportive	• Postoperative analgesia as needed. • Appetite stimulants and antinausea medications if chemotherapy used. • Nutritional support as required.

Tumors of the cardiovascular system are rare in dogs. Primary cardiac hemangiosarcoma is the most common tumor type and usually involves the right atrium, often in the auricular appendage.[1] Cardiac hemangiosarcoma is described in more detail in Chapter 56.

In a large series of 913 dogs with cardiac tumors and a histologic diagnosis, primary cardiac tumors were more common than metastatic lesions.[2] In that study, 56% of tumors were malignant and only 2% were benign; the rest were not specified. Hemangiosarcoma accounted for 69% of the lesions. The next most common diagnosis was aortic body tumor (8%). Lymphoma accounted for 4% of tumors and thyroid carcinoma for 1%.[2] The remaining tumors were other epithelial or mesenchymal tumors, often metastatic lesions from other sites in the body.[2,3] Theoretically, chemotherapy would be the best treatment for cardiac lymphoma, as described in Chapter 47.[4,5]

Benign cardiac masses were reported in two dogs (necrotic pericardial fat and a chronic cystic hematoma after trauma), but this condition is very rare.[6]

Chemodectoma

Chemodectoma is a term that encompasses aortic and carotid body tumors, both of which are uncommon in dogs. Other terms for these tumors are *extraadrenal* or *cardiac paraganglioma, glomus tumor,* and *heart-base tumor.*

Aortic Body Tumors
INCIDENCE, SIGNALMENT, AND ETIOLOGY

Most chemodectomas are aortic body tumors located at the heart base, usually between the pulmonary artery and ascending aorta.[1] Affected dogs are older (10–15 years of age). In one study, the risk of aortic body tumors rose until the age of 15 years and then declined.[2] Boxers and Boston terriers are predisposed,[7] although retriever breeds accounted for nearly half the dogs in one study.[8] Chronic hypoxemia is suspected of having a role in the etiology of aortic body tumors, which would explain the predisposition in brachycephalic breeds.[9] Male dogs are more likely to develop aortic body tumors; in one study, female intact dogs had the lowest incidence of aortic body tumors when compared with spayed females or all males.[2] It is possible that estrogens exert a protective effect.

CLINICAL PRESENTATION AND HISTORY

Aortic body tumors may be extremely large (up to 13 cm or more) and most commonly affect the heart base, but they

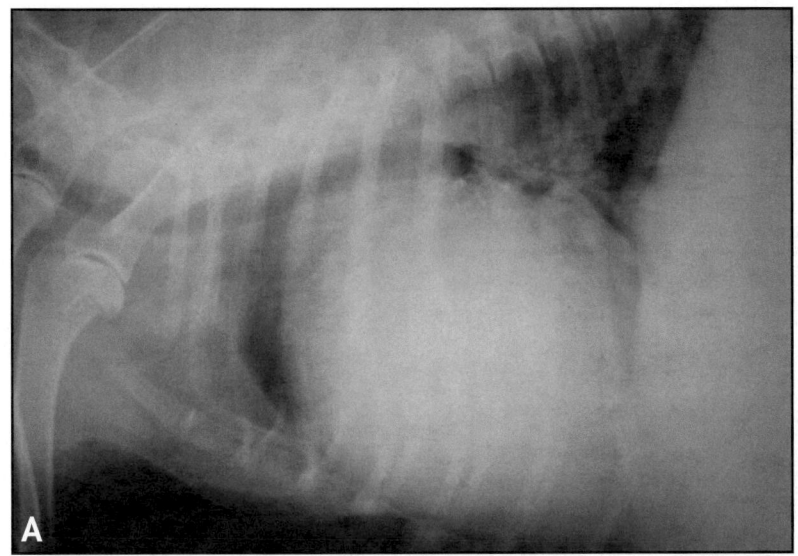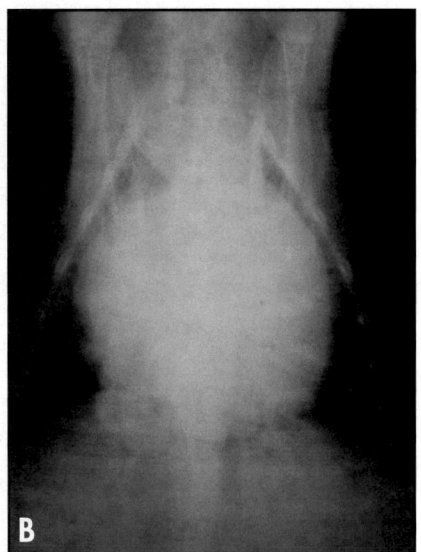

Figure 52-1. *Pericardial effusion has resulted in a radiographic globoid appearance of the heart in this dog with an aortic body tumor (**A** and **B**). (Courtesy of Nicole Northrup, DVM, University of Georgia College of Veterinary Medicine)*

STAGING AND DIAGNOSIS

Clinical signs associated with pericardial effusion may not allow the clinician to distinguish between neoplastic and nonneoplastic causes, and further imaging is required. Thoracic radiography may disclose a heart-base mass. Positive pericardiography may outline the mass more clearly,[12] although ultrasonography is less invasive and allows continued monitoring if therapy is undertaken.

On radiography, enlargement of the cardiac silhouette is seen in most dogs, with pulmonary edema and pleural effusion seen in nearly half the patients in one study[7] (Figure 52-1). On electrocardiography, electrical alternans (a sign of pericardial effusion) was seen in one-third of dogs. Echocardiography showed pericardial effusion in more than 80% of dogs, and more than half the dogs had cardiac tamponade[7] (Figures 52-2 and 52-3). Computed tomography (CT) is being used more commonly to evaluate the size of the primary tumor and to search for metastases.

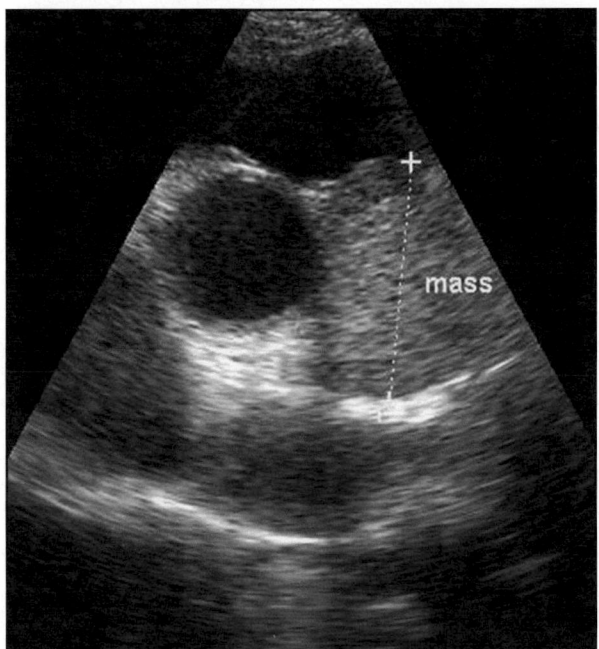

Figure 52-2. *A heart-base mass is easily visualized using echocardiography in this dog with an aortic body tumor. (Courtesy of Lenore A. Mohammadian, DVM, California Veterinary Specialists)*

> **Pericardial tamponade may be caused by a heart-base chemodectoma (aortic body tumor).**

can occasionally be found on the ventricle[10] or the mediastinum.[11] Aortic body tumors commonly cause signs of congestive heart failure. The most common signs in one study were abdominal distention and respiratory signs in nearly 50% of dogs, lethargy (40%), gastrointestinal signs (28%), weight loss (20%), and collapse (12%).[7] Pericardial fluid is a more common finding than peritoneal or pleural effusion.[7,8]

Malignant tumors are rare. When they occur, carcinomas are often larger than adenomas and may metastasize widely to the lungs, myocardium, liver, kidney, brain, and bone.[10] In one study, four of 24 dogs with aortic body tumors had pulmonary metastases at the time of diagnosis.[8] Local invasion by chemodectomas is common and may involve surrounding blood vessels. Local invasion into thoracic vertebrae has been reported.[13] Although studies have exam-

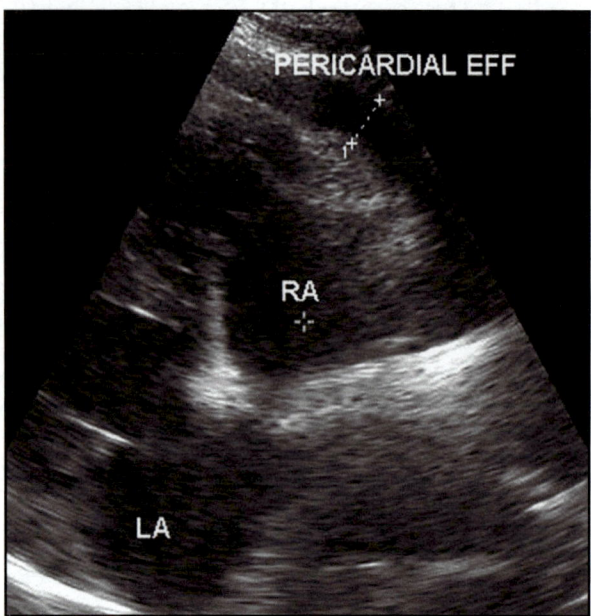

Figure 52-3. *Pericardial effusion can be clearly visualized in this dog with an aortic body tumor. (Courtesy of L. A. Mohammadian)*

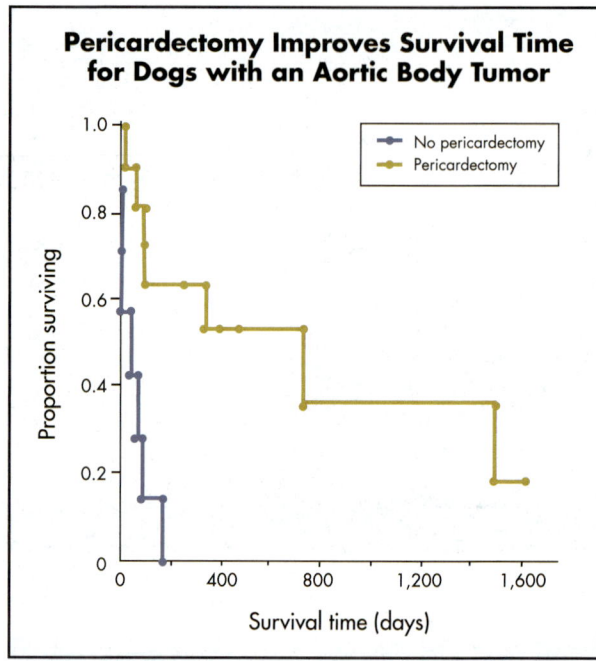

Figure 52-4. *Pericardectomy improves survival times for dogs with an aortic body tumor. (From Ehrhart N, Ehrhart EJ, Willis J, et al: Analysis of factors affecting survival in dogs with aortic body tumors. Vet Surg 31:44–48, 2002; with permission)*

ined the proliferative fraction in these tumors, no correlation with biologic behavior has been made.[11]

Canine chemodectoma seems to be associated with the presence of other endocrine tumors, such as pheochromocytoma. In one series of cases, thyroid tumors were present in 11 of 67 dogs with chemodectoma.[14]

TREATMENT

Treatment of aortic body tumors has rarely been described in animals. Surgery is difficult because of the invasive nature of these tumors. Complete resection of a chemodectoma of the ascending aorta was successful in one case report, and the dog was alive without evidence of disease 17 months after surgery.[12]

Pericardectomy has been described as a palliative procedure in dogs with aortic body tumors,[15] but it has recently been shown that there is a distinct survival advantage to this procedure. In one study, dogs treated with pericardectomy had a median survival time of 22 months compared with 4 months for dogs managed medically.[7] The difference was even more marked in another study, in which dogs treated with pericardectomy had a median survival of more than 2 years compared with less than 2 months for dogs not treated this way.[8] Survival was improved regardless of the presence of pericardial effusion (Figures 52-4 and 52-5).

KEY POINT

Pericardectomy improves survival in dogs with aortic body tumors, even in the absence of pericardial effusion.

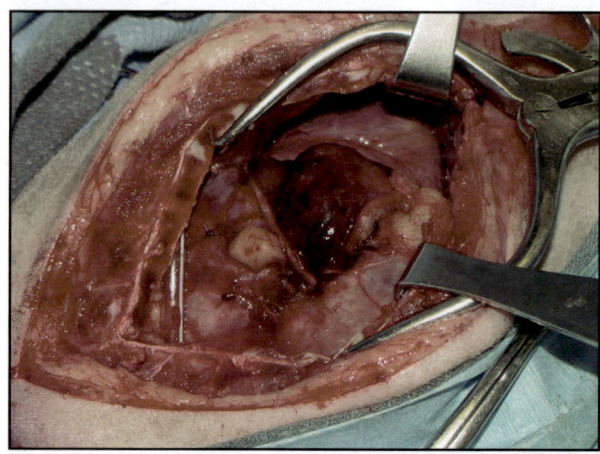

Figure 52-5. *Pericardectomy improves survival times for dogs with an aortic body tumor. (Courtesy of N. Northrup)*

Thoracoscopic partial pericardectomy has been described, but it is unclear whether this procedure confers the same survival benefit. It can relieve signs of pericardial effusion.[16]

Radiation therapy has been anecdotally recommended for aortic body tumors, but side effects (e.g., pneumonitis) may reduce its practicality.

Doxorubicin or platinum-based chemotherapy has been advocated by some; however, no data are available to document response to therapy.

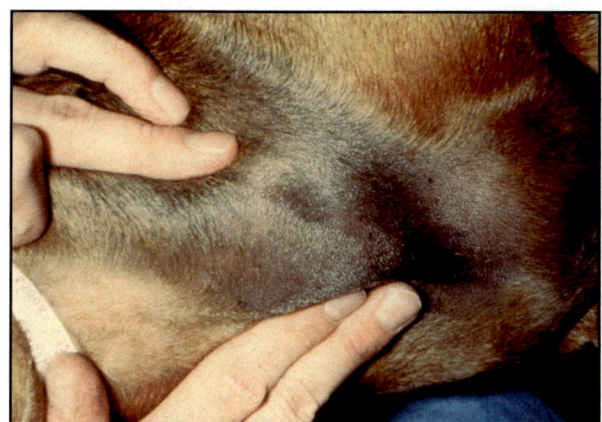

Figure 52-6. *A large palpable mass in the retropharyngeal area should be suspected of being a carotid body tumor. (Courtesy of John Berg, DVM, Tufts Cummings School of Veterinary Medicine)*

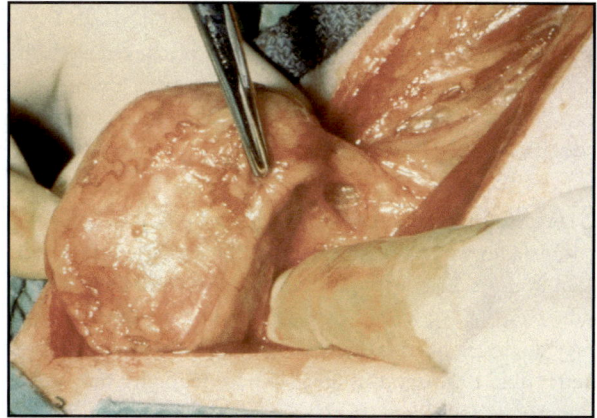

Figure 52-7. *At surgery for carotid body tumors, there is often considerable invasion of surrounding vasculature, making removal difficult (same tumor as in Figure 52-6). (Courtesy of J. Berg)*

Carotid Body Tumors
INCIDENCE, SIGNALMENT, AND ETIOLOGY

Carotid body tumors account for only 10% to 20% of chemodectomas.[9,14] There is no gender predilection reported for carotid body tumors. As for aortic body tumors, chronic hypoxemia is suspected of having a role in the etiology of carotid body tumors, and there is a predisposition for this tumor in brachycephalic breeds.[17]

CLINICAL PRESENTATION AND HISTORY

Dogs with carotid body tumors usually present with a palpable neck mass in the retropharyngeal area or just caudal to the angle of the jaw. They may also show dysphagia or dyspnea. Stridor and laryngeal paralysis have been described, presumably because of the locally invasive nature of this tumor.[18]

STAGING AND DIAGNOSIS

In one study, more than 40% of dogs with a carotid body tumor were found to have a concurrent aortic body tumor, which supports the contention that chronic hypoxemia has a role in the etiology of both tumor types.[17]

Metastases are common; early reports suggested that up to 30% of carotid body tumors may metastasize,[17,19] and more recent information suggests that up to 50% may metastasize when the local tumor is controlled.[18] Metastatic sites include the liver, mediastinum, brain, heart, and lungs. Two of 11 dogs had a concurrent mediastinal mass at diagnosis in one study.[18] Thoracic radiography and complete cardiac evaluation are recommended for dogs with a carotid body tumor.

Carotid body tumors may be imaged by ultrasonography before surgery to delineate margins and vessel involvement. Ultrasonography-guided fine-needle aspiration may be used to make a preoperative diagnosis. A CT scan may further delineate the tumor margins before surgical resection is attempted.[20] Carotid angiography was considered to be a useful preoperative imaging technique in one study because it clearly delineated the extent of the tumor.[18] Color-flow Doppler ultrasonography is also very effective in delineating the extent of the disease while quantifying the blood flow through the tumor.

TREATMENT

Mobile carotid body tumors in the neck may be amenable to successful surgical removal. In one series of 10 dogs with carotid body tumors, surgical excision was attempted, and perioperative mortality was 40%.[18] Postoperative Horner's syndrome and laryngeal paralysis were common in this series of dogs. Most tumors had invaded surrounding vessels. The more invasive tumors were associated with perioperative death or neurologic side effects (Figures 52-6 and 52-7). Four surviving dogs received no adjunctive treatment and survived a median of 25.5 months (range: 12–45 months); two dogs that received postoperative radiation therapy lived 6 and 27 months. Three of these six dogs died from distant metastases.

Cardiac Sarcomas
INCIDENCE, SIGNALMENT, AND ETIOLOGY

Cardiac sarcomas are rare. In a large study, they accounted for approximately 10% of cardiac tumors, with fibrosarcomas and rhabdomyosarcomas the most common diagnoses.[2] Rhabdomyomas, which have been reported less commonly, are often in a location that precludes treatment.[1,21] Chondrosarcoma has been reported.[22–24] Tumors may be of mixed histogenesis, showing areas of fibrosarcomatous, rhabdomyosarcomatous, liposarcomatous, and chondrosarcomatous differentiation.[25] A leiomyosarcoma of the pulmonary artery was described in one dog.[26]

CLINICAL PRESENTATION AND HISTORY

These tumors commonly cause signs of congestive heart failure such as abdominal distention (caused by ascites), exercise intolerance, and respiratory signs (e.g., dyspnea, cough).

STAGING AND DIAGNOSIS

On radiography, enlargement of the cardiac silhouette is seen in most dogs, with pulmonary edema and pleural effusion seen in nearly half of patients. Thoracic radiography may disclose a heart-base mass, although ultrasonography is better able to image this area. Ultrasonography may guide fine-needle aspiration to make a preoperative diagnosis.[22,27] CT or magnetic resonance imaging (MRI) may also be of value in imaging the tumor. Cardiac MRI is becoming a widely used tool in human cardiology.

Most tumors are malignant, although metastases may not be seen because most patients are euthanatized because of the primary tumor.[28] Most reports are of solitary tumors; occasionally, multiple masses are present.[29,30]

A pulmonary artery leiomyosarcoma that was shown on echocardiography to extend from the pulmonic valve along the pulmonary trunk to the left pulmonary artery was also found to have metastasized widely throughout the lung.[26]

TREATMENT

Treatment of cardiac sarcomas has rarely been described because the location and invasive nature of these tumors make surgery difficult. Pericardectomy was performed in one dog, but the ventricular mass, although pedunculated and outside the ventricular wall, was not resectable.[31] Atrial masses may benefit from atrial appendage removal as described for atrial hemangiosarcoma. In one dog that had a large, multilocular myxosarcoma within the pericardium, the mass was surgically excised from the left ventricular myocardium. Tumor recurrence with local metastasis was diagnosed 11 months after surgery when clinical signs of diarrhea and weight loss returned.[32] Removal of a myxosarcoma from the tricuspid valve in another dog was successful; however, the dog died in the perioperative period because of metastatic disease.[33]

REFERENCES

1. Girard C, Helie P, Odin M: Intrapericardial neoplasia in dogs. *J Vet Diagn Invest* 11:73–78, 1999.
2. Ware WA, Hopper DL: Cardiac tumors in dogs: 1982–1995. *J Vet Intern Med* 13:95–103, 1999.
3. Kirsch JA, Dhupa S, Cornell KK: Pericardial effusion associated with metastatic disease from an unknown primary tumor in a dog. *JAAHA* 36:121–124, 2000.
4. Ogilvie GK, Brunkow CS, Daniel GB, Haschek WM: Malignant lymphoma with cardiac and bone involvement in a dog. *JAVMA* 194:793–796, 1989.
5. MacGregor JM, Faria ML, Moore AS, et al: Primary cardiac lymphoma causing pericardial effusion in dogs: 12 cases (1997–2004). *JAVMA* 227:1449–1453, 2005.
6. Simpson DJ, Hunt GB, Church DB, Beck JA: Benign masses in the pericardium of two dogs. *Aust Vet J* 77:225–229, 1999.
7. Vicari ED, Brown DC, Holt DE, Brockman DJ: Survival times of and prognostic indicators for dogs with heart base masses: 25 cases (1986–1999). *JAVMA* 219:485–487, 2001.
8. Ehrhart N, Ehrhart EJ, Willis J, et al: Analysis of factors affecting survival in dogs with aortic body tumors. *Vet Surg* 31:44–48, 2002.
9. Hayes HM: An hypothesis for the aetiology of canine chemoreceptor system neoplasms, based upon an epidemiological study of 73 cases among hospital patients. *J Small Anim Pract* 16:337–343, 1975.
10. Cho KO, Park NY, Park IC, et al: Metastatic intracavitary cardiac aortic body tumor in a dog. *J Vet Med Sci* 60:1251–1253, 1998.
11. Brown PJ, Rema A, Gartner F: Immunohistochemical characteristics of canine aortic and carotid body tumours. *J Vet Med A Physiol Pathol Clin Med* 50:140–144, 2003.
12. Wykes PM, Rouse GP, Orton EC: Removal of five canine cardiac tumors using a stapling instrument. *Vet Surg* 15:103–106, 1986.
13. Blackmore J, Gorman NT, Kagan K, et al: Neurologic complications of a chemodectoma in a dog. *JAVMA* 184:475–478, 1984.
14. Patnaik AK, Liu SK, Hurvitz AI, McClelland AJ: Canine chemodectoma (extraadrenal paragangliomas)—A comparative study. *J Small Anim Pract* 16:785–801, 1975.
15. Kerstetter KK, Krahwinkel DJ Jr, Millis DL, Hahn K: Pericardiectomy in dogs: 22 cases (1978–1994). *JAVMA* 211:736–740, 1997.
16. Jackson J, Richter KP, Launer DP: Thoracoscopic partial pericardiectomy in 13 dogs. *J Vet Intern Med* 13:529–533, 1999.
17. Dean MJ, Strafuss AC: Carotid body tumors in the dog: A review and report of four cases. *JAVMA* 166:1003–1006, 1975.
18. Obradovich JE, Withrow SJ, Powers BE, Walshaw R: Carotid body tumors in the dog. Eleven cases (1978–1988). *J Vet Intern Med* 6:96–101, 1992.
19. Sander CH, Whitenack DL: Canine malignant carotid body tumor. *JAVMA* 156:606–610, 1970.
20. Fife W, Mattoon J, Drost WT, et al: Imaging features of a presumed carotid body tumor in a dog. *Vet Radiol Ultrasound* 44:322–325, 2003.
21. Mansfield CS, Callanan JJ, McAllister H: Intra-atrial rhabdomyoma causing chylopericardium and right-sided congestive heart failure in a dog. *Vet Rec* 147:264–267, 2000.
22. Albers TM, Alroy J, Garrod LA, et al: Histochemical and ultrastructural characterization of primary cardiac chondrosarcoma. *Vet Pathol* 34:150–151, 1997.
23. Greenlee PG, Liu SK: Chondrosarcoma of the mitral leaflet in a dog. *Vet Pathol* 21:540–542, 1984.
24. Southerland EM, Miller RT, Jones CL: Primary right atrial chondrosarcoma in a dog. *JAVMA* 203:1697–1698, 1993.
25. Machida N, Kobayashi M, Tanaka R, et al: Primary malignant mixed mesenchymal tumour of the heart in a dog. *J Comp Pathol* 128:71–74, 2003.
26. Callanan JJ, McCarthy GM, McAllister H: Primary pulmonary artery leiomyosarcoma in an adult dog. *Vet Pathol* 37:663–666, 2000.
27. Pérez J, Pérez-Rivero A, Montoya A, et al: Right-sided heart failure in a dog with primary cardiac rhabdomyosarcoma. *JAAHA* 34:208–211, 1998.
28. Briggs OM, Kirberger RM, Goldberg NB: Right atrial myxosarcoma in a dog. *J S Afr Vet Assoc* 68:144–146, 1997.
29. Krotje LJ, Ware WA, Niyo Y: Intracardiac rhabdomyosarcoma in a dog. *JAVMA* 197:368–371, 1990.
30. Camy G: Tumeur intracardiaque (rhabdomyosarcoma). *Pract Med Chirurgicale de L'animal Compagnie* 21:229–230, 1986.
31. Gonin-Jmaa D, Paulsen DB, Taboada J: Pericardial effusion in a dog with rhabdomyosarcoma in the right ventricular wall. *J Small Anim Pract* 37:193–196, 1996.
32. Foale RD, White RA, Harley R, Herrtage ME: Left ventricular myxosarcoma in a dog. *J Small Anim Pract* 44:503–507, 2003.
33. Machida N, Hoshi K, Kobayashi M, et al: Cardiac myxoma of the tricuspid valve in a dog. *J Comp Pathol* 129:320–324, 2003.

TUMORS OF THE GASTROINTESTINAL TRACT

Antony S. Moore and Gregory K. Ogilvie

CLINICAL BRIEFING

MDB (includes a CBC, biochemical profile, and urinalysis, and thoracic radiography [three views]).

Oral Tumors

Clinical factors
- Oral mass, halitosis, bleeding from the mouth, and dysphagia.
- Most common tumor types:
  — Benign: Fibromatous epulis, acanthomatous epulis (may invade bone; therefore, not strictly benign), ossifying epulis, giant-cell epulis.
    – Do not metastasize.
    – All ages.
  — Malignant:
    – Melanoma: High metastatic rate; older dogs.
    – SCC: Moderately metastatic; tonsillar SCC is highly metastatic; older dogs; locally invasive; oral papillary SCC in younger dogs.
    – Fibrosarcoma: Lower metastatic rate; younger dogs.

Staging and diagnosis
- MDB and lymph node assessment.
- Fine-detail radiography of affected area of mouth.
- CT if radiographs equivocal or if aggressive resection or radiation therapy planned.
- Metastatic rates as above.

Prognostic factors
All tumor types
- Small tumors and rostral location have a better prognosis.

SCC
- Dogs with maxillary tumors and young dogs have a better prognosis.
- Tonsillar location carries a poor prognosis.

Treatment
Initial
- Surgery.
- Local excision may be curative for epulides.
- Mandibulectomy or maxillectomy for local control of malignant tumors and acanthomatous epulis.

Adjunctive
- Radiation therapy:
  — Curative for acanthomatous epulis.
  — Coarse fractionation may be useful for melanoma.
  — Adjunctive for SCC and fibrosarcoma gives good control.
- Chemotherapy:
  — Platinum compounds best for melanoma but still have low efficacy.
  — Chemotherapy not usually required for other tumor types.
  — Cisplatin, mitoxantrone, and piroxicam may be effective for SCC.

Treatment *(cont.)*	
Supportive	• Pain relief after surgery. • Consider feeding tube for dogs with extensive oral surgery or radiation therapy.
Salivary Gland Tumors	
Clinical factors	• Cervical mass may cause anorexia or dysphagia. • Adenocarcinoma most common. • May be diffuse oral tumor rather than a mass. • Older animals affected.
Staging and diagnosis	• MDB. • Consider ultrasonography of accessible glands. • Assessment of tumor size and lymph nodes.
Prognostic factors	• Metastases confer a worse prognosis.
Treatment	
Initial	• Surgery alone • High rate of local recurrence.
Adjunctive	• Radiation therapy as an adjunct to surgery seems to improve local control.
Supportive	• Pain relief after surgery. • Consider feeding tube for dogs with extensive surgery or radiation therapy.
Stomach Tumors	
Clinical factors	• Chronic vomiting, weight loss, and inappetence because tumors cause ulceration. • Adenocarcinoma; less commonly, leiomyoma; most common in lower two-thirds of stomach. • Older male dogs.
Staging and diagnosis	• MDB. • Assessment of tumor size and lymph nodes using abdominal ultrasonography. • Abdominal ultrasonography to guide biopsy. • Commonly metastasize to perigastric lymph nodes or viscera.
Prognostic factors	• None identified. • Prognosis is generally poor.
Treatment	
Initial	• Tumors are usually diffuse and have metastasized at the time of diagnosis; therefore, aggressive surgery is rarely successful. • No reports of other therapies.
Supportive	• Pain and antinausea medications and fluid and nutritional support mandatory if treatment attempted. • Parenteral feeding or jejunostomy tube placement should be considered.

Intestinal Tumors

Clinical factors	• Signs: — Duodenum–jejunum: Vomiting, melena, weight loss. — Jejunum–ileum: Weight loss and diarrhea. — Colon–rectum: Tenesmus and hematochezia. • Adenocarcinoma. • Less commonly, leiomyosarcoma and lymphoma. • Leiomyosarcoma common in the cecum.
Staging and diagnosis	• MDB. • Abdominal ultrasonography to guide biopsy. • Adenocarcinoma more likely to metastasize than leiomyosarcoma, usually to regional lymph nodes.
Prognostic factors	
Small intestine	• Metastases of both carcinomas and leiomyosarcomas are worse.
Colorectal	• Dogs with annular lesions have poor survival times. • Other types of lesions have a better prognosis.
Treatment	
Initial	• Surgery: — Small intestine: Median survival for adenocarcinoma: 10 months; for leiomyosarcoma: 12 months. — Large intestine: Median survival for colorectal adenocarcinom: 15 months; for leiomyosarcoma: >1 year. • Radiation therapy: — Rectal adenocarcinoma may be controlled by high-dose fractions. — Median control: 6 months. • Cryotherapy: — Small, minimally invasive tumors of the rectum and distal colon.
Adjunctive	• Chemotherapy may delay metastases, but few reports; doxorubicin is investigational.
Supportive	• Pain and antinausea medications, and fluid and nutritional support mandatory after surgery. • Parenteral feeding or feeding tube placement should be considered postoperatively.

Adenocarcinoma of the Anal Sac

Clinical factors	• Tumors cause dyschezia, perianal mass, and polyuria and polydipsia attributable to hypercalcemia. • Older dogs. • Production of parathyroid hormone–like hormone causes hypercalcemia.
Staging and diagnosis	• MDB. • Abdominal ultrasonography to assess iliac lymph nodes. • Metastasis to regional lymph nodes is common and occurs early.

Prognostic factors	• Dogs with tumor size >10 cm² have shorter survival times. • Dogs with detectable lung metastases have shorter survival times. • Dogs with hypercalcemia have shorter survival times.
Treatment	
Initial	• Surgery usually resolves hypercalcemia. • Consider excision of sublumbar lymph nodes in addition to local excision of tumor.
Adjunctive	• Radiation therapy to regional nodes may delay metastases. • Chemotherapy with platinum derivatives, doxorubicin, mitoxantrone may be active. • Best treatment combination of surgery, radiation, and chemotherapy. • Median survival: 26 months.
Supportive	• Treatment of hypercalcemia before surgery. • Pain medication after surgery. • Nutritional support as needed. • Stool softeners if obstructed.

Oral Tumors

Before obtaining a biopsy or attempting surgical resection of an oral tumor, the veterinarian should confirm the patient's general good health with a minimum database (MDB), including blood work and urinalysis. Thoracic radiographs should be obtained to rule out macroscopic pulmonary metastases. Fine-detail radiographs of the affected area, including the dental arcade, can provide information on the aggressiveness of the tumor,[1] although computed tomography (CT) more accurately delineates bone involvement. Any local lymphadenopathy should be further investigated by fine-needle aspiration or biopsy performed at the same time as tumor biopsy.

The first surgical excision is the most likely to result in tumor control. The tumor should not be scraped or peeled from underlying bone because these actions ensure recurrence and enlarge the tumor bed. A definitive aggressive first surgery, such as maxillectomy or mandibulectomy, should be performed. Careful planning using CT imaging, radiation planning, and wide margins is required for radiation therapy.

EPULIDES
Incidence, Signalment, and Etiology

Despite their clinical appearance, epulides are intimately related to the dental arcade. There are three types: fibromatous and ossifying, which are benign, and acanthomatous, which arise from the periodontal ligament and may act aggressively by destroying bone and surrounding tissue. Giant-cell epulides are rare and less invasive than acanthomatous epulides. Acanthomatous epulis is also called *adamantinoma* and *ameloblastoma*, although ameloblastoma may be a distinct tumor in young dogs.[2]

Epulides affect both genders at equal rates.[3-5] Most affected dogs are middle aged, but the age range is wide, and epulides have been documented in dogs as young as 1 year and as old as 15 years. Younger dogs are more likely to have an acanthomatous epulis.[6] There is no difference in the signalment of any of the different types of epulides, with the exception that Shetland sheepdogs accounted for nearly 40% of dogs with acanthomatous epulis in one Japanese study.[6] Although boxers may be predisposed to developing gingival hyperplasia, this breed does not seem to be at excessive risk for developing epulides.[3]

One study found that dental plaque deposition was common in dogs with fibromatous and ossifying (but not acanthomatous) epulides; approximately half the affected dogs had severe dental tartar, and another 30% had moderate dental tartar.[6] Poor oral hygiene may be a predisposing factor for these tumors.

Clinical Presentation and History

Fibromatous and ossifying epulides are slow-growing, discrete masses that rarely exceed 2 cm in diameter. They are firm gingival tumors covered by oral epithelium. They may be single or multiple but are always discrete and located near teeth, particularly the premolars; they are most common in the maxilla. Ossifying epulides differ from fibromatous epulides only in osteoid production (Figure 53-1).[3,6]

Acanthomatous epulis is a more rapidly progressive tumor that has a high epithelial component and infiltrates readily into bone (Figure 53-2). It is usually found in the mandible, particularly around the canine teeth (Table 53-1).

As with other oral tumors, the most common signs are drooling, halitosis, and (occasionally) dysphagia.

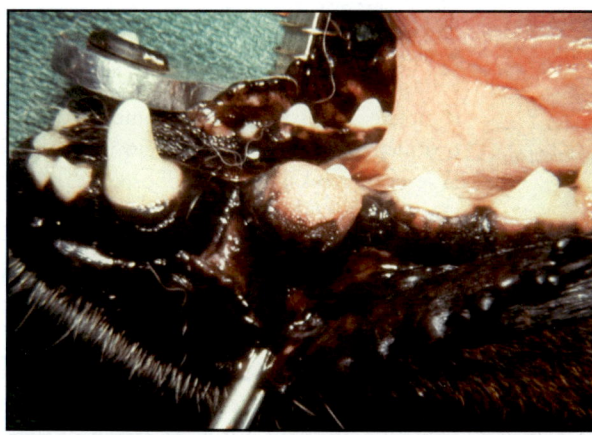

Figure 53-1. *Epulides, such as this fibromatous epulis in a 7-year-old dog, may be adequately excised by local surgical excision at the level of the gingiva, but regrowth is possible. (Courtesy of Gordon H. Theilen, DVM, University of California, Davis)*

Staging and Diagnosis

Staging should be performed as outlined in the Clinical Briefing. The proliferative capacity of acanthomatous epulides is more like a malignancy,[7] although metastases have not been reported. Thoracic radiographs should be obtained in any dog with an oral neoplasm as part of an MDB and before biopsy. Fibromatous and ossifying epulides are not invasive; therefore, high-detail radiographs of the affected bone are unlikely to identify changes in bone. Such radiographs may be helpful in assessing the degree of bony destruction caused by acanthomatous epulides. In one series of 39 dogs with an acanthomatous epulis, radiographic changes in bone were primarily osteolytic in 23 dogs and osteoblastic in eight dogs.[4]

Radiography should not be relied on for surgical margins because more than 50% of the bone must be replaced by tumor before lysis is evident radiographically. CT is a more accurate method of delineating the margins of tumor involvement and allows planning of surgery or radiation therapy. Technetium-99 nuclide scans tend to overestimate tumor margins by imaging peripheral reactive bone.

Caudally located tumors have been found to be larger than more rostrally located tumors, and larger tumors are more likely to recur.[8] This finding emphasizes the importance of instructing clients on good oral examination technique as part of preventive medicine.

Prognostic Factors

In one study, dogs younger than 8 years with acanthomatous epulides treated by radiation had a longer survival (median: 6 years) than older dogs (median: 3 years).[9]

Treatment

Local excision of a fibromatous or ossifying epulis may be all that is required. In one study, 104 dogs with fibromatous

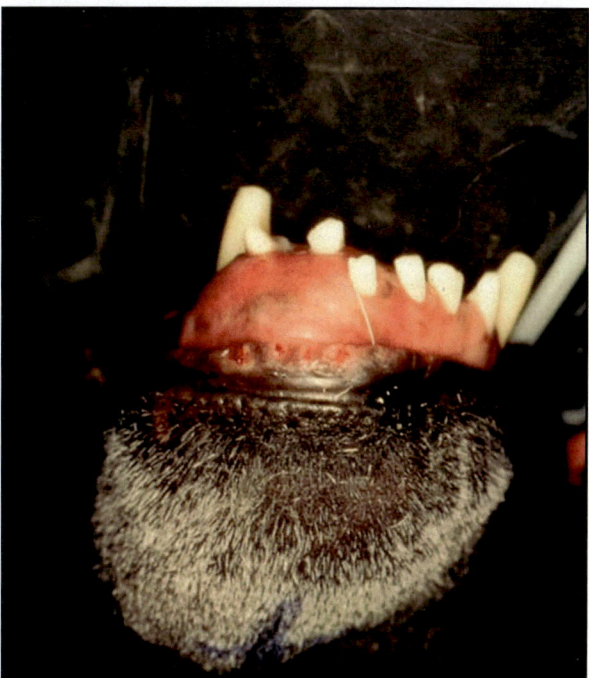

Figure 53-2. *Acanthomatous epulis is an invasive tumor that should not be considered benign. Note the displacement of incisors caused by mandibular invasion in this dog. Aggressive surgery or radiation is needed to control this tumor.*

epulides were treated by marginal excision; six dogs had a slow-growing recurrence between 6 and 7 months after surgery.[6] Similarly, 44 dogs with ossifying epulides had a simple excision, and four epulides recurred within 3 months. The rest of the dogs had no recurrence 1 year after surgery. In another study, one of eight dogs with fibromatous epulis had a recurrence after radiation therapy.[8]

Local gingival excision of acanthomatous epulides is rarely curative because these tumors arise from the periodontal ligament and therefore readily regrow from subgingival tumor tissue in the tooth socket. Of 23 dogs with a marginal excision, the tumor recurred in 21 (91%) within 1 month.[6] The

> *Epulides arise from the periodontal ligament; therefore, excision of an acanthomatous epulis at the level of the gingiva is incomplete, and the tumor will recur.*

excision is curative if surgical margins include the affected tooth root, as with mandibulectomy or maxillectomy. Wide surgical margins that include a section of normal bone encompassing the tooth root should be curative for small acanthomatous epulides. In a series of 37 dogs treated with aggressive surgery for acanthomatous epulis, only one had

Table 53-1 Distribution of 73 Acanthomatous and 151 Fibromatous or Ossifying Epulides in Relation to Dental Groupings[4,6]

Location	Acanthomatous		Fibromatous or Ossifying	
	Maxilla (n)	Mandible (n)	Maxilla (n)	Mandible (n)
Incisor	4	18	14	11
Canine	6	27	13	11
Premolar	3	4	65	17
Molar	3	8	13	7

local recurrence; all lived more than 1 year.[10] Adequate margins may be difficult to obtain for larger tumors.

Early reports indicated that long-term control of acanthomatous epulis could be achieved with adequate doses of radiation therapy.[11] In an early series of 39 dogs treated with orthovoltage radiation therapy instead of surgery, 27 dogs achieved a complete remission.[4] Tumors in the other dogs shrank or remained stable. Regrowth occurred in only three dogs at 8, 18, and 24 months after radiation, and two of these dogs responded to reirradiation. Overall median survival was 37 months. Malignant transformation, presumably as a consequence of radiation therapy, occurred in seven of the 39 dogs in this study and in two other dogs at a median of 47 months after radiation.[4,12] Malignant transformation and osteonecrosis are possible adverse effects of orthovoltage radiation. In another series of 39 dogs with

> **KEY POINT**
> *Wide surgical excision and radiation therapy have high cure rates for acanthomatous epulides in dogs.*

acanthomatous epulis, 85% were still free of tumor 1 year after cobalt-60 (^{60}Co) radiation therapy and 80% were free of tumor 3 years after treatment.[8] Tumor location within the oral cavity and bone involvement had no effect on outcome.

In two studies totaling 104 dogs with epulides treated with radiation therapy, malignant transformation was seen in four dogs (3.8%), with sarcomas occurring more than 5 years after treatment.[8,9]

Treatment of acanthomatous epulis should take into account the risks of recurrence and malignant transformation. Surgery may be the prudent treatment of choice in young dogs because of the risk, albeit low, of radiation-induced tumorigenesis. For old dogs, radiation preserves the normal oral architecture and may be better tolerated than surgery, and the low risk of new tumor induction is unlikely to affect longevity.

Chemotherapy is rarely warranted because systemic spread has not been reported for any epulis. In one young dog, an acanthomatous epulis recurred 6 weeks after treatment with 50 Gy of orthovoltage radiation therapy. This dog had almost complete regression of the tumor after 10 treatment courses of doxorubicin (30 mg/m^2 IV every 3 weeks) and cyclophosphamide (50 mg/m^2 PO q24h for 4 days every week) and remained stable for 20 months after starting chemotherapy.[5]

If access to radiation therapy is limited, intralesional chemotherapy may provide local control of acanthomatous epulides that cannot be resected. In one study, intralesional bleomycin (5 mg/dose) was used weekly to treat four dogs with acanthomatous epulis. Complete regression was seen in three dogs after six to 10 injections, and there was no recurrence 1 to 2 years later. The fourth dog had a partial response (PR) but was lost to follow up.[13]

Cryosurgery has been used for treatment of epulides, but recurrence is common, presumably because of poor ability to freeze bone and the restricted periodontal space.[14] This modality should not be used if it will delay more definitive treatments.

Ameloblastomas are seen in young dogs. Although they arise from odontogenic tissue, they are distinct from acanthomatous epulides. Two dogs younger than 1 year of age with ameloblastoma were treated with surgery; tumors recurred in both dogs within 6 months. A second surgery resulted in a cure for one dog, with no recurrence 9.5 years after surgery.[2]

Calcifying epithelial odontogenic tumors are rare in dogs but are probably benign. Recurrence may be seen after localized resection, but one dog treated by hemimandibulectomy had no recurrence 1 year later.[15]

MALIGNANT ORAL TUMORS

Surveys conducted in several countries have found that the most common malignant neoplasm in the canine oral cavity is melanoma (208 of 598 dogs; 35%).[16-18] The next most common is squamous cell carcinoma (SCC) (148 dogs; 25%), and fibrosarcoma is the third most common (95 dogs; 16%). Other tumors encountered include osteosarcomas and nerve sheath tumors (see Chapters 61 and 62).

SURGERY FOR MALIGNANT ORAL TUMORS

Surgery, including maxillectomy and mandibulectomy, is often described for oral tumors without discrimination of the histologic type. When possible, information on specific tumor types is provided below, but some observations about oral surgery are generally applicable.

Incomplete surgical resection is commonly associated with recurrence; therefore, making an early diagnosis and

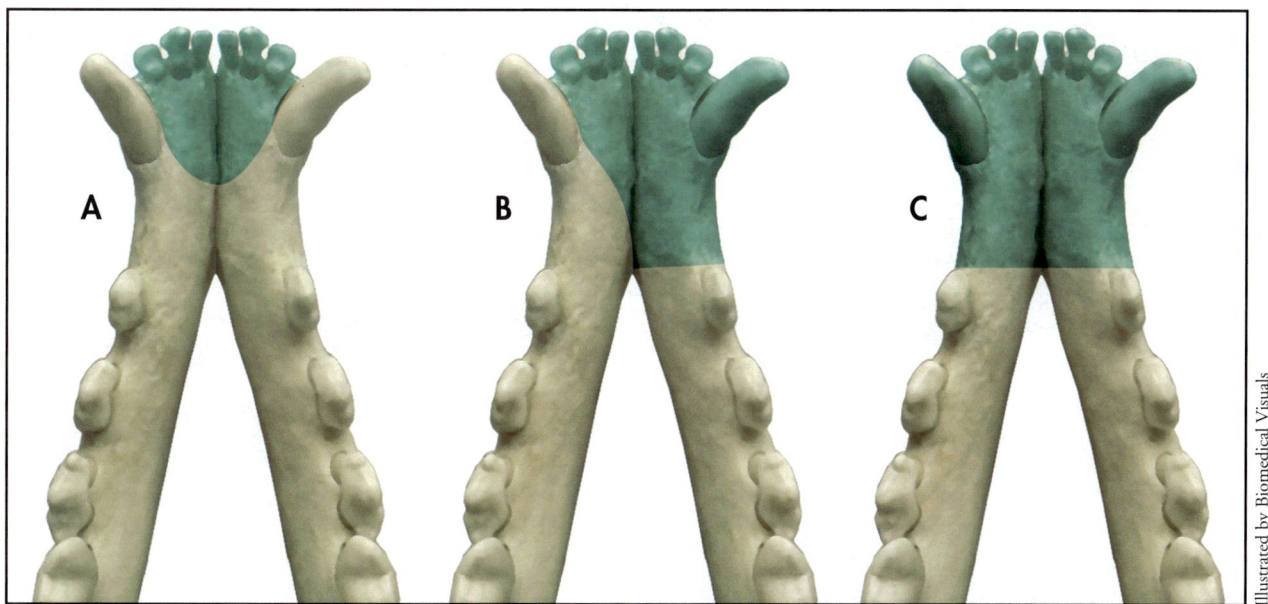

Figure 53-3. *Procedures for rostral mandibulectomy in dogs.* **(A)** *Partial,* **(B)** *unilateral, and* **(C)** *bilateral. (Adapted from White RA: Mandibulectomy and maxillectomy in the dog: Long term survival in 100 cases.* J Small Anim Pract *32:69–74, 1991; with permission)*

obtaining wide surgical margins by mandibulectomy or maxillectomy at the first surgery are very important. In one study, 65% of oral tumors treated by maxillectomy with incomplete margins recurred compared with 22% of tumors with complete histologic margins.[19] Similarly, 62% of oral tumors treated by mandibulectomy with incomplete margins recurred compared with 15% of tumors with complete histologic margins.[20]

Techniques for mandibulectomy and maxillectomy have been described in detail in surgical texts, and specific descriptions are beyond the scope of this book; however, schematic diagrams of oral surgeries are found in Figures 53-3 to 53-5. Pictures of dogs that have been treated with mandibulectomy or maxillectomy are found in Figures 53-6 to 53-9. A recent report of a technique for resection of tumors affecting the caudal maxilla (a difficult place to obtain clear surgical margins) found that more than 70% of resections had clear margins.[21] Although half of the tumors recurred, the median time to recurrence was 2 years. Another study described in detail an aggressive rostral maxillectomy and nasal planectomy in six dogs.[22] Complications included dehiscence, second surgery to enlarge the nasal orifice, hand feeding for 3 weeks after surgery, and lip reconstruction, each in one dog. Although the treatment was cosmetically aggressive, the appearance was acceptable to all owners (Figure 53-9).

The mandibular lymph nodes are regularly assessed when examining a dog with an oral tumor; however, metastases may involve other lymph nodes in the neck without involving the mandibular nodes. A single surgical approach was described that allowed biopsy of ipsilateral parotid, mandibular, and medial retropharyngeal lymph nodes.[23] Lymph nodes (parotid and medial retropharyngeal) that would have been difficult to evaluate by fine-needle aspiration provided useful diagnostic and prognostic information. The surgeon should also be aware that lymphatic drainage from the cranial mandible is commonly bilateral to mandibular nodes on both sides of the neck.[24]

Owner satisfaction with aggressive oral surgery remains a concern. A telephone survey of the caregivers of 27 dogs with oral tumors that had been treated with rostral mandibulectomy (nine dogs), partial mandibulectomy (seven dogs), or partial maxillectomy (11 dogs) assessed satisfaction with the respective surgical procedure.[25] Overall, 85% of owners were pleased with their decision to treat their dog, and the longer the dog lived afterward, the more likely the caregiver was to be satisfied. Although difficulty in eating was noted in 44% of the dogs (most commonly after maxillectomy; 64%), pain was thought to be less in most animals after surgery. All clients found the cosmetic appearance of their dog acceptable after facial hair regrew. The quality of the pet's life was perceived by the owner to be most improved after rostral mandibulectomy (100%) and least improved after partial mandibulectomy. Similar good reports came from owners of dogs in another study.[26]

ORAL MALIGNANT MELANOMA
Incidence, Signalment, and Etiology

Oral melanoma is the most common oral malignancy in dogs. Unlike cutaneous melanomas, which are often

432 MANAGING THE CANINE CANCER PATIENT

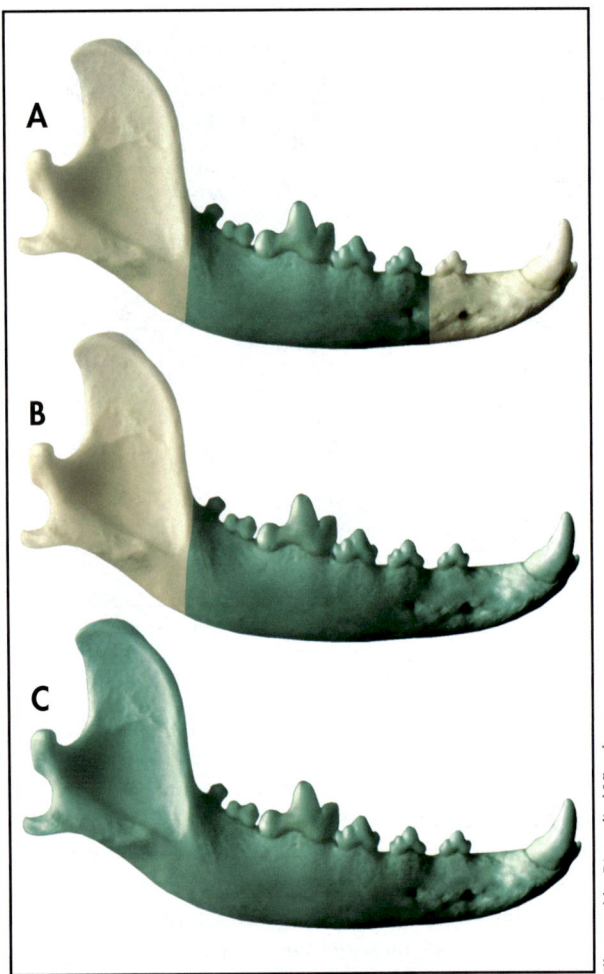

Figure 53-4. *Procedures for hemimandibulectomy in dogs. (**A**) Partial horizontal, (**B**) complete horizontal, and (**C**) total. (Adapted from White RA: Mandibulectomy and maxillectomy in the dog: Long term survival in 100 cases.* J Small Anim Pract 32:69–74, 1991; with permission)

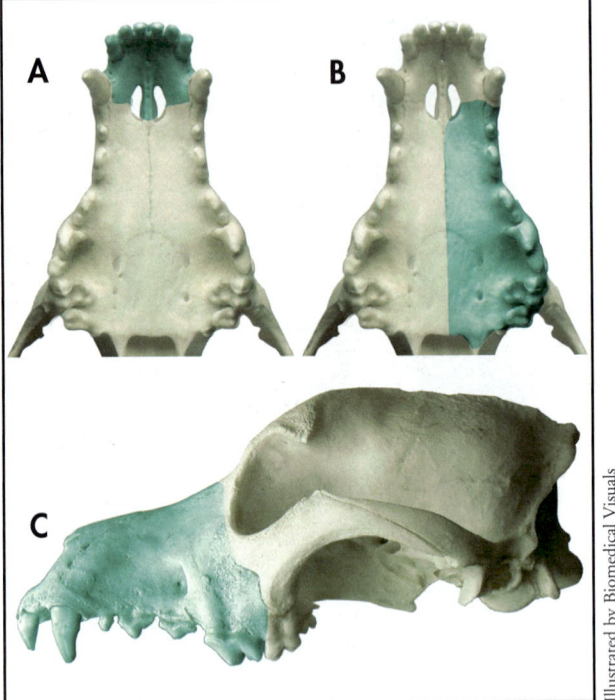

Figure 53-5. *Procedures for partial maxillectomy in dogs. (**A**) Rostral, (**B**) oral, and (**C**) nasal. (Adapted from White RA: Mandibulectomy and maxillectomy in the dog: Long term survival in 100 cases.* J Small Anim Pract 32:69–74, 1991; with permission)

benign, melanomas of the canine oral cavity are uniformly malignant. Oral melanomas are considered in detail in Chapter 54.

ORAL SQUAMOUS CELL CARCINOMA
Incidence, Signalment, and Etiology

SCC is the second most common oral malignancy in dogs. It is usually found in the gingival tissue. SCCs of the tongue and tonsils are addressed separately below. Tumors of the tonsil behave very differently from other SCCs.

SCC usually occurs in older dogs; the average age is 9 years.[20,27,28] There is no apparent breed or gender predilection. One study of SCC of the tongue found that 43% of affected dogs had a white haircoat and 30% were poodles.[29] This finding has not been corroborated. Papillary SCC occurs in dogs as young as 2 months.[30] Papillary SCC is a progressive disease with a high rate of lytic bone involvement and a low rate of metastasis.

Clinical Presentation and History

Most oral SCCs are rostral within the mouth; most occur in the maxilla (Table 53-2).[28] As with other oral tumors, the most common signs are drooling, halitosis, and (occasionally) dysphagia. Most dogs have shown signs for 3 months or less, but some dogs may show signs for 6 months to 1 year before diagnosis.

Staging and Diagnosis

As with most oral tumors, biopsy is required to differentiate SCC from amelanotic melanoma, ulcerated fibrosarcoma, and less common tumors (Figure 53-10). Staging should be performed as outlined in the Clinical Briefing. The size of the tumor is one of the most important prognostic factors.

SCC is highly invasive; high-detail radiographs of the skull often reveal extensive bony lysis.[29] However, bony lysis alone underestimates tumor size and should not be relied on for surgical margins or radiotherapy field size. CT scanning is recommended, particularly if radiation therapy is planned.

Metastasis of gingival SCC is uncommon, and metastasis to the lungs at the time of diagnosis is rare.[31] Regional lymph

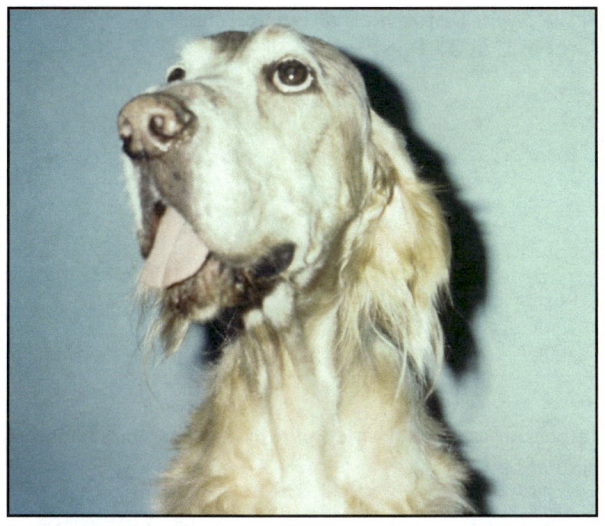

Figure 53-6. *This dog has been treated with a bilateral rostral mandibulectomy. When the dog is excited or hot, the tongue may protrude, but eating is normal, and quality of life is excellent.*

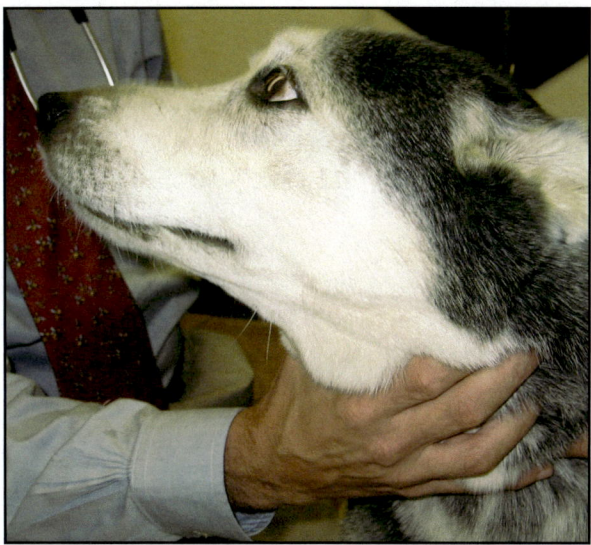

Figure 53-7. *This dog has been treated with a unilateral segmental mandibulectomy, resulting in a desired normal appearance.*

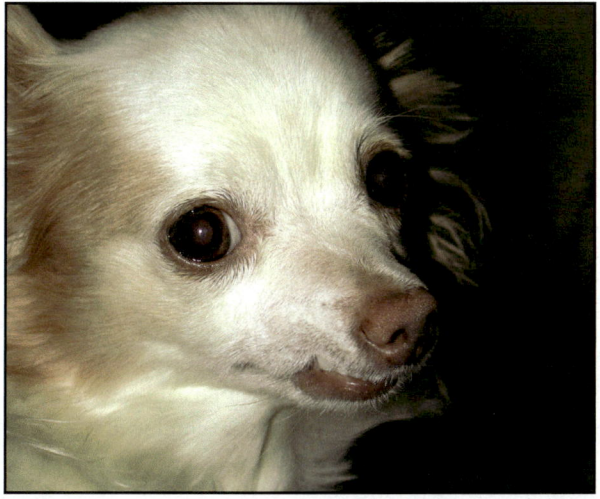

Figure 53-8. *This dog has been treated with a maxillectomy cranial to premolar 1 for an oral SCC. Cosmetics are only moderately affected, and function returns to normal soon after surgery.*

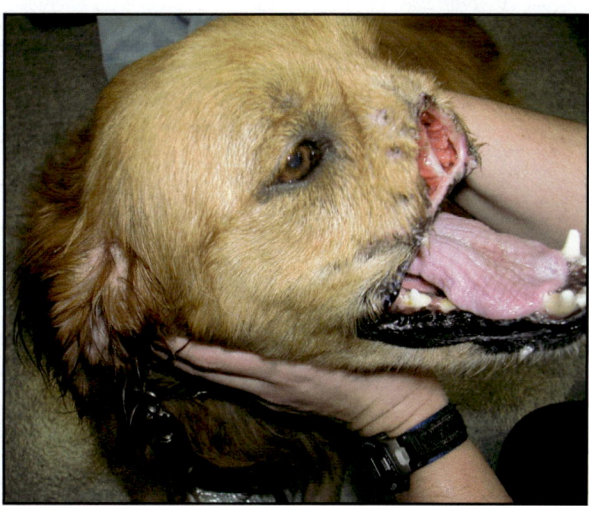

Figure 53-9. *This dog was treated for a fibrosarcoma with a caudal maxillectomy. Cosmetics are an issue, but after healing and hair regrowth, caregivers and dogs tolerate this procedure well.*

nodes are frequently enlarged at diagnosis and should be biopsied for cytology or histopathology; however, they usually do not contain metastases. In one study, 11 of 33 dogs had lymphadenopathy, and only three of these dogs had metastatic disease.[28] After therapy, regional lymph node metastasis was documented in six of 63 dogs (10%) in five case series.[19,20,27,32,33] Seven of 39 dogs developed distant metastases in another study.[32]

Prognostic Factors

In one report, dogs with maxillary tumors had a longer average response to radiation therapy (12 months) than did dogs with mandibular tumors (3.4 months) or soft tissue tumors (1.8 months).[28] In the same study, survival was influenced by tumor position within the oral cavity, radiation field size, and age of the dog. Eight dogs that were younger than 6 years lived for a median of 58 months after radiation; older dogs lived for a median of 6 months.[28] Similarly, another study of 14 dogs found younger dogs (<9 years of age) had longer disease-free periods and longer survival time than older dogs (15 and 35 months versus 7 and 10 months, respectively).[34]

Dogs with rostrally located tumors live longer than dogs with caudal tumors; dogs with tumors that extend both rostrally and caudally have significantly shorter survival times

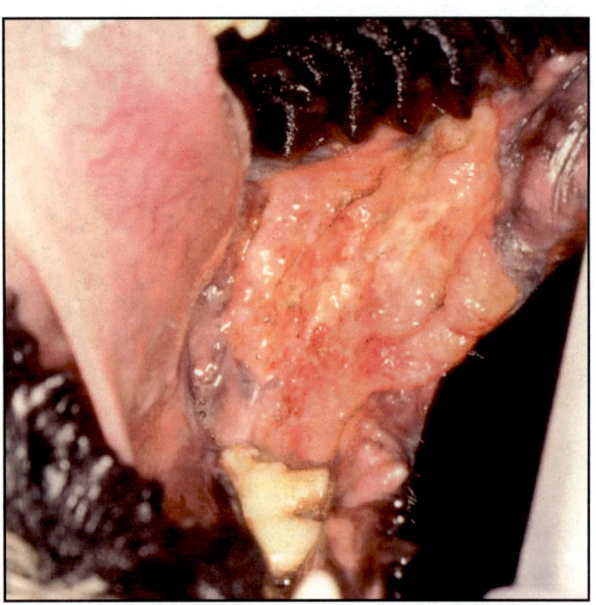

Figure 53-10. *SCC is often ulcerated and may affect the buccal mucosa, as in this dog.*

Table 53-2 **Distribution of Nontonsillar Oral SCC in 33 Dogs**[28]

Location	Site		
	Maxilla	Mandible	Soft tissue
Rostral	8	6	1
Caudal	7	—	3
Rostral and caudal	1	2	—
Tongue	—	—	5

important to survival time and tumor-free period in another study (Table 53-3).[32]

Treatment

The relatively low metastatic rate of rostral gingival SCC makes this malignancy a good candidate for local therapies such as surgery and radiation. Aggressive surgery is necessary to obtain adequate surgical margins; maxillectomy and mandibulectomy have been used (Figure 53-12). In 59 dogs from eight reports, median survival times ranged from 9 to 18 months.[10,19,20,27,31,33,35,36] Recurrence was more frequent than metastasis after surgery. Incomplete surgical resection is commonly associated with recurrence, which emphasizes the importance of making an early diagnosis and obtaining wide surgical margins by mandibulectomy or maxillectomy at the first surgery.[19,20] A combination of radiation and surgery gives the best control of gingival SCC, and postsurgical radiation should be considered for dogs with large tumors or with tumors that have incomplete margins on histopathology. One dog treated in this way had no evidence of disease 16 months after treatment.[27] This combined modality approach is the treatment of choice for larger, caudal, or incompletely excised SCC.

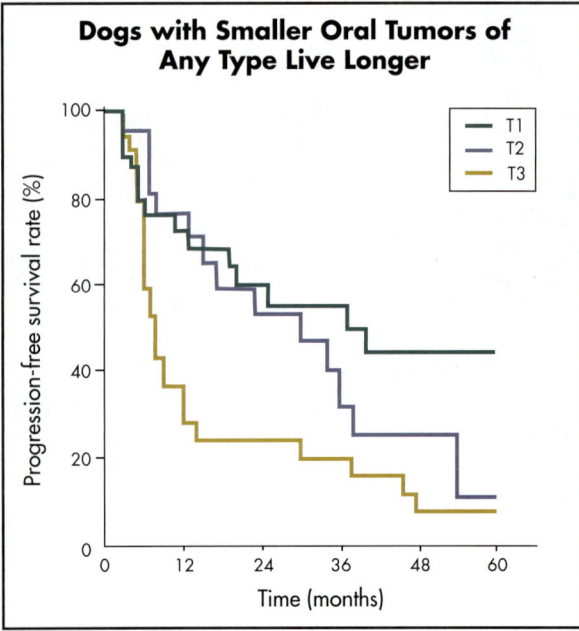

Figure 53-11. *Relationship between tumor size (T1, T2, T3) and tumor-free survival, regardless of tumor type (melanoma, SCC, and fibrosarcoma). (Adapted from Theon AP, Rodriguez C, Madewell BR: Analysis of prognosis factors and patterns of failure in dogs with malignant oral tumors treated with megavoltage irradiation. JAVMA 210:778–784, 1997; with permission)*

> **KEY POINT**
> *For oral SCCs, small rostral tumors (particularly of the maxilla) seem to have the best prognosis.*

For unresectable tumors, radiation therapy alone is the preferred treatment modality. Orthovoltage radiation therapy without surgery was used to treat 33 dogs to a total dose of approximately 40 Gy. Overall average survival time was approximately 14 months; however, the range was 6 to 58 months, depending on the size and location of the tumor and the age of the dog (see Prognostic Factors section, above).[28] There was recurrence in 15 dogs, metastasis in three dogs, and serious complications (e.g., bone necrosis) from radiation in two dogs. Orthovoltage is more likely than megavoltage to

than either.[28,32] Therefore, larger tumors (and concomitantly larger radiation fields) are associated with shorter survival (Figure 53-11). The size of the primary tumor was also

Table 53-3 Size of Primary Oral SCC Associated with Survival[32]

Tumor Size	Tumor Diameter (cm)	Median Progression-Free Survival (months)	1-Year Tumor-Free Survival (%)	3-Year Tumor-Free Survival (%)
Overall	—	36	72	55
T1	<2	*	89	74
T2	2–4	28	83	53
T3	>4	8	40	27

* More than 50% still tumor free; no median available.
T = primary tumor.

cause bone necrosis because the latter does not differentially deposit energy in bone. In a study of 14 dogs treated with megavoltage for nontonsillar SCC (no preradiation surgery), the median disease-free interval was 12 months and the median survival was 15 months.[34] In both studies, younger dogs had longer disease-free periods and longer survival times than older dogs.[28,34] In a third series, 31 dogs with SCC were treated with 48 Gy of ^{60}Co teletherapy.[32] Tumor recurred locally in 12 dogs. Nine dogs developed metastases: one dog developed metastases to regional lymph nodes, six dogs had distant metastases (two also had local recurrence), and two dogs developed metastases after salvage therapy. Dogs with rostrally located tumors and dogs with smaller tumors had longer remissions. Median progression-free survival time was approximately 17 months.

Local mucositis is the most common acute side effect of radiation therapy, and dogs may require antiinflammatory medications, antibiotics, pain relief with opioids (e.g., codeine, fentanyl), and appetite stimulants. It may be necessary to place a feeding tube in a dog undergoing radiation therapy for an oral tumor. Prophylactic tube placement is recommended for small dogs and dogs with a large radiation field. Ocular complications may occur if the field includes the orbit. Acute side effects rarely persist beyond 3 weeks after therapy.

Chemotherapy is rarely warranted for rostral gingival SCC in dogs because of the low metastatic rate for this tumor. Chemotherapy should always be considered for SCCs of the tongue, tonsil, and caudal location of the mouth because of the high metastatic rate of such tumors. Subcutaneous bleomycin treatment[37] and doxorubicin, cyclophosphamide, and chlorambucil treatment[27] failed to induce responses in two dogs with oral SCC. In early reports, cisplatin caused responses in dogs with metastatic subungual SCC[38]; however, no responses occurred in five dogs with oral SCC (including one tongue and one tonsillar tumor).[39] In another report, cisplatin caused a PR in three of five dogs with SCC for 2, 10, and 15 weeks, respectively.[40] Cisplatin has yet to be fully evaluated for oral SCC; however, it may be useful in combination therapy for this disease. Mitoxantrone (5 to 6 mg/m^2 IV q3wk) caused objective responses in four of nine dogs (45%) with SCC of various sites, including the oral cavity, for between 6 and 21 weeks.[41]

Piroxicam, a nonsteroidal inhibitor of cyclooxygenase-2 (COX-2), showed efficacy against canine oral SCC when given at a dose of 0.3 mg/kg PO sid. In a series of 17 dogs, one dog had a complete response (CR) and two dogs had a PR (tonsillar SCC and lingual SCC).[42] The median duration of response was 6 months. Stable disease was seen in another five dogs for a median of 3.5 months. Smaller tumors were more likely to maintain stable disease for a longer time. Concurrent misoprostol administration (6.5 μg/kg PO bid) may prevent gastrointestinal (GI) irritation. The mechanism by which piroxicam exerts its antitumor effects on SCC is still unclear, although it may affect tumor angiogenesis.

Combination cisplatin (50 mg/m^2) and piroxicam caused a remission in five of nine dogs with oral SCC; two dogs had a CR, and three dogs had a PR for a median of approximately 8 months. This cisplatin dosage was limited by renal toxicity, and dogs treated with this protocol should be monitored for renal damage before each treatment.[43]

In a preliminary report, combination carboplatin and piroxicam caused a complete remission in four of seven dogs with oral SCC for a median longer than 11 months.[44]

Papillary SCC in young dogs is a progressive disease. Conservative surgery alone is unlikely to be curative because of the high rate of bone involvement and the young age of the patient. Radiation therapy has a good success rate, although disruption of normal bone growth in young dogs may produce facial malformations. Radiation therapy to a total dose of 40 Gy was used to treat three puppies with this disease. There was no evidence of disease in any dog 39, 32, and 10 months after treatment; one dog had malformation of the affected jaw.[30]

TONSILLAR SQUAMOUS CELL CARCINOMA
Incidence, Signalment, and Etiology

Tonsillar SCC is considerably more aggressive than either gingival or lingual SCC. This tumor occurs in dogs at a

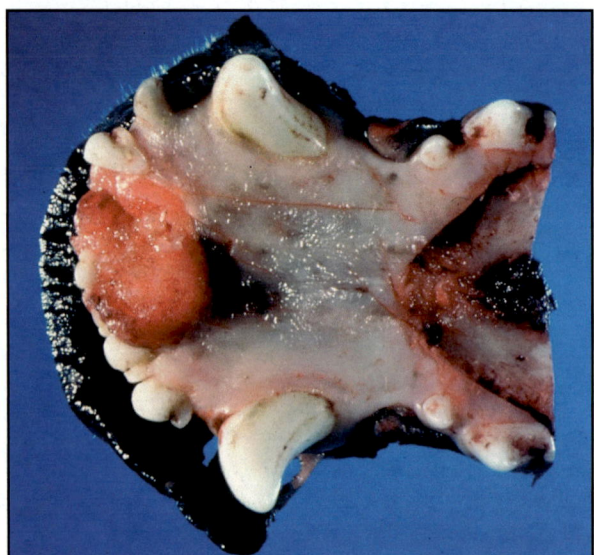

Figure 53-12. *Resected mandible from a dog with a rostrally located SCC. The prognosis for this dog is excellent after surgery alone.*

median age of 9 to 11 years.[37,45,46] There seems to be a male predisposition to developing tonsillar SCC. No breed predisposition has been described. Tonsillar SCC may occur bilaterally.[17]

A study conducted in the late 1930s showed that tonsillar SCC was one of the most common canine neoplastic diagnoses in the London area.[47] Further studies in France and England showed a high rate of this tumor in dogs from urban areas.[48,49] A study in the United States conducted in the late 1960s confirmed that the prevalence of tonsillar SCC was higher in urban areas than in rural areas,[50] and another study found a significant association between urban living and tonsillar SCC, with nearly 75% of affected dogs coming from an urban household.[51]

There has been some variation in the prevalence of this tumor over time; the prevalence of tonsillar SCC in London in the 1950s was four times greater than that in the 1980s and 15 times greater than that seen in Melbourne, Australia, at the same time. The rate in the United States was intermediate.[52] No more recent estimates of prevalence are available. Clearly, the tonsils are a target organ for industrial pollution, but it is less clear why the incidence has decreased over time.

Clinical Presentation and History

Most dogs with tonsillar SCC present with dysphagia, anorexia, and pain, and clients may have noticed a cervical swelling, which is usually lymph node metastasis rather than primary tumor. In fact, the primary tumor may be quite small, but lymphadenopathy may be marked (Figure 53-13). Most dogs have shown these signs for 1 month or less, although some may show signs for up to 3 months before presentation.[46]

> **KEY POINT**
> *Lymphadenopathy caused by metastasis from tonsillar SCC may be noticed by a caregiver long before a tonsillar tumor is suspected.*

As with other oral tumors, the most common signs are drooling, halitosis, and (occasionally) dysphagia.

Staging and Diagnosis

Both tonsils should be thoroughly examined in a dog with a large cervical mass. Aspiration cytology of the lymph node may confirm metastatic carcinoma. If no diagnosis can be reached, biopsy of the tonsil and the regional lymph node is warranted. Thoracic radiographs should be taken, although metastasis is unlikely to be seen at the time of diagnosis. If treatment is undertaken, radiographs should be repeated at regular intervals to screen for metastasis. In view of the high reported rate of intraabdominal metastases in one study,[45] abdominal radiography and ultrasonography should be conducted before any definitive treatment. They also may be useful for monitoring the patient for metastases after treatment.

Lymphadenopathy caused by metastasis from tonsillar SCC is common. In one group of 22 dogs, all had lymphadenopathy as well as infiltrative primary tumors at the time of diagnosis.[46] Despite early spread to the lymph nodes, pulmonary metastases are rarely noted at diagnosis. After treatment, nine of 27 dogs (33%) had evidence of distant metastases.[45,46] In two earlier studies, 77 of 91 dogs (85%) with tonsillar SCC had metastasis to regional lymph nodes at necropsy.[17] Systemic metastases were less common; they occurred in the lung, spleen, liver, and thyroid gland. In a smaller group of dogs, metastasis to the spleen and liver occurred more often than metastasis to the lungs.[45]

Treatment

Surgery alone is not generally effective for treating tonsillar SCCs because of the high rate of metastases, which manifest early in the course of the disease. A combination of surgery and radiation provided good local control at radiation doses of 35 to 42.5 Gy in one study; six of eight dogs showed a CR, and one dog showed a PR.[45] Recurrence was seen in only two of the seven responding dogs, although metastatic disease to the spleen, liver, bone, and lungs was seen or suspected in all seven. Survival ranged from 1.5 to 21 months, with a median of 3.5 months.

In an attempt to improve survival, dogs in another study were treated with a combination of surgery, orthovoltage radiation therapy, and chemotherapy that alternated doxorubicin (30 mg/m^2 IV q3wk) with cisplatin (60 mg/m^2 IV

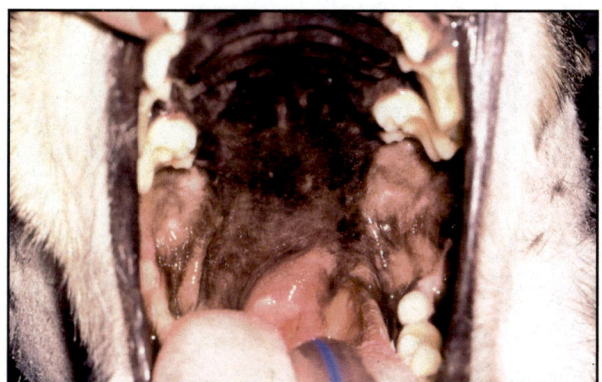

Figure 53-13. *A dog with unexplained mandibular lymphadenopathy should be examined for tonsillar SCC. This tumor may be much smaller than the nodal metastasis.*

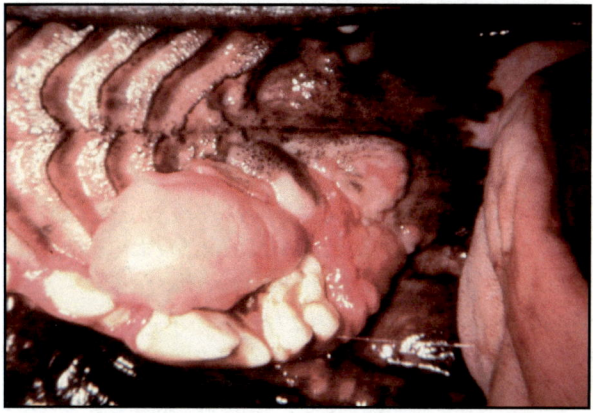

Figure 53-14. *Fibrosarcomas may arise in the maxilla and invade the hard palate by extension. They are often large and protruding.*

q3wk).[46] Of six dogs receiving this protocol, five achieved a CR with a median of 240 days. Four of these dogs developed tumor recurrence and metastatic disease. In comparison, 16 dogs had no response to treatment with this chemotherapy protocol (or combinations of doxorubicin, vinblastine, cisplatin, and cyclophosphamide) when it was administered without radiation therapy.[46] The median survival of these 16 dogs was 3.5 months.

Piroxicam, a nonsteroidal inhibitor of COX-2, given at a dose of 0.3 mg/kg PO sid, showed efficacy against canine tonsillar SCC. One of five dogs had a PR to piroxicam alone,[42] and two of three dogs had a PR to piroxicam and cisplatin.[43]

Clearly, the best results for this tumor can be obtained only if aggressive surgery and radiation therapy are combined with doxorubicin and cisplatin chemotherapy. Even then, tumor progression is difficult to control. The prognosis for dogs with tonsillar SCC is very poor.

ORAL FIBROSARCOMA
Incidence, Signalment, and Etiology

Fibrosarcomas are the third most common oral tumor in dogs. They occur in young dogs more commonly than melanoma or SCC.[17] The average age of dogs with oral fibrosarcoma is 7 years,[17,19,20,27,33,35,53] although these tumors have been reported in dogs as young as 6 months.[17,20,33] There do not seem to be any breed predilections, although four of 10 affected dogs in one study were golden retrievers.[53] There is an apparent male predilection for developing oral fibrosarcoma,[17,54] although this is not consistent in all studies.[53]

Clinical Presentation and History

Fibrosarcomas arise most commonly in the gingiva and are equally likely to be located around the maxilla or the mandible.[54] The hard palate is not commonly involved except by extension of a maxillary tumor (Figure 53-14). Tumors are usually large, with diameters of greater than 4 cm.[17,54]

As with other oral tumors, the most common signs are drooling, halitosis, and (occasionally) dysphagia.

Staging and Diagnosis

An MDB, including thoracic radiography, should be conducted before definitive surgery or radiation therapy. Before biopsy, dogs should be staged using blood work, thoracic radiography, lymph node evaluation, and fine-detail skull radiography. Fibrosarcomas frequently invade bone and may extend much farther than is obvious by external viewing. In addition, all soft tissue sarcomas have "tendrils" of tumor cells that extend deep into normal surrounding tissues, making complete excision very difficult without wide margins.

Before surgery is attempted, particularly when the tumor involves the maxilla, high-detail skull radiographs should be obtained to gain a better appreciation of tumor borders. Radiographs are superior to clinical examination in determining tumor borders but do not allow imaging of bony lysis until more than 50% of the bone has been destroyed (demineralized). Therefore, radiographs usually underestimate tumor margins. CT scanning is a more accurate method of assessing fibrosarcoma margins. A CT scan provides a spatial assessment of the tumor that may be useful for planning surgery as well as either presurgery or postsurgery radiation therapy. CT scanning may also indicate whether surgery is unlikely to benefit a patient, thereby protecting the animal from a poorly planned procedure.

Histologic reports of these tumors should be interpreted cautiously. Occasionally, a tumor may be termed a fibroma, which implies that the process is benign. In fact, all soft tissue sarcomas belong to a spectrum of disease, and fibromas of the oral cavity should be treated as aggressively as fibrosarcomas. A recent report described 25 dogs with tumors that were histologically diagnosed as fibromas, nodular fasciitis, or granulation tissue. Although all of these lesions are considered histologically benign, they invaded bone and metastasized in five dogs and are termed *histologically low-grade, biologically high-grade fibrosarcomas*.[55] Bony invasion should be interpreted as a sign of malignancy, regardless of the pathology report (Figure 53-15).

> **KEY POINT**
>
> *A histologic diagnosis of fibroma, nodular fascitis, or granulation tissue for an oral lesion, particularly if bony invasion is present, should be interpreted as fibrosarcoma and treated appropriately.*

Metastasis is uncommon in dogs with fibrosarcoma, particularly at the time of diagnosis.[17,54] Young dogs apparently have more aggressive tumors than old dogs. In a collected series totaling 135 dogs, metastasis was reported in 31 dogs (23%).[10,17,27,32,33,35,54] In most cases, metastasis was to regional lymph nodes.[33,35,54] Especially in young dogs, mandibular lymph nodes should be palpated and (if enlarged) subjected to fine-needle aspiration or biopsy. Systemic metastases from oral fibrosarcoma may be a late event, so the incidence may be higher as local tumor control improves.[17,32,33] Earlier reports with less effective therapies may have underestimated the metastatic rate because dogs died from inadequate local tumor control before metastasis occurred.

Prognostic Factors

The size of the primary tumor was important in determining tumor-free period and survival time in one study of 28 dogs with oral fibrosarcoma treated with radiation therapy (Table 53-4).[32]

Treatment

The optimum treatment of oral fibrosarcoma probably involves combined surgery and radiation therapy to doses that exceed 50 Gy. Chemotherapy is investigational but may improve survival rates by controlling metastases. Control rates similar to those seen with soft tissue sarcomas at other locations could be expected with this combined approach (see Chapter 62).

Surgery

The treatment of choice for fibrosarcoma of the oral cavity is complete surgical excision. Local or incomplete excisions lead to rapid recurrence[35]; therefore, early diagnosis and wide surgical margins at the first surgery are important.[19,20] Radical surgical techniques such as maxillectomy and mandibulectomy are necessary to obtain adequate surgical margins and are well tolerated by dogs. In six series totaling 68 dogs treated for oral fibrosarcoma with aggressive surgery,

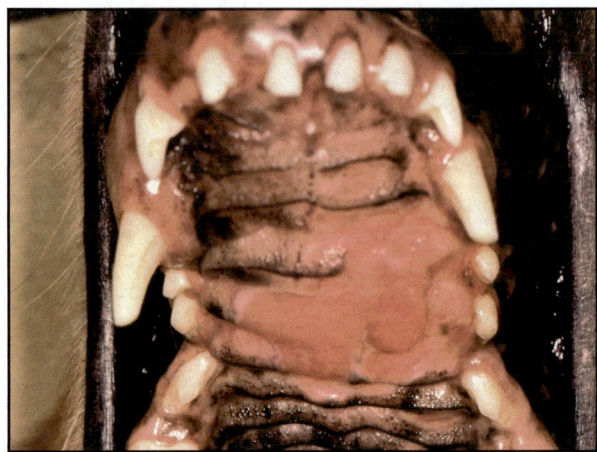

Figure 53-15. *A histologically low-grade, biologically high-grade fibrosarcoma in the maxilla of a dog. Histologic reports should always be interpreted in light of the clinical findings. Bony invasion is a sign of malignancy.*

the median survival was 12 months (range: 1.5 weeks to 33 months).[10,19,20,27,33,35] Even after mandibulectomy or maxillectomy, 20 of 54 dogs (37%) had local recurrence. However, tumor recurrence varied from 20%[33] to nearly 60%[35] between studies (and therefore surgeons) and occurred soon after surgery in studies with the highest rates of recurrence. In three dogs in one study, recurrence was treated by a second surgery (two dogs) or surgery plus radiation therapy (one dog), for second remissions of 2 months, 15 months, and 2 years, respectively.[27] Clearly, radiation therapy has an adjunctive role in the treatment of oral fibrosarcomas.

Radiation Therapy

The response of soft tissue sarcomas in the oral cavity is not as good as that of cutaneous soft tissue sarcomas. In one study, the median survival for dogs with oral tumors was 18 months compared with 75 months for dogs with tumors at other sites.[56]

Pretreatment with 50 to 56 Gy of radiation before surgery seemed to improve control rates in one study, although few dogs were involved.[35] Early results of radiation therapy as a single treatment modality were disappointing for canine oral fibrosarcoma, but this may reflect the source and dosage of radiation. Control of fibrosarcoma improves only at doses of 50 Gy or more.[50,53,54,57] Of 17 dogs treated with 40.0 to 54.5 Gy of orthovoltage, four died during or soon after radiation therapy. Survival times in the remaining 13 dogs ranged from 2 months to more than 27 months, with a median survival of 6 months. Tumors recurred in 12 dogs at an average of 3.9 months after radiation was complete.[54] In another study, radiation therapy without surgery was able to control tumor growth in three of 13 dogs.[57] A radioprotector used to reduce side effects also reduced response rate in another study.[58]

Table 53-4 Size of Primary Oral Fibrosarcoma Associated with Survival after Radiation Therapy[32]

Tumor Size	Tumor Diameter (cm)	Median Progression-Free Survival (months)	1-Year Tumor-Free Survival (%)	3-Year Tumor-Free Survival (%)
Overall	—	26	76	40
T1	<2	45	100	67
T2	2–4	31	100	36
T3	>4	7	38	13

T = primary tumor.

Megavoltage radiation may be more efficacious than orthovoltage in controlling oral fibrosarcomas. Of 28 dogs with fibrosarcoma treated with 48 Gy of ^{60}Co teletherapy, nine dogs had local recurrence. Eight dogs developed metastases: one dog developed metastases to regional lymph nodes, six dogs had distant metastases (two also had local recurrence), and one dog developed metastases after salvage therapy. Median progression-free survival was 26 months.[32] Dogs with smaller tumors had longer remissions (Table 53-4).

When used in combination with radiation, interstitial hyperthermia provides local control rates similar to those achieved by radiation alone. Interstitial hyperthermia to a temperature of either 50°C or 43°C for 30 seconds was administered to 10 dogs that also received between 32 and 48 Gy of orthovoltage.[53] Complete remission was obtained in nine dogs, and overall median survival was 12.9 months. Tumors recurred in four dogs between 38 days and 378 days after radiation. Complications of this combined modality include fistula formation and sepsis after tissue necrosis.

Chemotherapy

Little has been reported regarding chemotherapy in the treatment of oral cavity fibrosarcomas, although the metastatic rate of nearly 30% documented in one study shows that, with local control rates improving with more aggressive surgery and radiation therapy, as many dogs die from metastasis as from local recurrence.[32] Doxorubicin has been noted to produce objective responses in soft tissue sarcomas. Low dosages of doxorubicin (10 mg/m^2 IV every 7 days) appear to act as a "radiation sensitizer" and improve tumor response at lower radiation therapy dosages.

Intratumoral injections of cisplatin and bovine collagen matrix were given every week during a 48-Gy course of ^{60}Co teletherapy in five dogs with oral fibrosarcoma. Complete remission was seen in three dogs, and partial remission was seen in one dog for a median duration of 14 weeks. Tumors recurred in three of these dogs.[59] In these and other dogs treated with radiochemotherapy, recurrence often took place at the periphery of the chemotherapy site but still within the radiation field, implying that the combination is synergistic or additive in its effect on the tumor.

LINGUAL TUMORS

The most common tumors of the tongue are SCC, accounting for 37% of 57 lingual tumors in one study. Other tumors in this study were granular cell tumors (myoblastomas; 12%), melanomas (12%), and mast cell tumors (9%).[29]

SCC of the tongue is a more aggressive tumor than gingival SCC, and metastatic disease often determines survival; nine of 21 dogs (43%) in one study developed metastasis to lymph nodes, lung, or bone.[29] Surgery has variable results, and recurrence is common unless wide surgical margins are obtained. In some cases, complete removal of the tongue is indicated. Surprisingly, dogs adapt to this well (Figures 53-16 and 53-17). In one study, five dogs with small tumors were treated with surgery alone and had a median survival time of 8 months. Three of these dogs had local recurrence.[29] Recurrence of tongue tumors is also common after radiation therapy. Larger tumors in 10 dogs were treated with radiation therapy, and the dogs survived for a median of 4 months; nine of 10 dogs had recurrence.[29] The one dog that received radiation after surgery survived 26 months with no recurrence. A combined-modality approach seems warranted for local control of larger tumors, although metastasis occurs in approximately 50% of cases.[29]

A recent series evaluated subtotal to total glossectomy in a dog with a lingual SCC as well as dogs with other lingual tumors, lingual trauma, and inflammatory conditions of the tongue.[60] The two dogs in this series that were treated with subtotal and near-total glossectomy were able to eat and drink unassisted within 3 weeks of surgery. More aggressive removal of the tongue required that dogs have food supplemented with water or learned to suck water as a horse does. This surgery was well tolerated by owners and dogs.

Chemotherapy should be considered for lingual tumors as an adjuvant to surgery. Cisplatin has caused responses in

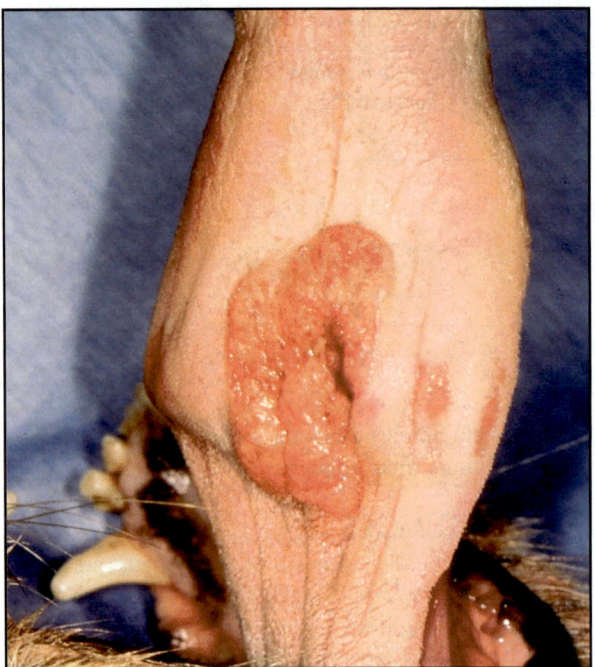

Figure 53-16. *SCC of the tongue is more likely to metastasize than gingival SCC.*

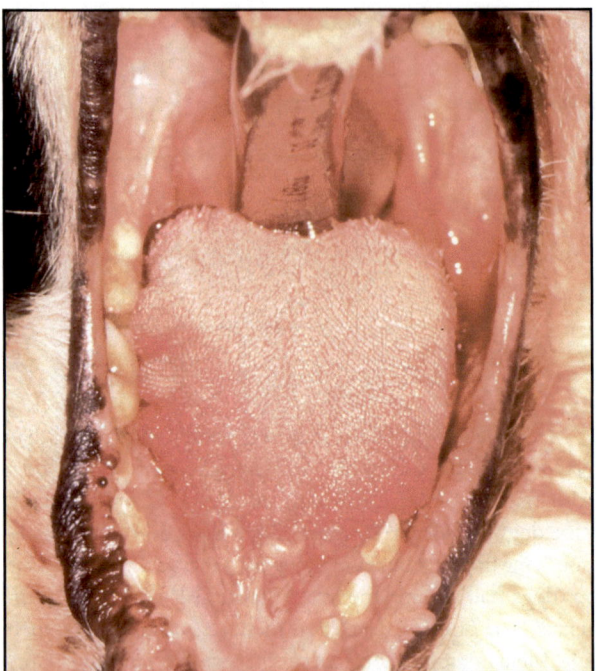

Figure 53-17. *The same dog as in Figure 53-16 after rostral glossectomy. Even after such radical procedures and adjuvant radiation therapy, local recurrence may be a problem. Dogs tolerate glossectomy surprisingly well.*

dogs with metastatic subungual SCC; however, no responses occurred in five dogs with oral SCC (including one tongue and one tonsillar tumor).[39]

Granular cell tumors are of uncertain histogenesis.[61] Dogs with lingual granular cell tumors have a good outcome after surgery, with five of seven affected dogs alive more than 2 years after surgery and no distant metastases noted in one study.[29] Two other dogs had no recurrence a year after surgery.[61,62] Very large tumors may prove more difficult to control, and early, wide excision should be performed.[63] Granular cell tumors have been reported at other oral locations.[64]

Aggressive lingual resection of more than 50% of the tongue lengthways was required to control a lingual hemangioma in a young dog.[65]

Salivary Gland Tumors

INCIDENCE, SIGNALMENT, AND ETIOLOGY

These tumors occur in older animals (median age: 10 years) with no obvious gender predilection. Poodles and possibly spaniel breeds[66] are at higher risk for developing this disease than other breeds.[67,68] More than 95% of reported salivary gland tumors are malignant.[67–69]

Carcinomas are the most common tumor type,[70] although salivary glands are occasionally invaded by fibrosarcomas or mast cell tumors. Enlargement of the salivary gland in a dog is more likely to be an inflammatory process than a tumor.[67,71]

CLINICAL PRESENTATION AND HISTORY

Most owners notice a swelling or mass in the neck; signs may also include anorexia, dysphagia, and pain on opening the mouth. In one study, the most commonly affected salivary gland was the parotid gland (50% of dogs).[72] Another study found that the mandibular glands were more likely to be affected than the parotid gland.[67] In this second study, tumor was often dispersed throughout the salivary tissue in the submucosa of the oral cavity, tongue, and oropharynx. Rarely, a salivary gland tumor will invade surrounding bone.[73]

STAGING AND DIAGNOSIS

Surgical excisional biopsy is warranted for localized tumors; however, more diffuse tumors may require incisional biopsy before a definitive procedure. Lymph node metastasis was confirmed in 17% of 24 affected dogs at presentation in one study.[72] Dogs with enlarged nodes should have a biopsy or a fine-needle aspiration. Pulmonary metastases are rare, occurring in 8% of dogs at presentation in one study,[72] and thoracic radiographs should be taken as part of a general health screen in older animals rather than with the expectation of seeing metastases. Occasionally, metastases are widespread at diagnosis.[74]

Ultrasonography may be helpful in examining the tumor and lymph nodes. One study found that although investigation of the mandibular gland was easily accomplished,

Table 53-5 Staging Scheme for Salivary Tumors in Dogs

Stage 1	T1	N0	M0
Stage 2	T2 or T3	N0	M0
Stage 3	Any T	N1	M0
Stage 4	Any T	Any N	M1

T: Primary tumor N: Regional node M: Distant metastasis
T1: <2 cm diameter N0: No metastasis M0: No metastasis
T2: 2–4 cm diameter N1: Metastasis M1: Metastasis
T3: 4 cm diameter

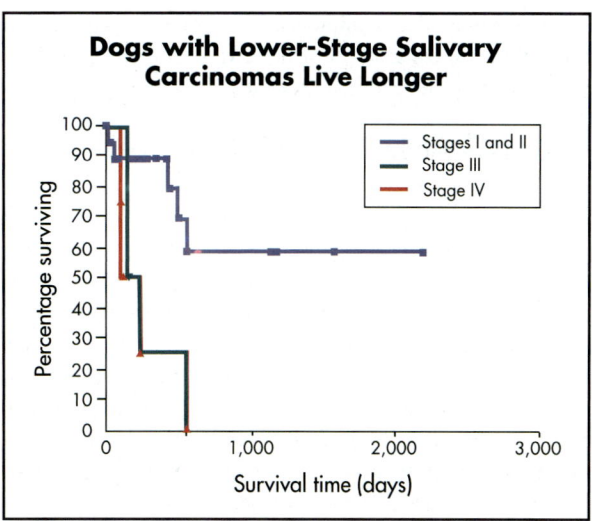

Figure 53-18. *Relationship between tumor stage and survival for dogs with salivary carcinomas. (Adapted from Hammer A, Getzy D, Ogilvie G, et al: Salivary gland neoplasia in the dog and cat: Survival times and prognostic factors. JAAHA 37:478–482, 2001; with permission)*

anatomic difficulties meant that only the oral section of the sublingual gland and the superficial rostrodorsal section of the parotid gland could be examined. The zygomatic gland was partly obscured by the zygomatic arch.[75] In dogs with tumors, some of these restrictions may not be as important because the affected gland will enlarge.

Paraneoplastic hypoglycemia has been associated with a salivary adenocarcinoma.[76]

PROGNOSTIC FACTORS

Staging (Table 53-5) has proven prognostic for dogs with salivary carcinoma. The presence of metastases gives a worse prognosis (Figure 53-18).[72]

TREATMENT

In two dogs, surgical excision resulted in local recurrence within 6 months.[67,68] One of these dogs and two other dogs received 45 Gy of orthovoltage radiation to the surgical site, and none of the three dogs had developed local recurrence or metastasis 12, 25, and 40 months after treatment.[68] Surgery alone and radiation therapy with surgery were the most successful modes of treatment in another study of 24 dogs. Both groups had median survival times of 2 years, with a number of animals alive beyond 4 years.[72] Radiation therapy should be considered as an adjunct to surgery for salivary gland tumors.[77]

Chemotherapy is rarely reported. One study reported a variety of protocols but no improved survival.[72] Cisplatin after incomplete surgery for a recurrent zygomatic salivary adenocarcinoma seemed to delay further recurrence in one dog that was free of tumor 9 months after a second surgery.[78]

Esophageal Tumors
INCIDENCE, SIGNALMENT, AND ETIOLOGY

Epithelial tumors of the esophagus are more common than mesenchymal tumors; however, they are considered very rare, at least in the United States. The only report specifically regarding esophageal tumors suggested that metastatic tumors to the esophagus (six dogs) were more common than primary tumors (two dogs).[79] Of 29 leiomyomas of the GI tract in one study, only four were found in the esophagus.[80]

Spirocerca lupi is a nematode parasite that primarily affects dogs living in the tropics and subtropics. Adult worms encyst in the esophagus, causing granulomas that precede neoplastic transformation in some dogs. The most common tumors seen are osteosarcomas, fibrosarcomas, and undifferentiated sarcomas.[81] In South Africa, more than 40% of practitioners reporting *Spirocerca* spp also reported neoplasia.[82] Granulomas that precede sarcoma formation may be treated successfully by doramectin (200 mg/kg SC q14d for three treatments; if no resolution, repeat at 500 mg/kg PO q24h for 6 weeks).[83]

Esophageal tumors are too diverse and rare for any signalment statements to be made.

CLINICAL PRESENTATION AND HISTORY

Clinical signs are consistent regardless of the histologic diagnosis. Most dogs appear eager to eat but regurgitate soon after eating. Liquids are usually not regurgitated. Intermittent postprandial regurgitation may precede regurgitation unrelated to eating, seen as the tumor progresses. Many of these signs are caused by motility disturbances rather than the mass itself and may persist even after successful surgery.[84,85] Most affected dogs show weight loss, are described as thin to emaciated, show lethargy and depression, and may be pyrectic. Tumors may infiltrate surrounding structures such as the trachea or adjacent lung lobes, causing respiratory signs.[86,87] Aspiration pneumonia is a common serious sequel to regurgitation and is the most common cause of death in affected dogs.[84,87,88] Hypertrophic osteopathy may occur.[87]

STAGING AND DIAGNOSIS

Most tumors are at the thoracic inlet or are intrathoracic. Plain radiography may demonstrate a soft tissue opacity if the lesion is intrathoracic or may show an air-filled and dilated megaesophagus.[84] In a study of 15 dogs with *Spirocerca*-associated tumors, caudal thoracic masses were demonstrated on survey radiographs of 13 dogs and thoracic spondylitis was detected in 12 dogs.[81] An esophagram may demonstrate megaesophagus and an irregular mucosal pattern and may outline a completely obstructive mass. Esophagoscopy is useful in visualizing the mass and obtaining a biopsy; however, superficial biopsies may be nondiagnostic because of severe ulceration and inflammatory changes.[84] Multiple biopsies are required to ensure a diagnosis.[88]

A CT scan was a useful pretreatment tool to rule out transmural invasion by the tumor in one report. Transmural invasion suggests that successful therapy would result in a leaking defect that could cause fatal complications.[88]

Metastasis to regional lymph nodes has not been reported, although tumors may infiltrate the trachea or adjacent lung lobes.

If *S. lupi* infection is suspected, eggs may be detected (two of eight patients in one study[81]).

TREATMENT

Treatment has rarely been reported for these tumors. If treatment is to be attempted, transtracheal aspirate should be obtained for bacteriologic culture and prophylactic antibiotics administered. The high proportion of affected dogs developing aspiration pneumonia implies that long-term antibiotic administration may be important for these patients. Also, if treatment is to be attempted, placement of a gastrostomy tube several days before definitive treatment allows the dog to be fully fed by tube before intervention.[84,88]

Gastroesophageal anastomosis has been attempted in two dogs, but both died from aspiration pneumonia.[84,87] Motility disorders persisted in another dog after resection of a 10-cm osteosarcoma, and the dog died.[85] An esophageal plasmacytoma was successfully resected.[89]

Photodynamic therapy was given twice to a dog with an esophageal SCC; tumor volume was partially reduced (50%), and the dog resumed eating. The response lasted 3 months, at which time a second lesion, 10 cm distal to the first, was diagnosed on esophagoscopy. The dog survived for 9 months after the first treatment.[88]

Six dogs with esophageal sarcomas (three fibrosarcomas, one undifferentiated sarcoma, and two osteosarcomas) were treated with partial esophagectomy. Esophageal masses were approached by thoracotomy and esophagotomy on the side opposite the mass and removed with 1-cm margins by full-thickness excision. Five of these dogs also received doxorubicin chemotherapy after surgery. The average survival time was 9 months (range: 2–16 months), with one dog alive 20 months after surgery.[90]

Stomach Tumors
INCIDENCE, SIGNALMENT, AND ETIOLOGY

The most common tumor of the stomach in dogs is gastric adenocarcinoma, and most reports of canine stomach cancer emphasize this neoplasm. The number of dogs affected by different tumor types has been studied.[91–93] In 89 dogs with stomach tumors, 51 (60%) had an adenocarcinoma and nine (10%) had an adenoma. Leiomyoma (19 dogs [20%]) was more common than leiomyosarcoma (four dogs [5%]). Mesenchymal tumors that are not derived from smooth muscle have been termed *GI stromal tumors* (GISTs) and occur mainly in the stomach and esophagus. GISTs uncommonly metastasize (30%), and their clinical distinction from leiomyosarcomas is probably not significant.[80] Lymphoma, either as a primary tumor or as part of systemic disease, occurred in six dogs (7% of total). A gastric carcinoid (neuroendocrine derived) has been described.[94]

Most carcinomas occur in the lower two-thirds of the stomach, particularly the pylorus. The lesser curvature is not usually affected except in Belgian shepherds.[95,96] Most affected dogs are older; the median age is 10 years. All studies report a male predominance ranging from 2:1 to 3:1. One study suggested that males were affected with gastric carcinoma up to seven times more often than females, depending on the histologic subtype.[97] Females may have benign gastric adenomas more often than male dogs.[92]

Belgian shepherds in Italy (of the Groenendael type)[95,96] and rough collies[98] are apparently at high risk for gastric adenocarcinoma. In one study, chow chows had a risk of gastric tumors that was more than 40 times the risk of the general population.[99] Two studies found a high incidence of gastric carcinoma (four of 13) and gastritis (all dogs) in Norwegian Lundehunds, suggesting a single pathogenetic process associated with increased numbers of mucous neck cells and metaplasia.[100,101]

Although gastric carcinomas can be experimentally induced in dogs by various compounds, no epidemiologic studies support a role for these compounds in naturally occurring disease.[102]

CLINICAL PRESENTATION AND HISTORY

Gastric tumors are consistently associated with vomiting, weight loss, and inappetence. Vomiting is often chronic and is rarely associated with eating. Hematemesis occurs in 20%

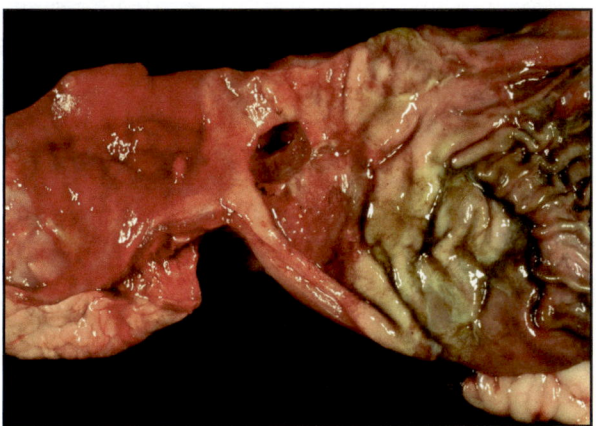

Figure 53-19. *Gastric carcinoma may involve a huge area of the stomach, often with extensive ulceration. These factors, combined with the poor condition of most affected dogs, make this a difficult tumor to treat.*

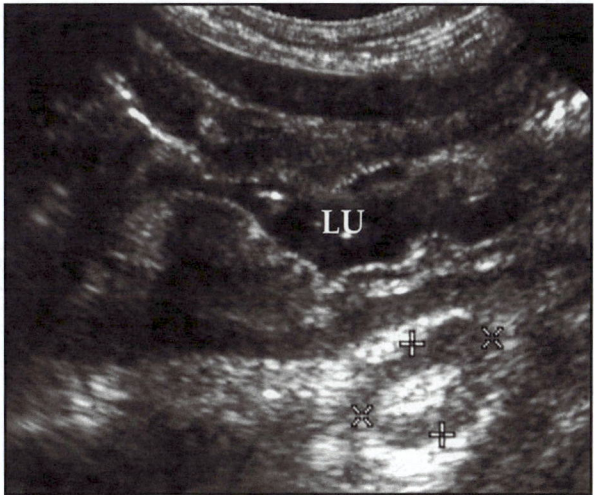

Figure 53-20. *Longitudinal sonogram of the stomach of a dog presented for vomiting and weight loss. The gastric wall is markedly and irregularly thickened. A small amount of fluid is present in the stomach. Despite the significant wall thickening, pseudolayering is noted. Gastric lymphadenopathy (between calipers) with a target pattern is also present. (LU = lumen) (Courtesy of Dominique G. Penninck, DVM, Tufts Cummings School of Veterinary Medicine)*

to 50% of dogs. Other signs include polydipsia, abdominal pain, melena, and anemia. Occasionally, ascites occurs as a result of carcinomatosis. Clinical signs, such as vomiting, are often chronic for 2 weeks to 18 months before presentation; the median duration is 2 months.

STAGING AND DIAGNOSIS

Gastric adenocarcinomas often involve a large area of the stomach wall, making them unresectable (Figure 53-19). They arise in the mucosa, but most extend to or through the serosa.[96] Ulceration is common and often deep and crater-like, causing hematemesis or melena.[91,98,103] Contrast radiography, particularly with fluoroscopy, may give indications of gastric tumor, but these indications are rarely definitive.[98]

An MDB should be obtained. Endoscopy can determine the location of most tumors, except when neoplasia is diffusely infiltrative, and may reveal tumor ulceration. Although endoscopy can be definitive,[98] it can also be inconclusive[96]; multiple biopsy specimens should be obtained, and deep biopsy specimens should be taken if the mucosa is not obviously involved. Endoscopy is ideal for evaluating the stomach, but ultrasonography should be used to assess epigastric lymph nodes and other abdominal viscera for evidence of metastasis.

Ultrasonography also can be used to define the borders of localized tumors and to identify ulcerations and diffuse infiltration.[103] Ultrasonographic features of gastric carcinomas that enable distinction from gastritis are loss of normal gastric layers, thickening of the stomach wall, and lymphadenopathy[99,104–106] (Figure 53-20). Pseudolayering may be a feature of carcinomas,[99] but it does not distinguish between lymphoma and carcinoma, and biopsy must still be performed.[106] Ultrasound-guided microcore biopsy has a high diagnostic sensitivity.[99,107,108] Operator experience is important in examining the gastric wall because this is a difficult area of the abdomen to image.[109] If ultrasonography alone does not diagnose a tumor in a patient with a history suggestive of carcinoma, endoscopy may be diagnostic.[110]

When the above modalities are unsuitable, exploratory laparotomy can be used to obtain biopsy specimens from affected sites. A therapeutic excisional biopsy may be possible for small localized tumors; however, incisional biopsy should be performed on larger tumors.

Gastric adenocarcinoma often metastasizes (>75% of cases in one review of 132 dogs[111]), particularly to the perigastric lymph nodes, peritoneum, liver, and other viscera, including the lungs.[91,96–98,111] Metastasis to the testes has also been described.[112] Extension of gastric adenocarcinoma through the serosa creates an intense scirrhous reaction in the mesentery and omentum, which may cause ascites.[113]

Histology of gastric adenocarcinomas varies, and "intestinal" types of tumors (e.g., papillary, acinar, solid) are less common than diffuse types (e.g., undifferentiated, glandular). No differences in biologic behavior have been ascribed to these different tumor types; all gastric adenocarcinomas are aggressive malignancies.

Leiomyomas and leiomyosarcomas are less common than epithelial tumors. One ultrasound study suggested that a focal mass in the antrum of the stomach had a very high likelihood of being either a leiomyoma or leiomyosarcoma.[106] Paraneoplastic hypoglycemia has been reported in five dogs that had large gastric leiomyosarcomas or leiomyomas; the tumors did not metastasize in any dog.[114–116]

TREATMENT

Parenteral nutrition is an integral part of the management of a dog with gastric carcinoma because any attempt at treatment is likely to require bypassing the stomach for a considerable period of time. IV parenteral nutrition can be used, although patient management is more intense than if a jejunostomy tube is placed at the time of surgery. Unfortunately, the poor response to therapies has meant that, even with nutritional support, most survival times have been short.[99,117]

The advanced stage at diagnosis, diffuse nature, and high rate of metastasis of gastric adenocarcinomas usually make surgery to remove them unsuccessful. Most tumors are too large or invasive for complete resection.[93,95] In these dogs, palliative side-to-side gastrojejunostomy may prolong survival, usually for less than 2 months.[111] Wide resection often requires gastroduodenostomy (Billroth I procedure); however, most dogs die from local recurrence and metastases within 4 months of surgery.[91,117-119] In two studies, two dogs were treated with gastroduodenostomy, cholecystoduodenostomy, and partial pancreatectomy, and neither dog lived longer than 2 months.[99,111] Earlier diagnosis occasionally allows successful surgical resection and long-term freedom from recurrence and metastasis.[95] Surgical excision (Billroth I) was attempted in another five dogs; these dogs lived a median of 6 weeks (range: 3 days to 10 months) which was no longer than the 4 and 5 weeks that 2 dogs treated palliatively for unresectable tumors survived.[111] Total gastrectomy with esophageal anastomosis to the antrum remnant, leaving the pylorus intact, was successful in resecting a huge gastric carcinoma in a small dog.[120] After initial use of jejunostomy feeding, maintaining adequate caloric density as well as a good appetite were challenges. The dog lived 8 months after surgery.

> **KEY POINT**
> *Adenocarcinoma of the stomach is usually large or diffuse, making complete surgical excision difficult.*

Results of chemotherapy for adenocarcinoma have rarely been reported; anecdotally, doxorubicin may prolong survival after surgery, but this is not consistent.[99,111] In one study, two dogs were treated with chemotherapy alone.[111] One treated with 5-fluorouracil and cyclophosphamide was euthanatized because of progression after 9 weeks. The other had an initial but inconsistent response to 5-fluorouracil, doxorubicin, and cyclophosphamide and finally received cisplatin. Survival in this dog was 7.5 months from diagnosis.

In one dog, an ulcerated, polypoid leiomyoma was removed from the pyloric antrum with narrow (5 mm) margins. Excision was complete, and the dog was free of disease 20 months later.[121] Two dogs with leiomyosarcomas underwent gastroduodenostomy, but metastases to liver and duodenum were diagnosed at surgery. Survival times were less than 3 months.[111]

In another dog, a gastric plasma cell tumor that had metastasized to a regional lymph node was resected completely, and doxorubicin chemotherapy was given. The dog was free of disease 30 months later.[122] Another dog with diffuse gastric plasmacytoma responded to treatment with melphalan, cyclophosphamide, and prednisone and was free of disease 33 months later.[123]

Small Intestinal and Cecal Tumors
INCIDENCE, SIGNALMENT, AND ETIOLOGY

Adenocarcinomas are the most common intestinal tumors in dogs. Leiomyosarcomas, although less common than adenocarcinomas, occur more frequently in the intestine than in the stomach. Intestinal leiomyomas are uncommon. Lymphoma may be found anywhere within the GI tract but is usually associated with systemic disease.[124,125] More information about lymphoma can be found in Chapter 47. Table 53-6 summarizes canine small intestinal tumor location. Less common tumor types include neurolemmoma, carcinoid,[126,127] and fibrosarcoma.[128]

Intestinal tumors occur in older dogs; the median age is 11 to 12 years, although the average age of dogs with lymphoma is younger.[125] There is no obvious breed predilection. Males are more frequently affected by intestinal tumors than females, although this trend is most marked for adenocarcinoma and is less obvious for smooth muscle tumors.[92,124,125,128-130]

CLINICAL PRESENTATION AND HISTORY

Clinical signs give very little indication of the type of neoplasm in a dog with an intestinal tumor. They may, however, direct the clinician to a particular area of the intestinal tract. For example, whereas vomiting is most often associated with tumors of the duodenum or jejunum, weight loss and diarrhea are usually seen in dogs with jejunal or ileal tumors.[126] Anorexia, depression, and lethargy may accompany tumors in any location. Hypochromic anemia is a less common sign; it may be caused by melena and iron deficiency.[126,131] Ascites, abdominal pain, and peritonitis from intestinal rupture may occur.[124,132] Clinical signs have often been present for weeks to months,[124,133-135] although dogs that are vomiting are usually presented by their owners more rapidly. Intussusception is rare but can be associated even with small, benign masses.[135]

On physical examination, an abdominal mass may be palpated, particularly if the tumor is in the upper small intestine.[128]

STAGING AND DIAGNOSIS

The first evaluation of a patient with a large intestinal tumor should be collection of an MDB. Abdominal radi-

Table 53-6 **Distribution of Small Intestinal Tumors in Dogs**[92,124,128]

Location	Dogs (%)
Jejunum	44
Duodenum	37
Ileum	19

ography, abdominal ultrasonography, and possibly endoscopy should be used to image the tumor and to identify metastasis.

Plain radiography may help delineate an abdominal mass and may also reveal other abnormalities, such as gas- and fluid-filled dilated loops of bowel, which are suggestive of obstruction. Pneumoperitoneum may indicate tumor rupture or septic peritonitis. Contrast radiography most often shows an "apple-core" lesion for tumors of the small intestine but may also show irregular filling defects or leakage caused by perforation.[124]

Ultrasonography is a rapid means of identifying intestinal tumors and provides a guide for obtaining biopsy specimens as well as a method of staging abdominal metastases.[103,107,108] (Figure 53-21). It is the staging method of choice for dogs with intestinal tumors. In a study of 15 dogs with small intestinal carcinoma, all lesions were poorly echogenic, had an irregular lumen, were transmural, and were associated with complete loss of wall layering. Lesions were localized (median length: 4 cm) and caused thickening of just over 1 cm and fluid accumulation proximal to the lesion in most dogs. Regional lymphadenopathy, nodular mesentery/omentum, or both were noted in 12 of 21 dogs.[136] Ultrasonography was useful in distinguishing enteritis from neoplasia in another study.[137] Dogs with neoplasia had larger lymph nodes and thicker intestinal walls than dogs with enteritis. Dogs with loss of intestinal wall layering were 50.9 times more likely to have a tumor than to have enteritis.

> **KEY POINT**
>
> *Ultrasonography is recommended when staging a dog with intestinal neoplasia because metastasis is more likely to occur to regional lymph nodes than to the lungs.*

Endoscopy can be used to obtain biopsy specimens and may provide a definitive diagnosis of duodenal tumor; however, multiple biopsy specimens should be taken because lesions beneath the mucosa may escape detection, and tumors that create ulcerated lesions may be obscured by inflammatory changes. Lesions beyond the duodenum are

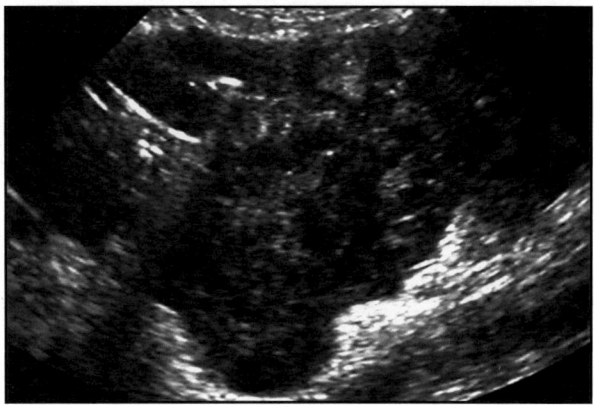

Figure 53-21. *A large, irregularly marginated, poorly echogenic, and exophytic intestinal leiomyosarcoma. A few small, bright interfaces associated with reverberation and shadowing artifacts are noted on the left of the image and represent gas within the distorted bowel segment. (Courtesy of D. G. Penninck)*

not approachable by endoscopy. In one study, endoscopic biopsy of intestinal lymphoma was confounded by the presence of inflammatory infiltrates in nearly 50% of the dogs.[125] Intestinal polyps have been documented to transform to a malignant state, so a diagnosis of intestinal polyp should still be treated with suspicion.[138] Biopsy of small intestinal tumors often requires exploratory laparotomy.

Metastasis is more commonly described for intestinal adenocarcinoma than for leiomyosarcoma.[126,128] In 28 of 40 dogs (70%) with small intestine adenocarcinoma, there was evidence of metastases to mesenteric lymph nodes; metastasis to liver and lung occurred in six (15%) and five (13%) dogs, respectively.[126,139]

In contrast, leiomyosarcoma metastases occur in less than 30% of affected dogs,[21,24,25] often long after definitive surgery.[116,130,131,133] The liver was the most common site of metastasis in one study.[139] Paraneoplastic diabetes insipidus has been associated with jejunal leiomyosarcoma,[140] and another report made an association between a cecal leiomyosarcoma and erythrocytosis.[141] Four dogs with jejunal or duodenal leiomyosarcomas had paraneoplastic hypoglycemia that resolved after surgery.[115,116]

Intestinal tumors of neuroendocrine derivation that may be hormonally active are described as *carcinoids*. Of eight reported intestinal carcinoids (four large intestinal and four small intestinal), all had metastases to the regional lymph nodes and liver at the time of diagnosis, and four dogs had additional sites of metastasis.[126,127,142–144]

PROGNOSTIC FACTORS

In one study, dogs with metastases detected at the time of surgery (regardless of tumor type) had a median survival time of 3 months (20% alive at 1 year) compared with 15 months (67% alive at 1 year) for those without metastases.[139]

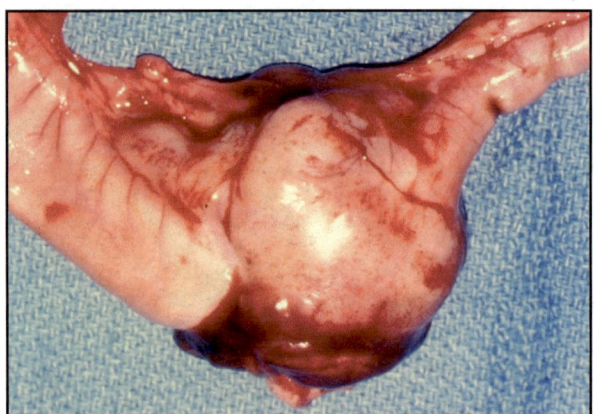

Figure 53-22. *Median survival after resection of a small intestinal carcinoma that has not metastasized is fair; median survival times of 10 months have been reported. Chemotherapy may improve survival, but literature is lacking.*

TREATMENT

Early reports of small numbers of dogs suggested that survival after surgery for a small intestinal carcinoma was poor, with occasional long survivors (Figure 53-22).[124,128] However, in two larger studies, the overall survival for 38 dogs with small intestinal carcinomas was 8 to 10 months; 41% were alive 1 year after surgery.[136,139] In one of these studies, female dogs lived a median of 1 month compared with 9 months for males.[136] Dogs with metastases detected at surgery had shorter survival times.[139]

In one study, there was no significant difference between the median survival for 23 dogs with carcinomas and 16 dogs with leiomyosarcomas (12 months; 40% alive 1 year after surgery). Dogs with metastases detected at surgery had shorter survival times.[139] In another study, fatal cecal rupture and peritonitis caused a perioperative mortality rate of 60% in 10 dogs with cecal smooth muscle tumors.[129,145] In a synopsis of studies, 27 (57%) of 47 dogs with GI leiomyosarcoma survived the perioperative period and had median survival times of 8 months (cecum), 13 months (stomach and small intestine), and 21 months.[129,130,145] Only five of these 27 dogs developed metastases. One dog had evidence of metastasis at the time of surgery and survived 3 years without adjuvant therapy.[130] One dog that developed two isolated pulmonary metastases 28 months after initial surgery had them removed and was free of disease 2 months later.[116]

Results of chemotherapy have rarely been reported for intestinal tumors in dogs. Doxorubicin may have efficacy in the treatment of carcinomas, although only anecdotal reports are available. Long-term regression of metastases from intestinal carcinomas in dogs treated with doxorubicin and its derivatives has been seen.[136]

Nearly half of the small intestinal carcinomas examined in one study showed marked expression of COX-2 in tumor cells.[146] This has led to speculation that nonsteroidal inhibitors of COX-2, such as piroxicam, may play a role in the treatment of intestinal carcinoma. No studies have tested this assumption.

Supportive care is important for dogs undergoing extensive GI surgery. Attention should be paid to nutritional requirements, and appropriate feeding tubes (jejunostomy tube) or IV parenteral nutrition used before weight loss and debilitation are essential. Supportive care is particularly important for dogs with evidence of septic peritonitis caused by rupture of the tumor and intestinal wall. Aggressive fluid therapy and treatment with broad-spectrum antibiotics while waiting for culture and sensitivity results are mandatory in these dogs. For dogs that survive this complication, particularly those with leiomyosarcomas, the prognosis is cautiously optimistic.

Large Intestinal Tumors
INCIDENCE, SIGNALMENT, AND ETIOLOGY

Adenocarcinomas are the most common tumor of the large intestine in dogs. Leiomyosarcomas occur more frequently in the small intestine and cecum than in the large intestine.[145,147] Lymphoma may be found anywhere within the GI tract but is usually associated with systemic disease.[125] Table 53-7 summarizes canine colorectal tumor location.

Intestinal tumors occur in older dogs; the median age is 11 to 12 years, although the average age of dogs with lymphoma is younger. There is no obvious breed predilection. Males are more frequently affected by intestinal tumors than females, although this trend is most marked for adenocarcinoma and is less obvious for smooth muscle tumors.[53,92,125,128,130,148]

In human patients, there is a clear clinical and molecular progression from colorectal polyps to colorectal carcinoma. There is evidence of similar progression in dogs with colorectal polyps, so these tumors should not be dismissed as purely benign lesions.[149,150] Mutations in the *p53* tumor suppressor gene are seen in preneoplastic, benign, and malignant colorectal epithelial lesions in dogs, but although this implies an early role in molecular progression, there is no prognostic significance to detection of *p53*.[151]

CLINICAL PRESENTATION AND HISTORY

Clinical signs give very little indication of the type or malignancy of a neoplasm in a dog with an intestinal tumor. They may, however, direct the clinician to a particular area of the intestinal tract. Anorexia, depression, and lethargy may accompany tumors in any location. Hypochromic anemia, a less common sign, may be caused by melena and iron deficiency.[126,131] Ascites, abdominal pain, and peritonitis from intestinal rupture may occur; the last condition is mainly seen with cecal leiomyosarcomas.[129,130] Clinical signs have often been present for weeks to months, and even benign tumors may have a history of years of hematochezia

Table 53-7 **Distribution of Colorectal Adenocarcinomas in Dogs**[53]

Location	Dogs (%)
Distal rectum	27
Midrectum	49
Proximal rectum	12
Colon	12

and tenesmus.[152,153] Tenesmus and hematochezia most often occur with colonic or rectal tumors.[53,126,128]

Colorectal polyps are usually solitary (80%) but can be multiple or diffuse. Polyps that are multiple or diffuse are more likely to show malignant transformation and to have recurrence of signs after treatment.[150]

Distal rectal carcinomas are mostly palpable as a single pedunculated mass; tumors located rostrally are more likely to be multiple ("cobblestone appearance") or appear as an annular constriction.[53] Carcinomas may extend to involve a few centimeters of the colon and occasionally involve most of the large intestine.[154] Dogs with rectal leiomyomas may be asymptomatic, presumably owing to the slow growth of these tumors; however, these tumors may become very large (up to 12 cm in one study).[148]

Rectal examination may reveal stricture, mass, or irregular rectal wall in more than 60% of dogs affected with adenomas and carcinomas.[53,148,150] The size of the tumor does not necessarily indicate whether the tumor is benign or malignant; some rectal polyps can be 3 to 7 cm in diameter.[153] Dogs with plasmacytomas of the rectal wall have masses that are usually between 2 and 3 cm in diameter, may be friable, and are sometimes pedunculated. These tumors may cause recurrent prolapse and tenesmus and may be multiple.[155]

STAGING AND DIAGNOSIS

The first evaluation of a patient with a large intestinal tumor should be collection of an MDB. Abdominal radiography, abdominal ultrasonography, and endoscopy should also be used to image the tumor and to identify metastasis.

Plain radiographs may help delineate an abdominal mass and may also reveal other abnormalities, such as gas- and fluid-filled dilated loops of bowel, which are suggestive of obstruction. Pneumoperitoneum may indicate tumor rupture or septic peritonitis.[62,128] Contrast enemas may show irregular filling defects or leakage caused by perforation.

Ultrasonography is a noninvasive and rapid means of identifying intestinal tumors and provides a guide for obtaining biopsy specimens and assessing organs for abdominal metastases, particularly sublumbar (iliac) lymph nodes[103,107,108] (Figure 53-23). Ultrasonography is the staging method of choice in dogs with large intestinal tumors.[136]

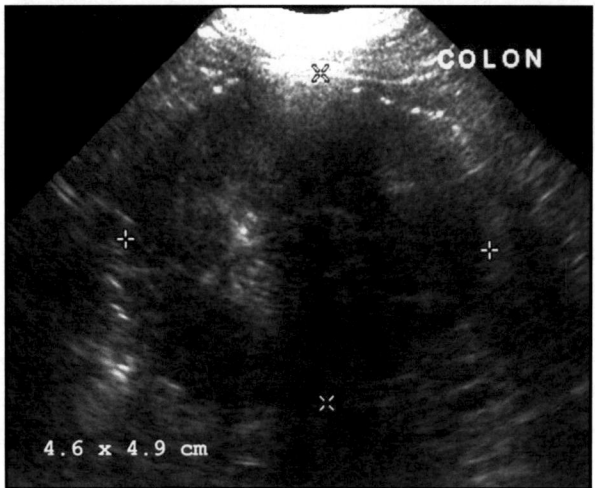

Figure 53-23. *Transverse sonogram of the distal portion of the descending colon with a colonic carcinoma. Marked transmural, asymmetric wall thickening with loss of layering is noted (between calipers). The irregular bright echoes within the mass represent the distorted lumen. (Courtesy of D. G. Penninck)*

The distal colon may not be accessible to ultrasonography, and endoscopy may be preferred for these tumors, either alone or in combination with ultrasonography. Endoscopy can be used to obtained biopsy specimens, which may provide a definitive diagnosis of rectal tumors; however, multiple biopsy specimens should be taken because lesions beneath the mucosa may escape detection and tumors that create ulcerated lesions may be obscured by inflammatory changes.[53,156,157] Endoscopy of the entire large bowel is particularly important when a distal rectal tumor is palpated because dogs may have additional proximal lesions that could otherwise remain undetected and continue to cause clinical signs after surgery.

Biopsy of rectal tumors may be achieved via proctoscopy or by prolapsing the rectum manually or with stay sutures.[53] The diagnosis of a rectal polyp should not be dismissed. Some rectal polyps have areas of carcinoma in situ, and complete histologic examination of any surgically removed tissue is important to detect such malignant transformation. Because diagnosis of small specimens may be difficult, complete excision and submission for histopathology are suggested.[150] Dogs with multiple lesions and those with diffuse disease were more likely to show malignant transformation in one study.[150]

Metastasis of colorectal adenocarcinoma is considered uncommon. There was no evidence of metastasis in 78 dogs with this disease, even after long survival times after surgery.[53] Similarly, metastasis from rarely encountered large intestinal leiomyosarcomas appears to be uncommon.

Paraneoplastic leukocytosis has been described in two dogs with rectal adenomatous polyps.[158,159] Resolution occurred after surgical excision in one dog, and reduction in counts occurred after piroxicam suppository treatment in another.

Carcinoid is used to describe intestinal tumors of neuroendocrine derivation that may be hormonally active. Of eight reported intestinal carcinoids (four large intestinal and four small intestinal), all had metastases to the regional lymph nodes and liver at the time of diagnosis, and there were additional sites of metastasis in four dogs.[126,127,142–144]

PROGNOSTIC FACTORS

In one study of colorectal adenocarcinomas, dogs with annular tumors had the shortest average survival time (1.6 months). Dogs with tumors that comprised multiple "cobblestone" nodules had an average survival time of 12 months. Dogs with a single pedunculated lesion had the longest survival time (32 months) after surgery.[53] These prognostic factors are probably related to the ease with which complete surgical excision may be performed.

TREATMENT

Most dogs with rectal polyps are cured by surgical excision. There is a clear clinical and molecular progression from colorectal polyps to colorectal carcinoma, so polyps should not be dismissed as purely benign lesions.[149] Localized excision, local excision followed by cryosurgery of the base, or full-thickness resection was used to treat 34 dogs with rectal polyps.[150] Only two of 12 dogs with adenomatous polyps had a recurrence at 9 and 12 months after surgery. In contrast, 12 of 22 dogs with areas of carcinoma in situ had recurrence, all within 3 months. Pathology aside, whereas eight of 27 dogs (30%) with solitary lesions had a recurrence, all but one dog with either multiple or diffuse masses had a recurrence. Invasive carcinoma (four dogs) or carcinoma in situ (two dogs) developed between 8 and 37 months after initial treatment; these six dogs represented 7% of dogs with solitary masses, 25% with multiple masses, and all dogs with diffuse disease.[150] Cryosurgery may help prevent recurrence in dogs with rectal polyps, and there were no adverse effects seen in this study.[150] Any dog with a colorectal polyp should have periodic examinations (preferably by endoscopy) after surgery to detect any new lesions, and lesions should be removed at the earliest possible time. An arbitrary 3- to 6-month period is suggested.[150]

Dogs with tumors that are surgically inaccessible or would require extensive surgery may be treated using endoscopic resection and cautery. This approach was successful in curing three of six dogs with rectal polyps, and two dogs had reduction in clinical signs; however, one dog died because of perforation of the rectal wall.[152] Multiple treatments (two to six) were needed in all dogs to achieve best results.

In contrast to the high levels of COX-2 expression seen in small intestinal carcinomas, few colorectal carcinomas show expression in tumor cells.[146] However, the peritumoral tissue around most colorectal adenomas showed COX-2 expression in one study.[146] This has led to speculation that nonsteroidal inhibitors of COX-2 may play a role in the treatment of colorectal polyps. Seven dogs with colorectal polyps (two with evidence of malignant transformation) were treated with piroxicam in suppository form (20 mg every 2 to 3 days) or oral form.[153,159] All but one dog had a reduction in size of the masses and reduced hematochezia, fecal tenesmus, and mucus production. There were no CRs, and it is uncertain if the reduction in size was attributable to antiinflammatory palliation or true antineoplastic effects.

Colorectal adenocarcinomas have a low rate of metastasis, and treated dogs may have long survival times after diagnosis. In one study, dogs with this disease that were treated palliatively with stool softeners lived an average of 15 months.[53] Of multiple treatment modalities, local excision gave the longest average survival time (22 months) with the lowest complication rate.[53] Recurrence after local excision of a solitary mass occurred in 11 of 21 dogs (50%). Radical surgical excision of annular colorectal adenocarcinoma resulted in wound dehiscence and septic peritonitis in all four dogs treated. In another study, 15 dogs treated by surgery for intestinal carcinoma had a median survival time of 8 months; whether the tumor was located in the small or in the large intestine did not influence outcome.[136]

Cryosurgery prolonged survival in 11 dogs with colorectal adenocarcinoma (average survival: 24 months). Recurrence was similar to that after local excision; however, additional complications, including stricture (five of 11 dogs), rectal prolapse, and perineal hernia, occurred after treatment.[53] Other techniques, such as electrocoagulation[53] and Nd:YAG laser-assisted surgery,[158] provide control similar to that of local excision.

Radiation therapy using a single high dose (15–25 Gy) of orthovoltage teletherapy may provide reasonable control for recurrent distal rectal adenocarcinomas. In six dogs, median tumor control duration was 6 months, and no complications were reported.[160] In another group of dogs, one dog treated with radiation therapy suffered a rectal perforation and died from peritonitis 2 months after treatment.[53]

Results of chemotherapy have not been reported for intestinal carcinomas in dogs.

Surgical excision of other intestinal and rectal tumors carries a fair prognosis. Thirteen (55%) of 23 dogs with leiomyosarcoma survived the perioperative period and had a median survival of 21 months (range: 2 months to 7 years). Only three of these 13 dogs developed metastases.[130] Unfortunately, leiomyosarcoma of the colorectum was not separated from tumors of other locations in the GI tract, so it is not possible to specifically report survivals for the large intestine. In a separate report, the median survival time after surgical resection of colorectal leiomyoma was 26 months.

Only one of five affected dogs died from tumor-related causes.[148] Excision of two small ganglioneuromas from the rectum of a dog was apparently successful; there was no evidence of recurrence 30 months after surgery.[161]

Excision of a rectal plasmacytoma and postoperative chemotherapy with melphalan and prednisone led to a dog being free of disease 22 months later.[123] Similar control was seen by Dr. Moore in another dog, but the tumor recurred after 16 months and was resistant to doxorubicin and cyclophosphamide (Figure 53-24). Radiation therapy may be another treatment option for unresectable or resistant rectal plasmacytomas.

Tumors of the Perianal (Hepatoid) Glands

INCIDENCE, SIGNALMENT, AND ETIOLOGY

The most common tumor arising from the hepatoid glands (also called *perianal* or *circumanal glands*) is adenoma. It is most common in older male intact dogs (63% of this tumor type) and appears to be stimulated by androgen secretion. Growth hormone may also play a role in tumor development, although it does not appear critical for progression to malignancy.[162] Female dogs that have perianal gland adenomas may have ectopic testosterone secretion from the adrenal gland.[163] These tumors may also arise in other areas: although the perineum was the site of 89% of these tumors, 7% arose on the tail, 3% on the abdomen, and another 1% at other locations.[164] In a series of 2,700 perianal tumors, Siberian huskies, Samoyeds, and Pekingese were found to be at increased risk for developing adenomas.[164]

The specific literature on hepatoid gland adenocarcinomas is sparse. The existing literature suggests that despite their sebaceous origin, these tumors, when malignant, act in the same manner as canine anal sac (apocrine) adenocarcinomas, except that they do not cause hypercalcemia.

Distribution appears to be similar to that described for adenomas. In one series of dogs, 70% of tumors occurred in the perineum, 16% on the abdomen, 8% on the tail, and 7% at other sites.[164] Although females were more likely to have carcinomas in one study,[165] two other studies found that males predominated. In one of those studies, 90% of 145 dogs with perianal gland carcinomas were male, with an average age of 11 years.[164] Similarly, perianal adenocarcinoma was only diagnosed in older male dogs in another study[166]; most dogs in both studies were intact males. Arctic Circle breeds, specifically, Alaskan malamutes and Siberian huskies, were overrepresented in both studies. Bulldogs and German shepherds were also suggested to be overrepresented.[164,166]

CLINICAL PRESENTATION AND HISTORY

Affected dogs are often presented to veterinarians because of an unrelated problem, because the client often notices a

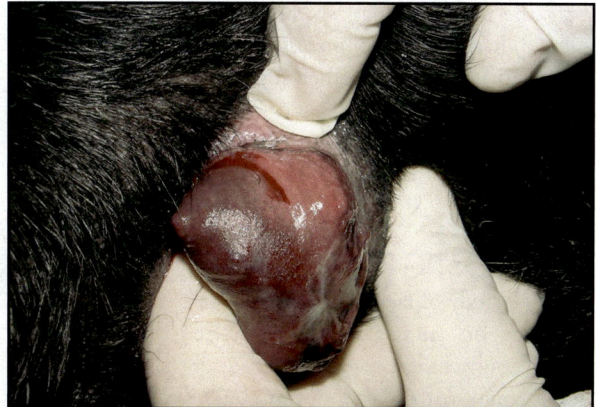

Figure 53-24. *A large colorectal plasmacytoma. Such tumors may respond to surgery when small, but chemotherapy or radiation therapy would be needed to treat this large tumor.*

swelling in the perineum that may be painful or irritating, or because there is ulceration of a lesion and tenesmus.[166] Tenesmus may be caused by the primary tumor or by sublumbar lymphadenopathy in cases of malignant tumors, which may be palpable rectally. The tumor may be an incidental finding, emphasizing the importance of including a rectal palpation on routine physical examinations.

STAGING AND DIAGNOSIS

In a study of 134 canine perineal gland tumors, most (58.3%) were classified as well-differentiated perianal gland tumors. Moderately or poorly differentiated perianal gland tumors (21.6%) and carcinomas without perianal gland differentiation (16.6%) were less common.[165] Tumors showing perianal gland differentiation almost invariably were benign. Carcinomas lacking any perianal gland differentiation often showed a distinct malignant behavior, with metastases to regional lymph nodes and internal organs. These malignant neoplasms showed morphologic and clinical features comparable with those of canine anal sac gland adenocarcinomas.[165] Perianal adenomas and adenocarcinomas are not clinically different in their appearance.[164] Most tumors are benign, but malignant tumors also occur in intact male dogs. Definitive diagnosis is best made by surgical biopsy. Histologic criteria of malignancy include invasiveness and a higher proportion of reserve cells as well as nuclear pleomorphism and increased mitoses.[166]

When perianal gland tumors are malignant, they appear to act in the same manner as canine anal sac (apocrine) adenocarcinomas; therefore, prognosis and treatment are often based on the literature for apocrine tumors. If perianal adenocarcinoma is suspected in a dog, an MDB should be conducted. Abdominal radiography or (preferably) ultrasonography should also be done to look for metastatic disease before proceeding with treatment because nodal metastases are common.

In one series of dogs, six of 41 dogs (14.6%) had evidence of metastasis at the time of diagnosis.[166] Another study estimated that between 10% and 30% of these tumors metastasize to regional (sublumbar, inguinal, and popliteal) lymph nodes.[164]

PROGNOSTIC FACTORS

In one study of factors studied for their influence on survival and disease-free interval, only clinical stage was statistically significant, with large tumors and metastatic tumors conferring a worse survival.[166]

TREATMENT

Most adenomas in male dogs regress after castration.[167] Perianal gland adenomas may be excised, but unless the source of androgen stimulation is removed, new tumors arise at other sites (Figures 53-25 and 53-26). Estrogens and antiandrogen drugs have been used; estrogens have bone marrow–suppressing properties that make them a poor choice for long-term management. Cryosurgery has been successful in the treatment of small adenomas, but again, unless the dog is castrated, new tumors arise. Radiation therapy causes tumor regression, although care must be taken not to irradiate deep around the colon because of the risk of late fibrosis and stricture. Testosterone production in a female dog with hyperadrenocorticism and perianal adenomas ceased when mitotane therapy was instituted for the adrenal disease.[163]

Surgical excision of perianal adenocarcinoma is often difficult because of the large size of these tumors and their invasive growth characteristics. Complications of surgery reflect the difficulties encountered in any surgical procedure involving the perineal area. Fecal incontinence can occur after surgery in up to 20% of dogs and may be permanent. Wound infection can occur and cause sepsis.

Local recurrence is a problem with some dogs; others develop metastasis to the regional lymph nodes. If the sublumbar nodes are enlarged at diagnosis, it may be possible to remove them surgically; however, tumor-invaded nodes are frequently friable and invade around the vessels and nerves in this area.

In one study, 32 dogs were treated for perianal adenocarcinomas.[166] A complete excision was performed in 16 dogs, and these dogs had a median survival of 23.5 months (22 months disease free). An additional 13 dogs, mostly with smaller carcinomas, also had cryosurgery after incomplete surgical excision; these dogs had a median survival time of 20 months (19 months disease free). Adjuvant radiation therapy should be considered for incompletely excised tumors, although the role of this therapy is undefined. Three dogs with very large carcinomas in one study received 40 Gy of radiation therapy after surgical debulking and survived a median of 18.5 months. Overall, in that study, dogs with very large tumors were less likely to have long disease control, although radiation therapy appeared to improve control rates.[166]

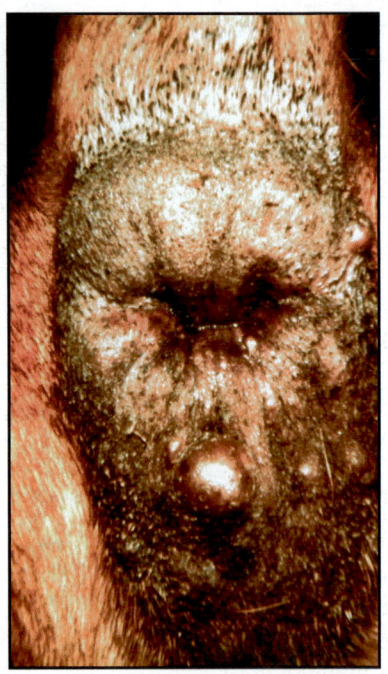

Figure 53-25. Small perianal adenomas may regress after castration.

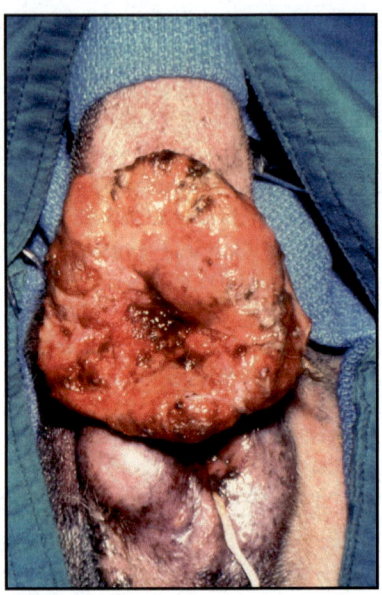

Figure 53-26. Large, ulcerated perianal adenomas may require surgical intervention or radiation therapy as well as castration. Biopsy should be performed to ensure that the tumor is not a carcinoma.

Chemotherapy might be promising as adjuvant therapy for this tumor, but little has been reported. Chemotherapy drug choices are the same as those for anal sac adenocarcinomas (see Adenocarcinoma of the Anal Sac section, below). Doxorubicin was ineffective in treating recurrence of carcinoma in two dogs in one study.[166] However, doxorubicin and platinum-derived drugs are most likely to be effective, either alone or in combination.

Adenocarcinoma of the Anal Sac
INCIDENCE, SIGNALMENT, AND ETIOLOGY

Early studies showed that anal sac adenocarcinoma occurs most commonly in old, female dogs, either intact or spayed.[165,168–170] Two larger studies have questioned that assumption, and a combined series of 351 dogs had no gender predilection, although neutered and spayed dogs of both genders had a higher incidence.[171,172] The age of affected dogs ranges from 5 to 17 years, with an average age of 10.5 years. In most reports, there is no obvious breed predilection, and crossbred and purebred dogs are affected equally. However, one European study reported that five of eight affected dogs were longhaired or wirehaired German shorthair pointers,[173] and a study from the United States showed that English cocker spaniels, dachshunds, and Alaskan malamutes were all more than four times as likely as the general population to develop these tumors.[171]

A characteristic feature of this tumor is production of a parathyroid hormone–related protein that causes hypercalcemia and hypophosphatemia, occurring in 25% to 30% of affected dogs.[172,174]

Rarely, SCC may arise from the lining of the anal sac. In a series of five dogs, these tumors infiltrated surrounding tissue but were not associated with hypercalcemia or metastasis.[175]

CLINICAL PRESENTATION AND HISTORY

Affected dogs are often presented because of an unrelated problem; because the owner notices a swelling in the perineum (Figure 53-27); or because of dyschezia, tenesmus, or ribbon-like stools.[168,170,172] Tenesmus may be caused by the primary tumor or by sublumbar lymphadenopathy, which may be palpable rectally. In one study, 30% of dogs had a history of licking or biting at the perineum.[172] Other signs were perianal bleeding (24% of dogs), polyuria and polydipsia (22%), scooting (21%), and hindlimb weakness (18%). Polydipsia and polyuria are common in hypercalcemic dogs. The identification of hypercalcemia on a biochemical profile warrants careful palpation of the anal sacs.[170] Signs may be present for up to 1 year before presentation.[169] In 40% to 60% of dogs in a reported series, the tumor was an incidental finding on rectal examination[168,169] or was found only after hypercalcemia had been identified.[170] This emphasizes the importance of including a rectal palpation in routine physical examinations. The tumor mass is usually between 1 and 10 cm in diameter, although smaller primary masses that are difficult to palpate may be present.[165,168] In one study, the product of tumor diameters was greater than 10 cm² in 43% of affected dogs.[172] Because the tumor may be bilateral, it is important to palpate both anal sacs.[168–170]

> **KEY POINT**
>
> *If hypercalcemia is detected on routine biochemistry, the anal sacs should be palpated for the presence of a tumor.*

STAGING AND DIAGNOSIS

If anal sac adenocarcinoma is suspected in a dog, routine biochemical profiles should be conducted to identify hypercalcemia and any secondary renal damage. Abdominal radiography or (preferably) ultrasonography should be conducted to look for metastatic disease before taking thoracic radiographs because pulmonary metastases are uncommon.

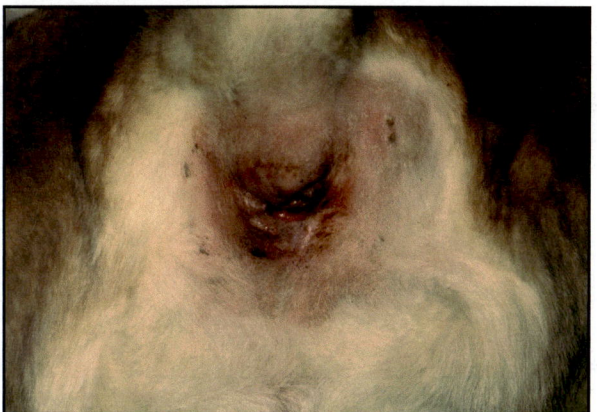

Figure 53-27. *Swelling on the right side of the rectum in this dog was caused by an anal sac carcinoma. Hypercalcemia should prompt examination of the anal sacs for a tumor.*

Hypercalcemia is common in dogs with apocrine gland adenocarcinoma of the anal sacs and may occur in males and females. In one small study, 90% of dogs with anal sac adenocarcinoma had elevated serum calcium levels (average: 16.1 mg/dl).[170] In two larger studies, serum calcium was elevated in 25% of affected dogs.[168,172] Hypophosphatemia occurred concurrently with hypercalcemia in some dogs.[170] If hypercalcemia is prolonged, calcium nephropathy may occur, terminating in renal failure.[176] Prompt treatment of hypercalcemic dogs is important (see below).

This neoplasm is highly malignant and infiltrates the surrounding perirectal soft tissues and even the rectal sphincter. Metastasis to the sublumbar and iliac lymph nodes occurs early in the course of the disease (Figure 53-28). Other affected regional lymph nodes are the inguinal and the popliteal nodes. All external nodes should be carefully palpated and fine-needle aspiration for cytology or biopsy for histopathology conducted. In two studies, 94% of dogs had metastases to the regional lymph nodes.[170,173] However, a larger study found that less than half the dogs (47%) had enlarged lymph nodes at the time of diagnosis; this may reflect earlier diagnosis.[172] Lateral abdominal radiographs are useful in identifying sublumbar lymphadenopathy, but ultrasonography is more accurate than radiography or digital rectal palpation in disclosing the extent of lymph node involvement.[177]

Less frequent sites of metastasis are the lungs, which may show a nodular or diffuse pattern radiographically, and (rarely) the lumbar vertebrae, spleen, liver, and kidneys.[168,171,173] Metastasis may occur when the primary tumor is very small, and clinical signs relating to the primary tumor may not be obvious.[168] Definitive diagnosis is made by surgical biopsy, although a high index of suspicion for this disease should follow detection of a perianal mass in an older dog with hypercalcemia.

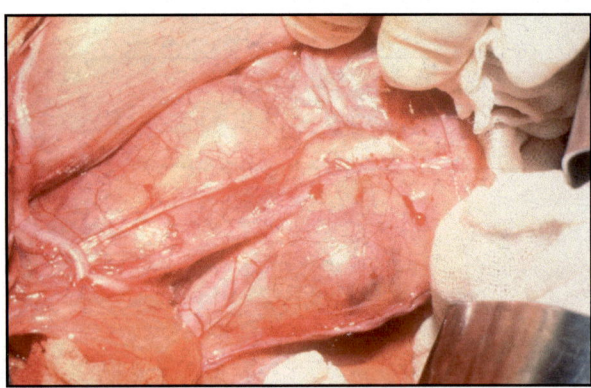

Figure 53-28. *Exploratory laparotomy reveals metastasis of an anal sac adenocarcinoma to the sublumbar nodes. These nodes are easily visualized with ultrasonography, and dogs with this tumor should be routinely examined for metastatic spread before definitive treatment. (Courtesy of John Berg, DVM, Tufts Cummings School of Veterinary Medicine)*

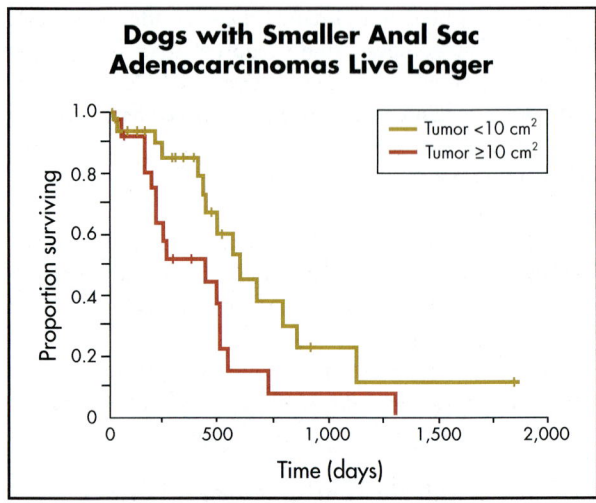

Figure 53-29. *Survival curves for dogs with anal sac adenocarcinomas 10 cm² or larger (n = 24) or smaller than 10 cm² (n = 32). (Adapted from Williams LE, Gliatto JM, Dodge RK, et al: Carcinoma of the apocrine glands of the anal sac in dogs: 113 cases (1985–1995). JAVMA 223:825–831, 2003; with permission)*

PROGNOSTIC FACTORS

A large study of 113 dogs found that dogs with tumors of an area greater than 10 cm² (product of two greatest diameters) had a shorter median survival than dogs with smaller tumors: 8 months and 19 months, respectively (Figure 53-29). This and another study[168] found that dogs with hypercalcemia had a shorter median survival time than dogs with normocalcemia: 9.6 months and 19 months, respectively (Figure 53-30). In the larger study, dogs with pulmonary metastases detected at surgery predictably had shorter median survival times (7 months) than dogs without metastases (18 months).[172] However, the finding of iliac lymphadenopathy did not affect prognosis (Figure 53-31).

TREATMENT

Dogs with anal sac adenocarcinomas should be treated surgically in an attempt to achieve complete excision of the primary mass. Sublumbar lymph nodes should be removed if they are enlarged, although this is a technically demanding surgery. Radiation therapy to the sublumbar (iliac) lymph nodes and chemotherapy using doxorubicin with or without platinum derivatives should be used adjunctively. If hypercalcemia is detected, treatment before and during surgery is important to ensure adequate hydration and urinary output. Sodium chloride is a good fluid of choice because it causes calciuresis. Bisphosphonates such as pamidronate (1–2 mg/kg IV given over 1–4 h) can be very helpful at reducing calcium levels. Furosemide and glucocorticoids may also be used in well-hydrated patients as soon as a histologic or cytologic diagnosis has been made.

In one study of 113 dogs that received multiple treatment modalities either alone or in combination, dogs that had surgery as part of their treatment (alone or in combination with radiation therapy, chemotherapy, or both) lived longer than dogs treated without surgery.[172] This retrospective study was limited by some selection bias (i.e., dogs in different treatment groups were prescribed different treatments based on their extent of disease). Dogs treated with surgery alone had 90% survival at 6 months, 65% survival at 1 year, and 29% survival at 2 years. Median survival time for 81 dogs treated with surgery, either alone or in combination with any other modality, was 18 months compared with 13 months for dogs treated without surgery.[172] Similar survival times have been reported in other smaller studies.[168,170]

> **KEY POINT**
>
> *Even with incomplete excision of an anal sac tumor, most dogs that are hypercalcemic become normocalcemic.*

Surgical excision of the primary tumor is often difficult because of the large size of these tumors and their invasive growth characteristics. Local recurrence is seen in approximately 25% of dogs.[168,169] However, even with incomplete surgical excision, most dogs that are hypercalcemic become normocalcemic after surgery. Hypercalcemia presumably reflects some critical tumor mass because even dogs with metastases may not show recurrence of hypercalcemia until the metastases become large.[173,178] Complications of surgery reflect the difficulties encountered in any surgical procedure involving the perineal area. Fecal incontinence can occur after surgery in up to 20% of dogs and may be permanent.[168] Wound infection can occur and cause dehiscence and sepsis.

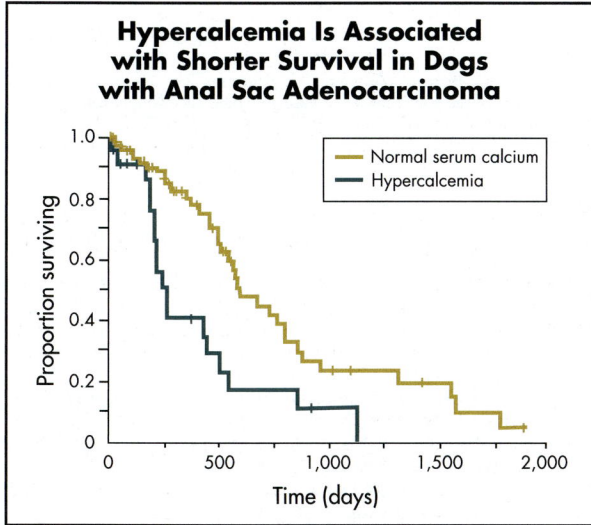

Figure 53-30. Survival curves for dogs with anal sac adenocarcinoma. Serum calcium was normal in 74 dogs and elevated in 26 dogs. (From Williams LE, Gliatto JM, Dodge RK, et al: Carcinoma of the apocrine glands of the anal sac in dogs: 113 cases (1985–1995). JAVMA 223:825–831, 2003; with permission)

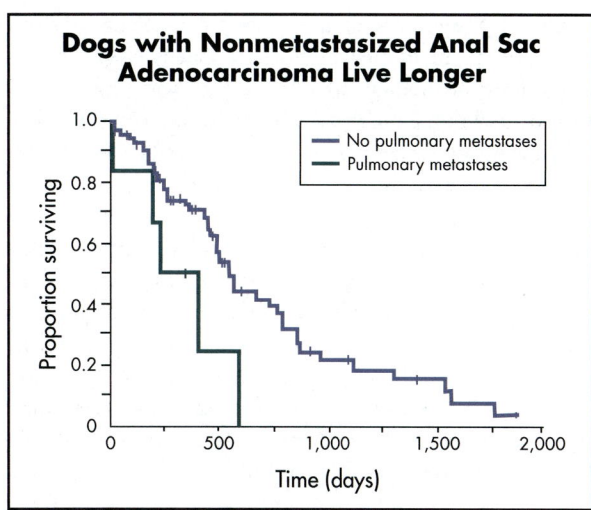

Figure 53-31. Survival curves for dogs with anal sac adenocarcinoma. Pulmonary metastases were seen in 7 dogs; 88 dogs had no evidence of pulmonary metastases. (From Williams LE, Gliatto JM, Dodge RK, et al: Carcinoma of the apocrine glands of the anal sac in dogs: 113 cases (1985–1995). JAVMA 223:825–831, 2003; with permission)

If the sublumbar nodes are enlarged at diagnosis, it may be possible to remove them surgically; however, tumor-invaded nodes are frequently friable and invade around the vessels and nerves in this area (Figure 53-28). The nodes were well encapsulated in 80% of dogs treated surgically in one study, but they were also well vascularized; thus, the surgeon should be prepared to encounter bleeding. In this study, complications during lymph node surgery caused the death of one-third of the dogs; almost one-third of the survivors developed transient urinary incontinence, presumably as a result of neurologic trauma. Overall, six of 27 dogs died within 2 weeks after undergoing surgery to remove either the primary tumor or its metastases.[168]

At presentation, most affected dogs have metastases only in regional lymph nodes, and further spread is rare. For this reason, radiation therapy might be expected to be palliative. In a large study, 10 dogs that received radiation alone had a median survival time of 22 months, but these dogs may have been selected based on more localized disease.[172] The median survival time was 26 months for 27 dogs that received radiation therapy alone or in combination with surgery, chemotherapy, or both. Clearly, radiotherapy may be worth adding to a multimodal approach to therapy. Of 27 dogs receiving radiation therapy as part of treatment, the only significant side effect was rectal stricture in four dogs (15%); most of these dogs received multimodal treatment.[172] In another study, radiation therapy and mitoxantrone chemotherapy gave symptomatic relief and tumor control for nearly 10 months to dogs that had only local disease or lymph node metastases. Survival times were considerably longer. None of the dogs in this study had distant (lung) metastases, and most of the improvement in survival was probably attributable to radiation therapy.[179]

Chemotherapy might be promising as adjuvant therapy, but relatively few data have been reported. A large retrospective study found that dogs with iliac lymphadenopathy were significantly more likely to receive chemotherapy. Dogs treated with surgery plus chemotherapy (most received a platinum agent, doxorubicin, or mitoxantrone) had 86% survival at 6 months, 69% at 1 year, 36% at 2 years, and 14% at 3 years (median: 18 months). This slightly longer survival in dogs with more extensive disease suggests that chemotherapy can have value as an adjunct. Dogs that received chemotherapy alone (usually because their tumors were too extensive to approach surgically) had 67% survival at 6 months, with a median survival time of 7 months.[172] GI toxicity was greatest in the group of dogs receiving surgery, radiation therapy, and chemotherapy. Another, smaller study showed that approximately one-third of dogs receiving platinum chemotherapy experienced a greater than 50% decrease in tumor size.[180]

Other information is anecdotal: three dogs treated with doxorubicin and cyclophosphamide, either alone or in combination with prednisone, vincristine, and L-asparaginase (for concurrent lymphoma), had survival times of 1, 2, and 14 months.[168] Another tumor did not respond to treatment with melphalan and cyclophosphamide.[169]

Supportive and Palliative Care

Often, the reason for euthanasia of a dog with anal sac carcinoma is obstruction caused by lymph node metastases that can be very large. One option is palliative radiation therapy to reduce the size of the lymph nodes. Late effects of fibrosis and colonic or urethral stricture are high with this form of treatment, although survival will probably be shorter than the time it would take to see such effects. Palliative omentalization of a cystic lymph node prevented signs of pelvic obstruction from recurring in a dog for 18 months.[178]

Palliative treatment of hypercalcemia may control clinical signs and delay renal damage in a dog that cannot be treated surgically (e.g., with massive lymph node metastases). Drugs that interfere with osteoclast activity (pamidronate, etidronate [10 mg/kg PO q24h], or prednisone) may provide long-term control of serum calcium, although as the tumor enlarges and hypercalcemia becomes refractory to control, dosages should be increased[178] (see also Chapter 36).

REFERENCES

1. Verstraete FJ, Kass PH, Terpak CH: Diagnostic value of full-mouth radiography in dogs. *Am J Vet Res* 59:686–691, 1998.
2. Poulet FM, Valentine BA, Summers BA: A survey of epithelial odontogenic tumors and cysts in dogs and cats. *Vet Pathol* 29:369–380, 1992.
3. Dubielzig RR, Goldschmidt MH, Brodey RS: The nomenclature of peridontal epulides in dogs. *Vet Pathol* 16:209–214, 1979.
4. Thrall DE: Orthovoltage radiotherapy of acanthomatous epulides in 39 dogs. *JAVMA* 184:826–829, 1984.
5. Gorman NT, Bright RM, Mays MB, Thrall DE: Chemotherapy of a recurrent acanthomatous epulis in a dog. *JAVMA* 184:1158–1160, 1984.
6. Yoshida K, Yanai T, Iwasaki T, et al: Clinicopathological study of canine oral epulides. *J Vet Med Sci* 61:897–902, 1999.
7. Yoshida K, Yanai T, Iwasaki T, et al: Proliferative potential of canine oral epulides and malignant neoplasms assessed by bromodeoxyuridine labeling. *Vet Pathol* 36:35–41, 1999.
8. Theon AP, Rodriguez C, Griffey S, Madewell BR: Analysis of prognosis factors and patterns of failure in dogs with periodontal tumors treated with megavoltage irradiation. *JAVMA* 210:785–788, 1997.
9. McEntee MC, Page RL, Theon A, et al: Malignant tumor formation in dogs previously irradiated for acanthomatous epulis. *Vet Radiol Ultrasound* 45:357–361, 2004.
10. White RA: Mandibulectomy and maxillectomy in the dog: Long term survival in 100 cases. *J Small Anim Pract* 32:69–74, 1991.
11. Langham RF, Mostosky UV, Schirmer RG: X-ray therapy of selected odontogenic neoplasms in the dog. *JAVMA* 170:820–822, 1977.
12. White RA, Jefferies AR, Gorman NT: Sarcoma development following irradiation of acanthomatous epulis in two dogs. *Vet Rec* 118:668, 1986.
13. Yoshida K, Watarai Y, Sakai Y, et al: The effect of intralesional bleomycin on canine acanthomatous epulis. *JAAHA* 34:457–461, 1998.
14. Werner RE Jr: Canine oral neoplasia: A review of 19 cases. *JAAHA* 17:67–69, 1981.
15. Ishikawa T, Yamamoto H: Case of calcifying epithelial odontogenic tumour in a dog. *J Small Anim Pract* 37:597–599, 1996.
16. Delverdier M, Guire F, Van Harverbeke G: Les tumeurs de la cavite buccale du chien: Etude anatomoclinique a partir de 117 cas. *Revue Med Vet* 142:811–816, 1991.
17. Todoroff RJ, Brodey RS: Oral and pharyngeal neoplasia in the dog: A retrospective study of 361 cases. *JAVMA* 175:567–571, 1979.
18. von Reiswitz A, Hörsting N, Meyer-Lindenberg A, et al: Orale und pharyngeale umfangsvermehrungen des hundeseine retrospektive kasuistische und pathohistologische untersuchung. *Kleintierpraxis* 45:745–759, 2000.
19. Schwarz PD, Withrow SJ, Curtis CR, et al: Partial maxillary resection as a treatment for oral cancer in 61 dogs. *JAAHA* 27:617–624, 1991.
20. Schwarz PD, Withrow SJ, Curtis CR, et al: Mandibular resection as a treatment for oral cancer in 81 dogs. *JAAHA* 27:601–610, 1991.
21. Lascelles BD, Thompson MJ, Dernell WS, et al: Combined dorsolateral and intraoral approach for the resection of tumors of the maxilla in the dog. *JAAHA* 39:294–305, 2003.
22. Lascelles BD, Henderson RA, Seguin B, et al: Bilateral rostral maxillectomy and nasal planectomy for large rostral maxillofacial neoplasms in six dogs and one cat. *JAAHA* 40:137–146, 2004.
23. Smith MM: Surgical approach for lymph node staging of oral and maxillofacial neoplasms in dogs. *JAAHA* 31:514–518, 1995.
24. Wright MA, Brawner WR, Smith AS, Henderson RA: Unexpected lymphatic drainage of the rostral mandible during sentinel node lymphoscintigraphy in normal dogs. *Proc 22nd Annu Conf Vet Cancer Soc*:45, 2002.
25. Fox LE, Geoghegan SL, Davis LH, et al: Owner satisfaction with partial mandibulectomy or maxillectomy for treatment of oral tumors in 27 dogs. *JAAHA* 33:25–31, 1997.
26. Kessler M: Mandibulectomy and maxillectomy for treatment of bone invasive oral neoplasia in the dog: A retrospective analysis in 31 patients. *Kleintierpraxis* 48:289–300, 2003.
27. Wallace J, Matthiesen DT, Patnaik AK: Hemimaxillectomy for the treatment of oral tumors in 69 dogs. *Vet Surg* 21:337–341, 1992.
28. Evans SM, Shofer F: Canine oral nontonsillar squamous cell carcinoma: Prognostic factors for recurrence and survival following orthovoltage radiation therapy. *Vet Radiol Ultrasound* 29:133–137, 1998.
29. Beck ER, Withrow SJ, McChesney AE, et al: Canine tongue tumors: A retrospective review of 57 cases. *JAAHA* 22:525–532, 1996.
30. Ogilvie GK, Sundberg JP, O'Banion K, et al: Papillary squamous cell carcinoma in three young dogs. *JAVMA* 192:933–936, 1988.
31. Bradley RL, MacEwen EG, Loar AS: Mandibular resection for removal of oral tumors in 30 dogs and 6 cats. *JAVMA* 184:460–463, 1984.
32. Théon AP, Rodriguez C, Madewell BR: Analysis of prognostic factors and patterns of failure in dogs with malignant oral tumors treated with megavoltage irradiation. *JAVMA* 210:778–784, 1997.
33. Salisbury SK, Lantz GC: Long term results of partial mandibulectomy for treatment of oral tumors in 30 dogs. *JAAHA* 24:285–294, 1988.
34. LaDue-Miller T, Price S, Page RL, Thrall DE: Radiotherapy of canine non-tonsillar squamous cell carcinoma. *Vet Radiol Ultrasound* 37:74–77, 1996.
35. Salisbury SK, Richardson DC, Lantz GC: Partial maxillectomy and premaxillectomy in the treatment of oral neoplasia in the dog and cat. *Vet Surg* 15:16–26, 1986.
36. Withrow SJ, Nelson AW, Manley PA, Biggs DR: Premaxillectomy in the dog. *JAAHA* 21:45–55, 1985.
37. Buhles WC Jr, Theilen GH: Preliminary evaluation of bleomycin in feline and canine squamous cell carcinoma. *Am J Vet Res* 34:289–291, 1973.
38. Himsel CA, Richardson RC, Craig JA: Cisplatin chemotherapy for metastatic squamous cell carcinoma in two dogs. *JAVMA* 189:1575–1578, 1986.
39. Knapp DW, Richardson RC, Bonney PL, Hahn K: Cisplatin therapy in 41 dogs with malignant tumors. *J Vet Intern Med* 2:41–46, 1988.
40. Shapiro W, Kitchell BE, Fossum TW, et al: Cisplatin for treatment of transitional cell and squamous cell carcinomas in dogs. *JAVMA* 193:1530–1533, 1988.
41. Ogilvie GK, Obradovich JE, Elmslie RE, et al: Efficacy of mitoxantrone against various neoplasms in dogs. *JAVMA* 198:1618–1621, 1991.
42. Schmidt BR, Glickman NW, DeNicola DB, et al: Evaluation of piroxicam for the treatment of oral squamous cell carcinoma in dogs. *JAVMA* 218:1783–1786, 2001.
43. Boria PA, Murry DJ, Bennett PF, et al: Evaluation of cisplatin combined with piroxicam for the treatment of oral malignant melanoma and oral squamous cell carcinoma in dogs. *JAVMA* 224:388–394, 2004.
44. de Vos JP, Burm AG, Focker BP, et al: Results of the combined treatment with piroxicam and carboplatin in canine oral non-tonsillar squamous cell carcinoma. *Proc 24th Annu Conf Vet Cancer Soc*:62, 2004.
45. MacMillan R, Withrow SJ, Gillette EL: Surgery and regional irradiation for treatment of canine tonsillar squamous cell carcinoma: Retrospective review of eight cases. *JAAHA* 18:311–314, 1982.
46. Brooks MB, Matus RE, Leifer CE, et al: Chemotherapy versus chemotherapy plus radiotherapy in the treatment of tonsillar squamous cell carcinoma in the dog. *J Vet Intern Med* 2:206–211, 1988.
47. Withers FW: Squamous-celled carcinoma of the tonsil in the dog. *J Pathol Bact* 49:429–432, 1939.
48. Wyers M, Irgens K, Parodi A-L: Le cancer de l'amygdale dans l'espece canine. *Rec Méd Vét* 145:333–351, 1969.
49. Cotchin E: Some tumours of dogs and cats of comparative veterinary and human interest. *Vet Rec* 71:1040–1054, 1959.
50. Ragland WL 3rd, Gorham JR: Tonsillar carcinoma in rural dogs. *Nature* 214:925–926, 1967.
51. Reif JS, Cohen D: The environmental distribution of canine respiratory tract neoplasms. *Arch Environ Health* 22:136–140, 1971.
52. Bostock DE, Curtis R: Comparison of canine oropharyngeal malignancy in various geographical locations. *Vet Rec* 114:341–342, 1984.
53. Brewer WG Jr, Turrel JM: Radiotherapy and hyperthermia in the treatment of fibrosarcomas in the dog. *JAVMA* 181:146–150, 1982.

54. Thrall DE: Orthovoltage radiotherapy of oral fibrosarcomas in dogs. *JAVMA* 179:159–162, 1981.
55. Ciekot PA, Powers BE, Withrow SJ, et al: Histologically low-grade, yet biologically high-grade, fibrosarcomas of the mandible and maxilla in dogs: 25 cases (1982–1991). *JAVMA* 204:610–615, 1994.
56. Forrest LJ, Chun R, Adams WM, et al: Postoperative radiotherapy for canine soft tissue sarcoma. *J Vet Intern Med* 14:578–582, 2000.
57. McChesney SL, Withrow SJ, Gillette EL, et al: Radiotherapy of soft tissue sarcomas in dogs. *JAVMA* 194:60–63, 1989.
58. McChesney SL, Gillette EL, Dewhirst MW, Withrow SJ: Influence of WR 2721 on radiation response of canine soft tissue sarcomas. *Int J Radiat Oncol Biol Phys* 12:1957–1963, 1986.
59. Theon AP, Madewell BR, Ryu J, Castro J: Concurrent irradiation and intratumoral chemotherapy with cisplatin: A pilot study in dogs with spontaneous tumors. *Int J Radiat Oncol Biol Phys* 29:1027–1034, 1994.
60. Dvorak LD, Beaver DP, Ellison GW, et al: Major glossectomy in dogs: A case series and proposed classification system. *JAAHA* 40:331–337, 2004.
61. Rallis TS, Tontis DK, Soubasis NH, et al: Immunohistochemical study of a granular cell tumor on the tongue of a dog. *Vet Clin Pathol* 30:62–66, 2001.
62. Giles RC Jr, Montgomery CA Jr, Izen L: Canine lingual granular cell myoblastoma: A case report. *Am J Vet Res* 35:1357–1359, 1974.
63. Lascelles BD, McInnes J, Dobson JM, White RA: Rhabdomyosarcoma of the tongue in a dog. *J Small Anim Pract* 39:587–591, 1998.
64. Patnaik AK: Histologic and immunohistochemical studies of granular cell tumors in seven dogs, three cats, one horse, and one bird. *Vet Pathol* 30:176–185, 1993.
65. Schoofs SH: Lingual hemangioma in a puppy: A case report and literature review. *JAAHA* 33:161–165, 1997.
66. Karbe E, Schiefer B: Primary salivary gland tumors in carnivores. *Can Vet J* 8:212–215, 1967.
67. Spangler WL, Culbertson MR: Salivary gland disease in dogs and cats: 245 cases (1985–1988). *JAVMA* 198:465–469, 1991.
68. Carberry CA, Flanders JA, Harvey HJ, Ryan AM: Salivary gland tumors in dogs and cats: A literature and case review. *JAAHA* 24:561–567, 1988.
69. Koestner A, Buerger L: Primary neoplasms of the salivary glands in animals compared to similar tumors in man. *Path Vet* 2:201–226, 1965.
70. Thomsen BV, Myers RK: Extraskeletal osteosarcoma of the mandibular salivary gland in a dog. *Vet Pathol* 36:71–73, 1999.
71. Bindseil E, Madsen JS: Lipomatosis causing tumour-like swelling of a mandibular salivary gland in a dog. *Vet Rec* 140:583–584, 1997.
72. Hammer A, Getzy D, Ogilvie G, et al: Salivary gland neoplasia in the dog and cat: Survival times and prognostic factors. *JAAHA* 37:478–482, 2001.
73. Louw GJ, van Schouwenburg SJ: A case of a highly invasive carcinoma of a salivary gland in a crossbred dog. *J S Afr Vet Assoc* 55:131–132, 1984.
74. Habin DJ, Else RW: Parotid salivary gland adenocarcinoma with bilateral ocular and osseous metastases in a dog. *J Small Anim Pract* 36:445–449, 1995.
75. Valentini S, Spinella G, Negrini J, Fedrigo M: Ultrasonography of the salivary glands in dogs and cats. *Summa* 20:51–56, 2003.
76. Leifer CE, Peterson ME, Matus RE, Patnaik AK: Hypoglycemia associated with nonislet cell tumor in 13 dogs. *JAVMA* 186:53–55, 1985.
77. Evans SM, Thrall DE: Postoperative orthovoltage radiation therapy of parotid salivary gland adenocarcinoma in three dogs. *JAVMA* 182:993–994, 1983.
78. Ratto A, Peiffer RL Jr, Peruccio C, Rossi L: Zygomatic salivary gland adenocarcinoma in a dog. *Vet Comp Ophthal* 1:59–62, 1991.
79. Ridgeway RL, Suter PF: Clinical and radiographic signs in primary and metastatic esophageal neoplasms of the dog. *JAVMA* 174:700–704, 1979.
80. Frost D, Lasota J, Miettinen M: Gastrointestinal stromal tumors and leiomyomas in the dog: A histopathologic, immunohistochemical, and molecular genetic study of 50 cases. *Vet Pathol* 40:42–54, 2003.
81. Ranen E, Lavy E, Aizenberg I, et al: Spirocercosis-associated esophageal sarcomas in dogs. A retrospective study of 17 cases (1997–2003). *Vet Parasitol* 119:209–221, 2004.
82. Lobetti RG: Survey of the incidence, diagnosis, clinical manifestations and treatment of *Spirocerca lupi* in South Africa. *J S Afr Vet Assoc* 71:43–46, 2000.
83. Berry WL: *Spirocerca lupi* esophageal granulomas in 7 dogs: Resolution after treatment with doramectin. *J Vet Intern Med* 14:609–612, 2000.
84. Matros L, Jergens AE, Miles KG, Kluge JP: Megaesophagus and hypomotility associated with esophageal leiomyoma in a dog. *JAAHA* 30:15–19, 1994.
85. Wilson RB, Holscher MA, Laney PS: Esophageal osteosarcoma in a dog. *JAAHA* 27:361–363, 1991.
86. Nohara H: Fibrosarcoma arising from the thoracic part of the esophagus in a dog. *J Jpn Vet Med Assoc* 44:227–229, 1991.
87. Randolph JF, Center SA, Flanders JA, Diters RW: Hypertrophic osteopathy associated with adenocarcinoma of the esophageal glands in a dog. *JAVMA* 184:98–99, 1984.
88. Jacobs TM, Rosen GM: Photodynamic therapy as a treatment for esophageal squamous cell carcinoma in a dog. *JAAHA* 36:257–261, 2000.
89. Hamilton TA, Carpenter JL: Esophageal plasmacytoma in a dog. *JAVMA* 204:1210–1211, 1994.
90. Ranen E, Shamir MH, Shahar R, Johnston DE: Partial esophagectomy with single layer closure for treatment of esophageal sarcomas in 6 dogs. *Vet Surg* 33:428–434, 2004.
91. Murray M, Robinson PB, McKeating FJ, et al: Primary gastric neoplasia in the dog: A clinico-pathological study. *Vet Rec* 91:474–479, 1972.
92. Patnaik AK, Hurvitz AI, Johnson GF: Canine gastrointestinal neoplasms. *Vet Pathol* 14:547–555, 1977.
93. Sautter JH, Hanlon GF: Gastric neoplasms in the dog: A report of 20 cases. *JAVMA* 166:691–696, 1975.
94. Albers TM, Alroy J, McDonnell JJ, Moore AS: A poorly differentiated gastric carcinoid in a dog. *J Vet Diagn Invest* 10:116–118, 1998.
95. Fonda D, Gualtieri M, Scanziani E: Gastric carcinoma in the dog: A clinico-pathological study of 11 cases. *J Small Anim Pract* 30:353–360, 1989.
96. Scanziani E, Giusti AM, Gualtieri M, Fonda D: Gastric carcinoma in the Belgian shepherd dog. *J Small Anim Pract* 32:465–469, 1991.
97. Patnaik AK, Hurvitz AI, Johnson GF: Canine gastric adenocarcinoma. *Vet Pathol* 15:600–607, 1978.
98. Sullivan M, Lee R, Fisher EW, et al: A study of 31 cases of gastric carcinoma in dogs. *Vet Rec* 120:79–83, 1987.
99. Penninck DG, Moore AS, Gliatto J: Ultrasonography of canine gastric epithelial neoplasia. *Vet Radiol Ultrasound* 39:342–348, 1998.
100. Kolbjornsen O, Press CM, Landsverk T: Gastropathies in the Lundehund. II. A study of mucin profiles. *APMIS* 102:801–809, 1994.
101. Kolbjornsen O, Press CM, Landsverk T: Gastropathies in the Lundehund. I. Gastritis and gastric neoplasia associated with intestinal lymphangiectasia. *APMIS* 102:647–661, 1994.
102. Sano T, Kobori O, Kuroki S, et al: Effect of experimental hypochlorhydria on the histological differentiation of adenocarcinomas in the canine stomach. *Jpn J Cancer Res* 84:495–500, 1993.
103. Penninck DG, Nyland TG, Kerr LY, Fisher PE: Ultrasonographic evaluation of gastrointestinal diseases in small animals. *Vet Radiol* 31:134–141, 1990.
104. Kaser-Hotz B, Hauser B, Arnold P: Ultrasonographic findings in canine gastric neoplasia in 13 patients. *Vet Radiol Ultrasound* 37:51–56, 1996.
105. Rivers BJ, Walter PA, Johnston GR, et al: Canine gastric neoplasia: Utility of ultrasonography in diagnosis. *JAAHA* 33:144–155, 1997.
106. Lamb CR, Grierson J: Ultrasonographic appearance of primary gastric neoplasia in 21 dogs. *J Small Anim Pract* 40:211–215, 1999.
107. Penninck DG, Crystal MA, Matz ME, Pearson SH: The technique of percutaneous ultrasound guided fine-needle aspiration biopsy and automated microcore biopsy in small animal gastrointestinal diseases. *Vet Radiol Ultrasound* 34:433–436, 1993.
108. Crystal MA, Penninck DG, Matz ME, et al: Use of ultrasound-guided fine-needle aspiration biopsy and automated core biopsy for the diagnosis of gastrointestinal diseases in small animals. *Vet Radiol Ultrasound* 34:438–444, 1993.
109. Easton S: A retrospective study into the effects of operator experience on the accuracy of ultrasound in the diagnosis of gastric neoplasia in dogs. *Vet Radiol Ultrasound* 42:47–50, 2001.
110. Hirt R: Endoskopisch diagnsostizierte magenkarzinome beim hund. *Kleintierpraxis* 45:33–43, 2000.
111. Swann HM, Holt DE: Canine gastric adenocarcinoma and leiomyosarcoma: A retrospective study of 21 cases (1986–1999) and literature review. *JAAHA* 38:157–164, 2002.
112. Esplin DG, Wilson SR: Gastrointestinal adenocarcinomas metastatic to the testes and associated structures in three dogs. *JAAHA* 34:287–290, 1998.
113. Roth L, King JM: Mesenteric and omental sclerosis associated with metastases from gastrointestinal neoplasia in the dog. *J Small Anim Pract* 31:28–31, 1990.
114. Bellah JR, Ginn PE: Gastric leiomyosarcoma associated with hypoglycemia in a dog. *JAAHA* 32:283–286, 1996.
115. Beaudry D, Knapp DW, Montgomery T, et al: Hypoglycemia in four dogs with smooth muscle tumors. *J Vet Intern Med* 9:415–418, 1995.
116. Bagley RS, Levy JK, Malarkey DE: Hypoglycemia associated with intra-abdominal leiomyoma and leiomyosarcoma in six dogs. *JAVMA* 208:69–71, 1996.
117. Elliott GS, Stroffregen DA, Richardson DC, et al: Surgical, medical and nutritional management of gastric adenocarcinoma in a dog. *JAVMA* 185:98–101, 1984.
118. Dorn AS, Anderson NV, Guffy MM, et al: Gastric carcinoma in a dog. *J Small Anim Pract* 17:109–117, 1976.

119. Sinclair CJ, Jones BR, Verkerk G: Gastric carcinoma in a bitch. *N Z Vet J* 27:16–18, 1979.
120. Sellon RK, Bissonnette K, Bunch SE: Long-term survival after total gastrectomy for gastric adenocarcinoma in a dog. *J Vet Intern Med* 10:333–335, 1996.
121. Beck JA, Simpson DS: Surgical treatment of gastric leiomyoma in a dog. *Austr Vet J* 77:161–163, 999.
122. Brunnert SR, Dee LA, Herron AJ, Altman NH: Gastric extramedullary plasmacytoma in a dog. *JAVMA* 200:1501–1502, 1992.
123. MacEwen EG, Patnaik AK, Johnson GF, Hurvitz AI: Extramedullary plasmacytoma of the gastrointestinal tract in two dogs. *JAVMA* 184:1396–1398, 1984.
124. Gibbs C, Pearson H: Localized tumours of the canine small intestine: A report of twenty cases. *J Small Anim Pract* 27:507–519, 1986.
125. Couto CG, Rutgers HC, Sherding RG, Rojko J: Gastrointestinal lymphoma in 20 dogs. A retrospective study. *J Vet Intern Med* 3:73–78, 1989.
126. Patnaik AK, Hurvitz AI, Johnson GF: Canine intestinal adenocarcinoma and carcinoid. *Vet Pathol* 17:149–163, 1980.
127. Giles RC Jr, Hildebrandt PK, Montgomery CA Jr: Carcinoid tumor in the small intestine of a dog. *Vet Pathol* 11:340–349, 1974.
128. Birchard SJ, Couto CG, Johnson S: Nonlymphoid intestinal neoplasia in 32 dogs and 14 cats. *JAAHA* 22:533–537, 1986.
129. Gibbons GC, Murtaugh RJ: Cecal smooth muscle neoplasia in the dog: Report of 11 cases and literature review. *JAAHA* 25:191–197, 1989.
130. Kapatkin AS, Mullen Hs, Matthiesen DT, Patnaik AK: Leiomyosarcoma in dogs: 44 cases (1983–1988). *JAVMA* 201:1077–1079, 1992.
131. Comer KM: Anemia as a feature of primary gastrointestinal neoplasia. *Compend Contin Educ Pract Vet* 12:13–19, 1990.
132. Laratta LJ, Center SA, Flanders JA, et al: Leiomyosarcoma in the duodenum of a dog. *JAVMA* 183:1096–1097, 1983.
133. Bruecker KA, Withrow SJ: Intestinal leiomyosarcomas in six dogs. *JAAHA* 24:281–284, 1988.
134. Chen HC, Parris LS, Parris RG: Duodenal leiomyosarcoma with multiple hepatic metastases in a dog. *JAVMA* 184:1506, 1984.
135. Watson DE, Mahaffey MB, Neuwirth LA: Ultrasonographic detection of duodenojejunal intussception in a dog. *JAAHA* 27:367–369, 1991.
136. Paoloni MC, Penninck DG, Moore AS: Ultrasonographic and clinicopathologic findings in 21 dogs with intestinal adenocarcinoma. *Vet Radiol Ultrasound* 43:562–567, 2002.
137. Penninck D, Smyers B, Webster CR, et al: Diagnostic value of ultrasonography in differentiating enteritis from intestinal neoplasia in dogs. *Vet Radiol Ultrasound* 44:570–575, 2003.
138. Brown PJ, Adam SM, Wotton PR, et al: Hamartomatous polyps in the intestine of two dogs. *J Comp Pathol* 110:97–102, 1994.
139. Crawshaw J, Berg J, Sardinas JC, et al: Prognosis for dogs with nonlymphatous, small intestinal tumors treated by surgical excision. *JAAHA* 34:451–456, 1998.
140. Cohen M, Post GS: Nephrogenic diabetes insipidus in a dog with intestinal leiomyosarcoma. *JAVMA* 215:1806,1818–1820, 1999.
141. Sato K, Hikasa Y, Morita T, et al: Secondary erythrocytosis associated with high plasma erythropoietin concentrations in a dog with cecal leiomyosarcoma. *JAVMA* 220:486–490, 2002.
142. Patnaik AK, Lieberman PH: Canine goblet-cell carcinoid. *Vet Pathol* 18:410–413, 1981.
143. Sako T, Uchida E, Okamoto M, et al: Immunohistochemical evaluation of a malignant intestinal carcinoid in a dog. *Vet Pathol* 40:212215, 2003.
144. Coughlin AS: Carcinoid in canine large intestine. *Vet Rec* 130:499–500, 1992.
145. Cohen M, Post GS, Wright JC: Gastrointestinal leiomyosarcoma in 14 dogs. *J Vet Intern Med* 17:107–110, 2003.
146. McEntee MF, Cates JM, Neilsen N: Cyclooxygenase-2 expression in spontaneous intestinal neoplasia of domestic dogs. *Vet Pathol* 39:428–436, 2002.
147. LaRock RG, Ginn PE: Immunohistochemical staining characteristics of canine gastrointestinal stromal tumors. *Vet Pathol* 34:303–311, 1997.
148. McPherron MA, Withrow SJ, Seim IHB, Powers BE: Colorectal leiomyomas in seven dogs. *JAAHA* 28:43–46, 1992.
149. McEntee MF, Brenneman KA: Dysregulation of beta-catenin is common in canine sporadic colorectal tumors. *Vet Pathol* 36:228–236, 1999.
150. Valerius KD, Powers BE, McPherron MA, et al: Adenomatous polyps and carcinoma in situ of the canine colon and rectum: 34 cases (1982–1994). *JAAHA* 33:156–160, 1997.
151. Wolf JC, Ginn PE, Homer B, et al: Immunohistochemical detection of p53 tumor suppressor gene protein in canine epithelial colorectal tumors. *Vet Pathol* 34:394–404, 1997.
152. Holt PE, Durdey P: Transanal endoscopic treatment of benign canine rectal tumours: Preliminary results in six cases (1992 to 1996). *J Small Anim Pract* 40:423–427, 1999.
153. Knottenbelt CM, Simpson JW, Tasker S, et al: Preliminary clinical observations on the use of piroxicam in the management of rectal tubulopapillary polyps. *J Small Anim Pract* 41:393–397, 2000.
154. Prater MR, Flatland B, Newman SJ, et al: Diffuse annular fusiform adenocarcinoma in a dog. *JAAHA* 36:169–173, 2000.
155. Trevor PB, Saunders GK, Waldron DR, Leib MS: Metastatic extramedullary plasmacytoma of the colon and rectum in a dog. *JAVMA* 203:406–409, 1993.
156. Leib MS, Fallin EA, Johnston SA: Endoscopy case of the month: Abnormally shaped feces in a dog. *Vet Med* 87:762–766, 1992.
157. Henry CJ, Lanevschi A, Marks SL, et al: Acute lymphoblastic leukemia, hypercalcemia, and pseudohyperkalemia in a dog. *JAVMA* 208:237–239, 1996.
158. Thompson JP, Christopher MM, Ellison GW, et al: Paraneoplastic leukocytosis associated with a rectal adenomatous polyp in a dog. *JAVMA* 201:737–738, 1992.
159. Knottenbelt CM, Simpson JW, Chandler ML: Neutrophilic leucocytosis in a dog with a rectal tumour. *J Small Anim Pract* 41:457–460, 2000.
160. Turrel JM, Theon AP: Single high-dose irradiation for selected canine rectal carcinomas. *Vet Radiol Ultrasound* 27:141–145, 1986.
161. Reimer ME, Leib MS, Reimer MS, et al: Rectal ganglioneuroma in a dog. *JAAHA* 35:107–110, 1999.
162. Petterino C, Martini M, Castagnaro M: Immunohistochemical detection of growth hormone (GH) in canine hepatoid gland tumors. *J Vet Med Sci* 66:569–572, 2004.
163. Dow SW, Olson PN, Rosychuk RA, Withrow SJ: Perianal adenomas and hypertestosteronemia in a spayed bitch with pituitary-dependent hyperadrenocorticism. *JAVMA* 192:1439–1441, 1988.
164. Goldschmidt MH, Shofer FS: Hepatoid gland tumors, in Goldschmidt MH, Shofer FS (eds): *Skin Tumors of the Dog and Cat*, ed 1, Tarrytown, NY, Pergamon Press, 1992, pp 66–74.
165. Berrocal A, Vos JH, van den Ingh TS, et al: Canine perineal tumours. *Zentralbl Veterinarmed A* 36:739–749, 1989.
166. Vail DM, Withrow SJ, Schwarz PD, Powers BE: Perianal adenocarcinoma in the canine male: A retrospective study of 41 cases. *JAAHA* 26:329–334, 1990.
167. Wilson GP, Hayes HM Jr: Castration for treatment of perianal gland neoplasms in the dog. *JAVMA* 174:1301–1303, 1979.
168. Ross JT, Scavelli TD, Matthiesen DT, Patnaik AK: Adenocarcinoma of the apocrine glands of the anal sac in dogs: A review of 32 cases. *JAAHA* 27:349–355, 1991.
169. Goldschmidt MH, Zoltowski C: Anal sac gland adenocarcinoma in the dog: 14 cases. *J Small Anim Pract* 22:119–128, 1981.
170. Meuten DJ, Cooper BJ, Capen CC, et al: Hypercalcemia associated with an adenocarcinoma derived from the apocrine glands of the anal sac. *Vet Pathol* 18:454–471, 1981.
171. Goldschmidt MH, Shofer FS: Anal sac gland tumors, in Goldschmidt MH, Shofer FS (eds): *Skin Tumors of the Dog and Cat*, ed 1. Tarrytown, NY, Pergamon Press, 1992, pp 103–108.
172. Williams LE, Gliatto JM, Dodge RK, et al: Carcinoma of the apocrine glands of the anal sac in dogs: 113 cases (1985–1995). *JAVMA* 223:825–831, 2003.
173. Rijnberk A, Elsinghorst TA, Koeman JP, et al: Pseudohyperparathyroidism associated with perirectal adenocarcinomas in elderly female dogs. *Tijdschr Diergeneeskd* 103:1069–1075, 1978.
174. Rosol TJ, Capen CC, Danks JA, et al: Identification of parathyroid hormone-related protein in canine apocrine adenocarcinoma of the anal sac. *Vet Pathol* 27:89–95, 1990.
175. Esplin DG, Wilson SR, Hullinger GA: Squamous cell carcinoma of the anal sac in five dogs. *Vet Pathol* 40:332–334, 2003.
176. Hause WR, Stevenson S, Meuten DJ, Capen CC: Pseudohyperparathyroidism associated with adenocarcinomas of anal sac origin in four dogs. *JAAHA* 17:373–379, 1981.
177. Llabres-Diaz FJ: Ultrasonography of the medial iliac lymph nodes in the dog. *Vet Radiol Ultrasound* 45:156–165, 2004.
178. Hoelzler MG, Bellah JR, Donofro MC: Omentalization of cystic sublumbar lymph node metastases for long-term palliation of tenesmus and dysuria in a dog with anal sac adenocarcinoma. *JAVMA* 219:1729–1731, 1708, 2001.
179. Turek MM, Forrest LJ, Adams WM, et al: Postoperative radiotherapy and mitoxantrone for anal sac adenocarcinoma in the dog: 15 cases (1991–2001). *Vet Comp Oncol* 1:94–104, 2003.
180. Bennett PF, DeNicola DB, Bonney P, et al: Canine anal sac adenocarcinomas: Clinical presentation and response to therapy. *J Vet Intern Med* 16:100–104, 2002.

MELANOMA 54
Antony S. Moore and Gregory K. Ogilvie

CLINICAL BRIEFING

MDB (includes a CBC, biochemical profile, urinalysis, and thoracic radiography [three views]).

Oral Melanoma

Clinical factors
- Friable, often pigmented, oral lesion in older dogs.

Staging and diagnosis
- MDB.
- Regional lymph node cytology.
- Metastasis common, usually regional lymph nodes or lungs.

Prognostic factors
- Melanoma of the lip may mean longer patient survival.
- Mitotic index not as predictive of behavior as for other sites.
- Size: Small tumors have a better prognosis.
- Location: Caudal is worse.
- Staging: Higher stage is worse.
- Histopathologic grade correlates with survival.

Treatment

Initial
- Surgery rarely curative because metastatic rate is high.

Adjunctive
- Radiation therapy may achieve local control for unresectable lesions.
- Cisplatin or carboplatin chemotherapy may be effective for metastatic tumors or as an adjunct to local therapies.
- Gene therapy may prove promising.

Supportive
- Analgesia postoperatively.
- Nutritional support as needed.

Cutaneous Melanoma

Clinical factors
- Darkly pigmented epidermal lesion in adult to senior dogs.
- Usually raised but not ulcerated.
- Most are well differentiated (benign).
- Subungual tumors are more aggressive.

Staging and diagnosis
- MDB, including lymph node assessment.
- Thoracic radiography especially important for subungual lesions or melanoma with high mitotic index.

Prognostic factors
- Mitotic index >2 per 10 hpf or high proliferative index (based on Ki67) associated with poor prognosis.
- 50% of subungual melanomas metastasize.
- For other cutaneous sites, metastasis is rare.

Treatment	
Initial	• Surgical excision curative for most cutaneous lesions.
Adjunctive	• Cisplatin or carboplatin chemotherapy for metastatic lesions (or possibly as an adjunct to surgery in subungual melanoma).
Supportive	• Analgesia postoperatively.
	• Nutritional support as needed.
Ocular Melanoma	
Clinical factors	• Ocular mass, often pigmented.
	• Anterior uveal tumors are most common.
	• May occur in young dogs.
	• German shepherds predisposed to limbal lesions.
Staging and diagnosis	• MDB and lymph node evaluation.
	• Metastasis is rare except for conjunctival lesions.
Prognostic factors	• Mitotic index <2 per 10 hpf consistent with benign behavior.
Treatment	
Initial	• Surgical excision curative for most tumors; enucleation for extensive tumors.
Adjunctive	• Rarely required; platinum drugs may be most effective for metastatic disease.
	• Analgesia postoperatively.
Supportive	• Nutritional support as needed.

Oral Malignant Melanoma

INCIDENCE, SIGNALMENT, AND ETIOLOGY

Oral melanoma is the most common oral malignancy in dogs[1,2] (Figure 54-1). Unlike cutaneous melanomas, which are often benign, melanomas of the canine oral cavity are uniformly malignant. Aggressive local growth and distant metastasis are usual. Even histologically benign melanomas of the oral cavity may act malignantly.[3] These tumors are most common in poodles, dachshunds, Scottish terriers, and golden retrievers.[1,4] In three large series totaling 193 dogs with oral melanoma, 94 dogs were male and 99 were female.[4–6] This is a disease of older dogs. In one study, the median age of affected dogs was 11 years (range: 4–16 years).[5] The molecular biology of melanomas in dogs is reviewed in other publications.[7,8]

CLINICAL PRESENTATION AND HISTORY

Most melanomas arise in the gingiva.[5,6] In descending order of frequency, melanomas are also found on the lips, tongue, and hard palate. A recent study found it most clinically relevant to describe tumors in relation to the underlying bone.[4] Of 41 dogs, 19 had tumors overlying the rostral maxilla, six in the caudal maxilla, seven in the rostral mandible, and seven in the caudal mandible. Two tumors were in the hard palate.

Owners may present dogs for an oral mass or (more frequently) for persistent halitosis, bleeding from the mouth, and (occasionally) dysphagia. Tumors may be large, measuring up to 64 cm^3 in volume in one study.[3] Although masses are frequently pigmented, amelanotic tumors are common (Figures 54-2 and 54-3). Oral melanomas are friable and invasive within the soft tissues of the mouth,[9] although an occasional tumor may show osteoid formation.[10] Because these tumors often surround bony structures and invade bone, surgical excision is often difficult.

STAGING AND DIAGNOSIS

Dogs with oral tumors of any type should be staged using blood work, radiography, and cytology or histopathology. Although histopathology is required for definitive diagnosis of oral melanoma, the index of suspicion for this tumor should be high in an old dog with a friable oral mass. The metastatic rate is very high for oral melanoma, but the time to metastasis varies. Some immunohistochemical markers have been

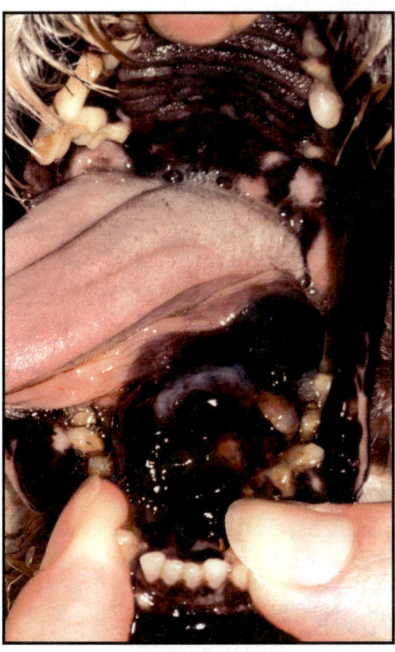

Figure 54-1. *Oral melanoma is the most common oral malignancy in dogs. It is usually heavily pigmented with melanin.*

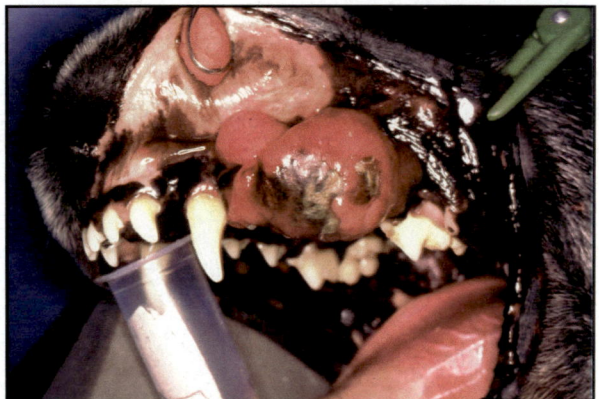

Figure 54-2. *Oral melanoma may be amelanotic, as in this 10-year-old Labrador retriever.*

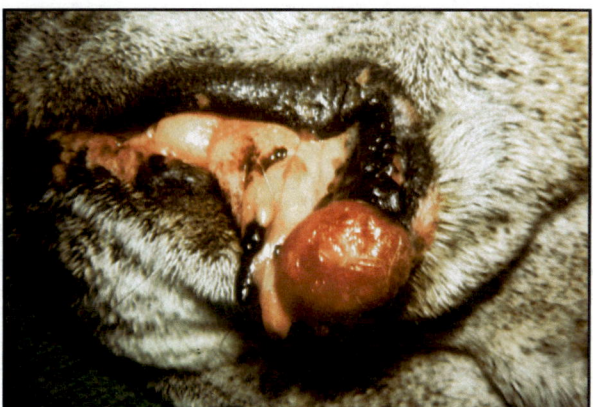

Figure 54-3. *Oral melanomas of the lip, as in this 9-year-old boxer, may be less aggressive than those arising from the oral mucosa.*

explored for their ability to diagnose melanoma when the tumor is poorly pigmented and poorly differentiated. No marker is absolutely specific for melanoma or for predicting behavior. Human melanosome-specific markers, when combined, may be positive in more than 80% of melanomas;[11] one study found Melan-A to be a sensitive and specific stain for canine melanomas of all sites.[12] Another study found that a panel of markers, including vimentin, S-100, and Melan-A, was helpful in the diagnosis of melanoma.[13] When the clinician suspects a tumor of being melanoma, requesting this panel of stains gives the greatest chance of reaching an accurate diagnosis. In another study, whereas S-100 was thought to be very sensitive but not very specific (i.e., it stains tumors other than melanomas), human melanoma marker HMB-45 was sensitive and specific.[14]

At diagnosis, the mandibular lymph nodes (both ipsilateral and contralateral) should be palpated and fine-needle aspiration conducted for cytologic examination. Evidence of atypical melanocytes or melanophages is suggestive of metastasis. Aspiration cytology that is suspicious should be confirmed by surgical biopsy. Although 60% of enlarged lymph nodes had cytologic evidence of metastases in one study of 100 dogs with oral melanoma, metastases were also detected in 40% of normal-sized lymph nodes[15]; thus, even normal-sized lymph nodes should be aspirated. In another study, only five of 41 dogs (12%) had metastatic disease in regional lymph nodes at diagnosis.[4] Although the mandibular nodes are the most commonly affected, other regional nodes may also contain metastases. Another study found that dissection of the lymph nodes at surgery increased the number of diagnoses of metastatic disease.[16]

Thoracic radiography may indicate pulmonary metastasis at the time of diagnosis. However, pulmonary metastasis frequently occurs late in the course of the disease. In one study, only three of 41 dogs (7%) had evidence of pulmonary metastasis at diagnosis,[4] but at the time of death, the metastatic rate for this tumor approximated 80%.[17] Melanoma may also spread systemically, and metastasis is reported in the kidneys, myocardium, and brain, as well as other sites.[3] The World Health Organization (WHO) staging scheme for oral melanoma is summarized in Table 54-1.

Metastasis of tumors is probably an early event, occurring during clinical stages I and II; however, metastases are often not detected until long after the primary melanoma is resected. The growth rate of metastases may vary, and it is this variation, rather than the time that metastasis occurs, that determines survival time.

Some investigators have found that the WHO staging system provides prognostic information,[5] but an alternative

Table 54-1 Clinical Stages of Canine Oral Melanoma (WHO)

Clinical Stage	Criteria			
	Tumor diameter (cm)	Node	Metastasis	Dogs (%)[5]
I	<2	-	-	43
II	2–4	-	-	44
III	>4 or any bone invasion	+	-	13
IV	Any	Any	+	Not available

- = absent; + = present.

T: Primary Tumor
- T_1 Tumor in situ or ≤2 cm maximum diameter (volume ≤8 cm^3)
- T_2 Tumor 2–4 cm maximum diameter (volume 8–64 cm^3)
- T_3 Tumor >4 cm maximum diameter (volume >64 cm^3)

Mitotic Index
- (a) ≤3 per hpf
- (b) >3 per hpf

Oral cavity or oropharyngeal location
- (1) Rostral mandible/caudal maxilla
- (2) Other

N: Regional Lymph Nodes
- N_0 No evidence of regional node involvement
- N_1 Histologic evidence of regional node involvement
- N_2 Fixed nodes

M: Distant Metastasis
- M_0 No evidence of distant metastasis
- M_1 Distant metastasis (including distant nodes)

Stage Grouping

	T	N	M
I	T_1a^1	N_0	M_0
II	T_1a^2, any T_1b, T_2a^1	N_0	M_0
	Any T	N_1	M_0
III	T_2a^2, any T_2b or T_3	N_0	M_0
	Any T	N_2	M_0
	Any T	Any N	M_1

Figure 54-4. *In dogs, a modified staging scheme has been proposed for oral melanoma that combines the traditional WHO scheme with other criteria, such as the location of the tumor within the oral cavity and the mitotic index as seen on histopathology. (Adapted from Hahn KA, DeNicola DB, Richardson RC, Hahn EA: Canine oral malignant melanoma: Prognostic utility of an alternative staging system. J Small Anim Pract 35:251–256, 1994; with permission)*

staging system that also offers prognostic information has been proposed.[4] This system includes the WHO criteria, the mitotic index from histopathology, and tumor location within the oral cavity (Figure 54-4).

Current recommendations for staging oral melanoma, therefore, include lymph node evaluation by cytology or biopsy, thoracic radiography, and tumor measurements, as well as anatomic location and evaluation of mitotic index as determined by histopathology.

Paraneoplastic hypercalcemia has been reported in a dog with oral melanoma.[18]

PROGNOSTIC FACTORS

The ability of the WHO staging scheme to prognosticate accurately for dogs with oral melanoma is controversial. Some studies found no utility for the scheme,[3,4] but other studies found significantly longer survival for dogs with stage I (small) tumors (median: 511 days) than for dogs with stage II or III tumors (median: 164 days).[5] Small melanomas were also associated with long survival times in another study (Table 54-2).[19]

One study found that the location of the tumor was not prognostic,[5] but two other studies indicated that tumors of the rostral mandible and the caudal maxilla had longer remissions and survival after surgery.[4,19] Another study found longer survival times for dogs with tumors that had fewer than 3 mitotic figures per high-power field (hpf; Figure 54-5).[4] In general, oral melanomas should be considered malignant regardless of their histologic appearance.

TREATMENT

Surgery remains the mainstay of treatment for oral melanoma and should consist of mandibulectomy or maxillectomy. Radiation has a role in local tumor control. Chemotherapy with platinum compounds, perhaps combined with immunotherapy, may offer the best adjunctive treatment for metastatic disease. Metastatic disease occurs in most patients, often within 6 months of treatment,[9] although metastases may not be visible until 1 year or more after surgery.[20,21] After metastases develop, dogs may still live a long time, depending on the growth rate.[21] Dogs may tolerate pulmonary metastatic disease with very little apparent effect on their quality of life.

Surgery

Oral melanomas in dogs have a high metastatic rate, but metastases frequently are not observed until late in the course

Table 54-2 Size of Oral Melanoma Associated with Survival[19]

	Tumor Diameter (cm)	Progression-Free Survival Median (months)	1 Year Tumor-Free (%)	3 Years Tumor-Free
Overall	—	8	36	20
T1	<2	19	71	54
T2	2–4	6	28	12
T3	>4	7	23	9

T = primary tumor.

of disease, occasionally more than 1 year after local therapy.[20] Most dogs are euthanatized because of progression or recurrence of local disease. If surgery is aggressive from the outset, it may prolong survival as well as provide palliation. Aggressive local therapy should include resection of underlying bone. In one early study, 34 of 49 dogs had local recurrence of tumor,[3] and 33 dogs developed metastases. The recurrence rate of 84% probably reflects the less aggressive nature of the surgery. More recent studies reported local recurrence rates of less than 15% for melanomas treated by mandibulectomy[9,22,23] to 48% for tumors treated by maxillectomy.[20,24] Both mandibulectomy and maxillectomy are tolerated well by dogs, with median hospitalization times ranging from 2 days for simple excision to 8 days for total hemimandibulectomy (see Chapter 53).[9] A recent study described a new technique of hemimandibulectomy that allowed a faster return to eating than other techniques.[25] In three studies, dogs treated with aggressive surgery had a median survival time of 7.3 to 9.1 months[6,9,20]; dogs that did not have surgery survived a median of 2 months.[6] Mandibulectomy or maxillectomy should be the first surgery used to treat oral melanoma in dogs. Less aggressive surgeries do not prolong survival and make subsequent surgery more difficult.

Surgical excision was used to treat five dogs with melanoma of the tongue and achieved local control in three dogs, with survival times ranging from 3 to 45 months (median: 19 months). Only one dog developed metastasis.[26] Long survival times (median: >2 years) were seen for dogs with tongue melanomas in another study.[27]

Radiation

Radiation therapy has a role in the treatment of melanoma, particularly for small tumors. Melanomas in 33 dogs were treated with 48 Gy of ^{60}Co teletherapy.[19] Five dogs had local recurrence. One dog had regional lymph node metastasis, and 14 developed distant metastasis. Dogs with rostrally located tumors and dogs with smaller tumors had longer remissions. Median progression-free survival was estimated to be 14 months.

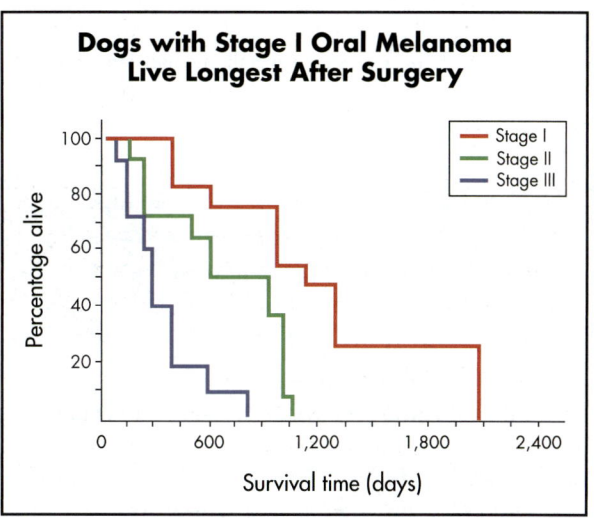

Figure 54-5. The staging scheme seen in Figure 54-4 influenced survival in 24 dogs with oral melanoma treated by surgery. Kaplan–Meier survival statistics showed a significant difference among melanoma stages I, II, and III. (Adapted from Hahn KA, DeNicola DB, Richardson RC, Hahn EA: Canine oral malignant melanoma: Prognostic utility of an alternative staging system. J Small Anim Pract 35:251–256, 1994; with permission)

In human patients, melanoma responds best when radiation therapy is delivered in large doses per fraction, and because metastatic disease is often the cause of death in dogs with melanoma, a palliative course of radiation is appealing from a quality-of-life perspective.

At least three reports examine radiation therapy for dogs with measurable oral melanomas. Delivery of three 8-Gy fractions given on days 0, 7, and 21 resulted in nine complete responses (CRs) and five partial responses (PRs) in 17 dogs (53% and 30%, respectively).[28] The median survival time was 8 months, and dogs with CRs lived longer. A similar protocol of four weekly treatments of 9 Gy resulted in 25 of 36 (75%) dogs having CRs; the remaining nine dogs had PRs.[29] Eight dogs had a local recurrence, and 22 had metastases (most commonly to the lung); some dogs had both. Dogs that had CRs lived a median of 37 weeks, which was significantly longer than dogs with PRs, who lived a median of 20 weeks. Dogs with small tumors (<5 cm^3) lived a median of 86 weeks, and dogs with larger tumors lived a median of 20 weeks. Late effects of bone necrosis or second malignancy were seen in five dogs. The third report compared three different protocols (four weekly treatments of 9 Gy; three weekly treatments of 10 Gy; conventional 2–4 Gy fractions given daily) in 140 dogs.[30] There was no effect of treatment protocol on the outcome for these dogs. There was measurable disease in 93 dogs, of which 51% had CRs and 31% had PRs. When all the dogs were evaluated, those with microscopic disease, those with no bony lysis on radiographs, and those with rostrally located tumors all had a lower chance of recurrence and lived longer. Overall median survival time was 7 months. Increasing numbers of negative prognostic factors correlated with shorter survival times (Table 54-3).[30]

Table 54-3 **Effect of Number of Negative Factors on Survival for 140 Dogs with Oral Melanoma**[30]

Poor Prognostic Factors (n)	Dogs (n)	Median Survival (months)
0	18	21
1	47	11
2	57	5
3	18	3

> **KEY POINT**
>
> *Dogs with rostrally located, small oral melanomas that have a low mitotic index probably have the best prognosis after treatment.*

Improvement in survival was seen in dogs with residual (rather than macroscopic) disease in another study in which the overall 1-year survival rate was 37.7% and the 2-year survival rate was 14.3%.[31] This study also found that 12 dogs with melanoma of the lip lived a median of 25 months (1-year survival: 57.4 %; 2-year survival: 34.3%), which was significantly longer than for 51 dogs with melanoma at other oral sites (median: 7 months). Another preliminary study found a similar survival advantage for dogs with lip melanoma when treated with multimodality therapy.[27]

Recent studies using radiation therapy have focused on treating dogs with microscopic disease. One study used doses of 6 Gy given weekly for 6 weeks (also given with weekly low doses of carboplatin or cisplatin) to dogs that had microscopic disease after surgery.[32] In this group of 39 dogs, recurrence was seen in six dogs a median of 4 months after treatment, and metastases were seen in 20 dogs a median of 10 months later. The median overall survival was more than 1 year.

In summary, coarsely fractionated radiation therapy causes a complete response in 50% to 75% of dogs with tumors that cannot be treated by surgery. If the melanoma can be reduced to microscopic disease, the prognosis is much better. In dogs with small, rostrally located melanomas, the risk of late effects of radiation therapy becomes greater because their survival times are likely to be long. For these dogs, the use of small doses per fraction, as is used in more conventional radiation therapy, should be considered.

Chemotherapy

Chemotherapy may improve survival times in dogs with oral melanoma when used as an adjunct to surgery but rarely when used to treat gross or metastatic disease. Drugs such as dacarbazine (1,000 mg/m^2 IV q3wk)[21,26] and doxorubicin (30 mg/m^2 IV q3wk) have not had repeatable success. Melphalan (0.5 mg/kg IV q4wk) caused responses in three of 11 dogs.[33] Platinum compounds may be more efficacious. Carboplatin (300–350 mg/m^2 IV q3wk) caused responses in seven of 25 dogs (28%) with unresectable oral melanoma, including one dog with a CR lasting nearly 3 years. Overall response duration was 5.5 months.[34] Higher dosages and the occurrence of gastrointestinal toxicity were associated with a higher likelihood for response. Cisplatin (60 mg/m^2 IV q3wk) caused a PR for a dog with metastatic melanoma.[35] In another trial, cisplatin and piroxicam caused a CR in two of 11 dogs with melanoma.[36]

Treatment of 11 oral melanomas using intralesional cisplatin mixed with bovine collagen matrix resulted in CRs in five dogs and PRs in another four dogs (total responders: 91%).[37] The combination of radiation therapy and intralesional cisplatin would seem a logical progression, but although the only reported dog treated this way had a CR, there was a local recurrence 3 months later.[38]

Other Therapies

Immunotherapy has a role in treating melanoma in other species. Cimetidine, which appears to inhibit suppressor T cells, has been shown to cause regression of melanoma in some horses,[39] although its role in the treatment of the disease in dogs is not defined. Immunotherapy with interleukin-2 (IL-2) has been beneficial in treating humans with melanoma. Combined with tumor necrosis factor, this treatment might be useful in dogs.[40] This combination was administered to 13 dogs with measurable oral melanoma. Five dogs showed reduction in tumor size, although only two had durable responses. One of these dogs had a CR for more than 3 years.

Immunotherapy with heat-inactivated *Corynebacterium parvum* (0.1 mg/kg IV per week) was used as an adjunct to surgery in 42 dogs.[5] *C. parvum* activates and increases the production of macrophages, which enhances the antibody response. Immunotherapy with *C. parvum* was found to benefit dogs with small tumors (stage I).

In another study, a more specific macrophage activator, liposome-encapsulated muramyl tripeptide-phosphatidyl-ethanolamine (L-MTP-PE), improved survival for a subset of dogs treated after surgery for oral melanoma.[41] L-MTP-PE was administered to 24 dogs after surgery, and 26 dogs received a placebo. Only dogs with stage I melanomas benefited, with 80% of these dogs alive 2 years after therapy. The addition of recombinant canine sargramostim (granulocyte–macrophage colony-stimulating factor [GM-CSF]) to the protocol did not improve these results.[41]

Gene therapy may also be effective in treating some dogs with melanoma. Treatment of 26 dogs with melanoma using lipid-complexed plasmid DNA encoding *Staphylococcus* enterotoxin-B and either GM-CSF or IL-2 was reported.[42] Tumor regression was seen in 13 dogs and was associated with tumor infiltration by CD4+ and CD8+ cells. Dogs with small tumors were most likely to respond to treatment; dogs with pulmonary metastases did not respond. Regression was seen over a period of 10 weeks in most dogs. When dogs with larger tumors and lymph node metastases were compared with similar dogs treated by surgery alone, dogs receiving gene therapy lived longer (four dogs were still alive nearly 2 years after treatment).[42]

Xenogeneic DNA vaccination with genes encoding human tyrosinase was used to treat nine dogs with advanced melanoma. Median survival was longer than 1 year, and one dog had complete regression of pulmonary metastases for nearly 1 year.[43] Clearly, immunotherapy has a role to play in the treatment of melanomas in dogs.

Cutaneous Melanoma
INCIDENCE, SIGNALMENT, AND ETIOLOGY

Cutaneous melanoma occurs in adult to senior dogs. There is no gender predilection for either benign or malignant melanomas of the skin. Cutaneous melanoma occurs most commonly on the head and limbs; tumors in these sites account for nearly 70% of benign melanomas and 60% of malignant melanomas in dogs.[44] Dog breeds that are more than three times as likely as the general population to develop benign cutaneous melanomas are toy Manchester, Irish, silky, and Australian terriers; miniature and standard schnauzers; vizslas; Doberman pinschers; Rhodesian ridgebacks; and Chesapeake Bay retrievers. Breeds more likely to develop malignant cutaneous melanomas include miniature and standard schnauzers and Scottish terriers.[44]

CLINICAL PRESENTATION AND HISTORY

Melanomas range from inconspicuous black macules to large, rapidly growing masses that may be either amelanotic or dark brown to gray or black in color. The appearance of a melanoma depends on its stage of development. Initially, melanomas can appear as flat, black macules. They may progress into elevated, firm nodules and can be smooth or rough.

Benign dermal melanomas usually range from 0.5 to 2.0 cm in diameter, are darkly pigmented and dome shaped, and have a smooth, hairless surface. On cut surface, the tumors are usually well defined but are seldom encapsulated (Figures 54-6 and 54-7). Malignant melanomas are normally large, and the overlying skin is frequently ulcerated and secondarily infected. Their color may vary from black to brown to light gray. Cutaneous melanomas are usually solitary, with multiple tumors occurring in 4% to 16% of dogs with benign melanomas and less than 1% of dogs with malignant melanomas.[44,45] The behavior of canine melanomas differs strikingly depending on their location. Most cutaneous melanomas are benign; of 1,116 melanomas in one series, only 143 (13%) were malignant. Melanoma of the subungual area (nail bed) is a notable exception and may be highly malignant; care must be taken to differentiate melanoma of the interdigital skin from a true subungual area because the former are usually benign (Figures 54-8 and 54-9). Subungual melanomas may invade the surrounding structures, although erosion of P3 is rare, occurring in 5% of dogs with subungual melanomas compared with 80% of dogs that have subungual squamous cell carcinoma.[46]

STAGING AND DIAGNOSIS

Malignant melanomas can metastasize via lymph channels and blood. Regional lymph nodes are commonly the first sites affected, and the lung is the most common site of visceral involvement. Therefore, thoracic radiography and blood work should be part of a minimum database (MDB), and cytologic evaluation of regional and enlarged lymph nodes is prudent, particularly for melanomas of the digits (Figure 54-10). In one study, six of 19 dogs with digital melanomas had pulmonary metastases at diagnosis, and another five dogs developed metastases after treatment, for a total of 58% affected.[46]

> *Most cutaneous melanomas are benign, although digital tumors are often highly malignant.*

Pathology is important in determining the likelihood of malignant behavior in cutaneous melanoma. Criteria of malignancy include nuclear pleomorphism, nuclear hyperchromasia, more than 2 or 3 mitotic figures per 10 hpf, and histologic evidence of invasion.[47,48] Specific pathology terms used to describe the histologic appearance of melanomas include *junctional activity*, which refers to the proliferation of nests of

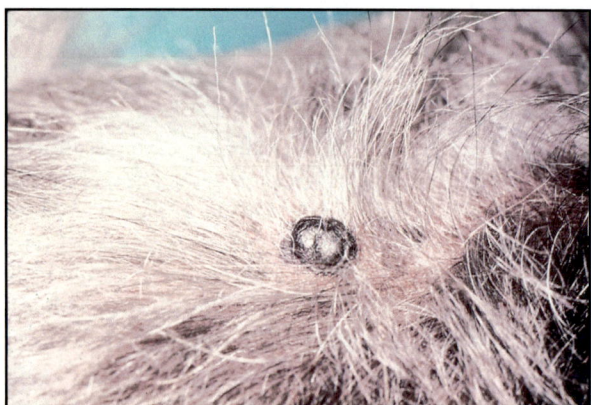

Figure 54-6. *Cutaneous melanomas, as in this 10-year-old schnauzer, are usually benign and can be resected for a cure.*

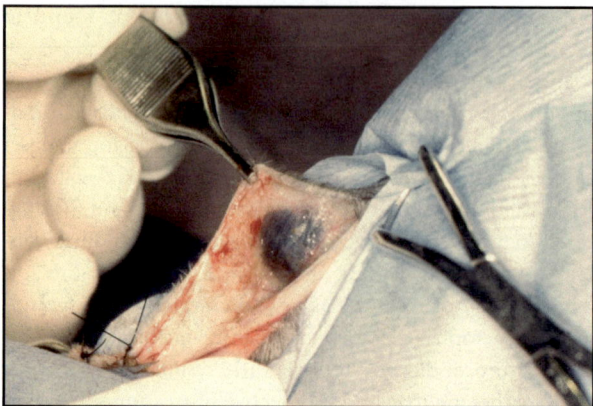

Figure 54-7. *Cutaneous melanomas are often located in the superficial dermis and can be cured at surgery.*

melanocytes along the dermoepidermal junction, and *compound melanoma*, which refers to junctional and intradermal components in the same tumor. Melanomas may also be described as spindle, epithelioid, and mixed, although none of these terms conveys any prognostic information over mitotic index alone. *Clear cell* (or *balloon cell*) *melanoma* is another pathologic term for a rare variant, but it appears to have little prognostic significance over other factors.[49] The importance of this variant is that it may be confused with other cutaneous tumors, such as liposarcoma or sebaceous carcinoma. Staining with melanocyte-specific markers should help in the differential diagnosis.[50-52] In one study, eight of 85 dogs with benign cutaneous melanoma had histologic criteria of malignancy (mitotic figures or cellular pleomorphism), so although histologic criteria do not provide a perfect system for prognosis, they predicted behavior in more than 90% of tumors.[45]

Other immunohistochemical markers have been explored for their ability to diagnose melanoma when the tumor is poorly pigmented and poorly differentiated. No marker is absolutely specific for melanoma or for predicting behavior (see also Oral Malignant Melanoma, above); however, one study found Melan-A to be a sensitive and specific stain for canine melanomas of all sites.[12] Another study found that a panel of markers, including vimentin, S-100, and Melan-A, was helpful in the diagnosis of melanoma.[13] When the clinician has a tumor suspected to be a melanoma, requesting this panel of stains gives the greatest chance of an accurate diagnosis.

PROGNOSTIC FACTORS

The intensity of Melan-A staining appeared to correlate inversely with malignant behavior in one study. Weak or negative staining was only seen in malignant melanomas.[13]

In a study that compared the prognostic value of clinical and pathologic variables for cutaneous melanoma, several factors independently predicted behavior.[48] Whereas high mitotic index, high proportion of dividing cells by Ki67 (MIB-1) staining, deep location, and ulceration were associated with a negative prognosis, heavy pigmentation and junctional activity were associated with a positive prognosis (Figures 54-11 and 54-12). Histology and mitotic index accurately predicted clinical behavior in 93% and 91% of dogs, respectively; Ki67 staining was accurate in predicting tumor behavior in 97% of dogs with melanomas. The study also identified a subset of patients with tumors that had histologic criteria of malignancy but low Ki67 staining; these dogs all had long survival times, further implying that Ki67 may be a helpful prognostic tool. Similar results for Ki67 were seen in two other studies.[47,53] Although not statistically significant, 56% of dogs with digital tumors were alive 2 years after surgery compared with 84% of dogs with tumors at other sites.[48] In contrast, the DNA content of a melanoma does not seem to correlate with prognosis.[54]

TREATMENT

Therapy includes wide surgical excision of any melanoma. Tumors arising in the subungual area and other mucocutaneous junctions always have a poor prognosis, and adjunctive therapy may be required.

Melanomas of the distal limbs in 28 dogs were reviewed.[55] Benign tumors were diagnosed in 14 dogs based on a mitotic index of fewer than 2 per 10 hpf and nuclear and nucleolar pleomorphism. There was no local recurrence or tumor-related death in this group. The tumor was more likely to be benign if it had been present for 6 months or more. Ulceration was equally common in malignant and benign groups in this study, and age, gender, location, size, and histologic type (spindle, epithelioid, mixed) did not influence survival.[55] The other 14 dogs in this study had malignant tumors. Two of 14 malignant melanomas recurred locally, and 10 of 14 metastasized to lymph nodes or lung. Lung metastasis occurred from 1 to 33 months after

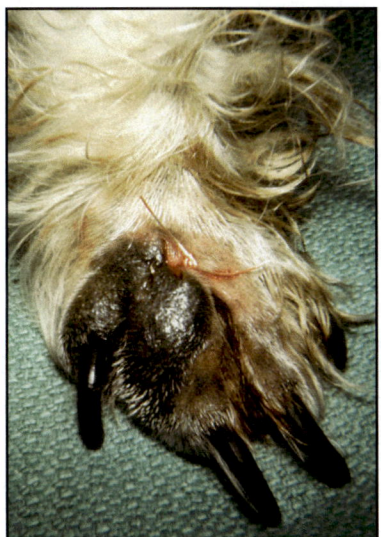

Figure 54-8. *Cutaneous melanomas of the interdigital skin, as in this 10-year-old schnauzer, may be less aggressive than those arising from the nail bed (see Figure 54-9) and may be cured by wide excision that may include a toe. (Courtesy of Gordon H. Theilen, DVM, University of California, Davis)*

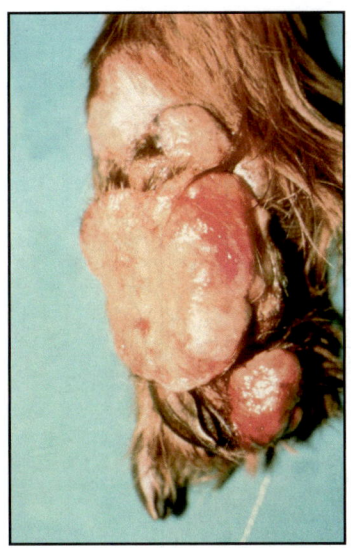

Figure 54-9. *Cutaneous melanomas of the nail bed (subungual) are invasive and very likely to metastasize. Adjuvant chemotherapy is probably warranted for these dogs. (Courtesy of Anne G. Evans, DVM, Veterinary Information Network)*

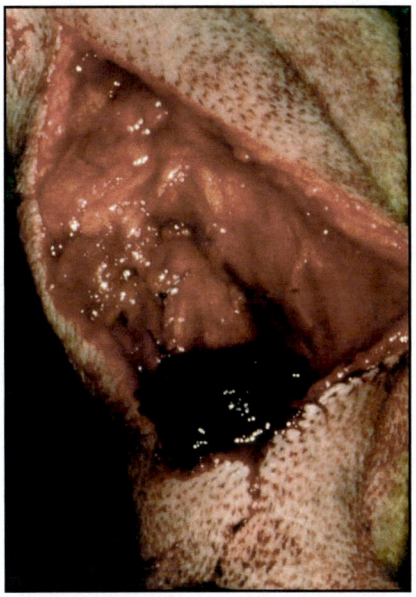

Figure 54-10. *This 9-year-old Doberman has a popliteal lymph node metastasis from a subungual melanoma. Chemotherapy with platinum drugs may have some efficacy in this dog.*

surgery; the mean time to metastasis was 13 months. Involvement of the nail bed in any dog suggested malignant melanoma, but histopathologic examination was the only reliable method of diagnosis. Dogs with stage I malignant disease had a longer survival time (average: 19.6 months).[55] In another study, the median survival after surgery for 19 dogs with digital melanoma was 12 months, with 42% of the dogs alive 1 year and 13% alive 2 years after surgery.[46]

The pads of the foot are another common site of melanoma; a technique has been described for digital pad transposition to provide a weight-bearing surface when the metacarpal or metatarsal pad is involved in melanoma.[56]

Radiation therapy has proven very effective in dogs with oral melanoma, but there are insufficient data to show efficacy for unresectable cutaneous lesions; however, this does not mean radiation is not a reasonable option. A coarsely fractionated approach, as described above for oral melanomas, may be effective, although more conventional fractionation may have fewer late effects. Radiation therapy can be palliative for painful or ulcerated lesions in dogs with metastatic disease (Figure 54-13).

Adjuvant chemotherapy may improve the long-term survival for dogs with malignant cutaneous melanoma. The role of adjuvant therapy in this disease is uncertain, but carboplatin and cisplatin are probably the most active agents (see Oral Malignant Melanoma section, above). Although immunotherapy may improve survival for dogs with oral melanoma,[5] clinical trials have not been conducted in dogs with cutaneous tumors. Cimetidine, which appears to inhibit suppressor T cells, has been shown to cause regression of melanoma in some horses,[39] although its role in the treatment of the disease in dogs is not defined.

Ocular Melanoma
INCIDENCE, SIGNALMENT, AND ETIOLOGY

Melanoma is the most common ocular tumor in dogs. In one study of 147 primary ocular tumors, more than half were melanoma.[57] Melanoma of the globe reportedly affects the limbus, choroid, iris, and other areas of the uvea.[58,59] Ocular melanoma occurs primarily in older dogs. Although affected dogs range in age from 2 months to 17 years, 70% are 7 years of age or older.[60] In one series, seven of 23 dogs were younger than 1 year of age.[61] Dogs with limbal tumors may be somewhat younger; most are younger than 7 years.[62,63] Most studies have not determined any breed predisposition for ocular melanoma,[60,64] although German shepherds accounted for 15 of 30 affected dogs in one study[63] and nearly 25% of dogs with limbal tumors in another.[65] In another study, German shepherds and boxers were overrepresented compared with the general population.[62] One author suggested that primary acquired melanosis, which occurs in some brachycephalic breeds and as a consequence of pannus in German shepherds, may be a premalignant change for ocular melanoma.[66] This hypothesis, however, requires further exploration.

Melanoma should be distinguished clinically from uveal cysts. Uveal cysts are pigmented and usually free floating in

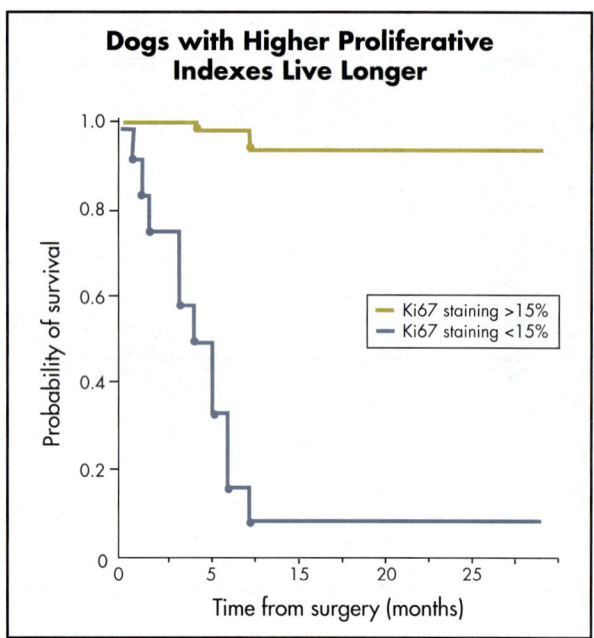

Figure 54-11. Survival curves for dogs with cutaneous melanoma showing the effect of proliferative index based on Ki67 staining of greater than 15% or less than 15%. (Adapted from Laprie C, Abadie J, Amardeilh MF, et al: MIB-1 immunoreactivity correlates with biologic behaviour in canine cutaneous melanoma. Vet Dermatol 12:139–147, 2001; with permission)

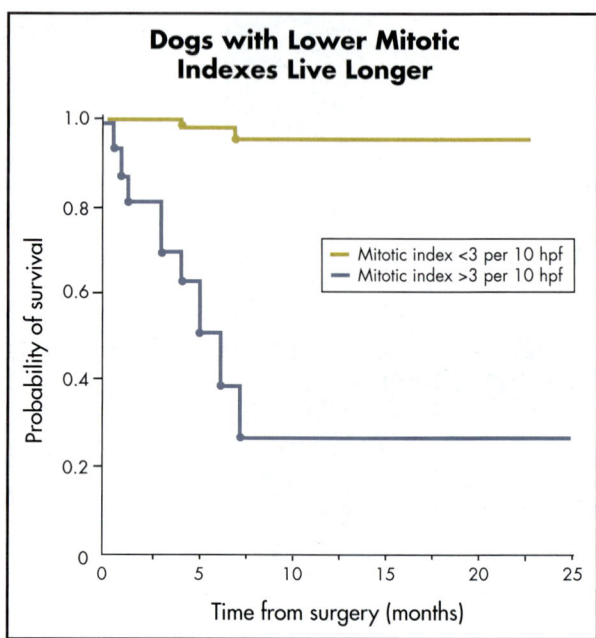

Figure 54-12. Survival curves for dogs with cutaneous melanoma showing the effect of mitotic index greater than 3 per 10 hpf or less than 3 per 10 hpf. (Adapted from Laprie C, Abadie J, Amardeilh MF, et al: MIB-1 immunoreactivity correlates with biologic behaviour in canine cutaneous melanoma. Vet Dermatol 12:139–147, 2001; with permission)

the anterior chamber; they are common in retrievers of any age.[67] If it is not possible to distinguish a uveal cyst from melanoma, the dog should be reexamined at a later date to check for growth of the lesion. Uveal cysts can be removed by fine-needle aspiration using a 25-gauge needle; a veterinary ophthalmologist should be consulted.[67]

Conjunctival melanoma, mostly (83%) arising from the nictitans, was reported in 12 dogs, of which eight were females and three were weimaraners.[68]

CLINICAL PRESENTATION AND HISTORY

The most common reasons for presentation of dogs with ocular melanoma are the presence of a mass, glaucoma, uveitis, and hyphema. Less common reasons are corneal edema, epiphora, and hyperemic conjunctivae. In 48 of 72 dogs (67%) with melanoma, an intraocular or scleral mass was visible, and in 34 of these dogs (47%), the mass was the only abnormality detected.[60] In contrast, nearly one-third of dogs with glaucoma caused by ocular melanoma have no visible tumor. The eye of any dog with unilateral glaucoma should be carefully examined for the presence of a mass.[64] Even when tumors are noticed, they may remain static for 1 year or more before definitive diagnosis.[62,63] Bilateral involvement with melanoma is very rare.[69]

Some authors have described melanomas with respect to the area of the eye involved: limbal (or epibulbar), anterior uveal (iris or ciliary body), or choroidal (Figure 54-14).

STAGING AND DIAGNOSIS

Any dog with unilateral glaucoma or an intraocular mass should be investigated for melanoma. Ultrasonography may be very helpful in delineating the extent of the mass and in guiding a needle aspirate for cytology.[70] Most melanomas arising from the uvea and corneoscleral limbus in dogs are not likely to metastasize; however, they may exhibit expansive growth patterns. Of 229 reported dogs[59,64,66,71,72] (including 190 dogs in one study[64]), ocular melanomas metastasized in only 10 cases (4%). Metastasis usually occurred between 2 and 5 months after enucleation,[60,66,71] although in one dog, metastases were seen nearly 2 years after excision of a "benign" choroidal melanoma.[73] When it occurs, metastasis is widespread, and metastases to the lungs, liver, kidney, spleen, bone, adrenal gland, heart, mandibular lymph nodes, and even the contralateral eye[74] have been reported.

A large study differentiated 188 benign and 56 malignant intraocular melanomas based on histologic criteria of mitotic index (>2 per 10 hpf), nuclear:cytoplasmic ratio greater than 1, and prominent nucleoli. The sizes of tumors in the two populations were similar, and whether they remained localized within the sclera, invaded the sclera, or demonstrated extrascleral extension was not different between the two groups. Malignant melanomas were more likely than benign tumors to arise from the anterior uveal tract (95% versus 79%).[65] Metastasis was observed or presumed in three of 129 dogs with benign melanoma and in 10 of 36 dogs with malignant melanoma.[65]

Many criteria are proposed as possible predictors of malignant behavior; however, most histologic features, such as necrosis, inflammation, degree of pigmentation, and growth pattern of cells, have no prognostic value.[60] The most valuable indicator of malignancy is the mitotic index of the tumor. In one study of 61 dogs with ocular melanomas, nine dogs (15%) had a mitotic index greater than 4, and four of these nine dogs developed metastases.[60] In contrast, in a series of 12 dogs with conjunctival melanoma, there was no obvious correlation between mitotic index and recurrence or metastases.[68] Not all tumors with high mitotic indexes metastasize.[59,60,64] Overall, ocular melanoma should be considered a benign tumor in dogs, although staging procedures should be used to establish the good health of the patient before treatment.

PROGNOSTIC FACTORS

Melanomas with a mitotic index greater than 4 may exhibit metastatic behavior, and a more guarded prognosis is warranted for dogs with this histologic finding.[60] Another study found that dogs with malignant melanoma lived a shorter time than those with benign melanoma, and the differentiation between the two groups was based on mitotic index and presence of anaplasia.[65] Dogs with malignant tumors lived for a shorter time than a control population of dogs, but dogs with benign melanoma did not have a shorter survival time than control dogs. Size of tumor and tumor extension into surrounding tissues were not predictive of survival in the same study.[65]

TREATMENT

Ocular melanoma in dogs is usually benign; therefore, observation alone may be a reasonable option for small, well-circumscribed lesions.[64,75] If the tumor grows, surgical resection of the tumor by enucleation should be curative. Tumors that involve the limbus or the conjunctiva warrant more aggressive treatment.

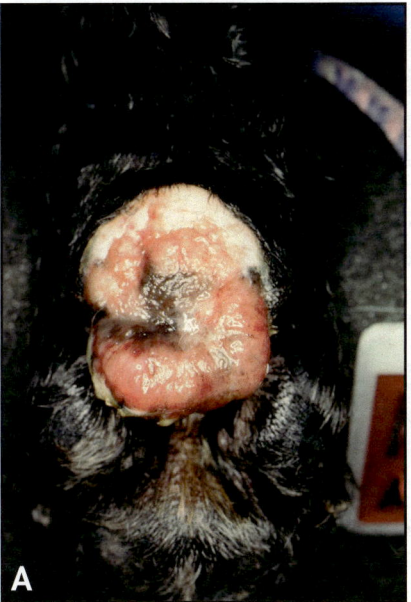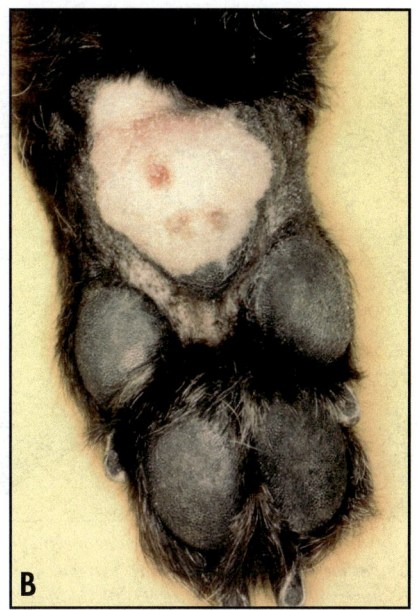

Figure 54-13. *Ulcerated melanoma. (A) This painful and ulcerated melanoma of the pad occurred in a Portuguese water dog that had pulmonary metastases. Palliative radiation therapy was performed to improve quality of life for this dog. (B) Regression of the tumor after three doses of radiation therapy.*

Local excision is an option for tumors of the limbus.[60] Partial iridectomy[60] and lamellar keratectomy[63] can also achieve local removal. Recurrence rates after local excision range from 30% to 40%.[60,63] Enucleation is curative for dogs whose tumors are not controlled by local excision or dogs that have ocular involvement and extensive tumor growth. After enucleation, more than 95% of dogs have no recurrence or metastases for 1 to 5 years.[60,62] Melanomas of the conjunctiva appear to be more aggressive tumors. In a series of nine dogs with conjunctival melanoma, the tumor was removed, often by excision of the nictitans.[68] Incomplete excision or lymphatic invasion based on histopathology was associated with recurrence in six dogs between 3 and 7 months after surgery (median: 5 months), and two of these dogs developed orbital melanoma. Four dogs developed metastatic disease. The authors suggested that cryosurgery

> *Ocular melanoma in dogs should almost always be considered a benign tumor that can be cured by enucleation.*

may improve local control of an incompletely excised lesion. Cryosurgery may reduce the chance of local recurrence after excision, but overzealous freezing can cause ocular damage.

Other methods of local treatment have been reported, including the unsuccessful use of a synthetic polytetrafluoroethylene graft[76] and partial regression of some melanomas after neodymium:yttrium–aluminum–garnet laser photoco-

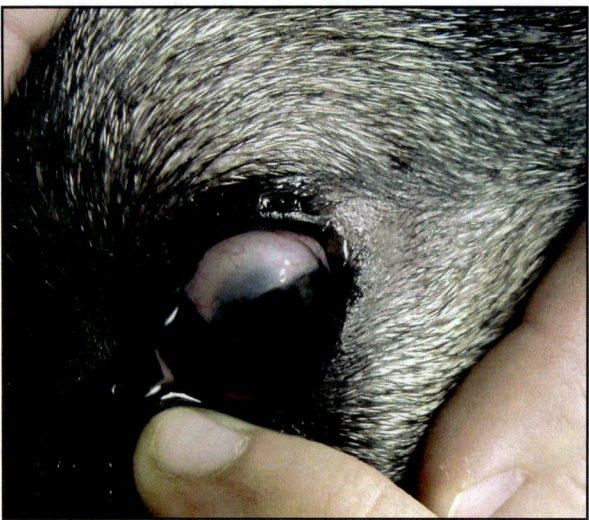

Figure 54-14. *Although most ocular melanomas in dogs are benign, limbal melanomas, as in this dog, warrant more aggressive treatment. (Courtesy of Nicole Northrup, DVM, University of Georgia College of Veterinary Medicine)*

agulation.[72] Laser photocoagulation was reported in 23 dogs with iris melanoma. One to three treatments resulted in shrinkage of the lesions, which remained static for a period of 6 months to 4.5 years (median: 2 years). No significant complications were reported.[61]

REFERENCES

1. Goldschmidt MH: Benign and malignant melanocytic neoplasms of domestic animals. *Am J Dermatopathol* 7:203–212, 1985.
2. Peiffer RL Jr: Primary intraocular tumors in the dog. Part I. *Mod Vet Pract* 60:383–387, 1979.
3. Bostock DE: Prognosis after surgical excision of canine melanomas. *Vet Pathol* 16:32–40, 1979.
4. Hahn KA, DeNicola DB, Richardson RC, Hahn EA: Canine oral malignant melanoma: Prognostic utility of an alternative staging system. *J Small Anim Pract* 35:251–256, 1994.
5. MacEwen EG, Patnaik AK, Harvey HJ, et al: Canine oral melanoma: Comparison of surgery versus surgery plus *Corynebacterium parvum*. *Cancer Invest* 4:397–402, 1986.
6. Harvey HJ, MacEwen EG, Braun D, et al: Prognostic criteria for dogs with oral melanoma. *JAVMA* 178:580–582, 1981.
7. Modiano JF, Ritt MG, Wojcieszyn J: The molecular basis of canine melanoma: Pathogenesis and trends in diagnosis and therapy. *J Vet Intern Med* 13:163–174, 1999.
8. Sulaimon SS, Kitchell BE: The basic biology of malignant melanoma: Molecular mechanisms of disease progression and comparative aspects. *J Vet Intern Med* 17:760–772, 2003.
9. Salisbury SK, Lantz GC: Long-term results of partial mandibulectomy for treatment of oral tumors in 30 dogs. *JAAHA* 24:285–294, 1988.
10. Chenier S, Dore M: Oral malignant melanoma with osteoid formation in a dog. *Vet Pathol* 36:74–76, 1999.
11. Berrington AJ, Jimbow K, Haines DM: Immunohistochemical detection of melanoma-associated antigens on formalin-fixed, paraffin-embedded canine tumors. *Vet Pathol* 31:455–461, 1994.
12. Ramos-Vara JA, Beissenherz ME, Miller MA, et al: Retrospective study of 338 canine oral melanomas with clinical, histologic, and immunohistochemical review of 129 cases. *Vet Pathol* 37:597–608, 2000.
13. Koenig A, Wojcieszyn J, Weeks BR, Modiano JF: Expression of S100a, vimentin, NSE, and melan A/MART-1 in seven canine melanoma cells lines and twenty-nine retrospective cases of canine melanoma. *Vet Pathol* 38:427–435, 2001.
14. Sulaimon S, Kitchell B, Ehrhart E: Immunohistochemical detection of melanoma-specific antigens in spontaneous canine melanoma. *J Comp Pathol* 127:162–168, 2002.
15. Williams LE, Packer RA: Association between lymph node size and metastasis in dogs with oral malignant melanoma: 100 cases (1987–2001). *JAVMA* 222:1234–1236, 2003.
16. Herring ES, Smith MM, Robertson JL: Lymph node staging of oral and maxillofacial neoplasms in 31 dogs and cats. *J Vet Dent* 19:122–126, 2002.
17. Todoroff RJ, Brodey RS: Oral and pharyngeal neoplasia in the dog: A retrospective study of 361 cases. *JAVMA* 175:567–571, 1979.
18. Pressler BM, Rotstein DS, Law JM, et al: Hypercalcemia and high parathyroid hormone-related protein concentration associated with malignant melanoma in a dog. *JAVMA* 221:263–265, 240, 2002.
19. Théon AP, Rodriguez C, Madewell BR: Analysis of prognostic factors and patterns of failure in dogs with malignant oral tumors treated with megavoltage irradiation. *JAVMA* 210:778–784, 1997.
20. Wallace J, Matthiesen DT, Patnaik AK: Hemimaxillectomy for the treatment of oral tumors in 69 dogs. *Vet Surg* 21:337–341, 1992.
21. Salisbury SK, Richardson DC, Lantz GC: Partial maxillectomy and premaxillectomy in the treatment of oral neoplasia in the dog and cat. *Vet Surg* 15:16–26, 1986.
22. White RA: Mandibulectomy and maxillectomy in the dog: long term survival in 100 cases. *J Small Anim Pract* 32:69–74, 1991.
23. Schwarz PD, Withrow SJ, Curtis CR, et al: Mandibular resection as a treatment for oral cancer in 81 dogs. *JAAHA* 27:601–610, 1991.
24. Schwarz PD, Withrow SJ, Curtis CR, et al: Partial maxillary resection as a treatment for oral cancer in 61 dogs. *JAAHA* 27:617–624, 1991.
25. Felizzola CR, Stopiglia AJ, de Araujo VC, de Araujo NS: Evaluation of a modified hemimandibulectomy for treatment of oral neoplasms in dogs. *J Vet Dent* 19:127–135, 2002.
26. Beck ER, Withrow SJ, McChesney AE, et al: Canine tongue tumors: A retrospective review of 57 cases. *JAAHA* 22:525–532, 1996.
27. Kudnig ST, Ehrhart N, Withrow SJ, et al: Survival analysis of oral melanoma in dogs. *Proc 23rd Annu Conf Vet Cancer Soc*:39, 2003.
28. Bateman KE, Catton PA, Pennock PW, Kruth SA: 0-7-21 radiation therapy for the treatment of canine oral melanoma. *J Vet Intern Med* 8:267–272, 1994.
29. Blackwood L, Dobson JM: Radiotherapy of oral malignant melanomas in dogs. *JAVMA* 209:98–102, 1996.
30. Proulx DR, Ruslander DM, Dodge RK, et al: A retrospective analysis of 140 dogs with oral melanoma treated with external beam radiation. *Vet Radiol Ultrasound* 44:352–359, 2003.
31. Azuma C, Ruslander DM, Brown MA, et al: Hypofractionated radiation therapy in the treatment of oral melanoma in dogs. Personal communication, 2004.
32. Freeman KP, Hahn KA, Harris FD, King GK: Treatment of dogs with oral melanoma by hypofractionated radiation therapy and platinum-based chemotherapy (1987–1997). *J Vet Intern Med* 17:96–101, 2003.
33. Page RL, Thrall DE, Dewhirst MW, et al: Phase I study of melphalan alone and melphalan plus whole body hyperthermia in dogs with malignant melanoma. *Int J Hyperthermia* 7:559–566, 1991.
34. Rassnick KM, Ruslander DM, Cotter SM, et al: Use of carboplatin for treatment of dogs with malignant melanoma: 27 cases (1989–2000). *JAVMA* 218:1444–1448, 2001.
35. Guptill L, Knapp DW, Hank K, et al: Retrospective study of cisplatin treatment for canine malignant melanoma. *Proc Vet Cancer Soc 13th Annu Conf*:65–66, 1998.
36. Boria PA, Murry DJ, Bennett PF, et al: Evaluation of cisplatin combined with piroxicam for the treatment of oral malignant melanoma and oral squamous cell carcinoma in dogs. *JAVMA* 224:388–394, 2004.
37. Orenberg EK, Luck EE, Brown DM, Kitchell BE: Implant delivery system: Intralesional delivery of chemotherapeutic agents for treatment of spontaneous skin tumors in veterinary patients. *Clin Dermatol* 9:561–568, 1992.
38. Theon AP, Madewell BR, Ryu J, Castro J: Concurrent irradiation and intratumoral chemotherapy with cisplatin: A pilot study in dogs with spontaneous tumors. *Int J Radiat Oncol Biol Phys* 29:1027–1034, 1994.
39. Goetz TE, Boulton CH, Ogilvie GK: Clinical management of progressive multifocal benign and malignant melanomas of horses with oral cimetidine. *Proc Annu Conv AAEP*:35:431–438, 1990.
40. Moore AS, Theilen GH, Newell AD, et al: Preclinical study of sequential tumor necrosis factor and interleukin-2 in the treatment of spontaneous canine neoplasms. *Cancer Res* 51:233–238, 1991.
41. MacEwen EG, Kurzman ID, Vail DM, et al: Adjuvant therapy for melanoma in dogs: Results of randomized clinical trials using surgery, liposome-encapsulated muramyl tripeptide, and granulocyte macrophage colony-stimulating factor. *Clin Cancer Res* 5:4249–4258, 1999.

42. Dow SW, Elmslie RE, Wilson AP, et al: In vivo tumor transfection with superantigen plus cytokine genes induces tumor regression and prolongs survival in dogs with malignant melanoma. *J Clin Invest* 101:2406–2414, 1998.
43. Bergman PJ, McKnight J, Novosad A, et al: Long-term survival of dogs with advanced malignant melanoma after DNA vaccination with xenogeneic human tyrosinase: A phase I trial. *Clin Cancer Res* 9:1284–1290, 2003.
44. Goldschmidt MH, Shofer FS: Melanoma and malignant melanomas, in Goldschmidt MH, Shofer FS (eds): *Skin Tumors of the Dog and Cat.* Tarrytown, NY, Pergamon Press, 1992, pp 131–151.
45. Bolon B, Calderwood Mays MB, Hall BJ: Characteristics of canine melanomas and comparison of histology and DNA ploidy to their biologic behavior. *Vet Pathol* 27:96–102, 1990.
46. Marino DJ, Matthiesen DT, Stefanacci JD, Moroff SD: Evaluation of dogs with digit masses: 117 cases (1981–1991). *JAVMA* 207:726–728, 1995.
47. Roels S, Tilmant K, Ducatelle R: PCNA and Ki67 proliferation markers as criteria for prediction of clinical behaviour of melanocytic tumours in cats and dogs. *J Comp Pathol* 121:13–24, 1999.
48. Laprie C, Abadie J, Amardeilh MF, et al: MIB-1 immunoreactivity correlates with biologic behaviour in canine cutaneous melanoma. *Vet Dermatol* 12:139–147, 2001.
49. Diters RW, Walsh KM: Canine cutaneous clear cell melanomas: A report of three cases. *Vet Pathol* 21:355–356, 1984.
50. Blanchard TW, Bryant NJ, Mense MG: Balloon cell melanoma in three dogs: A histopathological, immunohistochemical and ultrastructural study. *J Comp Pathol* 125:254–261, 2001.
51. Cangul IT, van Garderen E, van der Linde-Sipman JS, et al: Canine balloon and signet-ring cell melanomas: A histological and immunohistochemical characterization. *J Comp Pathol* 125:166–173, 2001.
52. Wilkerson MJ, Dolce K, DeBey BM, et al: Metastatic balloon cell melanoma in a dog. *Vet Clin Pathol* 32:31–36, 2003.
53. Millanta F, Fratini F, Corazza M, et al: Proliferation activity in oral and cutaneous canine melanocytic tumours: Correlation with histological parameters, location, and clinical behaviour. *Res Vet Sci* 73:45–51, 2002.
54. Roels SL, Van Daele AJ, Van Marck EA, Ducatelle RV: DNA ploidy and nuclear morphometric variables for the evaluation of melanocytic tumors in dogs and cats. *Am J Vet Res* 61:1074–1079, 2000.
55. Aronsohn MG, Carpenter JL: Distal extremity melanocytic nevi and malignant melanomas in dogs. *JAAHA* 26:605–612, 1990.
56. Olsen D, Straw RC, Withrow SJ, Basher AW: Digital pad transposition for replacement of the metacarpal or metatarsal pad in dogs. *JAAHA* 33:337–341, 1997.
57. Trucksa RC, McLean IW, Quinn AJ: Intraocular canine melanocytic neoplasms. *JAAHA* 21:85–88, 1985.
58. Dubielzig RR, Aguirre GD, Gross SL, Diters RW: Choroidal melanomas in dogs. *Vet Pathol* 22:582–585, 1985.
59. Collinson PN, Peiffer RL Jr: Clinical presentation, morphology and behavior of primary choroidal melanomas in eight dogs. *Prog Vet Comp Ophthalmol* 3:158–164, 1993.
60. Wilcock BP, Peiffer RL Jr: Morphology and behavior of primary ocular melanomas in 91 dogs. *Vet Pathol* 23:418–424, 1986.
61. Cook CS, Wilkie DA: Treatment of presumed iris melanoma in dogs by diode laser photocoagulation: 23 cases. *Vet Ophthalmol* 2:217–225, 1999.
62. Ryan AM, Diters RW: Clinical and pathologic features of canine ocular melanomas. *JAVMA* 184:60–67, 1984.
63. Diters RW, Ryan AM: Canine limbal melanoma. *Vet Med Small Anim Clin* 78:1529–1534, 1983.
64. Bussanich NM, Dolman PJ, Rootman J, Dolman CL: Canine uveal melanomas: Series and literature review. *JAAHA* 23:415–422, 1987.
65. Guiliano EA, Chappell R, Fischer B, Dubielzig RR: A matched observational study of canine survival with primary intraocular melanocytic neoplasia. *Vet Ophthalmol* 2:185–190, 1999.
66. Croxatto JO, Herrera HD, Lightowler CH: Malignant melanoma arising from primary acquired melanosis in a dog. *Canine Pract* 17:22–24, 1992.
67. Corcoran KA, Koch SA: Uveal cysts in dogs: 28 cases (1989–1991). *JAVMA* 203:545–546, 1993.
68. Collins BK, Collier LL, Miller MA, Linton LL: Biologic behavior and histologic characteristics of canine conjunctival melanoma. *Prog Vet Comp Ophthalmol* 3:135–140, 1993.
69. Roperto F, Restucci B, Crovace A: Bilateral ciliary body melanomas in a dog. *Prog Vet Comp Ophthalmol* 3:149–151, 1993.
70. Allgoewer I, Freiling E, Fritsche J, et al: Das choroidal melanom beim hund. *Kleintierpraxis* 45:361–369, 2000.
71. Minami T, Patnaik AK: Malignant anterior uveal melanoma with diffuse metastasis in a dog. *JAVMA* 201:1894–1896, 1992.
72. Nasisse MP, Davidson MG, Olivero DK, et al: Neodymium: YAG laser treatment of primary canine intraocular tumors. *Prog Vet Comp Ophthalmol* 3:152–157, 1993.
73. Hyman JA, Koch SA, Wilcock BP: Canine choroidal melanoma with metastases. *Vet Ophthalmol* 5:113–117, 2002.
74. Render JA, Ramsey DT, Ramsey CC: Contralateral uveal metastasis of malignant anterior uveal melanoma in a dog. *Vet Comp Ophthalmol* 7:263–266, 1997.
75. Weisse I, Frese K, Meyer D: Benign melanoma of the choroid in a beagle: Ophthalmological, light and electron microscopical investigations. *Vet Pathol* 22:586–591, 1985.
76. Wilkie DA, Wolf ED: Treatment of epibulbar melanocytoma in a dog, using full-thickness eyewall resection and synthetic graft. *JAVMA* 198:1019–1022, 1991.

TUMORS AFFECTING THE LIVER, PANCREAS, AND SPLEEN

Antony S Moore and Gregory K Ogilvie

CLINICAL BRIEFING

Liver Tumors

Clinical factors
- Nonspecific lethargy and weight loss.
- Dogs may be asymptomatic and may have a palpable mass.
- Primary hepatocellular carcinoma is most common; most appear as a solitary mass.
- Multiple nodular or diffuse involvement seen more with biliary tumors and carcinoids.
- Older dogs affected.

Staging and diagnosis
- Minimum database (MDB; includes a CBC, biochemical profile, urinalysis, and thoracic radiography [three views]).
- Abdominal ultrasonography or computed tomography or MRI and biopsy.
- Large solitary lesions have a low metastatic rate.

Prognostic factors
- Dogs with any size solitary hepatocellular carcinoma have a good prognosis after resection.

Treatment
Initial
- Surgery is the treatment of choice for solitary tumors.

Adjunctive
- Not described; gemcitabine chemotherapy anecdotally.

Supportive
- Analgesia postoperatively; nutritional support as needed.

Nonlymphoid, Nonangiogenic Splenic Tumors

Clinical factors
- Abdominal swelling and weakness; palpable abdominal mass.
- Leiomyosarcoma, osteosarcoma, and fibrosarcoma.
- Average age: 11 years.
- No breed or gender predilection.

Staging and diagnosis
- MDB.
- Abdominal ultrasonography and biopsy.
- Metastasis commonly occurs in abdominal sites.

Prognostic factors
- Mesenchymomas may have best prognosis.
- Mitotic index predicts survival regardless of histologic type.

Treatment
Initial
- Splenectomy may be palliative. Survival is often shortened by metastases.

Adjunctive
- Chemotherapy not described, but approach as hemangiosarcomas.

Supportive
- Analgesia postoperatively; nutritional support as needed.

Exocrine Pancreatic Tumors	
Clinical factors	• Nonspecific anorexia and weight loss. • Carcinoma is more common than adenoma. • Older dogs affected. • Spaniel breeds may be predisposed.
Staging and diagnosis	• MDB. • Abdominal ultrasonography and biopsy. • Metastasis occurs early and widely.
Prognostic factors	• None identified.
Treatment Initial Adjunctive Supportive	• Surgery may not be beneficial because of high metastatic rate. • Other modalities unreported. • Pain relief. • Nutritional support; possibly parenteral nutrition.

Primary Liver Tumors

INCIDENCE, SIGNALMENT, AND ETIOLOGY

In a study of 110 nonhematopoietic, nonvascular hepatic neoplasms, slightly more than 50% were primary hepatocellular tumors.[1] Cholangiocellular carcinomas and bile duct cystadenomas were diagnosed less frequently, together accounting for approximately 20% of tumors. Carcinoids and sarcomas each accounted for approximately 15%.[1] Dogs with liver tumors are generally older; the average age of affected dogs is 11 to 12 years.[2–4] In a study of primary hepatocellular tumors, the male:female ratio was 1.7:1.0.[2] Another study found that female dogs were more likely to have cholangiocellular carcinomas.[4] One study suggested that Labrador retrievers may have a predisposition to develop bile duct carcinomas.[5]

CLINICAL PRESENTATION AND HISTORY

Clinical signs associated with liver tumors are often nonspecific. Lethargy, weakness, anorexia, polyuria, polydipsia, and vomiting are the most common signs and occur in up to 65% of animals. Weight loss, seizures, ascites, diarrhea, jaundice, and hematochezia are less common. Infrequently, hypoglycemia accompanies very large tumors, inducing seizures.[6] In one study, five of 18 dogs with liver tumors were asymptomatic. On physical examination, most dogs have abdominal distention and palpable hepatomegaly.

STAGING AND DIAGNOSIS

Radiography can be helpful when attempting to confirm a diagnosis of hepatic tumor. The most common radiographically detected abnormality is a right cranioventral abdominal mass that displaces the gastric shadow caudally and to the left and displaces the small intestine caudally (Figure 55-1).[3,4] Peritoneal fluid from carcinomatosis may obscure radiographic detection of the mass.[4] Ultrasonography is more precise than radiography in detecting the site of origin of an abdominal mass and provides important information as to the extent of disease (Figure 55-2); however, it may not provide enough information to influence the decision of whether to attempt surgery. Ultrasonography is not helpful in determining the cell type of a neoplasm and does not help distinguish neoplastic from nonneoplastic lesions.[7–9] Magnetic resonance imaging (MRI) provides high soft tissue contrast and allows the differentiation of benign and malignant hepatic focal lesions in dogs. In one study, 27 hepatic lesions were characterized by MRI as malignant or benign, with an overall accuracy of 94%. The overall sensitivity and specificity were 100% and 90%, respectively. MRI classified malignant hepatic lesions as hepatocellular carcinoma in all confirmed cases and correctly predicted the histologic grade of five hepatocellular lesions.[10]

Diagnosis is best obtained by biopsy. Cytology of epithelial tumors was diagnostic and concurred well with biopsy results in one study.[11] Ultrasound-guided needle-core biopsy usually provides a definitive diagnosis. In one study, histologic diagnosis from 80% of needle biopsies concurred with a wedge biopsy of the lesion taken at the same time.[12] The size of the needle biopsy (more or less than 1 cm in length) made no difference. A coagulation profile should be obtained

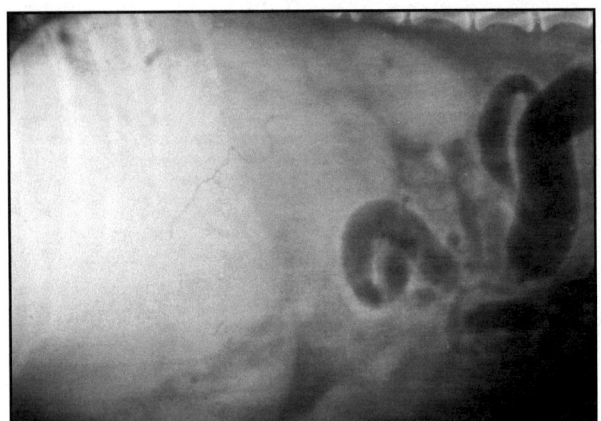

Figure 55-1. *Abdominal radiography may delineate a cranial abdominal mass, as shown in this 11-year-old dachshund; however, ultrasonography or exploratory laparotomy usually is required to confirm that a mass arises from the liver.*

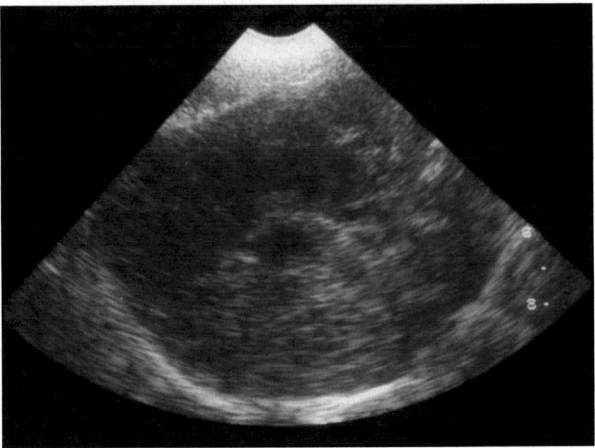

Figure 55-2. *Abdominal ultrasonography may confirm that a mass arises from the liver and whether it is a large solitary mass (as in this image) or is diffuse throughout all lobes.*

before a needle or wedge biopsy is performed, especially if liver function is abnormal. Fasting serum bile acids were elevated in approximately half the dogs with neoplasia in one study, implying liver dysfunction.[13]

Cholelithiasis may be diagnosed concurrently with obstructive tumors of the gallbladder (regardless of the histologic tumor type).[14,15]

Blood chemistry panels are rarely useful in diagnosing liver tumors. Alanine aminotransferase (ALT), alkaline phosphatase (ALP), and aspartate aminotransferase (AST) levels are elevated in 60% to 90% of dogs but are not specific for liver tumor.[1] ALP is the most commonly elevated parameter in dogs with liver tumors.[1,3,12,16] Fasting serum bile acid concentrations do not assist in detecting neoplasia.[13,16]

An enzymatic kit to detect α-fetoprotein (AFP) was used to distinguish different liver tumor types before biopsy.[16] Serum levels of AFP were highest in dogs with cholangiocarcinoma and hepatocellular carcinoma in one study[16] and in dogs with hepatocellular carcinoma only in another study.[17] Levels of AFP declined after surgical excision of hepatocellular carcinoma in three dogs, implying that this may be a helpful method of monitoring remission in selected dogs.[17] In contrast, only a poorly differentiated hepatic tumor expressed AFP in another study using immunohistochemical staining.[18] These tests are probably of limited diagnostic value to clinicians, and biopsy of the lesion should be performed when possible to obtain a definitive diagnosis.

Very large hepatocellular carcinomas have been associated with hypoglycemia. Clinical signs were related directly to adrenergic and neuroglucopenic effects of hypoglycemia and included collapsing episodes, tremors, restlessness, weakness, and grand mal seizures that were responsive to glucose administration. Surgical resection of the tumor achieved remission of clinical signs in three dogs.[6]

A paraneoplastic myelopathy has been reported in a dog with a metastatic hepatocellular carcinoma,[19] and myasthenia gravis was diagnosed in a dog with biliary carcinoma.[20]

Immunocytochemistry using monoclonal antibodies to hepatocyte paraffin 1 (Hep Par 1) and cytokeratin 7 (CK7) was conducted on 105 canine hyperplastic and neoplastic hepatic lesions. Hep Par 1 was detected in all hyperplastic nodules and hepatocellular adenomas and in 93% of hepatocellular carcinomas. In contrast, Hep Par 1 did not react with neoplastic biliary epithelium, other hepatic tumors, or tumors metastatic to the liver. The antibody to CK7 stained all hyperplastic biliary lesions and benign cholangiocellular tumors and nearly 80% of cholangiocellular carcinomas.[21] These markers may assist in distinguishing between hepatocellular and biliary neoplasms.

Hepatocellular Carcinoma

Three clinical forms of hepatocellular carcinoma have been described: massive, nodular, and diffuse.[2] A large mass lesion was the most common presenting sign of hepatocellular carcinoma in three studies.[3,4,22] In another study, 30 of 49 dogs (61%) with hepatocellular carcinoma had a massive lesion involving one hepatic lobe; however, 80% of these 30 dogs also had lesions in other lobes.[2] Nodular lesions involving more than one liver lobe and diffuse hepatocellular carcinoma accounted for 30% and 10% of other liver tumors, respectively.[2] Metastasis occurred in 35 of 57 dogs (60%) in this study, most frequently to regional lymph nodes or to lungs (14 dogs each). Metastasis also occurred to the peritoneal surfaces in approximately 20% of dogs.[2] Metastasis was more common for nodular and diffuse forms (nearly 100% for both) than for massive lesions (37%). Clear-cell carcinomas had a lower rate of metastasis than other histologic forms.[2] Large solitary hepatocellular carcinomas are less likely to

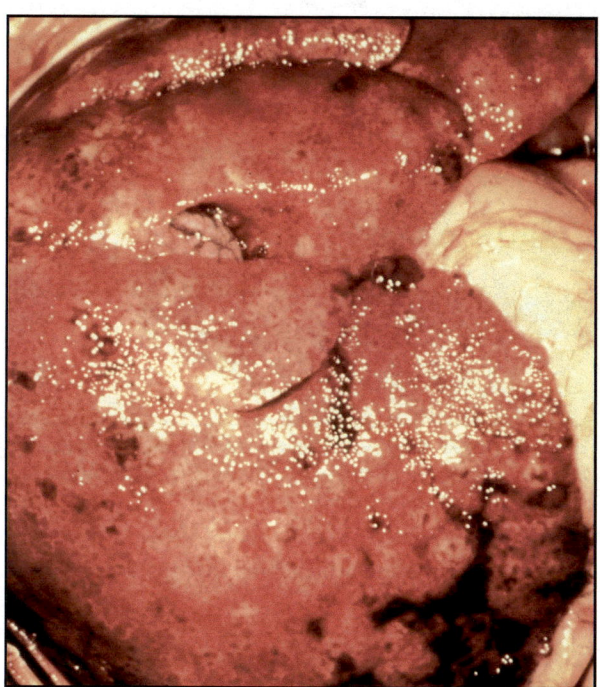

Figure 55-3. *Diffuse involvement of liver lobes, as in this biliary carcinoma, is not amenable to treatment. (Courtesy of John Berg, DVM, Tufts Cummings School of Veterinary Medicine)*

metastasize than are multiple lesions, but even some carcinomas that are multifocal throughout the liver are free of metastases.[3] In one study of 48 dogs with massive tumors, 42 dogs were treated surgically and lived a median of 48 months; only two dogs developed metastases (one lung and one liver).[22]

Biliary Carcinoma

As with hepatocellular carcinomas, bile duct carcinomas can be categorized as massive, nodular, or diffuse (Figure 55-3). Biliary carcinomas can also be categorized as arising from the intrahepatic bile ducts, extrahepatic bile ducts, or gallbladder. Those arising from intrahepatic bile ducts are the most common. Biliary tract carcinomas are a rare cause of biliary obstruction. In a study of causes of extrahepatic biliary obstruction, pancreatitis was nearly twice as common (42% of cases) as neoplasia (24% of cases), and only one neoplasia (a squamous cell carcinoma of the gallbladder) was attributable to the biliary system.[23] Distant metastases, most commonly involving the lungs, lymph nodes, and peritoneum, were seen in nearly 90% of dogs in one study.[24]

In one study, cystic bile duct adenomas were seen in association with bile duct cystadenocarcinomas, and transformation between the two tumor types was identified in 50%.[24] For this reason, biliary cystadenomas should not be dismissed as lesions that can be monitored instead of surgically removed, and dogs with a cystadenoma should be monitored by ultrasonography for development of other lesions.

Hepatic Carcinoids

These are epithelial tumors that appear to arise from the APUD (amine precursor uptake and decarboxylase) cells, also called *enterochromaffin* or *argentaffin cells*. These tumors appear only in the nodular or diffuse form, often causing adjoining hepatic necrosis and desmoplasia. The metastatic rate is more than 90%, and metastases occur most commonly to the peritoneal surface (carcinomatosis) and regional lymph nodes.[25]

Hepatic Mesenchymomas

Hepatic mesenchymomas (as described for splenic tumors below) are a rare primary tumor in dogs.[26,27]

TREATMENT

Dogs with primary liver tumors that are solitary mass lesions are probably the best candidates for treatment. Thoracic radiographs should be taken before surgery, and abdominal ultrasonography should be used to detect hepatic lymphadenopathy, other organ involvement, or lesions in multiple lobes. Dogs with hepatocellular carcinoma that involves a single liver lobe or, possibly, two lobes should be treated by lobectomy or partial hepatectomy. Dogs with lesions in multiple liver lobes have a poor prognosis.

Six dogs with massive liver hepatocellular carcinomas were treated supportively and survived a median of 9 months.[22] Dogs with these tumors have a good prognosis (Figures 55-4 and 55-5). In another study, hepatocellular carcinoma was resected in 18 dogs, and survival times were close to 1 year, with more than half the dogs still alive after surgery.[3] Only three dogs died because of hepatocellular carcinoma. In a larger study, 42 dogs were treated with aggressive resection; only four dogs had an incomplete excision.[22] Surgical complications occurred in approximately 30% of the dogs treated; two died from hemorrhage when the caudal vena cava was lacerated, and three others died in the first 5 days after surgery. Overall median survival for the 42 dogs

> **Dogs with large, solitary liver tumors usually have a good prognosis after surgery.**

was 48 months, with no recurrences. Whether the tumor was well differentiated or moderately differentiated did not influence outcome. Nearly 70% of these dogs had a left-sided tumor; dogs with right-sided tumors had a worse prognosis (40% died intraoperatively), and dogs with high serum ALT levels had a worse prognosis.[22]

Supportive care in the postoperative period and access to blood transfusion during surgery are very important. If the patient survives the perioperative period, prognosis is excellent.

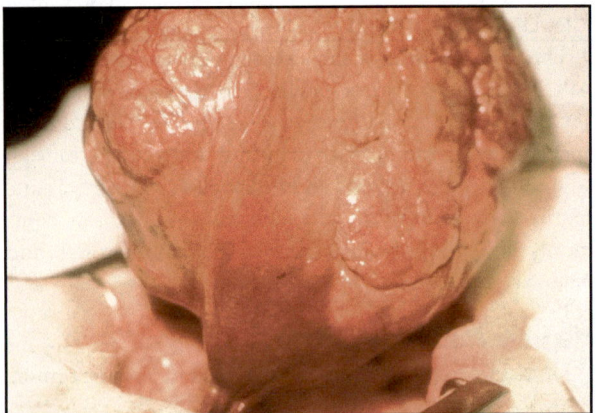

Figure 55-4. *This large solitary liver tumor is a hepatocellular carcinoma. If no other lobes are involved with the disease, prognosis after surgery should be good. (Courtesy of J. Berg)*

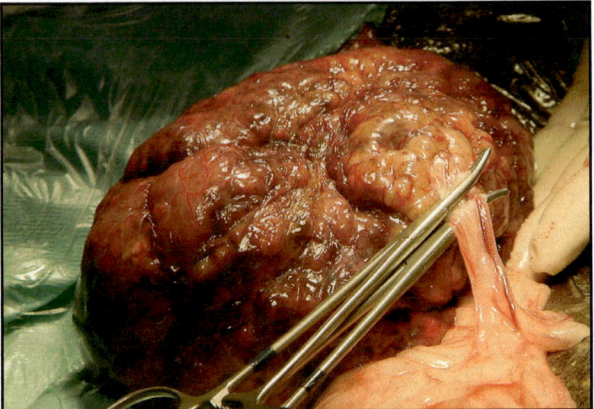

Figure 55-5. *This large solitary liver tumor had multiple omental adhesions but was resected completely. (Courtesy of Sarah Goldsmid, BVSc, Animal Referral Hospital)*

Arterial embolization has been attempted for palliation of unresectable hepatic tumors. Two dogs with unresectable nodular or massive hepatocellular carcinoma were treated by percutaneous arterial embolization for palliation.[28] Subjective palliation was seen in one dog for 4 months. A third dog that underwent chemoembolization with doxorubicin died from liver necrosis after 3 weeks. In another study, unresectable hepatic adenoma was treated by embolization in two dogs, but neither dog had a response.[29] This technique is very successful in human patients, but its use may be restricted to small tumors in dogs.

The success of surgical treatment for other types of hepatic neoplasms is less defined. In one report, one dog with cholangiocellular carcinoma and one dog with biliary adenocarcinoma had tumor recurrence 6 months after partial hepatectomy.[30] A well-differentiated adenocarcinoma of the gallbladder neck was resected with the gallbladder from a 9-year-old poodle. The dog had no evidence of recurrence 14 months later.[15] A carcinoid of the gallbladder was removed at cholecystectomy, and the dog survived an additional 8 months before developing signs of metastasis.[14] A hepatic mesenchymoma treated by excision had metastasized 4 months after surgery in another dog.[26]

Chemotherapy is generally not effective for treatment of human patients with primary liver tumors. This is likely the case for dogs, but there are no reports of adjunctive chemotherapy. Part of the difficulty with chemotherapy is the high prevalence of multidrug resistance protein in tumors derived from hepatic tissue, particularly tumors derived from the biliary tree.[31] This means that many of the commonly used drugs are ineffective. One dog with a hepatocellular carcinoma had a partial response to mitoxantrone chemotherapy.[32] Gemcitabine chemotherapy caused an anecdotal (not histologically confirmed) remission in a dog with hepatocellular carcinoma.[33] The ideal dose and schedule for gemcitabine in dogs is still under investigation.

Nonlymphoid, Nonangiogenic Splenic Tumors

INCIDENCE, SIGNALMENT, AND ETIOLOGY

In one study, hemangiosarcomas (57%) and lymphoma (9%) accounted for most malignant splenic tumors. In the same study, hemangiomas, lipomas, and leiomyomas accounted for 11% of tumors.[34] More details regarding lymphoma are found in Chapter 47; splenic hemangiosarcoma is discussed in Chapter 56.

After hemangiosarcoma and lymphoma, sarcomas are the predominant tumor in the canine spleen. Their mesenchymal differentiation varies. In three series of nonvascular, nonlymphomatous sarcomas of the spleen that involved 137 dogs,[34-36] the most common diagnosis was undifferentiated sarcoma (28%), followed by leiomyosarcoma (19%). The median age of all affected dogs was 11 years. There were no breed or gender predilections. Other tumors, in order of frequency, were fibrosarcoma, osteosarcoma, histiocytic sarcoma, mixed mesenchymal sarcoma, myxosarcoma, and liposarcoma. In 10 dogs, the tumor had mixed histogenesis with adipose, myxomatous, osseous, or chondroid components predominating; these tumors may be classified as mesenchymomas or mixed mesenchymal sarcomas. Mesenchymomas have the potential to differentiate and give rise to a variety of other sarcoma types, such as osteosarcoma.

In a separate report, histiocytic sarcomas were diagnosed in the spleen of six dogs.[37] Chapter 63 provides further details about these tumors.

CLINICAL PRESENTATION AND HISTORY

Clinical signs of splenic tumors are vague, consisting of lethargy, anorexia, weakness, weight loss, and abdominal

Table 55-1 Median Survival of Dogs Surviving Surgery for Splenic Sarcoma[39]

Pathologic Diagnosis	Dogs (n)	Mean Age (years)	Median Survival (months)
Mesenchymoma	7	13	12
Fibrosarcoma	11	12.5	2
Histiocytic sarcoma	4	11	2
Leiomyosarcoma	7	11	3
Myxosarcoma	6	12.5	2
Osteosarcoma	6	10	1
Undifferentiated sarcoma	12	13	4
All sarcomas (except mesenchymoma)	46	12	3

distention in some dogs. Tumors are often large (>15 cm); therefore, physical examination usually detects a splenic mass and may reveal abdominal pain.

In one study, the duration of clinical signs was longer than 1 week in 70% of dogs and longer than 1 month in 20% of dogs.[35]

STAGING AND DIAGNOSIS

Some splenic masses are benign or nonneoplastic. A dog with a splenic mass should be staged to exclude the common malignancies (hemangiosarcoma and lymphoma) and to identify macroscopic metastases. Procedures should include a complete blood count (CBC), biochemical profile, and urinalysis as well as more definitive procedures such as radiography and ultrasonography. Overall, ultrasonography is more effective than abdominal radiography for examining an enlarged spleen in a dog, identifying peritoneal effusion, and detecting sites of abdominal metastasis, including metastases in the liver and peritoneum. In one study,[38] a splenic mass was easily identified, although ultrasonographic findings ranged from anechoic to hyperechoic areas throughout the same lesion. These findings are not helpful in distinguishing splenic hemangiosarcoma from splenic hematoma, nodular hyperplasia, or another splenic sarcoma.[8] Care must be taken to distinguish hepatic regenerative nodules from metastases (which may be difficult). Needle biopsies, even when guided by ultrasonography, are often nondiagnostic, and definitive diagnosis usually occurs after exploratory laparotomy.

MRI allowed high soft tissue contrast and thus differentiation of benign from malignant splenic focal lesions in dogs in one study. The overall accuracy in differentiating malignant from benign lesions was 94%. The overall sensitivity and specificity were 100% and 90%, respectively.[13] This may be a helpful adjunct in patients considered to be at high risk for complications associated with splenectomy.

Thoracic radiographs should be taken before any definitive treatment is initiated. Thoracic radiographs were obtained in 53 of 57 dogs with different types of splenic tumors, and pulmonary metastases were present in four. Pleural effusion (two dogs) and enlarged sternal lymph nodes (one dog) were also detected. Metastatic disease at other sites was documented at surgery or necropsy in 40 dogs. Sites of metastasis varied; the liver was most commonly involved (35 dogs), but metastasis occurred in multiple visceral sites.[35]

Histopathologic estimates of mitotic index (number of mitoses per 10 high-power fields) appear to be prognostic and should be requested on splenectomy specimens.[39]

PROGNOSTIC FACTORS

One study found that dogs with mixed mesenchymal tumors (mesenchymomas) had better survival rates than dogs with any other splenic sarcomas, with median survival of 12 and 4 months, respectively (Table 55-1 and Figure 55-6).[39] In the same study, dogs with tumors that had a mitotic index of less than 9 had a median survival of 7 months compared with 1 to 2 months for all other groups (Figure 55-7).[39]

TREATMENT

Splenectomy is the treatment of choice for all splenic tumors except lymphoma. Dogs with benign tumors had a similar outcome to dogs with nonneoplastic splenic disease in one report; 20 of 29 dogs were alive 12 months after surgery.[34]

Splenectomy was performed in 27 of 57 dogs with splenic sarcomas.[35] Of these 27 dogs, 11 had obvious metastatic disease at the time of surgery. Five dogs died perioperatively, emphasizing the importance of postsurgical monitoring for signs of shock, blood loss, coagulopathies, and ventricular arrhythmias. Only five dogs lived more than 1 year. Overall median survival was 2.5 months. The median survival improved to 9 months for dogs without evidence of metastasis at the time of surgery. Survival times similar to those for dogs with hemangiosarcoma of the spleen (approximately 3 months) have been reported in smaller studies.[36]

The mitotic index of a splenic tumor is highly predictive of survival after splenectomy.

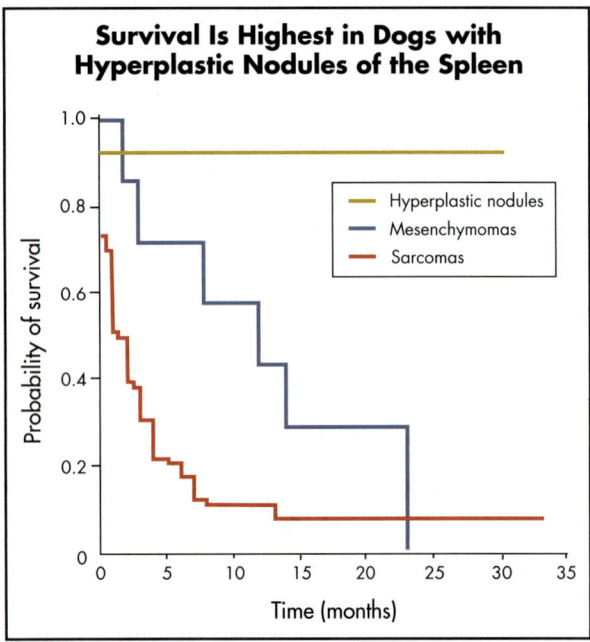

Figure 55-6. Survival curves for 136 dogs grouped by hyperplastic nodules, mesenchymomas, and other splenic sarcomas. (Adapted from Spangler WL, Culbertson MR, Kass PH: Primary mesenchymal (nonangiomatous/nonlymphomatous) neoplasms occurring in the canine spleen: Anatomic classification, immunohistochemistry, and mitotic activity correlated with patient survival. Vet Pathol 31:37–47, 1994; with permission)

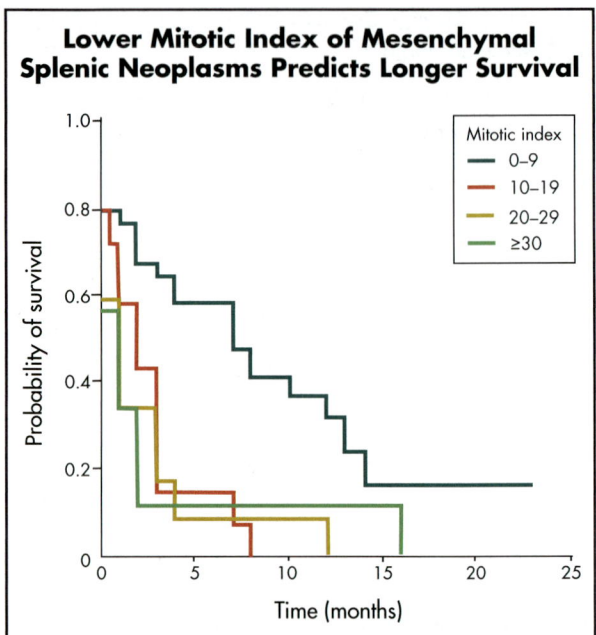

Figure 55-7. Survival curves for 68 dogs grouped by mitotic index: 0–9, 10–19, 20–29, or ≥30. (Adapted from Spangler WL, Culbertson MR, Kass PH: Primary mesenchymal (nonangiomatous/nonlymphomatous) neoplasms occurring in the canine spleen: Anatomic classification, immunohistochemistry, and mitotic activity correlated with patient survival. Vet Pathol 31:37–47, 1994; with permission)

In a group of 16 dogs with splenic leiomyosarcoma, five dogs had evidence of multiple-organ involvement at laparotomy and were euthanatized.[40] Splenectomy was performed in 11 dogs that survived for a median of 8 months after surgery (range: 1–21 months). Nine of these dogs developed liver metastases.

Chemotherapy should be considered investigational for these tumors but probably should follow guidelines for soft tissue sarcomas of other sites. Doxorubicin, platinum drugs, and possibly ifosfamide are the chemotherapy agents most likely to improve survival in the adjuvant setting.

Tumors of the Exocrine Pancreas

Tumors of the exocrine pancreas are rare in dogs. Insulinoma, a rare tumor of the islet cells of the pancreas, is discussed in Chapter 57.

INCIDENCE, SIGNALMENT, AND ETIOLOGY

Adenomas of the exocrine pancreas are rare, although hyperplastic nodules appear to be a normal aging change.[41,42] Exocrine pancreatic carcinomas show no obvious gender predilection. They are most common in old dogs, with a mean age of about 9 years.[43–45] In one report, cocker spaniels accounted for three of 14 dogs.[43] Only spaniel breeds were affected in another study.[44]

CLINICAL PRESENTATION AND HISTORY

Clinical signs are often nonspecific and include weight loss, depression, and anorexia. Although pancreatic tumors are commonly believed to cause emesis, vomiting is uncommon[44] and is a late, often terminal, occurrence.[43,45,46] A mass in the anterior abdomen may be palpable, and ascites may occur.[43] The owner may notice a swollen abdomen if ascites is present.[46] If the tumor is in the midportion of the pancreas, the clinical picture may be complicated by bile duct obstruction, jaundice, and other clinical signs.[42] In three dogs, a painful and debilitating syndrome of paraneoplastic steatitis manifesting as panniculitis caused subcutaneous swellings and shifting lameness over a period of months.[44] In these dogs, pancreatic carcinoma was an incidental necropsy finding, and no clinical signs directly attributable to the tumor were noted before death.

STAGING AND DIAGNOSIS

After a general health screen with blood work, urinalysis, and thoracic radiography, ultrasonography of the abdomen should be considered. In many animals, pancreatic carcinomas are thought to metastasize before clinical signs are apparent.[41] Pancreatic tumors are a solitary mass in 50% of affected dogs[43]; the other 50% may have numerous nodules throughout the pancreas. In one study of 13 dogs, metastases were present in the liver in 12 dogs, in the omentum and mesentery in six dogs, and in regional lymph nodes in four dogs.[43] Other visceral sites are less frequently affected.[43-46] Serum lipase levels may be extremely elevated in dogs with pancreatic tumors, and a level 25 times greater than normal is probably diagnostic of exocrine pancreatic carcinoma,[47] particularly if

> **KEY POINT**
>
> *Contrary to common belief, vomiting is rarely reported in dogs with exocrine pancreatic tumors.*

the serum amylase level is minimally increased.[48] A painful and debilitating syndrome of paraneoplastic steatitis that manifested itself in the subcutaneous fat (panniculitis) or omental fat was associated with very high levels of serum lipase in three spaniels. None of these dogs had metastatic disease, and one had no signs referable to pancreatitis despite marked elevations in serum lipase and amylase.[44]

Ultrasonography can be useful in detecting a pancreatic mass, although the pancreas is difficult to image because of shadowing from gas-filled gastrointestinal structures. Liver metastases may also be detected, although definitive diagnosis requires biopsy. In one study, cytology of samples obtained by ultrasound or fluoroscopic-guided fine-needle aspiration was helpful in establishing a diagnosis of pancreatic carcinoma. Histopathology of ultrasound or fluoroscopic-guided biopsies provided a definitive diagnosis in most cases and may be an alternative to exploratory laparotomy.[49]

TREATMENT

Treatment has not been described for this tumor, and surgical resection usually requires a Billroth II procedure. Chemotherapy is rarely helpful in human patients and has not been described in dogs. Gemcitabine is the most useful chemotherapy agent for this disease in human patients; however, its efficacy in dogs is unknown. The ideal dose and schedule for gemcitabine in dogs are still under investigation.[33]

Supportive care is very important for dogs with pancreatic carcinoma and may be the major influence a clinician can have on quality of life for the patient. Antiemetics and pain relief may make the patient more comfortable, and parenteral nutrition may avoid stimulating the gastrointestinal tract and exacerbating signs. All such procedures may not be effective, however, and many patients are euthanatized soon after diagnosis.

REFERENCES

1. Patnaik AK, Hurvitz AI, Lieberman PH: Canine hepatic neoplasms: A clinicopathologic study. *Vet Pathol* 17:553–564, 1980.
2. Patnaik AK, Hurvitz AI, Lieberman PH, Johnson GF: Canine hepatocellular carcinoma. *Vet Pathol* 18:427–438, 1981.
3. Kosovsky JE, Manfra-Marretta S, Matthiesen DT, Patnaik AK: Results of partial hepatectomy in 18 dogs with hepatocellular carcinoma. *JAAHA* 25:203–206, 1989.
4. Evans SM: The radiographic appearance of primary liver neoplasia in dogs. *Vet Radiol Ultrasound* 28:192–196, 1987.
5. Hayes HM Jr, Morin MM, Rubenstein DA: Canine biliary carcinoma: Epidemiological comparisons with man. *J Comp Pathol* 93:99–107, 1983.
6. Leifer CE, Peterson ME, Matus RE, Patnaik AK: Hypoglycemia associated with nonislet cell tumor in 13 dogs. *JAVMA* 186:53–55, 1985.
7. Voros K, Vrabely T, Papp L, et al: Correlation of ultrasonographic and pathomorphological findings in canine hepatic diseases. *J Small Anim Pract* 32:627–634, 1991.
8. Feeney DA, Johnston GR, Hardy RM: Two-dimensional, gray-scale ultrasonography for assessment of hepatic and splenic neoplasia in the dog and cat. *JAVMA* 184:68–81, 1984.
9. Biller DS, Kantrowitz B, Miyabayashi T: Ultrasonography of diffuse liver disease. A review. *J Vet Intern Med* 6:71–76, 1992.
10. Roth L: Comparison of liver cytology and biopsy diagnoses in dogs and cats: 56 cases. *Vet Clin Pathol* 30:35–38, 2001.
11. Cole TL, Center SA, Flood SN, et al: Diagnostic comparison of needle and wedge biopsy specimens of the liver in dogs and cats. *JAVMA* 220:1483–1490, 2002.
12. Center SA, Baldwin BH, Erb HN, Tennant BC: Bile acid concentrations in the diagnosis of hepatobiliary disease in the dog. *JAVMA* 187:935–940, 1985.
13. Clifford CA, Pretorius ES, Weisse C, et al: Magnetic resonance imaging of focal splenic and hepatic lesions in the dog. *J Vet Intern Med* 18:330–338, 2004.
14. Morrell CN, Volk MV, Mankowski JL: A carcinoid tumor in the gallbladder of a dog. *Vet Pathol* 39:756–758, 2002.
15. Brömel C, Smeak DD, Léveillé R: Porcelain gallbladder associated with primary biliary adenocarcinoma in a dog. *JAVMA* 213:1137–1139, 1998.
16. Lowseth LA, Gillett NA, Chang IY, et al: Detection of serum alpha-fetoprotein in dogs with hepatic tumors. *JAVMA* 199:735–741, 1991.
17. Yamada T, Fujita M, Kitao S, et al: Serum alpha-fetoprotein values in dogs with various hepatic diseases. *J Vet Med Sci* 61:657–659, 1999.
18. Martin de las Mulas J, Gomez-Villamandos JC, Perez J, et al: Immunohistochemical evaluation of canine primary liver carcinomas: Distribution of alpha-fetoprotein, carcinoembryonic antigen, keratins and vimentin. *Res Vet Sci* 59:124–127, 1995.
19. Duran ME, Ezquerra J, Roncero V, et al: Acute necrotizing myelopathy associated with a hepatocarcinoma. *Progress Vet Neurol* 3:35–38, 1998.
20. Krotje LJ, Fix AS, Potthoff AD: Acquired myasthenia gravis and cholangiocellular carcinoma in a dog. *JAVMA* 197:488–490, 1990.
21. Ramos-Vara JA, Miller MA, Johnson GC: Immunohistochemical characterization of canine hyperplastic hepatic lesions and hepatocellular and biliary neoplasms with monoclonal antibody hepatocyte paraffin 1 and a monoclonal antibody to cytokeratin 7. *Vet Pathol* 38:636–643, 2001.
22. Liptak JM, Dernell WS, Monnet E, et al: Massive hepatocellular carcinoma in dogs: 48 cases (1992–2002). *JAVMA* 225:1225–1230, 2004.
23. Fahie MA, Martin RA: Extrahepatic biliary tract obstruction: A retrospective study of 45 cases (1983–1993). *JAAHA* 31:478–482, 1995.
24. Patnaik AK, Hurvitz AI, Lieberman PH, Johnson GF: Canine bile duct carcinoma. *Vet Pathol* 18:439–444, 1981.
25. Patnaik AK, Lieberman PH, Hurvitz AI, Johnson GF: Canine hepatic carcinoids. *Vet Pathol* 18:445–453, 1981.
26. McDonald RK, Helman RG: Hepatic malignant mesenchymoma in a dog. *JAVMA* 188:1052–1053, 1986.
27. Haines DM, Doige CE, Matte G, Wilkinson AA: Multifocal telangiectatic osteosarcoma and malignant mixed hepatic tumor in a dog. *JAAHA* 23:509–513, 1987.
28. Weisse C, Clifford CA, Holt D, Solomon JA: Percutaneous arterial embolization and chemoembolization for treatment of benign and malignant tumors in three dogs and a goat. *JAVMA* 221:1430–1436, 1419, 2002.
29. Cave TA, Johnson V, Beths T, et al: Treatment of unresectable hepatocellular adenoma in dogs with transarterial iodized oil and chemotherapy with and without an embolic agent: A report of two cases. *Vet Comp Oncol* 1:191–199, 2003.
30. Fry PD, Rest JR: Partial hepatectomy in two dogs. *J Small Anim Pract* 34:192–195, 1993.
31. Ginn PE: Immunohistochemical detection of P-glycoprotein in formalin-fixed and paraffin-embedded normal and neoplastic canine tissues. *Vet Pathol* 33:533–541, 1996.
32. Ogilvie GK, Obradovich JE, Elmslie RE, et al: Efficacy of mitoxantrone against various neoplasms in dogs. *JAVMA* 198:1618–1621, 1991.
33. Moore AS, Kitchell BE: New chemotherapy agents in veterinary medicine. *Vet Clin North Am Small Anim Pract* 33:629–649, viii, 2003.
34. Spangler WL, Kass PH: Pathologic factors affecting postsplenectomy survival in dogs. *J Vet Intern Med* 11:166–171, 1997.
35. Weinstein MJ, Carpenter JL, Schunk CJ: Nonangiogenic and nonlymphomatous

sarcomas of the canine spleen: 57 cases (1975–1987). *JAVMA* 195:784–788, 1989.
36. Day MJ, Lucke VM, Pearson H: A review of pathological diagnoses made from 87 canine splenic biopsies. *J Small Anim Pract* 36:426–433, 1995.
37. Hendrick MJ, Brooks JJ, Bruce EH: Six cases of malignant fibrous histiocytoma of the canine spleen. *Vet Pathol* 29:351–354, 1992.
38. Wrigley RH, Park RD, Knode LJ, Lebel JL: Ultrasonographic features of splenic hemangiosarcoma in dogs: 18 cases (1980–1986). *JAVMA* 192:1113–1117, 1988.
39. Spangler WL, Culbertson MR, Kass PH: Primary mesenchymal (nonangiomatous/nonlymphomatous) neoplasms occurring in the canine spleen: Anatomic classification, immunohistochemistry, and mitotic activity correlated with patient survival. *Vet Pathol* 31:37–47, 1994.
40. Kapatkin AS, Mullen Hs, Matthiesen DT, Patnaik AK: Leiomyosarcoma in dogs: 44 cases (1983–1988). *JAVMA* 201:1077–1079, 1992.
41. Kircher CH, Nielsen SW: Tumours of the pancreas. *Bull World Health Organ* 53:195–202, 1976.
42. Rowlatt U: Spontaneous epithelial tumours of the pancreas of mammals. *Br J Cancer* 21:82–107, 1967.
43. Anderson NV, Johnson KH: Pancreatic carcinoma in the dog. *JAVMA* 150:286–295, 1967.
44. Brown PJ, Mason KV, Merrett DJ, et al: Multifocal necrotising steatitis associated with pancreatic carcinoma in three dogs. *J Small Anim Pract* 35:129–132, 1994.
45. Xu FN: Ultrastructural examination as an aid to the diagnosis of canine pancreatic neoplasms. *Aust Vet J* 62:197–198, 1985.
46. Ditchfield J, Archibald J: Carcinoma of the pancreas in small animals. A report of two cases. *Small Anim Clin* 1:173–176, 1961.
47. Fineman L, DeNicola D, Bruyette D, et al: Serum lipase concentrations in dogs with pancreatic carcinoma. *Proc 14th Annu Conf Vet Cancer Soc*:16–17, 1994.
48. Quigley KA, Jackson ML, Haines DM: Hyperlipasemia in 6 dogs with pancreatic or hepatic neoplasia: Evidence for tumor lipase production. *Vet Clin Pathol* 30:114–120, 2001.
49. Bennett PF, Hahn KA, Toal RL, Legendre AM: Ultrasonographic and cytopathological diagnosis of exocrine pancreatic carcinoma in the dog and cat. *JAAHA* 37:466–473, 2001.

TUMORS OF BLOOD AND LYMPH VESSELS

Antony S. Moore and Gregory K. Ogilvie

CLINICAL BRIEFING

Minimum database (MDB; includes a complete blood count, biochemical profile, urinalysis, and thoracic radiography [three views]).

Splenic Hemangiosarcoma

Clinical factors
- Palpable abdominal mass, hemoperitoneum, anemia, shock, and possibly collapse.
- Average age of affected dogs: 10 years.
- German shepherds predisposed.
- Metastases are often confined to abdominal cavity if no concurrent right atrial lesion exists.

Staging and diagnosis
- MDB.
- Abdominal ultrasonography.
- Coagulation profile.
- Cardiac ultrasonography (to rule out concurrent atrial lesion).

Prognostic factors
- Clinical stage; stage I better than stages II and III.
- Complete surgical excision improves survival after chemotherapy.
- Older dogs do better than younger dogs.
- Low-grade tumors better than intermediate grade.
- High-grade (highly anaplastic) tumors have poorest prognosis.

Treatment

Initial
- Surgery.
- Palliative for stage I or II, but survival is short.

Adjunctive
- Chemotherapy.
- Doxorubicin-based protocols prolong survival if disease is micrometastatic (low-stage tumors or achieved by surgery).
- Immunotherapy with biologic response modifier L-MTP-PE prolongs survival in dogs with micrometastatic disease.

Supportive
- Blood products as needed.
- Pain medications after surgery.
- Appetite stimulants and nutritional support as required.

Cardiac Hemangiosarcoma

Clinical factors
- Collapse and cardiac tamponade; hindlimb paresis.
- Right atrium is the most common location.
- Average age: 10 years.
- German shepherds predisposed.
- Metastasis may be widespread, commonly to lungs.

Staging and diagnosis	• MDB. • Cardiac ultrasonography. • Coagulation profile. • Abdominal ultrasonography (to rule out concurrent splenic lesion).
Prognostic factors	• Complete removal is better than incomplete removal.
Treatment	
Initial	• Surgery. • Palliative in dogs with resectable lesions.
Adjunctive	• Chemotherapy (doxorubicin based) as an adjunct improves survival over surgery alone
Supportive	• Blood products as needed. • Pain medications after surgery. • Appetite stimulants and nutritional support as required.

Cutaneous Hemangiosarcoma

Clinical factors	• Raised, red lesion; often in skin that is lightly pigmented. • Average age: 10 years. • Whippets and other dogs with lightly pigmented, lightly haired skin are predisposed.
Staging and diagnosis	• MDB. • Check regional lymph nodes. • Abdominal and cardiac ultrasonography (to rule out concurrent atrial or splenic lesion). • Coagulation profile. • Metastasis is uncommon.
Prognostic factors	• Histopathologic evidence of solar elastosis adjacent to tumor is good prognostic sign. • Tumors within epidermis and dermis (stage I) have a good prognosis. • Histologic grade is prognostic.
Treatment	
Initial	• Surgery may be curative in dogs with a localized lesion. • Histopathologic evidence of solar elastosis adjacent to tumor is good prognostic sign. • Tumors within epidermis and dermis (stage I) have a good prognosis. • Histologic grade is prognostic.
Adjunctive	• Chemotherapy. • Role of adjuvant therapy for subcutaneous hemangiosarcoma probably as for other anatomic sites (i.e., doxorubicin-based protocols).
Supportive	• Pain medications after surgery. • Appetite stimulants and nutritional support as required.

Lymphangioma and Lymphangiosarcoma

Clinical factors	• Most often in skin. • May be a sequela to chronic lymphatic obstruction. • Average age: 7 years; may occur in very young animals. • Beagles may be predisposed.

Staging and diagnosis	• MDB. • Check regional lymph nodes. • Abdominal ultrasonography. • Metastasis is uncommon; most reported tumors are benign.
Prognostic factors	• None reported.
Treatment	
Initial	• Surgery may be curative in dogs with a localized lesion.
Adjunctive	• Chemotherapy. • Role of adjuvant therapy for lymphangiosarcoma probably as for other hemangiosarcoma (i.e., doxorubicin-based protocols).
Supportive	• Radiation therapy may provide local control. • Pain medications after surgery. • Appetite stimulants and nutritional support as required.
Other Tumors Reviewed	
	• Hemangiosarcomas of the urogenital tract, bone, liver, muscle, central nervous system, and eye; retroperitoneal sarcomas.

Splenic Hemangiosarcoma
INCIDENCE, SIGNALMENT, AND ETIOLOGY

The spleen is the most common primary site of hemangiosarcoma in dogs. The tumor is characterized by rapid growth and widespread metastasis, presumably because of its tissue of origin, the vascular endothelium, and its resultant ready access to systemic circulation.

Older dogs are affected by this disease (average age: 9-11 years), and German shepherds are predisposed.[1-3] There is no clear gender predilection; male dogs are overrepresented in some studies[1,4] and females in others.[3,5] Splenic hemangiosarcoma can occur in conjunction with hemangiosarcoma of the right atrium, which may represent synchronous primary tumors rather than metastatic disease.[5] No etiologic agent has been identified in dogs; in humans, exposure to vinyl chloride appears to be a high risk factor.[6]

CLINICAL PRESENTATION AND HISTORY

Between one-third[3,5] and two-thirds[7] of all splenic masses are malignant tumors, and most malignant tumors of the spleen are hemangiosarcomas. It is critical to differentiate splenic hemangiosarcoma from other possible diagnoses, which include splenic hematoma, hyperplastic nodules, and other types of sarcoma. The important differential diagnosis for a dog presenting with a palpable splenic mass is the combination of splenic hematoma and hyperplastic nodules, which is as common as hemangiosarcoma on surgical biopsy and necropsy surveys.[3,5,8] It is impossible to differentiate between splenic hemangiosarcoma and hematoma on the basis of gross appearance using radiography or ultrasonography or at surgery. However, the distinction between these conditions is critical because their average survival times differ greatly (19 days for hemangiosarcoma versus 340 days for hematoma) (Figure 56-1).[3]

Certain clinical signs may help distinguish hematoma from hemangiosarcoma, although a definitive histopathologic diagnosis is necessary. Collapse (39% versus 17%), hemoperitoneum (76% versus 30%), and anorexia (68% versus 45%) are more common in dogs with splenic hemangiosarcoma than in dogs with splenic hematoma.[3] However, lethargy, enlarged abdomen, sensitive abdomen, vomiting, and diarrhea were equally common in dogs with hematoma and those with hemangiosarcoma of the spleen in one study.[3] Both diseases occur in a similar age group of dogs, although hematomas may be more common in small-breed dogs.[9]

Other signs noted on clinical examination of a dog with hemangiosarcoma are pale mucous membranes and general weakness owing to anemia, which results from chronic bleeding into either the tumor or abdomen. Hematologic data from dogs with splenic hemangiosarcoma may be useful in diagnosis. Abnormal red blood cell (RBC) morphologies, such as acanthocytes, schistocytes, and nucleated RBCs, are common in splenic hemangiosarcoma. Schistocytes are associated with RBC fragmentation, microangiopathy, and disseminated intravascular coagulopathy (DIC) in dogs; they may reflect an inability of the diseased spleen to remove them

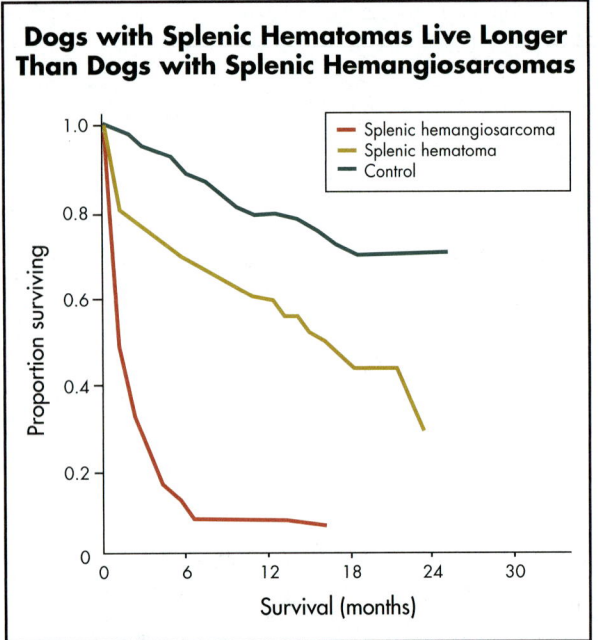

Figure 56-1. Survival time of 59 dogs with splenic hemangiosarcoma, 125 dogs with splenic hematoma, and 84 matched control dogs. (Adapted from Prymak C, McKee LJ, Goldschmidt MH, Glickman LT: Epidemiologic, clinical, pathologic, and prognostic characteristics of splenic hemangiosarcoma and splenic hematoma in dogs: 217 cases (1985). JAVMA 193:706–712, 1988; with permission)

Table 56-1 Staging of Canine Hemangiosarcoma

Stage	Clinical Description
T	T0: No tumor evident
	T1: Diameter <5 cm, confined to affected organ, does not invade beyond dermis (cutaneous lesions)
	T2: Diameter >5 cm, ruptured organ, or subcutaneous invasion
	T3: Invasive tumor
N	N0: No regional nodes involved
	N1: Regional nodes involved
	N2: Distant nodes involved
M	M0: No distant metastasis
	M1: Distant metastasis
I	T0 or T1, N0, M0
II	T1 or T2, N0 or N1, M0
III	T2 or T3, any N, M1

normally from circulation. DIC is more commonly identified in dogs with hemangiosarcoma than in most other cancers.[10]

STAGING AND DIAGNOSIS

Staging for suspected hemangiosarcoma should include a complete blood count (with careful attention to RBC morphology), biochemical profile, and urinalysis, as well as more definitive procedures, such as radiography and ultrasonogra-

> **KEY POINT**
>
> *Approximately one-third to two-thirds of splenic masses are malignant; however, collapse and hemoperitoneum seem to be more common in dogs with splenic hemangiosarcoma.*

phy. The staging system for canine hemangiosarcoma is shown in Table 56-1. Ultrasonography may be effective for examining an enlarged spleen, identifying peritoneal effusion, and detecting sites of abdominal metastasis. In one study,[11] a splenic mass was easily identified, although ultrasonographic findings ranged from anechoic to hyperechoic areas throughout the same lesion (Figure 56-2). Ultrasonography also aided in the detection of metastases in the liver and peritoneum.[11] Care must be taken to distinguish hepatic regenerative nodules from metastases (which may be difficult), and ultrasonography is not helpful in distinguishing splenic hemangiosarcoma from splenic hematoma or nodular hyperplasia. Overall, ultrasonography is more useful than abdominal radiography in detecting a primary lesion and its metastases (Figure 56-3). Abdominal fluid from bleeding may complicate a radiographic diagnosis.

Up to 25% of dogs with splenic hemangiosarcoma may also have a right atrial hemangiosarcoma[12]; therefore, it is important to examine the right atrial appendage by ultrasonography for the presence of a mass before making a firm recommendation for surgery or adjunctive therapy. Pulmonary metastases are much more common in dogs with both sites involved than in dogs in which the spleen is the only site of hemangiosarcoma at presentation. Splenic hemangiosarcoma and associated metastases are almost always confined to the peritoneal cavity.[12] This has important implications for monitoring for splenic hemangiosarcoma after treatment because thoracic radiographs would be expected to have a lower yield than abdominal ultrasonography, which may be the imaging modality of choice. In 19 dogs with splenic hemangiosarcoma without right atrial involvement, 15 (79%) had metastases. Of those 15 dogs, 13 had metastases to the liver, omentum (n = 8), and mesentery (n = 7). Metastases also occurred to the kidney, urinary bladder, small intestine, diaphragm, adrenal gland, and mesenteric lymph nodes.[12] Similar patterns have been reported in other studies.[13] In two studies of dogs with splenic hemangiosarcoma without right atrial involvement, fewer than 25% of dogs developed metastases outside the abdominal cavity.[12,14]

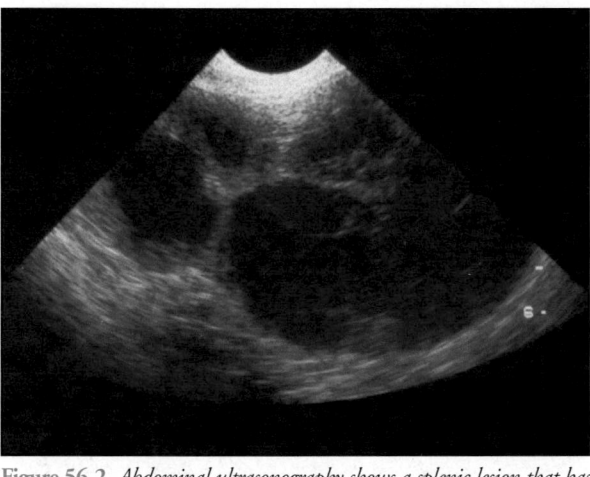

Figure 56-2. *Abdominal ultrasonography shows a splenic lesion that has multiple cavernous hypoechoic areas, consistent with a hemangiosarcoma or hematoma. Definitive diagnosis requires histopathology. (Courtesy of John Berg, DVM, Tufts Cummings School of Veterinary Medicine)*

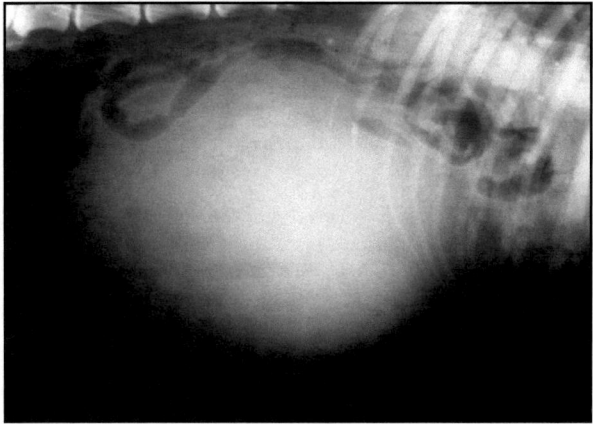

Figure 56-3. *Abdominal radiography confirms the presence of a mass in a dog with abdominal swelling. The mass is suspected of being splenic on the basis of dorsal, cranial, and caudal displacement of intestinal loops, but confirmation requires ultrasonography or exploratory laparotomy. (Courtesy of J. Berg)*

Definitive diagnosis of hemangiosarcoma requires histopathologic examination of surgically obtained biopsy specimens. The tumor contains mixed areas consisting of hematomas, fibrotic areas, and areas of extramedullary hematopoiesis, which means aspiration or needle biopsy rarely provides a definitive diagnosis.[15] In addition, the risk of bleeding is high in these patients after such procedures are performed.

> **KEY POINT**
>
> *Metastases associated with splenic hemangiosarcoma are mostly confined to the peritoneal cavity.*

Specific immunohistochemical staining for CD31 (platelet endothelial cell adhesion molecule) was positive in hemangiosarcomas and hemangiomas but not in any other sarcomas in one study.[16] This stain may be useful in determining the histogenesis of poorly differentiated hemangiosarcomas. Another endothelial cell-specific marker is factor VIII–related antigen.[17]

Vascular endothelial growth factor (VEGF) is a marker of angiogenesis that was proposed in one study to be a marker of hemangiosarcomas in dogs. In that study, plasma levels of VEGF were detectable in 13 of 17 dogs with hemangiosarcomas but in only one of 17 normal dogs.[18] VEGF level was not correlated with tumor burden nor with the presence of metastases, so it probably will not be useful as a clinical marker of disease progression in treated dogs.

PROGNOSTIC FACTORS

Clinical staging appears to be of prognostic benefit in some studies, particularly those in which adjuvant therapy is given after surgery. Stage I hemangiosarcomas are tumors confined to the spleen with no evidence of metastasis. Dogs with stage II disease may have a ruptured spleen with or without regional lymph node involvement. Stage III tumors are large, invasive tumors with distant metastases.[19] Dogs with stage I tumors were less likely to develop abdominal metastases after splenectomy in one study, and their median survival was 12 months compared with 5 months for dogs with stage II hemangiosarcoma.[14] Staging appeared prognostic in two other studies that involved dogs with hemangiosarcomas from all sites.[4,20] One study found that if a dog had a solitary hemangiosarcoma nodule in the spleen, the chance of long survival was greater; all 66 dogs with multiple lesions were dead 1 year after surgery compared with 41 of 49 dogs with a solitary hemangiosarcoma nodule.[21]

Another study proposed a histologic grading system for dogs with hemangiosarcomas.[22] The differentiation scheme is outlined in Table 56-2. The three histologic grades take into account cellular pleomorphism, percentage of necrosis, and the mitotic index (number per 10 high-power fields). Tumor grade (specifically, nuclear pleomorphism and mitotic index) appeared to predict the survival time of dogs treated with surgery and doxorubicin. To predict outcome, this grading scheme should be considered along with the stage of the disease, completeness of the excision, and age of the dog (older dogs did better) and whether doxorubicin-based chemotherapy is administered.[22]

TREATMENT
Surgery

Surgery is the treatment of choice for splenic hemangiosarcoma. Surgery relieves abdominal distention caused by a large tumor and provides palliation by stopping bleeding from the

Table 56-2 **Proposed Histologic Grading System for Canine Hemangiosarcomas**

Grade	Histologic Description
1	Well differentiated; numerous irregular vascular channels
2	Moderately differentiated with >50% of the tumor as well-defined vascular channels
3	Poorly differentiated; solid sheets with few vascular channels

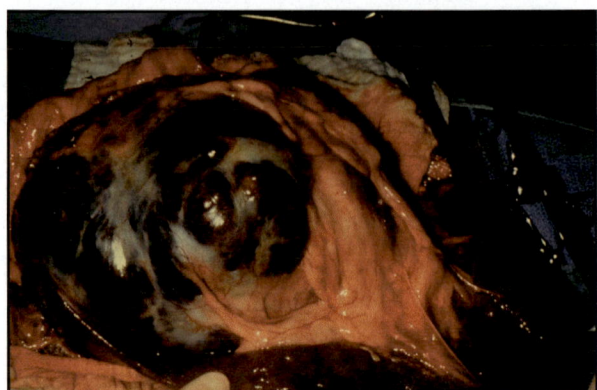

Figure 56-4. *The same dog shown in Figure 56-3. A vascular splenic mass has not ruptured, and micrometastases are not visible at surgery. The liver, however, should be examined and biopsied for evidence of gross or microscopic metastatic disease. (Courtesy of J. Berg)*

primary tumor (Figure 56-4). Surgery also prolongs survival because dogs would not survive continued bleeding. However, surgery does not prevent rapid growth of metastases. Survival data are distorted by the high rate of intraoperative euthanasia and perioperative mortality. In one study, one-third of dogs died in the first 2 weeks after surgery, most in the first 48 hours after surgery.[21] A group of 32 dogs with stage I or II splenic hemangiosarcoma that survived at least 2 weeks after surgery and received no further treatment had a median survival of 2.7 months (range: 0.5–15.5 months). Six months after surgery, 13% of dogs were alive, and only two dogs were alive 1 year after surgery. Metastatic disease was the overwhelming cause of death in all dogs. Factors such as whether the spleen had ruptured (stage I versus stage II), the presence of either anemia or postoperative arrhythmias, and whether the dog received a blood transfusion did not affect survival.[23]

Dogs undergoing splenectomy should be monitored electrocardiographically before, during, and after surgery. In a series of 59 dogs undergoing splenectomy for hemangiosarcoma, 14 developed ventricular arrhythmia after surgery.[24] None of these dogs had preexisting cardiac disease. Anemia was believed to cause these arrhythmias by decreasing myocardial oxygenation; only one dog developed arrhythmias that were not attributed to anemia. In the same series, metastatic myocardial disease was seen in 12 of 18 dogs, although only three of these dogs developed ventricular arrhythmias.[24] Treatment with drugs such as lidocaine and procainamide, along with continuous monitoring, should resolve arrhythmias within 1 to 5 days.

Chemotherapy

The effect of chemotherapy on malignancies such as osteosarcoma raised hopes that drug therapy may also improve the survival of dogs with hemangiosarcoma. Splenic hemangiosarcoma would appear to be very likely to respond positively to adjunctive therapy because the disease burden is often low after splenectomy. Thus far, however, the true impact of chemotherapy has been difficult to assess. Studies are often very small and include dogs with hemangiosarcomas from a variety of sites.

In one study, the tumor and accessible metastases were surgically resected from 46 dogs with metastatic (stage III) noncutaneous hemangiosarcoma (splenic = 14, cardiac = 5, subcutaneous = 9, other sites = 18) that were then treated with doxorubicin (30 mg/m^2 IV q3wk for up to five treatments).[22] Whereas the median survival time of dogs in which all visible disease was resected was 5.6 months, dogs that did not have complete resection lived an average of 2 months. This same study showed that the histologic grade of the tumor was highly prognostic: dogs with grade 1 tumors survived much longer than dogs with intermediate-grade (grade 2) tumors, which, in turn, survived longer than dogs with grade 3 tumors. Similarly, these investigators showed that older dogs survived longer than young dogs. Administration of doxorubicin at the same dosage every 2 weeks, thereby increasing dose intensity, may have improved slightly on these survival figures. In another study, whereas five dogs with stage I disease lived a median of 8.4 months (four of the five had subcutaneous hemangiosarcoma, which may have improved survival), six dogs with stage III disease lived a median of 3.5 months.[20] In a third study, liposome-encapsulated doxorubicin induced responses in hemangiosarcoma, but efficacy was not shown to be greater than that of nonencapsulated doxorubicin.[25] Combining doxorubicin with other chemotherapeutic drugs does not seem to appreciably improve survival times for dogs with splenic hemangiosarcoma over treatment with doxorubicin alone. In a series that included eight dogs with splenic hemangiosarcoma that received vincristine, doxorubicin, and cyclophosphamide followed by chlorambucil and methotrexate, overall median survival was 164 days (range: 10–>1,084 days).[19] In another group of dogs that received doxorubicin and cyclophosphamide, the median survival time was 179 days.[8] Many of these dogs had metastatic disease.[8,19] Toxicities in both studies included neutropenia and gastrointestinal signs that were severe enough to necessitate hospitalization in seven of 15 and three of 16 dogs, respectively. One dog in each study (two of 31 dogs) died from sepsis as a result of chemotherapy-induced neutropenia, and two dogs died from cardiomyopathy, presumably doxorubicin induced.

The alkylating agent ifosfamide is an active agent in human patients with sarcomas. In a series of six dogs with stage I or II splenic hemangiosarcoma treated after splenectomy with ifosfamide, median survival was 147 days[26] but was not significantly different from that of dogs treated with surgery alone (83 days[23]). The combination of doxorubicin alternating with ifosfamide was used to treat 13 dogs with stage II hemangiosarcoma after splenectomy.[27] These dogs had a median survival time of 123 days; 7.7% of dogs were alive 6 months after surgery. This was not significantly longer than dogs treated by surgery alone.[23]

Preliminary results of a protocol using vincristine, doxorubicin, and dacarbazine to treat 11 dogs with hemangiosarcoma of various sites found that four dogs were alive 2 weeks to 2 years after therapy.[28]

The effect of chemotherapy on this disease is still investigational, and assessment of response will only be meaningful if known prognostic factors such as clinical stage, histologic grade, age of dog, and completeness of surgical excision of tumor are included in the analysis. Future investigations of newer chemotherapeutic agents may provide more substantial improvements in survival. The confinement of metastatic disease to the abdominal cavity in most of these dogs has led some investigators to suggest that intracavitary chemotherapy may be a logical treatment for splenic hemangiosarcoma.[12] Intracavitary chemotherapy provides high levels of chemotherapy to the abdominal, visceral, and parietal surfaces as well as to the hepatic circulation, where splenic hemangiosarcoma most frequently metastasizes. To date, the success of this approach has not been reported.

Biologic Response Modifiers and Chemotherapy

An early study found trends in survival suggesting that dogs with splenic hemangiosarcoma may benefit from chemotherapy and treatment with biologic response modifiers after splenectomy.[29] In another study, dogs with splenic hemangiosarcoma without metastases were randomized to receive treatment with liposome-encapsulated muramyl tripeptide-phosphatidylethanolamine (L-MTP-PE) or a placebo after postoperative chemotherapy with doxorubicin and cyclophosphamide.[14] L-MTP-PE activates macrophages, enhancing their tumoricidal ability. The most impressive improvement in survival was seen in the group that received L-MTP-PE plus chemotherapy, in which the median survival was 277 days, significantly higher than the median survival of 143 days seen for dogs treated with chemotherapy alone. Dogs with stage II disease seemed to benefit most from immunotherapy; those receiving L-MTP-PE had a median survival of 162 days compared with 96 for those receiving chemotherapy alone. Dogs with stage I disease showed no benefit.

Angiogenesis may be an important component of any tumor, but there has been particular interest in strategies that target angiogenesis in canine hemangiosarcoma because it is an endothelium-derived tumor. Endostatin prevents angiogenesis and tumor growth by inhibiting endothelial cell proliferation and migration. Endogenous levels of endostatin were higher in dogs with hemangiosarcoma than in normal dogs and dogs with other tumors in one study.[30] Minocycline is an inhibitor of collagenase and therefore may be effective in preventing angiogenesis. In a small trial, the addition of minocycline to doxorubicin and cyclophosphamide chemotherapy did not improve survival.[4] This trial may not have had adequate statistical power to truly evaluate antiangiogenic therapy. Antiangiogenic strategies target proliferation of normal blood vessel growth, and hemangiosarcoma is a malignant endothelial process; therefore, it is uncertain whether hemangiosarcoma would be more responsive than other tumors to antiangiogenic therapy. Further studies are essential to explore these strategies.

Cardiac Hemangiosarcoma
INCIDENCE, SIGNALMENT, AND ETIOLOGY

The right atrium is the third most common site (after the spleen and skin) of hemangiosarcoma, accounting for three of 104 hemangiosarcomas,[4] 15 of 134 hemangiosarcomas,[1] and 31 of 61 hemangiosarcomas[31] in three separate studies. In a study of intrapericardial cancers, more than 40% were hemangiosarcoma.[32] In a large study of 633 dogs with cardiac tumors, nearly 70% had hemangiosarcoma.[33] In the same study, the risk of developing a cardiac hemangiosarcoma increased steadily to the age of 15 years and then declined.[33] Two series of dogs with cardiac hemangiosarcoma (totaling 69 dogs)[31,34] indicated that German shepherds are at high risk for developing this disease and account for 20% to 30% of affected dogs. The average age of affected dogs in both studies was 10 years (range: 2–15 years); all but one dog were 5 years of age or older. There was no obvious gender predilection in these two smaller studies, but, in a large study, intact males were three times more likely than intact females to develop hemangiosarcoma.[33] In this study, the predisposition of German shepherds was confirmed; additional breeds at high risk were Afghan hounds, American cocker spaniels, Doberman pinschers, English setters, golden and Labrador retrievers, and miniature poodles.[33]

CLINICAL PRESENTATION AND HISTORY

Most dogs are presented after a short duration of signs, which range from acute collapse and cardiac tamponade to

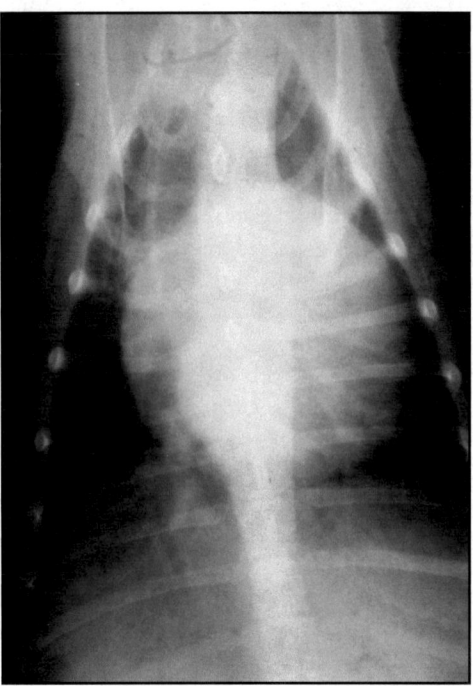

Figure 56-5. *A globoid heart shadow indicates pericardial effusion, caused by a bleeding right atrial hemangiosarcoma in this dog. (Courtesy of Dominique G. Penninck, DVM, Tufts Cummings School of Veterinary Medicine)*

nonspecific lethargy and generalized weakness.[35] Weakness is common and frequently affects the hindlimbs.[31] Most hemangiosarcomas of the right atrium are solitary, but they can be multiple within the atrium and auricle. Some are very large and invasive. Erosion of the endocardium may result in rupture of the atrial wall and subsequent cardiac tamponade. Sudden death follows in some dogs. In one study, hemangiosarcoma occurred most commonly in the right auricle. In the same study, there were metastases to the ventricle, left auricle, or both in nearly half of the dogs.[32]

In two studies, between 33% and 40% of dogs with pericardial effusion were found to have right atrial hemangiosarcoma; pericardial effusion in an old dog should increase suspicion for this tumor.[32,36]

STAGING AND DIAGNOSIS

In addition to the staging procedures outlined for dogs with splenic hemangiosarcoma, thoracic radiography and cardiac evaluation using ultrasonography provide valuable information. Abdominal ultrasonography should also be conducted to identify dogs with involvement of other organs.

Primary cardiac hemangiosarcoma has a very high rate of pulmonary metastases compared with splenic and cutaneous hemangiosarcoma. In two studies, pulmonary metastases were found at the time of presentation in 37 of 60 dogs (62%).[31,34] Metastases in the liver and spleen are less common. Metastases to abdominal viscera, skin, and brain are observed in some dogs.

Cardiac masses may be very difficult to see on thoracic radiographs, although findings of pericardial effusion, right heart enlargement, or specific right atrial enlargement may be suggestive of hemangiosarcoma of the right atrium (Figure 56-5). In one survey, these radiographic findings were recognized in fewer than 50% of dogs with cardiac hemangiosarcoma. Pulmonary metastases were less frequently overlooked in the same study, but because these metastases are small and miliary in distribution, both right and left lateral views are recommended to improve the chances of detection.[37]

Two-dimensional echocardiography is a noninvasive technique used to examine the right atrium and auricle. When it is used by a skilled operator, it can be helpful in detecting masses in this area.[38] Despite the utility of this imaging technique, necropsies in one study revealed atrial hemangiosarcomas in eight dogs that had not been detected on ultrasonography.[4] In one study, pneumopericardiography successfully outlined masses in the right atrium in seven of 12 dogs.[34]

> **KEY POINT**
> *Right atrial hemangiosarcoma is a common cause of pericardial effusion; ultrasonography should be used in these dogs to identify any suspicious mass.*

Cytology of pericardial fluid is rarely diagnostic of a right atrial hemangiosarcoma.[31] Definitive diagnosis usually requires thoracotomy and surgical biopsy, although a ventricular lesion may be accessible for endomyocardial biopsy.[39] Occasionally, a hematoma may be seen at this site,[40] but in an older dog with a right atrial mass and a hemorrhagic pericardial effusion, any diagnosis other than hemangiosarcoma is unlikely.

Cardiac troponin I (cTnI) and cardiac troponin T (cTnT) are markers of myocardial ischemia and necrosis. In one study, dogs with hemangiosarcoma had significantly higher concentrations of cTnI than dogs with idiopathic pericardial effusion, but there was no difference in the concentration of cTnT between the same two populations of dogs. Measurement of cTnI may be useful in helping to distinguish between pericardial effusion caused by hemangiosarcoma and idiopathic pericardial effusion.[41] Measurement of pericardial fluid pH was not found to be helpful in distinguishing malignant effusions from those resulting from benign or idiopathic conditions.[42]

TREATMENT

Most reported animals with cardiac hemangiosarcoma either died or were euthanatized at or shortly after diagnosis because of the high rate of metastasis. Cardiac supportive care is rarely successful for more than 1 month.[39]

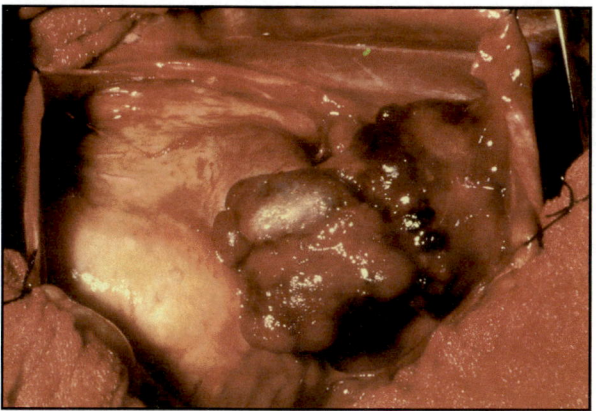

Figure 56-6. *A hemangiosarcoma of the right auricle may be clearly visible at exploratory thoracotomy. (Courtesy of J. Berg)*

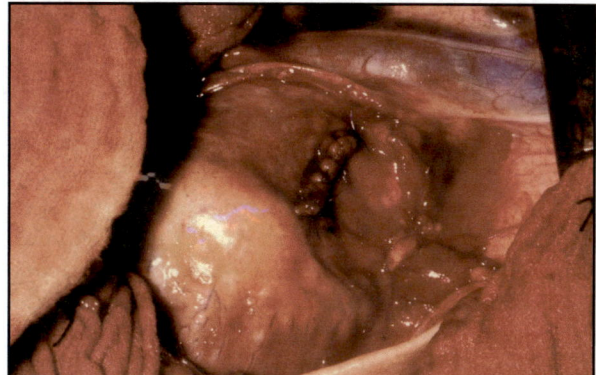

Figure 56-7. *Same dog as in Figure 56-6. The auricle may be resected with little patient morbidity; however, survival times are short. (Courtesy J. Berg)*

Surgery

Surgical resection of right atrial hemangiosarcoma was attempted in 13 dogs that lacked evidence of pulmonary metastasis on radiographs.[34,43] In 10 of these dogs, the primary tumor was confined to the right auricle and was completely resected. In the other three dogs, the tumor was more extensive and excision was incomplete. One of the latter dogs died in the perioperative period, and three other dogs that were found to have metastases at the time of surgery did not survive long. Survival times for all 13 dogs ranged from 2 days to 8 months (mean: 4 months); all dogs developed disseminated metastatic disease. In another study, three dogs that underwent a similar surgery died within 13 weeks of surgery[36] (Figures 56-6 and 56-7). Pericardectomy was performed to relieve the pericardial effusion in two dogs, but both died of metastatic disease 1 and 4 months after surgery.[44] Surgery may be palliative (as is splenectomy for dogs with splenic hemangiosarcoma), but the lungs should be carefully evaluated during surgery for evidence of pulmonary metastases (Figure 56-8). In a larger study, 21 dogs had a surgical resection of the right atrium or auricle. The median hospital stay after surgery was 3 days, and complications were few; median survival for 8 dogs with complete resection of the tumor and no gross metastases was 2 months.[35]

Chemotherapy

Early reports of chemotherapy for cardiac hemangiosarcoma were largely anecdotal. Doxorubicin after resection of auricular hemangiosarcomas in two dogs did not seem to improve survival compared with dogs that were treated with surgery alone.[43] One dog received doxorubicin, cyclophosphamide, and vincristine for 105 days. The size of the primary tumor was reduced, but pulmonary metastases developed during chemotherapy.[45] The dog developed cardiomyopathy, presumably because of the doxorubicin therapy, and died 140 days after starting chemotherapy. In another study, three dogs with disseminated hemangiosar-

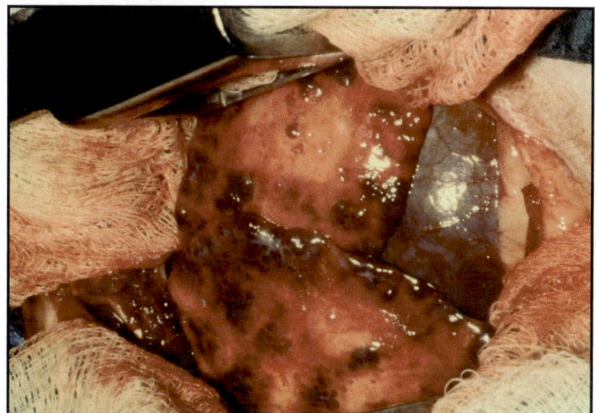

Figure 56-8. *Care should be taken at the time of surgery to evaluate the lungs for evidence of metastases, as are seen in this dog. (Courtesy J. Berg)*

coma that included the right atrium were treated with surgery (one dog) and the same chemotherapeutic protocol.[19] The three dogs lived 172, 173, and 218 days; the longest survivor died from cardiotoxicity. Other dogs with cardiac hemangiosarcoma were included in chemotherapy studies but were not identified by tumor site.[8,22,27]

In a larger study of 23 dogs, chemotherapy for cardiac hemangiosarcoma resulted in improvement in survival and quality of life. Doxorubicin-based chemotherapy was most commonly used.[35] Median survival for eight dogs that received adjunctive chemotherapy was 6 months, which was significantly better than the survival time of 2 months if no chemotherapy was given.[35]

Cutaneous Hemangioma
INCIDENCE, SIGNALMENT, AND ETIOLOGY

Hemangiomas are benign tumors of endothelial cells that occur in middle-aged dogs (mean age: 9 years) without gender predilection. Breeds that are more than twice as likely as the general population to develop cutaneous hemangiomas are Airedale terriers, Gordon setters, soft-coated wheaten terriers, and wirehaired fox terriers; boxers appear to be predisposed to developing multiple hemangiomas on the abdominal skin.[46] Cutaneous hemangiomas are more than four times as common than their malignant counterparts.[47] The increased incidence of dermal hemangioma and hemangiosarcoma on the ventral abdomen of dogs with glabrous (nonpigmented, lightly haired) skin suggests an association between these tumors and solar radiation in a manner similar to that described for squamous cell carcinoma.[47-49] Actinic dermatosis may precede tumor development by many years, and dogs may develop hemangiomas before or concurrent with hemangiosarcoma. Multiple benign angiomatous hemangiomas were documented in a 1-year-old dog. Over a period of 6 months, the number of lesions increased, and bleeding became continuous; metastases were seen on necropsy, implying that malignant transformation had occurred.[50]

CLINICAL PRESENTATION AND HISTORY

Hemangiomas are variably sized, usually solitary, well-circumscribed, nonencapsulated, dermoepidermal to subcutaneous, soft and spongy, and shaded red to black (Figure 56-9). Those in the superficial dermis may ulcerate and bleed; this is often the reason for an owner to present the dog for veterinary care. Hemangiomas in the subcutaneous tissue are usually larger, with little change to the overlying skin. Hemangiomas arise most commonly on the limbs, with more than 40% of 1,301 hemangiomas occurring on the limbs in one study.[46] Hemangiomas of the ventral abdomen are found in areas unprotected by hair and skin pigment.

TREATMENT

Surgical excision of cutaneous hemangioma should be curative. Dogs that develop many hemangiomas over years may show histologic evidence of progression to hemangiosarcoma.

Cutaneous Hemangiosarcoma
INCIDENCE, SIGNALMENT, AND ETIOLOGY

Cutaneous hemangiosarcoma occurs in older dogs (average age: 10 years) and is most common in intact males.[46] Unlike those with hemangiosarcoma of other sites, dogs with lightly haired, poorly pigmented skin are predisposed; Italian greyhounds, whippets, Irish wolfhounds, vizslas, American pit bull terriers, salukis, bloodhounds, and English pointers are at increased risk.[46,51] In one study, a colony of 991 beagles

> **KEY POINT**
> *Cutaneous hemangiosarcoma affects dogs with glabrous skin and is often a sunlight-induced tumor.*

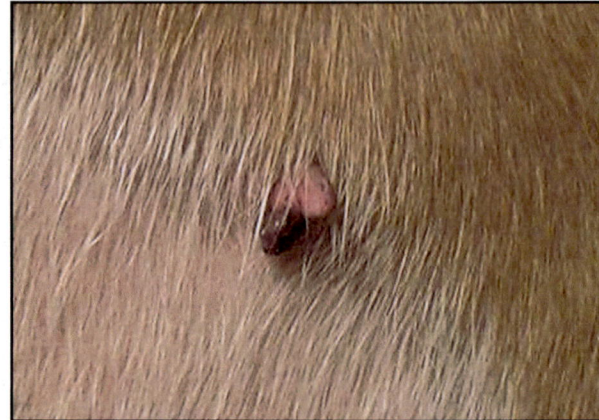

Figure 56-9. *Cutaneous hemangioma may arise in the nonpigmented abdominal skin because of actinic damage. This hemangioma is adjacent to the nipple and could be removed at surgery. (Courtesy of Kenneth M. Rassnick, DVM, Cornell University College of Veterinary Medicine)*

developed 48 cutaneous hemangiosarcomas.[48] Tumors in these breeds are often found in skin that shows histologic evidence of actinic (solar) dermatosis. These findings suggest that cutaneous hemangiosarcoma is a sunlight-induced tumor in many dogs. Actinic dermatosis may precede tumor development by many years, and dogs may develop hemangiomas long before malignancy is detected.

Cutaneous hemangiosarcoma may also be metastatic from systemic hemangiosarcoma, as found in one study, with a high rate of metastatic skin involvement from visceral sites.[52] Some authors make a distinction between cutaneous and subcutaneous hemangiosarcomas. Subcutaneous hemangiosarcoma is not associated with actinic exposure and has a more aggressive clinical course.

CLINICAL PRESENTATION AND HISTORY

Dogs may have cutaneous hemangiomas and hemangiosarcomas concurrently, and these may be clinically indistinguishable. Hemangiosarcomas are more likely to affect the dermis than the subcutis and have a predilection for the ventral abdominal skin as well as the limbs.[46] Of 48 dogs in one study, 42 had tumors in their abdominal skin.[47] Hemangiosarcomas are soft or spongy, poorly circumscribed, infiltrating, friable masses. The overlying epidermis is frequently thickened and ulcerated; it may be raised and red in appearance. Tumors below the dermis tend to be larger, possibly because owners detect them later.[53] Dogs with subcutaneous tumors often have a history of a rapidly enlarging tumor, possibly attributable to subcutaneous hemorrhage from the abnormal vasculature.

STAGING AND DIAGNOSIS

Cutaneous hemangiosarcoma may represent a metastasis from visceral sites; therefore, a thorough staging procedure should be performed.[13] Careful abdominal palpation to identify organomegaly, followed by abdominal ultrasonography, may help to eliminate the possibility of a splenic tumor. In addition, echocardiography to detect right atrial hemangiosarcoma should be conducted. Right and left lateral and ventrodorsal thoracic radiographs should be taken as well as routine blood work and urinalysis. If the skin is the primary site of the hemangiosarcoma, the prognosis is guarded but considerably better than for visceral hemangiosarcoma; many studies of hemangiosarcomas of all sites stage cutaneous hemangiosarcoma as stage I disease.[8,19] In one study, only two of 25 dogs developed distant metastases despite long survival times after surgery.[53]

The risk of developing DIC in dogs with primary cutaneous hemangiosarcomas seems low. In a series of 212 dogs with cutaneous hemangiomas or hemangiosarcomas, 11 dogs developed hemostatic defects that led to bleeding or petechiation and ecchymoses.[51] Six of these dogs had also had systemic hemangiosarcoma, and three had large, unresectable tumors.

Specific immunohistochemical staining for CD31 was positive in hemangiosarcomas and hemangiomas but not in any other sarcomas in one study.[16] This stain may be useful in determining the histogenesis of poorly differentiated hemangiosarcomas. Another endothelial cell–specific marker is factor VIII–related antigen.[17]

PROGNOSTIC FACTORS

Solar elastosis in the skin adjacent to hemangiosarcomas is related to long survival, implying that solar-induced cutaneous hemangiosarcomas may be less aggressive tumors than other hemangiosarcomas.[47] Clinically, a presumption of solar etiology may be made when the skin is lightly pigmented and lightly haired and a crusting dermatitis is present; however, histologic confirmation is required.

> **KEY POINT**
> *Histopathologic evidence of actinic changes in the skin adjacent to cutaneous hemangiosarcoma may be associated with a low chance of metastatic spread.*

In one study, dogs with subcutaneous tumors treated with chemotherapy had longer survival times than dogs with splenic hemangiosarcomas treated with the same chemotherapy, implying that subcutaneous tumors may respond better to therapy than visceral tumors.[27]

TREATMENT
Surgery

Surgery alone may be sufficient to resolve cutaneous hemangiosarcoma. Of 84 dogs with cutaneous hemangiosarcoma treated by surgical excision, 25 died of tumor-related causes, and only 11 had tumors that recurred at the site of surgery.[47] This is a considerably lower recurrence and mortality rate than is seen with hemangiosarcoma of systemic origin. Only four dogs with hemangiosarcoma concurrent with solar elastosis died from their tumors. In two of these dogs, the tumor had been present for 1.2 and 2.7 years before surgical removal. In another group of 48 beagles with cutaneous hemangiosarcomas, 11 dogs developed metastases and died from them.[48] Apparently, primary cutaneous hemangiosarcoma, particularly if found in association with solar-induced changes, is not as aggressive as hemangiosarcoma arising from other sites. In a series of 25 dogs, local recurrence after surgery was more common in dogs with subcutaneous hemangiosarcoma, and median survival for these dogs was significantly shorter than that for dogs with dermal tumors (307 days versus 780 days).[53] Dogs with subcutaneous hemangiosarcoma are still more likely to have stage I disease than dogs with hemangiosarcomas in other sites.[4,20]

Chemotherapy

In light of the long remissions that occur after surgery alone for cutaneous hemangiosarcoma, the contribution of chemotherapy to survival times is difficult to assess. Subcutaneous hemangiosarcoma is more likely to metastasize, but the rate of metastasis appears to be lower than that for hemangiosarcoma of the spleen or heart. Chemotherapy is warranted in dogs with subcutaneous hemangiosarcoma. In one study, six dogs received doxorubicin, cyclophosphamide, and vincristine as well as chlorambucil and methotrexate.[19] Responses in three dogs treated with chemotherapy alone were not impressive; two of the dogs developed progressive disease and died less than 4 months after treatment began, but one dog that maintained stable disease lived for 14 months. Survival times in three dogs that underwent surgical excision before chemotherapy ranged from 9 months to more than 34 months. In another study, administration of doxorubicin every 2 weeks instead of every 3 weeks led to a median survival of 8 months for four dogs with subcutaneous hemangiosarcoma.[20] In a third study, dogs with subcutaneous hemangiosarcoma that were treated with doxorubicin and cyclophosphamide also had a median survival of 8 months.[8] A dog with lymph node metastases from a primary subcutaneous hemangiosarcoma had a complete response to ifosfamide therapy and no evidence of recurrence 15 months after treatment.[26] In another study, the addition of ifosfamide to doxorubicin chemotherapy did not improve survival over doxorubicin alone, although dogs with subcutaneous hemangiosarcomas had longer median survival times (8 months) than dogs with splenic hemangiosarcomas treated with the same protocol (4 months).[27] Dogs with subcutaneous tumors were included in other studies but were not specifically identified by site of origin.[8,19,20,22,25]

Chemotherapy protocols that contain doxorubicin are warranted for dogs with subcutaneous hemangiosarcoma; a more favorable outcome than that seen for dogs with splenic hemangiosarcoma is probably likely.

HEMANGIOSARCOMA OF OTHER SITES

Hemangiosarcoma most commonly arises in the spleen, skin, or right atrium, but because blood vessels are ubiquitous, primary hemangiosarcoma may arise in any organ.

Any dog with hemangiosarcoma should be staged as described for cutaneous hemangiosarcoma to ascertain that the affected site is not a metastasis from more commonly affected sites, such as the spleen or right atrium. With the exception of some cutaneous hemangiosarcomas, the prognosis for any dog with hemangiosarcoma is poor. Adjunctive chemotherapy is investigational.

HEMANGIOSARCOMA OF THE UROGENITAL TRACT

Case reports of dogs with urogenital hemangiosarcoma show poor survival times. A primary prostatic hemangiosarcoma in an 11-year-old miniature poodle failed to respond to a course of radiation therapy and had metastasized widely at the time of euthanasia.[17] A middle-aged golden retriever had an incidental finding of an abdominal mass that arose from the dorsal surface of the bladder and left ureter. Partial cystectomy was able to completely resect the tumor. Bladder necrosis in the perioperative period was the cause of death.[54] A large urethral hemangiosarcoma in a boxer was found to have metastasized to the adjacent lumbar vertebrae.[55]

Four dogs with renal hemangiosarcoma had longer survival times (median: 6.4 months) than dogs with splenic hemangiosarcomas (median: 4 months) in a study that treated dogs with ifosfamide and doxorubicin.[27] In a preliminary report of 11 dogs with renal hemangiosarcoma, median survival was 9 months even though only three dogs received chemotherapy.[56]

HEMANGIOSARCOMA OF THE LIVER

Primary hepatic hemangiosarcoma is rarely reported but has a similar clinical course to splenic hemangiosarcoma.[57] Surgical excision is usually very difficult, so palliation of bleeding is often not possible (Figure 56-10). One experimental study found seven hepatic hemangiosarcomas in 55 dogs exposed to cesium radioisotopes.[58]

HEMANGIOSARCOMA OF MUSCLE

An 8-year-old bullmastiff presented for non–weight-bearing lameness was found on magnetic resonance imaging of the lumbosacral area to have a lesion of the iliopsoas muscle that was a hemangiosarcoma. Pulmonary metastases were present.[59]

A sublingual hemangiosarcoma in a different dog metastasized widely, including the lungs and spleen.[13]

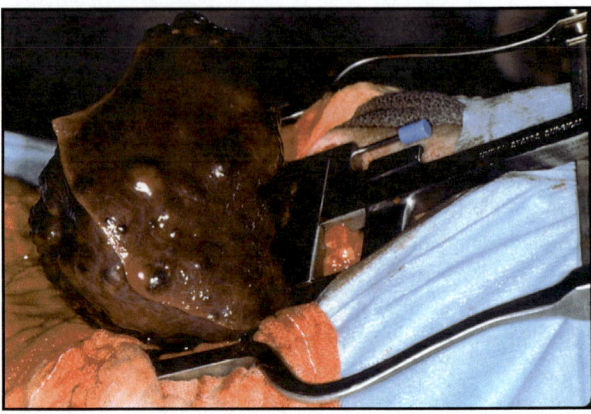

Figure 56-10. *Hemangiosarcoma may arise as a primary tumor in the liver; resection is often impossible.*

HEMANGIOSARCOMA OF THE CENTRAL NERVOUS SYSTEM AND EYE

A 10-year-old Great Dane presented for cervical and right forelimb pain and tetraparesis was found to have an extradural hemangiosarcoma. The tumor was removed by hemilaminectomy followed by doxorubicin chemotherapy. The dog developed splenic hemangiosarcoma and local recurrence 11 months after surgery.[60]

In two reports, hemangiosarcoma was excised from the limbal conjunctiva in two dogs and from the nictitans in five dogs; three dogs were English setters.[61,62] Of the seven dogs, two had recurrence: One dog treated with surgery for a nictitans tumor had recurrence after 14 months; the other tumor recurred after surgery and strontium-90 radiation therapy but was cured by enucleation. In the other five dogs, there was no evidence of recurrence between 6 and 17 months after surgery. No tumor metastasized. Hemangiosarcoma in this location may behave more like cutaneous hemangiosarcoma.

HEMANGIOSARCOMA OF BONE

Hemangiosarcoma as a primary bone tumor is rare. It most often affects young-adult, large-breed dogs and may be seen as a result of systemic metastases from a visceral site. Hemangiosarcomas are destructive lesions, and bony changes on radiographs are primarily lytic. The metastatic rate of this tumor is high.

There are several case reports of this tumor. Of seven dogs with hemangiosarcoma of the rib, one had metastases at diagnosis,[63] one had recurrence 1 month after surgery, two had metastatic disease within 5 months of surgery,[64] and three others lived 1 year or more (one was not treated).[65] Primary hemangiosarcoma of the vertebrae has been reported and was associated with rapid metastasis and short survival time.[66,67] One dog with appendicular hemangiosarcoma was treated with doxorubicin and cyclophosphamide after amputation and died 154 days later from metastatic disease[19]; hemangiosarcoma of the femur in another dog metastasized to the kidneys, lung, and spleen.[13] Two of three dogs with scapular hemangiosarcoma had metastases to the lungs noted at the time of diagnosis; the third dog was treated by partial scapulectomy and died from lung and vertebral metastases 7 months after surgery. These three dogs were all younger than 3 years.[68] A hemangiosarcoma that affected vertebra T9 was treated palliatively with corticosteroids for 3 months before the disease progressed to involve T9 to T11 and the dog was euthanatized.[66]

In a preliminary report of the only series of cases, 17 dogs with a median age of 12 years (range: 1.5–13.5 years) were reviewed.[69] Four dogs had axial lesions (mandible = 1, rib = 1, L4 = 2), and 13 had appendicular lesions (humerus = 5, femur = 5, tibia = 2, ulna = 1). Of 12 dogs with follow-up after diagnosis, the median survival was 4 months but ranged up to 2 years. Ten of 13 dogs had metastases confirmed at death.

RETROPERITONEAL SARCOMAS

The most common histologic type of retroperitoneal sarcoma is hemangiosarcoma, accounting for nine of 14 dogs in one study.[70] Most (57%) were grade 3 tumors. Median survival was 1 month. Chemotherapy with doxorubicin-based protocols was not completed in three dogs because of the onset of recurrence or metastases.[70]

CAVERNOUS HEMANGIOMA

This rare disorder was diagnosed in the cerebrum of a 13-month-old dog. The lesion affected the right olfactory lobe and caused seizures and progressive depression.[71]

A cavernous hemangioma was also diagnosed in a 12-month-old German shepherd with a 9-month history of ascites. The liver contained multiple 1-cm hemangiomas that appeared diffusely nodular on ultrasonographic examination.[72]

Cavernous hemangiomas were diagnosed in the popliteal lymph nodes of eight beagles and in one hepatic lymph node. They were an incidental finding, causing no clinically significant signs.[73]

NASAL ANGIOMATOUS PROLIFERATION

This inflammatory disease was diagnosed in 13 dogs with epistaxis.[74] Although tumors were histopathologically benign, there was radiographic evidence of extensive destruction by a mass that often invaded the sinuses or cranium. Six affected dogs were treated surgically, and five had no evidence of disease 4 years later; one dog had a recurrence 2 years after surgery. One dog had controlled disease after 2 years of corticosteroid treatment, and one dog that received no treatment developed neurologic disease 2 years after diagnosis.

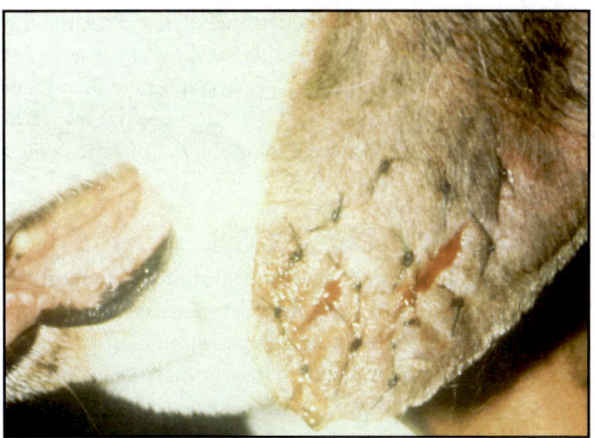

Figure 56-11. *Note the oozing serum from a lymphangiosarcoma of the pinna in this beagle. (Courtesy of Mark Hitt, DVM, Atlantic Veterinary Internal Medicine)*

Lymphangioma and Lymphangiosarcoma

INCIDENCE, SIGNALMENT, AND ETIOLOGY

Lymphangiomas and lymphangiosarcomas are tumors composed of lymph vessels forming capillary, cavernous, or cystic spaces. In a large study, lymphangioma was described in 57 dogs; 19 cases arose in the skin.[75] There was no gender predilection. The median age of affected dogs was 7 years. Golden retrievers accounted for seven cases. In another study, lymphangiomas were more common in neutered dogs of both genders, and beagles were seven times more likely to develop a cutaneous lymphangioma than dogs of other breeds.[76] This tumor may be associated with, and a sequela to, chronic lymphatic obstruction (i.e., after radical surgical procedures, such as a radical mastectomy for mammary tumors). Lymphangioma has also been seen as a sequela to congenital primary lymphedema.[77]

Lymphangiosarcoma is less common than lymphangioma and affects a wider variety of anatomic sites. Similar to lymphangioma, the malignant variant appears to be an uncommon sequela of congenital lymphedema. It has been reported in dogs ranging in age from 8 weeks[78] to 10 years.[79]

CLINICAL PRESENTATION AND HISTORY

Dogs with cutaneous lymphangiomas often have very large tumors. Lymphangiomas have a predilection for the abdominal skin and the hindlimbs.[76] Lymphangiomas are soft or spongy, poorly circumscribed, infiltrating masses that often have a persistent and severe pitting edema after digital palpation. The overlying epidermis may be eroded and ulcerated; lymph may ooze from the tumor, giving a moist appearance (lymphorrhea; Figure 56-11). Secondary infection may occur.[80] Less commonly, subepidermal vesicles and bullae may be seen because of accumulation of lymph in abnormal lymphatic channels.[76] If a mass lesion is present, there may be considerable swelling of the adjacent limb or of the head and neck.[81] Ulceration may be present for years before presentation.[80] The clinical appearance of lymphangiosarcoma is not distinguishable from the benign tumor.

STAGING AND DIAGNOSIS

Cutaneous lymphangioma can be diffuse throughout the lymphatics. Lymphangiography or lymphoscintigraphy may show evidence of lymphedema, but without biopsy it is not possible to determine whether it is primary or caused by lymphangioma.[77,81] Biopsy of the edematous tissue is very important.[81]

The endothelial cell–specific marker factor VIII–related antigen may be positive in hemangiosarcomas, lymphangiosarcomas, and lymphangiomas.[81] Immunohistochemical staining for different lectins may be able to distinguish between lymphangiosarcomas and hemangiosarcomas.[82]

Most reported cases are benign (lymphangioma), but lymphangiosarcomas often metastasize. Metastasis from an axillary lymphangiosarcoma to the mediastinal lymph nodes has been described in a 1-year-old dog.[82] A 2-year-old dog had widespread metastasis to the lungs, regional lymph nodes, kidney, bone marrow, and spleen.[83] Metastases to the lungs in another dog[84] and to lymph nodes in an 8-week-old puppy[78] were also reported. A lymphangiosarcoma that was apparently confined to the cranial mediastinum was reported in a 10-year-old dog. This dog was euthanatized because of persistent chylothorax that was not relieved by a pleuroperitoneal shunt.[79] Persistent chylothorax was the cause of death in another 8-year-old dog with lymphangiosarcoma localized to the pulmonary pleural surfaces.[85] Other lymphangiosarcomas have been reported and have varying lengths of clinical history, often prolonged.[86]

TREATMENT

There are few reports of treatment for these rare tumors in dogs. Nonetheless, a therapeutic approach similar to that described for hemangioma and hemangiosarcoma is recommended. Radiation therapy may control localized tumors.

For benign lesions, an aggressive surgical excision with 2- to 3-cm margins, as described for soft tissue sarcomas, may provide long-term control. A dog with lymphangiomas of the skin, subcutaneous tissues, mammary gland, and spleen was not treated after biopsy and had a waxing and waning course of swelling over a period of 22 months.[87] Progression of lymphangioma was seen over a period of 1 year in another dog that also had lymphangiectasia.[88]

Surgery is potentially curative in dogs with smaller lesions, but a large area is often involved. Surgical cure after recurrence was achieved in a 7-month-old dog with a 4-month history of cystic inguinal and mammary masses that appeared to follow the cutaneous lymphatic chain. Involvement of the inguinal lymph node was seen but was thought to be a synchronous primary rather than metastasis.[89] Multifocal involvement of the hindlimb was also seen in an 18-month-old dog.[90] Extensive inguinal involvement made it impossible to remove a lymphangioma secondary to primary lymphedema in a 4-year-old dog.[77] Removal and pad transposition was sufficient to control a lymphangioma of the digital pad in another dog for 1 year, but recurrence on the dorsal surface of the foot was not treated.[80] A wide excision (e.g., amputation), as described for other soft tissue sarcomas, may control otherwise localized lesions. In a review of previously published cases, surgery was the only treatment for five dogs with lymphangiomas.[87] Recurrence was seen in three dogs between 3 and 18 months, and two dogs had no recurrence between 6 and 9 months after surgery. Surgical marsupialization may provide palliation of a large fluid-filled lesion.[91]

There is a report of long-term control of a lymphangioma with radiation therapy to a total dose of 48 Gy after the tumor had recurred twice after surgery.[92]

Dogs with lymphangiosarcoma have either not been treated or died soon after surgery, except for a 9-year-old husky that had a recurrence 3 weeks after surgery but then responded completely after doxorubicin treatment. This dog had neither recurrence nor metastasis 9 months after treatment.[93]

REFERENCES

1. Srebernik N, Appleby EC: Breed prevalence and sites of haemangioma and haemangiosarcoma in dogs. *Vet Rec* 129:408–409, 1991.
2. Ng CY, Mills JN: Clinical and haematological features of haemangiosarcoma in dogs. *Aust Vet J* 62:1–4, 1985.
3. Prymak C, McKee LJ, Goldschmidt MH, Glickman LT: Epidemiologic, clinical, pathologic, and prognostic characteristics of splenic hemangiosarcoma and splenic hematoma in dogs: 217 cases (1985). *JAVMA* 193:706–712, 1988.
4. Sorenmo K, Duda L, Barber L, et al: Canine hemangiosarcoma treated with standard chemotherapy and minocycline. *J Vet Intern Med* 14:395–398, 2000.
5. Spangler WL, Culbertson MR: Prevalence, type, and importance of splenic diseases in dogs: 1,480 cases (1985–1989). *JAVMA* 200:829–834, 1992.
6. Popper H, Thomas LB, Telles NC, et al: Development of hepatic angiosarcoma in man induced by vinyl chloride, thorotrast, and arsenic. Comparison with cases of unknown etiology. *Am J Pathol* 92:349–369, 1978.
7. Johnson KA, Powers BE, Withrow SJ, et al: Splenomegaly in dogs. Predictors of neoplasia and survival after splenectomy. *J Vet Intern Med* 3:160–166, 1989.
8. Sorenmo KU, Jeglum KA, Helfand SC: Chemotherapy of canine hemangiosarcoma with doxorubicin and cyclophosphamide. *J Vet Intern Med* 7:370–376, 1993.
9. Wruck M: Milzhämatom bei einem rauhaardackel. *Kleintierpraxis* 44:773–779, 1999.
10. Maruyama H, Miura T, Sakai M, et al: The incidence of disseminated intravascular coagulation in dogs with malignant tumor. *J Vet Med Sci* 66:573–575, 2004.
11. Wrigley RH, Park RD, Konde LJ, Lebel JL: Ultrasonographic features of splenic hemangiosarcoma in dogs: 18 cases (1980–1986). *JAVMA* 192:1113–1117, 1988.
12. Waters DJ, Caywood DD, Hayden DW, Klausner JS: Metastatic pattern in dogs with splenic haemangiosarcoma: Clinical implications. *J Small Anim Pract* 29:805–814, 1988.
13. Wandera JG, Kamuau JA, Ngatia TA, et al: Haemangiosarcoma in dogs: Morphological and clinical findings. *Bull Anim Health Prod Afr* 38:301–308, 1990.
14. Vail DM, MacEwen EG, Kurzman ID, et al: Liposome-encapsulated muramyl tripeptide phosphatidylethanolamine adjuvant immunotherapy for splenic hemangiosarcoma in the dog: A randomized multi-institutional clinical trial.

Clin Cancer Res 1:1165–1170, 1995.
15. O'Keefe DA, Couto CG: Fine-needle aspiration of the spleen as an aid in the diagnosis of splenomegaly. J Vet Intern Med 1:102–109, 1987.
16. Ferrer L, Fondevila D, Rabanal RM, Vilafranca M: Immunohistochemical detection of CD31 antigen in normal and neoplastic canine endothelial cells. J Comp Pathol 112:319–326, 1995.
17. Hayden DW, Bartges JW, Bell FW, Klausner JS: Prostatic hemangiosarcoma in a dog: Clinical and pathologic findings. J Vet Diagn Invest 4:209–211, 1992.
18. Clifford CA, Hughes D, Beal MW, et al: Plasma vascular endothelial growth factor concentrations in healthy dogs and dogs with hemangiosarcoma. J Vet Intern Med 15:131–135, 2001.
19. Hammer AS, Couto CG, Filppi J, et al: Efficacy and toxicity of VAC chemotherapy (vincristine, doxorubicin, and cyclophosphamide) in dogs with hemangiosarcoma. J Vet Intern Med 5:160–166, 1991.
20. Sorenmo KU, Baez JL, Clifford CA, et al: Efficacy and toxicity of a dose-intensified doxorubicin protocol in canine hemangiosarcoma. J Vet Intern Med 18:209–213, 2004.
21. Spangler WL, Kass PH: Pathologic factors affecting postsplenectomy survival in dogs. J Vet Intern Med 11:166–171, 1997.
22. Ogilvie GK, Powers BE, Mallinckrodt CH, Withrow SJ: Surgery and doxorubicin in dogs with hemangiosarcoma. J Vet Intern Med 10:379–384, 1996.
23. Wood CA, Moore AS, Gliatto JM, et al: Prognosis for dogs with stage I or II splenic hemangiosarcoma treated by splenectomy alone: 32 cases (1991–1993). JAAHA 34:417–421, 1998.
24. Keyes ML, Rush JE, Autran B, et al: Ventricular arrhythmias in dogs with splenic masses. Vet Emerg Critical Care 3:33–38, 1994.
25. Vail DM, Kravis LD, Cooley AJ, et al: Preclinical trial of doxorubicin entrapped in sterically stabilized liposomes in dogs with spontaneously arising malignant tumors. Cancer Chemother Pharmacol 39:410–416, 1997.
26. Rassnick KM, Frimberger AE, Wood CA, et al: Evaluation of ifosfamide for treatment of various canine neoplasms. J Vet Intern Med 14:271–276, 2000.
27. Payne SE, Rassnick KM, Northrup NC, et al: Treatment of vascular and soft-tissue sarcomas in dogs using an alternating protocol of ifosfamide and doxorubicin. Vet Comp Oncol 1:171–179, 2003.
28. de Lorimier LP, Dhaliwal RS, Kitchell BE: The use of DAV, an aggressive combination chemotherapy protocol, in canine hemangiosarcoma and high-grade sarcomas. Proc 21st Annu Conf Vet Cancer Soc:40, 2001.
29. Brown NO, Patnaik AK MacEwen EG. Canine hemangiosarcoma: Retrospective analysis of 104 cases. JAVMA 186:56–58, 1985.
30. Rossmeisl JH Jr, Bright P, Tamarkin L, et al: Endostatin concentrations in healthy dogs and dogs with selected neoplasms. J Vet Intern Med 16:565–569, 2002.
31. Kleine LJ, Zook BC, Munson TO: Primary cardiac hemangiosarcomas in dogs. JAVMA 157:326–337, 1970.
32. Girard C, Helie P, Odin M: Intrapericardial neoplasia in dogs. J Vet Diagn Invest 11:73–78, 1999.
33. Ware WA, Hopper DL: Cardiac tumors in dogs: 1982–1995. J Vet Intern Med 13:95–103, 1999.
34. Aronsohn M: Cardiac hemangiosarcoma in the dog: A review of 38 cases. JAVMA 187:922–926, 1985.
35. Weisse C, Soares N, Beal MW, et al: Survival times in dogs with right atrial hemangiosarcoma treated by means of surgical resection with or without adjuvant chemotherapy: 23 cases (1986–2000). JAVMA 226:575–579, 2005.
36. Berg RJ, Wingfield W: Pericardial effusion in the dog: A review of 42 cases. JAAHA 20:721–730, 1984.
37. Holt D, Van Winkle T, Schelling C, Prymak C: Correlation between thoracic radiographs and postmortem findings in dogs with hemangiosarcoma: 77 cases (1984–1989). JAVMA 200:1535–1539, 1992.
38. de Madron E, Helfand SC, Stebbins KE: Use of chemotherapy for treatment of cardiac hemangiosarcoma in a dog. JAVMA 190:887–891, 1987.
39. Keene BW, Rush JE, Cooley AJ, Subramanian R: Primary left ventricular hemangiosarcoma diagnosed by endomyocardial biopsy in a dog. JAVMA 197:1501–1503, 1990.
40. Simpson DJ, Hunt GB, Church DB, Beck JA: Benign masses in the pericardium of two dogs. Aust Vet J 77:225–229, 1999.
41. Shaw SP, Rozanski EA, Rush JE: Cardiac troponins I and T in dogs with pericardial effusion. J Vet Intern Med 18:322–324, 2004.
42. Fine DM, Tobias AH, Jacob KA: Use of pericardial fluid pH to distinguish between idiopathic and neoplastic effusions. J Vet Intern Med 17:525–529, 2003.
43. Wykes PM, Rouse GP, Orton EC: Removal of five canine cardiac tumors using a stapling instrument. Vet Surg 15:103–106, 1986.
44. Kerstetter KK, Krahwinkel DJ Jr, Millis DL, Hahn K: Pericardiectomy in dogs: 22 cases (1978–1994). JAVMA 211:736–740, 1997.
45. de Madron E, Helfand SC, Stebbins KE: Use of chemotherapy for treatment of cardiac hemangiosarcoma in a dog. JAVMA 190:887–891, 1987.
46. Goldschmidt MH, Shofer FS: Cutaneous vascular tumors, in Goldschmidt MH, Shofer FS (eds): Skin Tumors of the Dog and Cat, ed 1. Tarrytown, NY, Pergamon Press, 1992, pp 204–215.
47. Hargis AM, Ihrke PJ, Spangler WL, Stannard AA: A retrospective clinicopathologic study of 212 dogs with cutaneous hemangiomas and hemangiosarcomas. Vet Pathol 29:316–328, 1992.
48. Nikula KJ, Benjamin SA, Angleton GM, et al: Ultraviolet radiation, solar dermatosis, and cutaneous neoplasia in beagle dogs. Radiat Res 129:11–18, 1992.
49. Er JC, Sutton RH: A survey of skin neoplasms in dogs from the Brisbane region. Aust Vet J 66:225–227, 1989.
50. Arp LH, Grier RL: Disseminated cutaneous hemangiosarcoma in a young dog. JAVMA 185:671–673, 1984.
51. Hargis AM, Feldman BF: Evaluation of hemostatic defects secondary to vascular tumors in dogs: 11 cases (1983–1988). JAVMA 198:891–894, 1991.
52. Oksanen A: Haemangiosarcoma in dogs. J Comp Pathol 88:585–595, 1978.
53. Ward H, Fox LE, Calderwood-Mays MB, et al: Cutaneous hemangiosarcoma in 25 dogs: A retrospective study. J Vet Intern Med 8:345–348, 1994.
54. Liptak JM, Dernell WS, Withrow SJ: Haemangiosarcoma of the urinary bladder in a dog. Aust Vet J 82:215–217, 2004.
55. Mellanby RJ, Chantrey JC, Baines EA, et al: Urethral haemangiosarcoma in a boxer. J Small Anim Pract 45:154–156, 2004.
56. Locke JE, Payne SE, Barber LG: Canine primary renal hemangiosarcoma: A retrospective study. Proc 24th Annu Conf Vet Cancer Soc:21, 2004.
57. Priester WA: Hepatic angiosarcomas in dogs: An excessive frequency as compared with man. J Natl Cancer Inst 57:451–454, 1976.
58. Hahn FF, Muggenburg BA, Boecker BB: Hepatic neoplasms from internally deposited 144CeCl3. Toxicol Pathol 24:281–289, 1996.
59. Tucker DW, Olsen D, Kraft SL, et al: Primary hemangiosarcoma of the iliopsoas muscle eliciting a peripheral neuropathy. JAAHA 36:163–167, 2000.
60. Jeffery ND: Treatment of epidural haemangiosarcoma in a dog. J Small Anim Pract 32:359–362, 1991.
61. Muhgannam AJ, Hacker DV, Spangler WL: Conjunctival vascular tumours in six dogs. Vet Comp Ophthalmol 7:56–59, 1997.
62. Liapis IK, Genovese L: Hemangiosarcoma of the third eyelid in a dog. Vet Ophthalmol 7:279–282, 2004.
63. Feeney DA, Johnston GR, Grindem CB, et al: Malignant neoplasia of canine ribs: Clinical, radiographic, and pathologic findings. JAVMA 180:927–933, 1982.
64. Pirkey-Ehrhart N, Withrow SJ, Straw RC, et al: Primary rib tumors in 54 dogs. JAAHA 31:65–69, 1995.
65. Baines SJ, Lewis S, White RA: Primary thoracic wall tumours of mesenchymal origin in dogs: A retrospective study of 46 cases. Vet Rec 150:335–339, 2002.
66. Parchman MB, Crameri FM: Primary vertebral hemangiosarcoma in a dog. JAVMA 194:79–81, 1989.
67. Mackenzie GB, Bellah JR, Threatte RM: What is your diagnosis? Hemangiosarcoma of the cervical vertebrae. JAVMA 222:1075–1076, 2003.
68. Erdem V, Pead MJ: Haemangiosarcoma of the scapula in three dogs. J Small Anim Pract 41:461–464, 2000.
69. Henry CJ, Selting KA, Turnquist SE, et al: Canine primary skeletal hemangiosarcoma: 17 cases. Proc 22nd Annu Conf Vet Cancer Soc:4, 2002.
70. Liptak JM, Dernell WS, Ehrhart EJ, et al: Retroperitoneal sarcomas in dogs: 14 cases (1992–2002). JAVMA 224:1471–1477, 2004.
71. Schoeman JP, Stidworthy MF, Penderis J, Kafka U: Magnetic resonance imaging of a cerebral cavernous haemangioma in a dog. J S Afr Vet Assoc 73:207–210, 2002.
72. Rallis TS, Tontis D, Adamama-Moraitou KK, et al: Hepatic haemangioma associated with ascites in a dog. Vet Rec 142:700–701, 1998.
73. HogenEsch H, Hahn FF: Primary vascular neoplasms of lymph nodes in the dog. Vet Pathol 35:74–76, 1998.
74. Burgess KE, Green E, Wood D, Dubielzieg RR: Angiomatous proliferation of the nasal cavity in 13 dogs. Proc 21st Annu Conf Vet Cancer Soc:69, 2001.
75. Lawler DF, Evans RH: Multiple hepatic cavernous lymphangiomas in an aged male cat. J Comp Pathol 109:83–87, 1993.
76. Goldschmidt MH, Shofer FS: Cutaneous lymphangioma, in Goldschmidt MH, Shofer FS (eds): Skin Tumors of the Dog and Cat, ed 1. Tarrytown, NY, Pergamon Press 1992, pp 217–221.
77. Webb JA, Boston SE, Armstrong J, Moens NM: Lymphangiosarcoma associated with

primary lymphedema in a Bouvier des Flandres. *J Vet Intern Med* 18:122–124, 2004.

78. Sagartz JE, Lairmore MD, Haines D, et al: Lymphangiosarcoma in a young dog. *Vet Pathol* 33:353–356, 1996.

79. Myers NC 3rd, Engler SJ, Jakowski RM: Chylothorax and chylous ascites in a dog with mediastinal lymphangiosarcoma. *JAAHA* 32:263–269, 1996.

80. Danielsson F: Lymphangioma in the metacarpal pad of a dog. *J Small Anim Pract* 39:295–298, 1998.

81. Voges AK, Ackerman N: MR evaluation of intra- and extracranial extension of nasal adenocarcinoma in a dog and cat. *Vet Radiol Ultrasound* 36:196–200, 1995.

82. Diessler ME, Castellano MC, Massone AR, et al: Cutaneous lymphangiosarcoma in a young dog: Clinical, anatomopathological and lectinhistochemical description. *J Vet Med A Physiol Pathol Clin Med* 50:452–456, 2003.

83. Kelly WR, Wilkinson GT, Allen PW: Canine angiosarcoma (lymphangiosarcoma). *Vet Pathol* 18:224–227, 1981.

84. Franklin RT, Robertson JJ, Thornburg LP: Lymphangiosarcoma in a dog. *JAVMA* 184:474–475, 1984.

85. Waldrop JE, Pike FS, Dulisch ML, et al: Chylothorax in a dog with pulmonary lymphangiosarcoma. *JAAHA* 37:81–85, 2001.

86. Barnes JC, Taylor SM, Clark EG, et al: Disseminated lymphangiosarcoma in a dog. *Can Vet J* 38:42–44, 1997.

87. Woods JP, Johnstone IB, Bienzle D, et al: Concurrent lymphangioma, immune-mediated thrombocytopenia, and von Willebrand's disease in a dog. *JAAHA* 31:70–76, 1995.

88. Fossum TW, Hodges CC, Scruggs DW, Fiske RA: Generalized lymphangiectasis in a dog with subcutaneous chyle and lymphangioma. *JAVMA* 197:231–236, 1990.

89. Belanger MC, Mikaelian I, Girard C, Daminet S: Invasive multiple lymphangiomas in a young dog. *JAAHA* 35:507–509, 1999.

90. Berry WL, Nesbit JW, Pearson J: Lymphangiomatosis of the pelvic limb in a Maltese dog. *J Small Anim Pract* 37:340–343, 1996.

91. Stambaugh JE, Harvey CE, Goldschmidt MH: Lymphangioma in four dogs. *JAVMA* 173:759–761, 1978.

92. Turrel JM, Lowenstine LJ, Cowgill LD: Response to radiation therapy of recurrent lymphangioma in a dog. *JAVMA* 193:1432–1434, 1988.

93. Itoh T, Mikawa K, Mikawa M, et al: Lymphangiosarcoma in a dog treated with surgery and chemotherapy. *J Vet Med Sci* 66:197–199, 2004.

TUMORS OF THE ENDOCRINE SYSTEM

Antony S. Moore and Gregory K. Ogilvie

CLINICAL BRIEFING

MDB (includes a CBC, biochemical profile, urinalysis, and thoracic radiography [three views]).

Hyperadrenocorticism

Clinical factors
- Hypercortisolism, polydipsia, polyuria, polyphagia (potbelly), and cutaneous changes.
- CNS dysfunction with large pituitary tumors.
- Pituitary adenomas of pars distalis lead to bilateral adrenal hyperplasia in 80% of dogs.
- Adrenal gland tumors (usually carcinomas) account for the remainder.
- Affects middle-aged to old dogs.
- Poodles, dachshunds, and boxers may be at higher risk; no gender predilection.

Staging and diagnosis
- MDB and urine culture.
- Metastasis of pituitary tumors rare.
- Adrenal tumors are locally invasive and commonly metastasize.
- Adrenal function testing to screen for hyperadrenocorticism and to aid in differentiation of PDH from adrenal tumor.
- Abdominal ultrasonography.
- CT scan if pituitary tumor suspected.

Prognostic factors
- None identified.

Treatment

Initial
- Surgery is the treatment of choice for adrenal tumors.
- Transsphenoidal hypophysectomy may be considered for pituitary tumors.
- Medical management is most common for pituitary tumors.
- Mitotane offers good long-term palliation by effects of adrenocortical destruction.
- Trilostane and ketoconazole inhibit steroid synthesis.
- Mitotane may be a useful agent at high doses for adrenal tumors.
- Trilostane may palliate signs in dogs with adrenal tumors.

Adjunctive
- Radiation therapy provides good palliation of neurologic dysfunction caused by large pituitary tumors and gives moderate control of cortisol levels.

Insulinoma	
Clinical factors	• Hypoglycemia and hyperinsulinemia caused by pancreatic islet cell tumor. • Weakness, lethargy, collapse, seizures, and peripheral neuropathies. • Signs are frequently intermittent. • Peripheral polyneuropathy may cause tetraparesis. • Most tumors are carcinomas. • Older dogs affected with no gender predisposition. • Large-breed dogs more commonly affected.
Staging and diagnosis	• MDB and high or "normal" fasting insulin level in the face of hypoglycemia. • Abdominal ultrasonography. • Most tumors are highly metastatic, primarily to the liver. • Assess lymph nodes and liver by biopsy during surgery.
Prognostic factors	• Surgery is more effective than medical management; both may be needed. • Dogs with tumors confined to pancreas have a longer symptom-free period and survival after surgery. • Dogs with only lymph node metastases live longer than dogs with distant metastases.
Treatment	
Initial	• Surgery is treatment of choice and provides palliation, even if metastases present.
Adjunctive	• Medical management using prednisone or diazoxide may maintain quality of life after surgery. • Chemotherapy with streptozocin may be effective in some dogs.
Supportive	• Dogs with peripheral neuropathy may benefit from corticosteroids. • Frequent feeding of a low glycemic-index food may help control hypoglycemia.
Thyroid Tumors	
Clinical features	• Most common reason for presentation is a mass in ventral neck. • Rarely, signs of hyperthyroidism. • Older dogs affected with no gender predilection. • Beagles, golden retrievers, and boxers predisposed.
Staging and diagnosis	• Local invasion is common; moderate metastatic rate. • MDB and lymph node assessment by physical examination and ultrasonography.
Prognostic factors	• Dogs with invasive tumors ("fixed" to underlying tissues) have worse survival rates. • Dogs with large tumors have worse survival rates. • Not correlated with histologic type, age, breed, or gender.
Treatment	
Initial	• Surgery may be curative for adenomas; may provide long-term control of small, noninvasive carcinomas, but these have potential to metastasize.
Adjunctive	• External-beam radiation may improve local control or reduce size of mass before surgery. • Radioiodine (^{131}I) may stabilize disease or cause regression. • Cisplatin and doxorubicin both have antitumor activity in adenocarcinomas, and both may have an adjunctive role with surgery.
Supportive	• Pain medication after surgery or radiation therapy; treatment of mucositis after radiation. • Appetite stimulants and nutritional support as needed.

> **Other Tumors Reviewed**
> - Gastrinomas, glucagonomas, pheochromocytomas, parathyroid tumors.

The major effect of most neoplasms is functional impairment of an organ or structure. Tumors of the endocrine system also affect the host by producing hormones at elevated levels.

Hyperadrenocorticism

PITUITARY-DEPENDENT HYPERADRENOCORTICISM

Incidence, Signalment, and Etiology

The clinical syndrome of hyperadrenocorticism is a result of adrenocorticotropic hormone (ACTH) secretion by pituitary tumors. Hyperadrenocorticism is the most common endocrinopathy in dogs. Affected dogs are middle aged to old (>6 years of age). Neither gender is predisposed. Poodles, dachshunds, and boxers are at increased risk. Adenoma of the pars distalis of the pituitary is the most common tumor in this disease, although pars intermedia tumors have also been described.

Most pituitary tumors in dogs produce ACTH; however, tumors that produce growth hormone (and cause secondary diabetes mellitus) have been reported.[1] Central diabetes insipidus may be associated with a pituitary tumor[2] and was associated with neurologic signs that developed many months after diagnosis in 10 of 20 dogs, most of which had a pituitary tumor on computed tomography (CT) or at necropsy.[3] Rarely, a pituitary tumor causes hypopituitarism.[4]

Clinical Presentation and History

Most dogs (80%–85%) with hyperadrenocorticism have a secretory tumor of the pituitary, usually a microadenoma. Dogs with hyperadrenocorticism show signs of polydipsia, polyuria, polyphagia, abdominal distention, muscle weakness, and biochemical abnormalities, as well as skin and haircoat changes. These signs are reviewed in detail in other publications.[5] Occasionally, the tumor is large and clinical signs are complicated by tumor expansion into the hypothalamus. Dogs with pituitary macroadenomas or macroadenocarcinomas may show central nervous system (CNS) signs of mental dullness, disorientation, ataxia, blindness, or convulsions (see Chapter 49).

Staging and Diagnosis

Clinical signs, dilute urine, a stress leukogram, and elevated serum alkaline phosphatase (ALP) level are classic findings in the disease. Screening tests for hyperadrenocorticism include a low-dose dexamethasone-suppression test (LDDST), a urine cortisol:creatinine ratio, and an ACTH stimulation test. In the LDDST, 0.01 mg/kg dexamethasone is injected intravenously. Pretreatment and 4- and 8-hour posttreatment serum samples are collected for cortisol levels. Failure to suppress cortisol levels at 8 hours indicates hyperadrenocorticism; concurrent suppression at 4 hours is supportive of pituitary-dependent hyperadrenocorticism (PDH).[6] The ACTH stimulation test is a shorter test that measures cortisol levels before and 1 hour after injection of ACTH. It differentiates naturally occurring from iatrogenic hyperadrenocorticism and is useful for monitoring response to therapy. The urine cortisol:creatinine ratio is a sensitive but nonspecific screening test that can be conducted on a single urine sample obtained at home. Figure 57-1 outlines the procedures for evaluating a dog with suspected hyperadrenocorticism (Cushing's syndrome).

Differentiation of pituitary-dependent disease from the less common adrenal-dependent disease can be aided by measuring the endogenous ACTH level, conducting a high-dose dexamethasone suppression test (HDDST; 0.1 mg/kg IV), and obtaining abdominal ultrasonographs.[5] Failure of cortisol suppression with the HDDST at 4 and 8 hours suggests adrenal-dependent hyperadrenocorticism. In dogs with adrenal tumors, measurement of plasma ACTH levels should be undetectable to low; however, ACTH is labile, and samples must be handled very carefully to ensure valid results.[5] In addition to routine blood work and thoracic radiographs as a general health screen, abdominal radiographs should be obtained to screen for metastatic disease, and a urine sample should be obtained for culture because there is a high incidence of occult urinary tract infection in these dogs.

Ultrasonography may be helpful in imaging the adrenal glands. Bilaterally symmetric adrenal hypertrophy is consistent with pituitary stimulation; asymmetric adrenal glands suggest an adrenal tumor (see Adrenocortical Tumors section, below).[7]

Macroadenoma of the pituitary gland, which can cause clinical signs of an intracranial mass as well as endocrinopathy, can be confirmed by CT or magnetic resonance imaging (MRI).[8] CT or MRI scanning should also be conducted if surgery is anticipated because either will allow localization of the pituitary relative to surgical landmarks, and dogs with macroadenomas can be identified and treated appropriately.[9,10] When dynamic contrast CT is conducted, localized microadenomas can also be identified, and diffuse pituitary involvement may be visualized.[10]

Occasionally, a dog has PDH and an adrenal tumor. Diagnostic testing for this rare condition is complicated, and ultrasonography as well as CT or MRI may be needed to diagnose these complicated cases.[11]

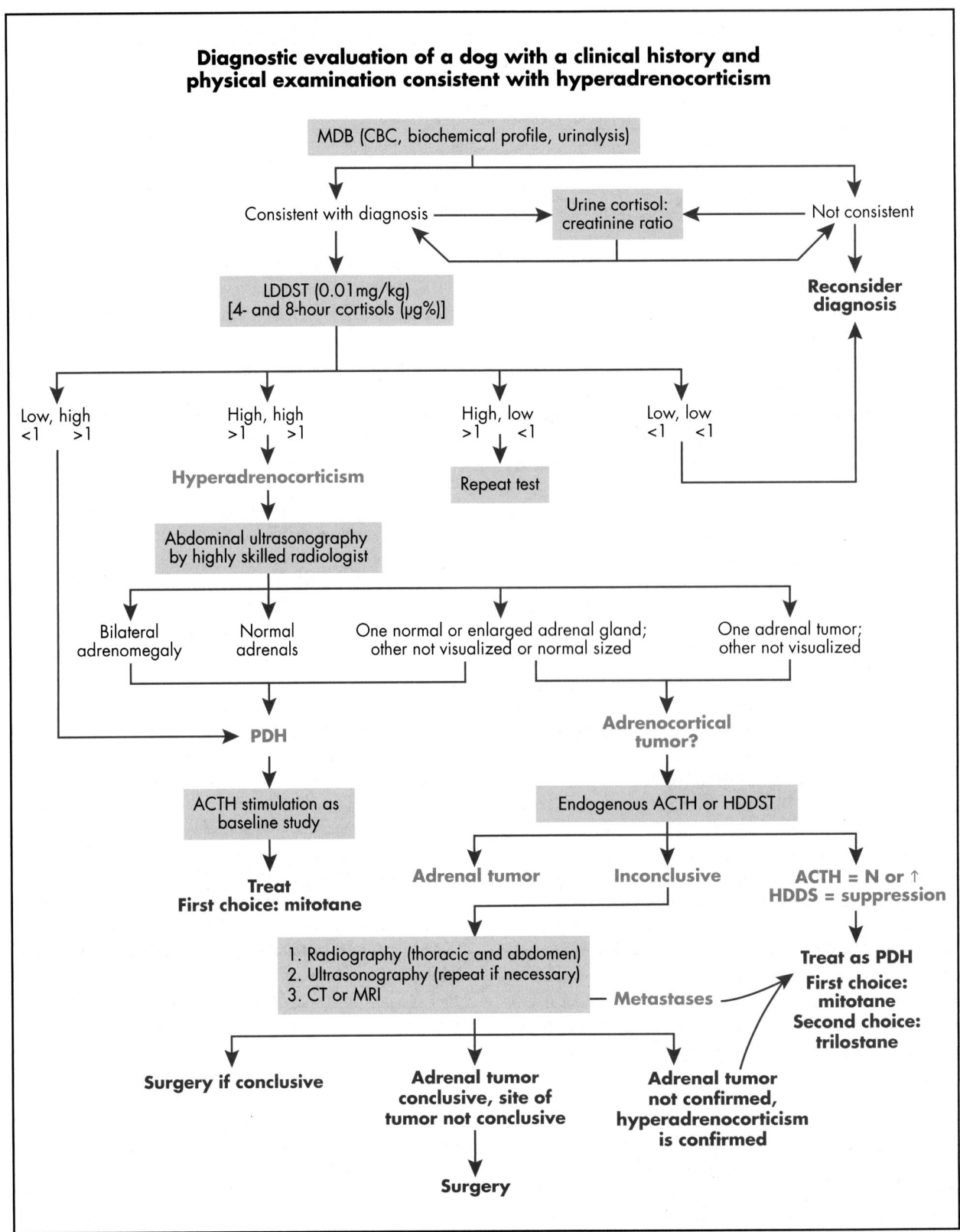

Figure 57-1. *A schematic flowchart for the diagnosis of a dog suspected to have hyperadrenocorticism. (Adapted from Feldman EC, Nelson RW: Canine and Feline Endocrinology and Reproduction, ed 3. Philadelphia, WB Saunders, 2003; with permission)*

Treatment
Surgery

Surgical hypophysectomy and bilateral adrenalectomy have been successful in treating PDH.[12] However, with either approach, excellent surgical skills, close postoperative monitoring, and lifelong hormonal supplementation are required; therefore, medical management is usually recommended. In a series of 52 dogs treated by transsphenoidal hypophysectomy, there were five surgery-related deaths and four dogs in which excision was grossly incomplete.[9] The remaining 43 dogs went into remission, and only five dogs had a relapse of hyperadrenocorticoid signs. Postsurgical CT scanning demonstrated hypophyseal remnants in 15 dogs. Only one of these dogs had a relapse of PDH; hence, postoperative CT was not helpful in predicting relapse. The 1-year survival rate was 84%, and the 2-year survival rate was 80%. Complications included transient hypernatremia and transient dry eye (18 dogs). Diabetes insipidus requiring vasopressin treatment was permanent in five dogs and prolonged in nine dogs (median duration: 4 months), and all dogs had secondary hypothyroidism requiring supplementation. In this study, experience in performing the procedure reduced the complication rate.

Medical Therapy

Mitotane (o,p'-DDD) is selectively cytotoxic to the adrenal cortex and is capable of causing hypoadrenocorticism. Mitotane is administered in two phases: a high induction dose and a lower maintenance dose. The induction dose is 50 mg/kg PO given in divided daily doses for up to 7 days until the first signs of decreasing appetite or thirst are noted. An ACTH stimulation test is then conducted to evaluate efficacy, the goal being subnormal pre- and poststimulation cortisol levels (1–5 µg/dl; 40–100 nmol/L). If control is incomplete, the induction dose is continued in weekly increments, with an ACTH stimulation test at the end of each week until control is achieved. Prednisone (0.2 mg/kg/day) can be given concurrently to help reduce toxic side effects; however, many endocrinologists find that it interferes with interpretation of test results and do not recommend it. If used, prednisone should be withheld on days when testing is conducted because it artificially elevates cortisol values. Anorexia, vomiting, and weakness are toxic effects that necessitate temporary cessation of mitotane therapy. After control is achieved, a maintenance dose of mitotane (50–200 mg/kg/wk) is given in divided doses with periodic ACTH stimulation tests to monitor the effectiveness of treatment.[5] The disease is considered well controlled if ACTH stimulation tests indicate that pre- and poststimulation cortisol levels are at or somewhat below normal levels. The urine cortisol:creatinine ratio has been suggested to be a good test to monitor dogs medically treated for PDH, but one study found that it consistently overestimated efficacy, thereby risking undertreatment with mitotane.[13]

An alternative protocol suggests destroying the adrenal cortices with high-dose mitotane, after which hypoadrenocorticism requires lifelong glucocorticoid and mineralocorticoid supplementation.[14] In one study of this protocol, recurrence of signs was uncommon, and investigators believed the protocol to be superior to conventional mitotane therapy for symptom and toxicity control. The protocol was also useful in treating adrenal tumors and occasionally resolved all evidence of grossly measurable tumor. Clinicians are advised to read the original article before using the protocol.[14] Briefly, mitotane (50–75 mg/kg PO) is given daily for 25 days in divided doses with meals. On the third treatment day, supplementation is started with cortisone acetate (2 mg/kg divided bid PO until 1 week after mitotane is stopped, then 1 mg/kg divided bid), fludrocortisone acetate (0.0125 mg/kg sid PO), and sodium chloride (0.1 mg/kg PO divided into two or three meals).[14] Strict owner compliance and good veterinary support are required, particularly in the early stages of mitotane therapy, when the risk of hypoadrenocorticism is highest. A repeat ACTH stimulation test 1 week after mitotane therapy has ended, particularly for adrenal tumors, ensures that functional adrenocortical tissue has been destroyed. Serum electrolytes should be measured and an ACTH stimulation test conducted at least every 3 to 6 months thereafter.

Ketoconazole is an antifungal agent that acts to block adrenal and gonadal steroid synthesis in dogs. Unlike mitotane, it is not cytotoxic and has been recommended to control the signs of hyperadrenocorticism in specific situations: (1) for medical management of dogs with malignant adrenal tumors or when surgery is not an option, (2) in dogs with hyperadrenocorticism that cannot be treated with mitotane because of drug toxicity, and (3) before surgery in dogs with an adrenal tumor. Ketoconazole is effective in rapidly reducing cortisol secretion (within 30 min of administration).[15] It is given at a dose of 5 mg/kg PO bid for 1 week. If side effects (e.g., vomiting, hepatopathy) are absent, the dose is doubled. If there is no improvement in the ACTH stimulation test after 14 days, the dose may be increased to 15 mg/kg PO bid. The ACTH stimulation test should be started within 1 to 3 hours of the last ketoconazole dose. In a series of 43 dogs, eight (20%) did not respond to ketoconazole therapy; however, toxicity was rare, and overdosage resulting in hypoadrenocorticism was unusual.[15] When overdosage occurred, ketoconazole was suspended and glucocorticoid supplementation was provided. The response was rapid, and within days, ketoconazole could be reinitiated.

Trilostane is a synthetic competitive blocker of steroid synthesis. This drug is emerging as a therapy for PDH and possibly for adrenal-dependent hyperadrenocorticism. Rarely, trilostane suppresses aldosterone production; hence, hypokalemia is a risk associated with this therapy. In a small study of 11 dogs with PDH, clinical signs resolved in nine dogs by

6 months of treatment.[8] Marked clinical improvement was seen in one of the other two dogs, and moderate improvement was reported in the other. Adverse side effects were mild transient lethargy and anorexia in one dog each. In a further study, trilostane doses ranged from 5 to 50 mg/kg (median: 16.7 mg/kg) and successfully controlled PDH in 29 of 30 dogs.[16] Control was durable in many dogs. The authors recommended starting trilostane at 5 mg/kg once daily and then reassessing after 2 and 4 weeks of therapy by evaluating clinical signs and conducting an ACTH stimulation test 4 hours after trilostane treatment. The dosage could then be adjusted if needed and the dog rechecked 2 weeks later. If clinical signs do not improve and there is minimal improvement in the ACTH stimulation test, then increasing the dosage to 10 mg/kg or giving the drug twice daily is recommended. Trilostane is an efficacious and apparently safe medication for treatment of dogs with PDH.

L-Deprenyl is a drug that indirectly acts to increase dopamine levels. It has been useful in controlling PDH in horses, in which tumors of the pars intermedia cause excess ACTH secretion. There is disagreement about whether dopamine exerts regulatory effects on ACTH secretion from pars distalis tumors in dogs. One study found that at a dose of 2 mg/kg PO daily, this agent caused significant clinical and biochemical improvement in 30 dogs with PDH.[17] Another study showed clinical control in only two of 10 dogs.[18]

Radiation Therapy

For dogs with confirmed macroadenoma of the pituitary, 40 to 45 Gy of megavoltage radiation to the tumor and 1 cm of surrounding normal tissue resolved neurologic signs within 6 months of therapy.[19] Resolution of clinical signs of hyperadrenocorticism was more variable. Radiation alone decreased ACTH levels in some dogs to normal, but others required concurrent mitotane therapy. Hypopituitarism was not noted in any of the dogs treated. Radiation therapy for the treatment of pituitary microadenomas in dogs has been reported in a small case series.[20] Of six dogs, three had resolution of clinical signs; this resolution was transient in two dogs. Signs improved but did not resolve in two other dogs, and one dog did not improve. Imaging showed marked reduction in the size of the tumor in five of six dogs. Radiation therapy is best used for dogs with tumors larger than 1 cm in height.

Radiation therapy was not successful in treating pituitary tumors in two dogs with diabetes insipidus and neurologic signs.[3]

See Chapter 49 for more information on pituitary tumors.

ADRENOCORTICAL TUMORS
Incidence, Signalment, and Etiology

Most dogs with hyperadrenocorticism have a secretory pituitary tumor. In 15% to 20%, however, the cause of hyperadrenocorticism is an adrenal tumor. Approximately half of adrenal tumors are carcinomas. Poodles may be overrepresented.[21] Some adrenal tumors appear to produce only minimal quantities of cortisol and varying amounts of progesterone and 17-hydroxyprogesterone.[22,23]

Clinical Presentation and History

Excessive cortisol produces classic signs of hyperadrenocorticism, including polydipsia, polyuria, cutaneous changes, and biochemical abnormalities. These abnormalities are reviewed in greater detail in other publications.[5] None of these clinical signs will allow the clinician to distinguish between PDH and hyperadrenocorticism caused by an adrenal tumor.

Staging and Diagnosis

In addition to a minimum database (MDB), dogs with hyperadrenocorticism should undergo the screening and differentiation tests outlined in the Pituitary-Dependent Hyperadrenocorticism section, above, to differentiate PDH from an adrenal tumor. When an adrenal tumor is suspected, thoracic radiographs and abdominal ultrasonographs are indicated.

A recent study found that an LDDST was able to distinguish between hyperadrenocorticism caused by an adrenal tumor and PDH. Of 181 dogs that underwent the LDDST, cortisol suppression was seen in 111 dogs, all of which had PDH; none of 35 dogs with an adrenal tumor showed suppression.[24] After an HDDST, 137 of the 181 dogs showed suppression (two had adrenal tumors and 135 had PDH). The authors concluded that the LDDST has value as a discrimination test to distinguish dogs with PDH from those with an adrenal tumor and that the HDDST is only indicated in dogs with hyperadrenocorticism that is not suppressed in response to the LDDST.

If an experienced abdominal ultrasonographer is available, most dogs that are suspected of having an adrenal tumor on the basis of an LDDST are best examined by ultrasonography as the next step in diagnosis. The finding of symmetrically enlarged bilateral glands is most consistent with PDH; a unilaterally enlarged gland is most likely to be an adrenal tumor.[25] Bilateral adrenocortical tumors are seen in approximately 20% of dogs.[26,27] If both adrenal glands are symmetrically enlarged, non–dexamethasone-suppressible PDH should be suspected before bilateral adrenal tumors. Biopsy of an adrenal gland may confirm this diagnosis if an endogenous ACTH level or cranial CT scan cannot be conducted. When test results are equivocal, referral to an internal medicine specialist is advised. Rarely, a dog may have PDH and a concurrent adrenal tumor.[11]

Radiography could detect adrenal gland enlargement in just over 50% of dogs in one study.[28] Normal sizes of the adrenal glands in dogs are well established, with a median

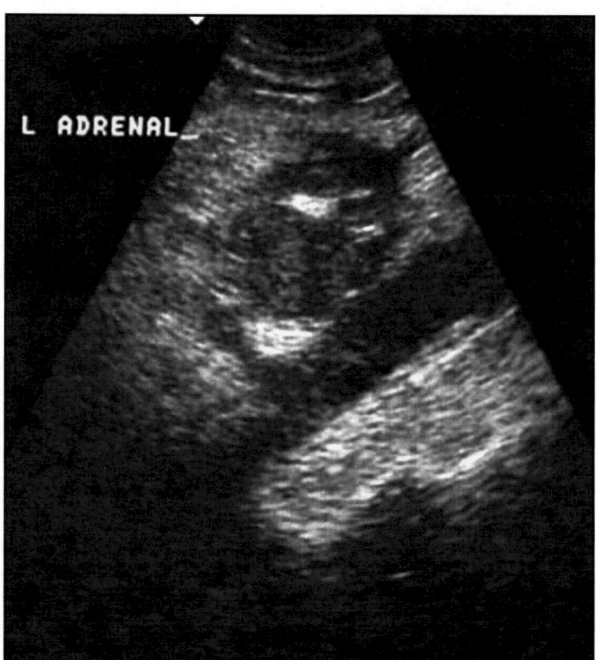

Figure 57-2. *Ultrasonography is more successful than radiography in detecting an adrenal tumor, and an experienced operator may discern not only the size and extent of the tumor but also whether the tumor has invaded the nearby caudal vena cava, as with this adrenal carcinoma. (Courtesy of Kenneth M. Rassnick, DVM, Cornell University College of Veterinary Medicine)*

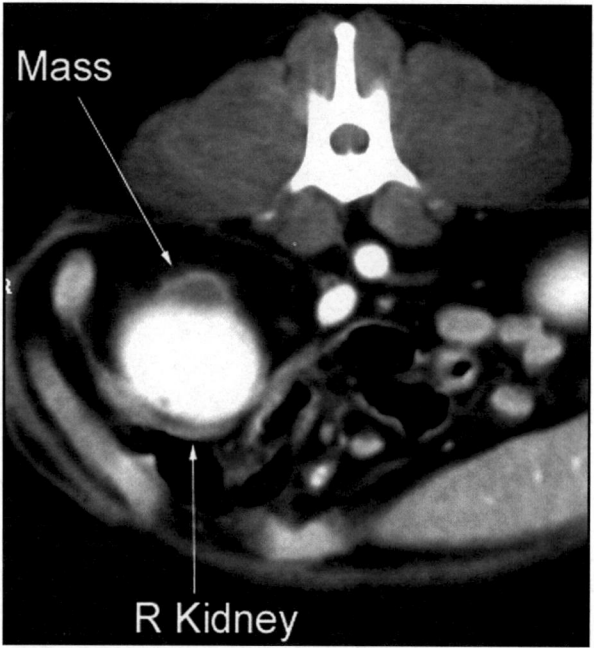

Figure 57-3. *A CT scan in this dog demonstrated a mass cranial to the kidney that compresses and possibly invades the caudal vena cava. The mass also causes ventral displacement of the right kidney and intestines. The diagnosis during surgery was an adrenal carcinoma and a renal cyst. (Courtesy of K. M. Rassnick)*

length of 17 mm and a median thickness of 4 mm; dimensions of adrenal tumors are at least twice these normal values.[27] A mineralized adrenal mass may be seen on radiographs in 25% to 50% of dogs with an adrenal tumor and can be associated with malignancy, but some benign tumors are mineralized.[29] In one study, an adrenal tumor was detected radiographically in only eight of 31 dogs.[21] Ultrasonography is a more sensitive diagnostic aid that may enable detection of an adrenal mass and invasion of adjacent blood vessels; it also allows visualization of other abdominal organs for lesions suggestive of metastases (Figure 57-2). Although one early study found that ultrasonography was successful in detecting only six of 13 adrenal masses,[21] ultrasonography is becoming the imaging modality of choice as the equipment improves and operators gain more experience.[27,29,30] Vascular invasion may be more difficult to discern.[29] Abdominal ultrasonography cannot distinguish between an adrenal adenoma and a carcinoma, although the finding of a large nonencapsulated mass is most suggestive of a carcinoma.[29]

CT and MRI are also very successful in visualizing adrenal masses, and CT obtained a positive finding in all 11 dogs in one study.[21] Anesthesia and expense are the major drawbacks of these imaging techniques (Figure 57-3).

Carcinomas commonly metastasize, usually to the liver but also to the lungs; however, metastases may not be clinically detectable for months to years after initial diagnosis. The overall metastatic rate was 14% in one study[31] but was 44% in a larger study.[21] Screening dogs with adrenal tumors for metastatic disease before surgery or mitotane therapy requires thoracic radiographs and abdominal ultrasonographs.

Treatment

Because it is not possible to distinguish between adrenal adenomas and carcinomas in dogs without metastatic disease, surgical removal is the treatment of choice for solitary adrenal tumors. Surgery is technically demanding, especially with vascular invasion, and referral to a specialist facility is recommended. Surgical excision of adenomas is often curative. Surgery may also be curative for carcinomas if metastasis has not occurred.

Atrophy of the contralateral adrenal gland is a consistent finding with adrenal tumors (Figure 57-4). The excess cortisol from the tumor provides negative feedback to the contralateral gland, which may take weeks to months to regain normal function after the tumor is removed. Exogenous glucocorticoids are required until the contralateral gland regains function.[32] On the morning before surgery, large doses of IV steroids should be given (5 mg/kg soluble hydrocortisone, 2.0 mg/kg prednisone sodium succinate or 0.1 to 0.2 mg/kg dexamethasone). Just before surgery, dogs with adrenal tumors should be treated with 15 mg/kg of keto-

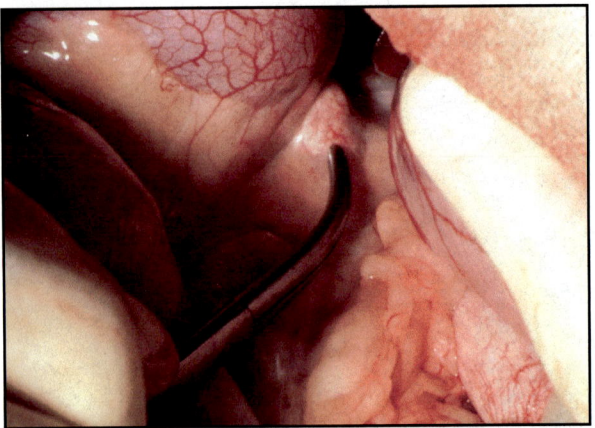

Figure 57-4. Surgical exploration may be necessary to demonstrate an adrenal mass, as pictured. The contralateral adrenal gland is usually atrophied as a result of cortisol secretion by the affected gland and consequent suppression of ACTH. (Courtesy of John Berg, DVM, Tufts Cummings School of Veterinary Medicine)

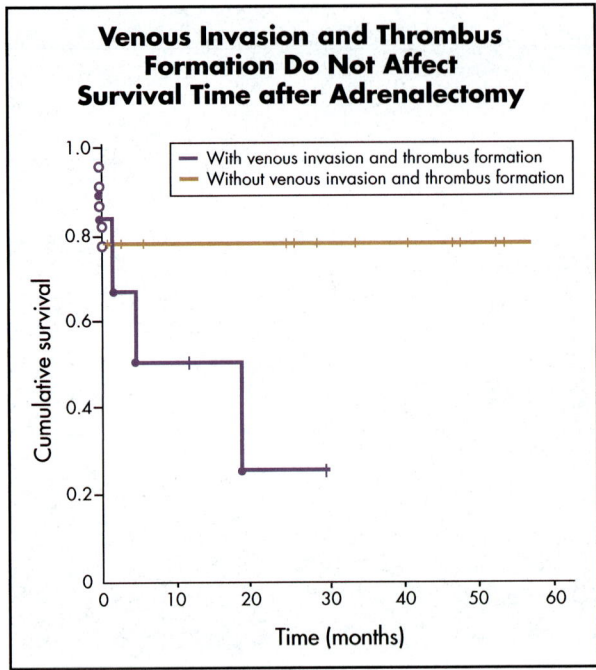

Figure 57-5. In a study of 28 dogs with adrenal tumors treated by adrenalectomy, there was no significant difference in survival times between dogs with (n = 6) and without (n = 22) venous invasion and thrombus formation. (Adapted from Kyles AE, Feldman EC, De Cock HE, et al: Surgical management of adrenal gland tumors with and without associated tumor thrombi in dogs: 40 cases (1994-2001). JAVMA 223:654–662, 2003; with permission)

conazole to normalize adrenocortical function and thereby improve surgical outcome. Ketoconazole reduces cortisol secretion within 30 minutes of administration. After surgery, the preoperative dose of steroids should be repeated. Starting on the first postoperative day, 0.5 mg/kg prednisolone or prednisone bid, 2.5 mg/kg cortisone bid, or 0.1 mg/kg dexamethasone sid should be given. After 7 to 10 days, the dose of steroids can be tapered; it can usually be discontinued by 2 months after surgery. Dogs with hyperadrenocorticism are at risk for pulmonary thromboembolic disease. A dose of 35 U/kg heparin given SC has been recommended by some authors during surgery and postoperatively bid, tapering to 10 U/kg bid SC over 3 to 4 days.[30]

> **KEY POINT**
>
> *Ketoconazole can control signs of hyperadrenocorticism before surgery in dogs with an adrenal tumor; heparin is required after surgery to reduce the risk of pulmonary thromboembolism.*

In a review of 25 dogs undergoing surgery for an adrenal tumor, 50% of the dogs that were not euthanatized during surgery developed serious complications, including cardiac arrest, pneumonia, pulmonary artery thromboembolism, pancreatitis, and acute renal failure.[32] Pancreatitis and peritonitis were the most common causes of perioperative mortality in eight of 36 dogs in another study.[33] However, in other reviews of dogs with adrenal tumors, complications after surgery were minimal, possibly because of the use of aggressive supportive care.[5,34] Of 183 dogs treated for adrenal tumors, 126 (69%) survived the postoperative period for reported medians of between 18 months and 3 years.[30-35] In one study, dogs with adrenal carcinomas had a median survival time of 26 months, but the median survival time for dogs with adenomas was not reached because no dog died of disease.[31] The difference in survival between the two groups was not significant. Other studies did not distinguish between adenomas and carcinomas. Some dogs with intraabdominal metastases are capable of long survival periods after surgery.[30]

Although invasion of the vena cava and thrombus formation is usually associated with pheochromocytomas, adrenocortical carcinomas may also invade this vessel.[30,36] In a study of 28 dogs with adrenal tumors treated by adrenalectomy, there was no difference in survival times between dogs with and without venous invasion and thrombus formation (Figure 57-5).[30]

Dogs with hyperadrenocorticism caused by adrenal tumors are generally more resistant to mitotane than those with pituitary tumors.[37] Treatment with mitotane results in fair to good control of cortisol levels in dogs with adrenocortical adenomas. For dogs with small carcinomas, similar results can be achieved with mitotane, but the duration of control is shorter. Mitotane was used to treat 32 dogs with adrenal tumors at doses that ranged from 27.5 to 75.0 mg/kg (average: 46.3 mg/kg) for 10 to 14 days.[21] After 2 weeks, hyperadrenocorticism was still present in 14 of 32 dogs. Higher doses of mitotane were required for a further period (median: 1 month) to control disease in these dogs. Signs were controlled in 30 dogs for periods ranging from 24 days to 4.9 years (median: 10.5 months), which is not as long as control after surgical excision. In dogs with large adrenocortical carcinomas or metastases, mitotane provides short-term palliation of signs; however, the high doses necessary to achieve these results are usually associated with unacceptable toxicity.[21,32] Mitotane may, however, be the only effective therapy in dogs with a recurrent adrenal carcinoma, and it can occasionally control signs for more than 1 year in these dogs.[33] Mitotane therapy is most useful in dogs with small tumors that are not candidates for surgery or as an adjunct to an incomplete surgery.

> **KEY POINT**
>
> *High doses of mitotane may be necessary to control signs in dogs with an adrenocortical carcinoma; surgery is the treatment of choice.*

Ketoconazole may provide control of clinical signs in dogs with adrenal tumors. In a small series, ketoconazole at a dose of 15 mg/kg q12h caused complete resolution of clinical signs of hyperadrenocorticism and reduced response to exogenous ACTH in all nine dogs with adrenal tumors.[15]

Trilostane is a synthetic competitive blocker of steroid synthesis. Suppression of aldosterone production and subsequent hypokalemia are risks with this drug. Trilostane at a dose of 4.4 mg/kg sid was able to manage signs for more than 20 months in a dog with an adrenal tumor.[38]

There are no reports of the efficacy of chemotherapy for adrenal tumors in dogs. There have been anecdotal responses, often of short duration, to doxorubicin- and cisplatin-based chemotherapy in about 20% of human patients.

Pheochromocytoma

INCIDENCE, SIGNALMENT, AND ETIOLOGY

Pheochromocytomas are functional tumors of the adrenal medulla that secrete catecholamines. These tumors are very rare and have been described in only a few dogs. Pheochromocytomas occur in old dogs with a median age of 11 years (range: 1–18 years). There is no obvious gender or breed predilection, although in one series of 98 dogs, miniature poodles and German shepherds each accounted for more than 10% of cases.[5] Rarely, pheochromocytoma may be bilateral.[39]

CLINICAL PRESENTATION AND HISTORY

Increased circulating catecholamines cause episodic or paroxysmal hypertension, with asymptomatic periods lasting from days to years. The resultant clinical signs may be vague; episodic panting, weakness, and restlessness are the predominant signs. In a series of 40 dogs, intermittent collapsing episodes, weakness, and panting or tachypnea each occurred in approximately one-third of dogs with pheochromocytomas.[5] Pheochromocytoma is frequently an incidental necropsy finding with no clinical history suggestive of its presence. In two studies, the diagnosis was an unexpected finding in 78 of 148 (53%) dogs.[5,39] In other dogs, diagnosis was made during anesthesia, or the tumor was found after sudden collapse and death. Pheochromocytoma was suspected before death in only 26% of dogs in one study.[39] CNS abnormalities, such as seizures attributable to brain metastasis or paraparesis attributable to aortic thrombus, were less common. Approximately 25% of dogs had clinical signs for more than 1 month and up to 3 years.[39]

It is rare that an abdominal mass is large enough to palpate, but two of 40 dogs in one series had a mass detected on abdominal palpation; a further four dogs had abdominal pain.[5]

STAGING AND DIAGNOSIS

In a dog with signs that could be compatible with a pheochromocytoma, abdominal ultrasonography is recommended to evaluate the adrenal glands. Some authors have suggested that dogs with clinical signs usually have a large tumor that is easily visualized (>80% had a tumor >2 cm in diameter); smaller tumors are usually incidental findings.[5,40] Abdominal ultrasonography is more sensitive than radiography in detecting an abdominal mass in the renal and adrenal region, particularly if the mass is small or if abdominal fluid is present. The contralateral adrenal gland should be of normal size. Although most tumors are localized to the adrenal gland, pheochromocytoma may obstruct the caudal vena cava and invade the vessel in about 40% of dogs.[41,42] Ultrasonography is usually able to detect vascular invasion.[30,40] Therefore, complete ultrasonographic evaluation of the vasculature adjacent to the tumor should be performed (Figure 57-2). Vascular invasion is suggestive of malignancy, although a venous thrombus may be seen with adrenal hyperplasia.[29] Rarely, a tumor may invade the spinal canal.[43]

Abdominal ultrasonography is such a good imaging modality for adrenal tumors that it is rarely necessary to conduct advanced imaging, but for dogs that are suspected to have a pheochromocytoma, CT may provide diagnostic and staging information.[44] As an adjunct to ultrasonography, renal caval contrast venography may outline venous thrombosis.[30]

Although the risk of catecholamine release would be suspected to be high, fine-needle aspiration of an adrenal pheochromocytoma without obvious complications has been reported; the cytologic diagnosis is usually carcinoma.[43]

In one study, thoracic radiographs showed nonspecific cardiovascular changes in many dogs. Although four of 50 dogs had pulmonary metastases, only two had radiographically detectable changes.[39] On necropsy, distant metastases to the lung, liver, spleen, kidney, and other sites were more common (12 of 50 dogs) than lymph node metastases (six of 50 dogs). Twenty-six of 50 dogs had local tumor invasion of surrounding tissue.[39]

Unlike dogs with adrenocortical tumors, dogs with pheochromocytomas rarely have any changes in biochemical profiles and complete blood count (CBC); this can be helpful in a dog with an unexpected adrenal mass diagnosed on abdominal ultrasonography.

High circulating levels of catecholamines and increased urinary excretion of their breakdown products are helpful in establishing the diagnosis; however, release is usually episodic, and the utility of such testing is usually low. Nuclear scintigraphy using iodine-123 metaiodobenzylguanidine (^{123}I-MIBG), a radioisotope that accumulates in chromaffin cells, may demonstrate accumulation in an adrenal mass first noted on ultrasonography. This is diagnostic for pheochromocytoma, and a negative scan reduces the chance of pheochromocytoma.[45]

Pheochromocytomas may be found in association with other endocrine tumors (multiendocrine neoplasia) as well as with other, unrelated tumors. Although uncommon, dogs with PDH or hyperadrenocorticism caused by an adrenal tumor may also have a pheochromocytoma. This should be suspected in a dog with an adrenal mass as well as PDH or if complications of hypertension arise during surgery for an adrenal cortical tumor.[40,46,47]

Staging of dogs with pheochromocytoma has been applied with possible prognostic value in one clinical study (Table 57-1). Of 13 dogs with a T0 tumor, none had metastases; of 24 dogs with a T1 tumor, two had metastases (one to lymph node and one distant); of six dogs with a T2 tumor, none had metastases; and of 18 dogs with a T3 tumor, seven had metastases (all distant, with three also to lymph node).[40]

TREATMENT

The treatment of choice for this rare tumor is surgery. However, surgery is technically demanding because many pheochromocytomas invade around the caudal vena cava and periaortic tissues. The situation is further complicated by the high risk of complications or death these patients face while undergoing anesthesia and surgery. Preoperative medical management to inhibit the effects of catecholamine is important. Phenoxybenzamine hydrochloride, an α-adrenergic–blocking agent, should be administered at a dosage of 0.5 to 2.5 mg/kg PO bid for 10 to 14 days before surgery, with dosing starting at the low end of the range and gradually increasing until the blood pressure is normal. Inhibition of catecholamine effects is also necessary for dogs that cannot undergo surgery.

The anesthesia used for dogs with pheochromocytoma must be selected carefully. Phenothiazines, such as acepromazine, should be avoided because they have α-blocking effects and could precipitate a hypotensive crisis. Narcotic agents may be used as preanesthetics. Because dogs with this tumor may show pronounced tachycardia after receiving atropine, its use should be avoided. Mask induction and maintenance anesthesia with isoflurane are recommended because isoflurane has low arrhythmogenic properties. Central venous pressure should be monitored throughout the surgery, and hypertensive episodes should be treated with IV phentolamine (constant rate infusion [CRI] of 1–2 μg/kg/min after a loading dose of 0.1 mg/kg), a short-acting competitive α-adrenergic blocker, or nitroprusside (CRI of 0.1–8.0 μg/kg/min). These drugs should be discontinued if intraoperative hypotension occurs.

Complications of surgery include hemorrhage, particularly if a venous thrombus must be resected, so blood products should be available (Figure 57-6). One study found that with careful surgery, the presence of caval invasion by the tumor did not increase the chances of postoperative complications or perioperative mortality.[30]

Table 57-1 **Staging Scheme Reflecting Tumor Size for Dogs with Pheochromocytoma**[40]

Tumor Stage	Description
T0	Microscopic tumor only
T1	Macroscopic tumor confined to the adrenal gland
T2	Local invasion of adjacent (nonvascular) structures
T3	Macroscopic vascular invasion

> *Appropriate supportive care before and after surgery can increase the likelihood of a successful outcome for a dog with a pheochromocytoma.*

In a series of 11 dogs with pheochromocytoma treated by excision, nine survived the perioperative period and none died of tumor-related causes over a median follow-up of 9 months (range: 1–36 months).[30] In another report of 12 dogs that had no metastases and were treated surgically with curative intent, most dogs died from unrelated causes, but one dog died because of metastatic pheochromocytoma 39 months after surgical excision.[40] Of the seven dogs with long-term follow-up, two dogs had a T1 tumor, three dogs had a T2 tumor, and two dogs had a T3 tumor; whether the tumor caused clinical signs or was an incidental finding did not appear to influence the prognosis.[40]

TUMORS OF THE ENDOCRINE SYSTEM

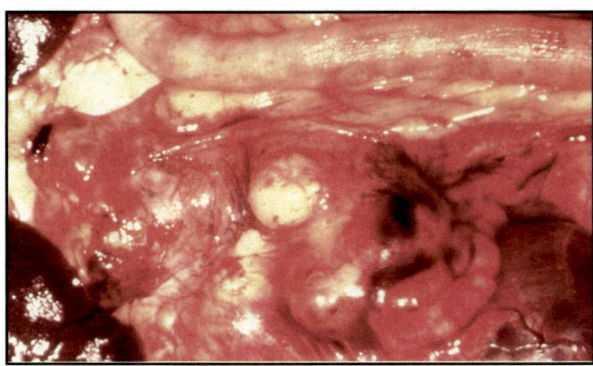

Figure 57-6. *This pheochromocytoma shows invasion around the perirenal tissue (kidney lower right of picture) as well as invasion of the vena cava.*

Chemotherapy for inoperable tumors in dogs has not been reported, although vincristine, dacarbazine, and cyclophosphamide are used in human patients and may be useful in dogs.

Pancreatic Tumors of the APUD System

The amine precursor uptake and decarboxylation (APUD) system comprises neuroendocrine-derived cells, most of which are found in the digestive system. Tumors derived from these cells are capable of producing active peptide hormones. In dogs, insulinomas are the most commonly diagnosed tumors of the APUD system, but gastrinomas, glucagonomas, and PPomas (tumors secreting pancreatic polypeptide [PP]) have all been described. Tumors derived from these cells are capable of producing any of a number of active peptide hormones, and one tumor may secrete multiple hormones at the same time. Therefore, it is not unusual for immunohistochemical staining to detect tumor cells secreting other hormones, which may be confusing to the clinician.[48,49] However, most tumors have a higher level of production of one hormone, and it is from this hormone production that their name is derived. In two studies of 43 dogs with a primarily insulin-secreting tumor, 18 tumors also had glucagon-secreting cells, 23 also secreted somatostatin, 28 also secreted PP, and two also secreted gastrin.[49,50] Additional hormones identified in studies include islet amyloid polypeptide, which is responsible for amyloid deposits seen mainly in tumors secreting insulin,[50,51] and ACTH.[52] There were no differences in metastatic rate for pancreatic endocrine tumors based on the presence of amyloid or the number of hormones contained within the tumor.[50]

Insulinoma
INCIDENCE, SIGNALMENT, AND ETIOLOGY

Insulinomas are functional, insulin-secreting β-cell tumors of the pancreas. Excessive insulin secretion by the tumor causes clinical signs of hypoglycemia. The mean age of onset of clinical signs in dogs with insulinoma is between 8 and 10 years (range: 4–14 years).[53-55] There is no apparent gender predisposition. Although insulinomas are reported in all sizes and many breeds of dog, large-breed dogs, such as Irish setters, golden retrievers, boxers, and German shepherds, are most frequently afflicted.[53,55]

CLINICAL PRESENTATION AND HISTORY

Clinical signs of hypoglycemia fall into two categories: adrenergic and neuroglycopenic. When glucose concentrations decrease rapidly, increased sympathetic tone may produce adrenergic signs such as tachycardia, nervousness, tremors, and hunger. With a more gradual decrease in blood glucose, neuroglycopenic signs may include seizures, dullness, weakness, confusion, and hypothermia. Signs may be episodic and may be related to events such as fasting, eating, or exercise. Studies indicate no correlation between stage of disease and clinical signs.[53]

A syndrome of peripheral polyneuropathy associated with canine (and human) insulinoma has been described, although the incidence is probably low.[56,57] Affected dogs may develop tetraparesis or paralysis after prolonged symptomatic hypoglycemia.[58,59] Affected dogs may also show muscle atrophy, hyporeflexia, or areflexia.[59] The pathophysiology of this paraneoplastic effect remains unclear. Current hypotheses explain this syndrome as (1) a metabolic defect of peripheral nerves that renders them susceptible to hypoglycemia, (2) an immune response arising from similarity between tumor and nerve tissue antigens, or (3) toxic effects on peripheral nerves caused by tumor-produced substances.

STAGING AND DIAGNOSIS

Insulinomas have been categorized as stage I (confined to the pancreas), stage II (confined to the pancreas and regional lymph nodes), and stage III (distant metastasis).[53] This staging system has some prognostic importance (see Prognostic Factors section, below). Insulinomas nearly always metastasize, even though they may lack histologic criteria of malignancy.

> **KEY POINT**
>
> *Prolonged hypoglycemia caused by insulinoma is associated with peripheral polyneuropathy.*

The only consistent abnormality seen on chemistry profiles is hypoglycemia; however, glucose concentrations may be within the normal range on an intermittent basis. Diagnosis is based on demonstration of inappropriately high insulin secretion concurrent with hypoglycemia. If initial testing for insulinoma fails to show simultaneous hypoglycemia and normal or increased insulin levels, the animal is retested. Glucose levels are monitored periodically during fasting until glucose decreases below a prescribed level, usually 60 mg/dl. At that time, serum insulin and glucose are measured. In normal animals, insulin levels should decrease as glucose concentration decreases.

Although controversial, results can be interpreted in light of the insulin:glucose ratio, glucose:insulin ratio, or amended insulin:glucose ratio (AIGR). An insulin:glucose ratio of greater than 0.3 or a glucose:insulin ratio of less than 2.5 supports the diagnosis of insulinoma. The AIGR is calculated as follows:

$$\frac{(\text{Serum insulin } [\mu U/ml] \times 100)}{(\text{Serum glucose } [mg/\mu l] - 30)} = \text{AIGR}$$

A result of greater than 30 indicates insulinoma.[54] The AIGR has been reported to be the most sensitive but least specific of these tests (i.e., it provides the fewest false-negative but the most false-positive results).[55,60] The test is particularly misleading when glucose concentrations are extremely low (<30 mg/dl). Therefore, the diagnosis of insulinoma should not be based solely on an abnormal AIGR. Dogs with low blood glucose should have a low blood–insulin level; any other finding (normal to high insulin level) must be considered abnormal. Provocative tests of insulin release can be used but are not usually necessary. In a fasted patient, glucose, glucagon, or tolbutamide is administered to release excess insulin from neoplastic cells. These tests are not without risk, however; tolbutamide, in particular, may cause severe and prolonged hypoglycemia and seizures.

> **KEY POINT**
>
> *Dogs with low blood glucose levels should have low blood insulin levels; any other insulin level must be considered abnormal.*

Radiography is rarely diagnostic of an insulinoma because the tumors are small even when clinical signs are advanced. In one study, one of 13 dogs with insulinoma had an enlarged liver as the only abnormality seen.[61] Because the tumors are small, ultrasonographic examination may not be revealing; however, when an experienced operator conducts the study, ultrasonography may reveal metastases to lymph nodes or other abdominal viscera. In one study, ultrasonography detected nine of 13 pancreatic insulinomas as a defined or possible pancreatic nodule that was spherical or lobulated and hypoechoic.[61] CT scans complement ultrasonography in human patients and could be useful in dogs when surgery is being contemplated but a tumor is not visualized. IV injection of methylene blue had been suggested as a method of detecting insulinomas and their metastases, but the risk of Heinz body anemia and the advances in ultrasonography have made this approach unnecessary.[62]

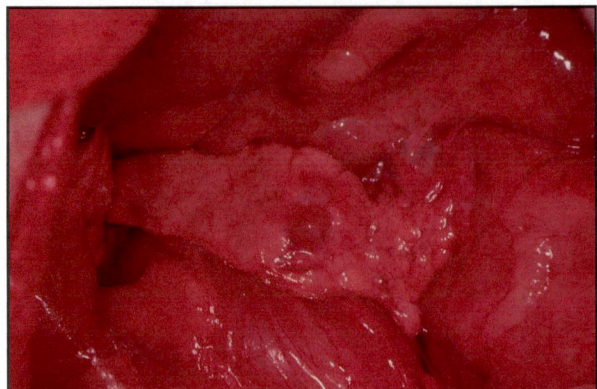

Figure 57-7. *Exploratory laparotomy is usually required to identify an insulinoma because these tumors are frequently very small. The regional lymph nodes and the liver should be examined carefully for evidence of metastatic spread. (Courtesy of J. Berg)*

One report documented the use of somatostatin receptor scintigraphy to diagnose a insulinoma.[63]

In dogs, definitive diagnosis is usually confirmed by exploratory laparotomy and histopathologic examination (Figure 57-7). Careful abdominal exploration, including abdominal lymph node palpation and gentle digital palpation of the pancreas, is important. Metastases are seen at the time of diagnosis in approximately half of insulinoma cases, and pancreatic masses may not be readily visualized. Pulmonary metastases are very rare.[61]

PROGNOSTIC FACTORS

In several studies, the mean survival time of all dogs with insulinoma has been estimated at about 12 months. Young dogs have shorter survival times than old dogs. For 52 dogs treated by surgery, dogs with stage I tumors had a mean hypoglycemia-free interval of 14 months, which was significantly longer than dogs with either lymph node or distant metastases; dogs with stage II tumors also lived longer than dogs that had distant metastases at the time of surgery[53] (Figure 57-8).

Another preliminary report found that 18 dogs that were hyperglycemic or normoglycemic after surgery had longer survival times (22 months) than eight dogs that were still hypoglycemic (3 months); this may reflect the stage of disease, which was not reported.[64]

TREATMENT
Surgery

The treatment of choice is wide surgical excision (partial pancreatectomy) in conjunction with preoperative or postoperative medical management. The mean survival is longer in dogs that undergo surgical resection than in dogs that receive medical management alone.[55,65] Masses are reportedly distributed approximately equally between the two lobes of the pan-

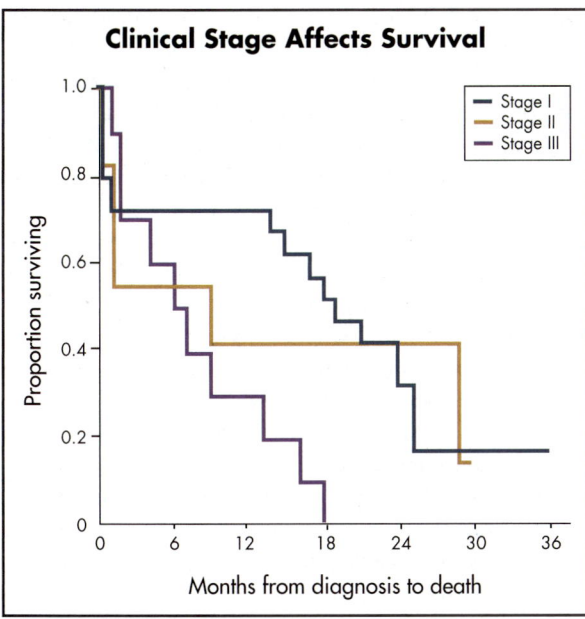

Figure 57-8. Dogs with stage I insulinoma (confined to the pancreas) have longer asymptomatic survival than dogs with metastases. Dogs with stage I or stage II (regional node metastasis) insulinoma live longer than dogs with distant metastases (stage III). (Adapted from Caywood DD, Klausner JS, O'Leary TP, et al: Pancreatic insulin-secreting neoplasms: clinical, diagnostic, and prognostic features in 73 dogs. JAAHA 24:577–584, 1988; with permission)

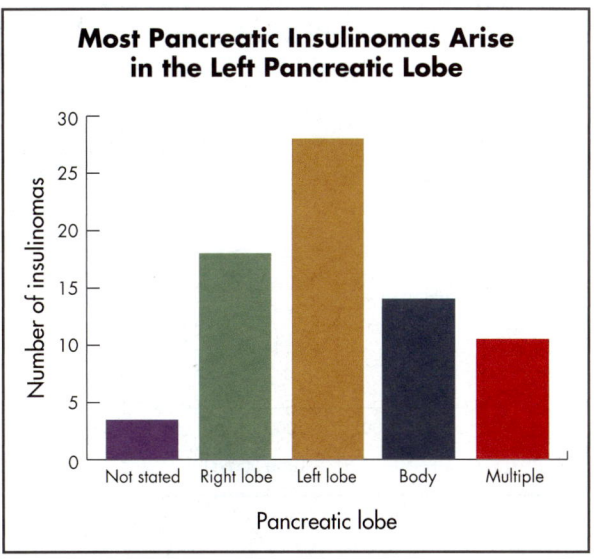

Figure 57-9. Distribution of pancreatic insulinomas in 73 dogs. (Adapted from Caywood DD, Klausner JS, O'Leary TP, et al: Pancreatic insulin-secreting neoplasms: clinical, diagnostic, and prognostic features in 73 dogs. JAAHA 24:577–584, 1988; with permission)

creas (Figure 57-9), and tumors are multiple in more than 10% of affected dogs.[53,64] Metastasis most commonly occurs to regional lymph nodes and liver, although metastases have also been reported in the mesentery, spleen, duodenum, and spinal cord. One source recommends removing one-half of the pancreas when the tumor is not visualized during surgery in an attempt to remove the portion that contains the tumor.[54]

A 5% glucose solution should be infused intravenously during and after surgery to prevent hypoglycemia. Preoperative and postoperative glucocorticoid therapy is also important. Adequate perioperative fluid therapy is necessary to prevent secondary pancreatitis by ensuring good circulation through the pancreatic microvasculature. A fluid rate of two times the maintenance levels has been recommended.

Postoperative complications include iatrogenic pancreatitis, diabetes mellitus that requires insulin therapy (for up to 1,118 days in one study),[55] hypoglycemia, and persistent seizures that continue despite resolution of hypoglycemia. Diabetes mellitus is believed to be caused by inadequate insulin secretion by atrophied normal β cells. Persistent seizures are attributed to cerebral laminar necrosis secondary to prolonged hypoglycemia.

The median survival reported for dogs treated by surgery with curative intent varies by study. An early study of 52 dogs treated with surgery found that 70% of dogs with stage I insulinoma, 55% of dogs with stage II insulinoma, and 42% of dogs with stage III insulinoma lived at least 1 month after surgery. There were some long survivors in all groups, although no dog with stage III insulinoma lived longer than 18 months.[53] The median survival of all dogs that were alive 1 month after surgery was 11.6 months, but dogs with metastases were less likely to survive.[53]

In another study, the median survival for dogs treated surgically was 12.5 months (not stratified by stage) compared with 2.4 months for dogs treated with dietary change with or without prednisone but no surgery[65] (Figure 57-10). Although medical management after surgery did help control hypoglycemia in some dogs, there was no difference in survival between dogs receiving and those not receiving medical management after surgery.[65]

> **Dogs with insulinoma confined to the pancreas during surgery have longer survival times than dogs with metastasis to the lymph nodes or distant sites.**

Medical Management

Medical management is indicated if surgery does not eliminate the insulin-secreting tumor or if surgery is not performed. Prolonged hypoglycemia may lead to neuronal necrosis and permanent damage to the CNS.[66] In some

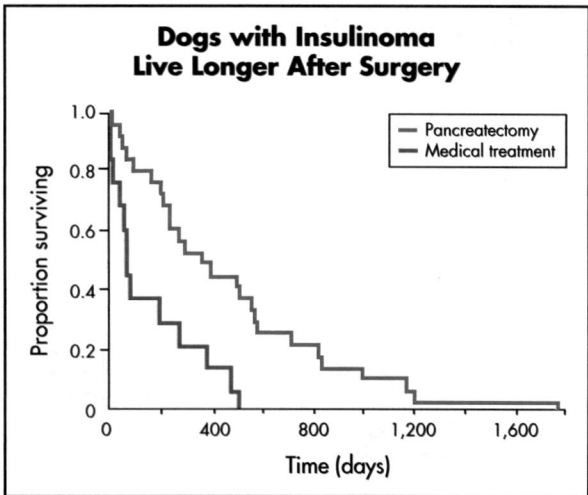

Figure 57-10. *Survival for 23 dogs with insulinoma treated by partial pancreatectomy versus survival for 13 dogs treated medically. The dogs treated with surgery lived significantly longer. (Adapted from Tobin RL, Nelson RW, Lucroy MD, et al: Outcome of surgical vs. medical treatment of dogs with beta cell neoplasia: 39 cases (1990-1997).* JAVMA 215:226–230, 1999; with permission)

dogs, frequent feedings of small, high-protein, low-carbohydrate meals, in addition to exercise restriction, may control hypoglycemia. If this fails, drug therapy must begin.

Corticosteroids cause peripheral insulin antagonism and gluconeogenesis, resulting in an increase in serum glucose levels and alleviation of clinical signs. Peripheral neuropathy may respond to prednisolone, even when hypoglycemia persists.[67] If prednisone is used as the initial treatment, a dosage of 0.5 mg/kg/day PO divided bid is given; this can be gradually increased to 4 mg/kg/day, if necessary. Prednisone can be administered in conjunction with diazoxide.

Diazoxide is a nondiuretic, benzothiadiazine antihypertensive drug with antiinsulin effects. It inhibits insulin secretion by blocking calcium mobilization, stimulates hepatic gluconeogenesis and glycogenolysis through stimulation of the β-adrenergic system, and decreases peripheral glucose utilization. It is expensive and sometimes difficult to obtain. In one study, diazoxide controlled hypoglycemia in 70% of dogs treated.[55] The recommended initial dosage is 10 mg/kg/day PO tid; the dosage may be increased gradually to 40 mg/kg/day.[55] The most common side effects are anorexia, vomiting, and diarrhea, which may be alleviated by administration with a meal. Sometimes control of hypoglycemia can be prolonged even at lower doses in individual animals; normoglycemia was maintained for 18 months in a dog with recurrent and metastatic insulinoma.[68]

Other drugs that have been used to treat insulinomas in dogs include somatostatin and its analogs (e.g., octreotide, propranolol, alloxan, streptozocin). Chemotherapy with streptozocin has been effective in human patients with insulinoma. Streptozocin is a nitrosourea alkylating agent that is selectively cytotoxic to β cells, although its clinical use in dogs has been limited by nephrotoxicity. Initial reports of toxicity with this drug were compromised by high dosages and lack of pretreatment hydration.[69-71] Streptozocin can be administered safely to dogs at a dose of 500 mg/m² every 3 weeks when combined with 0.9% NaCl diuresis, and it may have efficacy in the treatment of dogs with metastatic pancreatic islet cell tumors. In one study, 58 treatments were administered to 17 dogs with insulinoma. Only one dog developed renal disease. Elevations in serum alanine aminotransferase (ALT) levels were seen in some dogs and appeared to resolve with cessation of treatment. Hematologic toxicities were rare. Vomiting during administration was uncommon but occasionally severe despite the administration of butorphanol. Two dogs developed diabetes mellitus after receiving five treatments; these dogs were the longest survivors. Two dogs had rapid resolution of paraneoplastic peripheral neuropathy, and another two dogs had measurable reduction in the size of their tumors. The median normoglycemic survival for 14 evaluable dogs with stage II or III insulinoma treated with streptozocin was 163 days, which was longer than, but not significantly different from, 90 days for 15 historical control dogs that had been treated surgically and medically; there were long survivors in both groups.[72]

Serial measurement of fasting serum insulin and serum glucose levels is recommended as the best way to assess response in dogs treated with chemotherapy. Increases in insulin appear to precede hypoglycemia and may signal that a change of therapy is needed. Dogs treated with streptozocin should also have their renal function and serum liver enzyme activities checked at regular intervals.

Alloxan is also selectively cytotoxic to β cells. When this drug was administered once to normal dogs, two of five dogs developed hyperglycemia for many months.[73] Alloxan can be nephrotoxic. In limited clinical use, a dose of 65 mg/kg IV given once caused resolution of hypoglycemia after 3 to 5 days in four of eight dogs and lasted for several months. However, one dog died from acute renal failure, and two dogs died from acute respiratory distress syndrome or pulmonary edema within 24 hours of treatment.[5]

Octreotide is a long-acting somatostatin analogue that inhibits insulin synthesis and secretion. It effectively controlled clinical signs in two of five dogs for 1 and 9 months at a dose of 10 to 20 μg bid to tid SC.[74] In contrast, another report of octreotide showed no benefit in the three dogs that were treated.[75] More studies are needed before this treatment can be recommended.

Propranolol suppresses the insulin response to glucose and has been used in humans to induce hyperglycemia.

For dogs with acute episodes of hypoglycemia caused by uncontrolled insulinoma, acute and short-term control of seizures may be obtained by a CRI of glucagon. This method was used in one dog to stabilize signs while other methods of treatment were attempted. The dose used was 5 to 10 ng/kg/min.[76]

Gastrinoma
INCIDENCE, SIGNALMENT, AND ETIOLOGY

This tumor of the pancreas is notable for the production of gastrin and the resultant hypertrophic gastritis with peptic ulcers (Zollinger-Ellison syndrome). There are no breed or gender predilections noted for this rare tumor.[52,77,78]

CLINICAL PRESENTATION AND HISTORY

Similar to insulinomas, gastrinomas tend to be discrete and small within the pancreatic parenchyma, but occasionally they are only found as a metastatic lesion in the regional lymph node, and one dog had only a lesion in the root of the mesentery. Duodenal ulceration is common, seen in more than half of affected dogs; additional ulceration is seen in the stomach (45%) and, rarely, in the esophagus and jejunum.[5] Vomiting is the most common clinical sign, occurring in nearly all affected dogs. Hematemesis and melena are considerably less common, as is abdominal pain, which is usually a consequence of concurrent pancreatitis. Anorexia and weight loss are common sequelae to the gastric hyperacidity, and more than half the dogs are lethargic and depressed. Diarrhea is often watery and profuse, presumably because of hyperacidity and malabsorption.

STAGING AND DIAGNOSIS

In the few documented cases, 70% of gastrinomas were malignant.[5] Metastases were most commonly found in the liver (60%) and regional lymph nodes (30%) but were also found in the spleen and mesentery. Radiography rarely shows any abnormality unless a ruptured gastric ulcer and septic peritonitis are present. Ultrasonography is more likely to detect a tumor, although gastrinomas are often small and may be missed even by experienced operators. Liver metastases may be seen in dogs in which a pancreatic tumor is not visible. Gastroduodenoscopy cannot make a diagnosis of a gastrinoma, but the finding of hyperplastic gastric mucosa and ulceration may lead to a higher suspicion of this tumor. An elevated fasting gastrin level is supportive of, but not diagnostic for, a gastrinoma; serum gastrin may be elevated after treatment with H_2 blockers, such as cimetidine, corticosteroids, and proton pump inhibitors. Normal ranges of gastrin levels vary depending on the laboratory used but are usually in the range of 100 pg/ml; most affected dogs have a level two or more times the upper normal limit.

One report documented the use of somatostatin receptor scintigraphy to diagnose a gastrinoma.[79]

TREATMENT

Surgery can be used to resect a small, localized gastrinoma, but most gastrinomas have metastasized by the time diagnosis is confirmed. Surgery may also be needed if a gastric ulcer perforates the stomach. In a few reports of surgery in dogs, resection of the tumor and visible nodal metastases led to recurrence of signs within 1 to 2 months.[80] In a series of 16 dogs in which the location of the primary gastrinoma was known, most tumors (63%) occurred in the right lobe of the pancreas; 38% occurred in the pancreatic body, and only one dog had a gastrinoma in the left lobe. If there are no metastases and a tumor cannot be located, removal of the right lobe of the pancreas may resect the tumor.[5]

Chemotherapy has not been reported in treating this tumor, but an approach as for dogs with insulinoma may be successful.

Treatment with H_2 histamine-receptor blockers appears to benefit some patients; one dog was asymptomatic for 7 months when treated with cimetidine and sucralfate,[80] but others have had no response.[81]

Proton pump inhibitors (i.e., H^+, K^+, ATPase inhibitors), such as omeprazole, can relieve clinical signs of gastrinomas. One dog with an unresectable gastrinoma was refractory to treatment with H_2 blockers but was free of clinical signs for more than 2 years when treated with omeprazole (0.5–0.7 mg/kg PO sid).[81] However, another dog had no response when treated with omeprazole, metoclopramide, and ranitidine.[80] It seems that palliative therapy with omeprazole and an H_2 blocker (e.g., famotidine 0.5–1.0 mg/kg PO q12–24h) may be most successful in dogs with an unresectable or metastatic gastrinoma. Doses may need to be increased over time. Even for dogs with metastases, the clinical course may be prolonged by palliative therapy to decrease the stimulatory effect of gastrin on gastric acid secretion.

Alternative palliative treatments to decrease gastric acid secretion have been investigated. One dog with a gastrinoma was treated with octreotide at a dosage of 10 μg SC three times daily, as well as an H_2 blocker. Complete resolution of clinical signs was achieved for 20 months.[79] Attempts to discontinue therapy during this time resulted in recurrences of gastric ulceration and vomiting. Another dog treated with octreotide and omeprazole had resolution of signs that continued even when omeprazole was discontinued. Overall survival was 14 months after diagnosis.[79] Disadvantages of these treatments are the high cost and the need for frequent subcutaneous injections.

Glucagonoma
INCIDENCE, SIGNALMENT, AND ETIOLOGY

Glucagon is involved in the regulation of insulin release and stimulates catabolism of amino acids to glucose. Glucagonomas are very rare and appear to be without apparent gender or breed predisposition.

CLINICAL PRESENTATION AND HISTORY

The most startling clinical association in dogs with glucagonomas is superficial necrolytic dermatitis (canine metabolic epidermal necrosis). This dermatitis is characterized by hyperkeratosis of the footpads with painful fissuring. The mucocutaneous junctions on the head, perineum, and external genitalia and the surrounding skin are affected with an erythematous, erosive, crusting dermatitis. It is thought that low serum amino acids documented in affected dogs may lead to epidermal protein depletion and necrolysis of the keratinocytes. Some patients have a history of skin disease that is up to 1 year in duration.[82] Diarrhea (caused by reduced absorption of water and electrolytes) and hyperglycemia (potentially diabetes mellitus) are consequences of hyperglucagonemia. Other clinical signs are nonspecific and include lethargy, polydipsia and polyuria (presumably caused by secondary diabetes mellitus), and inappetence.[83]

STAGING AND DIAGNOSIS

Histologically, the skin lesions show superficial hydropic dermatitis and marked parakeratosis. This skin disease is very suggestive of a glucagonoma, but it has also been seen with liver disease and is not diagnostic. An MDB may show elevations in liver enzymes (ALP, ALT) and hyperglycemia.[5,83] If serum levels of amino acids are measured, all are usually markedly decreased.[83,84]

Radiographs rarely show any abnormality; ultrasonographs are more likely to detect a tumor, although glucagonomas are often small and may be missed even by experienced operators.[48,85] Liver metastases may be seen in dogs in which a pancreatic tumor is not visible. Concurrent pancreatitis was seen in one dog[83] and developed after surgery in other dogs.[85]

Plasma glucagon levels may be very high (normal levels reported are <80–250 pg/ml or 50 pmol/L) and are more than five times the upper limit in most affected dogs. A high plasma glucagon level combined with a tumor that demonstrates immunostaining for glucagon is diagnostic for a glucagonoma.

In the few dogs reported, metastases to the liver[82,83,86] and hepatic lymph nodes[84] seem to be common at diagnosis. Sometimes the primary tumor is not discernible and metastases are the only finding.[86] Some dogs appear to be free of metastases.[48]

TREATMENT

Surgery is probably the best approach to this disease; however, metastases to the liver and lymph nodes seem to be common at diagnosis. Two dogs treated surgically both died in the perioperative period, one because of pancreatitis.[85] One dog was treated by resection of a 2-cm pancreatic primary tumor and nodal metastases. Glucagon plasma levels were normal 1 day after surgery, and amino acid levels were improved by 1 month after surgery. The dog's skin improved starting 1 week after surgery, and all skin disease was resolved 1.5 months after surgery.[84] Although the initial report found the dog disease free 6 months after surgery, recurrence of signs apparently occurred 9 months after surgery.[5]

Palliative treatment of superficial necrolytic dermatitis may be achieved with highly available protein sources such as egg yolk[85] or Hill's Prescription Diet Canine a/d.[5] One dog responded briefly to corticosteroids (although care should be taken if the dog has diabetes)[82] and another to antibiotics, fish oil, and evening primrose oil.[83]

Chemotherapy has not been reported for this tumor, but an approach as for dogs with insulinoma may be successful.

PPoma

Tumors that stain for PP have been documented only twice in dogs. One report had no clinical details.[49] The other dog was detailed in two reports.[87,88] This dog had gastric mucosal hyperplasia and duodenal ulcers; however, the tumor cells and liver metastases did not stain for gastrin but rather for PP. This tumor also had some cells that secreted insulin, but the metastases only expressed PP. Clinical findings were indistinguishable from those of a gastrinoma, and there was some short-term clinical response to symptomatic treatment with cimetidine and metoclopramide.[88] Very high serum levels of PP may have produced the clinical picture in this dog. Many other APUD tumors express PP immunohistochemically in addition to another "primary" peptide.

Thyroid Tumors

Thyroid tumors are relatively uncommon and account for fewer than 2% of all canine tumors. Most of those reported are malignant (carcinomas), and approximately one-third have radiographically detectable metastases at the time of diagnosis. Between 40% and 80% of thyroid carcinomas metastasize at some point in their clinical course. When a thyroid tumor is detected, it is best to assume that it is malignant because adenomas are very rare.

INCIDENCE, SIGNALMENT, AND ETIOLOGY

Older dogs are most commonly affected (average age: 9.6 years). Beagles, boxers, and golden retrievers have been thought to be at greater risk for developing thyroid carcinomas than other breeds[89–91]; however, a series of 237 dogs with thyroid tumors found that mixed-breed dogs and retrievers were most commonly affected.[5] In one study of a beagle colony, the risk of developing thyroid neoplasia rose steadily until the age of 12 years, then accelerated; 67% of beagles over 17 years of age were affected.[92] Beagles are very likely as a breed to develop lymphocytic thyroiditis (26% of one population), and these dogs are likely to become hypothyroid. In one study, hypothyroid beagles were, in turn, more likely to develop a thyroid carcinoma (55% of hypothyroid dogs compared with 23% of euthyroid dogs).[93] This predisposition was though to result from chronic thyrotropin stimulation. It therefore seems possible that thyroid supplements may prevent cancer formation in hypothyroid beagles.

CLINICAL PRESENTATION AND HISTORY

Thyroid adenomas are rarely detected clinically and are usually an incidental necropsy finding. In contrast, 80% of thyroid carcinomas are recognized by the owner as a mass in the ventral neck. This mass may be unilateral or, rarely, bilateral (Figure 57-11). Occasionally, these masses may have been present for as long as 2 years.[91] Although most thyroid tumors are just below the larynx, larger tumors and ectopic tumors may be closer to the thoracic inlet. Other clinical concerns of owners include coughing, rapid breathing, dyspnea, and trouble swallowing, all occurring in more than 20% of affected dogs.[5]

Ectopic thyroid tumors have been seen in the heart and anterior mediastinum[94,95] and may account for up to 1% of all cardiac tumors in dogs.[96]

Most dogs with thyroid carcinoma are euthyroid, and some may be hypothyroid, presumably because pituitary thyrotropin secretion is inhibited by tumor production of biologically inactive thyroid hormones or because the normal thyroid tissue is destroyed. Rarely, canine thyroid carcinomas are hyperfunctional. Clinical signs most commonly observed in dogs with a hormonally active tumor include polydipsia, polyuria, and weight loss despite adequate caloric intake. Restlessness, heat intolerance, and panting are less common signs. In this way, affected dogs resemble cats with hyperfunctional thyroid adenomas.

> **KEY POINT**
>
> *Most dogs with thyroid carcinoma are euthyroid or even hypothyroid.*

STAGING AND DIAGNOSIS

A thyroid tumor may be suspected in any dog with a palpable mass in the neck. Radiographs of the cervical area are unlikely to be helpful because the tumor is rarely delineated. Careful palpation of the mass and assessment of its mobility and size are important in staging the tumor and predicting outcome after surgery. Pulmonary metastasis after invasion of the cranial and caudal thyroid veins occurs early in the course of the disease; this is followed by spread to regional lymph nodes (retropharyngeal or caudal cervical) and eventual invasion of the jugular veins and associated neck structures. Staging of a thyroid tumor should include an MDB, thoracic radiographs (dorsoventral and right and left lateral),

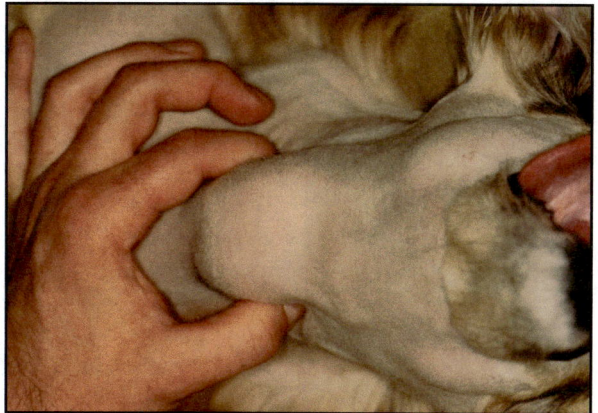

Figure 57-11. *A large palpable mass in the area of the thyroid should be suspected of being a thyroid carcinoma. Adenomas are rarely clinically detectable. (Courtesy of J. Berg)*

palpation of regional lymph nodes, and fine-needle aspiration of enlarged nodes. The lymph node spread is counterintuitive because lymphatic drainage is rostral, so retropharyngeal or caudal cervical (rather than prescapular) nodes should be examined and aspirated or biopsied if enlarged. This may require ultrasonography for the deeper retropharyngeal nodes. Metastasis is clinically detectable in 30% to 40% of dogs with thyroid carcinoma at the time of diagnosis.[90,97,98] The metastatic rate may be lower in dogs with small, movable tumors. In two studies, the metastatic rate was 15%.[99,100] This may reflect the slow progression of metastases; we have seen metastases more than 3 years after surgical excision of a thyroid tumor.

Ultrasonography or nuclear scintigraphy of the neck may be helpful in detecting an ectopic thyroid mass and in delineating a fixed mass. Ultrasonography is especially helpful in guiding a biopsy (particularly because these tumors are often very vascular). Thyroid carcinomas are rarely bilateral.

Functional canine thyroid carcinomas are rare. However, thyroxine (T_4) and triiodothyronine (T_3) tests are indicated before surgery. Nuclear scintigraphy of the thyroid may be useful in some cases. Even when resting T_3 and T_4 levels are within normal range, the thyroid malignancy may concentrate technetium Tc 99m (^{99m}Tc) pertechnetate and radioiodine[90] (Figure 57-12). Scintigraphy with ^{99m}Tc pertechnetate imaged benign and malignant thyroid tumors in 29 dogs regardless of their thyroid hormone status (i.e., euthyroid, hypothyroid, or hyperthyroid).[101] Heterogeneous uptake was associated with histologic evidence of capsular invasion in most cases. Pertechnetate scintigraphy is not as sensitive as radiography in detecting metastasis, so it is not a replacement for thoracic radiographs; in one study, scintigraphy was effective in identifying sites of ectopic thyroid tissue.[101] Lung metastases may occasionally be seen on scintigraphy but not on radiography or vice versa.[5,90] Accumulation of pertechnetate by a thyroid tumor does not

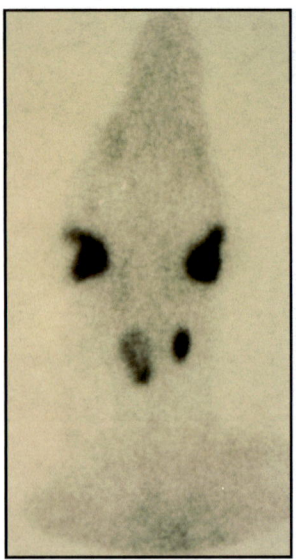

Figure 57-12. Thyroid carcinomas in dogs are usually nonfunctional, and a technetium scan may demonstrate a unilateral area of decreased nuclide uptake, or a "cold" scan, as seen in this figure. The contralateral thyroid is frequently normal in these dogs. This is a dorsoventral scan of a dog's head and neck. (Courtesy of Christopher R. Lamb, VetMB, Royal Veterinary College)

necessarily mean that the tumor will respond to treatment with radioiodine, although this is controversial. Therefore, in dogs with thyroid tumors, a pertechnetate scan is of most benefit as an ancillary aid to diagnosis of a cervical mass or as a screening test to look for ectopic tumor tissue. Radioiodine scans are more specific and provide more information regarding therapy; however, these studies require longer hospitalization because of the longer half-life of radioiodine compounds and thus create a radiation exposure hazard for hospital personnel.

Dogs that are suspected to have hyperfunctional thyroid tumors should be evaluated by cardiac ultrasonography because the potential for dysrhythmias and decreased function is high.

Thyroid carcinomas may arise from ectopic mediastinal thyroid tissue and have been reported at the heart base.[94–96] Ectopic thyroid tissue at the thoracic inlet, mediastinum, or cardiac muscle[95] may require ultrasonography, CT, or radionuclide imaging for detection. Dogs with thyroid neoplasms are apparently at higher risk of developing other primary tumors.[89] When staging dogs with thyroid carcinoma, the clinician should be aware that other tumor types may be encountered.

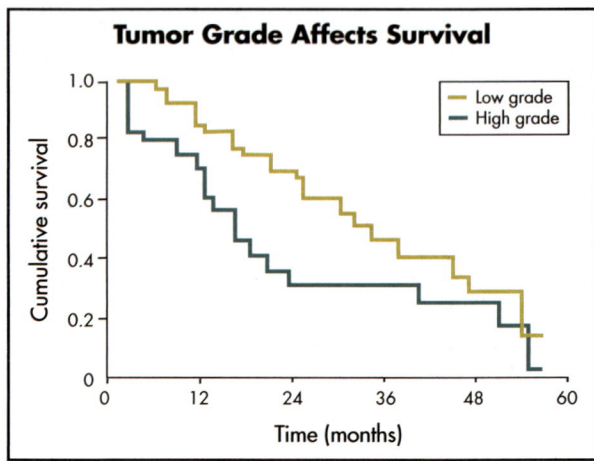

Figure 57-13. Histologic grading of thyroid carcinoma in 56 dogs took into account cellular and nuclear polymorphism, capsular and vascular invasion, and mitotic rate. Histologic grading was the most important prognostic factor for survival. Twenty-eight dogs with low-grade tumors lived longer than 24 dogs with high-grade tumors. (Adapted from Verschueren CP, Rutteman GR, Van Dijk JE, et al: Evaluation of some prognostic factors in surgically-treated canine thyroid cancer, in Clinico-pathological and Endocrine Aspects of Canine Thyroid Cancer. PhD Thesis, University of Utrecht, Netherlands, 1992, pp 11–25; with permission)

avoid "seeding" tumor cells into the tissue along the jugular furrow, where future excision would be difficult. Excisional biopsy is rarely complete, especially when the tumor is fixed (indicating invasion of associated structures).

Most studies do not ascribe prognostic significance to the histologic subtype of a thyroid carcinoma.[99,100] Immunohistochemistry using calcitonin, neuron-specific enolase, and synaptophysin has demonstrated that medullary carcinomas are more prevalent than once thought.[102] These medullary carcinomas may be more circumscribed and therefore more easily resectable than thyroid carcinomas with evidence of follicular patterns, and they may have a lower rate of metastasis, but survival times are no better for this subtype.[103]

PROGNOSTIC FACTORS

Large tumor size has been related to poor survival in many studies and may be an indication that larger tumors are more likely to invade surrounding structures.

Prognostic factors were evaluated in a series of 54 dogs treated surgically for thyroid carcinomas without evidence of metastases.[99] Histologic grading of the tumor, which took into account cellular and nuclear pleomorphism, capsular and vascular invasion, and mitotic rate, was the most important prognostic factor for survival (Figure 57-13). There were no differences in survival among different breeds, genders, or ages of dogs or histologic types of tumors. Plasma T_4 level and results of thyroid scintigraphy failed to predict survival. Dogs with invasive or fixed tumors that were unre-

> **KEY POINT**
>
> *Surgical biopsy or even fine-needle aspiration of a thyroid tumor may cause considerable bleeding; therefore, performing an excisional biopsy may be wise. If an incisional biopsy is done and excessive bleeding ensues, the surgeon should be prepared to perform a resection.*

Biopsy and even fine-needle aspiration may cause considerable bleeding, so care should be taken when obtaining a biopsy sample from thyroid masses; the surgeon should be prepared to perform a definitive resection if bleeding is excessive. Biopsy should be done via a midline approach to

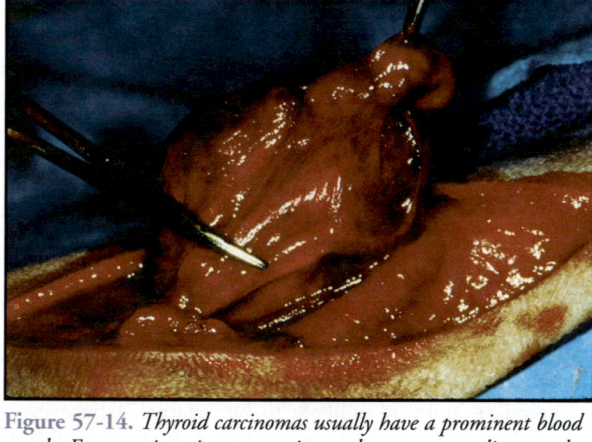

Figure 57-14. *Thyroid carcinomas usually have a prominent blood supply. For more invasive tumors, it may be necessary to ligate and remove carotid arteries* (pointed with forceps) *and jugular veins. (Courtesy of J. Berg)*

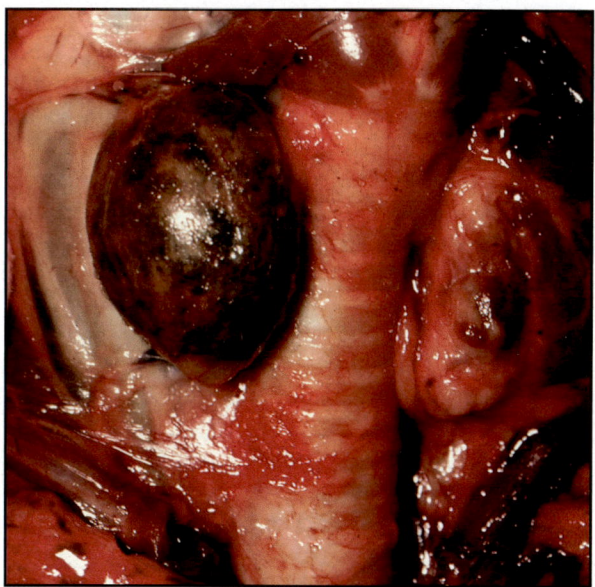

Figure 57-15. *Thyroid carcinomas may be bilateral, although the tumors may not be the same size. The contralateral gland should be examined and the surgeon prepared to perform a bilateral thyroidectomy.*

sectable had a poor survival (4 months) compared with dogs that had a surgically resectable tumor (12 months).[99]

Dogs with medullary carcinomas were more likely to have a movable tumor than dogs with a follicular carcinoma[103]; however, survival times were not different.

Dogs with bilateral tumors were 16 times more likely to develop metastases than dogs with a solitary tumor when treated with radiation therapy in one study.[104]

> **KEY POINT**
>
> *Dogs with freely movable thyroid tumors generally have a much better prognosis with surgical management than dogs with thyroid tumors that are fixed or invasive to surrounding tissues.*

TREATMENT

In one study, nine of 15 dogs with tumors considered inoperable because of invasiveness, distant metastases, or both were euthanatized within 1 week,[99] and in two studies, 13 dogs treated supportively survived a median of 3.5 months.[99,105]

Surgery

Complete surgical excision of thyroid *adenomas* should be curative. If the tumor is localized and not fixed to underlying tissue, surgical excision of a thyroid *carcinoma* also has the potential for cure, particularly for tumors of low histologic grade. For more invasive carcinomas, surgery is more complicated; it may be necessary to ligate and remove carotid arteries and jugular veins (Figure 57-14). For these dogs, hypoparathyroidism and bleeding are serious, potentially life-threatening complications; patients must be monitored after surgery and provided with supportive care.

Thyroid carcinomas can be bilateral (Figure 57-15). When bilateral thyroidectomy is performed, it is usually not possible to preserve the parathyroid glands; hypoparathyroidism is a frequent consequence. Hypocalcemia may cause signs of nervousness, irritability, panting, pyrexia, and, occasionally, convulsions or tetany. In a hypocalcemic crisis, 10% IV calcium gluconate should be administered at 1.0 to 1.5 ml/kg over 10 to 20 minutes and then 2.5 ml/kg as an IV infusion over 6 to 8 hours. In addition, oral vitamin D and calcium therapy should be started. Dihydrotachysterol may be administered at a loading dose of 0.05 mg/kg/day for 2 days and then 0.02 mg/kg/day for 2 days before starting maintenance therapy at 0.01 mg/kg/day. Calcium gluconate is given at 0.5 to 1.0 g/kg in divided doses, and the dose is adjusted according to weekly serum calcium determinations. Dogs with hypothyroidism should be treated with L-thyroxine at 20 to 30 µg/kg sid PO, with the dose tailored according to therapeutic monitoring.

The median survival times in dogs with movable (non-fixed) thyroid carcinomas have been studied. In three series totaling 58 dogs, the reported median survivals were 12, 36, and 50 months, and no dog developed local tumor recurrence.[99,100,105] In one of these studies, two of 20 dogs died from metastases, and five dogs died from complications of surgery (laryngeal paralysis, hypocalcemia, tracheostomy complications).[100] The authors postulated that wide surgical excisions were not necessary for these tumors and that more localized excision reduced the complication rate and did not increase the recurrence rate.

Another study found that dogs with medullary tumors were more likely to have a movable tumor; however, when we analyzed the reported survival times, we found no significant difference in survival between dogs with medullary and follicular carcinomas.[103]

Surgical excision of an ectopic thyroid carcinoma from the right ventricle was successful in one dog, and the dog had no recurrence 2 years after surgery.[95]

Radiation Therapy

For tumors that do not appear to have metastasized and cannot be completely excised, adjuvant external-beam radiation therapy to the surgical site gives local control. Distant metastases, however, require additional treatment. Thyroid tumors are highly sensitive to radiation, as indicated by the response to radionuclide therapy in humans and some dogs. In some dogs, external-beam radiation therapy may reduce the size of the tumor and form a fibrous capsule. Such a capsule enables surgery to be performed on a tumor once considered "inoperable."

Studies that report the efficacy of radiation therapy mostly comprise dogs that were not treated surgically. In one series, 25 dogs with invasive thyroid carcinomas but no evidence of metastases were treated with 48 Gy of radiation therapy given in 12 fractions of 4 Gy, three times a week.[104] Tumors shrank slowly after therapy, taking between 8 and 22 months to achieve maximum reduction. Progression-free survival was 80% at 1 year after treatment and 72% at 2 years. No factors affected survival. Acute radiation reactions included laryngeal, esophageal, and tracheal mucositis; these reactions were worse when larger treatment fields (larger tumors) were used. Chronic tracheitis developed in four dogs, and two dogs became hypothyroid, requiring supplementation. One of the latter two dogs also developed hypoparathyroidism.[104] A smaller series found similar results, although all tumors resolved completely.[106]

A third series used four once-weekly fractions of 9 Gy to treat 13 dogs with invasive thyroid carcinoma; most responses were partial, with only one complete remission seen. Four of the dogs died from progression of the primary disease, and four died from metastatic spread. The median survival time for all dogs was 22 months (range: 2–57 months).[107] Side effects were similar to those described above. Radiation therapy may be more effective when given in small fractions rather than in larger, "coarse" fractions.

In all three studies, metastases occurred in 14 of 46 dogs (30%), indicating a need for adjunctive chemotherapy in addition to radiation therapy.

Radioiodine

Functional thyroid tumors should accumulate iodine radioisotopes (as do thyroid adenomas in cats) and thus should be expected to be sensitive to radioiodine. The role of radioiodine in nonfunctional tumors is less clear. Radioactive iodine-131 (^{131}I) therapy has been documented in only a few canine cases. One dog had a tumor-free period of 17 months and received three treatments during that time.[108] In another series, follow-up was incomplete, but palliation of signs and shrinkage of the treated tumor were described. The median progression-free (stable disease) period was 15 months for three dogs treated with ^{131}I alone, but the upper end of the range was 27 months.[109] In human patients with functional thyroid carcinoma, the treatment of choice is extensive surgical debulking followed by radioiodine therapy in an attempt to ablate remaining tumor tissue. Radioiodine alone is unlikely to be curative. Surgery followed by radioiodine was reported in three dogs, and their median survival was 41 months, with one dog still alive at the end of follow-up.[109] The efficacy of ^{131}I therapy in dogs (compared with cats) is often compromised by the high doses required to treat the disease. If debulking of the tumor to reduce the required dose of radioiodine is not possible, hospitalization in isolation is often required for many weeks.

In the largest series reported to date, 43 dogs were treated with radioiodine either alone (32 dogs) or as an adjunct to incomplete surgical excision (11 dogs). Only 25% of the dogs in the ^{131}I-alone group, and none of the adjunctively treated group, had elevated serum T_4 levels. Median survival was 30 months for dogs treated with ^{131}I alone and 34 months for dogs treated adjunctively.[105] Stage of disease had no effect on survival, and nine dogs with stage IV disease (distant metastases) still had a median survival of 19 months. Thyroid supplementation was given if posttreatment hypothyroidism was observed.

Dogs with massive pulmonary metastases may not be good candidates for this therapy because accumulation of radioisotope could lead to fatal pneumonitis, as was seen in one dog.[90]

Chemotherapy

In cases of metastatic thyroid carcinoma in which radionuclide imaging provides no evidence of increased function, chemotherapy is the treatment of choice. Doxorubicin (30 mg/m^2 IV q3wk) has been recommended. In two studies, 22 dogs with measurable thyroid carcinoma received doxorubicin; one had a complete response and five showed partial responses.[110,111] Duration of response was not provided. In an anecdotal review of 64 cases from Colorado State University, doxorubicin given after surgery may have improved survival compared with surgery alone when the tumor was resected down to microscopic disease.[112] In another report, 10 dogs with thyroid carcinoma received mitoxantrone chemotherapy at various doses.[113] One dog had a short-term (21 days) partial response. Chemotherapeutics used as single agents in human patients with thyroid carcinoma include cisplatin. In one study, 13 dogs with thyroid carcinoma were treated every 21 days with 60 mg/m² of IV cisplatin.[114] One dog had a complete remission, and six had partial responses for a median of 7 months. Cisplatin and doxorubicin are the drugs of choice in the treatment of canine malignant thyroid tumors and may be useful as an adjuvant to surgery or radiation therapy.

Treatment Recommendations

For dogs with small (<3 cm diameter), movable tumors and no evidence of metastatic disease, surgical excision appears to be all that is required. If the tumor is fixed, external-beam radiation therapy may be used for palliation or to render the tumor smaller and surgically resectable. If radioiodine is available, it may be an alternative to external-beam radiation therapy. For larger tumors and for dogs with metastatic disease, chemotherapy with alternating doxorubicin and a platinum drug is suggested in combination with surgery, radiation therapy, or both. This approach has been used successfully in anecdotal reports.[115]

> **KEY POINT**
> *A combination of radiation therapy, surgery, and chemotherapy is needed for dogs with fixed, large thyroid carcinomas.*

Supportive Care

For dogs with a hyperfunctional tumor, pretreatment with methimazole may be successful in controlling clinical signs. Anecdotally, we have found that a dose of 1 mg/kg PO bid to tid given before surgery or radiation therapy results in control of clinical signs in 5 to 7 days.

Parathyroid Tumors
INCIDENCE, SIGNALMENT, AND ETIOLOGY

Parathyroid tumors are rare in dogs. Most affected dogs are middle aged to old (7 to 17 years). Although young dogs are occasionally reported with parathyroid tumors, dogs younger than 7 years accounted for only 4% of 168 patients in one series.[5] Parathyroid adenomas were observed in a litter of German shepherd puppies.[116] There is no gender predilection. In a series of 168 cases, keeshonds were overrepresented and accounted for 26% of dogs with this disorder.[5] Most reported cases involve parathyroid adenomas, although carcinomas can occur.[117] There may be a continuum of disease extending from hyperplasia to adenomatous change to carcinoma. These tumors are usually found in the cervical region, although an ectopic parathyroid adenocarcinoma was reported in the anterior mediastinum of one dog.[118]

CLINICAL PRESENTATION AND HISTORY

Although hypercalcemia is a consistent finding in dogs with a parathyroid tumor, clinical signs are often mild to absent. Most dogs in a series of 168 were diagnosed on a serum biochemical profile that had been collected for another reason or for nonspecific clinical signs. Some authors have postulated that dogs with primary hyperparathyroidism may have only slowly increasing serum calcium levels over time, implying that in some dogs, this may be a slowly progressive disease.[5] Dogs with clinical signs should be treated for the disease. Signs include polyuria, polydipsia, listlessness, muscle weakness, and lower urinary tract signs (e.g., urolithiasis).[5] Unlike dogs that are hypercalcemic with lymphoma or anal sac adenocarcinoma, signs of polyuria or polydipsia are rarely severe.[5] Parathyroid tumors are often small and, therefore, are rarely palpable on clinical examination.

STAGING AND DIAGNOSIS

The most common cause of canine hypercalcemia is lymphoma. Dogs with elevated serum calcium levels should have their lymph nodes palpated and aspirated. Thoracic radiography should be conducted, and the abdomen should be imaged by ultrasonography to rule out lymphoma. In addition, a careful rectal examination should be performed to detect possible adenocarcinoma of the anal sac, another cause of hypercalcemia. Lytic bone lesions on radiographs or an elevated globulin level may indicate multiple myeloma. After other neoplastic and metabolic causes have been eliminated, primary hyperparathyroidism can be considered, and cervical ultrasonography should be conducted and a serum parathyroid hormone (PTH) level obtained. IV injection of methylene blue had been suggested as a method of detecting parathyroid tumors, but the risk of Heinz body anemia and the advances in ultrasonography have made this approach less frequently used.[119]

Early studies with ultrasonography could not detect normal parathyroid glands; however, as technology and expertise have improved, this modality has assumed a role in the diagnosis of primary hyperparathyroidism. Results are still very operator dependent.[120] In one study, normal and abnormal parathyroid glands, regardless of disease process, were round and hypoechoic compared with the adjacent thyroid gland. Hyperplastic lesions were smaller than 4 mm in the same study, but adenomas and adenocarcinomas were larger.[121] In another series of 77 dogs, no dog had more than two parathyroid nodules observed on ultrasonography (Table 57-2).[5]

The serum level of PTH should be interpreted in conjunction with the serum calcium level. In a dog with normal parathyroid glands, an elevated calcium level should result in a low PTH level, so a finding of normal to increased PTH

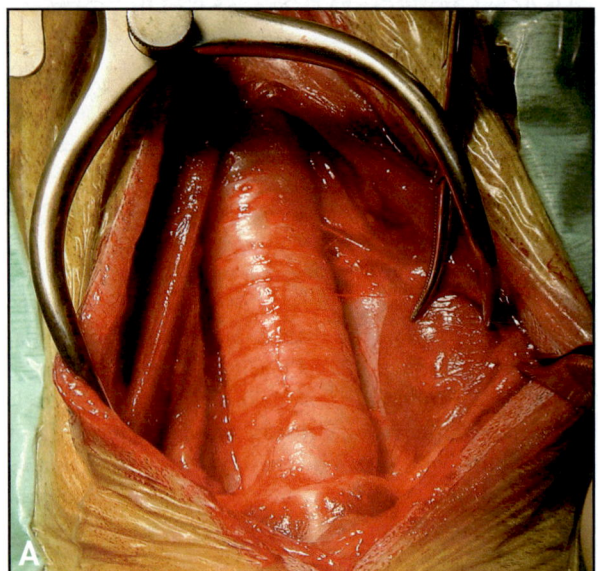 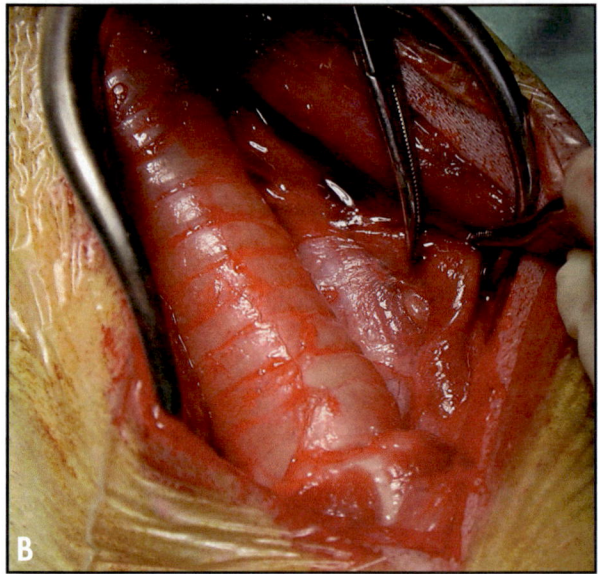

Figure 57-16. (**A**) *A parathyroid tumor may be very small and not easily visualized. At the right of this picture is the normal thyroid gland.* (**B**) *The same dog as in part A. The parathyroid adenoma is beneath the thyroid gland* (pointed with forceps). *All four glands should be identified by the surgeon because more than one gland may be affected. (Courtesy of Sarah Goldsmid, BVSc, Animal Referral Hospital)*

level in dogs with hypercalcemia is suggestive of parathyroid pathology. In addition, PTH-related peptide levels, which are elevated in dogs with hypercalcemia of malignancy, are undetectable in dogs with primary hyperparathyroidism.

Positive nuclear scintigraphy using ^{99m}Tc-sestamibi demonstrating uptake in the thyroid area may be suggestive of a parathyroid tumor.[122,123] A larger study, however, found that this technique of parathyroid scintigraphy was poorly sensitive and specific and could not be recommended for definitive identification of abnormal parathyroid glands.[124]

Although about 7% of 168 dogs with hyperparathyroidism had a diagnosis of carcinoma in one study,[5] no dog has been documented to have metastases. This may reflect the gradation of the disease between hyperplasia, adenoma, and carcinoma. The distinction between each histologic category is somewhat subjective, and some authors have suggested that primary hyperplasia of the parathyroid glands may actually be a multiple form of adenoma.[125]

TREATMENT

Surgical excision of the affected gland or glands should cure parathyroid adenoma. In one series, most dogs (92%) had a solitary tumor, and no dog had more than two tumors.[5] It is important to identify all abnormal parathyroid glands either by ultrasonography or during surgery before surgical removal (Figure 57-16). If all four glands are uniformly enlarged, secondary hyperparathyroidism should be considered.[5] It is not possible to distinguish hyperplasia from adenoma from carcinoma during surgery. In one series, the abnormal gland could not be identified during surgery in 5% of affected dogs; in these dogs, the entire thyroid–parathyroid complex corresponding to the abnormal ultrasonographic findings was removed.[5] This approach was successful in all dogs. In a series of 155 dogs that had a solitary parathyroid gland removed, 14 had recurrence of hypercalcemia more than 6 months later (in 12 of 14 dogs, recurrence was 12–30 months later).[5] Further control was achieved in each dog after identification and removal of another solitary gland. Periodic rechecks of serum calcium level are warranted in dogs treated for primary hyperparathyroidism. In the second series, six of the dogs with new tumors were keeshonds, implying rechecks may be even more important in this breed.[5]

> **KEY POINT**
> *Parathyroid tumors are usually solitary and are cured during surgery regardless of whether they are adenomas or carcinomas.*

After removal of a parathyroid tumor, the remaining normal parathyroid tissue may be atrophied from chronic hypercalcemia, and the dog should be treated for hypoparathyroidism, as outlined in the Thyroid Tumors section, above. Only about one-third of dogs in a large series had clinically significant hypocalcemia.[5] Most dogs that become hypocalcemic do so within 6 days of surgery, although occasionally, the delay is as long as 3 weeks after surgery.[5] If the pretreatment calcium level is less than 14 mg/dl, the risk of hypoparathyroidism is low; these dogs should be monitored in the hospital and treated with vitamin D if the serum calcium decreases below 8.5

mg/dL.[5] It is also acceptable to treat these dogs prophylactically. For dogs with higher serum calcium levels before surgery, prophylactic treatment starting the morning before surgery is mandatory. Treatment is usually required for 2 to 3 months until normal tissue regains function.[117] Vitamin D is withdrawn initially by reducing treatments every 2 weeks from bid to sid to eod, then to every third day, every fourth day, and finally weekly; the serum calcium is monitored at each reduction.[5] Calcium supplements can be withdrawn after vitamin D is withdrawn.

The success of ultrasonography in localizing abnormal parathyroid glands has allowed options other than surgery to be explored. Percutaneous ultrasound-guided radiofrequency heat ablation was successful in the treatment of 27 dogs with solitary parathyroid tumors.[5,126] Similarly, ultrasound-guided parathyroid tumor ablation using ethanol was successful in the treatment of dogs with solitary tumors.[126] Both techniques require considerable ultrasonographic experience to ensure that the procedure is performed successfully; otherwise, surgical excision is preferred.

Multiple Endocrine Neoplasia
INCIDENCE, SIGNALMENT, AND ETIOLOGY

In human patients, several combinations of endocrine neoplasms have been observed and appear to be genetically linked; they are collectively named *multiple endocrine neoplasia* (MEN) and divided into types 1, 2a, and 2b. In human MEN, the glands involved, in descending order of frequency, are the parathyroids, pancreas (PPomas [80%–100%], gastrinomas [50%], insulinomas [20%]), pituitary (adenomas often hormonally inactive, but 15% have acromegaly and 5% have hyperadrenocorticism), adrenal cortex, and thyroid (Table 57-3).

Similar syndromes have been seen in veterinary patients, but there are only eight reported cases that truly fit the human classification of MEN-2a syndrome: thyroid medullary carcinoma, parathyroid hyperplasia, and pheochromocytoma.[5,127] The possibility of a genetic trait as seen in humans has not been explored in dogs, but clinicians should be aware that dogs with one endocrine tumor may have others and should be staged accordingly.

CLINICAL PRESENTATION AND HISTORY

Clinical signs can be caused by any of the glands involved in MEN; in some dogs, hypercalcemia may be diagnosed before other endocrine abnormalities.[122] In other cases, a dog with hyperadrenocorticism may be found to have other tumors. The combinations of multiple endocrine tumors in 95 dogs are listed in Table 57-4.

STAGING AND DIAGNOSIS

Staging should be performed as described for individual tumor types in this chapter. Clinicians should be aware that some dogs may have multiple tumors. Some authors have recommended CT of the abdomen and thorax in dogs with thyroid tumors to assess the rest of the body for other endocrine neoplasms.[5] In one series of 237 dogs with thyroid tumors, 63 had one or more additional endocrine tumor,[5] and multiple endocrine tumors were seen in 26 (39%) of a series of 77 dogs with chemodectomas.[132]

TREATMENT

Treatment of dogs with multiple endocrine tumors should be approached from the perspective of treating the tumors that are most threatening to quality of life. Tumors that are

Table 57-2 Results of Biochemical Analyses and Ultrasonography in Dogs with Hyperparathyroidism[5]

Measurement	Dogs (n)	Range Normal	Range Measured (% of dogs)
Serum calcium (mg/dL)	168	9.6–11.7	12–14 (55) >16 (14)
Ionized calcium (mmol/L)	117	1.12–1.42	Normal (8) >1.66 (66)
PTH (pmol/L)	121	2–13	Normal (73) >20 (16)
Ultrasonographic size (mm)	77	<4	4–6 (60) >11 (14)

Table 57-3 Characteristics of MEN in Humans

Characteristic	MEN 1	MEN 2a	MEN 2b
Pheochromocytoma	No	70% bilateral	70% bilateral
Parathyroid hyperplasia	Yes	Yes	No
Pancreatic islet cell tumor	Yes	No	No
Thyroid medullary carcinoma	No	Bilateral	Bilateral
Pituitary tumor (%)	50–80		
Thyroid adenoma (%)	30		
Adrenal cortical tumor (%)	30		

Table 57-4 Distribution of Multiple Endocrine Neoplasms in 95 Dogs

Dogs (n)	Studies	Pheochromocytoma	Parathyroid Hyperplasia	Pancreatic Islet Cell Tumor	Thyroid Carcinoma
1	Thuróczy et al[128]	Yes			
1	Wright et al[122]	Yes	Yes		
1	Unterer et al[129]		Yes		Yes
1	Walker et al[130]		Yes		
2	Kiupel et al,[131] Patnaik et al[132]			Yes	
4	Patnaik et al,[132] Fife et al[133]				
1	Peterson et al[127]	Yes	Yes		Yes
6	van Sluijs et al,[33] von Dehn et al[46]	Yes			
4	von Dehn et al[46]	Yes			
2	Brewer and Crager[134]		Yes		
10	Feldman and Nelson,[5] Patnaik et al[132]				
3	Patnaik et al[132]			Yes	
8	Feldman and Nelson[5]				Yes
23	Feldman and Nelson[5]				Yes
12	Feldman and Nelson[5]		Yes		Yes
3	Feldman and Nelson[5]	Yes			
2	Feldman and Nelson[5]				
4	Feldman and Nelson[5]		Yes		Yes
7	Feldman and Nelson[5]	Yes	Yes		Yes

most easily controlled surgically should be removed, and other metabolic conditions may be controlled by chemotherapy. For example, a dog with a thyroid carcinoma and PDH may benefit from surgical excision of the thyroid nodule and mitotane chemotherapy.

One 10-year-old dog with adrenocortical adenomas, pheochromocytoma, and a pituitary ACTH-secreting adenoma was treated by bilateral adrenalectomy and remained well until neurologic complications of the pituitary macroadenoma led to euthanasia.[128] A 13-year-old dog with hypercalcemia was shown to have a pheochromocytoma and parathyroid hyperplasia. The dog was alive on corticosteroids 14 months after removal of the adrenal tumor.[122] A 15-year-old dog with a testicular seminoma and perianal adenomas also had a parathyroid adenoma, a thyroid carcinoma, and a thyroid adenoma detected during evaluation of the testicular disease.[129] The dog survived 2 months after surgical excision of the parathyroid adenoma and the thyroid carcinoma. A 12-year-old dog with hypercalcemia and hyperadrenocorticism was shown to have a parathyroid adenoma and a pituitary adenoma. The dog survived 14 months after removal of the parathyroid tumor while hyperadrenocorticism was controlled with mitotane therapy.[130]

REFERENCES

1. van Keulen LJ, Wesdorp JL, Kooistra HS: Diabetes mellitus in a dog with a growth hormone-producing acidophilic adenoma of the adenohypophysis. *Vet Pathol* 33:451–453, 1996.
2. Bilzer T: Hypophysentumoren als gemeinsame ursache von morbus Cushing und diabetes insipidus des hundes. *Teirartzl Prax* 19:276–281, 1991.
3. Harb MF, Nelson RW, Feldman EC, et al: Central diabetes insipidus in dogs: 20 cases (1986–1995). *JAVMA* 209:1884–1888, 1996.
4. Sato J, Sato R, Kinai M, et al: Pituitary chromophobe carcinoma with a low level of serum gonadotropin and an aspermatogenesis in a dog. *J Vet Med Sci* 63:183–185, 2001.
5. Feldman EC, Nelson RW: *Canine and Feline Endocrinology and Reproduction*, ed 3. Philadelphia, WB Saunders, 2003.
6. Feldman EC: Comparison of ACTH response and dexamethasone suppression as screening tests in canine hyperadrenocorticism. *JAVMA* 182:506–510, 1983.

Thyroid Adenoma	Adrenocortical Tumor	Chemodectoma	Pituitary Tumor
	Yes		Yes
Yes			
			Yes
	Yes	Yes	
		Yes	Yes
	Yes		
			Yes
			Yes
Yes		Yes	
		Yes	
	Yes		
			Yes
Yes			Yes
Yes	Yes		
			Yes

7. Grooters AM, Biller DS, Theisen SK, Miyabayashi T: Ultrasonographic characteristics of the adrenal glands in dogs with pituitary-dependent hyperadrenocorticism: Comparison with normal dogs. *J Vet Intern Med* 10:110–115, 1996.

8. Ruckstuhl NS, Nett CS, Reusch CE: Results of clinical examinations, laboratory tests, and ultrasonography in dogs with pituitary-dependent hyperadrenocorticism treated with trilostane. *Am J Vet Res* 63:506–512, 2002.

9. Meij BP, Voorhout G, van den Ingh TS, et al: Results of transsphenoidal hypophysectomy in 25 dogs with pituitary-dependent hyperadrenocorticism. *Vet Surg* 27:246–261, 1998.

10. van der Vlugt-Meijer RH, Meij BP, van den Ingh TS, et al: Dynamic computed tomography of the pituitary gland in dogs with pituitary-dependent hyperadrenocorticism. *J Vet Intern Med* 17:773–780, 2003.

11. Greco DS, Peterson ME, Davidson AP, et al: Concurrent pituitary and adrenal tumors in dogs with hyperadrenocorticism: 17 cases (1978–1995). *JAVMA* 214:1349–1353, 1999.

12. Meij B: Hypophysectomy in dogs: A review. *Vet Q* 21:134–141, 1999.

13. Angles JM, Feldman EC, Nelson RW, Feldman MS: Use of urine cortisol:creatinine ratio versus adrenocorticotropic hormone stimulation testing for monitoring mitotane treatment of pituitary-dependent hyperadrenocorticism in dogs. *JAVMA* 211:1002–1004, 1997.

14. Rijnberk A, Belshaw BE: An alternative protocol for the medical management of canine pituitary-dependent hyperadrenocorticism. *Vet Rec* 122:486–488, 1988.

15. Feldman EC, Bruyette DS, Nelson RW, Farver TB: Plasma cortisol response to ketoconazole administration in dogs with hyperadrenocorticism. *JAVMA* 197:71–78, 1990.

16. Braddock JA, Church DB, Robertson ID, Watson AD: Trilostane treatment in dogs with pituitary-dependent hyperadrenocorticism. *Aust Vet J* 81:600–607, 2003.

17. Bruyette DS, Ruehl WW, Smidberg TL: Canine pituitary-dependent hyperadrenocorticism: A spontaneous animal model for neurodegenerative disorders and their treatment with L-deprenyl. *Prog Brain Res* 106:207–215, 1995.

18. Reusch CE, Steffen T, Hoerauf A: The efficacy of L-deprenyl in dogs with pituitary-dependent hyperadrenocorticism. *J Vet Intern Med* 13:291–301, 1999.

19. Theon AP, Feldman EC: Megavoltage irradiation of pituitary macrotumors in dogs with neurologic signs. *JAVMA* 213:225–231, 1998.

20. Goossens MM, Feldman EC, Theon AP, Koblik PD: Efficacy of cobalt 60 radiotherapy in dogs with pituitary-dependent hyperadrenocorticism. *JAVMA* 212:374–376, 1998.

21. Kintzer PP, Peterson ME: Mitotane treatment of 32 dogs with cortisol-secreting adrenocortical neoplasms. *JAVMA* 205:54–61, 1994.

22. Syme HM, Scott-Moncrieff JC, Treadwell NG, et al: Hyperadrenocorticism associated with excessive sex hormone production by an adrenocortical tumor in two dogs. *JAVMA* 219:1725–1728, 2001.

23. Norman EJ, Thompson H, Mooney CT: Dynamic adrenal function testing in eight dogs with hyperadrenocorticism associated with adrenocortical neoplasia. *Vet Rec* 144:551–554, 1999.

24. Feldman EC, Nelson RW, Feldman MS: Use of low- and high-dose dexamethasone tests for distinguishing pituitary-dependent from adrenal tumor hyperadrenocorticism in dogs. *JAVMA* 209:772–775, 1996.

25. Barthez PY, Nyland TG, Feldman EC: Ultrasonographic evaluation of the adrenal glands in dogs. *JAVMA* 207:1180–1183, 1995.

26. Ford SL, Feldman EC, Nelson RW: Hyperadrenocorticism caused by bilateral adrenocortical neoplasia in dogs: Four cases (1983–1988). *JAVMA* 202:789–792, 1993.

27. Hoerauf A, Reusch C: Ultrasonographic characteristics of both adrenal glands in 15 dogs with functional adrenocortical tumors. *JAAHA* 35:193–199, 1999.

28. Penninck DG, Feldman EC, Nyland TG: Radiographic features of canine hyperadrenocorticism caused by autonomously functioning adrenocortical tumors: 23 cases (1978–1986). *JAVMA* 192:1604–1608, 1988.

29. Besso JG, Penninck DG, Gliatto JM: Retrospective ultrasonographic evaluation of adrenal lesions in 26 dogs. *Vet Radiol Ultrasound* 38:448–455, 1997.

30. Kyles AE, Feldman EC, De Cock HE, et al: Surgical management of adrenal gland tumors with and without associated tumor thrombi in dogs: 40 cases (1994–2001). *JAVMA* 223:654–662, 2003.

31. Anderson CR, Birchard SJ, Powers BE, et al: Surgical treatment of adrenocortical tumors: 21 cases (1990–1996). *JAAHA* 37:93–97, 2001.

32. Scavelli TD, Peterson ME, Matthiesen DT: Results of surgical treatment for hyperadrenocorticism caused by adrenocortical neoplasia in the dog: 25 cases (1980–1984). *JAVMA* 189:1360–1364, 1986.

33. van Sluijs FJ, Sjollema BE, Voorhout G, et al: Results of adrenalectomy in 36 dogs with hyperadrenocorticism caused by adrenocortical tumour. *Vet Q* 17:113–116, 1995.

34. Emms SG, Johnston DE, Eigenmann JE, Goldschmidt MH: Adrenalectomy in the management of canine hyperadrenocorticism. *JAAHA* 23:557–564, 1987.

35. Hill K, Scott-Moncrieff JC: Tumors of the adrenal cortex causing hyperadrenocorticism. *Vet Med*: 686–706, 2001.

36. Jaffe MH, Grooters AM, Partington BP, et al: Extensive venous thrombosis and hind-limb edema associated with adrenocortical carcinoma in a dog. *JAAHA* 35:306–310, 1999.

37. Feldman EC, Nelson RW, Feldman MS, Farver TB: Comparison of mitotane treatment for adrenal tumor versus pituitary-dependent hyperadrenocorticism in dogs. *JAVMA* 200:1642–1647, 1992.

38. Eastwood JM, Elwood CM, Hurley KJ: Trilostane treatment of a dog with functional adrenocortical neoplasia. *J Small Anim Pract* 44:126–131, 2003.

39. Gilson SD, Withrow SJ, Wheeler SL, Twedt DC: Pheochromocytoma in 50 dogs. *J Vet Intern Med* 8:228–232, 1994.

40. Barthez PY, Marks SL, Woo J, et al: Pheochromocytoma in dogs: 61 cases (1984–1995). *J Vet Intern Med* 11:272–278, 1997.

41. Bouayad H, Feeney DA, Caywood DD, Hayden DW: Pheochromocytoma in dogs: 13 cases (1980–1985). *JAVMA* 191:1610–1615, 1987.

42. Poffenbarger EM, Feeney DA, Hayden DW: Gray-scale ultrasonography in the diagnosis of adrenal neoplasia in dogs: Six cases (1981–1986). *JAVMA* 192:228–232, 1988.

43. Platt SR, Sheppard BJ, Graham J, et al: Pheochromocytoma in the vertebral canal of two dogs. *JAAHA* 34:365–371, 1998.

44. Rosenstein DS: Diagnostic imaging in canine pheochromocytoma. *Vet Radiol Ultrasound* 41:499–506, 2000.

45. Berry CR, DeGrado TR, Nutter F, et al: Imaging of pheochromocytoma in 2 dogs using p-[18F] fluorobenzylguanidine. *Vet Radiol Ultrasound* 43:183–186, 2002.
46. von Dehn BJ, Nelson RW, Feldman EC, Griffey SM: Pheochromocytoma and hyperadrenocorticism in dogs: Six cases (1982–1992). *JAVMA* 207:322–324, 1995.
47. Bennett PF, Norman EJ: Mitotane (o,p'-DDD) resistance in a dog with pituitary-dependent hyperadrenocorticism and phaeochromocytoma. *Aust Vet J* 76:101–103, 1998.
48. Cerundolo R, McEvoy F, McNeil PE, Lloyd DH: Ultrasonographic detection of a pancreatic glucagon-secreting multihormonal islet cell tumour in a dachshund with metabolic epidermal necrosis. *Vet Rec* 145:662–666, 1999.
49. Minkus G, Jutting U, Aubele M, et al: Canine neuroendocrine tumors of the pancreas: A study using image analysis techniques for the discrimination of metastatic versus nonmetastatic tumors. *Vet Pathol* 34:138–145, 1997.
50. O'Brien TD, Hayden DW, O'Leary TP, et al: Canine pancreatic endocrine tumors: Immunohistochemical analysis of hormone content and amyloid. *Vet Pathol* 24:308–314, 1987.
51. O'Brien TD, Westermark P, Johnson KH: Islet amyloid polypeptide and calcitonin gene-related peptide immunoreactivity in amyloid and tumor cells of canine pancreatic endocrine tumors. *Vet Pathol* 27:194–198, 1990.
52. Straus E, Johnson GF, Yalow RS: Canine Zollinger-Ellison syndrome. *Gastroenterology* 72:380–381, 1977.
53. Caywood DD, Klausner JS, O'Leary TP, et al: Pancreatic insulin-secreting neoplasms: Clinical, diagnostic, and prognostic features in 73 dogs. *JAAHA* 24:577–584, 1988.
54. Kruth SA, Feldman EC, Kennedy PC: Insulin-secreting islet cell tumors: Establishing a diagnosis and the clinical course for 25 dogs. *JAVMA* 181:54–58, 1982.
55. Leifer CE, Peterson ME, Matus RE: Insulin-secreting tumor: Diagnosis and medical and surgical management in 55 dogs. *JAVMA* 188:60–64, 1986.
56. Braund KG, Steiss JE, Amling KA, et al: Insulinoma and subclinical peripheral neuropathy in two dogs. *J Vet Intern Med* 1:86–90, 1987.
57. Braund KG, McGuire JA, Amling KA, Henderson RA: Peripheral neuropathy associated with malignant neoplasms in dogs. *Vet Pathol* 24:16–21, 1987.
58. Schrauwen E: Clinical peripheral polyneuropathy associated with canine insulinoma. *Vet Rec* 128:211–212, 1991.
59. Bergman PJ, Bruyette DS, Coyne BE, et al: Canine clinical peripheral neuropathy associated with pancreatic islet cell carcinoma. *Prog Vet Neurol* 5:57–62, 1994.
60. Thompson JC, Jones BR, Hickson PC: The amended insulin to glucose ratio and diagnosis of insulinoma in dogs. *N Z Vet J* 43:240–243, 1995.
61. Lamb CR, Simpson KW, Boswood A, Matthewman LA: Ultrasonography of pancreatic neoplasia in the dog: A retrospective review of 16 cases. *Vet Rec* 137:65–68, 1995.
62. Smeak DD, Fingeroth JM, Bilbrey SA: Intravenous methylene blue as a specific stain for primary and metastatic insulinoma in a dog. *JAAHA* 24:478–480, 1988.
63. Lester NV, Newell SM, Hill RC, Lanz OI: Scintigraphic diagnosis of insulinoma in a dog. *Vet Radiol Ultrasound* 40:174–178, 1999.
64. Trifonidou MA, Kirpensteijn J, Robben JH: A retrospective evaluation of 51 dogs with insulinoma. *Vet Q* 20(suppl 1):114–115, 1998.
65. Tobin RL, Nelson RW, Lucroy MD, et al: Outcome of surgical vs. medical treatment of dogs with beta cell neoplasia: 39 cases (1990–1997). *JAVMA* 215:226–230, 1999.
66. Shimada A, Morita T, Ikeda N, et al: Hypoglycaemic brain lesions in a dog with insulinoma. *J Comp Pathol* 122:67–71, 2000.
67. Van Ham L, Braund KG, Roels S, Putcuyps I: Treatment of a dog with an insulinoma-related peripheral polyneuropathy with corticosteroids. *Vet Rec* 141:98–100, 1997.
68. Parker AJ, O'Brien D, Musselman EE: Diazoxide treatment of metastatic insulinoma in a dog. *JAAHA* 18:315–318, 1982.
69. Meyer DJ: Temporary remission of hypoglycemia in a dog with an insulinoma after treatment with streptozotocin. *Am J Vet Res* 38:1201–1204, 1977.
70. Meyer DJ: Pancreatic islet cell carcinoma in a dog treated with streptozotocin. *Am J Vet Res* 37:1221–1223, 1976.
71. Huxtable CR, Farrow BR: Functional neoplasms of the canine pancreatic-islet β-cells: a clinico-pathological study of three cases. *J Small Anim Pract* 20:737–748, 1979.
72. Moore AS, Nelson RW, Henry CJ, et al: Streptozocin for treatment of pancreatic islet cell tumors in dogs: 17 cases (1989–1999). *JAVMA* 221:811–818, 2002.
73. Rossini AA, Arcangeli MA, Cahill GF Jr.: Studies of alloxan toxicity on the beta cell. *Diabetes* 24:516–522, 1975.
74. Lothrop CD Jr: Medical treatment of neuroendocrine tumors of the gastroenteropancreatic system with somatostatin, in Kirk RW (ed): *Current Veterinary Therapy*, vol X. Philadelphia, WB Saunders, 1989, pp 1020–1024.
75. Simpson KW, Stepien RL, Elwood CM, et al: Evaluation of the long-acting somatostatin analogue octreotide in the management of insulinoma in three dogs. *J Small Anim Pract* 36:161–165, 1995.
76. Fischer JR, Smith SA, Harkin KR: Glucagon constant-rate infusion: A novel strategy for the management of hyperinsulinemic-hypoglycemic crisis in the dog. *JAAHA* 36:27–32, 2000.
77. Happe RP, van der Gaag I, Lamers CB, et al: Zollinger-Ellison syndrome in three dogs. *Vet Pathol* 17:177–186, 1980.
78. Jones BR, Nicholls MR, Badman R: Peptic ulceration in a dog associated with an islet cell carcinoma of the pancreas and an elevated plasma gastrin level. *J Small Anim Pract* 17:593–598, 1976.
79. Altschul M, Simpson KW, Dykes NL, et al: Evaluation of somatostatin analogues for the detection and treatment of gastrinoma in a dog. *J Small Anim Pract* 38:286–291, 1997.
80. Green RA, Gartrell CL: Gastrinoma: A retrospective study of four cases (1985–1995). *JAAHA* 33:524–527, 1997.
81. Brooks D, Watson GL: Omeprazole in a dog with gastrinoma. *J Vet Intern Med* 11:379–381, 1997.
82. Torres S, Johnson K, McKeever P, Hardy R: Superficial necrolytic dermatitis and a pancreatic endocrine tumour in a dog. *J Small Anim Pract* 38:246–250, 1997.
83. Bond R, McNeil PE, Evans H, Srebernik N: Metabolic epidermal necrosis in two dogs with different underlying diseases. *Vet Rec* 136:466–471, 1995.
84. Torres SM, Caywood DD, O'Brien TD, et al: Resolution of superficial necrolytic dermatitis following excision of a glucagon-secreting pancreatic neoplasm in a dog. *JAAHA* 33:313–319, 1997.
85. Gross TL, O'Brien TD, Davies AP, Long RE: Glucagon-producing pancreatic endocrine tumors in two dogs with superficial necrolytic dermatitis. *JAVMA* 197:1619–1622, 1990.
86. Allenspach K, Arnold P, Glaus T, et al: Glucagon-producing neuroendocrine tumour associated with hypoaminoacidaemia and skin lesions. *J Small Anim Pract* 41:402–406, 2000.
87. Boosinger TR, Zerbe CA, Grabau JH, Pletcher JM: Multihormonal pancreatic endocrine tumor in a dog with duodenal ulcers and hypertrophic gastropathy. *Vet Pathol* 25:237–239, 1988.
88. Zerbe CA, Boosinger TR, Grabau JH, et al: Pancreatic polypeptide and insulin-secreting tumor in a dog with duodenal ulcers and hypertrophic gastritis. *J Vet Intern Med* 3:178–182, 1989.
89. Hayes HM Jr, Fraumeni JF Jr: Canine thyroid neoplasms: Epidemiologic features. *J Natl Cancer Inst* 55:931–934, 1975.
90. Mitchell M, Hurov LI, Troy GC: Canine thyroid carcinomas: Clinical occurrence, staging by means of scintiscans, and therapy of 15 cases. *Vet Surg* 8:112–118, 1979.
91. Brodey RS, Kelly DF: Thyroid neoplasms in the dog. A clinicopathologic study of fifty-seven cases. *Cancer* 22:406–416, 1968.
92. Haley PJ, Hahn FF, Muggenburg BA, Griffith WC: Thyroid neoplasms in a colony of beagle dogs. *Vet Pathol* 26:438–441, 1989.
93. Benjamin SA, Stephens LC, Hamilton BF, et al: Associations between lymphocytic thyroiditis, hypothyroidism, and thyroid neoplasia in beagles. *Vet Pathol* 33:486–494, 1996.
94. Stephens LC, Saunders WJ, Jaenke RS: Ectopic thyroid carcinoma with metastases in a beagle dog. *Vet Pathol* 19:669–675, 1982.
95. Ware WA, Merkley DF, Riedesel DH: Intracardiac thyroid tumor in a dog: Diagnosis and surgical removal. *JAVMA* 30:20–23, 1994.
96. Girard C, Helie P, Odin M: Intrapericardial neoplasia in dogs. *J Vet Diagn Invest* 11:73–78, 1999.
97. Birchard SJ, Roesel OF: Neoplasia of the thyroid gland in the dogs: A retrospective study of 16 cases. *JAAHA* 17:369–372, 1981.
98. Harari J, Patterson JS, Rosenthal RC: Clinical and pathologic features of thyroid tumors in 26 dogs. *JAVMA* 188:1160–1164, 1986.
99. Verschueren CP, Rutteman GR, Van Dijk JE, et al: Evaluation of some prognostic factors in surgically-treated canine thyroid cancer, in *Clinico-pathological and Endocrine Aspects of Canine Thyroid Cancer*. PhD Thesis, University of Utrecht, Netherlands, 1992, pp 11–25.
100. Klein MK, Powers BE, Withrow SJ, et al: Treatment of thyroid carcinoma in dogs by surgical resection alone: 20 cases (1981–1989). *JAVMA* 206:1007–1009, 1995.
101. Marks SL, Koblik PD, Hornof WJ, Feldman EC: 99mTc-pertechnetate imaging of thyroid tumors in dogs: 29 cases (1980–1992). *JAVMA* 204:756–760, 1994.
102. Patnaik AK, Lieberman PH: Gross, histologic, cytochemical, and immunocytochemical study of medullary thyroid carcinoma in sixteen dogs. *Vet Pathol* 28:223–233, 1991.
103. Carver JR, Kapatkin A, Patnaik AK: A comparison of medullary thyroid carci-

noma and thyroid adenocarcinoma in dogs: A retrospective study of 38 cases. *Vet Surg* 24:315–319, 1995.
104. Theon AP, Marks SL, Feldman ES, Griffey S: Prognostic factors and patterns of treatment failure in dogs with unresectable differentiated thyroid carcinomas treated with megavoltage irradiation. *JAVMA* 216:1775–1779, 2000.
105. Worth AT, Zuber RM, Hocking M: Radioiodide (131I) therapy for the treatment of canine thyroid carcinoma (65 cases). *Aust Vet J* 83:208–214, 2005.
106. Pack L, Roberts RE, Dawson SD, Dookwah HD: Definitive radiation therapy for infiltrative thyroid carcinoma in dogs. *Vet Radiol Ultrasound* 42:471–474, 2001.
107. Brearley MJ, Hayes AM, Murphy S: Hypofractionated radiation therapy for invasive thyroid carcinoma in dogs: A retrospective analysis of survival. *J Small Anim Pract* 40:206–210, 1999.
108. Peterson ME, Kintzer PP, Hurley JR, Becker DV: Radioactive iodine treatment of a functional thyroid carcinoma producing hyperthyroidism in a dog. *J Vet Intern Med* 3:20–25, 1989.
109. Adams WH, Walker MA, Daniel GB, et al: Treatment of differentiated thyroid carcinoma in 7 dogs utilizing [131]I. *Vet Radiol Ultrasound* 36:417–424, 1995.
110. Jeglum KA, Whereat A: Chemotherapy of canine thyroid carcinoma. *Compend Contin Educ Pract Vet* 5:96–98, 1983.
111. Ogilvie GK, Reynolds HA, Richardson RC, et al: Phase II evaluation of doxorubicin for treatment of various canine neoplasms. *JAVMA* 195:1580–1583, 1989.
112. Wheeler SL: Endocrine tumors, in Withrow SJ, MacEwen EG (eds): *Clinical Veterinary Oncology*. Philadelphia, JB Lippincott, 1989, pp 253–282.
113. Ogilvie GK, Obradovich JE, Elmslie RE, et al: Efficacy of mitoxantrone against various neoplasms in dogs. *JAVMA* 198:1618–1621, 1991.
114. Fineman LS, Hamilton TA, de Gortari A, Bonney P: Cisplatin chemotherapy for treatment of thyroid carcinoma in dogs: 13 cases. *JAAHA* 34:109–112, 1998.
115. Slensky KA, Volk SW, Schwarz T, et al: Acute severe hemorrhage secondary to arterial invasion in a dog with thyroid carcinoma. *JAVMA* 223:636, 649–653, 2003.
116. Thompson KG, Jones LP, Smylie WA, et al: Primary hyperparathyroidism in German shepherd dogs: A disorder of probable genetic origin. *Vet Pathol* 21:370–376, 1984.
117. Berger B, Feldman EC: Primary hyperparathyroidism in dogs: 21 cases (1976–1986). *JAVMA* 191:350–356, 1987.
118. Patnaik AK, MacEwen EG, Erlandson RA, et al: Mediastinal parathyroid adenocarcinoma in a dog. *Vet Pathol* 15:55–63, 1978.
119. Fingeroth JM, Smeak DD: Intravenous methylene blue infusion for intraoperative identification of parathyroid gland tumors in dogs. Part III: clinical trials and results in three dogs. *JAAHA* 24:673–678, 1988.
120. Feldman EC, Wisner ER, Nelson RW, et al: Comparison of results of hormonal analysis of samples obtained from selected venous sites versus cervical ultrasonography for localizing parathyroid masses in dogs. *JAVMA* 211:54–56, 1997.
121. Wisner ER, Penninck D, Biller DS, et al: High-resolution parathyroid sonography. *Vet Radiol Ultrasound* 38:462–466, 1997.
122. Wright KN, Breitschwerdt EB, Feldman JM, et al: Diagnostic and therapeutic considerations in a hypercalcemic dog with multiple endocrine neoplasia. *JAAHA* 31:156–162, 1995.
123. Matwichuk CL, Taylor SM, Wilkinson AA, et al: Use of technetium Tc 99m sestamibi for detection of a parathyroid adenoma in a dog with primary hyperparathyroidism. *JAVMA* 209:1733–1736, 1996.
124. Matwichuk CL, Taylor SM, Daniel GB, et al: Double-phase parathyroid scintigraphy in dogs using technetium-99M-sestamibi. *Vet Radiol Ultrasound* 41:461–469, 2000.
125. van Vonderen IK, Kooistra HS, Peeters ME, et al: Parathyroid hormone immunohistochemistry in dogs with primary and secondary hyperparathyroidism: The question of adenoma and primary hyperplasia. *J Comp Pathol* 129:61–69, 2003.
126. Pollard RE, Long CD, Nelson RW, et al: Percutaneous ultrasonographically guided radiofrequency heat ablation for treatment of primary hyperparathyroidism in dogs. *JAVMA* 218:1106–1110, 2001.
127. Peterson ME, Randolph JF, Zaki FA, Heath H 3rd: Multiple endocrine neoplasia in a dog. *JAVMA* 180:1476–1478, 1982.
128. Thuróczy J, van Sluijs FJ, Kooistra HS, et al: Multiple endocrine neoplasias in a dog: Corticotrophic tumour, bilateral adrenocortical tumours, and pheochromocytoma. *Vet Q* 20:56–61, 1998.
129. Unterer S, Grundmann S, Reiner B, et al: Ein fallbericht über einen hund mit mulitplen endokrinen neoplasien (MEN): Nebenschilddrüsenadenom, schilddrüsenadenom, schilddrüsenkarzinom, seminom und perianale adenome. *Kleintierpraxis* 47:577–636, 2002
130. Walker MC, Jones BR, Guildford WG, et al: Multiple endocrine neoplasia type 1 in a crossbred dog. *J Small Anim Pract* 41:61–70, 2000.
131. Kiupel M, Mueller PB, Ramos VJ, et al: Multiple endocrine neoplasia in a dog. *J Comp Pathol* 123:210–217, 2000.
132. Patnaik AK, Liu SK, Hurvitz AI, McClelland AJ: Canine chemodectoma (extraadrenal paragangliomas): A comparative study. *J Small Anim Pract* 16:785–801, 1975.
133. Fife W, Mattoon J, Drost WT, et al: Imaging features of a presumed carotid body tumor in a dog. *Vet Radiol Ultrasound* 44:322–325, 2003.
134. Brewer WG Jr, Crager CS: A syndrome similar to multiple endocrine neoplasia type I in two dogs. *Vet Cancer Soc Newsl* 15(3):10–11, 1991.

TUMORS OF THE REPRODUCTIVE SYSTEM

Antony S. Moore and Gregory K. Ogilvie

▶ TUMORS OF THE FEMALE REPRODUCTIVE TRACT

CLINICAL BRIEFING

Ovarian Tumors

Clinical factors	• Abdominal mass or swelling; unexplained or abnormal estrus or bleeding. • Usually adenomas and adenocarcinomas. • Old dogs most often affected (median age: 10 years); teratomas occur in young dogs.
Staging and diagnosis	• Minimum database (includes complete blood count, biochemical profile, urinalysis, and thoracic radiography [three views]) and abdominal ultrasonography. • Metastasis common, usually intraabdominal.
Prognostic factors	• None identified.
Treatment	
Initial	• Surgical excision curative for most tumors.
Adjunctive	• Adenocarcinomas may metastasize within the abdomen, causing carcinomatosis; cisplatin or bleomycin may be the drug of choice.
Supportive	• Analgesia postoperatively and nutritional support as needed.

Vaginal and Uterine Tumors

Clinical factors	• Vaginal mass, possibly tenesmus. • Usually leiomyoma and fibromas. • Old dogs affected (median age: 11 years).
Staging and diagnosis	• Minimum database and abdominal ultrasonography. • Evaluate regional lymph nodes. • Metastasis common, usually intraabdominal.
Prognostic factors	• None identified.
Treatment	
Initial	• Surgery is the treatment of choice. Most tumors are benign; therefore, complete excision may be curative. Rarely, ovariohysterectomy for hormonally induced vaginal tumors.
Adjunctive	• None reported.
Supportive	• Analgesia postoperatively and nutritional support as needed.

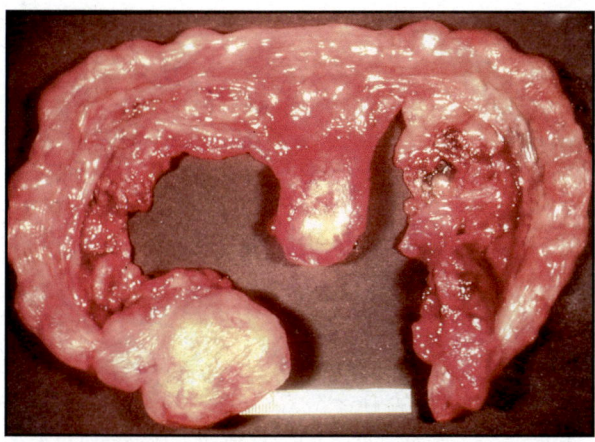

Figure 58-1. *There may be secondary cystic hyperplasia of the uterus in a dog with a Leydig cell tumor of the ovary, as in this 12-year-old cocker spaniel. (Courtesy of Gordon H. Theilen, DVM, University of California, Davis)*

Ovarian Tumors

INCIDENCE, SIGNALMENT, AND ETIOLOGY

Ovarian tumors are rare in dogs, partly because of early spaying. With the exception of teratomas, which usually affect young dogs (median age: 4 years), they tend to occur in older dogs (median age: 10 years). Boston terriers, German shepherds, and possibly poodles have a higher incidence of ovarian neoplasia than do other breeds.[1] In one study, adenomas and adenocarcinomas accounted for 33 (46%) of 71 ovarian tumors.[1] Sex-cord stromal tumors (i.e., granulosa cell tumors, Sertoli-Leydig tumors [luteal cell], and thecomas) have also been reported.[2] Large ovarian cysts may mimic ovarian neoplasms.[3,4]

Most ovarian tumors are unilateral regardless of tumor type. Adenocarcinomas and Sertoli-Leydig tumors are bilateral in about 30% of cases.[1,5] Secondary cystic changes are sometimes seen in the contralateral ovary and in the endometrium in dogs with ovarian tumors, particularly sex-cord stromal tumors (Figure 58-1).[2] Sex-cord stromal tumors are often associated with production of sex hormones.

Ovarian neoplasms should not be ruled out in a dog that has undergone ovariectomy. Ovarian remnants have been reported to give rise to granulosa cell tumors.[6,7]

Long-term treatment with mibolerone, a nonprogestational androgenic steroid, induces ovarian fibromas in dogs.[8]

CLINICAL PRESENTATION AND HISTORY

Ovarian tumors may be very large (up to 15,000 cm³). In one study, more than half of dogs with ovarian germ cell tumors, ovarian adenocarcinoma, or granulosa cell tumors had a mass that was larger than 125 cm³.[1] Therefore, most dogs with ovarian tumors are presented for abdominal distention, and the tumor is palpable on careful physical examination.

Dogs with ovarian neoplasia, particularly of sex-cord stromal origin, may present with vaginal bleeding, pyometra, or unusual frequency of estrus[9,10] related to endometrial hyperplasia, which is common with these tumors. One report described episodic depression, anorexia, and extreme timidity that resolved after surgical resection of a granulosa–theca cell tumor.[10] Rarely, a granulosa cell tumor produces sufficient estrogen over a prolonged period to cause bone marrow aplasia. These dogs may present with clinical signs, such as fever and sepsis due to neutropenia or bleeding due to thrombocytopenia. One dog had erythroid hypoplasia in addition to other signs of hyperestrogenism, including mammary hyperplasia and endocrine alopecia.[6]

Peritoneal carcinomatosis may follow seeding from the primary tumor, and malignant ascites may accumulate and be perceived by the owner as abdominal swelling. Visceral metastases outside the abdominal cavity are rare except with malignant teratomas.[1]

STAGING AND DIAGNOSIS

Ovarian tumors often metastasize. In one study, three of six ovarian teratomas and 10 of 21 adenocarcinomas had metastases, usually in the form of carcinomatosis.[11] Distant metastases in the kidneys, adrenal glands, lung, bone, and mediastinal lymph nodes were seen with teratomas. A dog with a dysgerminoma developed central vestibular disease 2 weeks after surgery due to brain metastasis.[12] Pleural effusion has been noted in some dogs with ovarian cancer; therefore, thoracic radiographs should be obtained in any dog with a suspected ovarian tumor.[5] Worsening effusion can compromise a patient if left untreated.

Ultrasonography may help determine the origin of a large abdominal mass and will disclose any ascites that might signal carcinomatosis. Some dogs have bilateral tumors; ultrasonography allows the clinician to detect these before surgery. Ultrasonography was also able to detect endometrial hyperplasia and pyometra in five dogs with granulosa cell tumors and other ovarian neoplasms.[5]

> *Most ovarian tumors are unilateral; however, adenocarcinomas and Sertoli-Leydig cell tumors are bilateral in about 30% of cases.*

Serum estrogen levels may be useful in making a diagnosis of ovarian tumor in a spayed animal. In one dog that had elevated serum estrogen with a normal progesterone level, the serum progesterone rose in response to a human chorionic gonadotropin (hCG) stimulation test, indicating a possible tumor.[6] Measurement of serum estrogen during therapy may also be used to monitor remission. Hyperadrenocorticism resolved after surgical removal of an ovarian steroid cell tumor (luteoma) in one dog.[13]

TREATMENT

Surgery is the treatment of choice for dogs that show no evidence of metastasis, and survival following surgery is usually long; however, there are few clinical reports of surgical resection of ovarian tumors. In three dogs with dysgerminoma, one dog survived 13 months and died of another cancer; the other two dogs survived 2 and 4 years, respectively.[11,14] Of nine dogs with teratoma, five survived more than 1 year. Two dogs died of metastatic disease 1 and 5 months after surgery, and one dog died intraoperatively.[9,11,15-17] Two dogs with granulosa cell tumors survived more than 2 years.[7,10]

Reports of therapy for metastatic ovarian tumors are few. In humans with ovarian carcinomatosis, long-term remissions and cures are sometimes obtained with cisplatin therapy. One dog with ovarian carcinomatosis was treated three times with 50 mg/m² of cisplatin intraperitoneally and was still alive 5 years after treatment.[18] Similar anecdotal successes indicate that cisplatin by intracavitary or possibly intravenous administration may give long-term control of ovarian carcinoma.[19] Cyclophosphamide was inactive alone in one dog[20] and in combination with chlorambucil and

> **KEY POINT**
> *Intracavitary cisplatin chemotherapy may give long-term control of ovarian carcinomatosis.*

lomustine in another dog.[21] In the latter dog, when abdominal fluid accumulated, intracavitary bleomycin was administered, and the dog had no evidence of tumor 10 months after surgery.

Vaginal Tumors

INCIDENCE, SIGNALMENT, AND ETIOLOGY

Tumors of the vulva and vagina are rare in dogs but are more common than ovarian and uterine neoplasms.[22] This may reflect spaying practices. More than 70% of tumors are benign and are derived from the supportive stroma of the vulva and vagina. The most common vulval and vaginal tumors are leiomyomas, fibromas, and lipomas. Leiomyomas accounted for 77% of tumors in one study[22]; in three other studies, they accounted for 12% to 50% of tumors.[23-25] In all four studies, 30% to 50% of tumors were fibromas[23,25] and 6% were lipomas.[22] Transmissible venereal tumor (TVT), the next most common tumor, is addressed below.

Malignant tumors are rare, accounting for less than 24% of tumors in one study[23] and less than 5% in another.[22] Leiomyosarcomas, mast cell tumors, and squamous cell car-

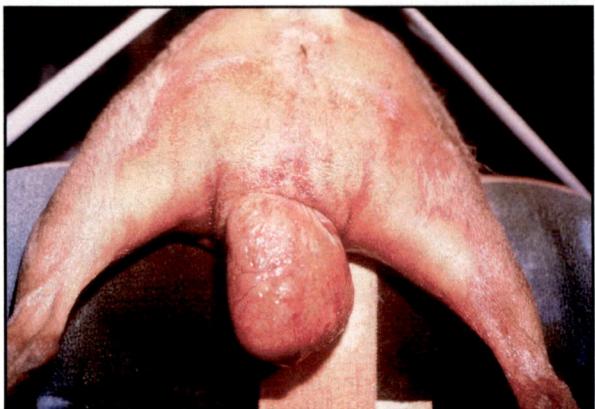

Figure 58-2. *The owner often first notes vaginal leiomyoma in a dog as a protruding mass.*

cinomas (SCCs) are the most common malignant vulval and vaginal tumors.[22,25]

The mean age of affected dogs is 11 years (range: 5–16 years). There is no obvious breed predilection, although poodles accounted for 17% of cases in two studies.[23,25] Cocker spaniels, German shepherds, and dachshunds were also commonly affected.[23] There is a reported association between leiomyomas and fibromas and hormonal influences in affected dogs.[25] Dogs that have been pregnant have a higher risk of developing these tumors. In one study, 39 of 40 affected dogs were intact.[24]

CLINICAL PRESENTATION AND HISTORY

Tumors that arise from the vestibule wall may protrude from the vulvar labia (Figure 58-2). Such tumors often produce a perineal mass and vulvar bleeding. Effects on micturition or defecation are rare and are usually associated with large tumors.[23] In one study, the most common reason for an owner seeking veterinary advice was the finding of a protruding tumor (58% of cases); less common reasons were bloody discharge (25%) and perineal swelling (11%).[23] An owner may mistake a protruding tumor for vaginal or uterine prolapse. Most tumors arise from the vagina (78%); 17% are classified as vulvar in origin.[23]

STAGING AND DIAGNOSIS

Routine staging with blood work, urinalysis, and thoracic radiography will provide a general health screen for affected dogs. Ultrasonography may be useful in determining whether intraabdominal extension or metastasis has occurred. Definitive diagnosis is made by biopsy; however, clinical findings of a pedunculated vaginal mass are most consistent with a benign tumor. Benign tumors are often slow growing and cause no clinical signs until they are very large. Malignant tumors vary in metastatic rate. In one study, metastasis was seen in 2 of 22 dogs with malignant tumors.[23]

TREATMENT

Surgery is the treatment of choice for benign and malignant tumors of the vagina and vestibule (Figure 58-3). For benign tumors, it is usually curative. One study had no recurrences 4 months to 4 years after surgery in 15 dogs.[24] In another study, the recurrence rate was 15%, with regrowth seen between 6 months and 3.5 years after surgery.[23] Surgical margins should be as wide as possible. Ovariohysterectomy at the time of excision of a benign vaginal tumor may reduce the risk of recurrence.[25]

Some vaginal tumors are nonpedunculated and grow toward the vestibule or the cervix. These tumors may cause urethral and rectal compression as well as local neurologic effects. Total and partial vaginectomy associated with urethroplasty was used to treat nonpedunculated vaginal tumors in four dogs.[26] The surgical procedure allowed complete resection of the tumor with little morbidity. There were no local recurrences or metastases.

Vulvovaginectomy and perineal urethrostomy may be required for malignant and some benign tumors, but palliative margins may be difficult to achieve.[27] Long-term survival after this surgery is often not reported, making it difficult to assess the efficacy of the procedure.[28]

There are few reports of surgery for malignant tumors. One dog with leiomyosarcoma of the vagina had four surgical excisions over a 2.5-year period.[22] Six dogs with vulvar leiomyosarcoma and two dogs with SCC survived an average of 11.3 and 15.5 months, respectively, after surgery. Recurrence was noted in only one dog with each tumor type.[25] A dog with vaginal fibrosarcoma was treated with carbon dioxide laser ablation and two doses of doxorubicin (30 mg/m^2 IV) and had no evidence of disease when it died 20 months later.[29]

Uterine Tumors

INCIDENCE, SIGNALMENT, AND ETIOLOGY

Most tumors of the reproductive tract originate in the vulva and vagina; relatively few are in the uterus (11 of 90 reproductive tract tumors in one study[22]). This may reflect spaying practices. The most common uterine tumors (leiomyomas [90%], leiomyosarcomas) are derived from the smooth muscle stroma, although carcinomas have also been reported. A uterine hemangiosarcoma has been reported.[30] Most tumors arise in the body of the uterus, although tumors originating from the oviduct[31] and the salpinx[32] have been described. There was a tenuous association between exogenous hormonal therapy and development of endometrial carcinoma in a dog treated with ethinylestradiol, methyltestosterone, and megestrol acetate.[33]

The mean age of affected dogs is 11 years (range: 5–16 years), although uterine carcinoma has been reported in young dogs.[33,34] There is no obvious breed predilection for these rare tumors.

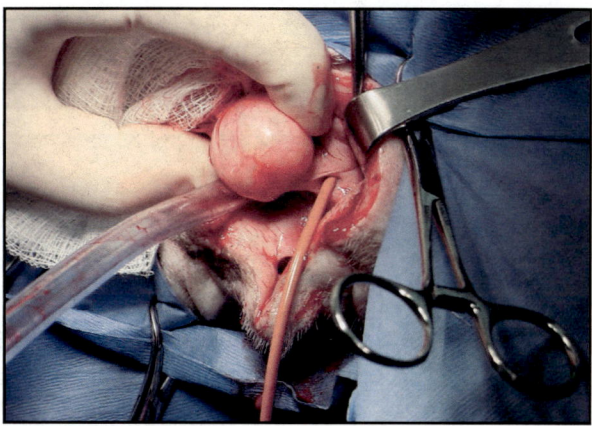

Figure 58-3. *Vaginal fibroleiomyoma may be completely resected, but before doing so, it is important to identify and catheterize the urethra. (Courtesy of Nicole Northrup, DVM, University of Georgia College of Veterinary Medicine)*

CLINICAL PRESENTATION AND HISTORY

Reports of specific clinical signs in dogs with uterine carcinomas are rare,[35] although the abdomen of one dog noticeably enlarged over several months as a result of a large adenomatous papilloma of the uterus.[31] A young dog with uterine carcinoma showed nonspecific signs of inappetence, occasional vomiting, and depression,[34] and anorexia and fever were the presenting signs in another dog with a benign uterine tumor.[36] An abdominal mass is often palpable.

STAGING AND DIAGNOSIS

Routine staging with blood work, urinalysis, and thoracic radiography will provide a general health screen for affected dogs. Abdominal ultrasonography should be conducted to determine the site of origin and whether metastasis has occurred. Benign tumors are often slow growing and cause no clinical signs until they are very large. Malignant tumors vary in metastatic rate. Leiomyosarcomas are not reported to metastasize; however, carcinomas of the uterine horns in three dogs metastasized to the lungs and kidney. In one of these dogs, metastases were also found in the liver and adrenal and thyroid glands.[35]

TREATMENT

Uterine carcinoma is a rare but highly metastatic tumor for which surgery is unlikely to be curative.

A dog with a uterine carcinoma was treated with 4 doses of epirubicin (30 mg/m^2 IV q3wk) and had no evidence of disease 2 years later.[34] Anecdotally, therefore, anthracycline-based chemotherapy seems to be the best approach for these tumors.

TUMORS OF THE MALE REPRODUCTIVE TRACT

CLINICAL BRIEFING

Testicular Tumors

Clinical factors
- Palpable mass in normal or atrophic testis.
- Tumors are seminomas, Sertoli cell tumors, and interstitial cell tumors.
- Many are not palpable.
- Feminization changes with some Sertoli cell tumors and seminomas.
- Seminomas and Sertoli cell tumors have a high incidence in retained testes.
- Old dogs affected; no breed predilection.

Staging and diagnosis
- Minimum database and abdominal ultrasonography.
- Metastasis rare, usually regional lymph nodes.

Prognostic factors
- Histologically diffuse seminomas may be more likely to metastasize.
- Seminomas with high AgNOR counts may be more likely to metastasize.

Treatment

Initial
- Usually curative; metastatic rate is low.

Adjunctive
- Radiation therapy may achieve long-term control for metastatic seminoma to sublumbar nodes. Cisplatin and bleomycin chemotherapy may be effective for metastatic tumors.

Supportive
- Analgesia postoperatively and nutritional support as needed.

Prostatic Tumors

Clinical factors
- Tenesmus, constipation, dyschezia, and (less commonly) dysuria and hematuria.
- Carcinoma arises from ducts, most commonly transitional cell carcinoma.
- Equal frequency in castrated and uncastrated dogs regardless of age at castration.
- Old dogs affected (median age: 10 years).

Staging and diagnosis
- Minimum database and abdominal ultrasonography.
- Metastasis common, usually regional lymph nodes and bone.

Prognostic factors
- May be more aggressive in castrated dogs (but highly malignant in both castrated and uncastrated).

Treatment

Initial
- Surgery difficult because of anatomy of canine prostate.

Adjunctive
- Radiation therapy palliative because of high metastatic rate. Chemotherapy as for transitional cell carcinoma may be effective. Piroxicam has some anecdotal efficacy. Hormonal therapy ineffective because of hormone independence of canine prostatic carcinoma.

Supportive
- Analgesia may be needed. If obstructed, may need transabdominal catheter. Nutritional support as needed.

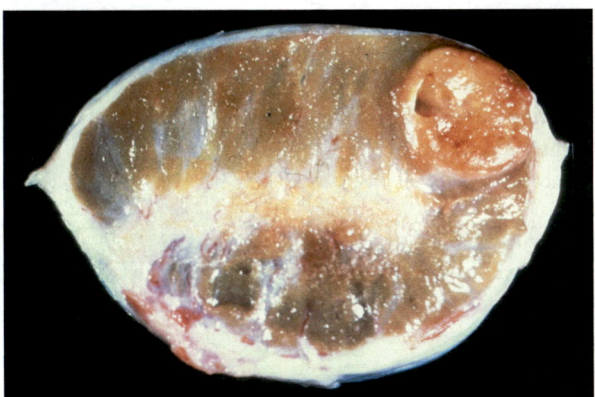

Figure 58-4. *Interstitial cell tumors, as seen here, arise within the testicular parenchyma and are rarely palpable.*

Testicular Tumors

INCIDENCE, SIGNALMENT, AND ETIOLOGY

Three types of testicular tumor are commonly diagnosed in dogs. Sertoli cell tumors and interstitial (Leydig) cell tumors are sex-cord, gonadal stromal tumors, and seminomas are germ cell tumors. Interstitial cell tumors account for approximately 40% of testicular tumors; seminomas and Sertoli cell tumors are the next most common types.[37-40] Dogs may have tumors that contain more than one cell population[37] and may have more than one tumor type in the same or contralateral testis. Some tumors are bilateral.

Approximately 20% of all testicular tumors and 30% to 50% of all Sertoli cell tumors occur in cryptorchid testes.[40,41] This may be a result of the higher temperature at which undescended testes are maintained compared with scrotal testes. A 2003 study found that although less than 7% of the dog population was cryptorchid, Chihuahuas accounted for 30% of cryptorchid dogs, boxers for 20%, and German shepherds for 14%.[42] Another study showed that approximately 6% of cryptorchid dogs will develop a testicular tumor.[43]

> **KEY POINT**
>
> *Dogs with cryptorchid testes or inguinal hernia are nine and four times more likely, respectively, to develop testicular tumors than dogs with normally descended testes.*

An elevated incidence of seminomas has been observed in military working dogs, possibly due to tetracycline treatment or exposure to pesticides.[44] The incidence of all canine testicular tumors increases with age. The average age at diagnosis for dogs with all tumor types was between 9 and 11 years, although dogs with tumors of cryptorchid testes are often younger than those with tumors of scrotal testes. No breed prevalence has been described for any tumor type.

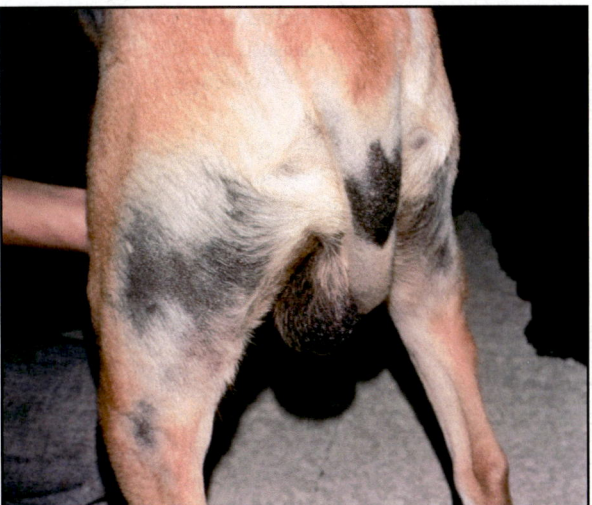

Figure 58-5. *Hormonal symmetric alopecia is seen in this dog with a Sertoli cell tumor.*

CLINICAL PRESENTATION AND HISTORY

Interstitial cell tumors are usually small (<1 cm diameter) and rarely palpable (Figure 58-4). They rarely cause hormonal effects.

Seminomas are larger than interstitial cell tumors and may be palpable as a mass in an otherwise normal testis. They are commonly found in undescended testicles and are often associated with interstitial and Sertoli cell tumors. Feminization changes have been described in dogs with seminoma, but they may have been due to undetected Sertoli cell tumors.

Sertoli cell tumors produce signs of feminization in approximately 30% of affected dogs, particularly in dogs with tumors of cryptorchid testes. Feminization may be concurrent with elevated serum estrogen levels and may be associated with suppression of pituitary gonadotropin secretion. Sertoli cell tumors are often large, and the contralateral testicle and normal testicular tissue in the affected testicle are often atrophic. Prostatic hyperplasia, gynecomastia, and haircoat changes, including bilaterally symmetric alopecia and epidermal atrophy due to atrophy of hair follicles and sebaceous glands, are common. Alopecic skin may be hyperpigmented (Figure 58-5). Prostatic hyperplasia due to squamous metaplasia may result in cyst and abscess formation. Affected dogs become attractive to other male dogs, which will attempt to mate with them.

STAGING AND DIAGNOSIS

Routine staging and health screening should be undertaken for all dogs with a testicular tumor. In certain cases, testicular and abdominal ultrasonography may be helpful. The risk of pulmonary metastasis is low, but thoracic radiographs should be taken for completeness and as part of a health screen in older dogs.

Although rare, bone marrow aplasia has been reported in a dog with an interstitial cell tumor,[45] and fatal bone marrow aplasia was seen in a dog with Sertoli cell tumor.[46]

Approximately half of interstitial cell tumors are bilateral. Malignant interstitial cell tumors have not been described.

> **KEY POINT**
>
> *Interstitial cell tumors are bilateral in approximately 50% of cases, whereas seminomas and Sertoli cell tumors are bilateral in only 10% of cases.*

Metastasis is seen in 5% to 10% of dogs with seminomas, primarily to the regional lymph nodes (i.e., inguinal, iliac, and sublumbar nodes) and occasionally to the lungs or other viscera. Metastases have been reported in the brain and eyes[47,48] and the skin.[48,49] Approximately 10% of seminomas are bilateral.

Sertoli cell tumors are reported to metastasize at about the same rate as seminomas and are bilateral in about 10% of cases. Metastasis occurs first to regional lymph nodes but may continue to paraaortic and mesenteric nodes. Paraneoplastic hypertrophic osteopathy was seen in one dog.[50] Metastatic tumors may be functional and may cause the return or continuation of feminization signs in a dog that has had the primary tumor removed.

Investigation of the molecular basis of these tumors has shown that seminomas and Sertoli cell tumors (but not interstitial cell tumors) express mutated *p53*, a tumor suppressor gene.[51] This expression may correlate with aggressive behavior in these tumors. Another study found that although estrogen receptors were present in benign testicular tumors, androgen, progesterone, and glucocorticoid receptors were more common in malignant tumors.[52]

Some histopathologic criteria may help identify "high-risk" seminomas. In one study,[53] seminomas with higher proliferation indexes, higher mitotic indexes, and increased numbers of argyrophilic nucleolar organizer regions (AgNORs) were classified as diffuse seminomas. Dogs with diffuse seminoma were more likely to develop metastatic disease, and AgNOR number appeared to be an independent predictor of metastasis.[53,54] A further study found that diffuse seminomas had more evidence of angiogenesis, which may increase the risk for metastasis.[55]

Ultrasonography and radiography of the abdomen may be useful in looking for a retained testicle or in evaluating abdominal lymph nodes and organs when metastasis of a seminoma or a Sertoli cell tumor is suspected. Ultrasonography of the testicle is useful in identifying and evaluating small testicular tumors for biopsy in breeding dogs for which castration is not an option and in identifying tumors in the contralateral testicle. In one study, all hypoechoic masses less than 3 cm in diameter were interstitial cell tumors.[56]

TREATMENT

Surgical castration cures most dogs with a testicular tumor. Unilateral castration may be an acceptable option for some dogs with a Sertoli cell tumor or seminoma, as these tumors are rarely bilateral and metastasis is rare. This technique allowed return to fertility (increased percentage of sperm and motility as well as successful mating in 6 to 10 months) in dogs made infertile by testicular tumors.[57] However, bilateral castration is preferred, particularly if the dog is not a valuable breeding animal and other diseases such as prostatic disease are present. Careful ultrasonography may help identify dogs with tumors in the contralateral testicle.

There are few reports of therapy for tumors that have metastasized. Four dogs with metastasis of a seminoma to the sublumbar lymph nodes but no other gross evidence of metastatic disease were treated with cesium-137 radiation therapy to a total dose of 17 to 40 Gy.[58] Lymph node metastases regressed in all four dogs. Three of the dogs died from apparently unrelated causes after survival times of 37, 43, and 57 months, respectively. The fourth dog died from transitional cell carcinoma of the urinary bladder with no evidence of seminoma 6 months after receiving radiation treatment.

There are few reports of chemotherapy for widespread metastatic testicular tumors in dogs. A dog with widespread cutaneous, ocular, and visceral metastases from a seminoma showed progression of the cancer despite vincristine and cyclophosphamide chemotherapy and died 4 months after initiation of treatment.[48] Another dog with cutaneous metastases from a seminoma had a partial (>50%) response to therapy (bleomycin 10 mg/m^2 SC daily for 4 days, then once weekly for 16 weeks). The residual tumor was excised, and the dog had no evidence of disease 12 months after diagnosis.[49] Cisplatin is a useful agent in human patients with testicular tumors, and a recent report implies that it may also have activity in dogs. In that report, cisplatin was administered to a bulldog with a metastatic Sertoli cell tumor; the dog was alive without evidence of tumor 31 months later. Other dogs mentioned in that report had shorter survival times.[59]

Penile Tumors

INCIDENCE, SIGNALMENT, AND ETIOLOGY

Penile neoplasms other than TVTs are rare. An early publication suggested that 1.5% of all reported carcinomas in dogs were associated with the penis and prepuce.[60] The most commonly reported penile tumor is SCC.[61,62] A mesenchymal chondrosarcoma of the os penis has also been described.[61]

CLINICAL PRESENTATION AND HISTORY

Stranguria and anuria were seen in one dog in which the SCC presumably arose from the urethra.[61] Another dog with SCC had a mass on the glans.[62] The dog with a chondrosarcoma was also dysuric.

STAGING AND DIAGNOSIS

Enlarged iliac lymph nodes identified at the time of diagnosis contained metastatic SCC in one dog.[61] That dog was not treated. No metastases were noted in the other dog with SCC.[62]

TREATMENT

Surgery is probably the initial treatment of choice for penile tumors and should be aggressive. Penile amputation and urethrostomy were performed in one dog with SCC and in the dog with chondrosarcoma. The dog with SCC was alive without evidence of recurrence or metastasis 9 months after surgery.[62] The chondrosarcoma recurred at the incision edge 4 months after initial surgery and was not treated further.[61]

Prostatic Tumors

INCIDENCE, SIGNALMENT, AND ETIOLOGY

Hyperplasia of the prostate is common in old dogs, and prostatic neoplasia is more common in dogs than in any other species except humans; however, prostatic tumors are rare in dogs. When they do occur, they are always malignant. Carcinoma is the most common histologic diagnosis. In humans, prostatic carcinoma arises from the acinar epithelium and is under androgenic hormone control. In contrast, canine prostatic tumors arise primarily from the ductular/urothelial epithelium and rarely express androgen receptors.[63] Studies using specific antibodies have found that while 25% of prostatic tumors were originally described as glandular (i.e., adenocarcinomas),[64] the true number appears to be much lower (one of 58 prostatic tumors in another study[65]).

A study found it was not possible to distinguish histologically between transitional cell carcinoma and prostatic carcinoma in dogs.[66] This suggests that many prostatic tumors

> **KEY POINT**
>
> *Prostatic carcinoma does not appear to arise from the glandular tissue but rather from the urothelial ducts and is therefore usually transitional cell carcinoma.*

are transitional cell carcinomas arising from the prostatic urothelium.[63,65] Prostatic sarcomas are rare; in one study, three of 79 dogs with prostatic tumors had sarcomas.[64]

Dogs with prostatic carcinoma tend to be 8 years of age or older,[67–70] with a median age of 10 years in some studies.[64,65,71] The only breed predilection demonstrated is in the Bouvier des Flandres, which had a more than eightfold increased risk of developing prostate carcinoma in one study.[72] German shepherds were the most commonly affected breed in another study.[65]

The progression to carcinoma appears to be stepwise, with one study showing foci of high-grade prostatic intraepithelial neoplasms (HGPINs) in 55% of older intact dogs but in only 8% of dogs younger than 4 years.[73] Other studies have not shown such a high incidence. In men, needle biopsy can be used to diagnose these early changes; however, no histologic evidence of HGPINs was detected in 20 normal canine prostates or in 95 dogs with benign prostatic hyperplasia, while seven of 20 dogs with prostatic carcinomas also had HGPINs.[74] In another study, HGPINs were seen in only 3% of dogs without prostate carcinoma and in 72% of dogs with prostatic adenocarcinoma.[75]

Two studies found that castration did not reduce the incidence of prostatic carcinoma, regardless of when surgery took place.[71,76] In one survey of 43 dogs, 19 (45%) had been castrated at least 3 years before developing prostatic carcinoma, including seven dogs that were castrated at less than 1 year of age.[76] In the other study, 10 (30%) of 31 dogs had been castrated 2 or more years before developing prostatic malignancy.[71] Another study found that dogs with diagnosed prostatic carcinoma were castrated at a median age of 5 years and that the median time from castration to cancer diagnosis was 7 years.[64] Although early castration was uncommon in this group of dogs, it did not prevent tumorigenesis. Castration actually increased the risk for prostatic carcinoma in a fourth study, with castrated dogs having a more than fourfold increase in the risk of prostatic carcinoma. The conclusion in this study was that castration may not initiate the development of carcinoma but may favor

> **KEY POINT**
>
> *Early castration of dogs does not reduce the risk of developing prostatic carcinoma.*

tumor progression.[72] These data are consistent with the fact that testosterone is not an etiologic factor in the development of prostatic carcinoma in dogs.

CLINICAL PRESENTATION AND HISTORY

The most frequent presenting signs relate to the lower bowel and include tenesmus, constipation, and dyschezia.

Dogs may also show anorexia, weight loss, and signs referable to the urinary tract, such as stranguria and hematuria. In one study, signs of inflammatory prostatic disease and neoplasia were similar, except that in dogs with carcinoma, weight loss and pain were more common and discharge and hematuria were less common.[77] Urinary tract signs, particularly in a castrated dog, should raise suspicion for prostatic neoplasia.[71] Lumbar pain and hindlimb weakness or lameness have been described, often in association with metastasis to the lumbar spine[78] or invasion of the rectal wall.[79] The duration of signs varies from weeks to years, although most affected dogs have signs for less than 1 month.[70,71] Secondary infections may lead to painful, debilitating abscessation.[80]

Prostatomegaly is not always noted on digital rectal examination. In one series, only 16 (50%) of 31 dogs had prostatic enlargement. In 10 of these dogs, enlargement was asymmetric. There were no differences in these findings between castrated and noncastrated dogs,[71] although prostatomegaly may be less frequently detected on digital rectal palpation in castrated dogs because of involution of normal prostatic tissue after castration. Approximately 30% of dogs show pain on rectal or abdominal palpation. The prostate tumor is often fixed to the floor of the pelvis and may cause narrowing of the pelvic canal[67] and invade surrounding bone in the pelvis and sacral spine.[78]

STAGING AND DIAGNOSIS

Definitive diagnosis is made by cytology or histopathology. Ultrasonographic guidance is very helpful in obtaining cytology samples by fine-needle aspiration (FNA). This method gives a high rate of positive diagnosis (80% in two studies[71,81]). False-negative results are more likely with prostatic wash or prostatic massage via a urethral catheter, which does not direct the sampler to a suspicious lesion.[82]

> **KEY POINT**
> *Adequate samples for diagnosis are best obtained by the use of FNA or needle biopsy.*

Transrectal biopsy with a Franzen transrectal needle guide rarely presents any complications.[71] The transrectal use of needle biopsy instruments is described in Chapter 18. However, if ultrasonography is available, the transabdominal approach is probably preferable for FNA and needle biopsy.

In a study that detailed diagnoses obtained by FNA and suction-catheter biopsy in dogs with prostatic disease, the sensitivity (true positive) and specificity (true negative) of each method used alone were 67% and 98%, respectively. The best results were obtained when both methods were used in combination, with a sensitivity of 73% and specificity of 98%. Insufficient material for diagnosis was

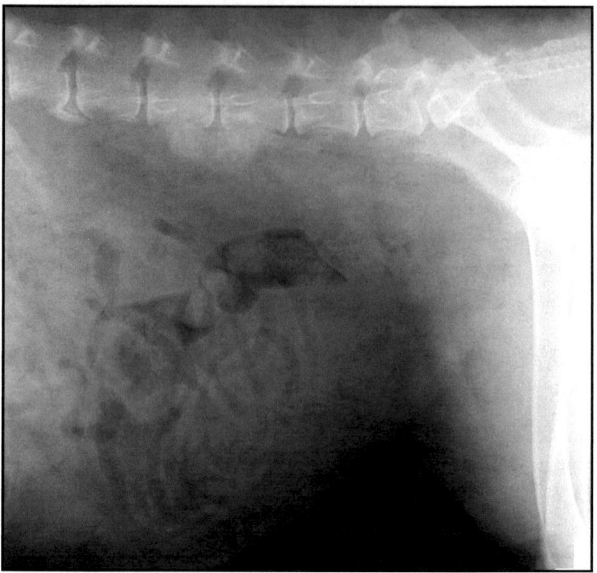

Figure 58-6. *Prostatic carcinoma may become large and invade regionally into the lumbar vertebrae.*

obtained in 7% of FNA samples and 18% of suction samples, but when the two techniques were used together, only 5% of cases had an insufficient sample. The combination of techniques therefore appears to be ideal.[77]

In human patients with prostatic carcinoma, serum levels of prostate-specific antigen (PSA) are often elevated, allowing screening for early tumors. In one study, PSA was not detected in the serum of any dog with prostatic carcinoma, which is consistent with the lack of immunohistochemical staining for the antigen.[65,83]

Hematology and a biochemical profile are rarely helpful in establishing a diagnosis. Urinalysis reveals pyuria and hematuria in 60% to 65% of dogs; however, secondary bacterial infections are rarely found on urine culture or on prostatic aspiration or massage.[71] Malignant cells were seen on urinalysis in 4 of 24 dogs with prostatic carcinoma.[71]

Metastasis is common in dogs with prostatic carcinoma, occurring in 80% of affected dogs in one study.[64] In another study, the most common sites were the iliac lymph nodes (43% of dogs) and the lungs (32% of dogs). Bone metastases (26% of dogs) and abdomen carcinomatosis (15% of dogs) were also common.[65] Spread through regional blood vessels to the penis has been reported.[84]

Radiography helps identify prostatomegaly and changes in the size or contour of the prostate (Figure 58-6). Prostatic mineralization is most frequently associated with neoplasia and occurred in approximately 40% of dogs in one study[71]; however, mineralization may also occur with chronic prostatitis.[85] A distention retrograde urethrocystogram may reveal distortion of the prostatic urethra and is a reliable indicator of neoplasia but does not distinguish between primary ure-

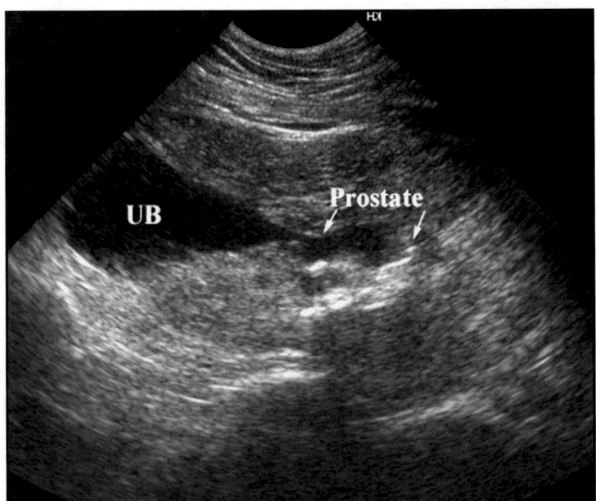

Figure 58-7. *Ultrasonography is preferred over radiography and may show multifocal areas of increased prostatic echogenicity suggestive of mineralization and neoplasia.*

thral and primary prostatic tumors. Thoracic radiographs should be obtained because pulmonary metastasis is found in more than 60% of dogs at necropsy[67,71] and is identified radiographically in nearly half of affected dogs.[71]

On ultrasonography, nearly 70% of dogs with prostatic neoplasia show multifocal areas of increased prostatic echogenicity (Figure 58-7).[86] Although not specific for prostatic carcinoma, this finding is strongly suggestive of a neoplastic process. Prostatic cysts are most frequently associated with prostatitis or hyperplasia, but they may also be seen with prostatic carcinoma. Conducting ultrasonography when the dog's bladder is full will aid in imaging the prostate.[86] Ultrasonography is also useful for evaluation of the sublumbar lymph nodes and other organs, such as the liver. Metastasis occurs to both sites in about one-third of cases.[71]

Bone metastasis of prostatic carcinoma occurs in 15% to 40% of affected dogs.[64,65,67,71,78] The most common sites are in the axial skeleton, with the pelvis and lumbosacral spine predominating.[64,78] The femur is the most common appendicular site.[65] Dogs with hindlimb weakness or lameness should be evaluated by radiography or bone scintigraphy for evidence of bony metastases to the pelvis and lumbar vertebrae or to distant bones (Figure 58-8). Bone scintigraphy may be more sensitive than radiography in detecting bony metastases from prostatic carcinoma.[78]

A case report of a dog with prostatic leiomyosarcoma described metastases that affected regional lymph nodes, the mesentery, the kidneys, and the lungs.[87]

PROGNOSTIC FACTORS

One study found a significantly higher rate of pulmonary metastasis for prostatic carcinoma in castrated dogs com-

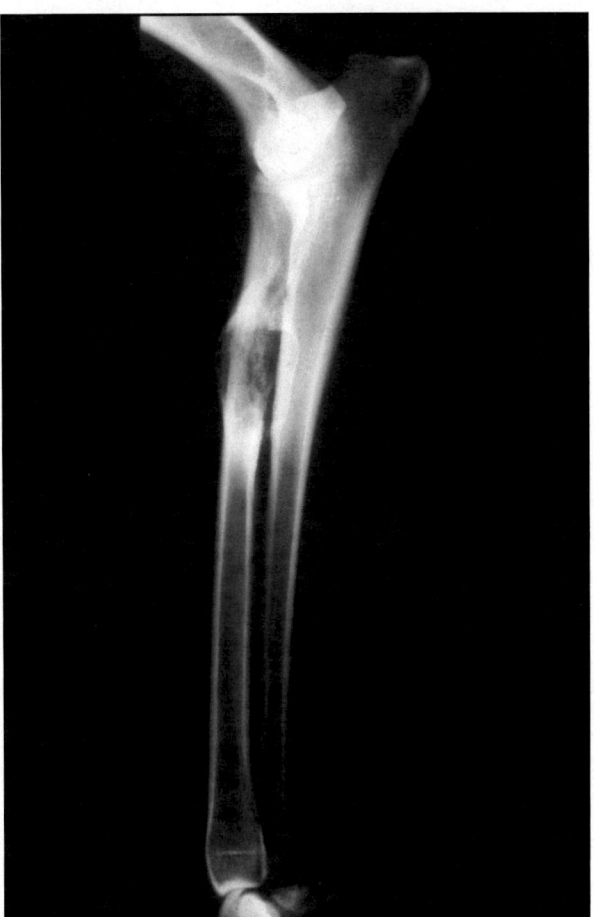

Figure 58-8. *A lytic bone metastasis from prostatic carcinoma affecting the radius in an Irish terrier. (Courtesy of Kenneth M. Rassnick, DVM, Cornell University College of Veterinary Medicine)*

pared with intact dogs (100% and 47%, respectively). There was no difference in overall metastatic rate.[71]

Positive staining for the ductular epithelial marker CK-7 was associated with a higher overall likelihood of metastasis, particularly bone metastasis, in one study.[65]

TREATMENT

In a series of 72 dogs with prostatic carcinoma, the median survival was 0 days, with 58 dogs euthanatized at the time of diagnosis.[64] This underscores the severity of clinical signs and the poor prognosis given by veterinarians to dog owners. For dogs that lived longer than 1 week, the median survival time was 30 days.[64]

Prostatectomy or subtotal prostatectomy is not recommended for prostatic carcinoma because of technical difficulties and the high rate of metastasis. When the prostate was surgically removed from six dogs with prostatic carcinoma, five dogs had survival times of less than 30 days, and the remaining dog died 60 days after surgery.[68] Metastasis was

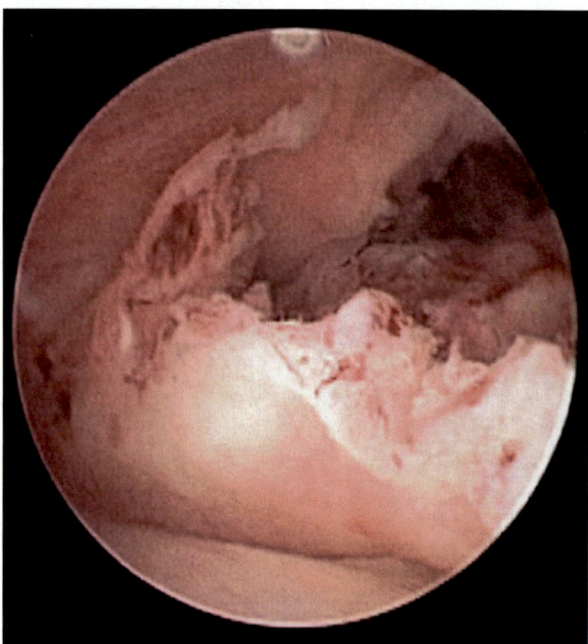

Figure 58-9. *Cystoscopic view of a prostatic carcinoma before TUR. (Courtesy of Julius M. Liptak, BVSc, Ontario Veterinary College, University of Guelph)*

common. A technique of transurethral prostatectomy has been described in normal dogs but has not been commonly evaluated in dogs with carcinomas.[88] Transurethral tumor tissue resection (TUR) performed through a cystoscope was found to give palliative results in male dogs with obstructive urinary disease.[89] TUR may be considered for rapid relief of urethral obstruction in male dogs (Figure 58-9).

Hormonal therapy in dogs with prostatic carcinoma has been limited to surgical castration and estrogen therapy. Neither approach has been useful, and these treatments give survival times of less than 30 days with no improvement in clinical signs.[68,70,71] Ketoconazole, which interferes with steroid synthesis, was used in two dogs in combination with external beam radiation therapy, with no effect.[71] The lack of effect of these hormonal manipulations is not surprising given the lack of influence of castration on development of this disease.

Radiation therapy may be palliative in the treatment of prostatic carcinoma, but the high rate of metastasis (85%–100%[36]) means that, as for surgery, overall survival statistics are unlikely to be greatly affected. Orthovoltage radiation therapy was given intraoperatively to 10 dogs with prostatic carcinoma.[90] Doses of 15 to 30 Gy were delivered to the prostate alone in seven dogs that had disease macroscopically confined to the prostate; the same dose was delivered to the sublumbar nodes of three dogs. The median survival time of all 10 dogs was 114 days (range: 41–750 days), despite a complete response to radiation in five dogs.

Other studies of radiation therapy had a maximum median survival time of 7 months.[71,91,92]

If radiation therapy is to be used, small, frequent fractions are more likely to avoid complications. In one study, dogs receiving more than 3.3 Gy per fraction to the pelvic area had an increased risk of developing severe colitis, and 60% of these dogs had intestinal perforation. Dogs treated with fractions of 2.7 Gy or less had mild to moderate self-limiting complications.[93]

> **KEY POINT**
>
> *If radiation therapy is used, small dose fractions will reduce the risk of complications.*

Photodynamic therapy was able to palliate urethral obstruction in one dog for 34 weeks, during which the tumor remained stable. Progression of prostatic disease and presumed distant metastases were the cause of death.[94] In another study, palliation was achieved in three dogs by using a retained urethral catheter, although urinary incontinence was a problem in all dogs.[91]

There are few reports of chemotherapy for prostatic carcinoma. Two dogs that underwent subtotal intracapsular prostatectomy received mitoxantrone (5 mg/m^2 IV q3wk) for two and three treatments.[91] Survival time in these two dogs was 5 and 3 months, respectively. Two dogs that received intraoperative radiation also received cyclophosphamide (50 mg/m^2 PO every other day) and 5-fluorouracil (100 mg/m^2 IV weekly), and one of these dogs also received doxorubicin (30 mg/m^2 IV q3wk). Survival time from the start of chemotherapy was 120 and 80 days, respectively.[90]

Further investigation is needed to define the role of chemotherapy in the treatment of prostatic carcinoma. Most prostatic carcinomas are ductular in origin; therefore, chemotherapy as described for transitional cell carcinoma may be the best approach. A recent study evaluated expression of cyclooxygenase (COX)-2 and the effect of COX-2 inhibitors on survival of dogs with prostatic carcinoma. Nearly 90% of the tumors expressed COX-2, and 16 dogs treated with either piroxicam (14 dogs) or carprofen (two dogs) lived longer than 15 untreated dogs: 7 months versus less than 3 weeks. This effect was more pronounced in dogs that did not have metastases when treatment was started; these dogs had a median survival time of more than 1 year.[95] These results echo those for transitional cell carcinoma of the urinary tract, and the role of COX-2 inhibitors in the treatment of prostatic carcinoma should be further investigated. Chapter 60 provides more information on the use of COX-2 inhibitors for tumors of the urinary tract.

TRANSMISSIBLE VENEREAL TUMOR

CLINICAL BRIEFING

Clinical factors	• Bleeding mass on external genitalia. • Spread by coitus and canine social behavior; females more susceptible than males. • Spontaneous regression in most cases after months, but not in immunosuppressed animals. • Metastasis rare.
Staging and diagnosis	• Minimum database and lymph node evaluation. • Metastasis rare, usually in immunosuppressed animals.
Prognostic factors	• Increase in the ratio of AgNOR area to nuclear area may correlate with poor prognosis.
Treatment	
Initial	• Chemotherapy with vincristine (0.5 mg/m^2) is treatment of choice. Surgery curative if wide excision and localized tumor. Radiation therapy at low doses (10–18 Gy) may be curative if localized.
Supportive	• Analgesia and nutritional support as needed.

Incidence, Signalment, and Etiology

TVT is readily transmitted during coitus by transfer of cells from diseased to healthy dogs, but it also may be spread by social behavior, such as sniffing or licking of genitalia. Any breed may be affected. This tumor most often affects young, sexually active dogs. It is most common in regions with many feral or stray dogs without breeding management. Females are more susceptible to TVT than males. Tumor behavior was studied in 40 generations of dogs, and implantation was found to occur in 68% of exposed animals.[96] The chromosomal complement of this tumor is constant worldwide, with 58 to 59 chromosomes found in the tumor (compared with 78 for normal dog cells).

Clinical Presentation and History

TVTs may be solitary or multiple and nearly always involve the external genitalia as firm, soft, or friable masses prone to ulceration and bleeding (Figure 58-10). Secondary bacterial infection may follow deeper mucosal involvement, resulting in serosanguineous or pure hemorrhagic discharge. Deformity of the genitalia, including marked swelling and ulceration, may follow. Dysuria or weakness occasionally occurs.[97] Occasionally, the nasal mucosa is the primary site of involvement.[98]

Staging and Diagnosis

Metastasis is uncommon and occurs in less than 5% of reported cases, mainly in immunosuppressed dogs or in puppies inoculated with the tumor. The tumor may spread by extension from the external genitalia to the uterus and oviducts in female dogs. The inguinal lymph nodes are the most likely site of lymphatic metastasis, and distant metastases have been seen in the abdominal viscera, skin, and central nervous system (Figure 58-11). In normal adult dogs, the tumor is infiltrated by T lymphocytes and regresses after approximately 2 to 4 months of progressive growth.[99,100] Definitive diagnosis is made by biopsy, but cytologic preparations from FNA or impression smears from the tumor surface characterize TVT. Tumor cells are discrete ("round cell tumor"), with nuclei that contain aggregated chromatin; the cytoplasm is pale blue or colorless with distinct clear vacuoles. Chapter 19 contains more information on cytology.

Dogs with TVT are at increased risk for developing urinary tract infections. Appropriate antibiotic therapy should be instituted and urine culture and sensitivity testing conducted concurrently with chemotherapy.[101]

Very few affected dogs have aggressive and metastasizing lesions that do not respond to therapy. One study tried to identify these dogs through AgNOR staining. In this study, an increase in the ratio of AgNOR area to nuclear area correlated with poor prognosis.[102]

Treatment

Surgery is not considered an effective treatment for this disease. In a study involving 35 dogs with primary or metastatic (nongenital) lesions, tumors recurred within 6 months after surgical excision in four dogs that had only genital lesions (locally in one dog and at other sites in three dogs) and in seven dogs with extragenital lesions.[103]

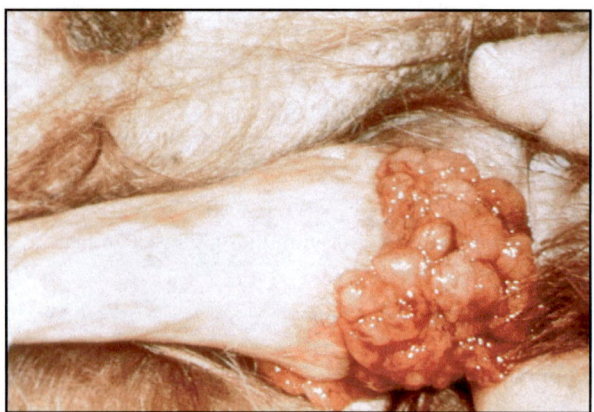

Figure 58-10. *Friable masses around the penis of a dog with TVT.*

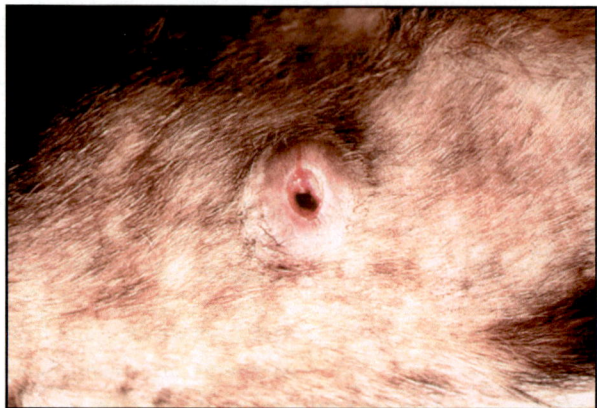

Figure 58-11. *A cutaneous metastasis in a dog with TVT. (Courtesy of Gordon H. Theilen, DVM, University of California, Davis)*

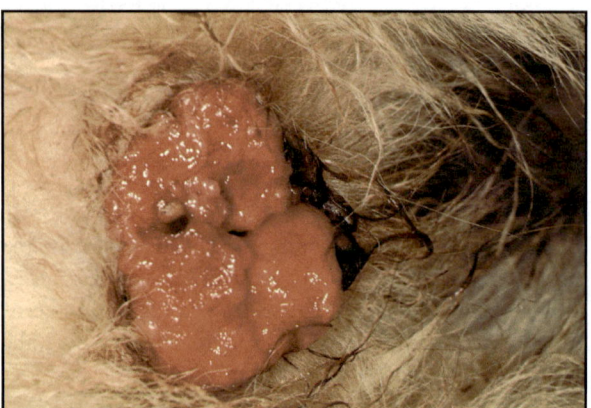

Figure 58-12. *TVT of the vulva in a 3-year-old mixed-breed dog before treatment with vincristine.*

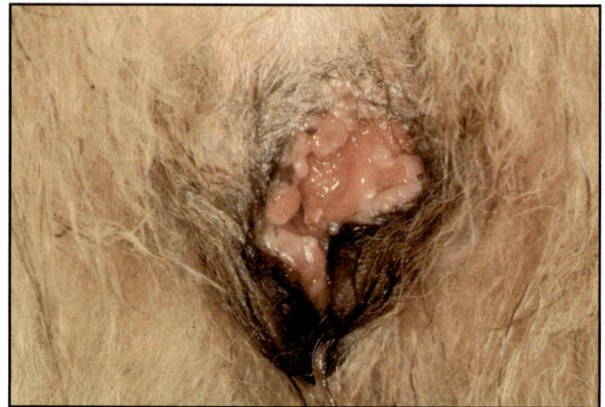

Figure 58-13. *The same dog as in Figure 58-14 after two weekly doses of vincristine at 0.5 mg/m² IV.*

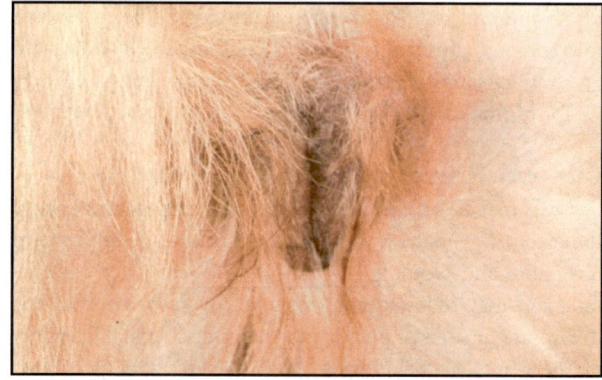

Figure 58-14. *The same dog as in Figure 58-12 after five weekly doses of vincristine at 0.5 mg/m² IV.*

Canine TVT is responsive to radiation therapy; 100% "cure" is obtained with a single therapeutic dose of 10 Gy as long as metastasis has not occurred.[104] Radiation therapy in three fractions (total dose: 10–18 Gy) was equally effective in one study.[98]

Because of the risk of metastasis, as well as the cost and limited availability of radiation therapy, chemotherapy is the most commonly used treatment for canine TVT. Vincristine is the treatment of choice. Vincristine at a dosage of 0.025 mg/kg (to a maximum dose of 1 mg) was administered to 41 dogs with TVT and resulted in complete remission in 39 dogs and partial remission in one dog.[105] The dogs received between two and seven treatments (mean: 3.3). Three dogs experienced vomiting, and two dogs had transient leukopenia. All 20 dogs receiving vincristine at a dose of 0.5 mg/m² IV achieved complete remission; only one dog relapsed in a period of 12 months. Vincristine at a dose of 0.6 mg/m² IV resulted in complete remission in 138 of 140 dogs with TVT. These responses occurred within 2 to 6 weeks.[97] Animals older than 5 years were more likely to show gastrointestinal toxicities.

One dog had regression of peripheral lesions, including lymph node metastases, but developed signs associated with brain and ocular metastases 4 months after vincristine chemotherapy,[106] and another dog developed bilateral eye metastases 1 month after successfully achieving cutaneous remission with vincristine chemotherapy.[107] The brain and eyes may be "sanctuary" sites from chemotherapy because of the blood–brain barrier; therefore, dogs with metastatic disease should be monitored for ocular and central nervous system changes after successful chemotherapy.

Single-agent treatment was compared using vincristine, methotrexate, or cyclophosphamide.[108] Two dogs treated with IV cyclophosphamide had partial responses. Tumors in all 20 dogs treated with vincristine completely resolved. Vinblastine caused complete regression of TVT in seven of seven dogs in one study.[109] In another trial, vincristine proved more rapidly effective than vinblastine.[110] Because of the higher risk of myelosuppression and apparently lower efficacy of vinblastine, vincristine is recommended over vinblastine. In two reports, two dogs that failed to respond to vincristine had a complete response to doxorubicin (one was treated at 30 mg/m^2 IV at 7-day intervals, which is a higher than normal dosage).[98,105] Radiation therapy to a total dose of 10 to 18 Gy was effective in treating four dogs that had a TVT resistant to vincristine (three dogs) or vincristine and doxorubicin (one dog) (Figures 58-12 through 58-14).[98]

> **KEY POINT**
>
> *Vincristine chemotherapy has a cure rate of nearly 100% for TVT and is the treatment of choice for this disease. Responses occur within 2 to 6 weeks.*

Owners of purebred dogs may be concerned about the potential loss of fertility in treated male dogs. In one report, sperm counts in a dog progressively decreased during the fourth and fifth weeks of a 6-week vincristine course; they returned to normal by week 10. There were no other effects on semen quality in this dog.[111]

REFERENCES

1. Patnaik AK, Greenlee PG: Canine ovarian neoplasms: A clinicopathologic study of 71 cases, including histology of 12 granulosa cell tumors. *Vet Pathol* 24:509–514, 1987.
2. Patnaik AK, Saigo PE, Lieberman PH, Greenlee PG: Morphology of canine ovarian Sertoli–Leydig cell neoplasms. A report of 12 cases. *Cancer* 62:577–584, 1988.
3. Ervin E, Homans P: Giant ovarian cyst in a bitch. *Compend Contin Educ Pract Vet* 8:698–700, 1986.
4. Faulkner RT, Johnson SE: An ovarian cyst in a West Highland white terrier. *Vet Med* 75:1375–1377, 1980.
5. Diez-Bru N, Garcia-Real I, Martinez EM, et al: Ultrasonographic appearance of ovarian tumors in 10 dogs. *Vet Radiol Ultrasound* 39:226–233, 1998.
6. Pluhar GE, Memon MA, Wheaton LG: Granulosa cell tumor in an ovariohysterectomized dog. *JAVMA* 207:1063–1065, 1995.
7. Sivacolundhu RK, O'Hara AJ, Read RA: Granulosa cell tumour in two speyed bitches. *Aust Vet J* 79:173–176, 2001.
8. Seaman WJ: Canine ovarian fibroma associated with prolonged exposure to mibolerone. *Toxicol Pathol* 13:177–180, 1985.
9. Jergens AE, Knapp DW, Shaw DP: Ovarian teratoma in a bitch. *JAVMA* 191:81–83,1987.
10. Cheng N: Aberrant behavior in a bitch with a granulosa–theca cell tumor. *Aust Vet J* 70:71–72, 1992.
11. Greenlee PG, Patnaik AK: Canine ovarian tumors of germ cell origin. *Vet Pathol* 22:117–122, 1985.
12. Fernández T, Díez-Bru N, Ríos A, et al: Intracranial metastases from an ovarian dysgerminoma in a 2-year-old dog. *JAAHA* 37:553–556, 2001.
13. Yamini B, VanDenBrink PL, Refsal KR: Ovarian steroid cell tumor resembling luteoma associated with hyperadrenocorticism (Cushing's disease) in a dog. *Vet Pathol* 34:57–60, 1997.
14. Jackson ML, Mills JHL, Fowler JD: Ovarian dysgerminoma in a bitch. *Can Vet J* 26:285–287, 1985.
15. Wilson RB, Cave JS, Copeland JS, Onks J: Ovarian teratoma in two dogs. *JAAHA* 21:249–253, 1985.
16. Nagashima Y, Hoshi K, Tanaka R, et al: Ovarian and retroperitoneal teratomas in a dog. *J Vet Med Sci* 62:793–795, 2000.
17. McCormick AE, McEntee M: Analyzing and unusual canine ovarian mass. *Vet Med* 83:368–373, 1988.
18. Moore AS, Kirk C, Cardona A: Intracavitary cisplatin chemotherapy experience with six dogs. *J Vet Intern Med* 5:227–231, 1991.
19. Olsen J, Komtebedde J, Lackner A, Madewell BR: Cytoreductive treatment of ovarian carcinoma. *J Vet Intern Med* 8:133–135, 1994.
20. McKee WM: Granulosa cell tumor and attempted chemotherapy in a 17 month old bitch. *Vet Rec* 117:501–502, 1985.
21. Greene JA, Richardson RC, Thornhill JA, Boon GD: Ovarian papillary cystadenocarcinoma in a bitch: Case report and literature review. *JAAHA* 15:351–356, 1979.
22. Brodey RS, Roszel JF: Neoplasms of the canine uterus, vagina and vulva: A clinicopathologic survey of 90 cases. *JAVMA* 151:1294–1307, 1967.
23. Münnic A, Grüssel T, Celzner J, Walter J: Untersuchungen zum auftreten von scheidenerkrankungen bei der hündin. *Kleintierpraxis* 44:831–842, 1999.
24. Kydd DM, Burnie AG: Vaginal neoplasia in the bitch: A review of forty clinical cases. *J Small Anim Pract* 17:255–263, 2004.
25. Thatcher C, Bradley RL: Vulva and vaginal tumors in the dog: A retrospective study. *JAVMA* 183:690–692, 1983.
26. Salomon JF, Deneuche A, Viguier E: Vaginectomy and urethroplasty as a treatment for non-pedunculated vaginal tumours in four bitches. *J Small Anim Pract* 45:157–161, 2004.
27. Bilbrey SA, Withrow SJ, Klein MK, et al: Vulvovaginectomy and perineal urethrostomy for neoplasms of the vulva and vagina. *Vet Surg* 18:450–453, 1989.
28. Hill TP, Lobetti RG, Schulman ML: Vulvovaginectomy and neo-urethrostomy for treatment of haemangiosarcoma of the vulva and vagina. *J S Afr Vet Assoc* 71:256–259, 2000.
29. Peavy GM, Rettenmaier MA, Berns MW: Carbon dioxide laser ablation combined with doxorubicin hydrochloride treatment for vaginal fibrosarcoma in a dog. *JAVMA* 201:109–110, 1992.
30. Murakami Y, Uchida K, Yamaguchi R, Tateyama S: Diffuse bilateral hemangiosarcoma of the uterus in a dog. *J Vet Med Sci* 63:191–193, 2001.
31. Sailasuta A, Tateyama S, Yamaguchi R, et al: Adenomatous papilloma of the uterine tube (oviduct) fimbriae in a dog. *Jpn J Vet Sci* 51:632–633, 1989.
32. Minoccheri F, Meluzzi A: Su di un tumore adenomatoide primitivo della salpinge. *Arch Vet Ital* 30:90–95, 1979.
33. Payne-Johnson CE, Kelly DF, Davies PT: Endometrial carcinoma in a young dog. *J Comp Pathol* 96:463–467, 1986.
34. Cave TA, Hine R, Howie F, et al: Uterine carcinoma in a 10-month-old golden retriever. *J Small Anim Pract* 43:133–135, 2002.
35. Vos JH: Uterine and cervical carcinomas in five dogs. *J Vet Med* 35:385–390, 1988.
36. Boisclair J, Dore M: Uterine angiolipoleiomyoma in a dog. *Vet Pathol* 38:726–728, 2001.
37. Patnaik AK: A clinicopathologic, histologic and immunohistochemical study of mixed germ cell-stromal tumors of the testis in 16 dogs. *Vet Pathol* 30:287–295, 1993.
38. Nielson SW, Lein DH: Tumours of the testis. *Bull World Health Organ* 50:71–78, 1992.
39. Hayes HM, Pendergrass TW: Canine testicular tumors. Epidemiologic features of 410 dogs. *Int J Cancer* 18:482–487, 1976.
40. Nieto JM, Pizarro M, Balaguer LM, Romano J: Canine testicular tumors in descended and cryptorchid testes. *Dtsch Tierarztl Wochenschr* 96:186–189, 1989.
41. Reif JS, Brodey RS: The relationship between cryptorchidism and canine testicular neoplasia. *JAVMA* 155:2005–2010, 1969.
42. Yates D, Hayes G, Heffernan M, Beynon R: Incidence of cryptorchidism in dogs and cats. *Vet Rec* 152:502–504, 2003.
43. Hayes HM Jr, Wilson GP, Pendergrass TW, Cox VS: Canine cryptorchism and subsequent testicular neoplasia: Case-control study with epidemiologic update. *Teratology* 32:51–56, 1985.
44. Hayes HM, Tarone RE, Casey HW, Huxsoll DL: Excess of seminomas observed in Vietnam service U.S. military working dogs. *J Natl Cancer Inst* 82:1042–1046, 1990.
45. Suess RP Jr, Barr SC, Sacre BJ, French TW: Bone marrow hypoplasia in a feminized dog with an interstitial cell tumor. *JAVMA* 200:1346–1348, 1992.
46. Sanpera N, Masot N, Janer M, et al: Oestrogen-induced bone marrow aplasia in a dog with a Sertoli cell tumour. *J Small Anim Pract* 43:365–369, 2002.

47. HogenEsch H, Whiteley HE, Vicini DS, Helper LC: Seminoma with metastases in the eyes and the brain in a dog. *Vet Pathol* 24:278–280, 1987.
48. Takiguchi M, Iida T, Kudo T, Hashimoto A: Malignant seminoma with systemic metastases in a dog. *J Small Anim Pract* 42:360–362, 2001.
49. Spugnini EP, Bartolazzi A, Ruslander D: Seminoma with cutaneous metastases in a dog. *JAAHA* 36:253–256, 2000.
50. Barrand KR, Scudamore CL: Canine hypertrophic osteoarthopathy associated with a malignant Sertoli cell tumour. *J Small Anim Pract* 42:143–145, 2001.
51. Inoue M, Wada N: Immunohistochemical detection of p53 and p21 proteins in canine testicular tumours. *Vet Rec* 146:370–372, 2000.
52. Golubeva VA, Kuz'mina ZV, Gershtein ES, et al: [Steroid hormone receptors in spontaneous testicular tumors in dogs]. *Vopr Onkol* 38:464–469, 1986.
53. De Vico G, Papparella S, Di Guardo G: Number and size of silver-stained nucleoli (Ag-NOR clusters) in canine seminomas: Correlation with histological features and tumour behaviour. *J Comp Pathol* 110:267–273, 1994.
54. Sarli G, Benazzi C, Preziosi R, Marcato PS: Proliferative activity assessed by anti-PCNA and Ki67 monoclonal antibodies in canine testicular tumours. *J Comp Pathol* 110:357–368, 1994.
55. Restucci B, Maiolino P, Paciello O, et al: Evaluation of angiogenesis in canine seminomas by quantitative immunohistochemistry. *J Comp Pathol* 128:252–259, 2003.
56. Johnston GR, Feeney DA, Johnston SD, O'Brien TD: Ultrasonographic features of testicular neoplasia in dogs: 16 cases (1980-1988). *JAVMA* 198:1779–1784, 1991.
57. England GC: Ultrasonographic diagnosis of non-palpable Sertoli cell tumor in infertile dogs. *J Small Anim Pract* 36:476–480, 1995.
58. McDonald RK, Walker M, Legendre AM, et al: Radiotherapy of metastatic seminoma in the dog: Case reports. *J Vet Intern Med* 2:103–107, 1988.
59. Dhaliwal RS, Kitchell BE, Knight BL, Schmidt BR: Treatment of aggressive testicular tumors in four dogs. *JAAHA* 35:311–318, 1999.
60. Kast VA: Probleme der präputial- und Zervixkarzinome bei tieren. *Geburtshilfe Frauenheilkd* 19:1080–1086, 1959.
61. Patnaik AK, Matthiesen DT, Zawie DA: Two cases of canine penile neoplasm: Squamous cell carcinoma and mesenchymal chondrosarcoma. *JAAHA* 24:403–406, 1988.
62. Wakui S, Furusato M, Nomura Y, et al: Testicular epidermoid cyst and penile squamous cell carcinoma in a dog. *Vet Pathol* 29:543–545, 1992.
63. Leav I, Schelling KH, Adams JY, et al: Role of canine basal cells in postnatal prostatic development, induction of hyperplasia, and sex hormone-stimulated growth; and the ductal origin of carcinoma. *Prostate* 48:210–224, 2001.
64. Cornell KK, Bostwick DG, Cooley DM, et al: Clinical and pathologic aspects of spontaneous canine prostate carcinoma: A retrospective analysis of 76 cases. *Prostate* 45:173–183, 2000.
65. Sorenmo KU, Goldschmidt M, Shofer F, et al: Immunohistochemical characterization of canine prostatic carcinoma and correlation with castration status and castration time. *Vet Comp Oncol* 1:48–56, 2003.
66. LeRoy BE, Nadella MV, Toribio RE, et al: Canine prostate carcinomas express markers of urothelial and prostatic differentiation. *Vet Pathol* 41:131–140, 2004.
67. Leav I, Ling GV: Adenocarcinoma of the canine prostate. *Cancer* 22:1329–1345, 1968.
68. Hargis AM, Miller LM: Prostatic carcinoma in dogs. *Compend Contin Educ Pract Vet* 5:647–653, 1983.
69. O'Shea JD: Studies on the canine prostate gland II. Prostatic neoplasms. *J Comp Pathol* 73:244–252, 1963.
70. Weaver AD: Fifteen cases of prostatic carcinoma in the dog. *Vet Rec* 109:71–75, 1981.
71. Bell FW, Klausner JS, Hayden DW, et al: Clinical and pathological features of prostatic adenocarcinoma in sexually intact and castrated dogs: 31 cases (1970–1987). *JAVMA* 199:1623–1630, 1991.
72. Teske E, Naan EC, van Dijk EM, et al: Canine prostate carcinoma: epidemiological evidence of an increased risk in castrated dogs. *Mol Cell Endocrinol* 197:251–255, 2002.
73. Waters DJ, Bostwick DG: Prostatic intraepithelial neoplasia occurs spontaneously in the canine prostate. *J Urol* 157:713–716, 1997.
74. Madewell BR, Gandour-Edwards R, deVere White RW: Canine prostatic intraepithelial neoplasia: Is the comparative model relevant? *Prostate* 58:314–317, 2004.
75. Aquilina JW, McKinney L, Pacelli A, et al: High grade prostatic intraepithelial neoplasia in military working dogs with and without prostate cancer. *Prostate* 36:189–193, 1998.
76. Obradovich JE, Walshaw R, Goulland E: The influence of castration of the development of prostatic carcinoma in the dog: 43 cases (1978–1985). *J Vet Intern Med* 1:183–187, 1987.
77. Teske E, Nickel RF: Zur aussagekraft der zytologie bei der diagnostik des prostatakarzinoms beim hund. *Kleintierpraxis* 41:239–247, 1996.
78. Durham SK, Deitze AE: Prostatic adenocarcinoma with and without metastasis to bone in dogs. *JAVMA* 188:1432–1436, 1986.
79. Swinney GR: Prostatic neoplasia in five dogs. *Aust Vet J* 76:669–674, 1998.
80. Rohleder JJ, Jones JC: Emphysematous prostatitis and carcinoma in a dog. *JAAHA* 38:478–481, 2002.
81. Nickel RF, Teske E: Diagnosis of canine prostatic carcinoma. *Tijdschr Diergeneeskd* 117 (Suppl 1):32S, 1992.
82. Barsanti JA, Finco DR: Evaluation of techniques for diagnosis of canine prostatic diseases. *JAVMA* 190:48–52, 1987.
83. Bell FW, Klausner JS, Hayden DW, et al: Evaluation of serum and seminal plasma markers in the diagnosis of canine prostatic disorders. *J Vet Intern Med* 9:149–153, 1995.
84. Rogers L, Lopez A, Gillis A: Priapism secondary to penile metastasis in a dog. *Can Vet J* 43:547–549, 2002.
85. Feeney DA, Johnston GR, Klausner J, et al: Canine prostatic disease—Comparison of radiographic appearance with morphologic and microbiology findings in 30 cases (1981–1985). *JAVMA* 190:1018–1026, 1987.
86. Feeney DA, Johnston GR, Klausner JS, et al: Canine prostatic disease—Comparison of ultrasonographic appearance with morphologic and microbiologic findings: 30 cases (1981–1985). *JAVMA* 190:1027–1034, 1987.
87. Hayden DW, Klausner JS, Waters DJ: Prostatic leiomyosarcoma in a dog. *J Vet Diagn Invest* 11:283–286, 1999.
88. Cromeens DM, Johnson DE, Price RE: Transurethral canine prostatectomy with the Nd:YAG laser. *J Invest Surg* 6:97–103, 1993.
89. Liptak JM, Brutscher SP, Monnet E, et al: Transurethral resection in the management of urethral and prostatic diseases in 6 dogs. *Vet Surg* 33:1–12, 2004.
90. Turrel JM: Intraoperative radiotherapy of carcinoma of the prostate gland in ten dogs. *JAVMA* 190:48–52, 1987.
91. Mann FA, Barrett RJ, Henderson RA: Use of a retained urethral catheter in three dogs with prostatic neoplasia. *Vet Surg* 21:342–347, 1992.
92. Proulx DR, Ruslander DM, Hauck ML, et al: Canine prostatic neoplasia: A retrospective analysis of 10 dogs treated with external beam radiation (1989–2001). *Proc 22nd Annu Conf Vet Cancer Soc* 40, 2002.
93. Anderson CR, McNiel EA, Gillette EL, et al: Late complications of pelvic irradiation in 16 dogs. *Vet Radiol Ultrasound* 43:187–192, 2002.
94. Lucroy MD, Bowles MH, Higbee RG, et al: Photodynamic therapy for prostatic carcinoma in a dog. *J Vet Intern Med* 17:235–237, 2003.
95. Sorenmo KU, Goldschmidt MH, Shofer FS, et al: Evaluation of cyclooxygenase-1 and cyclooxygenase-2 expression and the effect of cyclooxygenase inhibitors in canine prostatic carcinoma. *Vet Comp Oncol* 2:13–23, 2004.
96. Karlson AG, Mann FC: The transmissible venereal tumor of dogs: Observations on forty generations of experimental transfers. *Ann N Y Acad Sci* 54:1197–1213, 1952.
97. Boscos C: Canine transmissible venereal tumor: Clinical observations and treatment. *Anim Fam* 3:10–15, 1988.
98. Rogers KS, Walker MA, Dillon HB: Transmissible venereal tumor: A retrospective study of 29 cases. *JAAHA* 34:463–470, 1998.
99. Yang TJ: Immunobiology of a spontaneously regressive tumor, the canine transmissible venereal sarcoma (review). *Anticancer Res* 8:93–96, 1988.
100. Yang TJ, Palker TJ, Harding MW: Tumor size, leukocyte adherence inhibition and serum levels of tumor antigen in dogs with the canine transmissible venereal sarcoma. *Cancer Immunol Immunother* 33:255–262, 1991.
101. Batamuzi EK, Kristensen F: Urinary tract infection: The role of canine transmissible venereal tumour. *J Small Anim Pract* 37:276–279, 1996.
102. Harmelin A, Zuckerman A, Nyska A: Correlation of Ag-NOR protein measurements with prognosis in canine transmissible venereal tumour. *J Comp Pathol* 112:429–433, 1995.
103. Amber EI, Henderson RA: Canine transmissible venereal tumor: Evaluation of surgical excision of primary and metastatic lesions in Zaria-Nigeria. *JAAHA* 1882:350–352, 1982.
104. Thrall DE: Orthovoltage radiotherapy of canine transmissible venereal tumors. *Vet Radiol* 23:217–219, 1998.
105. Calvert CA, Leifer CE, MacEwen EG: Vincristine for treatment of transmissible venereal tumor in the dog. *JAVMA* 181:163–164, 1982.
106. Ferreira AJ, Jaggy A, Varejao AP, et al: Brain and ocular metastases from a transmissible venereal tumour in a dog. *J Small Anim Pract* 41:165–168, 2000.
107. Pereira JS, Silva AB, Martins AL, et al: Immunohistochemical characterization of intraocular metastasis of a canine transmissible venereal tumor. *Vet Ophthalmol* 3:43–47, 2000.
108. Amber EI, Henderson RA, Adeyanju JB, Gyang EO: Single-drug chemotherapy of canine transmissible venereal tumor with cyclophosphamide, methotrexate or vincristine. *J Vet Intern Med* 4:144–147, 1990.
109. Wasecki A, Mazur O: Zastosowanie preparatu vinblastin w leczeniu gozow Stickera. *Med Weter* 33:142–143, 1977.
110. Singh J, Rana JS, Sood N, et al: Clinico-pathological studies on the effect of different anti-neoplastic chemotherapy regimens on transmissible venereal tumours in dogs. *Vet Res Commun* 20:71–81, 1996.
111. Gobello C, Corrada Y: Effects of vincristine treatment on semen quality in a dog with a transmissible venereal tumour. *J Small Anim Pract* 43:416–417, 2002.

MAMMARY NEOPLASIA
Antony S. Moore and Gregory K. Ogilvie

CLINICAL BRIEFING

Clinical factors	• Presence of a mass in the mammary chain. • 50% of tumors are multiple. • Approximately 50% are benign (e.g., fibroadenomas, simple adenomas, benign mixed mammary tumors). • Approximately 50% are malignant (e.g., solid carcinomas; tubular or papillary adenocarcinomas; rarely, inflammatory carcinomas). • Most common neoplasm in females. • Average age, 10 to 11 years. • Poodles, terriers, cocker spaniels, and German shepherds are overrepresented. • Early ovariohysterectomy is protective.
Staging and diagnosis	• MDB, including a CBC, biochemical profile, urinalysis, and thoracic radiography (three views). • Lungs and lymph nodes are most common sites of metastasis.
Prognostic factors Poor prognosis	• Stage (increasing tumor size). • Metastasis. • Ulceration. • Degree of invasion. • Increasing degree of malignancy, proliferative indices, solid or ductular tumors. • Histologic margins. • Inflammatory carcinomas. • Lack of hormone receptors. • Diet (fat and protein). • Ovariectomy status.
No effect on prognosis	• Type of surgery. • Number of tumors. • Tumor location. • History of parity, estrous cycles.
Treatment Initial	• Regional surgical resection of tumor is as effective as mastectomy of the entire chain for localized tumor(s). • Removal of lymph node may be of prognostic value. • Ovariohysterectomy may be of value in preventing recurrence.
Adjunctive	• Doxorubicin- or mitoxantrone-based chemotherapy protocols may be effective in some cases. Taxanes and 5-fluorouracil possible.
Supportive	• Analgesia postoperatively and nutritional support as needed.

Mammary Tumors
INCIDENCE, SIGNALMENT, AND ETIOLOGY

Mammary tumors are the most common neoplasms in intact female dogs and account for approximately half of all neoplasms in the bitch. Fewer than 1% of mammary neoplasms occur in male dogs. The incidence of mammary tumors in dogs is higher than in any other domesticated animal and is three times the incidence in humans.[1,2] Approximately half of the tumors are malignant, and half of these have metastasized by the time they are initially diagnosed.[1-3] The average age of affected dogs is 10 to 11 years (range: 2–16 years). Dogs with benign tumors tend to be younger than dogs with malignant tumors.[4] In one study of mammary tumors, all dogs younger than 6 years had benign tumors.[3] Dogs that develop a benign mammary tumor are at greater risk for developing a malignant mammary tumor than dogs with no history of mammary cancer.[5,6]

There is no consensus about which breeds have the highest incidence. Poodles, terriers, cocker spaniels, and German shepherds are commonly noted as being overrepresented in early studies[1,2] but were not in a recent European study.[7] Chihuahuas and boxers reportedly have less risk of developing mammary tumors than other breeds.

Much research has examined risk factors that may be associated with the development of canine mammary neoplasia. Many risk factors associated with mammary tumors in humans do not seem to be significant in dogs. Factors that are not associated with increased risk in female dogs include estrus irregularity, stage of pregnancy, age at first litter, number of puppies born, and history of abnormal estrous cycles and of pseudopregnancy.[8-11]

However, sex hormones do play a role in the development of mammary tumors in the bitch. Intact females have a sevenfold increased risk of developing mammary cancer compared with spayed females. The age at which ovariohysterectomy takes place is directly related to the risk of developing mammary cancer (Table 59-1).[11] Data clearly indicate the preventive role of ovariectomy before the second estrus. Ovariectomies performed later in life, while not as protective, should not be discouraged (see Ovariectomy Status section, below).

Prolonged treatment with progesterone or its derivatives resulted in a dose-related incidence of mammary tumors in one study.[12] In a study from Norway, where ovariectomy is illegal, nearly 40% of dogs with mammary cancer compared with 20% of controls were treated with low doses of medroxyprogesterone acetate for reproductive management.[13]

Obesity may be a factor in mammary neoplasia in dogs. In one case-controlled study, the risk of mammary carcinoma was reduced by 40% in ovariectomized dogs that had been thin at 9 to 12 months of age. Risk of mammary cancer was not reduced among intact dogs that were thin at 9 to 12 months.[14] Another study showed that obesity at 1 year of age almost tripled the incidence of mammary cancer in intact dogs.[8] In this study, dogs with a higher intake of red meat in their diet were also at higher risk for developing mammary cancer. Feeding a high-fat diet and obesity in the year before mammary cancer diagnosis had no influence on tumor development.[14,15]

TABLE 59-1 Relationship Between Time of Ovariohysterectomy and Risk of Mammary Neoplasia[11]

Time of Ovariohysterectomy	Risk of Developing Mammary Tumor (%)
Before first estrus	0.05
Between first and second estrus	8
After second estrus	26

> **KEY POINT**
> *Intact females have a sevenfold increased risk of developing mammary cancer compared with neutered females. In dogs, ovariectomy before the second estrus reduces the risk of mammary tumor development.*

There is evidence of a familial tendency to develop mammary cancer in unspayed beagles. One lifetime study of this breed found that 57 female dogs in a susceptible family line developed 149 benign and 39 malignant tumors, while 95 beagles from another line developed only 70 benign and 20 malignant mammary tumors. The susceptible family was approximately 100 times more likely to develop mammary cancer.[16] Although germ-line mutations in tumor suppressor genes or oncogenes would be suspected to play a role in this phenomenon, such mutations are rare even in susceptible populations.[16-18]

CLINICAL PRESENTATION AND HISTORY

Mammary neoplasia may be suspected in dogs with a history that includes factors such as postponed ovariectomy, progesterone therapy, irregular estrous cycles, unexplained lactation, and the presence of a lump within the mammary chain. The owner may detect a mass when grooming the dog, or it may be an incidental finding on physical examination. All intact adult female dogs should have their mammary glands palpated thoroughly at wellness examinations. It may also be worthwhile to instruct caregivers on proper examination techniques.

Mammary masses can range in size from a few millimeters to many centimeters. At least 50% of dogs with mammary

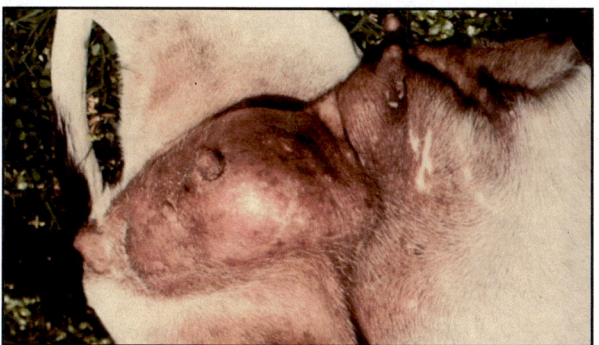

Figure 59-1. *Mammary tumors may be large and are multiple in more than half of affected dogs. The earlier the tumor is diagnosed and treated, the better the prognosis. (Courtesy of Gordon H. Theilen, DVM, University of California, Davis)*

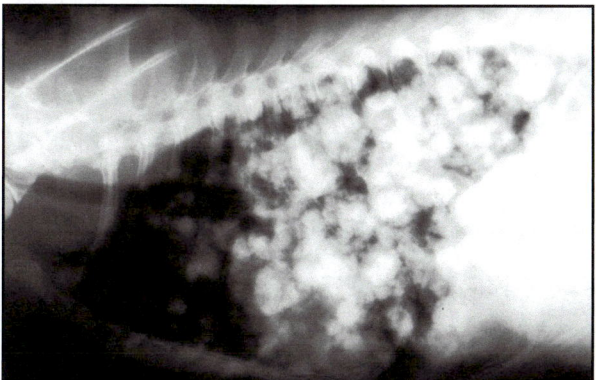

Figure 59-2. *Pulmonary metastases are often multiple and diffuse throughout the lungs. The prognosis is poor for these dogs.*

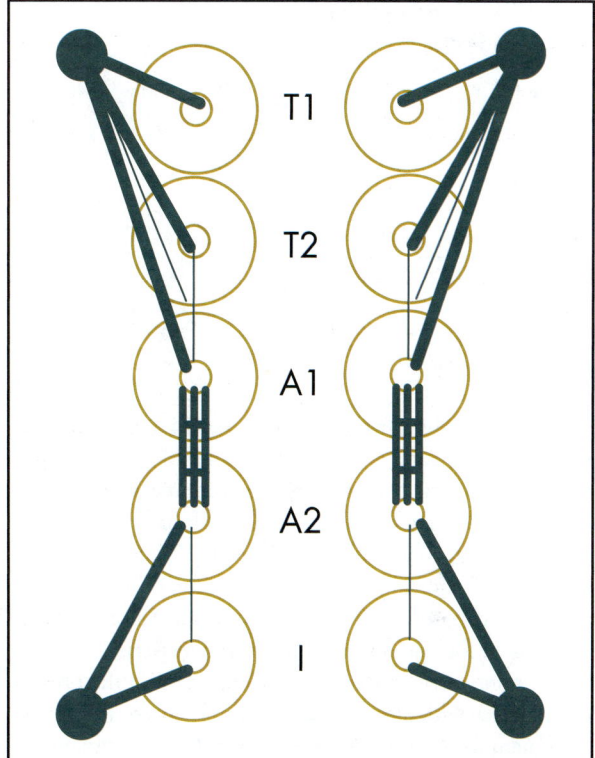

Figure 59-3. *A schematic showing the lymphatic drainage from the mammary glands of the dog. The axillary lymph nodes drain both cranial pairs of glands; the caudal two pairs drain to the inguinal node; the second abdominal gland can drain in either direction. Because mammary tumors are so frequently multiple, all lymph nodes should be palpated.) From Gutberlet K, Rudolph R: Angiosis carcinomatosa bei mammatumoren der hündin—häufigkeit und verbindung mit prognostisch wichtigen faktoren. Kleintierpraxis 41:473-482, 1996, with permission)* A1 = *first abdominal;* A2 = *second abdominal;* I = *inguinal;* T1 = *first thoracic;* T2 = *second thoracic*

gland tumors have multiple masses; however, the prognosis for dogs with mammary cancer is not influenced by location or number of tumors. Some studies[3,5,7,10] suggest that tumors are more common in the caudal mammary glands, whereas others report a uniform distribution throughout mammary tissue (Figure 59-1).

Inflammatory carcinoma, a rapidly progressive disease, is detailed separately later in this chapter.

STAGING AND DIAGNOSIS

The two most common sites of metastases are the lungs and regional lymph nodes. Therefore, staging should include a minimum database (MDB) of thoracic radiographs (three views), complete blood count (CBC), biochemical profile, and urinalysis and evaluation of regional lymph nodes by palpation, fine-needle aspiration cytology, and (if indicated) biopsy. Thoracic radiographs have a sensitivity of 65%, specificity of 97%, and diagnostic accuracy of 87% (Figure 59-2).[19] Lymphatic drainage in dogs is less complex than in cats; the axillary node and the inguinal nodes should be palpated and aspirated for cytologic examination if enlarged (Figure 59-3). The staging scheme for dogs with a mammary tumor is detailed in Table 59-2.

Excisional or incisional biopsy should always be used to confirm a suspected diagnosis. Ultrasonography was used to image primary tumors in one study[21] and found significant differences in appearance between malignant and benign tumors. Malignant tumors had irregular borders, heterogeneous echogenicity, and acoustic shadowing, while benign tumors were spherical or ovoid with regular margins, were homogenous in echogenicity, had edge shadowing, and showed acoustic enhancement.[21] However, while this information may be helpful in the early evaluation of a mammary mass, ultrasonography does not replace biopsy for a definitive diagnosis.

Fine-needle aspiration cytology may help make a definitive diagnosis in some cases; however, the results of cytology can be misleading. False-positive results from cytology are rare, but as many as one-third of cases of mammary neoplasia evaluated cytologically have false-negative results.[22]

Table 59-2 **Staging Scheme for Mammary Tumors in Dogs**[20]

Stage 1	T1	N0	M0
Stage 2	T2	N0	M0
Stage 3	Any T	N1	M0
Stage 4	Any T	Any N	M1

T: Primary tumor
T1: <3 cm diameter
T2: 3–5 cm diameter
T3: >5 cm diameter
N: Regional node
N0: No metastasis
N1: Metastasis
M: Distant metastasis
M0: No metastasis
M1: Metastasis

Table 59-3 **Effect of Tumor Stage on Survival**[20]

Stage	Alive 1 Year after Surgery (%)	Alive 2 Years after Surgery (%)
1	97.9	97.9
3	75.8	66.4
4	13.6	13.6

Table 59-4 **Effect of Tumor Stage on Survival**[36]

Stage	Number of Dogs	Median Survival Time (months)
1	8	17
2	7	14
3	14	7
4	6	3

Hemostatic abnormalities may be seen in dogs with mammary carcinoma and are most common in dogs with stage 3 or 4 disease, particularly dogs with distant metastases, tumor necrosis, invasive and fixed tumors, and inflammatory carcinomas.[23] Most abnormalities do not alter therapy, but evaluation of a clotting profile is warranted in dogs with advanced disease. Disseminated intravascular coagulation was seen in four dogs with pulmonary metastases.

Hormone-receptor status is very important in the prognosis of women with breast cancer, but this is not so clear in dogs with mammary cancer. Approximately 50% of canine mammary tumors are estrogen-receptor positive, and 44% are estrogen- and progesterone-receptor positive.[11,24–26] Receptor concentrations are variable and heterogeneously distributed through the tumor tissue.[27] Most studies agree that increased malignancy is associated with loss of hormone receptors so that precancerous lesions have the highest concentrations and benign lesions the next highest. Malignant tumors rarely express hormonal receptors.[27,28] In addition, tumors that have metastasized to lymph node or distant sites are almost all free of receptors.[29] Another study found that loss of hormonal receptors was correlated with a higher proliferation rate (stained for Ki67), supporting the notion that progression toward malignancy is accompanied by a decrease in hormonal steroid dependency.[30]

Other reported sites of metastases include the liver, kidney, adrenal glands, spleen, pancreas, diaphragm, ovaries, heart, and urethra. Although bone metastases may be common in the later stages of the disease, one study using radionuclide bone imaging showed that bone metastases are rare at initial presentation of dogs with mammary cancer, occurring in only one of 30 dogs.[31] Metastases to the central nervous system have been described.[32]

> **KEY POINT**
>
> *Fine-needle aspiration cytology may be helpful in making a definitive diagnosis in some cases; however, the results of cytology can be misleading. Excisional or incisional biopsy is always recommended.*

PROGNOSTIC FACTORS

The prognosis for dogs with mammary cancer is not influenced by tumor location or the number of tumors.[15,33] Other factors that are not prognostic are the number of pregnancies, age at first pregnancy, and occurrence of pseudopregnancies. The following prognostic factors have been shown in studies to predict survival or disease-free interval.[34]

Stage

Dogs with stage 1 tumors tend to survive longer than dogs with any other stage tumor.[15] This effect of tumor stage is detailed in Tables 59-3 and 59-4 (Figure 59-4).[20,35,36]

Tumor Size

This is one of the most important prognostic factors for a dog with a mammary mass. Dogs with mammary tumors less than 3 cm in diameter have a significantly better prognosis than dogs with larger tumors (Figure 59-5).[3,20,37,38] Tumor size is also a factor in the staging of mammary tumors (Table 59-2).

Metastasis

Metastasis to regional lymph nodes has been associated with an increased risk for tumor recurrence and with decreased overall survival.[3,29,39] Tumor stage, specifically the presence of distant metastases, was found to be prognostically important in other studies (Figure 59-6).[20,36] Dogs without metastases were more than three times as likely to survive 1 year from diagnosis as dogs with metastases.[15]

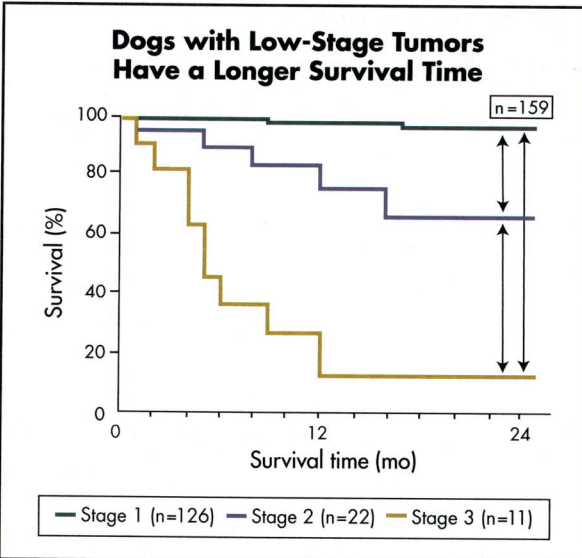

Figure 59-4. Survival curves for dogs with mammary carcinomas treated with surgery, according to tumor stage (TNM). (From Yamagami T, Kobayashi T, Takahashi K, Sugiyama M: Prognosis for canine malignant mammary tumors based on TNM and histologic classification. J Vet Med Sci 58: 1079-1083, 1996, with permission)

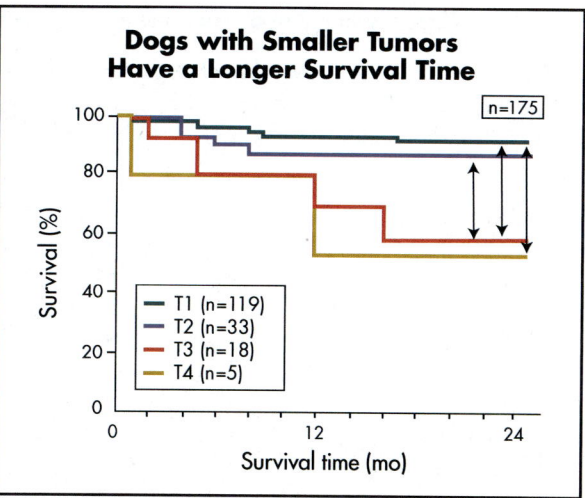

Figure 59-5. Survival curves for dogs with mammary carcinomas treated with surgery, according to tumor size. Dogs with tumors smaller than 5 cm (T1-T2) survive longer. (From Yamagami T, Kobayashi T, Takahashi K, Sugiyama M: Prognosis for canine malignant mammary tumors based on TNM and histologic classification. J Vet Med Sci 58: 1079-1083, 1996, with permission)

Age

Older dogs have a worse prognosis in some studies.[11,40] It is unclear whether this is due to tumor-related factors or to competing risks.[15,29]

Diet and Body Weight

One study has shown that dietary fat and protein together influence survival after surgery for mammary carcinoma.[41] Dogs were categorized by the percentage of total calories they derived from fat and protein in the year before diagnosis. The median survival time for dogs fed a low-fat diet (<39%) with protein greater than 27%, 23% to 27%, and less than 23% was 3 years, 1.2 years, and 6 months, respectively. One-year survival of dogs on a low-fat diet with 15%, 25%, and 35% of total calories derived from protein was 17%, 69%, and 93%, respectively. There was no difference in survival for the different intake levels of dietary protein in dogs fed a high-fat diet (>39%). Body conformation 1 year before diagnosis also affected survival. This study does not account for the type of fat consumed (e.g., n-3 versus n-6 long-chain fatty acid content) or for the carbohydrate content of the diet, both of which may influence outcome (see Chapter 31).

Invasion and Ulceration

Dogs with tumors that ulcerate overlying skin have a worse prognosis (shorter overall survival times) than dogs with tumors without ulceration.[35,42] Rapid and invasive growth correlates with a worse prognosis, which may be rec-

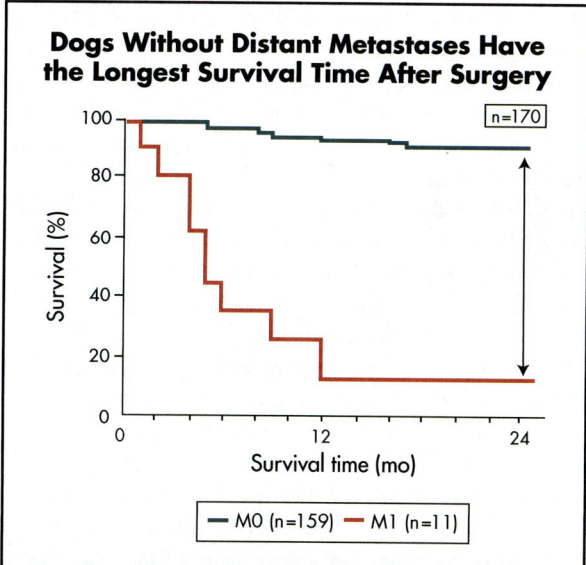

Figure 59-6. Survival curves for dogs with mammary carcinomas treated with surgery, according to detection of distant metastases, including distant nodes (M1). (From Yamagami T, Kobayashi T, Takahashi K, Sugiyama M: Prognosis for canine malignant mammary tumors based on TNM and histologic classification. J Vet Med Sci 58:1079–1083, 1996; with permission)

ognized as fixation of the tumor to the underlying tissue.[34,42] Vascular or lymphatic invasion is a poor prognostic factor; dogs with histologic evidence of invasion have a shorter median survival time (Figure 59-7).[20]

Table 59-5 Histopathology and Prognosis for Dogs with Malignant Mammary Tumors[46]

	Number of Dogs	Metastases (no.; %)	Recurrence (no.; %)	Died (no.; %)
Adenocarcinoma				
All	578	194 (32)	23 (4.0)	20 (3.5)
Simple	260	85 (33)	11 (4.2)	—
Complex	254	87 (34)	9 (3.5)	—
In mixed tumor	64	22 (34)	3 (4.7)	—
Ductular carcinoma	211	96 (46)	9 (4.3)	48 (23)
Carcinosarcoma	5	5 (100)	0	4 (80)
Squamous cell carcinoma	5	1 (20)	0	—
Total	799			

Histopathology

When reviewing a histopathology report, the clinician should look for information regarding completeness of the surgical excision, invasion into lymphatics or blood vessels, differentiation of the tumor, and ductular differentiation.

Several histologic grading schemes are of prognostic significance. Important factors include histologic classification, degree of nuclear differentiation, and presence of lymphoid accumulation.[3,37,42-44] In general, the more highly differentiated the tumor, the better the prognosis. Poorly differentiated tumors are much more likely to recur than well-differentiated tumors.[3] The chance of recurrence for poorly differentiated canine mammary tumors is 90%; for moderately differentiated tumors, 68%; and for well-differentiated tumors, 24%.[3] Dogs with mammary cancer but no evidence of lymphoid cellular reactivity at the time of initial mastectomy have a threefold increased risk of recurrence within 2 years compared with dogs that have such reactivity. Dogs with precancerous lesions have a ninefold increased risk of developing mammary cancer.[44] Thus, precancerous lesions should not be dismissed as benign.

Dogs with mammary sarcomas have a very poor prognosis compared with those with carcinomas or mixed malignant mammary tumors. Dogs with inflammatory carcinomas also have a poor prognosis (see Inflammatory Mammary Carcinoma section, below).

The histologic subtype of epithelial malignancy may influence the prognosis. Dogs with solid carcinomas may have a worse prognosis than those with adenocarcinomas.[16,20,41,45] In one study, dogs with anaplastic tumors survived a median of 2.5 months compared with 21 months for dogs with adenocarcinomas.[15]

Another study[46] reclassified mammary tumors as ductular carcinomas (also called *solid* or *lobular carcinomas*) that arise from the interlobular or intralobular ducts and adenocarcinomas (simple, complex, or part of a mixed tumor). Previous studies described adenocarcinomas as tubular, papillary, or complex, but these investigators found that the proportion of cells that fitted these descriptions varied within a single tumor, depending on the area examined. Recurrence after surgery was similar between groups, but metastases and death due to tumor were significantly higher in dogs with ductular carcinomas and carcinosarcomas (Table 59-5).[46]

Dogs with evidence of infiltration into adjacent tissue or with permeation into lymphatics or blood vessels have been shown to have a worse prognosis, whereas dogs with tumors that showed myoepithelial proliferation had a better prognosis.[20,41] Myoepithelial cells may be identified by a specific marker, p63.[47]

The ability of a mammary tumor to develop new blood vessels (angiogenesis) may be important to its ability to grow, invade adjoining tissue, and metastasize. In one study, total vascular density (determined by staining for factor VIII) was higher in tumors that recurred after surgery.[48] This stain also seemed able to differentiate malignant from benign tumors even when the tumors were small (T1; <3 cm diameter).

Hormone-Receptor Activity

Dogs with tumors that are estrogen- or progesterone-receptor positive have a better prognosis than dogs with tumors that do not have receptors, with longer disease-free and overall survival times. Receptor-positive tumors are likely to be benign.[24,25,29]

Proliferative Activity

Dogs with tumors that showed a high proportion of Ki67 staining (an immunohistochemical marker for cellular proliferation) were more likely to develop metastases in three studies.[29,35,49] Ki67 staining was also inversely related to survival time.[35,36,49] Another study found that Ki67 staining could be conducted on cytologic specimens as well as histopathologic specimens, with a high degree of correlation between the two.[49]

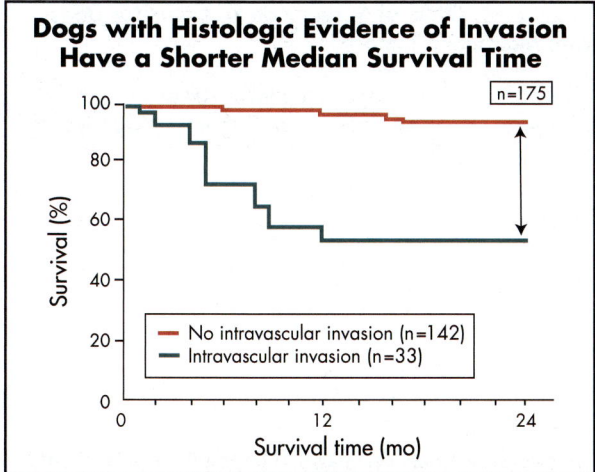

Figure 59-7. Survival curves for dogs with mammary carcinomas treated with surgery according to whether there was histologic evidence of tumor invasion into lymphatic or blood vessels; those with invasion fared worse. (From Yamagami T, Kobayashi T, Takahashi K, Sugiyama M: Prognosis for canine malignant mammary tumors based on TNM and histologic classification. J Vet Med Sci 58:1079–1083, 1996; with permission)

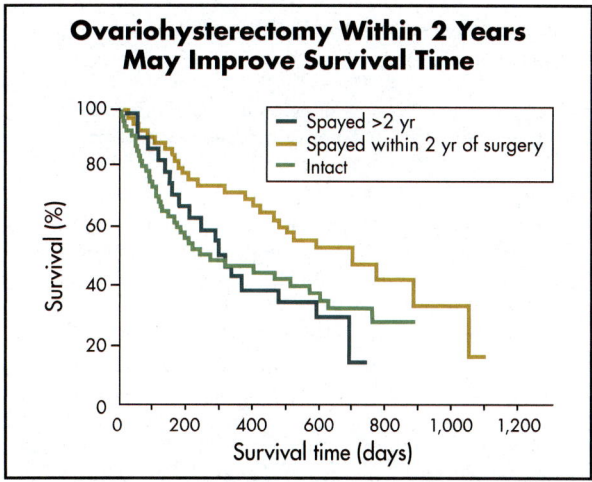

Figure 59-8. Survival curves for dogs with mammary carcinomas according to when they were spayed before surgery. Those spayed within 2 years of surgery fared best. (From Sorenmo KU, Shofer FS, Goldschmidt MH: Effect of spaying and timing of spaying on survival of dogs with mammary carcinoma. J Vet Intern Med 14:266–270, 2000; with permission)

Proliferating cell nuclear antigen (PCNA) index (another method of measuring proliferation) was higher in malignant tumors than in benign tumors but did not correlate with other clinical factors and is probably inferior to Ki-67 staining.[35,50]

Silver staining of nucleolar organizing regions (AgNORs) has proven predictive of behavior and prognosis for other canine tumors; however, there does not appear to be any prognostic value in studies conducted to date.[39,51]

Ovariectomy Status

In one study, dogs that were intact at the time of surgery for a mammary carcinoma survived a shorter time (median survival: 9.5 months) compared with dogs ovariectomized within the 2 years before surgery (median survival: 25 months).[33] Dogs ovariectomized more than 2 years before mammary tumor surgery did not benefit to the same extent. In addition, dogs that were intact had a higher proportion of solid and anaplastic carcinomas than either group of ovariectomized dogs (80% solid carcinomas in intact dogs compared with 20% [<2 years] and 7% [>2 years]) (Figure 59-8).[33] In contrast, ovariohysterectomy at the time of tumor removal had no effect on survival in another study in which approximately 60% of dogs with malignant tumors died within 2 years of surgery regardless of whether they were spayed at the time of mammary tumor removal.[6]

Male Dogs

Mammary cancer is rare in male dogs. In one study,[52] nine male dogs with benign (three dogs) or malignant (six dogs) tumors were treated by surgery alone. Most of the malignant tumors were low grade. No dogs developed metastases, and only one dog developed a new tumor. Based on this small study, mammary tumors in male dogs may have a nonaggressive clinical course.[52]

Breed

One author suggested that German shepherds with mammary cancer had a poorer prognosis than other breeds.[53] Other studies have found no effect of breed on prognosis.[15]

Extent of Surgery

The extent of surgery does not influence survival or disease-free interval; however, the histologic completeness of surgical margins as assessed by histopathology has been shown to be prognostic for survival. Therefore, the best surgery to achieve complete margins is the surgery that should be offered.[24,33,38,41,54]

TREATMENT
Prevention

Clients should be counseled to ovariectomize their dogs before the first estrus and to control the weight of their dogs in at least the first year of life. Because one study showed that dogs with a higher intake of red meat in their diet were at higher risk for developing mammary cancer, it may be better to feed a commercial food that ensures calories are primarily from other sources. Red meat contains n-6 long-chain polyunsaturated fatty acids known to be associated with an enhanced risk of cancer and more rapid tumor

> **Surgical Procedures for Excision of Mammary Tumors**
>
> **Lumpectomy:** This surgical procedure is performed by incising the skin and bluntly dissecting the mammary tissue that surrounds the tumor. It generally is indicated for tumors that are smaller than 1 cm.
>
> **Mammectomy:** The removal of one gland is indicated for tumors larger than 1 cm. Because glands four and five are often confluent, they are usually removed together. The body wall and skin are removed if they are involved or if the tumor approaches these structures.
>
> **Regional or total mastectomy:** Several glands can be removed if multiple glands contain tumors. For localized tumors, mastectomy does not prolong the disease-free interval or survival compared with lumpectomy or mammectomy.
>
> **Lymph node removal:** Because dogs with lymph node tumors have a poorer prognosis than those without such involvement, removal of an adjoining (regional) lymph node at surgery is recommended to gain prognostic information.
>
> **Ovariohysterectomy:** Most studies show that concurrent ovariohysterectomy fails to alter survival and disease-free interval.[3,42,43,55] One study, however, documented that ovariohysterectomy with tumor removal produced a mean survival of 18.5 months compared with 6.1 months for mastectomy alone.[56] Two other studies showed that after a malignant mammary tumor develops, there is no effect of ovariectomy on tumor progression.[6,54]

Table 59-6 **Effect of Surgery on Outcome for Dogs with Mammary Tumors**[54]

Type of Surgery	Number of Dogs	Number Alive at 2 Years	2-Year Survival (%)
Mass removal	56	52	92.9
Mammectomy	64	56	87.5
Ipsilateral mastectomy	25	21	84.0
Bilateral mammectomy	24	21	87.5

growth compared with n-3 long-chain polyunsaturated fatty acids.

Because tumor size is important to prognosis after treatment, all adult female dogs, particularly those that are intact, should have their mammary glands palpated thoroughly at regular intervals in order to detect tumors at the earliest time possible. Owners should be instructed in proper examination techniques.

Surgery

Surgery is the treatment of choice for localized mammary tumors. The extent of surgery influences neither survival nor disease-free interval but rather the histologic completeness of the excision.[24,33,38,54] Various surgical techniques are possible (see the box on this page). The results of several studies suggest that lumpectomy or regional mastectomy of affected glands with resection of available nodes for staging may be the best choice. The tumor and a surrounding "cuff" of normal tissue should be removed. As a general rule, there should be enough normal tissue around the tumor to remove any unseen "fingers" of tumor tissue that can extend from the primary lesion. All resected tissue should be submitted for histologic examination with the margins clearly inked for easy identification. The completeness of surgical margins as assessed by histopathology has been shown to be prognostic for survival, so the best surgery to achieve complete margins is the surgery that should be offered.[41]

One Japanese study compared 2-year survival rates for 175 dogs with mammary cancers; most were T1 tumors (<3 cm in diameter), and predominantly toy breeds were affected.[54] The most common diagnosis was adenocarcinoma (77%). The type of surgery did not influence outcome, as shown in Table 59-6.

Systemic Chemotherapy

Dogs with large, invasive, or metastatic mammary tumors may benefit from systemic chemotherapy. In particular, the population of dogs with ductular carcinomas could benefit from systemic therapy. In vitro studies using canine tumor cultures found that carboplatin inhibited growth of canine mammary carcinoma at clinically relevant levels (i.e., levels that could be achieved with systemic treatment in dogs).[57] Another in vitro study indicated that cisplatin and cyclophosphamide may have activity against a canine mammary tumor.[58] Anecdotally, cisplatin may cause regression of pulmonary metastases. Appropriate clinical studies to document the efficacy of chemotherapy have not yet been reported; however, several preliminary trials and case reports have reported increased survival or partial response in dogs treated with various chemotherapeutic agents.

In one report, a combination of 5-fluorouracil (150 mg/m^2 IV) and cyclophosphamide (100 mg/m^2 IV) was

> **KEY POINT**
>
> *Excisional biopsy of regional lymph nodes at the time of surgery is of prognostic but not therapeutic value. Metastasis to regional lymph nodes indicates a poor prognosis, but there is no evidence that removal of affected lymph nodes increases survival or disease-free interval.*

given once a week postoperatively for 4 consecutive weeks to eight dogs with stage 3 mammary carcinomas. The median survival in this group was 24 months compared with 6 months for eight dogs that did not receive chemotherapy.[59] Toxicity was considered mild.

Doxorubicin has been associated with partial remission of mammary tumors in dogs in preliminary trials.[60-62] Although not proven in large clinical trials, the combination of doxorubicin (30 mg/m² IV on day 1 of a 21-day cycle) and cyclophosphamide (50 mg/m² PO on days 3 to 6 of each 21-day cycle) has been recommended as an effective adjunctive treatment for malignant mammary neoplasia.[56]

A partial response to mitoxantrone, a drug that is effective in women with breast cancer, was seen in one of six treated dogs.[63]

Preliminary results of docetaxel following surgery for mammary tumors that showed lymphatic or blood vessel invasion also seemed to question efficacy; eight dogs that received docetaxel had a median survival of 6 months compared with 12 months if no chemotherapy was given. There were long-term survivors in each group, and the difference was not significant.[62]

In another preliminary study, the related taxane drug paclitaxel (132 mg/m² IV q3wk with appropriate pretreatment with dexamethasone, diphenhydramine, and cimetidine) caused partial responses in two of three dogs with mammary carcinomas.[64]

The finding that normal mammary tissue has no evidence of cyclooxygenase (COX)-2 expression and that 24% of benign and 56% of malignant mammary tumors express COX-2 has led to speculation that nonsteroidal COX-2 inhibitors may play a role in the treatment of mammary carcinoma and, possibly, the prevention of new lesions.[65-67]

Tamoxifen, an antiestrogen drug, has been anecdotally reported as effective for treating dogs with mammary adenocarcinoma, but trials have been hindered by estrogenic side effects.[68] Tamoxifen has antiangiogenic properties that may explain reports of effectiveness, but because estrogen receptors are rare in malignant tumors and their metastases, efficacy is likely to be low.

Other Local Therapies

Other reported local therapies include percutaneous laser placement in a mammary tumor to create interstitial hyperthermia, which in one study resulted in a partial response (>50% shrinkage in volume) in treated dogs.[69] It is difficult to see the utility of this approach over more conventional surgery.

Radiation therapy plays a role in preservation of breast tissue in women with mammary cancer, but its use in the treatment of canine mammary cancer has not been reported. It is possible that radiation therapy may help reduce the risk of local recurrence of tumors that are aggressive, (e.g., inflammatory carcinomas) or that cannot be completely removed.

Biologic Response Modifiers

Immunotherapy has been disappointing in the treatment of mammary cancer in dogs. Studies of levamisole, heat-inactivated *Propionibacterium acnes (Corynebacterium parvum)*, and liposome-encapsulated muramyl tripeptide-phosphatidylethanolamine (L-MTP-PE) showed no benefit in survival rate or time to tumor recurrence.[38,70,71]

Adoptive transfer of human TALL-104 killer cells into a dog with metastatic mammary adenocarcinoma resulted in 50% reduction of the largest lung metastasis and stabilization of other lesions for 10 weeks. However, tumor response appeared to require continued therapy because the dog developed new lung lesions soon after treatment was discontinued. This case report may indicate a role for immunotherapy.[72]

A preliminary trial of a multitargeted, orally administered, indolinone receptor tyrosine kinase inhibitor, SU11654, was reported in a variety of spontaneous tumors in dogs. SU11654 has both antitumor and antiangiogenic activity. Objective responses were seen in two of five mammary carcinomas, and the remaining three dogs had stabilization of growth.[73] This product may become commercially available in the future.

Gene therapy may have future prospects in the treatment of canine mammary carcinoma. Preliminary in vitro studies have shown it is possible to kill mammary tumor cells using an adenoviral vector that expresses canine p53.[74]

Supportive Therapy

Dogs with mammary carcinoma may benefit from a low-fat, high-protein diet after surgery (see Prognostic Factors, above). Pain relief after surgery is mandatory, particularly if the surgery is extensive.

Inflammatory Mammary Carcinoma
INCIDENCE, SIGNALMENT, AND ETIOLOGY

Inflammatory mammary carcinoma is an aggressive, painful, and debilitating form of mammary carcinoma that accounts for less than 10% of all mammary tumors in dogs.[75,76] It appears to occur with a similar breed predisposition as other mammary tumors, although most reported cases have been in larger-breed dogs. Older dogs are affected, with a mean age of 11 years in one study, which was significantly older than dogs with other malignant mammary tumors.[76] Of 43 cases reported, 40 occurred in intact females.[75,76] Inflammatory carcinomas appeared to arise sooner after an estrous cycle than did other malignant mammary tumors.[76]

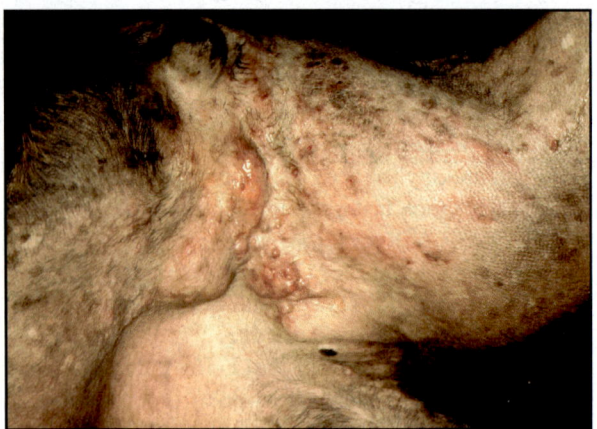

Figure 59-9. *Inflammatory carcinoma causes vesicular eruptions in the inguinal regions of affected dogs, as in this Doberman pinscher. The tumor causes pain and edema and metastasizes widely and early. Prognosis is poor for these dogs.*

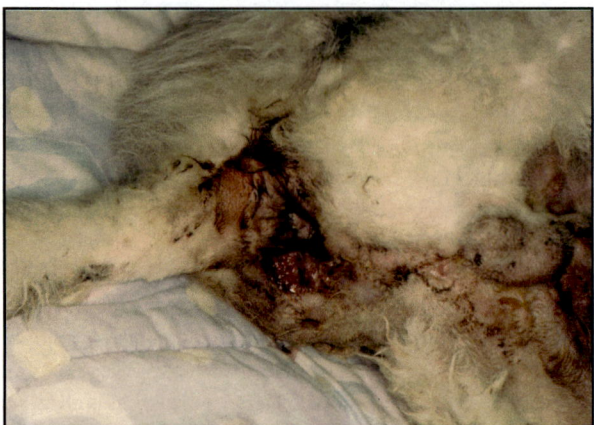

Figure 59-10. *Inflammatory carcinoma causes ulcerations that can spread to the perineal regions of affected dogs, as in this Samoyed. Pain management is mandatory. (Courtesy of Kim E. Knowles, DVM, Veterinary Neurological Center)*

In one study, inflammatory carcinoma was categorized as primary (tumors arising de novo as the first mammary tumor in a dog; 42% of cases) or secondary (tumors arising in dogs with a history of mammary carcinoma; 58% of cases).[76] About half of the dogs with secondary inflammatory carcinoma had a mammary nodule that had been present for an average time of more than 1 year and had a slow rate of growth until suddenly developing features of inflammatory carcinoma. The other dogs with secondary inflammatory carcinoma had a mass removed and recurrence an average of 1.5 months later.[76]

CLINICAL PRESENTATION AND HISTORY

Dogs with inflammatory mammary carcinoma usually have hot, swollen mammary glands that may be misdiagnosed as mastitis. The dermatitis can be severe, and vesicles and pustules may be part of the clinical picture.[77] Most dogs have neoplastic infiltration of multiple glands, often with bilateral involvement. These animals may have edema of the mammary tissue and a nearby limb due to invasion and embolization of dermal lymphatics by the tumor cells and obstruction of lymphatics by enlarged lymph nodes. The inflammation can be severe and suppurative, and most dogs exhibit pain when the mammary glands, axillae, perineum, or inner aspects of the limbs are touched (Figures 59-9 and 59-10). Affected dogs are more likely to be depressed, weak, and anorectic than dogs with other mammary carcinomas and are more likely to be thin at diagnosis.[76]

STAGING AND DIAGNOSIS

Diagnosis of an inflammatory carcinoma is made by biopsy along with the observation of an inflamed mammary gland. Affected dogs often have widespread microscopic or measurable metastatic disease. In two studies, 14 of 32 dogs had pulmonary metastases detected on radiographs. Nodal metastases were seen in 32 of 34 dogs. The inguinal or axillary nodes were most commonly affected.[75,76]

Hemostatic abnormalities such as disseminated intravascular coagulation have been seen in affected dogs at a higher incidence than in dogs with other mammary carcinomas.

Diagnosis using fine-needle aspiration cytology is often successful, although secondary inflammatory changes may obscure the diagnostic accuracy.[75] Histologically, most of these tumors correspond to ductular carcinomas (solid and tubular),[76] although histology in another study found several types of carcinomas to be present (including solid, tubular, papillary, and adenosquamous).[78] In dogs with secondary inflammatory carcinoma, dermal lymphatic invasion was recognized in the previously resected tumor specimens, even though clinical signs of inflammatory carcinoma were absent at the time of resection.[76]

Two histologic patterns of neoplastic dermal infiltration were observed: tubular/papillary and sarcomatous.[78] Dogs that had received progesterone treatment were more likely to have primary inflammatory carcinomas and to show dermal sarcomatous infiltration that was related to extreme local pain. All tumors were estrogen receptor negative. Progesterone receptor expression was significantly higher in secondary inflammatory carcinomas, whereas tumors without progesterone receptors were more likely to have pulmonary metastases.[78] In another study, hormone levels of progesterone, 17β-estradiol, androstenedione, dehydroepiandrosterone, and estrone sulphate in tumor tissue were all significantly higher in inflammatory carcinoma compared with other malignant and benign mammary tumors, dysplasias, and normal mammary tissue. Levels of dehydroepiandrosterone and estrone sulfate were two to three times higher in inflammatory carcinoma compared with other groups. These results suggested that development of canine inflammatory carcinoma could be autocrine.[79]

PROGNOSTIC FACTORS

The prognosis is very poor. Many dogs are euthanatized at the time of diagnosis.[76] In one study, inflammatory carcinomas without progesterone receptors were more likely to have pulmonary metastases.[78]

TREATMENT

Treatment has not been described for inflammatory carcinoma in dogs. Palliation of pain is probably the most important contribution a veterinarian can make to the quality of life of an affected dog. Response to NSAIDs or antibiotics is usually minimal. Corticosteroids improved pain in one affected dog.[77] Opioids may be more effective; the use of codeine or sustained release fentanyl may be necessary for intractable pain. Radiation therapy may also be palliative for pain but is not reported for this tumor type.

The prognosis after surgery was worse for dogs with inflammatory carcinoma than for dogs with any other carcinoma in one study.[20] Chemotherapy would be needed, as the disease is systemic in most dogs at the time of diagnosis, and the drugs listed for treatment of mammary tumors would be the best choices. COX-2 inhibitors, such as piroxicam (0.3 mg/kg PO sid), may have some palliative effect.

REFERENCES

1. Dorn CR, Taylor DO, Schneider R, et al: Survey of animal neoplasms in Alameda and Contra Costa Counties, California. II. Cancer morbidity in dogs and cats from Alameda county. *J Natl Cancer Inst* 40:307–318, 1968.
2. Priester WA, Mantel N: Occurrence of tumors in domestic animals. Data from 12 United States and Canadian colleges of veterinary medicine. *J Natl Cancer Inst* 47:1333–1344, 1971.
3. Kurzman ID, Gilbertson SR: Prognostic factors in canine mammary tumors. *Sem Vet Med Surg (Small Anim)* 1:25–32, 1986.
4. Misdorp W: Canine mammary tumors: Protective effect of late ovariectomy and stimulating effect of progestins. *Vet Q* 10:26–33, 1988.
5. Bender AP, Dorn RC, Schneider R: An epidemiological study of canine multiple primary neoplasia involving the female and male reproductive systems. *Preventive Vet Med* 2:715–731, 1984.
6. Morris JS, Dobson JM, Bostock DE, O'Farrell E: Effect of ovariohysterectomy in bitches with mammary neoplasms. *Vet Rec* 142:656–658, 1998.
7. Wey N, Kohn B, Gutberlet K, et al: Mammatumore bei der hündin: Klinische verlaufsstudie (1995–1997). *Kleintierpraxis* 44:565–578, 1999.
8. Alenza DP, Rutteman GR, Peña L, et al: Relationship between habitual diet and canine mammary tumors in a case-control study. *J Vet Intern Med* 12:132–139, 1998.
9. Brodey RS, Fidler IJ, Howson AE: The relationship of estrous irregularity, pseudopregnancy, and pregnancy to the development of canine mammary neoplasms. *JAVMA* 149:1049, 1966.
10. Allen SW, Mahaffey EA: Canine mammary neoplasia: Prognostic indications and response to surgical therapy. *JAAHA* 25:540–546, 1989.
11. Schneider R, Dorn CR, Taylor DO: Factors influencing canine mammary cancer development and postsurgical survival. *J Natl Cancer Inst* 43:1249–1261, 1969.
12. Frank DW, Kirton KT, Murchison TE, et al: Mammary tumors and serum hormones in the bitch treated with medroxyprogesterone acetate or progesterone for four years. *Fertil Steril* 31:340–346, 1979.
13. Stovring M, Moe L, Glattre E: A population-based case-control study of canine mammary tumours and clinical use of medroxyprogesterone acetate. *APMIS* 105:590–596, 1997.
14. Sonnenschein EG, Glickman LT, Goldschmidt MH, McKee LJ: Body conformation, diet, and risk of breast cancer in pet dogs: A case-control study. *Am J Epidemiol* 133:694–703, 1991.
15. Philibert JC, Snyder PW, Glickman N, et al: Influence of host factors on survival in dogs with malignant mammary gland tumors. *J Vet Intern Med* 17:102–106, 2003.
16. Schafer KA, Kelly G, Schrader R, et al: A canine model of familial mammary gland neoplasia. *Vet Pathol* 35:168–177, 1998.
17. Muto T, Wakui S, Takahashi H, et al: p53 Gene mutations occurring in spontaneous benign and malignant mammary tumors of the dog. *Vet Pathol* 37:248–253, 2000.
18. Mayr B, Dressler A, Reifinger M, Feil C: Cytogenetic alterations in eight mammary tumors and tumor-suppressor gene p53 mutation in one mammary tumor from dogs. *Am J Vet Res* 59:69–78, 1998.
19. Tiemessen I: Thoracic metastases of canine mammary gland tumors. A radiographic study. *Vet Radiol* 30:249–252, 1989.
20. Yamagami T, Kobayashi T, Takahashi K, Sugiyama M: Prognosis for canine malignant mammary tumors based on TNM and histologic classification. *J Vet Med Sci* 58:1079–1083, 1996.
21. Gonzalez de Bulnes A, Garcia Fernandez P, Mayenco Aguirre AM, Sanchez dela Muela M: Ultrasonographic imaging of canine mammary tumours. *Vet Rec* 143:687–689, 1998.
22. Allen SW, Prasse KW, Mahaffey EA: Cytologic differentiation of benign from malignant canine mammary tumors. *Vet Pathol* 23:649–655, 1986.
23. Stockhaus C, Kohn B, Rudolph R, et al: Correlation of haemostatic abnormalities with tumour stage and characteristics in dogs with mammary carcinoma. *J Small Anim Pract* 40:326–331, 1999.
24. Sartin EA, Barnes S, Kwapien RP, Wolfe LG: Estrogen and progesterone receptor status of mammary carcinomas and correlation with clinical outcome in dogs. *Am J Vet Res* 53:2196–2200, 1992.
25. MacEwen EG, Patnaik AK, Harvey HJ, Panko WB: Estrogen receptors in canine mammary tumors. *Cancer Res* 42:2255–2259, 1982.
26. Rutteman GR, Misdorp W, Blankenstein MA, Van den Brom WE: Oestrogen (ER) and progestin receptors (PR) in mammary tissue of the female dog: Different receptor profile in non-malignant and malignant states. *Br J Cancer* 58:594–599, 1988.
27. Wey N, Gutberlet K, Kohn B, et al: Mammatumore bei der hündin: Hormonelle abhängigkeit unter besonderer berücksichtigung von 17ß-östradiol und progesteron. *Kleintierpraxis* 45:19–31, 2000.
28. Donnay I, Rauis J, Devleeschouwer N, et al: Comparison of estrogen and progesterone receptor expression in normal and tumor mammary tissues from dogs. *Am J Vet Res* 56:1188–1194, 1995.
29. Nieto A, Peña L, Pérez-Alenza MD, et al: Immunohistologic detection of estrogen receptor alpha in canine mammary tumors: Clinical and pathologic associations and prognostic significance. *Vet Pathol* 37:239–247, 2000.
30. Geraldes M, Gartner F, Schmitt F: Immunohistochemical study of hormonal receptors and cell proliferation in normal canine mammary glands and spontaneous mammary tumours. *Vet Rec* 146:403–406, 2000.
31. Ogilvie GK, Allhands RV, Reynolds HA: Use of radionuclide imaging to identify malignant mammary tumor bone metastases in dogs. *JAVMA* 195:220–222, 1989.
32. Pumarola M, Balasch M: Meningeal carcinomatosis in a dog. *Vet Rec* 138:523–524, 1996.
33. Sorenmo KU, Shofer FS, Goldschmidt MH: Effect of spaying and timing of spaying on survival of dogs with mammary carcinoma. *J Vet Intern Med* 14:266–270, 2000.
34. Pérez-Alenza MD, Peña L, del Castillo N, Nieto AI: Factors influencing the incidence and prognosis of canine mammary tumours. *J Small Anim Pract* 41:287–291, 2000.
35. Peña L, Nieto AI, Pérez-Alenza MD, et al: Immunohistochemical detection of Ki-67 and PCNA in canine mammary tumors: Relationship to clinical and pathologic variables. *J Vet Diagn Invest* 10:237–246, 1998.
36. Mellin A, Simon D, Wasielewski RV, et al: Different criteria and their prognostic relevance for malignant canine mammary tumors. *Proc 21ˢᵗ Annu Conf Vet Cancer Soc*: 2, 2001.
37. Fidler IJ, Brodey RS: A necropsy study of canine malignant neoplasms. *JAVMA* 151:710–715, 1967.
38. MacEwen EG, Harvey HJ, Patnaik AK, et al: Evaluation of effects of levamisole and surgery on canine mammary cancer. *J Biol Response Mod* 4:418–426, 1985.
39. Löhr CV, Teifke JP, Failing K, Weiss E: Characterization of the proliferation state in canine mammary tumors by the standardized AgNOR method with postfixation and immunohistologic detection of Ki-67 and PCNA. *Vet Pathol* 34:212–221, 1997.
40. Hellmen E, Bergstrom R, Holmberg L, et al: Prognostic factors in canine mammary tumors: A multivariate study of 202 consecutive cases. *Vet Pathol* 30:20–27, 1993.
41. Shofer FS, Sonnenschein EG, Goldschmidt MH, et al: Histopathologic and dietary prognostic factors for canine mammary carcinoma. *Breast Cancer Res Treat* 13:49–60, 1989.
42. Misdorp W, Hart AA: Canine mammary cancer. I. Prognosis. *J Small Anim Pract*

20:385–394, 1979.
43. Fowler EH, Wilson GP, Koestner A: Biologic behavior of canine mammary neoplasms based on a histogenetic classification. *Vet Pathol* 11:212–229, 1974.
44. Gilbertson SR, Kurzman ID, Zachrau RE, et al: Canine mammary epithelial neoplasms: Biologic implications of morphologic characteristics assessed in 232 dogs. *Vet Pathol* 20:127–142, 1983.
45. Bostock DE: The prognosis following the surgical excision of canine mammary neoplasms. *Eur J Cancer* 11:389–396, 1975.
46. Benjamin SA, Lee AC, Saunders WJ: Classification and behavior of canine mammary epithelial neoplasms based on life-span observations in beagles. *Vet Pathol* 36:423–436, 1999.
47. Gama A, Alves A, Gartner F, Schmitt F: p63: A novel myoepithelial cell marker in canine mammary tissues. *Vet Pathol* 40:412–420, 2003.
48. Griffey SM, Verstraete FJM, Kraegel SA, et al: Computer-assisted image analysis of intratumoral vessel density in mammary tumors from dogs. *Am J Vet Res* 59:1238–1242, 1998.
49. Zuccari DA, Santana AE, Cury PM, Cordeiro JA: Immunocytochemical study of Ki-67 as a prognostic marker in canine mammary neoplasia. *Vet Clin Pathol* 33:23–28, 2004.
50. Funakoshi Y, Nakayama H, Uetsuka K, et al: Cellular proliferative and telomerase activity in canine mammary gland tumors. *Vet Pathol* 37:177–183, 2000.
51. Bratulic M, Grabarevic Z, Artukovic B, Capak D: Number of nucleoli and nucleolar organizer regions per nucleus and nucleolus—Prognostic value in canine mammary tumors. *Vet Pathol* 33:527–532, 1996.
52. Saba CF, Rogers KS, Mauldin GE, Vail DM: Mammary tumors in male dogs: A retrospective study. *Proc 23rd Annu Conf Vet Cancer Soc*:27, 2003.
53. Withrow SJ: Symposium on surgical techniques in small animal practice. Surgical management of canine mammary tumors. *Vet Clin North Am* 5:495–506, 1975.
54. Yamagami T, Kobayashi T, Takahashi K, Sugiyama M: Influence of ovariectomy at the time of mastectomy on the prognosis for canine malignant mammary tumours. *J Small Anim Pract* 37:462–464, 1996.
55. Misdorp W, Hart AA: Canine mammary cancer. II. Therapy and causes of death. *J Small Anim Pract* 20:395–404, 1979.
56. Johnston SD: Reproductive systems, in Slatter D (ed): *Textbook of Small Animal Surgery*, ed 2. Philadelphia, WB Saunders, 1993, pp 2177–2200.
57. Simon D, Knebel JW, Baumgärtner W, et al: In vitro efficacy of chemotherapeutics as determined by 50% inhibitory concentrations in cell cultures of mammary gland tumors obtained from dogs. *Am J Vet Res* 62:1825–1830, 2001.
58. Yamashita A, Maruo K, Suzuki K, et al: Experimental chemotherapy against canine mammary cancer xenograft in SCID mice and its prediction of clinical effect. *J Vet Med Sci* 63:831–836, 2001.
59. Karayannopoulou M, Kaldrymidou E, Constantinidis TC, Dessiris A: Adjuvant post-operative chemotherapy in bitches with mammary cancer. *J Vet Med A Physiol Pathol Clin Med* 48:85–96, 2001.
60. Ogilvie GK, Reynolds HA, Richardson RC, et al: Phase II evaluation of doxorubicin for treatment of various canine neoplasms. *JAVMA* 195:1580–1583, 1989.
61. Hahn KA, Richardson RC, Knapp DW: Canine malignant mammary neoplasia: Biological behavior, diagnosis, and treatment alternatives. *JAAHA* 28:251–256, 1992.
62. Simon D, Schoenrock D, Nolte I, Baumgartner W: Adjuvant treatment of canine malignant invasive mammary gland tumors with doxorubicin and docetaxel. *J Vet Intern Med* 18:790–791, 2004.
63. Ogilvie GK, Obradovich JE, Elmslie RE, et al: Efficacy of mitoxantrone against various neoplasms in dogs. *JAVMA* 198:1618–1621, 1991.
64. Poirier VJ, Hershey AE, Burgess KE, et al: Efficacy and toxicity of paclitaxel (Taxol) for the treatment of canine malignant tumors. *J Vet Intern Med* 18:219–222, 2004.
65. Dore M, Lanthier I, Sirois J: Cyclooxygenase-2 expression in canine mammary tumors. *Vet Pathol* 40:207–212, 2003.
66. Heller DA, Clifford CA, Goldschmidt MH, et al: COX-2 expression in canine hemangiosarcoma, histiocytic sarcoma, mast cell tumor and mammary carcinoma. *Proc 23rd Annu Conf Vet Cancer Soc*:10, 2003.
67. Knapp DW, Richardson RC, Bottoms GD, et al: Phase I trial of piroxicam in 62 dogs bearing naturally occurring tumors. *Cancer Chemother Pharmacol* 29:214–218, 1992.
68. Morris JS, Dobson JM, Bostock DE: Use of tamoxifen in the control of canine mammary neoplasia. *Vet Rec* 133:539–542, 1993.
69. Schmidt I, Allgoewer I, Walter J, et al: Laser-induzierte thermotherapie (LITT) an mammatumoren von hunden - in-vitro und in-vivo-untersuchungen. *Kleintierpraxis* 41:871–880, 1996.
70. Parodi AL, Misdorp W, Mialot JP, et al: Intratumoral BCG and *Corynebacterium parvum* therapy of canine mammary tumours before radical mastectomy. *Cancer Immunol Immunother* 15:172–177, 1983.
71. Teske E, Rutteman GR, vd Ingh TS, et al: Liposome-encapsulated muramyl tripeptide phosphatidylethanolamine (L-MTP-PE): A randomized clinical trial in dogs with mammary carcinoma. *Anticancer Res* 18:1015–1019, 1998.
72. Visonneau S, Cesano A, Jeglum KA, Santoli D: Adoptive therapy of canine metastatic mammary carcinoma with the human MHC non-restricted cytotoxic T-cell line TALL-104. *Oncol Rep* 6:1181–1188, 1999.
73. London CA, Hannah AL, Zadovoskaya R, et al: Phase I dose-escalating study of SU11654, a small molecule receptor tyrosine kinase inhibitor, in dogs with spontaneous malignancies. *Clin Cancer Res* 9:2755–2768, 2003.
74. Yazawa M, Setoguchi A, Hong SH, et al: Effect of an adenoviral vector that expresses the canine p53 gene on cell growth of canine osteosarcoma and mammary adenocarcinoma cell lines. *Am J Vet Res* 64:880–888, 2003.
75. Susaneck SJ, Allen TA, Hoopes J, et al: Inflammatory mammary carcinoma in the dog. *JAAHA* 19:971–976, 1983.
76. Pérez-Alenza MD, Tabanera E, Peña L: Inflammatory mammary carcinoma in dogs: 33 cases (1995–1999). *JAVMA* 219:1110–1114, 2001.
77. Ginel PJ, Perez J, Lucena R, Mozos E: Vesiculopustular dermatitis associated with cutaneous metastases of an inflammatory mammary carcinosarcoma in a bitch. *Vet Rec* 147:550–552, 2000.
78. Peña L, Pérez-Alenza MD, Rodriguez-Bertos A, Nieto A: Canine inflammatory mammary carcinoma: Histopathology, immunohistochemistry and clinical implications of 21 cases. *Breast Cancer Res Treat* 78:141–148, 2003.
79. Peña L, Silvan G, Pérez-Alenza MD, et al: Steroid hormone profile of canine inflammatory mammary carcinoma: A preliminary study. *J Steroid Biochem Mol Biol* 84:211–216, 2003.

TUMORS OF THE URINARY TRACT

Antony S. Moore and Gregory K. Ogilvie

CLINICAL BRIEFING

Renal Tumors

Common presentation
- Often no clinical signs; hematuria with tumors of the renal pelvis and hemangioma.
- Most commonly carcinomas and adenocarcinomas.
- Older dogs, usually males; nephroblastoma in young dogs.
- German shepherds often present with dermatologic disorders because they develop cystoadenocarcinomas and nodular dermatofibrosis on an inherited basis.

Staging and diagnosis
- MDB (including complete blood count, biochemical profile, urinalysis, and thoracic radiography [three views]), abdominal radiography, or ultrasonography.

Prognostic factors
- None identified.

Treatment

Initial
- Carcinomas have high metastatic rate; therefore, surgical cure is unlikely
- Early removal of nephroblastoma may be curative.

Adjunctive
- Chemotherapy only reported for nephroblastoma.
- Vincristine, doxorubicin, and actinomycin D may be effective.

Supportive
- Analgesia may be needed.
- Appetite stimulants and antinausea medications if chemotherapy used.
- Nutritional support as required.

Lower Urinary Tract Tumors

Common presentation
- Mimic infection: hematuria, stranguria, and pollakiuria; often have secondary infections.
- Most common tumor is TCC, usually in old female dogs.
- Obesity, exposure to insecticides (other than spot-on medications) or herbicides may be associated with increased risk of developing bladder tumors.

Staging and diagnosis
- MDB and abdominal ultrasonography.

Prognostic factors
- Dogs with histologic grade 1 tumors live longer.
- Glandular differentiation and TCC invading adjacent structures are both associated with poor response to chemotherapy.
- Dogs with small tumors are less likely to develop either lymph node or distant metastases.
- Dogs with small tumors are more likely to respond to therapy.

Treatment	
Initial	• Surgery palliative only; most tumors involve trigone of bladder.
Adjunctive	• Radiation therapy provides local control, but fibrosis of bladder may occur as late effect.
	• Chemotherapy mostly palliative; best results with combination of mitoxantrone and piroxicam. Responses also seen to piroxicam alone, cisplatin, and possibly doxorubicin and cyclophosphamide in combination.
Supportive	• Analgesia may be needed. If obstructed, may need transabdominal catheter to relieve obstruction and pain. Nutritional support as required.

Renal Tumors

INCIDENCE, SIGNALMENT, AND ETIOLOGY

Renal tumors are rare in dogs. The most common types are carcinomas and adenocarcinomas, which constituted more than 60% of 243 renal tumors in three extensive studies.[1-3] Fibrosarcomas, fibromas (also called *interstitial cell tumors*[4,5]), adenomas, hemangiosarcomas, neurofibromas,[6] and an oncocytoma[7] have also been reported.

Tumors of the renal pelvis are most often squamous cell carcinomas, transitional cell carcinomas (TCCs), papillomas, and fibrosarcomas. Most dogs with renal tumors are older (average age: 8–9 years) males. Nephroblastomas, which often occur in younger dogs, seem to have a unique biologic behavior and response to treatment and, therefore, are discussed separately in this chapter. German shepherds, the only breed known to be at increased risk, develop renal cystadenocarcinomas and multifocal nodular dermatofibrosis (see Renal Cystadenocarcinoma Complex section, below).

CLINICAL PRESENTATION AND HISTORY

For many renal tumors, particularly benign tumors such as fibromas,[6] adenomas, and papillomas,[2] there are no clinical signs noted other than a palpable abdominal mass.[2,6,8] Some dogs with malignant tumors are also free of signs.[3] In a series of 31 dogs with renal carcinoma, 14 had a palpable abdominal mass.[2] Most of these masses were between 10 and 20 cm (range: 1–22 cm) in diameter.[2]

Some dogs present with weight loss, and a few present with hematuria. Hematuria is common in dogs with TCCs or papillomas of the renal pelvis,[2,9] renal hemangiomas,[10-13] and hemangiosarcomas.[9] Signs referable to the urinary tract, such as hematuria,[14] dysuria[15] and pollakiuria,[2] are rarely described with other tumor types. Renal failure is uncommonly described in dogs with renal tumors, except in German shepherds with renal cystadenocarcinomas. Two dogs with renal tubular adenocarcinoma[11,16] and one dog with renal TCC[17] had extreme paraneoplastic neutrophilic leukocytosis (128,000–238,000 cells/μl), presumably as a result of tumor-derived colony-stimulating factors. One of these dogs[17] had tumor cells that expressed granulocyte–macrophage colony-stimulating factor. Polycythemia may also occur, presumably as a result of tumor-induced erythropoietin secretion[18,19] (see Chapter 37). Hypertrophic osteopathy has been described in dogs with nephroblastoma, cystadenocarcinomas, and TCC.[17] Dogs with bone metastases may present with lameness and stiff gait.[9,15,16]

> **KEY POINT**
> *Renal failure is rare in dogs with renal tumors, and dogs with tumors other than TCC rarely show hematuria.*

STAGING AND DIAGNOSIS

Abdominal ultrasonography should be used to evaluate both kidneys and to look for visceral metastases. Thoracic radiographs should be obtained because pulmonary metastases are common, even at presentation.[14] Routine blood work should be conducted as part of a minimum database (MDB), although azotemia caused by renal tumors is uncommon.

Large renal tumors may be obvious on abdominal palpation. For smaller tumors, ultrasonography is the diagnostic tool of choice[3,9] because it enables examination of renal architecture and needle-guided biopsy of suspected renal masses and of intraabdominal viscera that may contain metastases. Plain radiographs may outline an irregular kidney but may miss more subtle lesions, particularly in the contralateral kidney.[9] Contrast studies, such as arteriography and excretory urography, may outline an abnormal area but do not distinguish cystic structures from soft tissue densities.[10]

Renal carcinomas may occur bilaterally and may, rarely, be multicentric within the same kidney.[20] Renal tumors most commonly metastasize to the lungs, liver, and serosal surfaces.[3] Tumors that spread through lymphatics commonly spread to paraaortic and cranial-sternal lymph nodes, but popliteal lymph nodes may also be affected.[15] Metastases to bone are rare[3,9,15,16]; however, vertebrae may be involved by local extension.[16] Hypertrophic osteopathy has been reported in dogs with renal carcinoma.[14] Renal carcinomas are usually histologically classified as tubular, papillary, or solid and commonly contain more than one histologic pattern; however, histologic pattern does not correlate with biologic behavior.[2]

TREATMENT

Surgical excision of renal tumors is rarely reported; however, nephrectomy has been used to treat dogs with various types of renal tumors (Figure 60-1). One dog with a spindle cell sarcoma was free of disease 9 months after nephrectomy.[8] One dog with hemangioma was free of disease 6 months after nephrectomy, and another two dogs were free of disease 1 year after nephrectomy.[10,12,13] One of these three dogs had a marginal creatinine clearance; a "nephron-sparing" surgery was performed to enucleate the mass and part of the renal pelvis but preserve the rest of the kidney in this dog.[12] Another dog with renal fibrosarcoma was free of disease 20 months after surgery.[18] Two dogs with renal tubular adenocarcinoma were treated with nephrectomies.[11] One dog with apparently localized disease died from an unknown cause 9 months after surgery after resolution of its leukemoid response. The second dog had evidence of bone metastases and was treated with cobalt-60 (^{60}Co) palliatively; however, there was no response, and the dog died 7 weeks after surgery.

In one report, nephrectomy was performed in 29 dogs; 11 dogs died in the immediate postoperative period. For 15 dogs that survived the first 3 weeks, survival times ranged from 1 to 25 months.[3] In another literature review and report of dogs with renal carcinoma, eight dogs were treated by nephrectomy and survived between 10 days and 4 years; four dogs lived longer than 1 year.[14] The dog that lived 4 years eventually developed metastases from the renal tumor. A dog with renal TCC was alive without evidence of tumor 18 months after a unilateral nephrectomy.[17]

In dogs with carcinoma, which is the most common tumor type and has a high metastasis rate, surgery alone is unlikely to be curative; however, there are a few reports of successful adjunctive chemotherapy. In a recent report of 22 dogs treated by nephrectomy, the median survival time for dogs with carcinomas was 8 months.[21] For dogs with sarcomas, the median survival time was 5 months. Chemotherapy with doxorubicin-based protocols did not appear to improve survival in a small series of dogs.[21] In human patients, this tumor is commonly resistant to chemotherapy.

A recent study found that two of three renal cell carcinomas expressed cyclooxygenase (COX)-2, presumably as part of a return to a more embryonal state.[22] This may mean that strategies that target the COX-2 receptor, such as piroxicam, may show efficacy in the treatment of renal cell carcinoma. Piroxicam can be nephrotoxic; therefore, caution should be used with this drug, especially in dogs with preexisting marginal renal function.

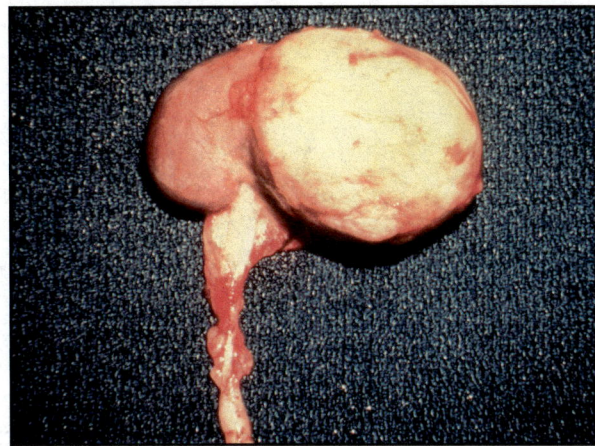

Figure 60-1. Solitary renal adenocarcinoma is best treated by nephrectomy; however, the high metastatic rate means that even with complete excision, the possibility of a cure is remote. (Courtesy of John Berg, DVM, Tufts Cummings School of Veterinary Medicine)

Paraneoplastic syndromes such as cancer cachexia, anemia of chronic disease, and hypertrophic osteopathy are possible. In one dog, hypertrophic osteopathy started to resolve 2 weeks after nephrectomy, and there was no evidence of hypertrophic osteopathy 18 months after surgery.[17]

Renal Cystadenocarcinoma Complex
INCIDENCE, SIGNALMENT, AND ETIOLOGY

A syndrome of multifocal renal cystadenocarcinomas, renal cysts, and nodular dermatofibrosis was first described in detail in 43 German shepherds in the early 1980s.[23] At this time, the disease was identified in 3.7% of all German shepherds autopsied in Norway.[23] Subsequent studies have focused on the heritability of this disease, which has been described in Europe,[24] the United States,[25] and Australia[26] in closely related dogs. Pedigree analysis suggests an autosomal dominant mode of inheritance, and a tumor suppressor gene on canine chromosome 5 has been identified as a possible genetic source for the disease.[27] The average age of dogs at presentation is 8 years, with very few dogs younger than 5 years being reported. There does not seem to be a gender predilection.

> **KEY POINT**
> *German shepherds may have concurrent multifocal nodular dermatofibrosis, uterine leiomyomas, and renal cystadenocarcinomas as a hereditary disorder.*

The disease has also been described in German shepherd cross-bred dogs,[24,28] a golden retriever,[29] and a boxer.[28]

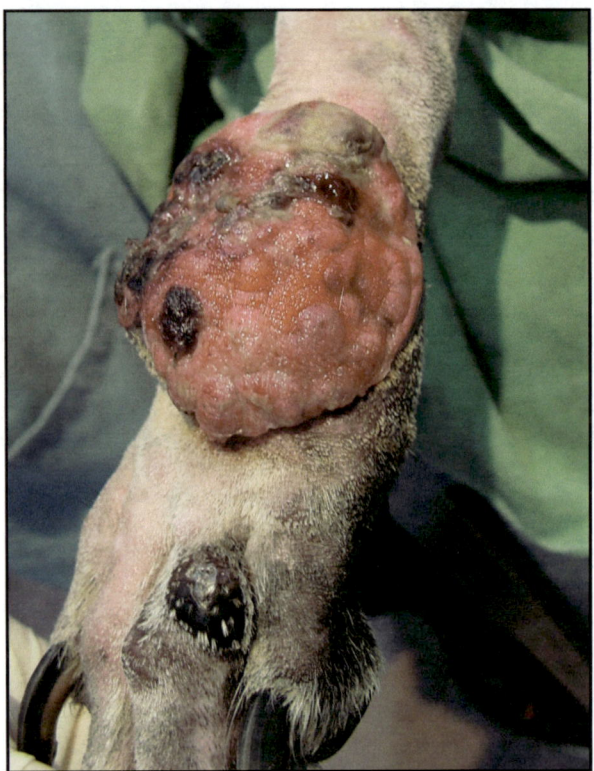

Figure 60-2. *Large ulcerative skin lesions (dermatofibrosis) are associated with bilateral renal cystadenocarcinomas in German shepherds and are often a source of considerable morbidity. (Courtesy of Sarah Goldsmid, BVSc, Animal Referral Hospital)*

CLINICAL PRESENTATION AND HISTORY

Dogs with this syndrome usually present with numerous very firm skin nodules (30% of cases; Figure 60-2). Abdominal distention, polyuria, hematuria, fever, depression, and inappetence are the other most common reasons owners seek veterinary care. The nonspecific signs may have been evident for weeks to months.[24] Female German shepherds with renal cystadenocarcinomas and nodular dermatofibrosis also develop multiple uterine leiomyomas. In one series of dogs,[24] enlarged and irregular kidneys were palpated in 60% of affected dogs; the largest kidney weighed 7 kg (Figure 60-3). Hyperplastic polyps were found in the small intestinal mucosa of approximately 10% of dogs, but these did not cause clinical signs.[24] Ascites developed over the course of the disease in approximately 20% of dogs, and pleural effusion developed in 10%.[24] A lesion on the tongue has been reported in one dog.[28] Secondary nephritis was the cause of death in one dog. Clinicians should be alert to the possibility of secondary bacterial infections.[26]

STAGING AND DIAGNOSIS

Both kidneys are always affected, although not always to the same degree. Routine blood work should be conducted

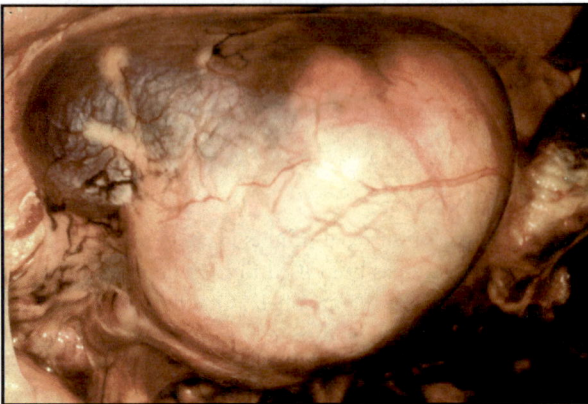

Figure 60-3. *Renal cystadenocarcinomas in German shepherds are inherited in a dominant fashion.*

as part of an MDB. Eight of 17 dogs were azotemic in one study of this tumor type.[23] Many dogs are euthanatized or die as a result of the cutaneous manifestations of the syndrome, but the clinical course is often protracted over a number of years. In one study, nearly half of the dogs showed metastases from the renal tumors.[24] The most common sites of metastases were the sternal and abdominal lymph nodes, liver, and lung; the pleura and peritoneum were less common sites.

Radiography can detect abnormal kidneys in dogs with advanced disease (dogs were older than 9.5 years in one study[24]), but there may be no detectable abnormalities in the early stages of the disease. Ultrasonography can detect cysts larger than 3 mm in diameter,[25,30] and computed tomography (CT) can detect cysts as small as 2 mm in diameter. No changes were detected by CT in dogs younger than 4 years.[31] Renal biopsy was able to detect microscopic cysts in two dogs at 9 months and 13 months of age and therefore may be the most sensitive method of identifying affected dogs before breeding.[32]

TREATMENT

The average time from diagnosis to death in a group of 51 dogs (including some diagnosed as part of a screening program) was 2.5 years. Renal and cutaneous complications were the cause of death or reason for euthanasia in 30%, and depression (23%), lameness (from lesions on the feet and pads; 10%) and other skin complications (8%) were the next most common.[24] With the often long clinical course of the disease, it may be necessary to palliate the cutaneous lesions to maintain quality of life. Surgical excision of skin lesions (10 dogs), unilateral nephrectomy to relieve obstructive disease or a space-occupying mass (four dogs), and ovariohysterectomy (two dogs) were palliative in one study.[24] Intermittent cryosurgery and surgical excision were used to palliate lesions in one dog over a period of 32 months.[25]

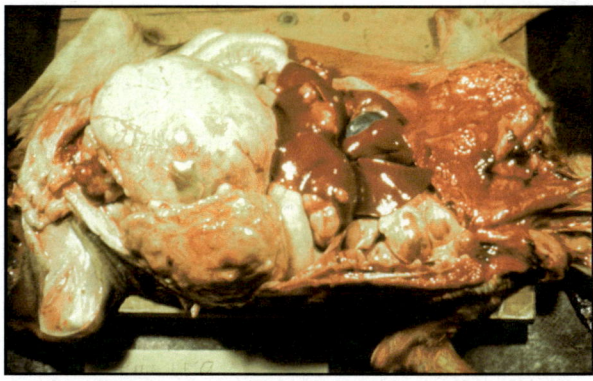

Figure 60-4. *Nephroblastoma can be huge at diagnosis, as seen in this Great Dane at necropsy. (Courtesy of Gordon H. Theilen, DVM, University of California, Davis)*

Table 60-1 **Staging System for Nephroblastoma in Dogs**

Stage	Description
1	Renal capsule intact, completely excised
2	Infiltrating neoplasm or vascular invasion, completely excised
3	Infiltrating neoplasms, peritoneal involvement or lymph node involvement
4	Hematogenous metastasis
5	Bilateral renal involvement

Because the cause of death in many affected dogs is the cutaneous manifestation of the syndrome and because the cutaneous lesions act in a malignant way despite their histologic appearance, the clinician should be prepared to resect lesions that could cause pain before they become large.

Prednisolone had no effect on the clinical course of cutaneous disease in one large study,[24] but in case reports, intralesional[33] and systemic[28] corticosteroids appeared to soften cutaneous lesions and temporarily relieve pain.

Radiation therapy may be palliative for cutaneous lesions but has not been reported. Chemotherapy has not been reported for this disease.

Nephroblastoma
INCIDENCE, SIGNALMENT, AND ETIOLOGY

Nephroblastoma (or embryonal nephroma) is rare in dogs. This kidney tumor is unilateral, congenital, and often very large. It is mostly described in young dogs with a mean age of 11 months,[2,9,34–42] although it may occur in older dogs.[3,9,43–45] Male dogs seem to be predisposed.[2] This is a congenital tumor, but there is no evidence that it is hereditary, although most reported cases have occurred in purebred dogs.

CLINICAL PRESENTATION AND HISTORY

Some dogs present with hematuria,[2,9,41] but most owners observe abdominal swelling.[2] Two dogs with hypertrophic osteopathy and nephroblastoma presented with lameness.[38,45] Two dogs with paraneoplastic polycythemia caused by nephroblastoma have also been described.[38,46] Paraparesis was the presenting sign in a dog with spinal metastasis.[47]

STAGING AND DIAGNOSIS

Nephroblastoma should be suspected in young dogs with a large unilateral tumor. Nephroblastoma can be highly invasive locally and often grows large (Figure 60-4). Postsurgical follow-up examinations of dogs with nephroblastoma often document metastases. Metastasis is primarily to the liver, mesentery, and lungs; however, metastases to the mesenteric, mediastinal, and bronchial lymph nodes have also been observed. The contralateral kidney, adrenal gland, thyroid, urinary bladder, and bone are also commonly affected. The spinal cord may be involved with metastases,[47] but spinal nephroblastoma, which presumably arises from embryonic tissue isolated within the dura during fetal development, has also been described in dogs.

Complete staging of dogs with renal tumors is outlined above. A staging system adapted from human patients has been used to characterize nephroblastoma in dogs (Table 60-1). However, too few cases have been reported to assess the prognostic value of this system.

TREATMENT

Surgical excision of nephroblastoma has been reported in a few dogs. Of four dogs treated with surgery alone, two developed metastases. One of these dogs was euthanatized 1 month after surgery, and the other was euthanatized 6 months after surgery.[36,37] The other two dogs had no evidence of recurrence between 6 and 21 months after surgery.[9,38,48] It seems that unless surgical excision is performed early in the course of the disease, surgery alone is unlikely to be curative. However, surgery may have some benefit for clinical signs. Hypertrophic osteopathy started to resolve 5 weeks after nephrectomy in one dog, and there was no evidence of hypertrophic osteopathy 7 months after surgery.[45]

Adjuvant treatment was prescribed for five dogs that were discovered to have either metastases or grossly unresectable tumors at surgery. One dog was treated with mithramycin after developing pulmonary metastases 6 weeks after surgery.[37] The metastases partially regressed; however, the dog died as a result of drug-induced myelosuppression.[49] The second dog had no response to vincristine and cyclophosphamide chemotherapy.[44] Another dog received 21 Gy of radiation to the surgical site and chemotherapy with actinomycin D.[43] Treatment was continued intermittently even after metastases were discovered 40 weeks after surgery. The dog died 69 weeks after surgery. Another dog with stage 3 nephroblastoma received actinomycin D, vincristine, and doxorubicin after an incomplete surgery and remained stable

> **KEY POINT**
> *When a nephroblastoma is small, nephrectomy may be curative. Large tumors, however, have frequently metastasized, and adjuvant chemotherapy should be considered.*

until chemotherapy was discontinued.[40] The dog had widespread metastases and was euthanized 16 weeks after surgery. The fifth dog had a complete excision of a stage 1 tumor with anaplastic histology and received a protocol of vincristine and doxorubicin every 3 weeks.[45] That dog was alive without evidence of disease 25 months after surgery.

Ureteral Tumors

The presentation and treatment of four older dogs with ureteral fibroepithelial polyps have been reported.[50] The dogs presented with urinary incontinence, urinary tract infection, polydipsia, and pollakiuria. Three dogs were male and intact. Unilateral hydronephrosis was seen, and the ureter was dilated proximal to an intraluminal polypoid mass attached to the ureteral wall by a thin stalk. Unilateral ureteronephrectomy was performed in three dogs with proximal ureter lesions, and ureteral resection and anastomosis were performed in one dog with a distal ureter polyp. These polyps appeared to be either benign neoplasms or chronic inflammatory reactions and had a good prognosis with surgical removal.

Bladder and Urethral Tumors
INCIDENCE, SIGNALMENT, AND ETIOLOGY

In dogs, tumors of the lower urinary tract are more common than renal neoplasia. One report suggests that lower urinary tract tumors have become more common in recent years.[51] In five series totaling 453 dogs with primary tumors of the bladder and urethra, 90% to 97% of tumors were epithelial; most were malignant and categorized as TCCs.[52–56] Benign tumors, such as fibromas and papillomas, are often associated with chronic urinary tract disease and calculi.[54,57] In one series of dogs, only 3% of tumors were benign.[53]

Most tumors originate in the bladder urothelium, but some arise from the urethra. However, the point of origin is not clinically significant because these tumors frequently involve multiple areas of the urinary tract. Most tumors that have been termed "prostatic carcinomas" are likely to be TCCs.[58,59] Rhabdomyosarcomas can occur in the urinary bladder, and most occur in young dogs (1–2 years of age).[60] These tumors are discussed in more detail below.

Female dogs are predisposed to developing TCC, perhaps because they urinate less frequently than males, thereby maintaining contact between the bladder wall and any carcinogens that are excreted in the urine.[52,54,61] Many such carcinogens have been identified in experimental studies, but their role in natural disease is uncertain. Two studies have not found any gender predilection,[53,55] although neutered animals seemed to be at increased risk of tumor formation.[53] In one study, males outnumbered females 11 to two in the development of urethral TCC, and the prostatic urethra was a predilection site.[62] These dogs were beagles, which are considered to be predisposed to development of lower urinary tract tumors, thus confounding the gender issue.[52] Other breeds at high risk are Scottish terriers,[52,53] Shetland sheepdogs, collies, and Airedales.[52] In one study, dogs that weighed less than 10 kg were at higher risk for developing bladder tumors.[53] Affected dogs are older (average age: 9.5 years).[53–55] In one study, only two of 114 dogs with tumors were younger than 2 years.[53]

Other epidemiologic factors increasing the risk for bladder cancer in dogs include the application of insecticidal "dips" (but not powders, sprays, or collars). In one study, dogs that were dipped once or twice a year had 1.6 times the risk of developing a bladder tumor compared with dogs that were never dipped; for dogs that were treated more than twice a year, the risk increased 3.5 times.[63] Dogs that lived near marshes were also at high risk, possibly as a result of insecticidal spraying for mosquitoes. Risks were higher in overweight or obese animals in one study,[63] although only nine of 70 dogs (13%) in another survey of bladder tumors were categorized as obese.[54]

In two refinements of that study,[63] 83 Scottish terriers with TCC were compared with a control group of Scottish terriers. Dogs with TCC were more likely to be neutered (95% versus 82% of controls) and to have had signs of urinary tract disease in the 2 years before diagnosis (33% versus 5% of controls). The latter finding implies that earlier diagnosis would be possible in these dogs. The risk of developing TCC was higher in Scottish terriers older than 8 years.

> **KEY POINT**
> *Exposure to herbicides and insecticides (other than "spot-on" medications) appears to increase the risk of developing bladder cancer in dogs.*

Most notably, this study demonstrated that exposure to herbicides and insecticides increased the risk of developing TCC. Scottish terriers that were exposed to lawns treated with herbicides alone had a nearly fourfold increased risk of developing TCC, and those exposed to lawns treated specifically with phenoxy herbicides had a more than fourfold increased risk of developing TCC.[64] The risk of developing TCC was more than seven times greater in Scottish terriers that were exposed to lawns treated with both herbicides and insecticides.[64] Phenoxy herbicides have also been implicated as a potential risk factor in the development of lymphoma in dogs.[65]

In another study of the same dogs, Scottish terriers exposed to flea control products such as dips, powders, and collars were more than five times as likely as unexposed dogs to develop TCC.[66] Spot-on flea control products had no effect on TCC incidence, with the exception of fipronil-containing products, which decreased the risk by more than threefold compared with dogs not exposed to flea-control products at all.[66]

Although tobacco smoke has been associated with TCC in humans, there was no association between living with a human smoker and dogs developing TCC in one study.[63] There is a tenuous but unlikely association between cyclophosphamide treatment and the development of TCC in dogs.[67,68]

Table 60-2 lists tumor types diagnosed in a group of 422 dogs.

CLINICAL PRESENTATION AND HISTORY

Although signs referable to the urinary tract are rare in dogs with renal tumors, they are common with tumors of the lower urinary tract. Most presenting signs are identical to those in animals with infections or inflammatory conditions of the bladder or urethra, which may coexist with a tumor. The most common presenting signs are hematuria, stranguria, and pollakiuria for both malignant[53,54,69] and benign[57] tumors. Less common signs are polyuria and polydipsia, urinary incontinence, and tenesmus. Treatment with antibiotics may result in temporary clinical improvement. Signs can occur in affected dogs for up to 2.5 years before definitive diagnosis, but in most dogs, signs have been present for 4 weeks.[53,54] Occasionally, a dog with bony metastasis presents with lameness.[52,53] Similarly, hypertrophic osteopathy is possible in dogs with a bladder TCC and without pulmonary metastatic disease.[70] Pulmonary metastases are rarely associated with dyspnea despite diffuse involvement of the lungs.[52]

Even though most TCCs are advanced and invasive at the time of diagnosis (>98% in one study[71]), physical examination may not be rewarding. In one group of 115 dogs, 35 had no obvious abnormalities.[52] More commonly, however, rectal or vaginal examination reveals a urethral mass or urethral thickening, prostatomegaly, and (possibly) a distended bladder (Figure 60-5). A mass in the region of the urinary bladder may be palpated abdominally. In one study, urethral involvement was associated with a higher likelihood of metastasis, and prostate involvement was associated with a shorter survival time.[71]

Table 60-2 Tumors of the Lower Urinary Tract in 422 Dogs[52-55]

Epithelial Tumors	Dogs (n)	Mesenchymal Tumors	Dogs (n)
Transitional cell carcinoma	278	Leiomyosarcoma	11
Squamous cell carcinoma	20	Leiomyoma	13
Adenocarcinoma	23	Fibrosarcoma	7
Papilloma	30	Fibroma	5
Undifferentiated carcinoma	18	Hemangiosarcoma	4
Adenoma	1	Hemangioma	3
		Rhabdomyosarcoma	1
		Undifferentiated sarcoma	8

STAGING AND DIAGNOSIS

Dogs with suspected urinary bladder cancer should have routine blood work and urinalysis conducted. Abdominal ultrasonography should also be conducted to examine the entire urinary tract because other sites are frequently involved. Thoracic radiographs should be obtained before reaching a definitive diagnosis.

Routine blood work is helpful to establish a baseline for anesthesia, surgery, and chemotherapy. Urinalysis may reveal hematuria and active inflammatory sediment. Neoplastic cells may be seen on urinalysis; however, the yield is 30% or less.[53,72] Extreme care should be taken in interpreting cytology of sediment because severe chronic inflammatory changes in transitional epithelium may be difficult to distinguish from neoplastic changes.[53]

Cystoscopy may allow visualization and direct biopsy of the lesion. This is particularly helpful when ultrasonography is unable to visualize the intrapelvic urethra in dogs with urethral tumors. A closed biopsy technique that uses a urinary catheter and negative pressure while moving the catheter in a suspicious area (catheter biopsy; see Chapter 17) may result in a better diagnostic yield than sediment cytology. The accuracy of this technique approaches 80%; occasional false-positive diagnoses occur.[53,56,73] Aspiration cytology was diagnostic in more than 90% of cases in one study and is preferred to cytology of urethral washes or urine sediment.[53] Surgical biopsy should be performed if a definitive diagnosis is required. Caution should be used when performing surgical or fine-needle aspiration biopsy because both techniques have been associated with "seeding" of tumor cells along the biopsy tract.[74,75]

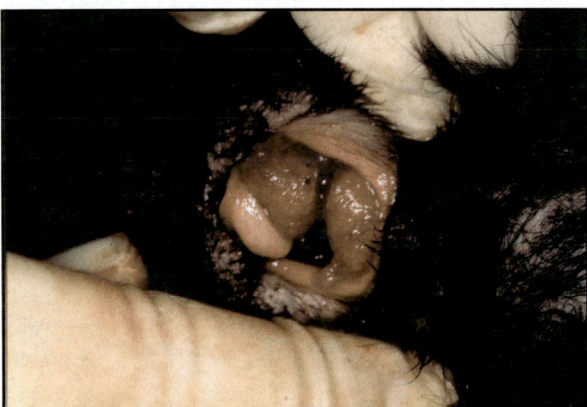

Figure 60-5. *A vaginal mass may be an extension of a urethral TCC, as in this Labrador cross.*

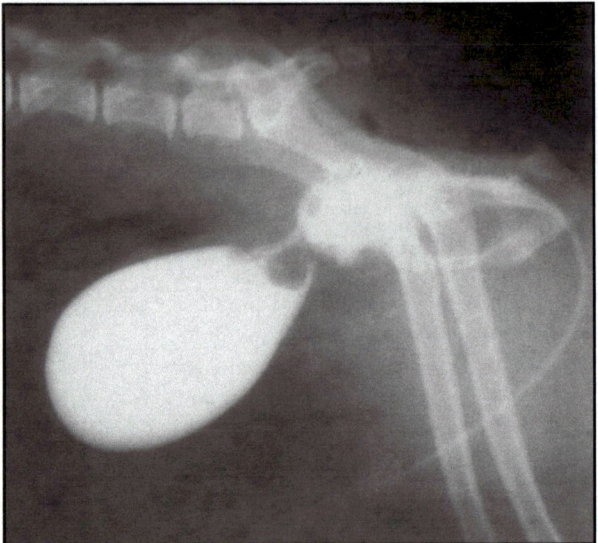

Figure 60-6. *TCC of the bladder is frequently trigonal in location and is well visualized on contrast cystography. (Courtesy of Dominique G. Penninck, DVM, Tufts Cummings School of Veterinary Medicine)*

Abdominal plain radiography may reveal prostatomegaly, sublumbar lymphadenopathy, and (occasionally) evidence of vertebral body metastasis.[53] Double-contrast cystourethrography is more helpful in outlining irregularities or mass lesions in the bladder or urethra (Figure 60-6).[53,54] Care is necessary in interpreting radiographs, particularly of urethral lesions, because chronic urethritis may be difficult to distinguish from neoplasia on the basis of urethrography alone.[56] Ultrasonography has largely replaced cystography, particularly because it does not require catheterization. However, contrast urethrography is still useful because the pelvic bones shield the urethra from ultrasonographic examination.

Extension of the primary tumor to other areas of the urinary tract is common with TCC, and dogs may present with involvement of the bladder, urethra, and vagina[76] or with ureteral and renal involvement. Although positive-contrast urethrography remains the imaging technique of choice for suspected urethral tumors, abdominal ultrasonography provides a noninvasive method of examining the urinary bladder, cranial urethra, and prostate and is useful in obtaining measurements to assess the efficacy of treatment modalities (Figure 60-7). Abdominal ultrasonography also allows examination of regional lymph nodes and other abdominal organs for metastases or tumor extension. Careful evaluation of the entire urinary tract is warranted before definitive treatment is undertaken.

Ultrasonographic appearance alone is not sufficient to make a diagnosis of TCC because dogs with severe ulcerative cystitis may have a similar appearance, and a biopsy is warranted.[77] Although ultrasonography is useful in obtaining needle-guided biopsy specimens or aspirates, the same caution regarding transplantation of tumor cells and seeding the biopsy tract should be observed.[78] It may be safer to use ultrasonography to guide a suction-catheter biopsy.[77,79] This guidance may improve on the accuracy of the same technique performed "blindly."[73]

Differentiating dogs with a primary diagnosis of urinary tract infection from those with an underlying neoplasm can be difficult. In one study, testing for levels of basic fibroblast growth factor (bFGF) in the urine (Quantikine kit; R&D Systems, Minneapolis, MN) showed that 90% of dogs with TCC had an elevated bFGF level. Only one dog with a primary infection had the same level of elevation.[80] A urine bladder tumor antigen test (bladder tumor-associated antigen; Bard Diagnostic Sciences, Inc., Redmond, CA) has been evaluated in dogs, with an overall sensitivity of 90% and a specificity of 78% in one study.[81] Another study showed similar sensitivity but lower specificity.[82] False-positive results were seen in dogs with glucosuria, proteinuria, pyuria, or hematuria, which are common with almost all neoplastic and nonneoplastic disorders of the canine urinary tract. This test would be an excellent noninvasive screening method for dogs known to be at high risk for developing TCC (e.g., Scottish terriers). Negative results would be conclusive, and positive results could be followed by ultrasonographic examination. Early diagnosis may improve the prognosis for these patients.

The incidence of metastases appears to increase with longer survival, so the percentage of dogs that have metastatic disease increases with successful treatment. In a study of 102 dogs with TCC, only 16% had lymph node metastases at the time of diagnosis, and a further 14% had systemic metastases; nearly half the dogs had metastases after treatment.[71] The most common sites are the lungs and regional lymph nodes (iliac or sublumbar nodes), but widespread metastases have also been reported.[71,83] Thoracic radiographs

TUMORS OF THE URINARY TRACT

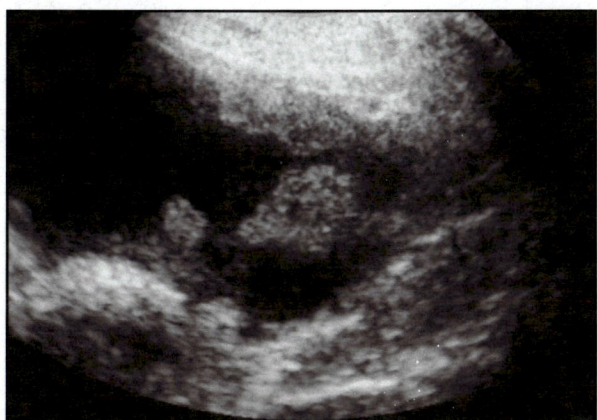

Figure 60-7. *Ultrasonography is technically easier to perform than contrast cystography and allows examination of the rest of the urinary tract (except for the distal urethra). (Courtesy of D.G. Penninck)*

Table 60-3 **Histologic Grading System for Urinary Bladder Tumors in Dogs**[83]

Grade	Dogs (%)	Description
1	22	Regular nuclear placement Nuclei round with mild anisokaryosis Nucleoli small or inapparent
2	57	Regular nuclear placement Nuclei round with mild anisokaryosis Nucleoli small or inapparent
3	21	Marked variation in cell and nuclear size and shape Irregular nuclear crowding and molding Deeply stained, irregularly distributed chromatin Nucleoli frequently multiple and variably located

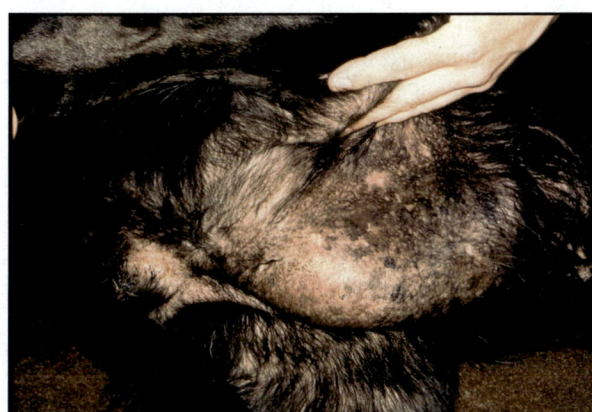

Figure 60-8. *Massive inguinal lymph node metastasis from a urethral TCC was associated with hindlimb edema in this 8-year-old dog.*

Table 60-4 **Histopathologic Grading of TCC of the Lower Urinary Tract in 98 Dogs**[83]

Survival (months)	Grade (n)			Dogs (n)
	1	2	3	
<1	7	36	17	60
1–6	5	18	1	24
7–12	4	3	1	8
>12	2	3	1	6
Total	18	60	20	98

occasionally show evidence of metastasis at the time of diagnosis.[53] The pulmonary metastatic pattern has been described as interstitial nodular and as diffuse unstructured interstitial opacity and may appear similar to chronic aging changes. Metastasis to the lumbar vertebrae and pelvis has been described, and regional lymph node metastasis is observed in up to 60% of dogs at diagnosis.[54,55,84] Metastasis to the sternal, mediastinal, tracheobronchial, hepatic, retropharyngeal, and popliteal nodes has also been reported.[62,85] Intralymphatic and massive lymph node metastasis may lead to mechanical edema of one or both hindlimbs (Figure 60-8).[86] In one study, 22% of dogs with bladder or urethral tumors had a second, third, or fourth primary malignancy.[53]

PROGNOSTIC FACTORS

Tumor stage is an important prognostic factor (see box on page 558). Dogs with a large (T3) tumor developed nodal metastases and distant metastases in 35% of cases compared with 11% and 8% of dogs with T1 or T2 tumors, respectively.[71] Distant metastases were seen in 56% of dogs with evidence of lymph node metastases but in only 6% of dogs without lymph node metastases.[71]

Histopathologic grading (Table 60-3) appears to correlate with prognosis.[83] Specifically, one study[83] showed a correlation between tumor grade and survival, with dogs with grade 1 tumors living longer (Table 60-4). TCCs that showed glandular or squamous differentiation were more likely to be grade 3 tumors. There was also a correlation between peritumoral desmoplasia and the occurrence of metastasis.[83] In another study, the presence of vascular invasion correlated with a higher likelihood of lymph node and distant metastases, and glandular differentiation was associated with a poor response to chemotherapy.[71]

Response to therapy is more likely in dogs with smaller tumors. Response to piroxicam or chemotherapy was seen in

Staging of Urinary Bladder Tumors in Dogs

T: Primary Tumor
- Tis: In situ
- T1: Superficial papillary
- T2: Invading bladder wall
- T3: Invading neighboring organs

N: Regional Node
- N0: No metastasis
- N1: Regional node metastasis
- N2: Regional and juxtaregional

M: Distant Metastasis
- M0: No metastasis
- M1: Metastasis

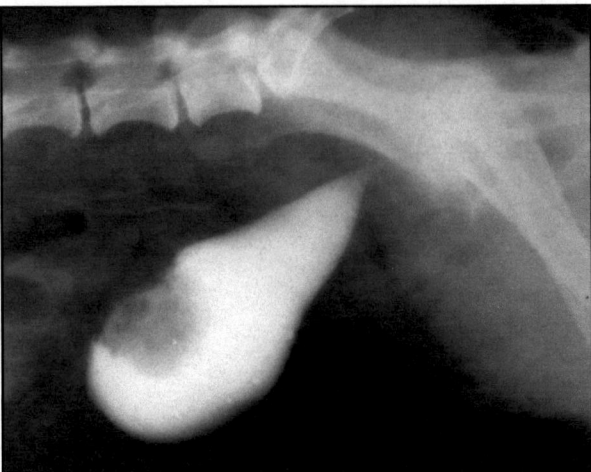

Figure 60-9. *A TCC located in the dorsal bladder wall away from the trigone may be resectable, as in this 14-year-old Brittany.*

30% of dogs with T1 or T2 tumors but in only 5% of dogs with T3 tumors.[71]

Attempts to correlate DNA ploidy with prognosis have not shown any correlation.[87] Immunohistochemical staining for TAG-72 antigen showed positive results in all TCC specimens and negative results in hyperplastic or inflamed urothelial tissues, proving to be an excellent way of distinguishing a neoplastic process, but did not correlate with prognosis.[88]

TREATMENT

Most dogs are euthanatized or die from the primary tumor. If the primary tumor is controlled by therapy and clinical signs abate, survival is prolonged despite metastasis in more than 50% of dogs.

The most effective treatment for TCC has yet to be determined. For tumors located a distance from the trigone in which surgical margins are possible, surgical excision is the treatment of choice; the second choice is adjuvant chemotherapy using piroxicam and mitoxantrone, with cisplatin or carboplatin as further options. For large tumors, particularly those that involve the trigone, surgical debulking may be palliative, but the primary treatment modality should be chemotherapy. The role of radiation therapy is still investigational.

Surgery

The trigonal location of most tumors of the bladder and urethra means that surgical excision is impossible unless the ureters are sacrificed or translocated. However, surgery for benign bladder tumors is potentially curative. In one study, 11 dogs with benign bladder tumors had postsurgical survival times of 6 months to more than 5 years.[54] Similarly, 41 of 43 dogs with surgically removed fibromas were asymptomatic for 3 to 52 months.[57] Ten of the 43 dogs had local recurrence. In contrast, in an early study of 44 dogs with TCC, only four dogs lived more than 4 months, and only one was alive 7 months after surgery.[54]

Local therapies, such as surgery, are unlikely to cure a patient with TCC unless the tumor is located in the bladder away from the trigone (Figure 60-9). In these animals, complete tumor resection is possible; one study reported a median survival of 12 months.[53] Surgical transplantation of tumor cells into the incision line has been reported in five dogs with TCC and was the cause of death in one dog[74]; therefore, care should be taken to "flush" the surgical area after surgery. A different instrument pack should always be used for laparotomy closure (Figure 60-10).

In one report of dogs undergoing surgery for urethral tumors, sagittal pubic osteotomy was performed and surgical excision of the tumor included a section of the urethra.[61] Three of 10 dogs died perioperatively. The median survival for all dogs was 5.5 months. Local recurrence, metastasis, and incontinence were reasons for euthanasia. Aggressive surgical techniques, including trigonal colonic anastomosis[89] and ureterocolonic anastomosis,[90,91] have been used to allow removal of the bladder and urethra in dogs with TCC. Survival times ranged from 1 to 5 months[89–91]; one dog lived 2.7 years.[89] Complications of these surgeries were hyperchloremic acidosis, which was controlled in some dogs with oral sodium bicarbonate (0.5–1.0 g bid)[91]; pyelonephritis (30%–50% of dogs)[89,91]; hydroureter; hydronephrosis; ureteral stenosis; and urinary incontinence. Despite these complications, most owners reported that their dogs had an acceptable quality of life.[91] Surgical complications were the cause of death or reason for euthanasia in most cases, but local recurrence[90] and metastasis[91] were also common causes.

Cystectomy and ureterourethral anastomosis was performed in six dogs.[92] Complete resection was achieved in four

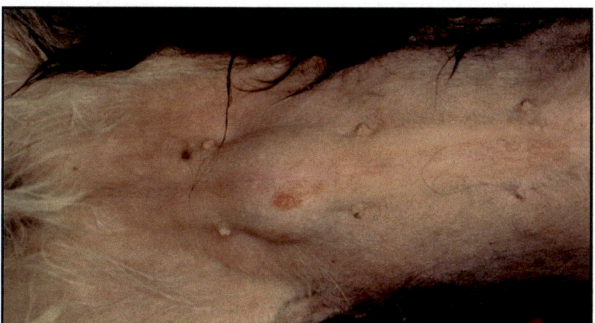

Figure 60-10. *Subcutaneous seeding of TCC after cystostomy, as seen in this dog, can be avoided by paying scrupulous attention to flushing the surgical site and changing surgical instrument packs before closing surgical incisions.*

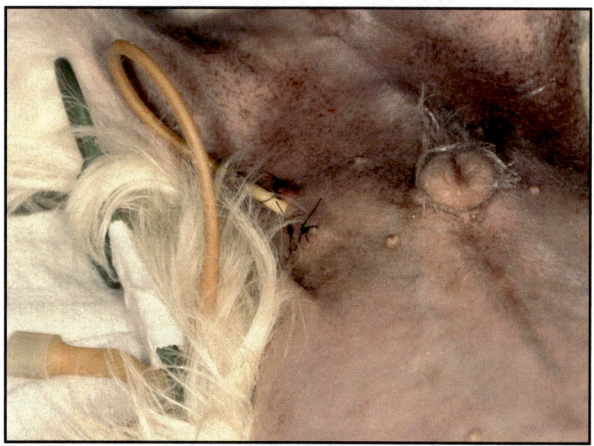

Figure 60-11. *A transabdominal Foley catheter can provide palliative support while other treatment modalities are attempted.*

dogs. After surgery, the dogs needed to wear diapers; survival was between 6 and 25 months. Partial cystectomy of between 40% and 70% of the bladder was reported in 10 dogs.[84] Reimplantation of the ureter was performed when necessary. Seven dogs received adjunctive chemotherapy with cisplatin or carboplatin; two of these dogs also received radiation therapy. Despite the aggressive resection, tumor resection was incomplete in 30% of dogs, and two dogs had dehiscence of the surgery site. The other major complication was pollakiuria (60% of dogs), which was persistent in two dogs (20%). Despite these problems, the median survival in this group of dogs was 13 months (range: 2–48 months), and the longest survivor had two partial cystectomies 2 years apart.

In another study, dogs that had a debulking surgery as part of their combination therapy lived longer (median survival: 350 days) than dogs that did not have a debulking surgery (207 days), regardless of tumor location.[93]

Transurethral resection (TUR) may be considered for rapid relief of urethral obstruction in male dogs. TUR can be performed through a cystoscope. The results of this palliative approach were found to be better in males than in females because of the higher risk of complete urethral thickness invasion in females, leading to potential urethral perforation and tumor seeding.[94]

Palliative surgery to relieve urinary obstruction may prolong comfortable survival. In one study, a permanent transabdominal cystostomy catheter was placed to relieve obstruction caused by TCC (Figure 60-11). Survival ranged from 1 to 5 months, and quality of life appeared to improve.[95] The major problem with this palliative approach is that the catheter is bulky and requires limiting the patient's mobility to prevent dislodgment. To address this issue, one study used a low-profile gastrostomy port to create a cystostomy.[96] The tube was less than 4 cm long, and patients with TCC were successfully managed for up to 7.5 months after tube placement. Owners that had experience with both this and the larger cystostomy catheters preferred the appearance of the low-profile device and the extra mobility it allowed their pets.

Radiation Therapy

Localized radiation therapy has been used for bladder tumors, but most reports have used large fractions given intraoperatively, which increases the likelihood of severe late radiation effects. Intraoperative radiation using cesium-137 (^{137}Cs) for a single treatment of 22 to 29 Gy (median: 27 Gy) was delivered to 11 dogs with TCC.[97] The median survival for these dogs was 15 months (range: 3–67 months). Complications of radiation therapy included the same clinical signs that were associated with the tumor: pollakiuria and incontinence in 50% of dogs, cystitis in 40%, and stranguria in 15%. Hydronephrosis caused by ureteral fibrosis was common. Local recurrence occurred in six dogs (46%), and two of these dogs had distant metastases. Two dogs had metastases without local recurrence. In an attempt to reduce local recurrence, nine dogs with TCC received a median dose of 30 Gy intraoperatively to the tumor bed and a further median dose of 30 Gy in fractions as external-beam radiation using a 6 MeV linear accelerator.[98] Despite these high dosages, tumor recurrence was still common (seven of nine dogs); six dogs also had distant metastases. Most dogs became incontinent within 1 month of radiation therapy because of bladder fibrosis that rendered the organ nondistensible. Survival was for a median of 4 months (range: 1–15 months). Nine dogs treated with surgery and radiation therapy as intraoperative and/or external-beam radiation had a median survival of 3.5 months (range: 1–21 months).[53]

If radiation therapy is used, small, frequent fractions are more likely to avoid complications. In one study,[99] dogs receiving more than 3.3 Gy per fraction to the pelvic area had an increased risk of developing severe colitis, and 60% of these dogs had intestinal perforation. In contrast, dogs treated with fractions of 2.7 Gy or less had mild to moderate self-limiting complications.[99]

Pilot studies that used combination radiation therapy and chemotherapy to treat bladder tumors in dogs have not shown improved survival times over the use of either therapy alone. One pilot study using ^{60}Co teletherapy (44 and 48 Gy) and preradiation cisplatin chemotherapy (50 mg/m^2 twice, divided into three doses before first three and last three radiation treatments) found a minor shrinkage in tumor volume but fewer severe side effects. Survival times were 6 and 7 months.[100] Eight dogs in a group of 15 treated with mitoxantrone and piroxicam also received radiation therapy. The response rate was higher (75%) in the group receiving radiation therapy than in the group treated with chemotherapy alone (60%), although survival times were not different.[101] In another pilot study of 10 dogs, the addition of once-weekly coarse fraction radiation therapy (six fractions of 5.75 Gy weekly) to mitoxantrone and piroxicam did not improve on survival times seen with mitoxantrone and piroxicam chemotherapy alone.[102]

Chemotherapy

Because of the high metastatic rate and difficulties of surgery and radiation therapy, chemotherapy has often been used alone to treat TCC of the lower urinary tract.

Cisplatin, one of the earliest chemotherapeutic agents studied, caused one complete remission (CR) and two partial remissions (PRs) in three dogs in one study. In a more extensive study of 15 dogs, cisplatin (50 mg/m^2 IV q4wk) caused no CRs but resulted in three PRs for a median of 147 days. Three dogs had a minimal response to cisplatin. Median survival time was 6 months, and dogs with any tumor response survived longer, implying that even minor tumor shrinkage may drastically improve clinical signs and therefore delay euthanasia.[103] Renal toxicity was more common in this series of dogs than in dogs with other tumor types treated with cisplatin, presumably because the subclinical renal disease in these dogs predisposed them to cisplatin-induced renal damage. Further evaluation of higher dosages of cisplatin has failed to show any improvement on these data, with only three of 25 dogs having a PR for a median of 130 days.[71,104] Smaller dogs were more likely to have a response or stable disease, implying that further increases in dosage may improve response rate; however, the risk of renal toxicity makes this unlikely to be easily achieved. Dogs that received further chemotherapy or piroxicam after failing to respond to cisplatin lived five times longer than those that received no further treatment.[71,104] This implies that it is worth attempting other treatments even if the first approach is not successful.

Carboplatin, which is not a significant renal toxin, did not have efficacy in the treatment of TCC in one small study. In a group of 12 dogs, one dog had tumor progression after one treatment, 10 dogs had progression after two treatments, and one dog had progression after three treatments, with a median time to progression of 41 days.[105] Carboplatin is cleared by the kidneys, and dogs with azotemia had worse gastrointestinal (GI), but not hematologic, toxicoses than dogs without azotemia. Despite anecdotal responses to carboplatin in dogs with TCC, this drug is unlikely to be markedly better than cisplatin in the treatment of dogs with TCC. Similar to findings with cisplatin, dogs that received further chemotherapy or piroxicam after failing to respond to carboplatin lived eight times longer than those that received no further treatment.[71]

Piroxicam, a nonsteroidal inhibitor of COX-2, given at 0.3 mg/kg PO sid, showed efficacy against TCC in 34 dogs that was superior to results with single-agent chemotherapy.[106,107] In a study of 62 dogs, two dogs had a CR, and four dogs had a PR for between 4 months and 11 months (median: 7 months); the two dogs with CR were free of disease between 2 and 3 years after treatment.[51] In an update from the same group, there were two CRs (3%), nine PRs (15%), and 35 dogs with stable disease (56%).[51] Piroxicam was also effective in achieving remission in dogs that did not respond to carboplatin therapy.[105] Concurrent misoprostol administration (6.5 µg/kg PO bid) may prevent GI irritation. The mechanism by which piroxicam exerts its antitumor effects on TCC is still unclear, although it may affect tumor angiogenesis. In one study, there were correlations between the proportion of apoptotic cells, the urinary concentration of bFGF, and tumor response in dogs treated with piroxicam.[108] There was no correlation between COX-2 staining in the tumor and response, despite the finding that expression of COX-2 was high in bladder tumor tissue and not in normal bladder cells.[109] Although results are only preliminary, other, more potent inhibitors of COX-2, such as deracoxib, have failed to show better than stabilization of TCC in dogs.[110]

Combination therapy using chemotherapy with piroxicam has had various results. One study compared dogs receiving cisplatin alone with dogs receiving cisplatin and piroxicam.[111] The response rate was higher for the combination, with two CRs and eight PRs in 10 of 14 dogs in the cisplatin–piroxicam combination group. However, the renal toxicity of cisplatin and piroxicam was significant and precludes recommendation of the protocol despite the im-

> **KEY POINT**
>
> *Even minor tumor shrinkage may drastically reduce clinical signs and therefore improve length and quality of life for dogs with bladder cancer.*

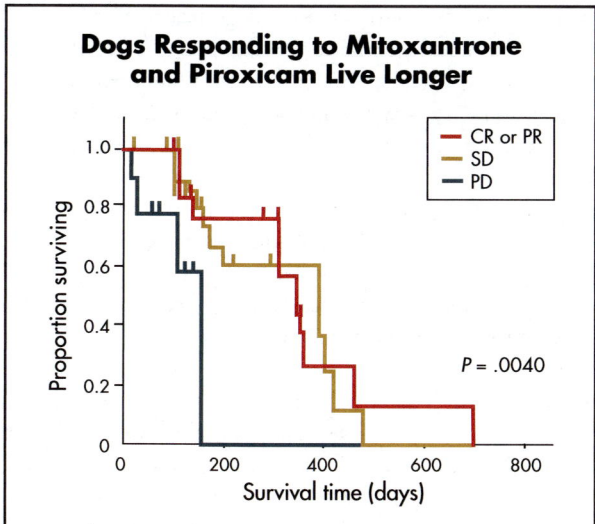

Figure 60-12. Survival curves for dogs with TCC treated with mitoxantrone and piroxicam therapy and having an objective response. (Adapted from Henry CJ, McCaw DL, Turnquist SE, et al: Clinical evaluation of mitoxantrone and piroxicam in a canine model of human invasive urinary bladder carcinoma. Clin Cancer Res 9:906–911, 2003; with permission)

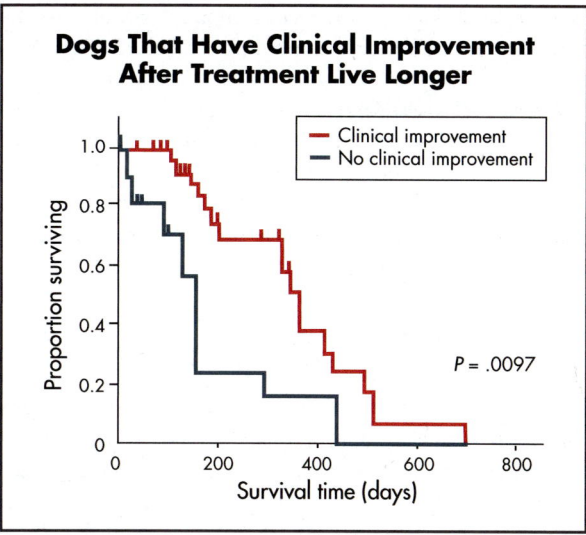

Figure 60-13. Survival curves for dogs with TCC having either subjective clinical improvement or none with mitoxantrone and piroxicam therapy. (Adapted from Henry CJ, McCaw DL, Turnquist SE, et al: Clinical evaluation of mitoxantrone and piroxicam in a canine model of human invasive urinary bladder carcinoma. Clin Cancer Res 9:906–911, 2003; with permission)

proved response rate. In a preliminary report, renal toxicity was still prevalent even when the dosage of cisplatin was reduced to between 40 and 50 mg/m^2.[112] Carboplatin and piroxicam showed an increased response rate of 37%, but the responses were of short duration, and the median survival time was less than 6 months.[113] GI toxicity was seen in 80% of dogs and was moderate or severe in most. The protocol is not recommended.

> **KEY POINT**
>
> *Mitoxantrone and piroxicam in combination is the chemotherapeutic protocol of choice for dogs with TCC.*

One of six dogs with TCC treated with mitoxantrone chemotherapy had a PR for 63 days.[114] Subsequently, a trial of mitoxantrone combined with piroxicam in 48 dogs documented one CR, 16 PRs, 22 dogs with stable disease (SD), and nine dogs with progressive disease (PD) for an overall response rate of 35.4%.[115] Subjective clinical improvement was seen in 36 dogs (75%) and was associated with tumor response. Both measurable and subjective responses were associated with improved survival, as has been seen in other studies (Figures 60-12 and 60-13). The median time to tumor progression was 7 months, and the median survival time was 12 months, the longest recorded for adjunctive therapy of this disease. The most notable toxicities were GI and occurred in nearly 20% of dogs. GI toxicity was rarely severe and often responded to the addition of misoprostol to the protocol and continuation of therapy. Hematologic side effects were rare. Renal failure was seen in five dogs (10%); it was regarded as a protocol-related toxicity in three dogs. The addition of radiation therapy to mitoxantrone and piroxicam chemotherapy did not improve survival times in two studies.[101,102]

Ifosfamide is an active agent in the treatment of TCC in humans, but it has not been shown to have efficacy in dogs. Kenneth M. Rassnick, DVM, observed that in one series of 16 dogs treated with ifosfamide, only two had a PR to treatment.

Drugs used anecdotally without response include cyclophosphamide, interferon, megestrol acetate, and doxorubicin.[53,72] In one trial, 11 dogs treated with doxorubicin and cyclophosphamide had longer survival times (mean: 259 days) than did 14 dogs treated with surgery alone (86 days) and six dogs treated with intravesicular thiotepa (57 days).[74,116] Intravesicular 5-fluorouracil caused regression of bladder TCC in some treated dogs.[117] Intravesicular therapy is less likely to be of significant benefit for large tumors. Tumors invading adjacent structures were less likely to respond to chemotherapy in one study and were associated with shorter survival times.[71] Glandular differentiation of TCC was also associated with a poor response to chemotherapy.[71]

Other Therapy

A pilot study found that 5-aminolevulinic acid–based photodynamic therapy gave short-term symptomatic relief to six treated dogs for a median tumor control of 6 weeks. One dog was treated four times for a total of 48 weeks.[118]

Supportive Therapy

Palliative and supportive therapy for dogs with tumors of the lower urinary tract includes antibiotics based on bacterial culture and sensitivity testing, pain relief (if the patient is receiving piroxicam, then other nonsteroidal drugs should be avoided), and appetite stimulants and nutritional care as needed.

Bladder Rhabdomyosarcomas
INCIDENCE, SIGNALMENT, AND ETIOLOGY

Rhabdomyosarcomas of the lower urinary tract are rare, and most occur in young dogs (1–2 years of age). These tumors seem to be more commonly reported in large-breed dogs, including St. Bernards,[60,119] rottweilers,[120] Great Danes,[120] and Newfoundlands.[121]

CLINICAL PRESENTATION AND HISTORY

As for dogs with TCC, signs referable to the urinary tract are common with rhabdomyosarcomas of the lower urinary tract. Most presenting signs are identical to those in animals with infections or inflammatory conditions of the bladder or urethra, which may coexist with the tumor. Tumors may be very large (≤17 cm in one series of cases).[60] The most common presenting signs are hematuria, dysuria, stranguria, and pollakiuria.[60,120,122,123] Signs can occur in affected dogs for up to 6 months before definitive diagnosis.[124] Occasionally, a dog with hypertrophic osteopathy presents with lameness.[124]

STAGING AND DIAGNOSIS

Dogs with suspected rhabdomyosarcoma of the urinary bladder should have routine blood work and urinalysis conducted. Abdominal ultrasonography should be conducted to examine the bladder (this tumor may be multifocal in the bladder itself)[121] as well as the entire abdomen; the only metastases reported were to the liver.[125] Although metastases to the lungs are not reported, thoracic radiographs should be obtained as part of an MDB before initiating definitive treatment. Routine blood work is helpful to establish a baseline for anesthesia, surgery, and chemotherapy. Urinalysis may reveal hematuria and active inflammatory sediment. Neoplastic cells are rarely seen on urinalysis.[126]

An undifferentiated sarcoma of the bladder may be more clearly diagnosed as rhabdomyosarcoma by using the immunohistochemical marker desmin.[120]

TREATMENT

The paucity of reported metastases makes surgery an attractive option; however, surgical excision is difficult because, like TCCs, rhabdomyosarcomas arise near the trigone of the bladder. Local recurrence was seen within 3 weeks, 5 weeks, 3 months, and 5 months in four dogs treated with surgery alone.[60,84,121] Local recurrence was also seen in a dog that had more than 50% of the bladder resected.[84] Adjunctive therapy appears to be necessary for long-term tumor control.

Intraoperative radiation using ^{137}Cs for a single treatment of 22 to 29 Gy (median: 27 Gy) was delivered to one dog with rhabdomyosarcoma and one dog with leiomyosarcoma.[97] These two dogs lived 12 and 25 months, respectively. One of the dogs was euthanatized because of incontinence, and the other was euthanatized because of tumor recurrence.

A postoperative chemotherapy protocol of four cycles of doxorubicin (30 mg/m^2) given on day 1 of a 3-week cycle and cyclophosphamide (75 mg/m^2) given on days 4 through 7 of the same cycle was used in a dog that was still free of disease 21 months later.[127] The same protocol with higher dosages appeared to prevent local tumor recurrence in another study, but another tumor arose in the abdomen adjacent to the bladder 8.5 months after treatment.[122]

Ifosfamide is an active agent in the treatment of soft tissue sarcomas in human patients. In a preliminary evaluation in dogs, a CR was seen in a dog with leiomyosarcoma of the bladder.[128]

REFERENCES

1. Hayes HM Jr, Fraumeni JF Jr: Epidemiological features of canine renal neoplasms. *Cancer Res* 37:2553–2556, 1977.
2. Baskin GB, De Paoli A: Primary renal neoplasms of the dog. *Vet Pathol* 14:591–605, 1977.
3. Klein MK, Cockerell GL, Harris CK, et al: Canine primary renal neoplasms: A retrospective review of 54 cases. *JAAHA* 24:443–452, 1988.
4. Diters RW, Wells M: Renal interstitial cell tumors in the dog. *Vet Pathol* 23:74–76, 1986.
5. Picut CA, Valentine BA: Renal fibroma in four dogs. *Vet Pathol* 22:422–423, 1985.
6. Zwicker GM, Cronin NS: Naturally occurring renal neurofibroma in a laboratory beagle. *Toxicol Pathol* 20:112–114, 1992.
7. Buergelt CD, Adjiri-Awere A: Bilateral renal oncocytoma in a greyhound dog. *Vet Pathol* 37:188–192, 2000.
8. Rudd RG, Whitehair JG, Leipold HW: Spindle cell sarcoma in the kidney of a dog. *JAAHA* 198:1023–1024, 1991.
9. Konde LF, Wrigley RH, Park RD: Sonographic appearance of renal neoplasia in the dog. *Vet Radiol* 26:74–81, 1985.
10. Widmer WR, Carlton WW: Persistent hematuria in a dog with renal hemangioma. *JAVMA* 197:237–239, 1990.
11. Lappin MR, Latimer KS: Hematuria and extreme neutrophilic leukocytosis in a dog with renal tubular carcinoma. *JAVMA* 192:1289–1292, 1988.
12. Mott JC, McAnulty JF, Darien DL, Steinberg H: Nephron sparing by partial median nephrectomy for treatment of renal hemangioma in a dog. *JAVMA* 208:1274–1276, 1996.
13. Eddlestone S, Taboada J, Senior D, Paulsen DB: Renal haemangioma in a dog. *J Small Anim Pract* 40:132–135, 1999.
14. Lucke VM, Kelly DF: Renal carcinoma in the dog. *Vet Pathol* 13:264–276, 1976.
15. Arai C, Ono M, Une Y, et al: Canine renal carcinoma with extensive bone metastasis. *J Vet Med Sci* 53:495–497, 1991.
16. Madewell BR, Wilson DW, Hornof WJ, Gregory CR: Leukemoid blood response and bone infarcts in a dog with renal tubular adenocarcinoma. *JAVMA* 197:1623–1625, 1990.
17. Peeters D, Clercx C, Thiry A, et al: Resolution of paraneoplastic leukocytosis and hypertrophic osteopathy after resection of a renal transitional cell carcinoma producing granulocyte-macrophage colony-stimulating factor in a young bull terrier. *J Vet Intern Med* 15:407–411, 2001.
18. Gorse MJ: Polycythemia associated with renal fibrosarcoma in a dog. *JAVMA* 192:793–794, 1998.
19. Crow SE, Allen DP, Murphy CJ, Culbertson R: Concurrent renal adenocarci-

noma and polycythemia in a dog. *JAAHA* 31:29–33, 1995.
20. Ghosh AK, Bhattacharjee GC: Primary multicentric carcinomas of kidney. *J Indian Med Assoc* 90:69–70, 1992.
21. Bryan J, Jackson T, Henry CJ, et al: Canine renal neoplasms: a retrospective of 30 cases. *Proc 22nd Annu Conf Vet Cancer Soc*:26, 2002.
22. Khan KN, Stanfield KM, Trajkovic D, Knapp DW: Expression of cyclooxygenase-2 in canine renal cell carcinoma. *Vet Pathol* 38:116–119, 2001.
23. Llum B, Moe L: Hereditary multifocal renal cystadenocarcinomas and nodular dermatofibrosis in the German shepherd dog: Macroscopic and histopathologic changes. *Vet Pathol* 22:447–455, 1985.
24. Moe L, Lium B: Hereditary multifocal renal cystadenocarcinomas and nodular dermatofibrosis in 51 German shepherd dogs. *J Small Anim Pract* 38:498–505, 1997.
25. Atlee BA, DeBoer DJ, Ihrke PJ, et al: Nodular dermatofibrosis in German Shepherd dogs as a marker for renal cystadenocarcinoma. *JAAHA* 27:481–487, 1991.
26. Perry W: Generalised nodular dermatofibrosis and renal cystadenoma in a series of 10 closely related German shepherd dogs. *Aust Vet Practit* 25:90–93, 1995.
27. Jonasdottir TJ, Mellersh CS, Moe L, et al: Genetic mapping of a naturally occurring hereditary renal cancer syndrome in dogs. *Proc Natl Acad Sci USA* 97:4132–4137, 2000.
28. White SD, Rosychuk AW, Schultheiss P, Scott KV: Nodular dermatofibrosis and cystic renal disease in three mixed-breed dogs and a boxer dog. *Vet Dermatol* 9:119–126, 1998.
29. Marks SL, Farman CA, Peaston A: Nodular dermatofibrosis and renal cystadenomas in a golden retriever. *Vet Dermatol* 4:133–137, 1994.
30. Vilafranca M, Fondevila D, Marlasca MJ, Ferrer L: Chromophilic-eosinophilic (oncocyte-like) renal cell carcinoma in a dog with nodular dermatofibrosis. *Vet Pathol* 31:713–716, 1994.
31. Moe L, Lium B: Computed tomography of hereditary multifocal renal cystadenocarcinomas in German shepherd dogs. *Vet Radiol Ultrasound* 38:335–343, 1997.
32. Moe L, Gamlem H, Jonasdottir TJ, Lingaas F: Renal microcystic tubular lesions in two 1year-old dogs—An early sign of hereditary renal cystadenocarcinoma? *J Comp Pathol* 123:218–221, 2000.
33. Cosenza SF, Seely JC: Generalized nodular dermatofibrosis and renal cystadenocarcinomas in a German shepherd dog. *JAVMA* 189:1587–1590, 1986.
34. Jones TL: Embryonal nephroma in a dog. *Can J Comp Med* 164:153–154, 1952.
35. Savage A, Isa JM: Embryonal nephroma with metastasis in a dog. *JAVMA* 124:185–186, 1954.
36. Medway W, Nielsen SW: Canine renal disorders II. Embryonal nephroma in a puppy. *North Am Vet* 35:920–923, 1954.
37. Coleman GL, Gralla EJ, Knirsch AK, Stebbons RB: Canine embryonal nephroma: A case report. *Am J Vet Res* 31:1315–1320, 1970.
38. Simpson RM, Gliatto JM, Caseey HW, Henk WG: The histologic, ultrastructural, and immunohistochemical features of a blastema-predominant canine nephroblastoma. *Vet Pathol* 26:281–282, 1989.
39. Takeda T, Makita T, Nakamura N, Horie H: Congenital mesoblastic nephroma in a dog: A benign variant of nephroblastoma. *Vet Pathol* 26:281–282, 1989.
40. Frimberger AE, Moore AS, Schelling SH: Treatment of nephroblastoma in a juvenile dog. *JAVMA* 207:596–598, 1995.
41. Caywood DD, Osborne CA, Stevens JB, et al: Hypertrophic osteoarthropathy associated with an atypical nephroblastoma in a dog. *JAAHA* 16:855–865, 1980.
42. Abrahamsson K, Uhlhorn M, Lamb CR: What is your diagnosis? Embryonal nephroma. *J Small Anim Pract* 37:154–184, 1996.
43. Sagartz JW, Ayers KM, Cashell IG, Robinson FR: Malignant embryonal nephroma in an aged dog. *JAVMA* 161:1658–1660, 1972.
44. Nakayama H, Hayashi T, Takahashi R, Fujiwara K: Nephroblastoma with liver and lung metastases in an adult dog. *Nippon Juigaku Zasshi* 46:897–900, 1984.
45. Seaman RL, Patton CS: Treatment of renal nephroblastoma in an adult dog. *JAAHA* 39:76–79, 2003.
46. Hartmann M, Steidel T: Sekundäre polyzythämie infolge neophroblastom bei einem beutschen schäferhund. *Kleintierpraxis* 42:577–588, 1997.
47. Gasser AM, Bush WW, Smith S, Walton R: Extradural spinal, bone marrow, and renal nephroblastoma. *JAAHA* 39:80–85, 2003.
48. Seibold HR, Hoerlein BF: Embryonal nephroma (nephroblastoma) in a dog. *JAVMA* 130:82–85, 1957.
49. Coleman GL, Gralla EJ, Knirsch AK, Stebbins RB: Mithramycin treatment of metastatic canine embryonal nephroma (radiographic evidence of regression was associated with histopathologic changes). *Fed Proc* 28:686, 1969.
50. Reichle JK, Peterson RA, Mahaffey MB, et al: Ureteral fibroepithelial polyps in four dogs. *Vet Radiol Ultrasound* 44:433–437, 2003.
51. Mutsaers AJ, Widmer WR, Knapp DW: Canine transitional cell carcinoma. *J Vet Intern Med* 17:136–144, 2003.
52. Hayes HM Jr: Canine bladder cancer: Epidemiologic features. *Am J Epidemiol* 104:673–677, 1976.
53. Norris AM, Laing EJ, Valli VE, et al: Canine bladder and urethral tumors: A retrospective study of 115 cases (1980–1985). *J Vet Intern Med* 6:145–153, 1992.
54. Burnie AG, Weaver AD: Urinary bladder neoplasia in the dog; A review of seventy cases. *J Small Anim Pract* 24:129–143, 1983.
55. Osborne CA, Low DG, Perman V, Barnes DM: Neoplasms of the canine and feline urinary bladder: Incidence, etiologic factors, occurrence and pathologic features. *Am J Vet Res* 29:2041–2055, 1968.
56. Moroff SD, Brown BA, Matthiesen DT, Scott RC: Infiltrative urethral disease in female dogs: 41 cases (1980–1987). *JAVMA* 199:247–251, 1991.
57. Esplin DG: Urinary bladder fibromas in dogs: 51 cases (1981–1985). *JAVMA* 190:440–444, 1987.
58. Leav I, Schelling SH, Adams JY, et al: Role of canine basal cells in postnatal prostatic development, induction of hyperplasia, and sex hormone-stimulated growth; and the ductal origin of carcinoma. *Prostate* 48:210–224, 2001.
59. Sorenmo KU, Goldschmidt M, Shofer F, et al: Immunohistochemical characterization of canine prostatic carcinoma and correlation with castration status and castration time. *Vet & Comp Oncol* 1:48–56, 2003.
60. Kelly DF: Rhabdomyosarcoma of the urinary bladder in dogs. *Vet Pathol* 10:375–384, 1973.
61. Davies JV, Read HM: Urethral tumours in dogs. *J Small Anim Pract* 31:131–136, 1990.
62. Nikula KJ, Benjamin SA, Angleton GM, Lee AC: Transitional cell carcinomas of the urinary tract in a colony of beagle dogs. *Vet Pathol* 26:455–461, 1989.
63. Glickman LT, Schofer FS, McKee LJ, et al: Epidemiologic study of insecticide exposure, obesity, and risk of bladder cancer in household dogs. *J Toxicol Environ Health* 28:407–414, 1989.
64. Glickman LT, Raghavan M, Knapp DW, et al: Herbicide exposure and the risk of transitional cell carcinoma of the urinary bladder in Scottish terriers. *JAVMA* 224:1290–1297, 2004.
65. Hayes HM, Tarone RE, Cantor KP, et al: Case-control study of canine malignant lymphoma: Positive association with dog owners use of 2, 4-dichlorophenoxyacetic acid herbicides. *J Natl Cancer Inst* 83:1226–1231, 1991
66. Raghavan M, Knapp DW, Dawson MH, et al: Topical flea and tick pesticides and the risk of transitional cell carcinoma of the urinary bladder in Scottish terriers. *JAVMA* 225:389–394, 2004.
67. Macy DW, Withrow SJ, Hoopes J: Transitional cell carcinoma of the bladder associated with cyclophosphamide administration. *JAAHA* 19:965–969, 1983.
68. Samma S, Uemura H, Tabata S, et al: Rapid induction of carcinoma in situ in dog urinary bladder by sequential treatment with N-methyl-N'-nitrosourea and N-butyl-N-(4-hydroxybutyl)-nitrosamine. *Gann* 75:385–387, 1984.
69. Osborne CA, Low DG, Perman V: Neoplasms of the canine and feline urinary bladder: Clinical findings, diagnosis and treatment. *JAVMA* 152:247–259, 1968.
70. Fontaine J, Coignoul F, Moureau P, Penninck D: Un cas d'ostéoarthropathie hypertrophique. *Ann Med Vet* 128:545–554, 1984.
71. Knapp DW, Glickman NW, DeNicola DB, et al: Naturally occurring canine transitional cell carcinoma of the urinary bladder. A relevant model of human invasive bladder cancer. *Urologic Oncol* 5:47–59, 2000.
72. Rozengaurt N, Hyman WJ, Berry A, et al: Urinary cytology of a canine bladder carcinoma. *J Comp Pathol* 96:581–585, 1986.
73. Holt PE, Lucke VM, Brown PJ: Evaluation of a catheter biopsy technique as a diagnostic aid in lower urinary tract disease. *Vet Rec* 118:681–684, 1986.
74. Gilson SD, Stone EA: Surgically induced tumor seeding in eight dogs and two cats. *JAVMA* 196:1811–1815, 1990.
75. Anderson WI, Dunham BM, King JM, Scott DW: Presumptive subcutaneous surgical transplantation of a urinary bladder transitional cell carcinoma in a dog. *Cornell Vet* 7989:263–266, 1989.
76. Magrie ML, Hoopes PJ, Kainer RA, et al: Urinary tract carcinomas involving the canine vagina and vestibule. *JAAHA* 21:767–772, 1985.
77. Hanson JA, Tidwell AS: Ultrasonographic appearance of urethral transitional cell carcinoma in ten dogs. *Vet Radiol Ultrasound* 37:293–299, 1996.
78. Nyland TG, Wallack ST, Wisner ER: Needle-tract implantation following US-guided fine-needle aspiration biopsy of transitional cell carcinoma of the bladder, urethra, and prostate. *Vet Radiol Ultrasound* 43:50–53, 2002.
79. Lamb CR, Trower ND, Gregory SP: Ultrasound-guided catheter biopsy of the lower urinary tract: Technique and results in 12 dogs. *J Small Anim Pract* 37:413–416, 1996.

80. Allen DK, Waters DJ, Knapp DW, Kuczek T: High urine concentrations of basic fibroblast growth factor in dogs with bladder cancer. *J Vet Intern Med* 10:231–234, 1996.
81. Borjesson DL, Christopher MM, Ling GV: Detection of canine transitional cell carcinoma using a bladder tumor antigen urine dipstick test. *Vet Clin Pathol* 28:33–38, 1999.
82. Billet JP, Moore AH, Holt PE: Evaluation of a bladder tumor antigen test for the diagnosis of lower urinary tract malignancies in dogs. *Am J Vet Res* 63:370–373, 2002.
83. Valli VE, Norris A, Jacobs RM, et al: Pathology of canine bladder and urethral cancer and correlation with tumour progression and survival. *J Comp Pathol* 113:113–130, 1995.
84. Stone EA, George TF, Gilson SD, Page RL: Partial cystectomy for urinary bladder neoplasia: Surgical technique and outcome in 11 dogs. *J Small Anim Pract* 37:480–485, 1996.
85. Walter PA, Haynes JS, Feeney DA, Johnston GR: Radiographic appearance of pulmonary metastases from transitional cell carcinoma of the bladder and urethra of the dog. *JAVMA* 185:411–418, 1984.
86. Weber KO, Willimzik HF: Mechanisches gliedmaßenödem durch eine lymphangiosis carcinomatosa infolge eines metastasierenden übergangszellkarzinoms der harnblase bein einem hund. *Kleintierpraxis* 44:35–41, 1999.
87. Clemo FA, DeNicola DB, Carlton WW, et al: Flow cytometric DNA ploidy analysis in canine transitional cell carcinoma of urinary bladders. *Vet Pathol* 31:207–215, 1994.
88. Clemo FA, DeNicola DB, Carlton WW, et al: Immunoreactivity of canine transitional cell carcinoma of the urinary bladder with monoclonal antibodies to tumor-associated glycoprotein 72. *Vet Pathol* 32:155–161, 1995.
89. Bove KC, Pass MA, Wardley R, et al: Trigonal-colonic anastomosis: A urinary diversion procedure in dogs. *JAVMA* 174:184–191, 1979.
90. Montgomery RD, Hankes GH: Ureterocolonic anastomosis in a dog with transitional cell carcinoma of the urinary bladder. *JAVMA* 190:1427–1429, 1987.
91. Stone EA, Withrow SJ, Page RL, et al: Ureterocolonic anastomosis in ten dogs with transitional cell carcinoma. *Vet Surg* 17:147–153, 1988.
92. Kadosawa T, Takagi S, Osaki T, Fujinaga T: Total cystectomy and ureteroourethral anastomosis in dogs 6 dogs with transitional cell carcinoma of bladder. *Proc 23rd Annu Conf Vet Cancer Soc*:18, 2003.
93. Josel JR, Pagor CA, Glickman NW, et al: The role of surgical debulkment in dogs with transitional cell carcinoma of the urinary bladder: A retrospective study of 122 dogs. *Proc 22nd Annu Conf Vet Cancer Soc*:5, 2002.
94. Liptak JM, Brutscher SP, Monnet E, et al: Transurethral resection in the management of urethral and prostatic neoplasia in 6 dogs. *Vet Surg* 33:1–12, 2004.
95. Smith JD, Stone EA, Gilson SD: Placement of a permanent cystostomy catheter to relieve urine outflow obstruction in dogs with transitional cell carcinoma. *JAVMA* 206:496–499, 1995.
96. Stiffler KS, McCrackin Stevenson MA, Cornell KK, et al: Clinical use of low-profile cystostomy tubes in four dogs and a cat. *JAVMA* 223:325–329, 2003.
97. Walker M, Breider M: Intraoperative radiotherapy of canine bladder cancer. *Vet Radiol* 28:200–204, 1987.
98. Withrow SJ, Gillette EL, Hoopes PJ, McChesney SL: Intraoperative irradiation of 16 spontaneously occurring canine neoplasms. *Vet Surg* 18:7–11, 1989.
99. Anderson CR, McNiel EA, Gillette EL, et al: Late complications of pelvic irradiation in 16 dogs. *Vet Radiol Ultrasound* 43:187–192, 2002.
100. McCaw DL, Lattimer JC: Radiation and cisplatin for treatment of canine urinary bladder carcinoma: A report of two case histories. *Vet Radiol* 29:264–268, 1988.
101. Turner AI, Hahn KA, King GK, Carreras JK: Mitoxantrone, piroxicam and external beam radiation therapy in the treatment of canine bladder tumors, 15 cases (2001–2003). *Proc 23rd Annu Conf Vet Cancer Soc*:20, 2003.
102. Poirier VJ, Forrest LJ, Adams WM, Vail DM: Piroxicam, mitoxantrone, and coarse fraction radiotherapy for the treatment of transitional cell carcinoma of the bladder in 10 dogs: A pilot study. *JAAHA* 40:131–136, 2004.
103. Moore AS, Cardona A, Shapiro W, Madewell BR: Cisplatin (cisdiamminedichloroplatinum) for treatment of transitional cell carcinoma of the urinary bladder or urethra. A retrospective study of 15 dogs. *J Vet Intern Med* 4:148–152, 1990.
104. Chun R, Knapp DW, Widmer WR, et al: Cisplatin treatment of transitional cell carcinoma of the urinary bladder in dogs: 18 cases (1983–1993). *JAVMA* 209:1588–1591, 1996.
105. Chun R, Knapp DW, Widmer WR, et al: Phase II clinical trial of carboplatin in canine transitional cell carcinoma of the urinary bladder. *J Vet Intern Med* 11:279–283, 1997.
106. Knapp DW, Richardson RC, Bottoms GD, et al: Phase I trial of piroxicam in 62 dogs bearing naturally occurring tumors. *Cancer Chemother Pharmacol* 29:214–218, 1992.
107. Knapp DW, Richardson RC, Chan TC, et al: Piroxicam therapy in 34 dogs with transitional cell carcinoma of the urinary bladder. *J Vet Intern Med* 8:273–278, 1994.
108. Effects of the cyclooxygenase inhibitor, piroxicam, on tumor response, apoptosis, and angiogenesis in a canine model of human invasive urinary bladder cancer. *Cancer Res* 62:356–358, 2002.
109. Kahn KN, Knapp DW, DeNicola DB, Harris RK: Expression of cyclooxygenase-2 in transitional cell carcinoma of the urinary bladder in dogs. *Am J Vet Res* 61:478–481, 2000.
110. Boria PA, Biolsi SA, Greenberg CB, et al: Preliminary evaluation of deracoxib in canine transitional cell carcinoma of the urinary bladder. *Proc 23rd Annu Conf Vet Cancer Soc*:17, 2003.
111. Knapp DW, Glickman NW, Widmer WR, et al: Cisplatin versus cisplatin combined with piroxicam in a canine model of human invasive urinary bladder cancer. *Cancer Chemother Pharmacol* 46:221–226, 2000.
112. Greene SN, Lucroy MD, Greenberg CB, et al: Evaluation of cisplatin (40–50 mg/m^2) and piroxicam in dogs with transitional cell carcinoma of the urinary bladder. *Proc 24th Annu Conf Vet Cancer Soc*:9, 2004.
113. Boria PA, Mutsaers AJ, DiBernardi L, et al: Carboplatin and piroxicam therapy in 31 dogs with transitional cell carcinoma. *Proc 22nd Annu Conf Vet Cancer Soc*:25, 2002.
114. Ogilvie GK, Obradovich JE, Elmslie RE, et al: Efficacy of mitoxantrone against various neoplasms in dogs. *JAVMA* 198:1618–1621, 1991.
115. Henry CJ, McCaw DL, Turnquist SE, et al: Clinical evaluation of mitoxantrone and piroxicam in a canine model of human invasive urinary bladder carcinoma. *Clin Cancer Res* 9:906–911, 2003.
116. Helfand SC, Hamilton TA, Hungerford L, et al: Comparison of three treatments for transitional cell carcinoma of the bladder in the dog. *JAAHA* 30:270–275, 1994.
117. Harrold MW, Edwards CN, Gravey FK: Treatment of bladder tumors by direct instillation of 5-fluorouracil. Experimental observations in dogs. *Invest Urol* 15:47–51, 1964.
118. Lucroy MD, Ridgway TD, Peavy GM, et al: Preclinical evaluation of 5-aminolevulinic acid-based photodynamic therapy for canine transitional cell carcinoma. *Vet Comp Oncol* 1:76–85, 2003.
119. Pletcher JM, Dalton L: Botryoid rhabdomyosarcoma in the urinary bladder of a dog. *Vet Pathol* 18:695–697, 1981.
120. Andreasen CB, White MR, Swayne DE, Graves GN: Desmin as a marker for canine botryoid rhabdomyosarcomas. *J Comp Pathol* 98:23–29, 1988.
121. Kuwamura M, Yoshida H, Yamate J, et al: Urinary bladder rhabdomyosarcoma (sarcoma botryoides) in a young Newfoundland dog. *J Vet Med Sci* 60:619–621, 1998.
122. Kriegleder H: Behandlung eines botryoiden rhabdomyosarkoms der harnblase bei einme hund. *Kleintierpraxis* 43:117–126, 1998.
123. Stamps P, Harris DL: Botryoid rhabdomyosarcoma of the urinary bladder of a dog. *JAVMA* 153:1064–1068, 1968.
124. Halliwell WH, Ackerman N: Botryoid rhabdomyosarcoma of the urinary bladder and hypertrophic osteoarthropathy in a young dog. *JAVMA* 165:911–913, 1974.
125. Takiguchi M, Watanabe T, Okada H, et al: Rhabdomyosarcoma (botryoid sarcoma) of the urinary bladder in a Maltese. *J Small Anim Pract* 43:269–271, 2002.
126. Roszel JF: Cytology of urine from dogs with botryoid sarcoma of the bladder. *Acta Cytol* 16:443–446, 1972.
127. Senior DF, Lawrence DT, Gunson C, et al: Successful treatment of botryoid rhabdomyosarcoma in the bladder of a dog. *JAAHA* 29:386–390, 1993.
128. Rassnick KM, Frimberger AE, Wood CA, et al: Evaluation of ifosfamide for treatment of various canine neoplasms. *J Vet Intern Med* 14:271–276, 2000.

TUMORS OF BONE
Antony S. Moore and Gregory K. Ogilvie

61

CLINICAL BRIEFING

MDB includes a complete blood count, biochemical profile, and urinalysis, as well as thoracic radiography (three views).

Osteosarcoma of the Appendicular Skeleton

Clinical factors
- Lameness and pain at metaphyseal sites, particularly the distal radius, proximal humerus, proximal tibia, and distal femur.
- Lytic and productive bone lesion on radiography.
- Most commonly osteoblastic osteosarcoma.
- Affects large- to giant-breed dogs with no gender predilection.
- Usually middle-aged to older dogs.

Staging and diagnosis
- MDB; note serum T-ALP particularly (prognostic).
- High-detail radiographs of lesion.
- Serum B-ALP if available.
- Metastasis occurs early but is usually not clinically evident.
- Biopsy for grading.
- Scintigraphy may assist in identifying bone metastases.

Prognostic factors
- Adjunctive chemotherapy improves survival markedly.
- Serum T-ALP above normal confers worse prognosis.
- Low-grade osteosarcoma confers better prognosis.
- When chemotherapy is used, smaller dogs have better prognosis.

Treatment

Initial
- With amputation alone, median survival is 162 days; 11% of dogs alive at 1 year.
- Limb sparing provides good limb function for distal radial tumors.

Adjunctive
- Chemotherapy
  - Cisplatin: Median survival: 10.5 months; 1-year survival: 46%.
  - Doxorubicin: Median survival: 9.5 months; 1-year survival: 40%.
  - Carboplatin: Median survival: 10.5 months; 1-year survival: 35%.
  - Combinations may improve on single agent.
- Radiation therapy
  - Palliative for painful bony lesions.

Supportive
- Pain relief with radiation therapy, bisphosphonates, nonsteroidal drugs, and possibly opioids.
- Nutritional support as needed.

Osteosarcoma of the Axial Skeleton (including MLO)	
Clinical factors	• Tumors of the appendicular skeleton are four times more common than axial tumors. • Older dogs (except rib tumors, which often affect young dogs). • No breed predilection; more females may be affected.
Staging and diagnosis	• MDB. • High-detail radiography of lesion. • CT or MRI of lesion. • Highly metastatic, but local recurrence usually occurs earlier. • Mandibular osteosarcoma may have lower metastatic rate.
Prognostic factors	• Complete excision confers longer survival. • Smaller dogs may live longer than larger dogs. • Mandibular osteosarcoma appears to confer better prognosis than any other site.
Treatment	
Initial	• Surgery difficult because of location of tumors. • Mandible and rib tumors can be resected.
Adjuvant	• Cisplatin chemotherapy is recommended for osteosarcoma of all sites. • Radiation therapy may be useful adjunct to surgery to reduce local recurrence.
Supportive	• Pain relief with radiation therapy, bisphosphonates, nonsteroidal drugs, and possibly opioids. • Nutritional support as needed.
Nonosteosarcoma Bone Tumors	
Clinical factors	• More often affect axial skeleton than appendicular skeleton. • Usually chondrosarcoma, fibrosarcoma, and hemangiosarcoma. • Older dogs, except oral fibrosarcoma, which predominantly affects younger dogs.
Staging and diagnosis	• MDB. • High-detail radiography of the lesion. • CT or MRI. • Metastases occur at a lower rate than osteosarcoma and may occur late in the course of the disease. • Care required in interpreting incisional biopsy specimens because small biopsies may miss osteosarcoma.
Treatment	
Initial	• Surgery palliative; may be curative in some dogs, although metastases may arise even months to years after surgery.
Adjunctive	• Chemotherapy not known to be effective. • Radiation therapy may improve tumor control.
Supportive	• Pain relief with radiation therapy, bisphosphonates, nonsteroidal drugs, and possibly opioids. • Nutritional support as needed.

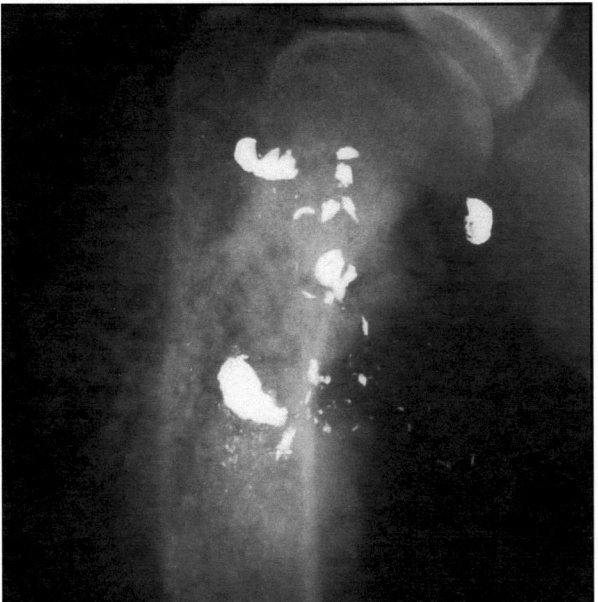

Figure 61-1. *Radiograph of a proximal humeral osteosarcoma showing lysis and "sunburst" periosteal reaction. This dog was shot 5 years previously, and the bullet remains in situ. Trauma and inflammation may play a role in osteosarcoma formation, but the occurrence is rare. (Courtesy of Nicole Northrup, DVM, University of Georgia College of Veterinary Medicine)*

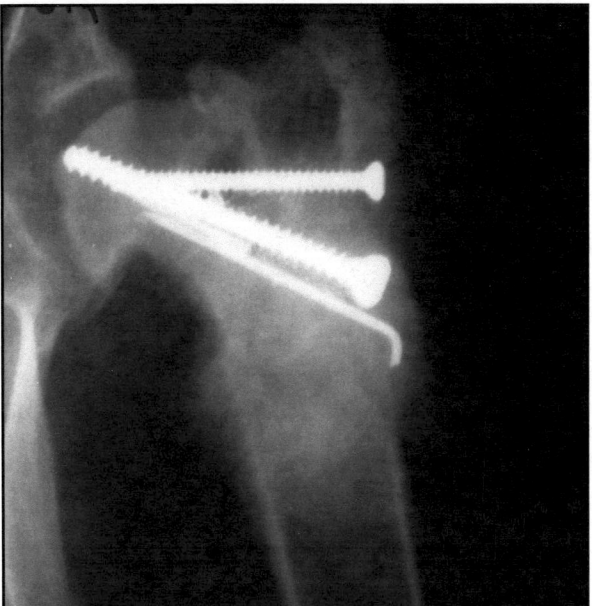

Figure 61-2. *An osteosarcoma with a classic radiographic appearance occurred at the site of a femoral head osteotomy performed 6 years previously. (Courtesy of Randy Boudrieau, DVM, Tufts Cummings School of Veterinary Medicine)*

Osteosarcoma of the Appendicular Skeleton

INCIDENCE, SIGNALMENT, AND ETIOLOGY

Osteosarcoma of the limbs is more common in dogs than in any other species and accounts for more than 80% of malignant bone tumors in dogs. These tumors are believed to arise from the medullary cavity, usually at a metaphysis, and expand outward, destroying cortex and disrupting periosteum.

Large- to giant-breed dogs with a body weight of more than 20 kg are most often affected. Compared with dogs that weigh less than 10 kg, giant-breed dogs (>35 kg) are 60 times more likely and large-breed dogs (20–35 kg) are eight times more likely to develop osteosarcoma.[1] A case-control study of more than 3,000 dogs with osteosarcoma confirmed that the risk of osteosarcoma increased with increasing age, increasing weight, and increasing height.[2] The effect of weight was greatest on increasing risk of forelimb osteosarcomas. Compared with dogs weighing less than 23 kg, dogs weighing more than 45 kg had 16 and eight times the risk of developing forelimb and hindlimb tumors, respectively.[2] The effect of height was similar: Compared with dogs that were shorter than 35.5 cm, dogs that were taller than 54 cm had approximately 25 times the risk of developing forelimb osteosarcoma and nine times the risk of hindlimb osteosarcoma.[2]

Osteosarcoma was shown to be hereditary in a family of Saint Bernard dogs,[3] and another study found that Irish wolfhounds, Saint Bernards, and great Danes had the highest breed risks (21, 12, and five times the average risk, respectively).[2] Scottish deerhounds appear to have an autosomal recessive mode of inheritance of susceptibility to this tumor.[4] Rapid early growth and increase in stress on weight-bearing limbs have been hypothesized to lead to multiple minor trauma to the predilection sites. However, one study failed to find histologic evidence of such trauma.[5]

Dogs with osteosarcoma have a median age of 8 years (range: 8 months–13 years),[2] although giant-breed dogs are affected at a younger age. One study found that risk increased with age, then plateaued at the age of 10 years.[2] There is no gender predilection; however, neutered dogs of both genders appear to be at twice the risk of intact dogs.[2,6–8] This association of increased risk for neutered dogs was most noticeable in rottweilers, particularly those neutered before the age of 1 year.[9]

Osteosarcoma has been associated with sites of healed fractures or internal-fixation devices, implying that chronic irritation may play a role in tumor development. A specific and strong example of this association has been seen with the Jonas pin.[10] A number of case reports, including some of osteosarcoma formation after total hip arthroplasty, have appeared in the veterinary literature.[11–13] The association with other internal fixation devices is controversial because one study found that there was actually a reduced risk of developing osteosarcoma after internal fracture fixation compared with external fixation.[14] Most veterinarians agree

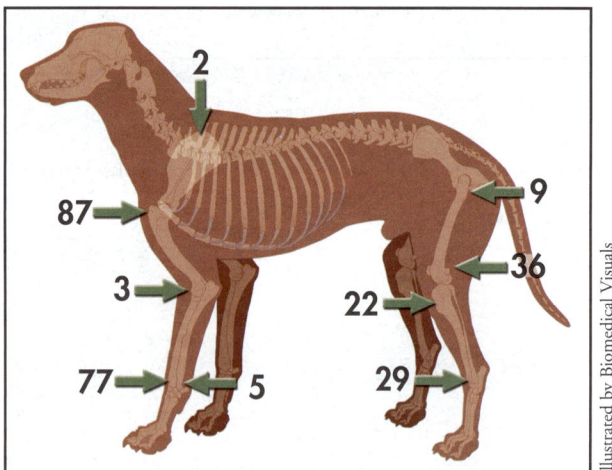

Figure 61-3. The distribution of appendicular osteosarcoma in 270 dogs.

that if there is a risk, it is low and is possibly outweighed by the benefit of internal fixation of a fracture (Figures 61-1 and 61-2). In contrast, there is no controversy over the finding that osteosarcoma may occur in sites that are irradiated for treatment of other tumors. These tumors occur in fewer than 5% of dogs between 1.5 and 5 years after irradiation. High single-dose radiation (i.e., coarse fractionation) in one study increased the risk of tumor formation.[15]

Mutations in the *p53* tumor suppressor gene result in high levels of the abnormal gene product that can be detected on immunohistochemistry. Inactivation of normal function results in cellular progression to the malignant state.[16] Overexpression of *p53* is seen in 70% to 80% of appendicular osteosarcomas, 40% to 55% of axial osteosarcomas, and 20% of multilobular osteochondrosarcomas (MLOs) of bone.[17,18] This overexpression is thought by some to be a result of germline mutations and may explain the breed-related increase in the incidence of osteosarcoma. Overexpression of mutated *p53* is higher in high-grade tumors and may correlate with more aggressive clinical behavior.[18]

CLINICAL PRESENTATION AND HISTORY

Osteosarcoma most commonly affects the appendicular skeleton. Osteosarcomas arise in the long-bone metaphyses of limbs that receive the greatest load associated with daily activity. The most common sites are the distal radius and the proximal humerus ("away from the elbow") (Figure 61-3). Less common sites are the proximal tibia and distal femur ("toward the knee").[6,7] Lameness is often intermittent early in the course of the disease and may be exacerbated by or associated with a traumatic event. Lameness then becomes chronic, and the limb can no longer bear weight. The early fluctuating course is believed to be partly attributable to

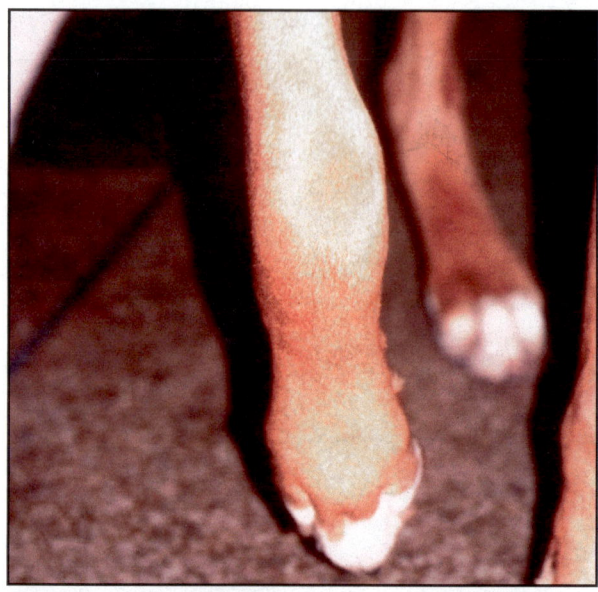

Figure 61-4. This 1-year-old boxer has classic signs of a primary bone tumor. The distal radius is swollen and painful, and the dog is reluctant to touch its foot to the ground. (Courtesy of Kenneth M. Rassnick, DVM, Cornell University College of Veterinary Medicine)

subperiosteal bleeding and microfractures of the weakened cortex. Initially, there may be no clinically apparent lesion on palpation, and radiographs of the limb may show only subtle radiographic changes. As the disease progresses, swelling and lameness may rapidly worsen and the lesion may become painful to the touch (Figure 61-4). If the tumor is untreated, progressive erosion of the cortex may cause a pathologic fracture of the affected limb (Figure 61-5). The duration of clinical signs may be very short and often ranges from 1 to 3 months.

In small dogs (<15 kg) in one study, about 25% of bone tumors were metastases, and only 46% of tumors were osteosarcomas.[19] Osteosarcomas frequently affected the axial skeleton (50%). In dogs with appendicular osteosarcomas, the femur was most commonly affected; the distal radius was affected in only 12%. Appendicular osteosarcomas in small dogs still appear to have a high metastatic rate.[19]

STAGING AND DIAGNOSIS

Suspected primary bone tumors should be imaged on high-detail radiographs. Routine blood work, urinalysis, and thoracic radiographs should also be part of a minimum database (MDB) in these dogs. Primary bone tumors may have a lytic, productive, or mixed appearance on high-detail radiographs. The signs most suggestive of neoplasia include cortical bone lysis in a lesion that does not cross a joint. Classically, tumor extension and mineralization form periosteal spicules in the surrounding soft tissues, imparting a "sunburst" appearance on radiographs (Figures 61-1, 61-2, and 61-6).

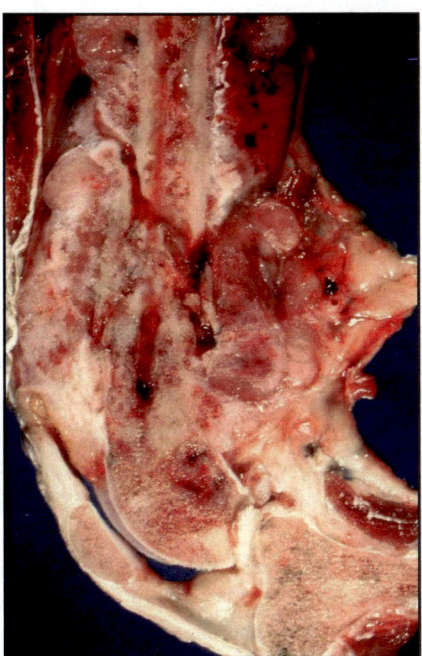

Figure 61-5. *This amputation pathology specimen shows cortical disruption, periosteal new bone production, and a pathologic fracture resulting from an osteosarcoma in the left distal femur. Note that despite the severity of the lesion, it does not cross the joint. (Courtesy of Scott H. Schelling, DVM, Wyeth Research)*

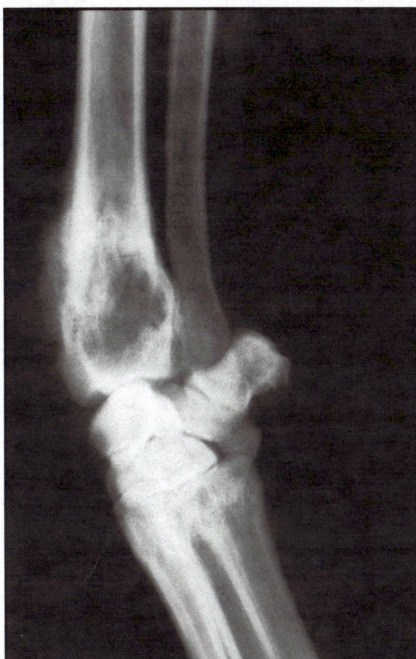

Figure 61-6. *Radiograph of a distal radial osteosarcoma showing lysis and medullary extension. Note that the lesion does not cross the joint.*

Tumor margins are important if limb salvage, rather than amputation, is contemplated. Bony lysis is not radiographically apparent until more than 50% of mineral has been removed; therefore, the margins or extent of neoplastic disease in osteosarcoma may be difficult to define on radiographs. Computed tomography (CT) or magnetic resonance imaging (MRI) scans may be more accurate than radiographs, but this is controversial.[20,21] Bone scintigraphy overestimates tumor margins by delineating the tumor plus surrounding reactive bone[22] and may detect other lesions in bone and soft tissue sites.[23] In a group of 66 dogs with appendicular osteosarcoma that underwent technetium scintigraphy, none manifested other bony lesions.[24] However, in 7.8% of 399 dogs, scintigraphy detected suspicious lesions that also appeared on radiographs.[25] It was unclear how many of these dogs also had pulmonary metastases and whether scintigraphy improves the staging procedure. The difficulties in conducting scans in private practice, combined with the relatively low yield, mean that routine use of scintigraphy is probably not warranted.

> **KEY POINT**
>
> *A radiographic bone lesion that includes bone lysis but does not cross a joint space is very suggestive of neoplasia.*

Based on studies of survival after amputation, the metastatic rate of appendicular osteosarcomas is 98%, and the most commonly detected site of metastases is the lungs.[6] Although pulmonary metastases are rarely detectable at the time of diagnosis, thoracic radiographs should still be taken because the finding of measurable metastases profoundly and negatively influences the effectiveness of adjuvant therapy and, hence, survival time. Right and left lateral views and a dorsoventral view should be obtained to improve the likelihood of detection.[26] Dogs with clinically detectable pulmonary metastases rarely respond to treatment. Some investigators have suggested that CT of the lungs might improve the detection of pulmonary metastases that are just below the detection level of radiographs. Identifying dogs that have metastatic disease with CT may result in enhanced patient comfort by directing the care toward palliative procedures such as pain control rather than using chemotherapy with curative intent. Regional lymphadenopathy from tumor metastasis is observed in less than 3% of dogs at the time of presentation, which approximates the incidence of pulmonary metastases.[27]

Fine-needle aspiration cytology may be suggestive of an osteosarcoma, but more than 50% of dogs will have a nondiagnostic sample.[28] Ultrasound-guided aspiration may increase the percentage of diagnostic samples; however, histopathology is still preferred for definitive diagnosis. For older animals with a large lytic metaphyseal bone lesion, osteosarcoma is the most common diagnosis. Differential diagnoses include other neoplastic conditions and fungal and bacterial infections. A preoperative biopsy is recommended with a confirmatory biopsy at the time of amputation. However, if the dog's age, breed, and weight and the tumor's metaphyseal location and radiographic appearance are strongly suggestive of osteosarcoma, an excisional biopsy taken at the time of amputation is not only diagnostic but also therapeutic. Unlike soft tissue tumors, diagnostic biopsy samples of bone tumors are best obtained from the center of the lesion. Multiple biopsy specimens increase the chance of diagnosis.[29] A Jamshidi bone marrow biopsy needle is an excellent instrument for this purpose (see Chapter 16).

Table 61-1 Survival in Dogs Treated by Amputation and Doxorubicin Chemotherapy[35]

	Normal T-ALP	High T-ALP	Normal B-ALP	High B-ALP
Dogs (n)	202	91	168	72
Median survival (months)	8.7	5.9	10.3	5.9
Dogs alive at 1 year (%)	39	26	42	16
Dogs alive at 2 years (%)	20	10	23	3
Dogs alive at 3 years (%)	11	2	14	0

> **KEY POINT**
>
> *Unlike soft tissue tumors, in bone tumors, biopsy samples are most likely to be diagnostic if obtained from the center of the lesion.*

Osteosarcoma frequently includes areas of cartilage and fibrous tissue as well as osteoid and is often surrounded by new bone. Therefore, a histopathologic diagnosis of chondrosarcoma, fibrosarcoma, or reactive bone should be considered suspect, and further samples obtained at amputation or limb-sparing surgery should be submitted for histopathologic examination. Tumor histologic grade has been identified as an important prognostic factor in dogs with appendicular osteosarcoma, and the ability to assign such a grade is a benefit of preoperative biopsy. Tumors that invade vessels or lymphatics are classified as grade 3. Grade 3 tumors are also characterized by a high number of mitoses, increased cellular pleomorphism, small amounts of tumor matrix, and more than 50% necrosis in the tumor biopsy. These tumors account for more than 75% of osteosarcomas in dogs and have a worse prognosis.[30]

Histologic subtypes of osteosarcomas have been described, depending on the proportion of other tissues in addition to osteoid-producing cells. For example, a chondroblastic osteosarcoma may have a high proportion of tumor cells producing cartilage matrix in addition to osteoid. Telangiectatic osteosarcomas have a high proportion of blood vessels and cavernous blood-filled spaces and may be confused with hemangiosarcoma of bone. These subtypes appear to have little clinical significance, although one study found some differences in *p53* expression among them.[18]

PROGNOSTIC FACTORS

Prognostic factors that do not influence survival after amputation are gender, tumor site (i.e., distal or proximal; forelimb or hindlimb), and whether a presurgical biopsy was performed.[6]

Recent studies have shown that the level of serum total alkaline phosphatase (T-ALP) is highly prognostic for dogs undergoing amputation and chemotherapy; dogs with a T-ALP greater than the upper limit of normal have a worse prognosis than dogs with a normal level, regardless of the chemotherapy used.[30-34] In one study, whereas dogs with normal T-ALP that were treated with cisplatin and doxorubicin had a median survival of 12.5 months, dogs that had an elevated T-ALP and were treated with the same protocol had a median survival of 5.5 months.[32] In another study, 293 dogs treated with doxorubicin alone also lived longer if they had a normal T-ALP. Because T-ALP activity consists of isoenzymes derived from liver and steroid as well as bone, some investigators have explored the prognostic significance of bone alkaline phosphatase (B-ALP).[32,35] Measuring B-ALP may further predict dogs that are unlikely to respond to chemotherapy, allowing caregivers to choose more aggressive treatments or palliative options (Table 61-1).

The other very important prognostic factor identified for dogs with appendicular osteosarcoma is the histologic grade. In one study, grade 3 tumors accounted for more than 75% of osteosarcomas; dogs with low-grade tumors had a better prognosis.[30] Low-grade tumors may be controlled with less aggressive treatments.[36] In another study, mitotic index alone was a predictor of survival, with increasing numbers of mitoses correlating with a poor prognosis.[35]

Early studies indicated a relatively favorable prognosis for dogs with the fibrosarcomatous variant of osteosarcoma[7]; however, this has not been recently substantiated. In two studies, age at time of diagnosis was important for determining survival in dogs treated with amputation alone. In one study, dogs between the ages of 7 and 10 years had the longest survival times, and both old and young dogs fared less well.[6] In the other study, survival times decreased with increasing age.[35]

Two studies that used adjuvant single-agent chemotherapy (carboplatin[37] and doxorubicin[38]) retrospectively showed that smaller dogs had longer survival times. This may be because of a higher dose-per-kilogram delivered to these dogs, and it argues for increasing dosages in dogs that do not have toxicity after initial doses.

In studies of adjuvant therapy for appendicular osteosarcoma, the percentage of tumor necrosis after doxorubicin chemotherapy correlated with survival.[39] The percentage of necrosis after preoperative cisplatin or radiation correlated with local tumor control after limb-sparing surgery but not with survival.[40]

TREATMENT
Amputation

Surgical treatment of osteosarcoma by amputation is palliative and increases survival by pain relief, thereby delaying euthanasia. Amputation usually eliminates the primary tumor and causes little to no reduction in mobility and quality of life for the dog. Although most clients do not initially embrace the concept that their dog will have three legs, the procedure is very acceptable to caregivers after amputation. In two studies conducted in the United States and Europe, dogs learned to walk well on three legs within a month, which exceeded most clients' expectations.[41,42] It is also our experience, after sending many hundreds of dogs to amputation, that clients are very happy with their decision; the veterinarian should be confident in offering amputation to these clients. For lesions in the forelimbs, complete forequarter amputation, including the scapula, provides cosmetically and functionally good results. For distal hindlimb tumors, amputation at the proximal third of the femur is performed. For distal femoral tumors, a hip disarticulation is performed; proximal femoral lesions are treated by hemipelvectomy.

In one study, the median survival of 65 dogs treated with amputation was 126 days; only 10.7% of dogs were alive 1 year after surgery.[43] A larger study of 162 dogs treated with amputation corroborated these data.[6] Surgery of any type is only palliative, and dogs with appendicular osteosarcoma should receive chemotherapy.

Limb-Sparing Surgery

Limb-sparing surgery is important in human patients, for whom cosmetic appearance and function are impaired by amputation. This procedure may be appropriate in dogs that are poor candidates for amputation (e.g., very large dogs, dogs with other orthopedic or neurologic problems) or dogs whose owners refuse amputation.[44,45] Caution is advised because dogs that are not good candidates for amputation may not be good candidates for limb-sparing surgery because of the prolonged period of postoperative recovery.

During limb-sparing surgery, a cortical bone graft is used to replace the widely excised tumor, and arthrodesis of the nearby joint is usually performed. The best results are obtained with distal radial lesions or lesions of the ulna (Figures 61-7 and 61-8). It is possible to perform limb salvage for proximal humeral or scapular lesions, but function is poor, and the rate of postoperative complications is high, including a high rate of incomplete resection.[46] Good functional results have been reported for partial or complete scapulectomy in dogs with osteosarcoma.[47]

Limb salvage is not an option for large lesions that involve more than 50% of the bone, tumors that invade adjacent soft tissue, and tumors of the hindlimb. Complications of limb salvage include allograft rejection and implant failure. Complications occurred in 86 (55%) of 145 dogs treated with limb salvage in one study.[45] Implant failure was seen in 12 dogs (8%) and infection in 71 (49%). Infection required allograft removal or limb amputation in 16 dogs (11%).[45] Local recurrence of osteosarcoma is a frequent problem with limb salvage procedures and affects up to 40% of dogs. Even at institutions that perform limb salvage frequently and use adjunctive chemotherapy, recurrence rates of 17% to 27% are seen.[45,48] Local recurrence is not a significant problem when amputation is performed.

Another disadvantage of limb-sparing procedures is the need for allografts from normal donors (usually dogs euthanatized for another disease). These grafts must be stored, and fitting to the patient is always approximate. Pasteurized excised tumor has been used as an autograft for dogs with distal radial osteosarcoma. Local recurrence and infection rates were similar to those from the use of an allograft.[49]

Some surgeons use surgical metallic "spacers" attached to the surgical plate. These devices fill the space where the tumor is excised. Benefits include the lack of need for a bone bank and, potentially, a lower complication rate. Another technique adapted by surgeons at Colorado State University has been used on a small number of dogs with osteosarcoma that does not involve the bone or cartilage at or near a joint. In this procedure, the involved bone is stripped of attachments to soft tissues. A cut is made distal to the tumor, and the bone containing the tumor is exteriorized surgically. The tumor in the bone is given very high dosages of external-beam radiation therapy and then replaced in its normal position and fixed in place with a surgical plate. Dr. Ogilvie has observed that complication rates with this technique may be higher than with more routine limb-sparing procedures.

Before limb salvage is performed, intraarterial cisplatin, with or without radiation therapy, often increases tumor necrosis and reduces the risk of local recurrence.[40,50] In addition, a locally implanted polymer impregnated with cisplatin (open polylactic acid–cisplatin or OPLA–Pt) can be used. OPLA–Pt releases cisplatin slowly into the tumor bed,

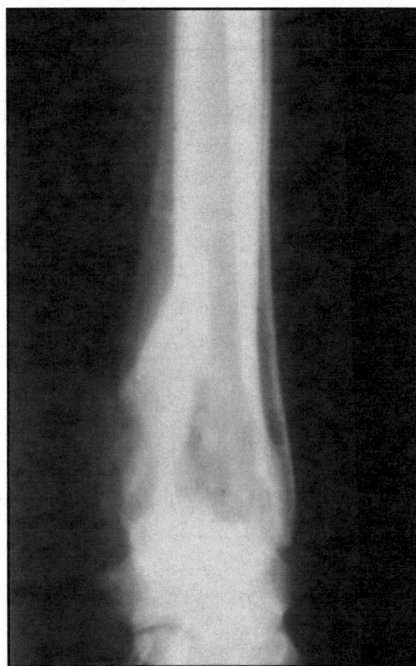

Figure 61-7. *An osteosarcoma of the distal radius in a dog with a severe arthropathy that precluded amputation as a treatment. Treatment options are radiation therapy and limb-sparing surgery.*

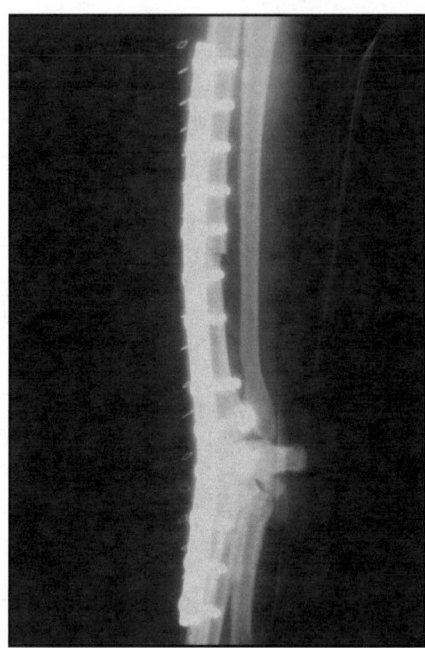

Figure 61-8. *Same dog as Figure 61-7 after resection of the primary tumor and arthrodesis of the carpal joint, with an allograft plated in position. Complications are common, and the procedure is very operator dependent.*

and its use reduces local recurrence rates from 27% to 17%. The survival time and disease-free interval in dogs treated with OPLA–Pt are similar to those of dogs receiving systemic cisplatin, presumably because locally implanted cisplatin is dispersed systemically. Because cisplatin release is slow, systemic toxicity is reduced.

A limb-salvage technique that abrogates the need for any graft is the use of bone transport osteogenesis.[51] This technique slowly transports a small portion of normal bone adjacent to the defect caused by tumor resection into the defect (0.25 mm every 6 hours) while new bone forms behind the distracted bone. The resultant bone is a well-vascularized autogenous graft. The limb is held with the ends of the defect distracted by an external fixation device. A report of this method in six dogs found that local recurrence was a problem, but some long-term survivors were seen.[51] Radiation therapy may have contributed to graft failure in one dog. Chemotherapy was also used in this report and did not appear to impair new bone formation.[51,52]

Chemotherapy

Survival of dogs with osteosarcoma can be significantly prolonged by adjuvant chemotherapy. When chemotherapy protocols for the treatment of osteosarcoma are evaluated, median survival times are often very similar, and the use of 1-, 2- and 3-year survival rates will provide more information as to the likelihood of long-term control and even cure.

Dog owners often understand these figures better than median survival times.

Single Agents

Methotrexate was given intravenously to five dogs with osteosarcoma at doses ranging from 3 to 6 g/m^2. Treatment was preceded by vincristine at 1 mg/m^2. Leucovorin rescue was used. Myelosuppression was the dose-limiting toxicity, and no clinical response was seen.[53] In another study, 17 dogs with osteosarcoma were treated by local resection and implantation of acrylic cement containing methotrexate at total doses ranging from 1.6 mg/kg to 16 mg/kg.[54] Gastrointestinal (GI) toxicities were seen in four dogs receiving more than 4 mg/kg of methotrexate, and one of these dogs died. Four dogs showed delayed wound healing and sepsis. At 8 months, 10 of 17 dogs were alive without metastases; however, no further follow-up examination was reported. With the toxicity and uncertain efficacy of methotrexate and the availability of proven alternatives, we cannot recommend treatment with methotrexate at this time.

Cisplatin markedly improves survival rates to a median survival of between 6 and 13 months and 1-year survival rates to between 30% and 62%; 2-year survival rates are between 7% and 21% (Table 61-2 and Figure 61-9).[55–59] Whether the drug is administered intravenously or intraarterially does not appear to affect efficacy.

Table 61-2 Survival Times and Rates for Dogs with Osteosarcoma of the Appendicular Skeleton Treated with Surgery and Cisplatin Chemotherapy

Dogs (n)	Cisplatin (mg/m²)	Treatment Interval (days)	Courses (n)	1-Year Survival (%)	2-Year Survival (%)	Median Survival (months)	Study
17	70 (postoperatively)	21	2	38.0	18.0	7.4	Straw et al[56]
19	70 (pre- and perioperatively)	21	2	43.0	16.0	5.8	Straw et al[56]
5	40–50 (postoperatively)	28	2–6	Not reported	Not reported	10.0	Shapiro et al[55]
15	60 (postoperatively)	14 and 35	2	30.0	7.0	9.5	Thompson and Feguent[57]
16	50 (postoperatively)	28	6+	62.0	19.0	13.6	Kraegel et al[58]
22	60 (postoperatively)	21	1–6	45.0	21.0	10.7	Berg et al[59]
162	Surgery only	—	—	11.5	2.0	4.3	Spodnick et al[6]

Other methods of administration have also been investigated. OPLA–Pt appears to release a controlled amount of cisplatin over a prolonged period as well as provide high local concentrations in the site of limb-sparing surgery. OPLA–Pt was implanted in the surgical wounds of 39 dogs that had an amputation. The median survival time was 8 months, and the 1-year survival rate was 41%, which was similar to that achieved with systemic chemotherapy.[60] In another study, OPLA–Pt was related to nonunion of limb salvage grafts.[61] OPLA–Pt is not readily obtainable, so another study evaluated the utility of subcutaneously administered cisplatin and saline for slow-release chemotherapy. Renal, GI, and bone marrow toxicities and local tissue reaction were seen in five of six dogs; this treatment is not recommended.[62] Intramedullary cisplatin administration led to resolution of osteosarcoma in one dog with apparent survival benefit but was not so successful in three other dogs.[63] Cisplatin is best given intravenously with saline diuresis.

Early reports of doxorubicin failed to show efficacy.[64] Larger studies have shown benefit for the use of doxorubicin given as five biweekly doses at a dosage of 30 mg/m². In one study, two or three doses were given before surgery; subsequent doses were given the day after surgery and 2 weeks later. The median survival time was 12 months, and the efficacy approached that of cisplatin; 50% of the dogs were alive at 1 year, and 10% were alive at 2 years.[38] Another group of more than 300 dogs received five doses of doxorubicin every 2 weeks, starting 2 weeks after amputation. Median survival time was 8 months, and 1-, 2-, and 3- survival rates were 35%, 17%, and 9%, respectively, which is very similar to results from cisplatin chemotherapy.[35] Survival times were greater in younger dogs, lighterweight dogs, and dogs with normal T-ALP and B-ALP.

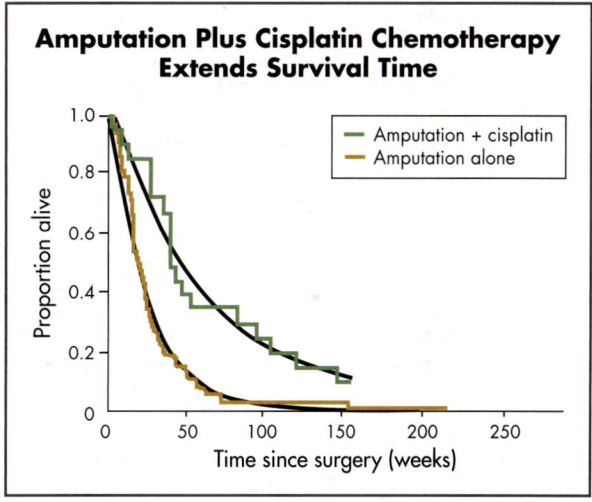

Figure 61-9. Survival curves for dogs with osteosarcoma treated by amputation alone (162 dogs) or with adjuvant cisplatin chemotherapy (22 dogs). (From Berg RJ, Weinstein MJ, Schelling SH, Rand MW: Treatment of dogs with osteosarcoma by administration of cisplatin after amputation or limb-sparing surgery: 22 cases (1987–1990). JAVMA 200:2005–2008, 1992; with permission)

Carboplatin (300 mg/m² IV) was given adjunctively after surgery to 48 dogs.[37] Median survival time was 10.5 months; 35% of the dogs were alive 1 year after surgery. In this study, smaller dogs had longer survival times. Slightly lower survival rates were seen in a smaller group of dogs,[34] but overall results are similar to that achieved with other drugs.

Lobaplatin (35 mg/m² IV) was given adjunctively after surgery to 28 dogs.[33] The median survival was not reported, but 32% of the dogs were alive 1 year after surgery. In this

Table 61-3 Dose Intensity and Survival Rates for Different Adjuvant Chemotherapy Protocols

Protocol	Dogs (n)	Dose Intensity	Median Survival (months)	1-Year Survival (%)	2-Year Survival (%)	3-year Survival (%)
Surgery alone	162	—	4.3	12	2	Not reported
Cisplatin	100	0.71-1.0	10.5	46	11	Not reported
Doxorubicin	303	1.0	9.5	40	21	10
Carboplatin	48	1.0	10.5	35	Not reported	Not reported
Lobaplatin	28	1.0	Not reported	32	Not reported	Not reported
Cisplatin and doxorubicin alternating	19	0.76	10	37	26	Not reported
Cisplatin and doxorubicin together	102	1.19–1.3	11	48	28	19
Carboplatin and doxorubicin together	24	0.91	7.8	Not reported	Not reported	Not reported
Carboplatin and doxorubicin alternating	32	1.0	10.5	48	18	Not reported
Carboplatin and cisplatin together	17	1.19	9	Not reported	Not reported	Not reported

study, dogs with grade 1 tumors and with normal T-ALP had longer survival times.

Liposome encapsulation of cisplatin did not improve survival times compared with carboplatin in another randomized study.[34]

Single-agent treatment with carboplatin or doxorubicin seems to be as effective as cisplatin in treating canine appendicular osteosarcoma, and the choice of which drug to offer may depend on other factors. For example, doxorubicin may be less expensive than either of the platinum drugs; however, doxorubicin causes a cumulative cardiotoxicity, the risk of which is higher in breeds predisposed to cardiomyopathy. Many dogs with osteosarcoma are also breeds that are at risk for cardiomyopathy (e.g., Dobermans, Great Danes), so doxorubicin may not be a good choice for these dogs. Even with prescreening of prospective patients and elimination of those with early cardiac changes or significant breed risk, more than 7% of patients developed cardiomyopathy in one study of more than 300 dogs treated with five doses of doxorubicin.[35] Similarly, the fluid diuresis required to prevent renal toxicity of cisplatin may make it unsuitable for a dog with clinical or subclinical heart disease. Dogs that cannot be admitted as day patients for fluid diuresis and cisplatin treatment may be better treated with carboplatin or doxorubicin because these drugs can be given on an outpatient basis.

Table 61-3 summarizes various protocols applied to osteosarcoma of the appendicular skeleton in dogs.

Combination Chemotherapy

Combinations of drugs that show activity as single agents should, in theory, be more effective than single agents alone because of their effects on dose intensity (combined mg/m^2 of drugs per week). A dose intensity of 1 is a drug given at the prescribed maximum dosage at the prescribed interval; in combinations, the dose intensity of each drug is proportional according to dosage and interval, and the results for each drug are added together. Thus, it is possible to have a dose intensity of greater than 1 with combination chemotherapy. It is also possible to have a dose intensity of less than 1 because combination requires either reductions in dosages or lengthening of the intertreatment interval between individual drugs, particularly when both drugs cause similar toxicities. For example, doxorubicin and cisplatin each have a dose intensity of 1 when given at maximum dosage every 3 weeks. Because they have the same dose-limiting toxicity (myelosuppression), combination of these two agents requires significant dose reduction for each. When they are combined by giving each drug on its own, alternating every 3 weeks, the dose intensity of each drug is effectively halved because the drug is given every 6 weeks. Thus, the combined dose intensity would be 1. Cisplatin is limited by nephrotoxicity, but it is mildly myelosuppressive, so maintaining close to full dosages in combination therapy may be possible. Combining cisplatin and doxorubicin on the same day would require a

> **KEY POINT**
>
> *Cisplatin, carboplatin, and doxorubicin are active agents in the adjuvant treatment of canine osteosarcoma with approximately equal efficacy.*

reduction in the dosage of one or both drugs, but both could be given every 3 weeks, so the dose intensity may be increased. An increased dose intensity should, in theory, be associated with improved efficacy.

A protocol alternating cisplatin (60 mg/m²) with doxorubicin (30 mg/m²) every 21 days for two cycles was delivered after amputation to 19 dogs with appendicular osteosarcoma. The median survival was 10 months, with 37% of dogs alive at 1 year and 26% alive at 2 years. Despite the lower dose intensity (0.76) of the two drugs compared with single-agent protocols, survival rates were comparable with those for cisplatin chemotherapy alone.[65]

Another study delivered doxorubicin (15–25 mg/m²) and cisplatin (60 mg/m²) on the same day (doxorubicin in post-diuresis fluids) to 102 dogs with osteosarcoma. Median survival was 11.5 months, and 1-, 2-, and 3-year survival rates were 47%, 28%, and 17%, respectively (Figure 61-10).[66] The dose intensity of this protocol (1.19–1.30) was greater than that of either single agent. A later evaluation of toxicity showed that a 20-mg/m² dose of doxorubicin was well tolerated in these dogs.[67] A small pilot study of 19 dogs that used lower doses of doxorubicin and cisplatin (15 mg/m² and 50 mg/m², respectively; dose intensity: 1.04) showed a greater median survival,[68] but as more dogs were added to the study, the median survival decreased, illustrating the need for larger numbers to adequately assess efficacy.

Carboplatin (175 mg/m²) and doxorubicin (15 mg/m²) were given on the same day every 3 weeks after amputation to 24 dogs with osteosarcoma. The dose intensity was 0.91 because lower dosages of these drugs were needed to avoid myelosuppression. The median survival time was 8 months; the 1-year survival rate was not reported.[69]

Carboplatin (300 mg/m²) and doxorubicin (30 mg/m²) were given in an alternating protocol every 3 weeks for three cycles for a dose intensity of 1.0. Median survival time was 10.5 months, and 1- and 2-year survival rates were 48% and 18%, respectively.[70] The dogs that finished the protocol had a median survival of 18 months. Clients often want to know how their pet is likely to do after completing a course of chemotherapy; this finding serves as encouraging news for dogs that have not developed metastatic disease during chemotherapy.

Carboplatin (100 mg/m²) and cisplatin (60 mg/m²) were combined to assess the influence of increased platinum compounds (dose intensity: 1.19) on osteosarcoma. Median survival time was 9 months in this preliminary report by Dr. Moore, and the 1-year survival rate was not reported.

In conclusion, the best reported long-term survival rates have been reported for doxorubicin and cisplatin given together on the same day. Dosages of 60 mg/m² cisplatin and 20 mg/m² doxorubicin should be well tolerated by this population of mainly large dogs.

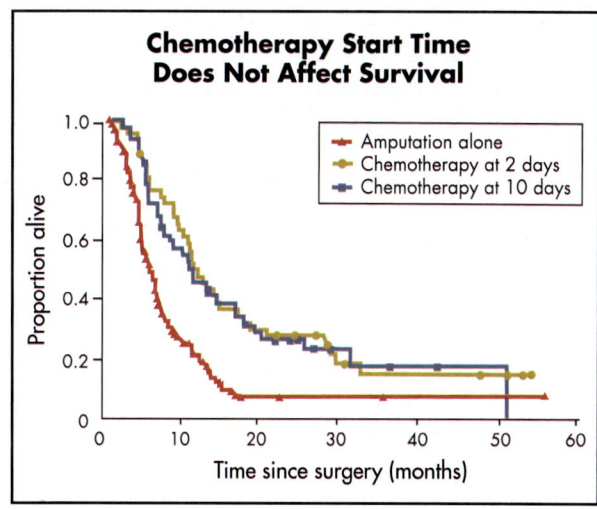

Figure 61-10. Survival curves for dogs with osteosarcoma treated by amputation alone or with adjuvant cisplatin and doxorubicin chemotherapy starting either 2 or 10 days after surgery. Both treatment groups lived longer than controls (see text) but no longer than each other. (From Berg J, Gebhardt MC, Rand WM: Effect of timing of postoperative chemotherapy on survival of dogs with osteosarcoma. Cancer 79:1343–1350, 1997; with permission)

Number of Doses and Timing of Chemotherapy

There are trends toward longer survival times with increasing the number of doses of cisplatin, but statistical evaluation is lacking.[45,58] More than two doses of cisplatin may improve survival.[45,59]

Theoretical data suggest that chemotherapy very soon after amputation may take advantage of a "growth spurt" that renders micrometastases more sensitive to chemotherapy. To test this hypothesis, one study randomized 100 dogs to receive cisplatin and doxorubicin (together on the same day) starting either 2 days or 10 days after amputation. There was no difference in survival, but dogs treated 2 days after surgery were more likely to show myelosuppression, presumably because the bone marrow had been stimulated by postoperative inflammation.[66] It is recommended that because efficacy is not improved, and because toxicity is increased, chemotherapy should be delayed until wound healing has occurred, usually 10 to 14 days after surgery (Figure 61-10).

Biologic Response Modifiers

In early studies, nonspecific immunostimulation appeared to improve survival. Median survival was 10 months for dogs treated with bacillus Calmette-Guérin after surgery.[71] More recent studies have been conducted on small numbers of dogs, using biologic response modifiers that are not commercially available. It seems, however, that immunotherapy may have a future role to play in multimodality treatment of canine osteosarcoma.

Liposome-encapsulated muramyl tripeptide-phosphatidylethanolamine (L-MTP-PE) is a nonspecific activator of monocytes and macrophages that induces tumoricidal activity in these cells. Dogs treated with L-MTP-PE showed prolonged median survival (7 months) over dogs receiving liposomes alone (2.5 months).[72] In another study, 11 dogs that had received four doses of cisplatin (70 mg/m² every 28 days) after amputation were treated with L-MTP-PE. These dogs had a median survival of 14.4 months, and three dogs did not develop metastases.[73] Clinical data from small numbers of dogs may be misleading, and further studies to confirm these results have not been conducted.

In another study, 23 dogs treated by surgical excision of the osteosarcoma, chemotherapy, and human cytotoxic T cells from a cultured cell line lived a median of 11.5 months, which is not much different than survival after chemotherapy alone; however, approximately 40% of dogs were alive 2 years after surgery.[74]

Interleukin-2 (IL-2) is a lymphocyte-derived stimulator of natural killer cells and macrophage/monocytes; hence, it is a potent immunostimulant. IL-2 was delivered in liposomes via aerosol to four dogs with pulmonary metastases from osteosarcoma. Two dogs had complete regression of metastases that was ongoing 12 and 20 months later.[75]

Antiangiogenic therapy is a new area of interest in veterinary medicine. Angiogenesis is a complex, multifactorial process by which new blood vessels sprout from existing vessels and then dissolve surrounding matrix to extend further into tumors. New blood vessel growth is rarely needed in existing normal tissue (except during pregnancy and wound healing), so inhibiting aspects of the angiogenic pathway should target tumors specifically. Without new blood vessels, tumors cannot expand beyond a size that allows passive diffusion of nutrients and oxygen to the tumor cells, and existing tumors may shrink. Blood vessel density has been found to be highest in osteosarcomas that metastasize early.[76] Tumors also need to dissolve surrounding cellular matrix in order to invade blood vessels and to form metastases. Osteosarcomas have been found to contain matrix metalloproteinases that are important in the dissolution of collagen, allowing angiogenesis to occur and tumor invasion to proceed.[77] Various drugs may target angiogenesis and matrix dissolution through various pathways. The antibiotic doxycycline has been found to inhibit collagenase (metalloproteinase) activity by canine osteosarcoma cells,[78] although clinical activity has not been documented. Three of four dogs that had presumed spontaneous regression of osteosarcoma had been treated with the antiinflammatory drug carprofen.[79] It is possible that the antiinflammatory drug played a role in tumor regression. It has been suggested that inhibitors of cyclooxygenase-2 (COX-2) may also inhibit tumor growth and angiogenesis; only three of 13 tumors expressed COX-2 in one preliminary study,[80] but 79% expressed COX-2 in a larger study, and expression appeared to correlate with poorer survival.[81] Definitive treatment is still preferred, and clinicians are cautioned against relying on COX-2 inhibitors as sole treatment.

A large, multiinstitutional, randomized clinical trial found no survival benefit to the oral administration of an inhibitor of metalloproteinases 2 and 9 (MMP-2 and MMP-9) in conjunction with amputation and doxorubicin chemotherapy, despite the finding that serum levels of MMP-2 and MMP-9 activity influenced survival.[35]

Metastatic Disease

After osteosarcoma metastases are clinically or radiographically evident, good response to chemotherapy is rare. In one study, two of three dogs with metastatic osteosarcoma responded partially to cisplatin chemotherapy.[82] In another report, 45 dogs with osteosarcoma metastases were treated with cisplatin, doxorubicin, mitoxantrone, or sequential combinations of these drugs every 3 weeks. Only one dog experienced a partial remission for 21 days with doxorubicin.[83] Cisplatin had been given before the development of metastases in 29 of the 45 dogs.

Pulmonary metastatectomy seems to prolong survival only if the animal develops clinically evident metastases more than 10 months after the initial diagnosis and if fewer than three nodules are radiographically apparent. Median survival time after metastatectomy was 6 months in one study.[84] Median survival of dogs with few metastases that are not treated with metastatectomy is uncertain.

In 90 dogs with metastatic osteosarcoma at the time of diagnosis (dogs euthanatized at diagnosis were excluded), the median survival time was 2.5 months. Dogs that were treated with either surgery or adjuvant therapy lived longer than those treated supportively.[85]

Palliative Radiation Therapy

If caregivers refuse definitive treatment for a pet with osteosarcoma or if an animal is not considered eligible for amputation or limb-sparing surgery, consideration may be given to palliation of tumor pain with radiation therapy (Figure 61-11).

Radiation delivered in two to four weekly fractions of 8 to 10 Gy has been reported as a palliative treatment for 125 dogs with pain or other clinical signs related to osteosarcoma. Improved limb function was seen in approximately 75% of dogs treated with either 8 Gy on days 0, 7, 14, and 21; 10 Gy on days 0, 7, and 21; or 8 Gy on days 0 and 7. Improvement lasted for a median of 2 to 3 months regardless of the protocol, and toxicities were rare and acute.[86-88] Chemotherapy appeared to improve response rate and dura-

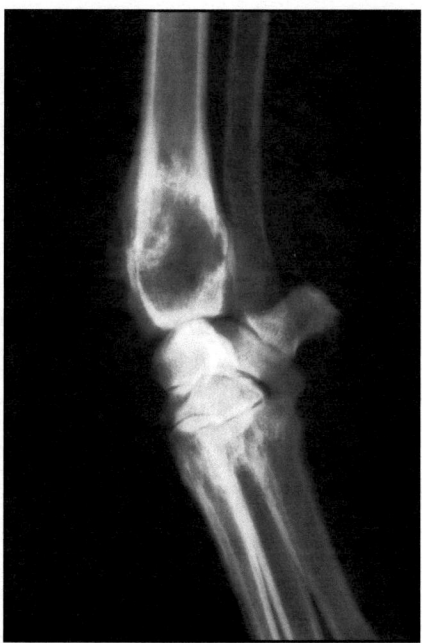

Figure 61-11. *Same dog as in Figure 61-6 after radiation therapy. Note the smoothing of the periosteal reaction, concurrent with pain relief in this patient, despite minimal resolution of lysis.*

tion. Dogs with large lesions extending to involve a greater length of limb were less likely to respond for long.[87,88] Many radiation therapists agree that a reasonable clinical approach may be to deliver a single large dose to the affected site and then to repeat a single dose as necessary to maintain pain control.

Targeted stereotactic "radiosurgery" may offer some advantages in delivering a single high dose of 30 Gy to the tumor alone. Preliminary results are encouraging.[89]

Samarium-153-ethylene diamine tetramethylene phosphonate (EDTMP) emits β particles and accumulates in areas of increased bony activity, thereby providing high-dose localized radiation therapy. This compound was given to 28 dogs with osteosarcoma of the appendicular (n = 20) or axial (n = 8) skeleton.[90] Many dogs showed functional improvement, and the average survival time for dogs with appendicular osteosarcoma was 8 months. This treatment may palliate in a manner similar to that of external-beam radiation. Another study found that with the exception of one dog that had a long-lasting complete response, pain relief was poor in a series of nine dogs with presumed osteosarcoma; survival was for a median of 4 months.[91] There are anecdotal reports of long survival after surgery and samarium therapy.[36,92]

Other Palliative Therapy

Bisphosphonates are inhibitors of osteoclast activity that have been used in human patients with osteolytic disease, including metastatic neoplasia. Pamidronate is an intravenously administered drug that has anecdotally been associated with decreased pain from osteosarcoma. Unpublished observations by Dr. Moore suggest that the improvement is subjective but not associated with increased weightbearing as measured by force-plate analysis. Alendronate is an orally administered bisphosphonate that was reported to reduce pain in two dogs for 10 to 12 months, despite neither dog being treated with amputation.[93] The dose used was approximately 0.25 mg/kg.

Pamidronate has also been used in combination with radiation therapy; it is difficult to decide whether the subjective improvement is attributable to the combination or the individual components.

Supportive Therapy

Palliation of pain as described above should be considered supportive. Dogs with osteosarcoma have alterations in energy expenditure and are in negative nitrogen balance.[94] Nutritional support with a high percentage of calories from protein may be beneficial to dogs with osteosarcoma.

TUMORS OF NONWEIGHTBEARING APPENDICULAR SITES

Owners of dogs with osteosarcoma of unusual appendicular sites often seek guidance as to prognosis. There is little published literature, but what exists suggests that osteosarcoma of these sites still exhibits a high metastatic rate.

Patella

Of two reported dogs, one had metastases at diagnosis, and the other was not followed.[95,96]

Distal to Antebrachial or Tarsocrural Joint

Of 10 dogs with osteosarcomas in this location, nine were treated by surgery alone or with chemotherapy and six developed metastases, primarily to the lungs.[97,98] The median survival time was 15.3 months, indicating that the prognosis was better than that associated with other appendicular sites but that the metastatic rate was still very high.

Ulna

In a series of 12 dogs, 11 were treated by surgery and adjuvant therapy.[99] The median survival for treated dogs was 8.5 months, and 11 dogs developed metastases. Osteosarcoma of the ulna should be treated as osteosarcoma of any other appendicular site.

Radial Carpal Bone

Dr. Moore observed a solitary case that metastasized despite chemotherapy (Figure 61-12).

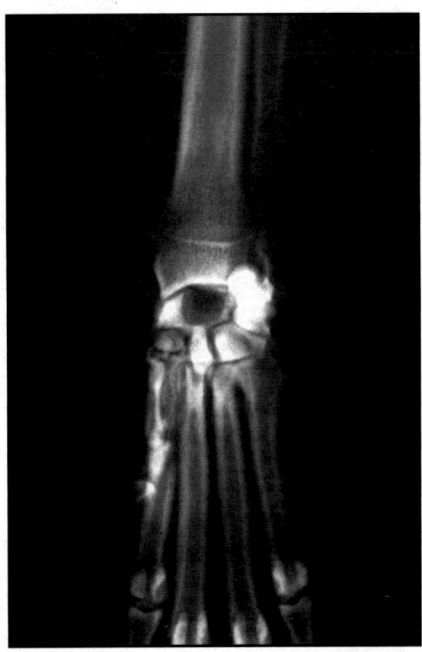

Figure 61-12. *Solitary lytic lesion affecting the radial carpal bone. Despite chemotherapy, this dog developed pulmonary metastases after amputation. Appendicular osteosarcoma is a highly metastatic tumor regardless of location, and chemotherapy is recommended.*

Osteosarcoma of the Axial Skeleton
INCIDENCE, SIGNALMENT, AND ETIOLOGY

In a large series of 116 dogs with osteosarcoma of the axial skeleton,[100] 31 lesions (27%) were located in the mandible, 26 (22%) in the maxilla, 17 (15%) in the spine, 14 (12%) in the cranium, 12 (10%) in the ribs, 10 (9%) in the nasal bones, and six (5%) in the pelvis. In this study, medium to large dogs were most commonly affected, but there was no specific breed predilection. Older dogs were affected (mean age: 9 years), with the exception of rib tumors, which occurred in younger dogs (median age: 7 years). The ratio of males to females varied with the site of the osteosarcoma. Overall, these tumors are more common in female dogs than in males; the trend is most pronounced for maxillary and pelvic osteosarcomas, which occur primarily in female dogs.[100] Axial skeleton osteosarcomas accounted for approximately 20% to 25% of all cases of osteosarcoma in dogs.[2,100]

Some of the risk factors for developing appendicular osteosarcoma also increase the risk for axial osteosarcoma, although the effects are less pronounced. In a large epidemiologic study, neutered dogs of both genders appeared to be at twice the risk of intact dogs for developing axial skeleton osteosarcomas.[2] The effect of weight was greatest on increasing risk for appendicular osteosarcomas, but dogs weighing more than 45 kg were more than twice as likely to develop an axial osteosarcoma.[2] The effect of height was similar: dogs that were taller than 54 cm had approximately twice the risk of developing axial osteosarcoma than dogs that were less than 35.5 cm in height.[2]

CLINICAL PRESENTATION AND HISTORY

The average duration of signs was 10 weeks in 54 of 116 dogs with axial osteosarcoma, but the range was from days to 2 years. Signs varied depending on the site affected.[100]

> **KEY POINT**
>
> *Osteosarcoma of the axial skeleton in dogs should, with few exceptions, be considered to act as aggressively as appendicular osteosarcoma.*

STAGING AND DIAGNOSIS

At the time of presentation, 10% to 18% of dogs may have evidence of pulmonary metastasis, which is a slightly higher rate than that for osteosarcoma of appendicular sites.[100–103] Metastases are more common later in the course of disease; metastatic rates around 45% have been reported.[101,102] It is possible that more dogs would develop metastases if local disease could be controlled longer, but local recurrence causes death in most treated dogs.

The ability to obtain complete surgical margins is associated with a better prognosis. Additional imaging using CT or MRI assists in planning a surgical approach and may allow the clinician to identify tumors that cannot be excised and that may require adjunctive radiation therapy.

PROGNOSTIC FACTORS

In one study, the ability to achieve complete surgical margins was associated with longer survival. Whereas dogs that had histologically complete excisions lived a median of 7.4 months, those with an incomplete excision lived a median of less than 2 months.[101] In the same study, smaller dogs lived longer (5 months) compared with dogs that weighed more than 30 kg (3 months).[101]

T-ALP levels are clearly associated with prognosis in dogs with appendicular osteosarcoma, but no studies have evaluated the influence of elevated T-ALP on dogs with axial skeleton osteosarcomas.

TREATMENT

In most dogs with axial osteosarcoma, tumors recur after surgery and before metastases are clinically evident. This contrasts with appendicular osteosarcoma, in which surgical margins are easily obtained but the metastatic rate is very high. Reported local recurrence rates of axial osteosarcoma are between 55%[102] and 64%.[101] Recurrence rates are lower in dogs with mandibular osteosarcoma, presumably because complete resection is easier.[104]

The overall median survival time for 38 dogs that underwent attempted surgical removal of an axial osteosarcoma was 22 weeks. At 1 year, 25% of the dogs were still alive, and nearly 20% were alive at 2 years.[100] Untreated dogs died within 1 month.

In another study, 22 large dogs with axial osteosarcoma were evaluated; 20 received radiation therapy as part or all of their therapy. Palliative radiation was used in 12 dogs with gross disease, and their median survival time was 2.5 months. This was significantly shorter than for eight dogs (five with gross disease) that lived a median of 9 months after definitive radiation therapy.[102] Similar results were seen in another study of spinal osteosarcomas.[105] It appears that daily, small-fraction radiation therapy may be a more successful approach to dogs with nonresectable axial skeleton osteosarcomas.

For supportive therapy, palliation by radiation therapy may be an option in some dogs. Although the survival times for dogs treated palliatively were not as long as those associated with definitive treatment, they were identical to those achieved for palliation of dogs with osteosarcoma of appendicular sites.[102] Pain relief and improved quality of life may still be achieved with palliative radiation therapy.

MANDIBULAR OSTEOSARCOMA
Incidence, Signalment, and Etiology

Two studies of axial skeletal tumors found that mandibular osteosarcoma has a statistically better prognosis than osteosarcoma of other axial sites, although the median survival times differ.[101,104] The one large study that probably best defines this tumor found no obvious breed predilection among 51 dogs with mandibular osteosarcoma, including seven small dogs (<15 kg).[104] There were 33 female and 18 male dogs, which accords with dogs with axial skeletal osteosarcoma of other sites.[100]

Staging and Diagnosis

Of 51 dogs studied, 17 (33%) developed metastases, of which most were pulmonary metastases. Other metastatic sites were the ribs, skull, subcutaneous tissue, muscle, and lymph nodes. In another study, only one of 19 dogs had metastatic disease at the time of diagnosis.[100] Mandibular osteosarcoma may not be as aggressive as osteosarcoma of the appendicular skeleton. Histologic grading has been used for dogs with mandibular osteosarcoma and is similar to the scheme used for appendicular osteosarcoma (Table 61-4).[104]

Prognostic Factors

Mandibular osteosarcomas were graded according to similar criteria used for appendicular osteosarcomas, and dogs with grade 1 tumors had significantly longer survival times.[104]

Table 61-4 Variables Used to Determine the Histologic Grade of Canine Mandibular Osteosarcoma[104]

Score	Parameter		
	Nuclear pleomorphism	Mitotic index	Tumor necrosis
0	None	—	None
1	Mild	1–10	<15%
2	Moderate	11–20	15–50%
3	Marked	21–30	>50%
4	—	>30	—

Grade Description
1 Cumulative score of 1–5
2 Cumulative score of 6–8
3 Cumulative score of 9–10

Treatment

Overall survival 1 year after surgery was 60% for the 51 dogs with mandibular osteosarcoma.[104] When the tumor is localized, mandibulectomy alone may provide good control of this tumor. Recurrence rates after aggressive resection are low compared with less aggressive local excision. Of 32 dogs with mandibular osteosarcoma treated with surgery alone, nine had a local recurrence and nine developed metastases; however, the 1-year survival rate was 71%, implying that metastases were often identified long after surgery.[104] A second surgery for locally recurrent disease may occasionally be successful.[104]

For mandibular osteosarcoma, the success of therapy adjunctive to mandibulectomy is unclear. Additional therapy using chemotherapy with cisplatin and doxorubicin (10 dogs), radiation therapy (external beam or samarium; five dogs), or a combination (three dogs) did not seem to improve survival significantly over mandibulectomy alone.[104] However, dogs often received additional treatment modalities because they had a worse prognosis (i.e., radiation because the tumor was incompletely excised or chemotherapy because metastases were detected). With a metastatic rate of approximately 33%, adjuvant chemotherapy as used for osteosarcoma of appendicular sites would seem appropriate, particularly for dogs with higher-grade tumors. For dogs with grade 1 mandibular osteosarcoma and no evidence of metastases, surgery with complete margins may be sufficient.

In case reports, radiation therapy alone provided long-term control (1,229 days) in one dog but failed to control the tumor in another. One dog with mandibular osteosarcoma was treated with samarium-153-EDTMP.[90] The lesion remained static for more than 3 years after treatment.

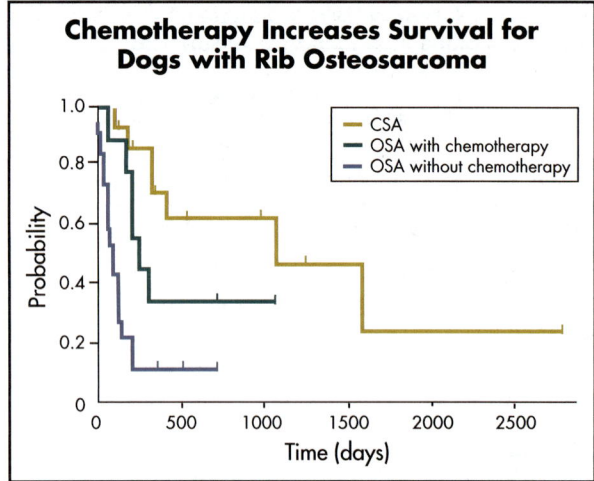

Figure 61-13. *Survival curves for dogs with rib tumors. Nine dogs with osteosarcoma (OSA) treated with adjuvant chemotherapy and 15 dogs with chondrosarcoma (CSA) lived longer than 20 dogs with osteosarcoma that did not receive chemotherapy. (From Pirkey-Ehrhart N, Withrow SJ, Straw RC, et al: Primary rib tumors in 54 dogs. JAAHA 31:65–69, 1995; with permission)*

OSTEOSARCOMA OF THE RIB
Incidence, Signalment, and Etiology

Although primary rib tumors are much less common than appendicular osteosarcomas, they behave equally aggressively. Osteosarcoma of the rib was seen primarily in dogs that weighed at least 20 kg.[106] The median age of affected dogs was 7 years. There was no gender predilection.

Clinical Presentation and History

Tumors of the rib are often large at the time of presentation. The median tumor volume is 500 cm^3; not surprisingly, finding a mass is the most common reason that owners seek veterinary advice.[106,107] Lameness may be caused by pain, interference with function, or hypertrophic osteopathy.[107] In one study, pleural effusion was seen in four of 10 dogs with osteosarcoma of the rib.[108]

Staging and Diagnosis

The metastatic rate of osteosarcoma of the ribs is higher than that of other flat bones,[101] and metastases may be seen in up to 50% of dogs at diagnosis, possibly because of the long interval until diagnosis.[108] Thus, if osteosarcoma of the rib is suspected, thoracic radiographs, along with preoperative blood work and a surgical biopsy, should be routine. Additionally, the thoracic cavity should be examined at the time of surgery. In one series of dogs, pulmonary metastases that were not suspected on thoracic radiographs were detected at surgery in four dogs.[107] In another study, all 20 dogs with rib osteosarcomas had metastases after surgical treatment alone.[109]

Prognostic Factors

Complete resection as determined by histologic examination is an important prognostic factor for dogs with rib tumors of any histologic type.[106] Dogs with incomplete resection are six times more likely to die from their disease.[106] Dogs that receive chemotherapy live longer than dogs treated by surgery alone.[106]

Treatment

In two series of 47 dogs with rib osteosarcomas, 13 were not treated and lived a median of 2 to 5 weeks after diagnosis.[106,107]

Surgical excision of a rib tumor may require removal of more than one rib. In one series of dogs, seven of 27 dogs had four ribs resected. Most closures were achieved with polypropylene mesh or diaphragmatic advancement.[107]

Local recurrence was only seen in dogs with incomplete margins and occurred in six of 57 dogs.[106,107,109]

Osteosarcoma of the rib develops aggressively, but adjuvant cisplatin chemotherapy seems to prolong survival. In one trial, nine dogs received adjuvant chemotherapy after surgery with cisplatin or an alternating schedule of cisplatin and doxorubicin, as described previously for osteosarcoma of the appendicular skeleton. Median survival for this group of nine dogs was 8 months, which was significantly longer than that for 20 dogs treated with surgery alone (3 months; Figure 61-13).[106]

SPINAL OSTEOSARCOMA
Incidence, Signalment, and Etiology

This is a rare tumor despite being the most common tumor of the canine vertebrae.[105] Neurologic changes in affected dogs range from mild ataxia to paresis or paralysis; the severity of these signs may be prognostic because poor quality of life may lead to a decision to euthanatize.

Staging and Diagnosis

Most spinal osteosarcomas are solitary; occasionally, they are multicentric. In one study, more than half the dogs developed metastases, despite often short survival times caused by local tumor recurrence.[105] One dog had an osteosarcoma in every vertebra from L3 to L7 as well as the sacrum and pulmonary metastases.[110] Spinal osteosarcomas may also be metastatic from another (appendicular) site.[105]

Prognostic Factors

Postoperative neurologic status was the only prognostic factor in a series of dogs with spinal osteosarcoma. Whereas those with only pain or weakness after treatment had a median survival of 4.4 months, those with ataxia, loss of proprioception, paralysis, or motor loss had a median survival of 2 weeks.[105] Dogs with pain as the only presenting sign had a median survival of 11 months compared with 4 months for dogs with more advanced neurologic problems, but the difference was not statistical.

Treatment

Five dogs with spinal osteosarcoma had tumor resection by laminectomy and curettage of three extradural tumors, debulking of a ventral lumbosacral tumor, or removal of a coccygeal vertebra by tail amputation.[100] The dog with tail amputation survived for 2.5 years and died of unrelated causes. None of the other dogs survived more than 3 days.

In another series, the use of radiation therapy increased survival times, but not statistically.[105] Overall survival for the 10 dogs with primary spinal osteosarcoma in that study was 4 months, and 50% developed metastases.

MAXILLARY OSTEOSARCOMA

Aggressive resection is warranted for osteosarcoma of the maxilla because recurrence, not metastasis, is usually the cause of death. Local recurrence is common if a limited surgery is performed, and even with partial maxillectomy, recurrence rates are still high.[100,111] The skill of the surgeon and preoperative planning are important to the success of surgery. Recurrence rates as low as 25%, with up to 45% of dogs alive 1 year after surgery, have been reported.[112] Resection of the hard palate followed by carboplatin was successful in controlling osteosarcoma in a dog for more than 33 months.[113] Samarium-153-EDTMP was used as an adjunct to surgery in a dog with a recurrent maxillary osteosarcoma, and the dog had no recurrence 21 months later.[92]

Distant metastases may be a late occurrence, with rates of 35% to 50%; however, rates may be higher in dogs that do not have local tumor recurrence and therefore live longer.[111,112] Cisplatin chemotherapy alone or in combination with radiation therapy did not reduce recurrence rates in one study of 10 dogs.[100]

ZYGOMATIC ARCH AND ORBITAL OSTEOSARCOMA

Because the zygomatic arch is a resectable structure, it would seem that osteosarcoma at this site should be resectable. In one series of four dogs, two were treated with surgery alone and two were treated with surgery plus radiation therapy.[114] Of the two dogs that underwent surgery alone, one had recurrence 2 months after surgery and the other had no evidence of disease 2 years later; both dogs that received radiation lived 6 months until recurrence.

In contrast, four of six dogs with orbital osteosarcoma survived more than 1 year after surgery.[115]

Surgical excision with wide margins followed by radiation therapy is probably the treatment of choice. Preoperative CT should be used for surgical planning. Chemotherapy as described for appendicular osteosarcoma is recommended.

NASAL OSTEOSARCOMA

Surgical excision was attempted in three dogs; the tumor recurred within 6 weeks in two dogs.[100] One dog that received 48 Gy of orthovoltage radiation with low-dose cisplatin (10 mg/m^2 IV) instead of surgery remained tumor-free for 12 months and died of unrelated causes (see Chapter 51).[100]

PELVIC OSTEOSARCOMA

The pelvis was the least common site of axial skeleton osteosarcomas in one study.[100] Hemipelvectomy is the treatment of choice for pelvic osteosarcoma; however, the metastatic rate may be high. Although no metastases were seen at presentation in two dogs with pelvic osteosarcoma in one study,[100] another study found that two of three dogs lived longer than 1 month after hemipelvectomy and cisplatin chemotherapy, and both developed metastases 1.6 and 3.5 months after surgery.[116] Tumors from this site may behave more like appendicular osteosarcoma.

MULTILOBULAR OSTEOCHONDROSARCOMA
Incidence, Signalment, and Etiology

MLO is considered the most common tumor of the canine skull and has been described using several names, including *chondroma rodens, multilobular osteoma, multilobular osteosarcoma, multilobular chondroma,* and *multilobular tumor of bone.*

MLO is a tumor of middle-aged to older dogs (median age: 8 years) with no breed or gender predilection. The tumor is usually found in medium to large dogs (median weight: 29 kg).

This disease should be distinguished from the benign osteochondromas that can occur singly or in multiple sites, including the ribs, vertebrae, and appendicular skeleton.[117] Those tumors may transform to a malignant state (osteosarcoma or chondrosarcoma) in older animals.[117,118]

Clinical Presentation and History

MLO usually grows slowly, and the progression of signs may also be gradual. Most dogs present with a palpable mass or swelling noticed by their owner. Dogs may also present with dysphagia and pain in opening the mouth, exophthalmia, or neurologic signs. Most MLOs occur in the calvarium (parietal crest, temporooccipital region, and zygomatic arch), from which tumors may extend into the sinuses, orbit, or cranial vault; the maxilla and mandible are the next most common sites (Figure 61-14).[119] Tumor diameter ranged from 1 cm to 11 cm (median: 4 cm) in one study.

Staging and Diagnosis

Radiographs of the thorax and tumor site are recommended before treatment, and thoracic radiographs should be used to

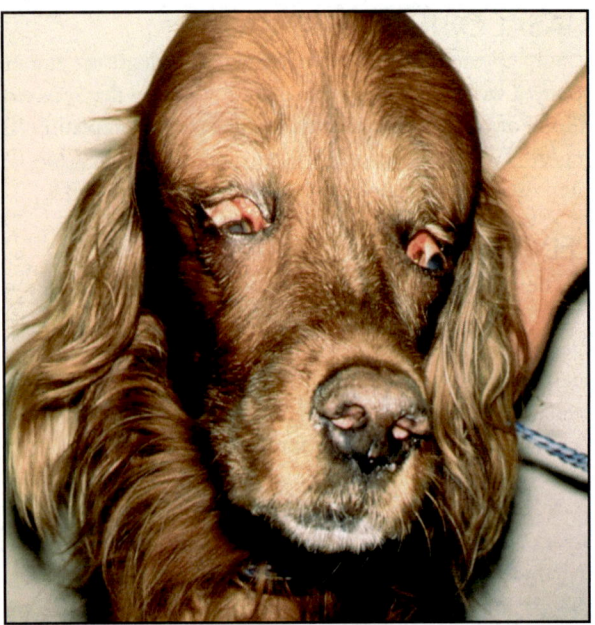

Figure 61-14. *Massive multilobular osteochondrosarcoma involving the skull of a Irish setter. This tumor was considered inoperable because of the size and amount of calvarium that would have needed to be resected. (Courtesy of John Berg, DVM, Tufts Cummings School of Veterinary Medicine)*

monitor patients after surgery. Radiographically, the lesion is sharply delineated with a lobulated appearance, and margins are usually indistinct. CT or MRI will assist the surgeon in planning surgery and may assist if radiation therapy is planned after incomplete excision. MRI may be more helpful in delineating soft tissue and brain involvement.[120,121]

Metastasis at the time of presentation is unusual and was reported in only three of 39 dogs in one study[119] and rarely in case reports.[122] However, metastasis occurred a median of 18 months after surgical excision in 19 of 34 (56%) dogs.[119] The median time from detection of metastasis to death was 11 months (range: 5–33 months) in one study,[123] which concurs with other case reports of long survival even after metastasis occurs.[124,125]

The histologic grade of MLO has been shown to be prognostic. The scheme for grading is outlined in Table 61-5.[119]

Prognostic Factors

Surgical margins as determined by histology were very important in one study in which 8 of 19 dogs with a complete excision had a local recurrence compared with 10 of 13 dogs that had a local recurrence after incomplete excision.[119] Similarly, 19 dogs with complete resection had not reached a median survival 44 months after surgery, while the median survival was 10.5 months if excision was incomplete.[119]

Grading as described above was important in determining local recurrence, survival, and time to metastasis (Table 61-6).[119]

Treatment

Surgery is the treatment of choice for MLO, although complete excision is often difficult. In one study, complete resection was accomplished in 19 of 32 dogs with MLO; recurrence and survival were related to margins (Figure 61-15).[119] Local recurrence was seen in 47% of dogs at a median time of 26 months after surgery.[119] Because margins are so important, wider resections are advisable. For dogs with larger tumors, excision may reduce the skull below the horizon of the brain. In these dogs, reconstruction of the calvarium may be achieved using a molded polymethylmethacrylate prosthesis. Exposure to the nasal cavity may increase the risk of implant infection, and resection of the dorsal orbital rims may not allow prosthesis stabilization.[126]

Treatment of MLO with radiation therapy as an adjunct to surgical excision seems justified on the basis of limited data. Four dogs that received adjuvant radiation therapy (with or without chemotherapy) at the time of surgery for MLO had good tumor control; in two dogs, this was for more than 2 years. In this small number of cases, this was no better than aggressive surgery alone.[119] Orthovoltage radiation therapy (45 Gy) resulted in more than 9 months of control of a tumor that had been resected three times in 8 months.[127]

Although cisplatin seems to give the best chance of preventing metastasis, there are only preliminary data at this time. More anaplastic MLO tumors are likely to metastasize and thus may warrant adjunctive therapy. In one study, 10 dogs received cisplatin either as a slow-release formulation (OPLA-Pt) or in addition to radiation therapy, and no survival benefit over surgery alone was seen; however, three of these dogs had metastases at the time of chemotherapy, so they were at a considerably more advanced stage than other dogs.[119] Further studies are necessary to define the role of chemotherapy and radiation therapy for MLO.

SURFACE OSTEOSARCOMA
Incidence, Signalment, and Etiology

Other terms for this disease in the veterinary literature, in order of increasing aggressive behavior, are *extraosseous osteosarcoma, parosteal osteosarcoma (juxtacortical osteosarcoma), periosteal osteosarcoma,* and *high-grade surface osteosarcoma*. All are rare in dogs. These tumors are best described as osteosarcomas that do not disrupt the cortex of the underlying bone.

Clinical Presentation and History

Despite the lack of cortical involvement, pain is characteristic of these tumors. Depending on the site, lameness or a mass lesion may be noted.

Table 61-5 **Variables Used to Determine the Histologic Grade of Canine MLO**[119]

Score	Parameter					
	Cellular pleomorphism	Borders	Mitotic index	Size of lobules	Tumor necrosis	Organization
0	Monomorphic	—	—	—	None	—
1	Mild	Pushing	1–5	Small and medium	Present	Well
2	Moderate	Pushing and invasive	6–10	Large	—	Moderate
3	Marked	Invasive	>10	—	—	Poor

Grade	Description
1	Cumulative score of ≤7
2	Cumulative score of 8–12
3	Cumulative score of ≥13

Staging and Diagnosis

Tumors have been reported at mostly axial sites; even histologically benign parosteal osteosarcomas may metastasize to lungs, although time to metastasis may be prolonged.[128,129] One dog with a high-grade surface osteosarcoma developed metastases within 1 month of diagnosis.[130]

Treatment

Treatment of parosteal osteosarcomas has been reported infrequently. Even histologically benign parosteal osteosarcomas may not be resectable if they involve a vertebral body.[131] One dog with a parosteal osteosarcoma of the distal radius was treated with 80 Gy of radiation over an 18-month period with palliation until pulmonary metastases were diagnosed 2 years after initial diagnosis.[128]

It would seem that surgical resection should be aggressive. Two dogs had no metastases at diagnosis, so long-term control may be possible if complete excision is achieved.[131,132]

EXTRASKELETAL OSTEOSARCOMA
Incidence, Signalment, and Etiology

Osteosarcomas may affect sites other than bone. In these situations, they are probably differentiated mesenchymal tumors. In one study of 169 dogs, the most common sites of extraskeletal osteosarcoma were the mammary gland (101 dogs), GI tract, skin, spleen, liver, kidney, bladder, muscle, thyroid, and eye.[133] Extraskeletal osteosarcomas accounted for 11% of all osteosarcoma diagnoses at the pathology service used in the study. Other studies have reported the spleen as a common site.[134,135] Dogs with extraskeletal osteosarcoma are older (median age: 11 years).[133,136] Some studies have suggested that there may be a higher incidence in female dogs,[134,136] although if mammary tumors are removed from analysis, there is no gender predisposition.[133] There was a breed predilection for beagles and rottweilers to develop nonmammary extraskeletal osteosarcoma in one study; the same study found miniature poodles and German shepherds to have a higher risk of mammary osteosarcoma.[133]

Osteosarcoma has been associated with retained surgical sponge in two dogs; both tumors metastasized.[137,138]

Table 61-6 **Grade as a Prognostic Factor for 34 Dogs with MLO**[119]

Grade	Dogs (n)	Dogs with Local Recurrence (n [%])	Median Survival (months)
1	10	3 (30)	>29
2	15	7 (47)	17
3	9	7 (78)	13

Clinical Presentation and History

Clinical signs vary with the site of involvement. In dogs with mammary or cutaneous tumors, the caregiver usually detects a mass.[133,136] In dogs with splenic tumors, anorexia, lethargy, and abdominal distention are most common, as is true in dogs with any other sarcoma of the spleen.[135]

Staging and Diagnosis

Staging other than an MDB depends on the site affected. Ultrasonography may be helpful in detecting abdominal metastases to organs or regional lymph nodes. CT or MRI may assist in planning surgery. Metastatic disease is common, and most tumors metastasize to the liver, lungs, and omentum.[134,136] In one study, eight of 14 dogs (57%) had metastases at diagnosis, and by the time of death, 85% had metastases.[136] Other extraskeletal osteosarcomas, particularly those of the mammary gland, may spread by local extension only.[133]

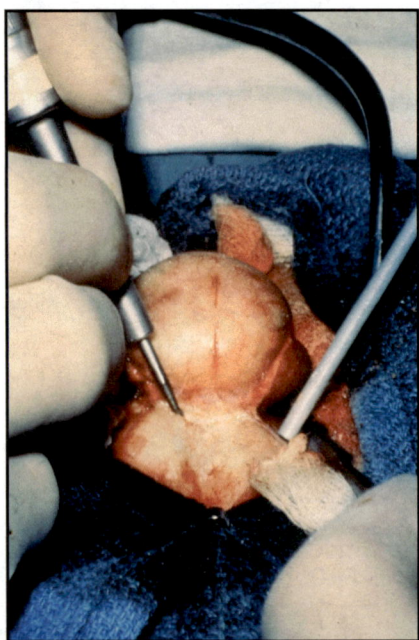

Figure 61-15. *Surgical excision of a multilobular osteochondrosarcoma smaller than the unresectable one seen in Figure 61-14. Wide surgical margins may provide long-term control; however, if the tumor has an anaplastic histology or if margins cannot be ensured, adjuvant radiation therapy should be considered. (Courtesy of J. Berg)*

Prognostic Factors

Chemotherapy with doxorubicin or cisplatin improved survival in one study.[136] The median survival time for five dogs treated with surgery and chemotherapy was 5 months compared with 1 month for dogs treated with surgery alone.

Treatment

Surgical excision is the principal method of treatment for dogs with extraskeletal osteosarcoma.

Local recurrence was the cause of death for most dogs with soft tissue osteosarcoma (92%); the median survival time of these dogs was less than 1 month. Dogs with mammary osteosarcoma fared better, with a median survival of 3 months, but most developed pulmonary metastasis (63%).[133] Median survival was 3 months for 20 dogs with mammary osteosarcoma of the cranial glands and 7.4 months for dogs with tumors of the caudal glands. Dogs with subcutaneous osteosarcoma appeared to have longer survival times than dogs with other extraskeletal osteosarcoma.[133] This study was hindered by lack of follow-up for many patients. In another study, the use of chemotherapy improved survival for dogs with extraskeletal osteosarcoma.[136]

Splenectomy may not have a good outcome in dogs with splenic osteosarcoma, even if evidence of metastatic disease at the time of surgery is lacking (see Chapter 55).[135]

Nonosteosarcoma Bone Tumors

Primary bone tumors that are not osteosarcomas are rare in dogs, but those most commonly described are fibrosarcomas, chondrosarcomas, and hemangiosarcomas. Chondrosarcoma probably predominates in the axial skeleton.[139] Affected dogs are mostly large breeds. There is no gender predilection, and older dogs (average age: 9 years) are most often affected.[140] Less common tumors include giant-cell tumors, liposarcomas, and synovial cell sarcomas. Synovial cell tumors are not strictly bone tumors and are described separately in Chapter 62.

FIBROSARCOMA OF BONE
Incidence, Signalment, and Etiology

Fibrosarcomas of bone are rare and usually involve the axial skeleton.[141,142] These tumors primarily affect mature male dogs. The outlook for a dog with fibrosarcoma of the bone is better than that for a dog with osteosarcoma, but the prognosis is still guarded.

Staging and Diagnosis

Complete staging for any dog with a bone tumor should include blood work, urinalysis, fine-detail radiographs of the lesion, thoracic radiographs, and careful evaluation of regional lymph nodes.

Histopathology from incisional or needle biopsies of bone lesions must be viewed with some skepticism because osteosarcomas frequently have localized areas that do not contain osteoid and are composed of purely fibrous or cartilaginous tissue. For this reason, a definitive diagnosis should be delayed until a larger biopsy specimen is obtained (e.g., at amputation). In one retrospective study, six of 11 dogs initially diagnosed with fibrosarcoma were found on further histologic sectioning to have osteosarcoma.[142] This point is particularly important if adjuvant therapy is being considered.

In a series of five dogs with mandibular fibrosarcoma, metastasis to the regional lymph node was confirmed in one dog and suspected in two dogs at 13, 7, and 10 months after mandibulectomy, respectively.[143] In another series of 14 dogs with fibrosarcoma of the maxilla (n = 7) or mandible (n = 7), metastasis occurred in only 14%.[112] Two dogs with fibrosarcoma of the rib developed systemic metastases 120 and 450 days after surgical resection.[106]

Metastases were seen in the cardiac muscle and pericardium, skin, and patella in three of five dogs with appendicular fibrosarcomas treated by amputation.[142] Metastasis of fibrosarcomas of the axial skeleton may be less prevalent than at appendicular sites and may occur late in the course of the disease.

Treatment

For five dogs with appendicular fibrosarcoma, survival after amputation ranged from 4 to 40 months; three dogs developed metastatic disease.[142] Three of the dogs also received adjuvant cisplatin (70 mg/m² IV or intraarterially every 3 weeks). Two of these dogs developed metastasis, and one had no evidence of disease 17 months later. One dog that did not receive chemotherapy had no evidence of disease 40 months after surgery. Two dogs with pelvic fibrosarcoma were treated by hemipelvectomy. One with complete margins had no evidence of disease more than 37 months after surgery, and the other died of local recurrence and metastases 2.5 months after incomplete surgery.[116] From this small number of cases, it is difficult to make recommendations. Amputation followed by doxorubicin-based chemotherapy may be the best treatment for appendicular fibrosarcoma, but further studies are needed to define the role of adjuvant chemotherapy.

Of six dogs with fibrosarcoma of the rib, the median survival was 6 months; 33% were alive 1 year after rib resection, and none was alive 2 years after surgery.[106,107] Two dogs developed metastases. A case report of a dog with a fibrosarcoma of vertebra L5 in which the vertebral body was resected documented survival of more than 2 years.[144] As with appendicular fibrosarcoma, it is difficult to make strong recommendations above adjuvant chemotherapy.

Median survival for 34 dogs treated for fibrosarcoma by mandibulectomy or maxillectomy was 12 months.[112,143] Local recurrence was seen in 11 dogs. Local recurrence may be more of a problem with maxillectomy than with mandibulectomy (see Chapter 53).

Local control rates may be improved by using radiation therapy as an adjuvant to surgery. This approach has improved survival times for dogs with soft tissue sarcomas and may play a similar role for dogs with fibrosarcoma of bone if surgical margins cannot be ensured (see Chapter 62).

CHONDROSARCOMA OF BONE
Incidence, Signalment, and Etiology

Chondrosarcomas were found in 41 of 394 bone tumors or tumor-like lesions in dogs. Older dogs were mostly affected in two studies (mean age: 8–9 years; age range: 1–15 years).[140,145] Chondrosarcomas most commonly involve the axial skeleton and ribs, nasal turbinates, and pelvis.[139,140,145] These tumors are most common in large-breed dogs, and golden retrievers were overrepresented in one study.[140]

Chondrosarcomas of the appendicular skeleton are uncommon, accounting for 16 of 97 cases in one study, and seem to involve the hindlimb more frequently (14 of 16).[140] Transformation of an aneurysmal bone cyst into a chondrosarcoma was documented in one dog.[146]

Staging and Diagnosis

Staging should be performed as described for all bone tumors. Tumors of the ribs may be visualized best by CT,

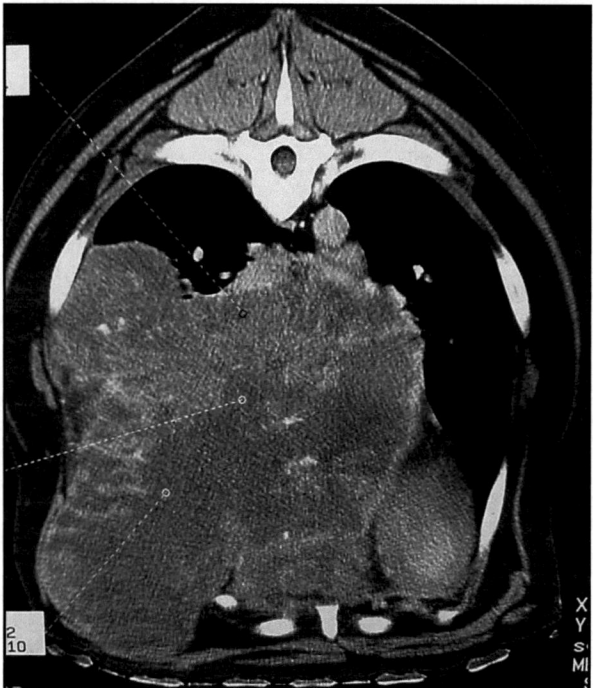

Figure 61-16. *A CT scan from a dog that had a comparatively small external rib chondrosarcoma with massive intrathoracic extension. (Courtesy of John Chretin, DVM, VCA West Los Angeles Animal Hospital)*

which can also provide information about the size and invasiveness of the tumor before surgical removal (Figures 61-16 to 61-19).

Histopathology from incisional or needle biopsies of bone lesions must be interpreted with caution because osteosarcomas frequently have localized areas that do not contain osteoid and are composed of purely fibrous or cartilaginous tissue. For this reason, a definitive diagnosis should be delayed until a larger biopsy specimen is obtained (e.g., at amputation). This point is particularly important if adjuvant therapy is being considered.

Chondrosarcoma is believed to have a low metastatic rate compared with osteosarcoma. The metastatic rate may depend on the primary site. Overall metastatic rate appears to be low at diagnosis for this tumor type. In three studies, 27 of 135 dogs (20%) with chondrosarcoma of all sites had systemic metastases, most commonly to the lungs.[139,140,145]

Chondrosarcoma of the appendicular skeleton has been associated with widespread systemic metastases[140] and had the highest metastatic rate in one study.[147] In five series of 47 dogs with chondrosarcoma of the rib, 22 dogs developed metastases.[106,107,109,139,140] However, these metastases often occurred long (i.e., years) after surgical excision of the primary tumor. Thoracic radiographs to monitor for pulmonary metastasis are warranted, particularly in dogs with appendicular and rib chondrosarcomas.

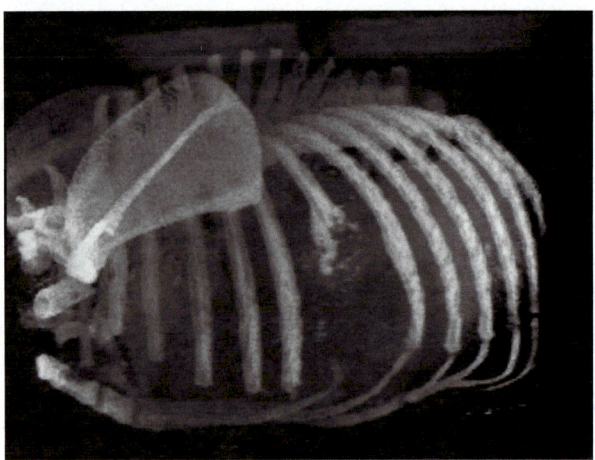

Figure 61-17. *CT technology allows reconstruction of CT images into a three-dimensional image that is helpful to clients in understanding the extent of disease and to surgeons in planning surgery. This is the same dog as in Figure 61-16. (Courtesy of J. Chretin)*

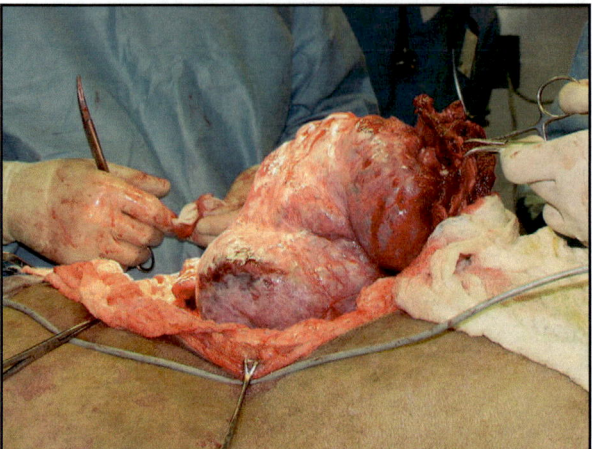

Figure 61-18. *The same dog in Figure 61-16 at surgery. Even a very large tumor such as this may be removed completely, although the defect may need to be closed with a mesh (see Figure 61-19). (Courtesy of J. Chretin)*

In a study of 55 dogs with chondrosarcoma, metastasis was noted from all sites except the nasal passages.[147] Only one of 12 dogs with a nasal chondrosarcoma developed metastases in another study.[103]

Treatment

The prognosis for dogs with appendicular chondrosarcoma is controversial. In two studies, 60% of 13 dogs with appendicular chondrosarcoma treated by amputation alone died from metastatic disease; however, the median survival time varied from 5 months[147] to 18 months.[140] Case reports support the shorter survival times.[148] Amputation alone is possibly a good option for treatment of dogs with appendicular chondrosarcoma compared with those with osteosarcoma; however, this surgery cannot necessarily be considered curative. Three dogs with digital chondrosarcoma treated by amputation survived between 4.5 months and 3.6 years.[140] Two dogs with pelvic chondrosarcoma were treated by hemipelvectomy with complete margins; neither had evidence of disease more than 42 months after surgery.[116] It is possible that other prognostic factors such as tumor grading may be helpful for this tumor type, but there are no studies to examine this presumption.

In three studies, the survival for dogs with chondrosarcoma of the rib was found to be significantly longer than that for dogs with osteosarcoma of the rib (Figure 61-13).[106,109,149] Contrary to earlier reports that may have included dogs treated with less aggressive surgeries,[109,149] surgical resection of rib chondrosarcomas seems to result in long-term control and survival. In three series totaling 28 dogs that survived the perioperative period, the median survival was more than 3 years, even though three dogs (11%) had local recurrence and 12 dogs (43%) developed metastatic disease. No adjunctive chemotherapy was administered to these dogs.[106,107,140] The longest survivor was free of disease 7 years after surgery. Wide surgical margins are important in prolonging the survival of dogs with rib chondrosarcomas. Complete resection as determined by histologic examination was an important prognostic factor in dogs with rib tumors of any histologic type; dogs with incomplete resection were six times more likely to die from the disease.[106] Metastases tend be detected late in the course of disease, so the effect of adjuvant chemotherapy would be difficult to assess.

Radiation may be a useful adjunct to treatment of chondrosarcomas. In one series of 55 dogs with chondrosarcoma, the longest median survival (500 days) was in dogs with nasal chondrosarcoma that received radiation therapy.[147] In another study, two of four dogs that received orthovoltage radiation as an adjunct to surgery for nasal chondrosarcoma lived more than 2 years.[140] Dogs with nasal chondrosarcoma have a better prognosis than dogs with nasal carcinomas (see Chapter 51).[150]

> **KEY POINT**
> *Metastases from chondrosarcoma of the rib are often not evident for a long time after surgical resection of the primary tumor.*

> **KEY POINT**
> *Fibrosarcomas and chondrosarcomas of the axial skeleton in dogs seem less likely to metastasize than those of the appendicular skeleton.*

PLASMA CELL TUMOR OF BONE

Vertebral plasma cell tumors not associated with multiple myeloma were diagnosed in five dogs. Of two dogs treated

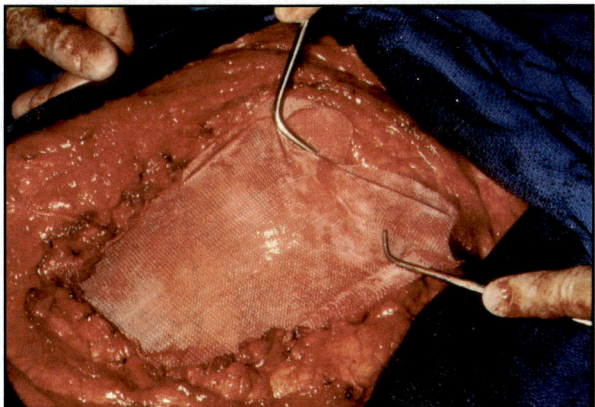

Figure 61-19. *Marlex mesh being used to close a large defect in the thoracic wall of a dog with multiple ribs resected. The dog recovered well from surgery.*

by chemotherapy with melphalan and prednisone as well as radiation therapy, survival was 4.5 months (4 treatments of 9 Gy; dog died from radiation myelopathy) and 65 months (3 Gy to a total dose of 48 Gy; dog developed multiple myeloma).[151] Radiation therapy to the spine should not be given as a coarsely fractionated series.

HEMANGIOSARCOMA

Hemangiosarcoma as a primary bone tumor is rare (see Chapter 56).

REFERENCES

1. Tjalma RA: Canine bone sarcoma: Estimation of relative risk as a function of body size. *J Natl Cancer Inst* 36:1137–1150, 1966.
2. Ru G, Terracini B, Glickman LT: Host related risk factors for canine osteosarcoma. *Vet J* 156:31–39, 1998.
3. Bech-Nielsen S, Haskins ME, Reif JS, et al: Frequency of osteosarcoma among first-degree relatives of St. Bernard dogs. *J Natl Cancer Inst* 60:349–353, 1978.
4. Phillips JC, Dillberger J, Rizzo C, et al: Genetic analysis of osteosarcoma in the Scottish deerhound. *Proc 23rd Annu Conf Vet Cancer Soc*:9, 2003.
5. Gellasch KL, Kalscheur VL, Clayton MK, Muir P: Fatigue microdamage in the radial predilection site for osteosarcoma in dogs. *Am J Vet Res* 63:896–899, 2002.
6. Spodnick GJ, Berg J, Rand W, et al: Prognosis for dogs with appendicular osteosarcoma treated by amputation alone: 162 cases (1978–1988). *JAVMA* 200:995–999, 1992.
7. Misdorp W, Hart AA: Some prognostic and epidemiologic factors in canine osteosarcoma. *J Natl Cancer Inst* 62:537–545, 1979.
8. Brodey RS, Riser WH: Canine osteosarcoma: A clinicopathy study of 194 cases. *Clin Orthop Rel Res* 62:54–64, 1969.
9. Cooley DM, Beranek BC, Schlittler DL, et al: Endogenous gonadal hormone exposure and bone sarcoma risk. *Cancer Epidemiol Biomarkers Prev* 11:1434–1440, 2002.
10. Sinibaldi KR, Pugh J, Rosen H, Liu SK: Osteomyelitis and neoplasia associated with use of the Jonas intramedullary splint in small animals. *JAVMA* 181:885–890, 1982.
11. Roe SC, DeYoung D, Weinstock D, Kyles A: Osteosarcoma eight years after total hip arthroplasty. *Vet Surg* 25:70–74, 1996.
12. Murphy ST, Parker RB, Woodard JC: Osteosarcoma following total hip arthroplasty in a dog. *J Small Anim Pract* 38:263–267, 1997.
13. Marcellin-Little DJ, DeYoung DJ, Thrall DE, Merrill CL: Osteosarcoma at the site of bone infarction associated with total hip arthroplasty in a dog. *Vet Surg* 28:54–60, 1999.
14. Li XQ, Hom DL, Black J, Stevenson S: Relationship between metallic implants and cancer: A case-control study in a canine population. *Vet Comp Orthop Traumatol* 2:70–74, 1993.
15. McChesney-Gillette S, Gillette EL, Powers BE, Withrow SJ: Radiation-induced osteosarcoma in dogs after external beam or intraoperative radiation therapy. *Cancer Res* 50:54–57, 1990.
16. Mendoza S, Konishi T, Dernell WS, et al: Status of the *p53, Rb* and *MDM2* genes in canine osteosarcoma. *Anticancer Res* 18, 4449–4454, 1998.
17. Sagartz JE, Bodley WL, Gamblin RM, et al: *p53* tumor suppressor protein over-expression in osteogenic tumors of dogs. *Vet Pathol* 33:213–221, 1996.
18. Loukopoulos P, Thornton JR, Robinson WF: Clinical and pathologic relevance of p53 index in canine osseous tumors. *Vet Pathol* 40:237–248, 2003.
19. Cooley DM, Waters DJ: Skeletal neoplasms of small dogs: A retrospective study and literature review. *JAAHA* 33:11–23, 1997.
20. Wallack ST, Wisner ER, Werner JA, et al: Accuracy of magnetic resonance imaging for estimating intramedullary osteosarcoma extent in pre-operative planning of canine limb-salvage procedures. *Vet Radiol Ultrasound* 43:432–441, 2002.
21. Davis GJ, Kapatkin AS, Craig LE, et al: Comparison of radiography, computed tomography, and magnetic resonance imaging for evaluation of appendicular osteosarcoma in dogs. *JAVMA* 220:1171–1176, 2002.
22. Lamb CR, Berg J, Bengston AE: Preoperative measurement of canine primary bone tumors, using radiography and bone scintigraphy. *JAVMA* 196:1474–1478, 1990.
23. Daniel GB, Avenell JS, Young K, et al: Scintigraphic detection of subcutaneous metastasis in a dog with appendicular osteosarcoma. *Vet Radiol Ultrasound* 37:146–149, 1996.
24. Berg J, Lamb CR, O'Callaghan MW: Bone scintigraphy in the initial evaluation of dogs with primary bone tumors. *JAVMA* 196:917–920, 1990.
25. Jankowski MK, Uhriteyn PF, Lana SE, et al: Nuclear scanning with 99mTc-HDP for the initial evaluation of osseous metastasis in canine osteosarcoma. *Vet Comp Oncol* 1:152–158, 2003.
26. Lang J, Wortman JA, Glickman LT, et al: Sensitivity of radiographic detection of lung metastases in the dog. *Vet Radiol* 27:74–78, 1986.
27. Hillers KR, Lana SE, Lafferty MH, et al: A retrospective study: The incidence and significance of lymph node metastasis in canine osteosarcoma. *Proc 23rd Annu Conf Vet Cancer Soc*:13, 2003.
28. Samii VF, Nyland TG, Werner LL, Baker TW: Ultrasound-guided fine-needle aspiration biopsy of bone lesions: A preliminary report. *Vet Radiol Ultrasound* 40:82–86, 1999.
29. Wykes PM, Withrow SJ, Powers BE, Park RD: Closed biopsy for diagnosis of long bone tumors: Accuracy and results. *JAAHA* 21:489–494, 1985.
30. Kirpensteijn JK, Kik M, Rutteman GR, Teske E: Prognostic significance of a new histologic grading system for canine osteosarcoma. *Vet Pathol* 39, 240–246, 2002.
31. Ehrhart N, Dernell WS, Hoffmann WE, et al: Prognostic importance of alkaline phosphatase activity in serum from dogs with appendicular osteosarcoma: 75 cases (1990–1996). *JAVMA* 213:1002–1006, 1998.
32. Garzotto CK, Berg J, Hoffmann WE, Rand WM: Prognostic significance of serum alkaline phosphatase activity in canine appendicular osteosarcoma. *J Vet Intern Med* 14:587–592, 2000.
33. Kirpensteijn J, Teske E, Kik M, et al: Lobaplatin as an adjuvant chemotherapy to surgery in canine appendicular osteosarcoma: A phase II evaluation. *Anticancer Res* 22:2765–2770, 2002.
34. Vail DM, Kurzman ID, Glawe PC, et al: STEALTH liposome-encapsulated cisplatin (SPI-77) versus carboplatin as adjuvant therapy for spontaneously arising osteosarcoma (OSA) in the dog: A randomized multicenter clinical trial. *Cancer Chemother Pharmacol* 50:131–136, 2002.
35. Moore AS, Dernell WS, Ogilivie GK, et al: Doxorubicin for osteosarcoma treatment in dogs. *21st Annu ACVIM Forum Proc*:309–310, 2003.
36. Cooper S, Black AP, Smith BA, et al: Low grade osteosarcoma in a dog. *Aust Vet Pract* 32:104, 2002.
37. Bergman PJ, MacEwen EG, Kurzman ID, et al: Amputation and carboplatin for treatment of dogs with osteosarcoma: 48 cases (1991–1993). *J Vet Intern Med* 10:76–81, 1996.
38. Berg J, Weinstein MJ, Rand WM: Results of surgery and doxorubicin chemotherapy in dogs with osteosarcoma. *JAVMA* 206:1555–1560, 1995.
39. Weinstein MJ, Berg J, Kusazaki K, et al: In vitro assays of nuclear uptake of doxorubicin hydrochloride in osteosarcoma cells of dogs. *Am J Vet Res* 52:1951–1955, 1991.
40. Powers BE, Withrow SJ, Thrall DE: Percent tumor necrosis as a predictor of treatment response in canine osteosarcoma. *Cancer* 67:126–134, 1991.
41. Kirpensteijn J, van Den Bos R, Endenburg N: Adaptation of dogs to the amputation of a limb and their owner's satisfaction with the procedure. *Vet Rec* 144:115–118, 1999.

42. Carberry CA, Harvey HJ: Owner satisfaction with limb amputation in dogs and cats. *JAAHA* 23:227–232, 1987.
43. Brodey RS: Results of surgical treatment in 65 dogs with osteosarcoma. *JAVMA* 168:1032–1035, 1993.
44. Straw RC, Withrow SJ: Limb-sparing surgery versus amputation for dogs with bone tumors. *Vet Clin North Am Small Anim Pract* 26:135–143, 1996.
45. O'Brien MG, Straw RC, Withrow SJ: Recent advances in the treatment of canine appendicular osteosarcoma. *Compend Contin Educ Pract Vet* 15:939–947, 1993.
46. Kuntz CA, Asselin TL, Dernell WS, et al: Limb salvage surgery for osteosarcoma of the proximal humerus: Outcome in 17 dogs. *Vet Surg* 27:417–422, 1998.
47. Trout NJ, Pavletic MM, Kraus KH: Partial scapulectomy for management of sarcomas in three dogs and two cats. *JAVMA* 207:585–587, 1995.
48. LaRue SM, Withrow SJ, Power BE, et al: Limb-sparing treatment for osteosarcoma in dogs. *JAAHA* 195:1734–1744, 1989.
49. Morello E, Vasconi E, Martano M, et al: Pasteurized tumoral autograft and adjuvant chemotherapy for the treatment of canine distal radial osteosarcoma: 13 cases. *Vet Surg* 32:539–544, 2003.
50. Withrow SJ, Thrall DE, Straw RS: Intra-arterial cisplatin with or without radiation in limb sparing for canine osteosarcoma. *Cancer* 71:2484–2490, 1993.
51. Degna MT, Ehrhart N, Feretti A, Buracco P: Bone transport osteogenesis for limb salvage. *Vet Comp Orthop Traumatol* 13:18–22, 2000.
52. Ehrhart N, Eurell JA, Tommasini M, et al: Effect of cisplatin on bone transport osteogenesis in dogs. *Am J Vet Res* 63:703–711, 2002.
53. Cotter SM, Parker LM: High-dose methotrexate and leucovorin rescue in dogs with osteogenic sarcoma. *Am J Vet Res* 39:1943–1945, 1978.
54. Hernigou P, Thiery JP, Benoit J, et al: Methotrexate diffusion from acrylic cement. Local chemotherapy for bone tumours. *J Bone Joint Surg Br* 71:804–811, 1989.
55. Shapiro W, Fossum TW, Kitchell BE, et al: Use of cisplatin for treatment of appendicular osteosarcoma in dogs. *JAVMA* 192:507–511, 1988.
56. Straw RC, Withrow SJ, Richter SL, et al: Amputation and cisplatin for treatment of canine osteosarcoma. *J Vet Intern Med* 5:205–210, 1991.
57. Thompson JP, Feguent MJ: Evaluation of survival time after limb amputation, with and without subsequent administration of cisplatin, for treatment of appendicular osteosarcoma in dogs: 30 cases (1979–1990). *JAVMA* 200:531–533, 1992.
58. Kraegel SA, Madewell BR, Simonson E, Gregory CR: Osteogenic sarcoma and cisplatin chemotherapy in dogs: 16 cases (1986–1989). *JAVMA* 199:1057–1059, 1991.
59. Berg RJ, Weinstein MJ, Schelling SH, Rand MW: Treatment of dogs with osteosarcoma by administration of cisplatin after amputation or limb-sparing surgery: 22 cases (1987–1990). *JAVMA* 200:2005–2008, 1992.
60. Withrow SJ, Straw RC, Brekke JH: Slow-release adjuvant cisplatin for the treatment of metastatic canine osteosarcoma. *Eur J Musculoskel Res* 4:110, 1995.
61. Liptak JM, Dernell WS, Straw RC, et al: Intercalary bone grafts for joint and limb preservation in 17 dogs with high-grade malignant tumors of the diaphysis. *Vet Surg* 33:457–467, 2004.
62. Dernell WS, Withrow SJ, Straw RC, Lafferty MH: Adjuvant chemotherapy using cisplatin by subcutaneous administration. *In Vivo* 11:345–350, 1997.
63. Hahn KA, Richardson RC, Blevins WE, et al: Intramedullary cisplatin chemotherapy: Experience in four dogs with osteosarcoma. *J Small Anim Pract* 37:187–192, 1996.
64. Madewell BR, Leighton RL, Theilen GH: Amputation and doxorubicin for treatment of canine and feline osteogenic sarcoma. *Eur J Cancer* 14:287–293, 1978.
65. Mauldin GN, Matus RE, Withrow SJ, Patnaik AK: Canine osteosarcoma. Treatment by amputation versus amputation and adjuvant chemotherapy using doxorubicin and cisplatin. *J Vet Intern Med* 2:177–180, 1988.
66. Berg J, Gebhardt MC, Rand WM: Effect of timing of postoperative chemotherapy on survival of dogs with osteosarcoma. *Cancer* 79:1343–1350, 1997.
67. DeRegis CJ, Moore AS, Rand WM, Berg J: Cisplatin and doxorubicin toxicosis in dogs with osteosarcoma. *J Vet Intern Med* 17:668–673, 2003.
68. Chun R, Kurzman ID, Couto CG, et al: Cisplatin and doxorubicin combination chemotherapy for the treatment of canine osteosarcoma: A pilot study. *J Vet Intern Med* 14:495–498, 2000.
69. Bailey D, Erb H, Williams L, et al: Carboplatin and doxorubicin combination chemotherapy for the treatment of appendicular osteosarcoma in the dog. *J Vet Intern Med* 17:199–205, 2003.
70. Kent MS, Strom A, London CA, Seguin B: Alternating carboplatin and doxorubicin as adjunctive chemotherapy to amputation or limb-sparing surgery in the treatment of appendicular osteosarcoma in dogs. *J Vet Intern Med* 18:540–544, 2004.
71. Bech-Nielsen S, Brodey RS, Fidler IJ, et al: The effect of BCG on in vitro immune reactivity and clinical course in dogs treated surgically for osteosarcoma. *Eur J Cancer* 13:33–41, 1977.
72. MacEwen EG, Kurzman TD, Rosenthal RC, et al: Therapy for osteosarcoma in dogs with intravenous injection of liposome encapsulated muramyl tripeptide. *J Natl Cancer Inst* 81:935–938, 1989.
73. Kurzman ID, MacEwan EG, Rosenthal RC, et al: Adjuvant therapy for osteosarcoma in dogs: Results of randomized clinical trials using combined liposome-encapsulated muramyl tripeptide and cisplatin. *Clin Cancer Res* 1:1595–1601, 1995.
74. Visonneau S, Cesano A, Jeglum KA, Santoli D: Adjuvant treatment of canine osteosarcoma with the human cytotoxic T-cell line TALL-104. *Clin Cancer Res* 5:1868–1875, 1999.
75. Khanna C, Anderson PM, Hasz DE, et al: Interleukin-2 liposome inhalation therapy is safe and effective for dogs with spontaneous pulmonary metastases. *Cancer* 79:1409–1421, 1997.
76. Coomber BL, Denton J, Sylvestre A, Kruth S: Blood vessel density in canine osteosarcoma. *Can J Vet Res* 62:199–204, 1998.
77. Lana SE, Ogilvie GK, Hansen RA, et al: Identification of matrix metalloproteinases in canine neoplastic tissue. *Am J Vet Res* 61:111–114, 2000.
78. Cakir Y, Hahn KA: Direct action by doxycycline against canine osteosarcoma cell proliferation and collagenase (MMP-1) activity in vitro. *In Vivo* 13:327–332, 1999.
79. Mehl ML, Withrow SJ, Seguin B, et al: Spontaneous regression of osteosarcoma in four dogs. *JAVMA* 219:614–617, 2001.
80. Greenberg, C. B., Snyder, P. W., Khan, K. N., et al: Cyclooxygenase-2 expression in naturally-occurring canine osteosarcoma: A preliminary report. *Proc 23rd Annu Conf Vet Cancer Soc*:11, 2003.
81. Mullins MN, Ehrhart EJ, Lana SE, et al: Cyclooxygenase-2 expression in canine appendicular osteosarcomas. *Proc 23rd Annu Conf Vet Cancer Soc*:15, 2003.
82. Knapp DW, Richardson RC, Bonney PL, Hahn K: Cisplatin therapy in 41 dogs with malignant tumors. *J Vet Intern Med* 2:41–46, 1988.
83. Ogilvie GK, Straw RC, Jameson VJ: Evaluation of single agent chemotherapy for treatment of clinically evident osteosarcoma metastasis in dogs: 45 cases (1987–1991). *JAVMA* 202:304–306, 1993.
84. O'Brien MG, Straw RC, Withrow SJ: Resection of pulmonary metastases in canine osteosarcoma: Thirty-one cases (1983–1992). *Vet Surg* 22:105–109, 1993.
85. Boston, S., Ehrhart, N., Dernell, W., et al: Retrospective evaluation of survival time of dogs with stage III osteosarcoma that undergo treatment. *Proc 24th Annu Conf Vet Cancer Soc*:38, 2004.
86. McEntee MC, Page RL, Novotney CA, Thrall DE: Palliative radiotherapy for canine appendicular osteosarcoma. *Vet Radiol Ultrasound* 34:367–370, 1993.
87. Green EM, Adams WM, Forrest LJ: Four fraction palliative radiotherapy for osteosarcoma in 24 dogs. *JAAHA* 38:445–451, 2002.
88. Ramirez O, III, Dodge RK, Page RL, et al: Palliative radiotherapy of appendicular osteosarcoma in 95 dogs. *Vet Radiol Ultrasound* 40:517–522, 1999.
89. Farese JP, Milner R, Thompson M, et al: Stereotactic radiosurgery for the treatment of lower extremity canine appendicular osteosarcoma. *Proc 23rd Annu Conf Vet Cancer Soc*: 69, 2003.
90. Lattimer JC, Corwin LA, Stapleton J, et al: Clinical and clinicopathologic response of canine bone tumor patients to treatment with samarium-153-EDTMP. *J Nucl Med* 31:1316–1325, 1990.
91. Milner RJ, Dormehl I, Louw WK, Croft S: Targeted radiotherapy with Sm-153-EDTMP in nine cases of canine primary bone tumours. *J S Afr Vet Assoc* 69:12–17, 1998.
92. Moe L, Boysen M, Aas M, et al: Maxillectomy and targeted radionuclide therapy with 153Sm-EDTMP in a recurrent canine osteosarcoma. *J Small Anim Pract* 37:241–246, 1996.
93. Tomlin JL, Sturgeon C, Pead MJ, Muir P: Use of the bisphosphonate drug alendronate for palliative management of osteosarcoma in two dogs. *Vet Rec* 147:129–132, 2000.
94. Mazzaferro EM, Hackett TB, Stein TP, et al: Metabolic alterations in dogs with osteosarcoma. *Am J Vet Res* 62:1234–1239, 2001.
95. Lucroy MD, Peck JN, Berry CR: Osteosarcoma of the patella with pulmonary metastases in a dog. *Vet Radiol Ultrasound* 42:218–220, 2001.
96. Maute AM, Grundmann S, Grest P, von Werthern CJ: Osteosarkom der patella beim hund. *Kleintierpraxis* 45:295–298, 2000.
97. Sukhiani HR, Gains MJ: Osteosarcoma of the talus in a dog. *Can Vet J* 34:624–626, 1993.
98. Gamblin RM, Straw RC, Powers BE, et al: Primary osteosarcoma distal to the antebrachiocarpal and tarsocrural joints in nine dogs. *JAAHA* 31:86–91, 1995.

99. Straw RC, Withrow SJ, Powers: Primary osteosarcoma of the ulna in 12 dogs. *JAAHA* 27:323–326, 1991.
100. Heymann SJ, Diefender DL, Goldschmidt MH, Newton CD: Canine axial skeletal osteosarcoma. A retrospective study of 116 cases (1986 to 1989). *Vet Surg* 21:304–310, 1992.
101. Hammer AS, Weeren FR, Weisbrode SE, Padgett SL: Prognostic factors in dogs with osteosarcomas of the flat or irregular bones. *JAAHA* 31:321–326, 1995.
102. Dickerson ME, Page RL, LaDue TA, et al: Retrospective analysis of axial skeleton osteosarcoma in 22 large-breed dogs. *J Vet Intern Med* 15, 120–124. 2001.
103. Patnaik AK, Lieberman PH, Erlandson RA, Liu SK: Canine sinonasal skeletal neoplasms: Chondrosarcomas and osteosarcomas. *Vet Pathol* 21:475–482, 1984.
104. Straw RC, Powers BE, Klausner J, et al: Canine mandibular osteosarcoma: 51 cases (1980–1992). *JAAHA* 32:257–262, 1996.
105. Dernell WS, Van Vechten BJ, Straw RC, et al: Outcome following treatment of vertebral tumors in 20 dogs (1986–1995). *JAAHA* 36:245–251, 2000.
106. Pirkey-Ehrhart N, Withrow SJ, Straw RC, et al: Primary rib tumors in 54 dogs. *JAAHA* 31:65–69, 1995.
107. Baines SJ, Lewis S, White RA: Primary thoracic wall tumours of mesenchymal origin in dogs: A retrospective study of 46 cases. *Vet Rec* 150:335–339, 2002.
108. Feeney DA, Johnston GR, Grindem CB, et al: Malignant neoplasia of canine ribs: Clinical, radiographic, and pathologic findings. *JAVMA* 180:927–933, 1982.
109. Matthiesen DT, Clark GN, Orsher RJ, et al: Enbloc resection of primary rib tumors in 40 dogs. *Vet Surg* 21:201–204, 1992.
110. Moore GE, Mathey WS, Eggers JS, Estep JS: Osteosarcoma in adjacent lumbar vertebrae in a dog. *JAVMA* 217:1008, 1038–1040, 2000.
111. Wallace J, Matthiesen DT, Patnaik AK: Hemimaxillectomy for the treatment of oral tumors in 69 dogs. *Vet Surg* 21:337–341, 1992.
112. White RA: Mandibulectomy and maxillectomy in the dog: Long term survival in 100 cases. *J Small Anim Pract* 32:69–74, 1991.
113. Beck JA, Strizek AA: Full-thickness resection of the hard palate for treatment of osteosarcoma in a dog. *Aust Vet J* 77:163–165, 1999.
114. Withrow SJ, Doige CE: Enbloc resection of a juxtacortical and three intraosseous osteosarcoma of the zygomatic arch in dogs. *JAAHA* 16:867–872, 1980.
115. Hendrix DV, Gelatt KN: Diagnosis, treatment and outcome of orbital neoplasia in dogs: A retrospective study of 44 cases. *J Small Anim Pract* 41:105–108, 2000.
116. Straw RC, Withrow SJ, Powers BE: Partial or total hemipelvectomy in the management of sarcomas in nine dogs and two cats. *Vet Surg* 21:183–188, 1992.
117. Doige CE: Multiple cartilaginous exostoses in dogs. *Vet Pathol* 24:276–278, 1987.
118. Green EM, Adams WM, Steinberg H: Malignant transformation of solitary spinal osteochondroma in two mature dogs. *Vet Radiol Ultrasound* 40:634–637, 1999.
119. Dernell WS, Straw RC, Cooper MF, et al: Multilobular osteochondrosarcoma in 39 dogs: 1979–1993. *JAAHA* 34:11–18, 1998.
120. Hathcock JT, Newton JC: Computed tomographic characteristics of multilobular tumor of bone involving the cranium in 7 dogs and zygomatic arch in 2 dogs. *Vet Radiol Ultrasound* 41:214–217, 2000.
121. Lipsitz D, Levitski RE, Berry WL: Magnetic resonance imaging features of multilobular osteochondrosarcoma in 3 dogs. *Vet Radiol Ultrasound* 42:14–19, 2001.
122. Johnston TC: Osteosarcoma of the canine skull (a case report). *Vet Med Small Anim Clin* 71:629–631, 1976.
123. Straw RC, LeCouter RA, Power BE, Withrow SJ: Multilobular osteosarcoma of the canine skull: 16 cases (1978–1988). *JAVMA* 195:1764–1769, 1989.
124. Mclain DL, Hill JR, Pulley LT: Multilobular osteoma and chondroma (chondroma rodeus) with pulmonary metastasis in a dog. *JAAHA* 19:359–362, 1983.
125. Losco DL, Hill JR, Pulley LT: Canine multilobar osteosarcoma of the skull with metastasis. *J Comp Pathol* 94:621–624, 1984.
126. Bryant KJ, Steinberg H, McAnulty JF: Cranioplasty by means of molded polymethylmethacrylate prosthetic reconstruction after radical excision of neoplasms of the skull in two dogs. *JAVMA* 223:67–72, 59, 2003.
127. Pletcher JM, Koch SA, Stedham MA: Orbital chondroma rodens in a dog. *JAVMA* 175:187–190, 1979.
128. Banks WC: Parosteal osteosarcoma in a dog and a cat. *JAVMA* 158:1412–1415, 1971.
129. Brogdon JD, Brightman AH, Helper LC, et al: Parosteal osteosarcoma of the mandible in a dog. *JAVMA* 194:1079–1081, 1989.
130. Moores AP, Beck AL, Baker JF: High-grade surface osteosarcoma in a dog. *J Small Anim Pract* 44:218–220, 2003.
131. Thomas WB, Daniel GB, McGavin MD: Parosteal osteosarcoma of the cervical vertebra in a dog. *Vet Radiol Ultrasound* 38:120–123, 1997.
132. Cook JL, Huss BT, Johnson GC: Periosteal osteosarcoma in the long head of the triceps in a dog. *JAAHA* 31:317–320, 1995.
133. Langenbach A, Anderson MA, Dambach DM, et al: Extraskeletal osteosarcoma in dogs: A retrospective study of 169 cases (1986–1996). *JAAHA* 34:113–120, 1998.
134. Patnaik AK: Canine extraskeletal osteosarcoma and chondrosarcoma: A clinicopathologic study of 14 cases. *Vet Pathol* 27:46–55, 1990.
135. Weinstein MJ, Carpenter JL, Schunk CJ: Nonangiogenic and nonlymphomatous sarcomas of the canine spleen: 57 cases (1975–1987). *JAVMA* 195:784–788, 1989.
136. Kuntz CA, Dernell WS, Powers BE, Withrow S: Extraskeletal osteosarcoma in dogs: 14 cases. *JAAHA* 34:26–30, 1998.
137. Pardo AD, Adams WH, McCracken MD, Legendre AM: Primary jejunal osteosarcoma associated with a surgical sponge in a dog. *JAVMA* 196:935–938, 1990.
138. Bradley WA: Extraskeletal soft tissue compound osteosarcoma intimately associated with a retained surgical sponge. *Aust Vet Pract* 25:172–175, 1995.
139. Brodey RS, Misdorp W, Riser WH, van der Heul RO: Canine skeletal chondrosarcoma: A clinicopathological study of 35 cases. *JAVMA* 165:68–78, 1974.
140. Popovitch CA, Weinstein MJ, Goldschmidt MH, Shofer FS: Chondrosarcoma: A retrospective study of 97 dogs (1987– 1990). *JAAHA* 30:81–85, 1994.
141. Gibbs C, Denny HR, Lucke VM: The radiological features of non osteogenic malignant tumors of bone in the appendicular skeleton of the dog. *J Small Anim Pract* 26:537–553, 1985.
142. Wesselhoeft-Albin L, Berg J, Schelling SH: Fibrosarcoma of the canine appendicular skeleton. *JAAHA* 27:303–309, 1991.
143. Salisbury SK, Lantz GC: Long term results of partial mandibulectomy for treatment of oral tumors in 30 dogs. *JAAHA* 24:285–294, 1988.
144. Chauvet AE, Hogge GS, Sandin JA, Lipsitz D: Vertebrectomy, bone allograft fusion, and antitumor vaccination for the treatment of vertebral fibrosarcoma in a dog. *Vet Surg* 28:480–488, 1999.
145. Liu SK, Dorfman HD, Hurvitz AI, Patnaik AK: Primary and secondary bone tumors in the dog. *J Small Anim Pract* 18:313–326, 1977.
146. Barnhart MD: Malignant transformation of an aneurysmal bone cyst in a dog. *Vet Surg* 31:519–524, 2002.
147. Obradovich, JE, Straw, RC, Powers, BE, Withrow, SJ: Canine chondrosarcoma: A clinicopathologic review of 55 cases. *Proc 10th Annu Conf Vet Cancer Soc*:29–30, 1990.
148. Boudrieau RJ, Schelling SH, Pisanelli ER: Chondrosarcoma of the radius with distant metastasis in a dog. *JAVMA* 205:580–583, 1994.
149. The Veterinary Cooperative Oncology Group: Retrospective study of 26 primary tumors of the osseous thoracic wall in dogs. *JAAHA* 29:68–72, 1993.
150. Theon AP, Madewell BR, Harb MF, Dungworth DL: Megavoltage irradiation of neoplasms of the nasal and paranasal cavities in 77 dogs. *JAVMA* 202:1469–1475, 1993.
151. Rusbridge C, Wheeler SJ, Lamb CR, et al: Vertebral plasma cell tumors in 8 dogs. *J Vet Intern Med* 13:126–133, 1999.

SOFT TISSUE SARCOMAS

Antony S. Moore and Gregory K. Ogilvie

CLINICAL BRIEFING

MDB includes a complete blood count, biochemical profile, and urinalysis, as well as thoracic radiography (three views).

Clinical factors	• Firm, often irregular mass that appears (but is not) encapsulated. • Often subcutaneous. • Ulceration may occur in larger tumors. • Common histologic types include fibrosarcoma, hemangiopericytoma, nerve sheath tumor, rhabdomyosarcoma, leiomyosarcoma, myxosarcoma, liposarcoma, and histiocytic sarcoma.
Staging and diagnosis	• MDB and possibly abdominal ultrasonography. • CT scan or MRI and biopsy before definitive treatment. • Tumor grade and mitotic index. • Lymph node cytology if lymphadenopathy. • Metastasis relatively uncommon, usually to lungs.
Prognostic factors	• Tumor grade is an important predictor of recurrence after surgery and development of metastases. • Mitotic index is an independent predictor of metastases.
Treatment	
Initial	• Wide surgical excision (3-cm margins) alone for grade 1 tumors. • If wide surgery not possible, consider preoperative or postoperative radiation therapy.
Adjunctive	• Adjuvant external-beam radiation therapy of >60 Gy gives control of 80%–90% at 4 years for grade 1–2 tumors. • Chemotherapy with doxorubicin-based protocols for grade 3 tumors.
Supportive	• Analgesia postoperatively.
Other soft tissue sarcomas detailed in this book	• Hemangiomas and hemangiosarcomas (Chapter 56). • Lymphangiomas and lymphangiosarcomas (Chapter 56). • Lipomas, infiltrative lipomas, and liposarcomas (Chapter 64). • Histiocytic sarcomas (Chapter 63).

The soft tissue sarcomas are grouped together because of their apparent similarities in biologic and therefore clinical behavior. The nomenclature for individual tumors largely depends on microscopic appearance. Histologic distinction may be difficult.[1] For example, confirmation of muscle origin (rhabdomyosarcoma) requires immunohistochemical staining for the intermediate filament desmin, and histologic differentiation of neurofibrosarcoma from schwannoma is possible only by using electron microscopy or by identifying small bundles and palisades of cells called *Antoni type A pattern*. Soft tissue sarcomas with a highly mucinous stroma are called *myxofibrosarcomas* or *myxosarcomas*. Because microscopic appearance may change depending on the site of biopsy or stage of growth, the same tumor may be given different names at different stages. This is initially frustrating to clinicians; however, there is very little difference in the biologic behavior of these tumors. Thus, whether a tumor is labeled fibroma, fibrosarcoma, hemangiopericytoma, neurofibroma, neurofibrosarcoma, schwannoma, rhabdomyoma, rhabdomyosarcoma, leiomyoma, leiomyosarcoma, or histiocytic sarcoma may not matter as much as the site and grade of tumor and the thoroughness of excision. Some of these tumors may initially be characterized as benign, but it is more clinically correct to consider them as histologic "gradations" of a single tumor type and to treat them in the same aggressive manner as tumors described as sarcomas.

The first section of this chapter discusses soft tissue sarcomas as a group; following sections address the incidence, signalment, and etiology of each sarcoma subtype (e.g., peripheral nerve sheath tumor of the brachial plexus), as well as any specific details of treatment. The treatment of all soft tissue sarcomas is otherwise identical and is outlined in the first section.

Incidence, Signalment, and Etiology

A definitive cause for soft tissue sarcomas in dogs has not been identified. In cats, injection-site sarcomas, particularly at the site of rabies and FeLV vaccinations, have been recognized. Recently, a study found an increased incidence of vaccine site sarcomas in dogs.[2] These 15 fibrosarcomas from presumed injection sites (back, shoulder, and thoracic wall) were mostly high grade and showed lymphocytic inflammatory infiltration located at the tumor periphery in a pattern similar to that of feline postvaccinal fibrosarcomas. Aluminum deposits that were conjectured to come from vaccine adjuvant were detected in eight tumors. A myxoma arose at the subcutaneous site of pacemaker implantation in another dog.[3] It is possible that chronic inflammation could play a role in the genesis of these tumors.

Clinical Presentation and History

Soft tissue sarcomas are often dermal in origin, so the most common reason for presentation is a mass detected by the owner while grooming or petting the dog. Tumors can vary in size and are typically not well demarcated. Ulceration is rare but may occur secondary to pressure necrosis of the overlying skin (Figure 62-1). Most tumors are firm; cystic or mucinous tumors can feel soft. Soft tissue sarcomas can be slow to enlarge, and owners may delay seeking veterinary advice for years after first detecting a mass.

Tumors that infiltrate the underlying bone may cause lameness, and those arising from the nerve sheath may cause weakness and pain.

Staging and Diagnosis

Soft tissue sarcomas infiltrate far beyond the clinically palpable borders, and those affecting the nerve sheath may extend along nerve roots to involve the spinal dura, particularly at the brachial plexus. Therefore, wide surgical excision is needed to ensure that adequate tissue margins are obtained, and adjunctive radiation therapy is often necessary. Because wide surgical margins in all directions are essential for cure, a preoperative biopsy can be of great value

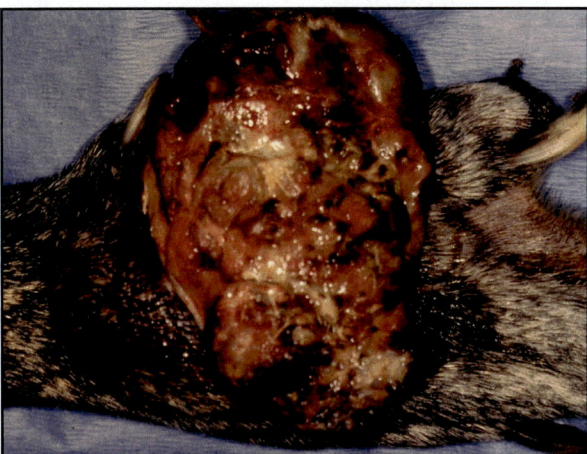

Figure 62-1. *Soft tissue sarcomas can expand to cause pressure necrosis of the overlying skin. Palliation of this distal tumor would be difficult, and amputation may be the best option, particularly if it is a low-grade tumor.*

in planning surgery. Preoperative biopsy also allows tumor grading. One study has established the value of tumor grading based on mitotic index, percentage of necrosis, and differentiation (Table 62-1).[4] However, the biopsy tract must be considered contaminated with tumor tissue and must be included in the planned treatment area with margins of 2 to 3 cm; therefore, the biopsy itself must be planned with consideration of the effect on future surgery or radiation therapy.

Needle-core, punch, or incisional biopsy is preferred over fine-needle aspiration (FNA) or excisional biopsy. FNA may fail to give a diagnosis, particularly if the tumor has necrotic areas or if there is a lot of blood in the aspirate and may thereby delay progress to definitive treatment. In one study, only 62% of FNA samples gave a correct diagnosis.[5] Excisional biopsy may compromise definitive treatment by altering tissue architecture and seeding surrounding unaffected tissues. Therefore, needle-core or punch biopsy is preferred.

A needle-core biopsy is generally safe and rapid and can be performed with the patient lightly sedated, using a local anesthetic block. Histologic examination is more accurate than needle aspiration but not as accurate as punch or incisional biopsy because the tissue sample obtained is small. The small tissue fragments must be handled with care to avoid damage.

Punch biopsy often requires only light sedation, a local anesthetic block, and little suturing and yields a larger tissue specimen than needle biopsy. A limitation of this technique is that subcutaneous or deep-seated tissues may not be adequately biopsied. Punch biopsies are best taken from a dermal mass at the junction of normal and abnormal tissue. A 3- or 6-mm diameter punch biopsy instrument is ideal.

An incisional biopsy may be preferred over a punch biopsy when a larger piece of tissue is needed or when the

Table 62-1 Variables Used to Determine Histologic Grade of Canine Soft Tissue Sarcomas[4]

Score	Degree of Differentiation	Mitotic Figures per 10 High-Power Fields	Necrosis
1	Resemble normal adult mesenchymal tissue	<10	None
2	Specific histologic type	10-19	<50%
3	Undifferentiated	>19	>50%

Grade	Description
1	Cumulative score of <5
2	Cumulative score of 5 or 6
3	Cumulative score of >6

tumor is subcutaneous. This technique usually requires general anesthesia and is best performed using a scalpel blade. An incisional biopsy also provides the pathologist with a larger specimen for assessment of invasion and malignancy.

After obtaining an incisional, punch, or needle-core biopsy, the clinician is advised to consult with an experienced surgeon or radiation oncologist. If aggressive surgery or radiation therapy is planned, further pretreatment staging should include computed tomography (CT) or magnetic resonance imaging (MRI) to delineate the margins of the tumor.

> **KEY POINT**
>
> *After obtaining an incisional, punch, or needle-core biopsy, the clinician is advised to consult with an experienced surgeon or radiation oncologist.*

Metastasis appears to be uncommon (range: 8%–17%), regardless of the subtype of soft tissue sarcoma.[4-6] Recent studies have included dogs treated with more radical surgical procedures and, often, adjunctive therapies such as radiation therapy. In these studies, local tumor control has improved, which may increase the chances for occurrence and, therefore, detection of metastases. In one study, metastases were seen in 17% of dogs; the lungs were involved as the only site in 11%, the lungs and lymph nodes in 5%, and the lymph nodes alone in 1% (Table 62-2).[4] All dogs with metastases at diagnosis had grade 3 tumors. Thoracic radiographs do not usually disclose evidence of metastasis at the time of presentation; however, they should be included as part of the minimum database (MDB) in staging procedures. Although lymph node involvement is uncommon, the nodes should be palpated and FNA conducted for cytologic evaluation if they are enlarged.

Prognostic Factors

One study found that the median survival after surgery was longer for dogs with hemangiopericytoma than for 84 dogs with fibrosarcomas; however, when the effect of the tumor mitotic index was investigated, the effect of subtype disappeared.[6] The median survival for dogs with a mitotic index greater than 9 per 10 high-power fields (hpf) was 11 months; for dogs with a mitotic index less than 9 per 10 hpf, it was 27 months. The recurrence rate after surgery in these two groups of dogs was 62% and 25%, respectively. The metastatic rate was also affected by the mitotic index.

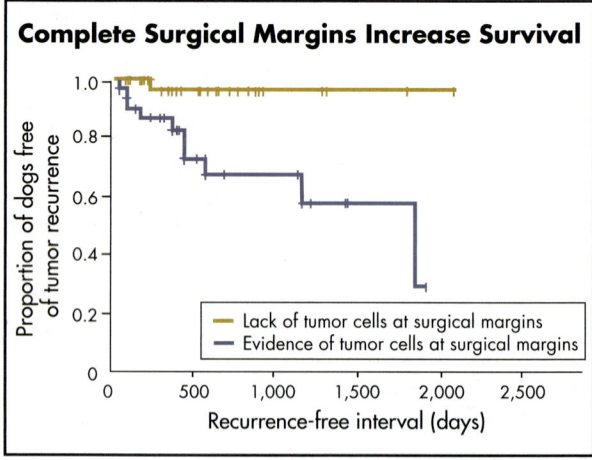

Figure 62-2. Survival curves for 39 dogs with complete surgical margins (median not reached) and 36 dogs with incomplete excision (median: 61 months). (From Kuntz CA, Dernell WS, Powers BE, et al: Prognostic factors for surgical treatment of soft-tissue sarcomas in dogs: 75 cases (1986–1996). JAVMA 211:1147–1151, 1997, with permission)

> **KEY POINT**
>
> *Tumor grade of a soft tissue sarcoma is probably the single most important factor in determining the prognosis and optimal treatment course.*

In one study, dogs with a histologically incomplete excision were more than 10 times as likely to develop a recurrence as dogs with complete margins; the recurrence rate was 28% in dogs with incomplete margins (Figure 62-2).[4] The grade of the tumor was related to metastatic rate, and mitotic index was related to median survival after surgery alone (Figure 62-3 and Table 62-2).[4] In the same study, the increasing percentage of tumor necrosis was a poor prognostic sign. In another study of surgery and intralesional chemotherapy, tumor grade also predicted recurrence.[7]

One study showed that the longer a soft tissue sarcoma was present before definitive surgical excision, the more likely it was to recur.[8] Surgical excision should not be delayed after a diagnosis is made.

Dogs with high-grade sarcomas and metastasis to the regional lymph node had a median survival time of 3 months compared with 10 months for dogs without nodal metastases in one study.[9] In another study of surgery and radiation therapy, dogs with hemangiopericytoma of the front limb had significantly shorter survival times than those with hemangiopericytoma of the hindlimbs.[10]

Table 62-2 Grade and Mitotic Index as Prognostic Variables[4,6]

	Dogs (n)	Median Survival (months)	Metastases (%)
Overall		46.5	17
Grade			
1	31	Not given	13
2	27	Not given	7
3	17	Not given	41
Mitotic index (per hpf)		**Kuntz et al[4]**	**Bostock and Dye[6]**
<10	46	47.5	27	2
10–19	18	17.5	11[a]	15[a]
>19	11	8		

[a]Value is for mitotic index >10 per hpf.

Treatment
SURGERY

In contrast to many other malignancies, soft tissue sarcomas rarely metastasize. If metastasis occurs, it is usually late in the course of disease. Therefore, local therapies such as surgery and radiation are potentially curative if used appropriately and early. A preoperative incisional, punch, or needle-core biopsy can be of great value in planning definitive treatment (see Staging section, above). After obtaining a biopsy, the clinician should consult with an experienced surgeon or radiation oncologist. If aggressive surgery is planned, further pretreatment staging should include CT or MRI to help delineate tumor margins.

> **KEY POINT**
> *Soft tissue mesenchymal tumors are rarely biologically benign, and wide surgical margins should be taken regardless of histologic appearance.*

Excision of soft tissue sarcomas is frequently incomplete because the extent of disease is underestimated preoperatively. Excision should be wide and deep because sarcomas are surrounded by a pseudocapsule of tumor cells, some of which are undergoing pressure necrosis. Despite the pressure, many cells are viable and are capable of forming local recurrent tumors. Soft tissue sarcomas also send microscopic, finger-like projections into tissue surrounding the pseudocapsule, increasing the likelihood of incomplete excision. If possible, surgical margins should include one fascial plane below the clinically detectable tumor or 2 to 3 cm of tissue in all surgical planes around the palpable tumor. The first attempt at surgical removal should be the definitive one, and margins should include bone, muscle, and other structures in order to obtain wide excision. The aim should be to remove the tissue en bloc without incising tumor tissue itself.

Because the completeness of surgical excision has been shown to be prognostic, the entire sample should be submitted for histopathology. Margins should be inked by the surgeon where they are suspected to be close. Indelible dyes that do not alter tissue architecture can be used to determine whether resection is complete and are preferred to the use of sutures or multiple random sectioning by the pathologist. One study found that alcian blue, India ink in acetone, and a commercial kit (Davidson Marking System, Bradley Products, Inc., Bloomingdale, MN) were all superior to correction fluid. The commercial kit has the advantage of including multiple dyes that can used to anatomically localize the margins for later clinical assessment.[11] One preliminary study found that recurrence was more likely if the closest surgical margin was 10 mm or less. The only exception seemed to be when a fascial plane was included, in which case margins of 1 mm were sufficient.[12]

Tumors that involve the limb often recur after attempted local excision. Amputation greatly increases the likelihood of long-term control (Figure 62-4). Procedures that are less aggressive than amputation, such as scapulectomy, need to be carefully evaluated by examination of surgical margins because the chance of local recurrence is high.[13] For extensive limb tumors that approach the pelvis, a hemipelvectomy may be required, but if complete margins cannot be obtained, rapid recurrence should be expected. In one study,

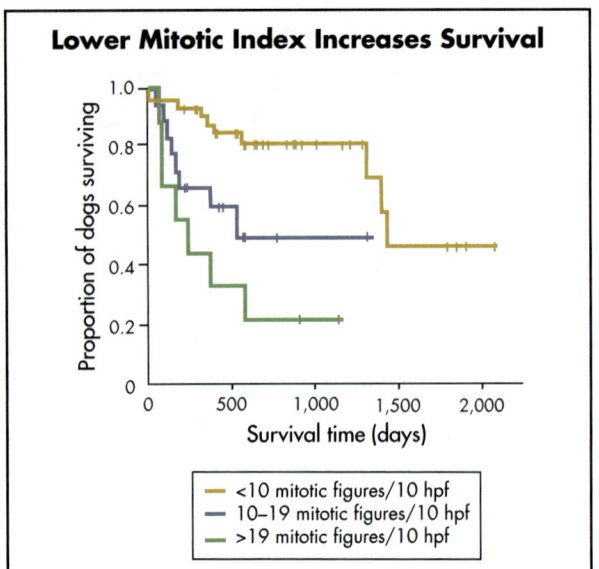

Figure 62-3. Recurrence-free survival curves for 46 dogs with a mitotic index of less than 10, 18 dogs with a mitotic index of 10 to 19, and 11 dogs with a mitotic index greater than 19; see text for details. (From Kuntz CA, Dernell WS, Powers BE, et al: Prognostic factors for surgical treatment of soft tissue sarcomas in dogs: 75 cases (1986–1996). JAVMA 211:1147–1151, 1997, with permission)

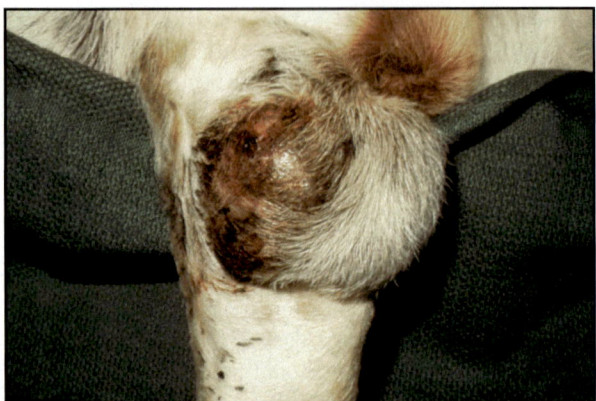

Figure 62-4. Soft tissue sarcomas are highly invasive and often recur after surgery. The metastatic rate for low-grade soft tissue sarcomas is low, and wide surgical margins may provide a cure. The hemangiopericytoma on the elbow of this 8-year-old dog is best treated by amputation. (Courtesy of Gordon H. Theilen, DVM, University of California, Davis)

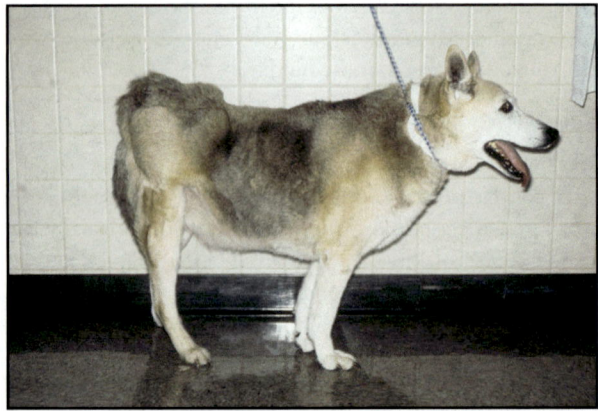

Figure 62-5. After multiple incomplete surgical excisions, soft tissue sarcomas may recur throughout the previous surgical sites, creating a huge, unresectable tumor, as in this aged crossbreed dog. (Courtesy of John Berg, DVM, Tufts Cummings School of Veterinary Medicine)

four dogs with a soft tissue sarcoma in the biceps femoris had the entire muscle belly removed with no effect on mobility 4 to 33 months later.[14] Margins were clear after surgery, and no dog had a recurrence.

Aggressive surgical excisions in areas other than the limb may lead to long-term tumor control, even after other methods have failed. However, the first surgery should be considered definitive; second or third surgeries should not be relied on for salvage (Figure 62-5). Wide resection on the chest wall of flank may require rib or body wall removal and the use of polypropylene mesh. Even with extensive surgery and reconstructive attempts, recurrences are possible.

The effect of aggressive surgical resection alone has been studied in dogs with sarcomas at sites other than the limbs. Grade 1 tumors (Table 62-1) may recur after surgery, but approximately 90% of dogs with grade 1 tumors were tumor-free at 12 months after an aggressive excision in one study.[4] Most importantly, grade 1 tumors showed very low metastatic rates (13%) compared with grade 3 tumors (41%). In addition, dogs that had tumors with a low mitotic index had a median survival of 4 years. This means that with aggressive therapy, the likelihood of long-term control is very high for dogs with grade 1 tumors. Dogs with grade 3 tumors probably benefit from adjunctive systemic therapy.

RADIATION THERAPY

Most early studies reported very little efficacy for radiation therapy in reducing recurrence rates for soft tissue sarcoma.[15-17] A combination of minimal surgical excision and low doses of radiation therapy probably contributed to these results. Soft tissue sarcomas are relatively resistant to low doses of radiation. For two groups of dogs, a total dose of 45 Gy controlled tumor growth in 48% to 60% of dogs for 1 year; 67% of dogs treated with 50 Gy experienced similar control.[10,18] By 2 years, only 50% of the dogs treated with 50 Gy still experienced tumor control.[18]

More recent studies suggest that aggressive surgery in combination with high doses of radiation therapy either before or after surgery is the treatment of choice for soft tissue sarcoma. In one study, 75% of dogs treated at a dose of 55 Gy had local control of disease 1 year after surgery and radiation.[19]

Doxorubicin is believed to be a radiation sensitizer and may increase the effect of radiation on cancer cells when given at low dosages. Doxorubicin (10 mg/m² IV) was given weekly 1 hour before 51 Gy of orthovoltage radiation in 39 dogs with incompletely excised soft tissue sarcomas. Seven dogs (18%) developed local recurrence a median of 7 months after treatment; recurrence was more likely in dogs with grade 2 or 3 tumors. Six (15%) dogs developed distant metastases, two without local recurrence. The 1-, 2-, and 4-year survival rates were 85%, 79%, and 72%, respectively. Tumor control and patient survival were longer in dogs with grade 1 tumors.[20] This control was similar to that seen with higher doses of radiation therapy.

> **KEY POINT**
>
> *The response of soft tissue sarcomas to radiation therapy depends on the total dose delivered. Higher doses give longer control.*

With higher doses of radiation and with accelerated fractionation (i.e., more frequent treatments), response rates for soft tissue sarcoma continue to improve. In a study using a total dose of 63 Gy of megavoltage (cobalt-60) radiation delivered to the surgical site of incompletely excised soft tissue sarcomas, only eight of 48 (17%) tumors recurred a median of 23 months after treatment. These recurrences were at the margins of or just outside the radiation field, emphasizing the importance of pretreatment staging with CT or MRI to delineate tumor margins, which was not done on all dogs in this study. Another 8% of dogs developed metastases.[21] Median disease-free interval was 35.5 months. The 1- and 2-year survival rates were 87%, and the 5-year survival rate was 76%. Radiation doses of greater than 60 Gy apparently controlled soft tissue sarcoma effectively in dogs that could not be treated with radical surgery.

Recurrence after radiation therapy may be able to be successfully treated surgically. Three dogs that underwent surgical excision of a recurrence had a second remission of between 22 and 53 months.[21]

Adjunctive high-dose radiation therapy after an incomplete excision of a low-grade sarcoma has a high likelihood of long-term control. In some dogs, this provides an excellent, functionally better alternative to amputation (Figure 62-6).

The side effects of radiation are mainly limited to acute reactions that subside with supportive care, topical preparations, and pain medication.

CHEMOTHERAPY

For rare cases in which these tumors metastasize, or for dogs with grade 3 sarcomas, chemotherapy should be considered. Unfortunately, there are few published data regarding efficacy. In human patients with soft tissue sarcoma, doxorubicin is the adjunctive treatment of choice. Doxoru-

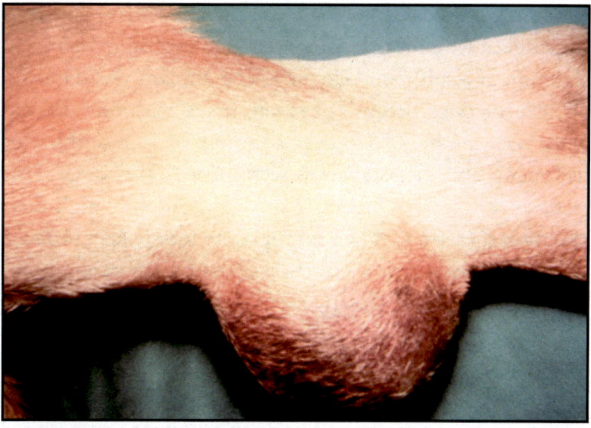

Figure 62-6. *This low-grade soft tissue sarcoma cannot be excised with adequate margins unless an amputation is performed. Narrow excision followed by radiation therapy provides a high likelihood of long-term control.*

bicin treatment caused three complete responses (CRs) and two partial responses (PRs) in 29 dogs with soft tissue sarcomas.[22] Another anecdotal remission was also seen.[23] In a preliminary report, 60 dogs with grade 3 soft tissue sarcomas were treated with surgery and doxorubicin.[9] Overall survival was greater if dogs received doxorubicin (7 months with doxorubicin versus 3 months without). The effect was not seen when 27 dogs with complete excisions were analyzed separately; the 23 dogs with an incomplete excision benefited most from adjuvant chemotherapy.

Mitoxantrone was used to treat 16 dogs with soft tissue sarcomas. Two dogs achieved CRs, and two dogs had PRs; these responses were for a median of 21 days (range: 16–63 days).[24]

Ifosfamide is an active agent in the treatment of soft tissue sarcomas in human patients. In a preliminary evaluation in dogs, CR was seen in a dog with leiomyosarcoma of the bladder.[25] A further study evaluated a combination of alternating ifosfamide and doxorubicin given to 12 dogs with soft tissue sarcomas; most were treated in the adjuvant setting, so no response rate was reported.[26]

An anecdotal partial remission was seen in a metastatic sarcoma after systemic cisplatin therapy.[27]

> **KEY POINT**
>
> *Adjuvant doxorubicin chemotherapy improves survival after surgery for dogs with* **high-grade, incompletely excised** *soft tissue sarcomas.*

In intralesional chemotherapy, the chemotherapeutic agent is mixed with a depot agent. This formulation may provide higher levels of chemotherapy in the tumor while releasing only small amounts of drug into the circulation. This approach has been successful in cats and horses.[28] Cisplatin in a degradable polymer (OPLA–Pt) was implanted in the surgical wounds of 30 dogs that had incomplete surgical resection of a soft tissue sarcoma. The implant was removed in 28% of dogs because of severe tissue reactions. Recurrence was seen in 30% of dogs a median of 21 months after treatment, and metastasis was seen in two (7%) dogs. This recurrence rate was higher than that seen with high-dose radiation therapy. Grade 3 tumors were more likely to recur (Figure 62-7).[7] Intralesional cisplatin treatment in combination with radiation therapy seemed to enhance antitumor response compared with radiation alone.[29]

Doxorubicin, possibly in combination with a platinum chemotherapy agent, is likely the best chemotherapy for dogs with metastatic lesions or as an adjunct to surgery for dogs with high-grade tumors.

BIOLOGIC RESPONSE MODIFIERS

A novel, orally administered, multitargeted indolinone receptor tyrosine kinase inhibitor, SU11654, appears to cause both direct antitumor and antiangiogenic effects. Measurable objective responses were observed in two dogs with soft tissue sarcomas.[30]

OTHER THERAPIES

A photosensitizing agent was given to 16 dogs with hemangiopericytomas, followed by surgical removal of the tumor and photodynamic therapy. Nine dogs (56%) had recurrence of tumor from 2 to 29 months (median: 9 months) after treatment. These results are not as good as those of other forms of therapy.[31]

SUPPORTIVE CARE

Supportive care is critical to successful treatment of soft tissue sarcomas and should include appropriate analgesia, nutritional support (including placement of gastrostomy or esophagostomy tubes if needed), and antiemetic therapy if needed. The placement of a vascular access port may be helpful in small dogs if radiation or chemotherapy is used because the multiple anesthesia and chemotherapy treatments result in poor peripheral vascular integrity.

Specific Subtypes of Soft Tissue Sarcomas

FIBROMAS AND FIBROSARCOMAS

Fibrosarcomas are relatively common in adult and aged dogs. There are no gender predilections. Breeds that were found to have a higher incidence in a series of 452 fibrosarcomas were Gordon setters, Irish wolfhounds, Brittanys, golden retrievers (neck and abdomen), and Doberman pinschers (on the back).[32] Fibrosarcomas may occur anywhere but are most common on the limbs (46%), head and neck (23%), and trunk (28%); they are rare on the tail and perineum, and fewer than 1% are multiple.[32] They vary in size and are usually poorly circumscribed, irregular, nonencapsulated, firm to fleshy nodules, with soft, friable, or ulcerated areas. They may be located subcutaneously or dermoepidermally. On cut surface, there may be a pattern of interweaving bands of white tissue with foci of hemorrhage and necrosis. They cannot be clinically distinguished from any other soft tissue sarcoma.

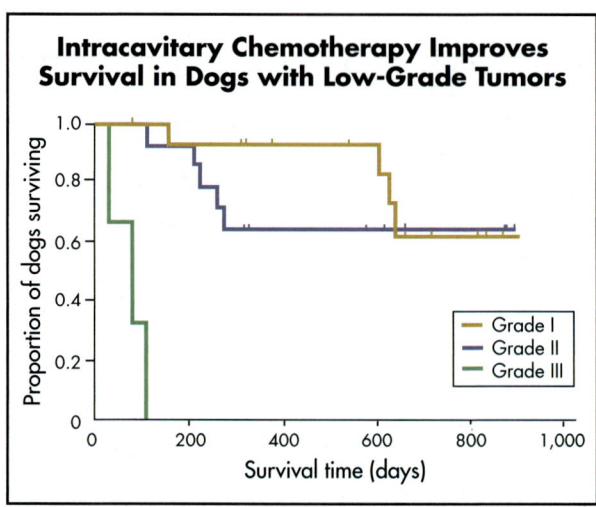

Figure 62-7. *Recurrence-free survival curves for 15 dogs with grade 1 tumors, 13 dogs with grade 2 tumors, and three dogs with grade 3 tumors treated using intracavitary cisplatin released from a polymer device (OPLA–Pt). The effect is the same as that seen with surgery alone. (From Dernell WS, Withrow SJ, Straw RC, et al: Intracavitary treatment of soft tissue sarcomas in dogs using cisplatin in a biodegradable polymer. Anticancer Res 17:4499–4505, 1997, with permission)*

HEMANGIOPERICYTOMAS (SPINDLE CELL SARCOMAS, DERMATOFIBROSARCOMAS)

Hemangiopericytomas were originally thought to derive from the pericytes of vessels; however, this theory of histogenesis is under debate.[33–35] Hemangiopericytomas tend to occur in adult to older animals. In one series of 1,939 hemangiopericytomas, females were twice as likely as males to develop a hemangiopericytoma.[33] Mixed-breed dogs were predisposed, with Siberian huskies the only pure breed at higher risk, particularly for tumors on the forelimb. In another study, boxers appeared to be overrepresented.[6] These tumors frequently occur over the joints of the limbs (68%; 38% of all affect forelimb) as masses that are solitary, subcutaneous, smooth to lobulated, firm, slow growing, and poorly circumscribed (Figure 62-4).[33] The other common location is the thoracic wall. Only 0.6% of 1,939 dogs had multiple tumors. As with other soft tissue sarcomas, the metastatic rate is low.

A number of histologic patterns have been described, of which the perivascular whorl pattern is the most common; hemangiopericytomas can also have a storiform pattern, myxoid foci, or an epithelioid pattern. None of these patterns was shown to have clinical or prognostic significance in one study,[33] although another, smaller study found that the epithelioid pattern was associated with a higher rate of metastasis.[35]

MYXOMAS AND MYXOSARCOMAS

These rare tumors consist of mucin-producing altered fibroblasts and act clinically like all soft tissue sarcomas. They usually occur in adult or aged animals (median age: 10 years). There are no gender predilections. Breeds that were found to be at higher risk for myxosarcomas in a study of 175 dogs were basset hounds and Doberman pinschers.[36] Most myxosarcomas occurred on the limbs (42%); 30% occurred on the thorax and abdomen. Multiple tumors are rare.[36]

In one series of 184 myxoid tumors, only nine (5%) were histologically benign.[36] Myxosarcomas usually are infiltrative growths with no definite shape (e.g., soft, slimy, and nonencapsulated). They are often grayish-white, with clear, viscid, honey-like areas visible on the cut surface. The tumors are difficult to remove completely but rarely metastasize.

LEIOMYOMAS AND LEIOMYOSARCOMAS

These tumors are extremely rare in the cutaneous tissues; benign or malignant tumors arise from arrector pili muscles. In a series of 29,150 cutaneous tumors, only 10 were piloleiomyomas.[37] Most were less than 1 cm in diameter and located on the back and neck of older dogs.

OTHER RARE SKIN MESENCHYMAL TUMORS

In a series of 29,150 skin tumors, there were six chondrosarcomas (rear limb and thorax, surgically excised), five osteosarcomas, one osteoma (surgically cured), and one chondroma (surgically cured).[37]

Cutaneous Nerve Sheath Tumors

Nerve sheath tumor, or neurofibrosarcoma, is the most common tumor of peripheral nerve tissue in dogs. It is sometimes termed schwannoma, neurilemmoma, or perineural fibroblastoma. Primary cutaneous nerve sheath tumors are rare. They occur in adult to aged animals without gender predilection. In a series of 124 dogs, only golden retrievers were found to be at increased risk of developing cutaneous nerve sheath tumors. These tumors are most common on the limbs (51%, with 35% in the forelimb); another 30% occur in the skin of the head.[38] Nerve sheath tumors tend to be solitary but can be multiple (tortuous and nodular enlargement of nerve or "chains of nodes," called *neurofibromatosis*). They often grow large rapidly and tend to be firm, poorly demarcated, adherent to overlying skin, and ulcerative. As with all soft tissue sarcomas, the clinical behavior is similar regardless of whether the diagnosis is neurofibroma or neurofibrosarcoma. They are prone to regrowth and are invasive but rarely metastasize.

Nerve Sheath Tumors of the Nerve Roots
INCIDENCE, SIGNALMENT, AND ETIOLOGY

In dogs, nerve sheath tumors commonly arise from fibrous nerve sheaths and usually involve spinal or cranial nerve roots (most commonly the brachial plexus). Clinically, they behave like any soft tissue sarcoma (i.e., the probability of metastasis and aggressive local invasion of surrounding tissue is low). Middle-aged dogs (median: 7 years; range: 4–9 years) are predisposed to cervical neurofibrosarcomas; there is no obvious breed or gender predilection. Large-breed dogs have been reported to be commonly affected,[39] although small dogs accounted for 10 of 13 cases in one study[40] and dog sizes were randomly distributed in another large study.[41] Neurofibrosarcomas also occur in the thoracolumbar region as intradural–extramedullary tumors (see Chapter 49).

CLINICAL PRESENTATION AND HISTORY

The most common clinical sign of nerve sheath tumor in dogs is forelimb lameness that progresses slowly because of brachial plexus involvement. Neurologic deficits are minimal, but severe muscle atrophy, particularly of the scapular musculature, is common (Figure 62-8). Depending on the nerves involved, Horner's syndrome may be present. The tumors occasionally extend through the intervertebral foramen to compress the spinal cord, resulting in neurologic deficits in the ipsilateral pelvic limb. The history of lameness is usually chronic, extending over many months. A large mass may be palpated deep within the axilla, but small tumors may not be detectable on palpation; only 14 of 71 dogs in two series had a palpable mass.[41,42] Pain is an inconsistent finding, although when present, it may be marked, especially on palpation around the affected area.[41]

A series of 10 dogs with nerve sheath tumors of the trigeminal nerve were described. Affected dogs had no signalment predispositions, and all had ipsilateral atrophy of the temporalis and masseter muscles (Figure 62-9). Some dogs had decreased facial and corneal sensation as well as other signs consistent with trigeminal nerve damage. Invasion of the brain stem was seen in three dogs.[43]

STAGING AND DIAGNOSIS

After a general health screen is completed and other causes of lameness and muscle wasting are ruled out, if a tumor of the brachial plexus is suspected, staging should include advanced imaging. Survey radiographs are rarely helpful because bony lysis is rare. CT or MRI should be conducted before treating brachial plexus neurofibrosarcomas

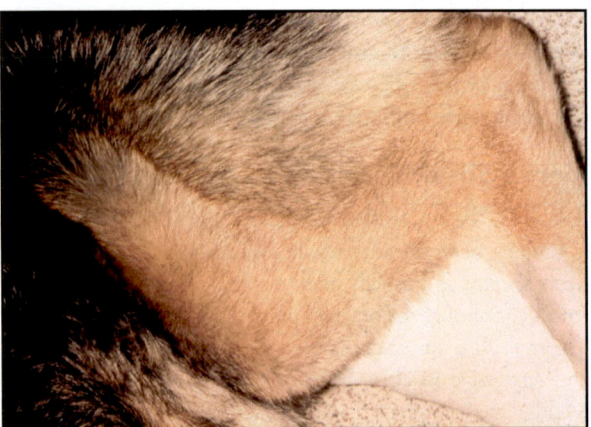

Figure 62-8. *The most common clinical sign of nerve sheath tumor in dogs is forelimb lameness that progresses slowly because of brachial plexus involvement. Neurologic deficits are minimal, but severe muscle atrophy, particularly of the scapular musculature, is common.*

because of the propensity of these tumors to invade the intervertebral foramen, even if the dog shows no hindlimb signs. When 51 cases were classified according to their location, eight tumors were localized distal to the brachial or lumbosacral plexus, 20 dogs had a tumor that involved the plexus (nine had a palpable mass), and 23 tumors invaded the intervertebral foramen (three dogs had a palpable mass).[41] The tumor involved a single nerve in 27 dogs and multiple nerves in 17 dogs.[41]

Electromyography may localize a lesion to a particular nerve but is not specific for a nerve sheath tumor.

CT scanning and MRI are the most accurate ways to image these tumors (Figure 62-10). One study characterized the CT appearance of 24 masses of the brachial plexus and contributing nerve roots in dogs and determined the minimum detectable mass size. Masses ranged from 1.0 to 6.5 cm in diameter. The presence or absence of contrast enhancement, the margin character, the size, the extent of local invasion, and the presence of vertebral canal or spinal cord involvement did not appear to correlate with histology or clinical behavior.[42] For smaller nerves (e.g., the sciatic), MRI may be more able to detect a small mass.

One dog that had two surgical resections of a brachial plexus neurofibrosarcoma developed pulmonary metastases 20 months after the first surgery,[39] but this is rare. Of 51 affected dogs in another study, none died from detectable metastases.[41]

TREATMENT

Peripheral nerve tumors are locally invasive and rarely metastasize; thus, the treatment of choice is surgical excision. For small tumors that involve only one or two nerves, excision of affected nerves close to the intervertebral foramen may allow complete resection.[44] For large tumors that involve multiple nerves, or for dogs with severe neurologic

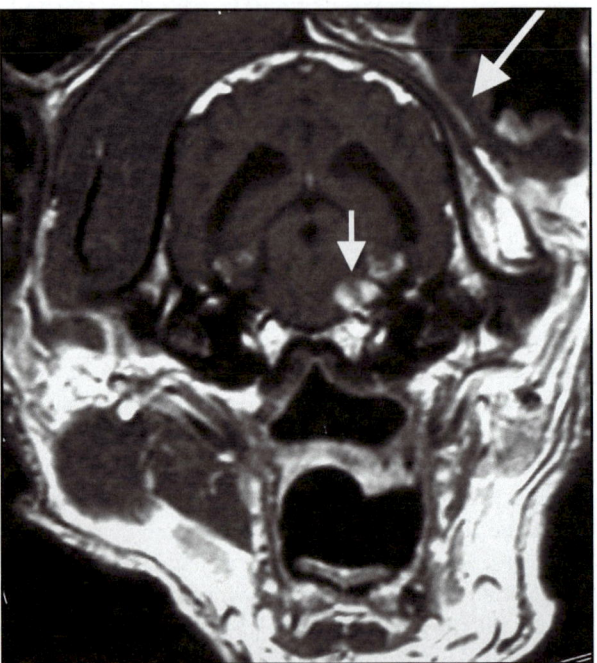

Figure 62-9. *A transverse T1-weighted postcontrast MRI image of the brain of a dog evaluated for unilateral atrophy of the temporalis and masseter muscles. At the level of the pons, the trigeminal nerve is enlarged and strongly contrast enhanced* (small arrow). *The diagnosis was nerve sheath tumor affecting the trigeminal nerve. Note the atrophy of the temporalis and masseter muscles* (large arrow). *(Courtesy of Marc Kent, DVM, University of Georgia College of Veterinary Medicine)*

deficits in the forelimb, amputation should be considered. If the tumor extends into the spinal canal, the prognosis is guarded because surgical excision (even with laminectomy) is unlikely to be complete. The owner of an animal with any neurofibrosarcoma should be warned that excision may not be complete and local recurrence is possible.

In a series of 47 dogs that were treated by one or more surgeries (local resection, 30 dogs; amputation, 14 dogs; hemilaminectomy, 21 dogs), those with a peripheral tumor had the longest survival times, with only one of nine dogs having a recurrence.[41] Median relapse-free survival was 7.5 months (range: 0–43 months) for dogs with plexus tumors and 1 month (range: 0–14 months) for dogs with tumors invading the intervertebral foramen. Corresponding survival times were 12 months and 5 months. Only six dogs with plexus or invasive tumors were tumor free 1 year after surgery, echoing a previous, smaller study.[39]

For a small series of dogs with trigeminal nerve sheath tumors, surgical exposure of the tumor required a craniotomy to expose the tumor in the calvarium; in two of three dogs, the tumor could not be completely resected.[43]

Because nerve sheath tumors respond poorly to surgery alone and yet have a low metastatic rate, radiation therapy is warranted to decrease local recurrence. There are no spe-

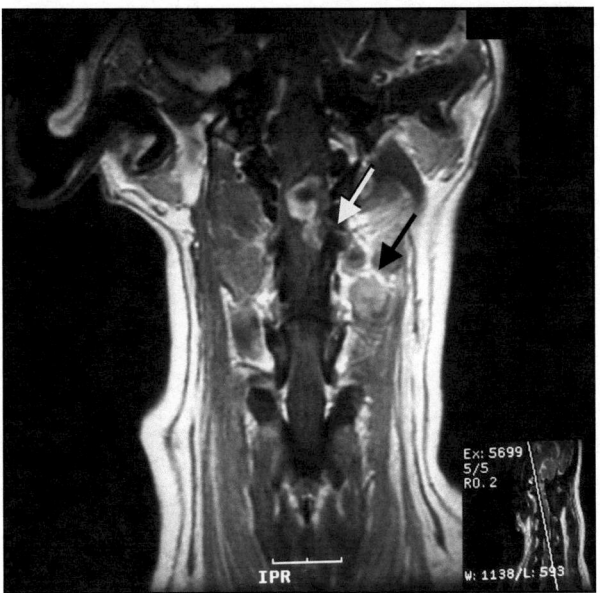

Figure 62-10. *A dorsal T1-weighted postcontrast MRI image of the cranial cervical vertebral column of a dog. There is an intraaxial mass affecting the spinal cord at the atlantoaxial articulation. The mass is a nerve sheath tumor originating from the C2 spinal nerve. It can be seen traversing the vertebral foramen* (white arrow) *and extending into the paravertebral musculature* (black arrow). *(Courtesy of M. Kent)*

cific reports of the efficacy of adjunctive radiation therapy for brachial plexus nerve sheath tumors, although responses similar to those reported for other soft tissue sarcomas are likely. Remission durations and cure rates for dogs with soft tissue sarcomas treated with radiation therapy largely depend on the dose of radiation delivered (see Radiation Therapy section, above). Radiation therapy is probably the adjunctive therapy of choice in the treatment of peripheral nerve sheath sarcomas in dogs; however, irradiation of the spinal cord may limit the dose of radiation able to be safely delivered.

Unless access to aggressive surgery and radiotherapy is limited, chemotherapy for brachial plexus neurofibrosarcoma is rarely justified because the metastatic rate is low. For metastatic tumors, an approach as outlined above for soft tissue sarcomas is recommended.

Retroperitoneal Sarcomas

Although retroperitoneal sarcomas are comparatively rare tumors and are not expected to have a biologic behavior that differs from that of soft tissue sarcomas at other locations, the retroperitoneal space offers a unique set of therapeutic challenges because of the visceral structures found in close proximity to this area.

The most common histologic type of retroperitoneal sarcoma is hemangiosarcoma, accounting for nine of 14 dogs in one study. Osteosarcoma was described in two dogs, and leiomyosarcoma, nerve sheath tumor, and hemangiopericytoma were each described in one dog.[45] Most tumors (57%) were grade 3. Median survival was 1 month. The only long-term survivor was a dog with a grade 2 leiomyosarcoma (13 months). Case reports of mesenchymoma and chondrosarcomas have detailed similar poor survival.[46–48]

Chemotherapy with doxorubicin-based protocols was not completed in four dogs because of recurrence or metastases.[45,46]

Synovial Cell Sarcoma and Other Joint Sarcomas

INCIDENCE, SIGNALMENT, AND ETIOLOGY

Synovial cell sarcoma is rare in dogs. It arises from the synovioblastic mesenchymal tissue deep in the connective tissue adjacent to joints. In four reviews totaling 110 reported cases, this tumor was found to occur primarily in male dogs (male:female ratio: 1.5:1.0) at a median age of 7 to 9 years (range: 1–14 years).[49,50] There was no obvious breed predisposition, although the disease is most common in large-breed dogs (median weight: 22 kg).

Synovial cell sarcoma occurred in the stifle in 41 of 96 dogs; the next most commonly affected sites were the elbow and hock (17 and 14 dogs, respectively). Tumors were also diagnosed in the shoulder, carpus, metatarsus, digit, radius, hip, and femur.[49–51] One study found a 3:1 predilection for the right side among 35 dogs with synovial sarcoma[50]; this was not seen in other smaller studies.[51]

What was originally thought to be an only mildly heterogeneous group of tumors may actually represent a wide range of histologic subtypes. Two large studies found that only 13 of 65 joint-associated tumors (20%) were synovial sarcomas.[52,53] In one of these studies, an additional six dogs had synovial myxomas, and most of the remainder (20 dogs; 57%) had histiocytic sarcomas based on positive immunostaining for CD18 (histiocytic cell marker).[53] Rottweilers accounted for more than 60% of this group. The most commonly affected site was the stifle.[53] Histiocytic sarcomas are recognized as being aggressive, often high-grade tumors (see Chapter 63). Another study found that of 30 dogs with tumors involving the joint, only six were true synovial sarcomas, with fibrosarcomas and rhabdomyosarcomas the next most common.[52] Biopsy is required to make a definitive diagnosis.

STAGING AND DIAGNOSIS

Evaluation of a patient with a joint soft tissue sarcoma includes an MDB as well as high-detail radiographs of the affected joint. Dogs with synovial sarcomas often have considerable lysis of bone on both sides of the joint space, unlike those with primary bone tumors, which are limited to one bone (Figures 62-11 and 62-12).[54] Ultra-

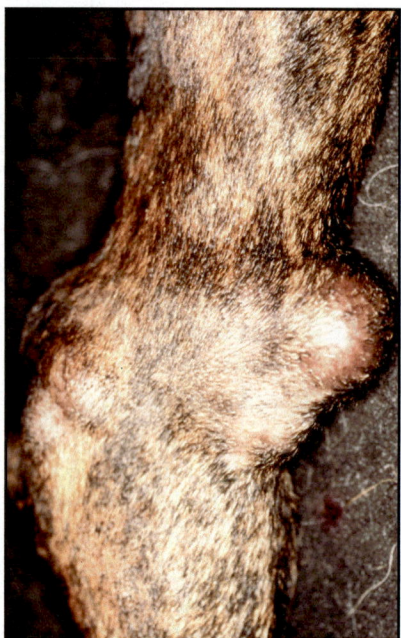

Figure 62-11. *A synovial sarcoma surrounding the hock of a dog presented with lameness and obvious masses around the joint. (Courtesy of J. Berg)*

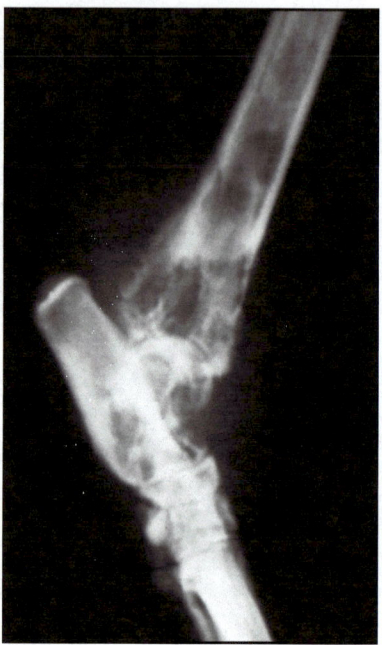

Figure 62-12. *The same dog as in Figure 62-9. Note the radiographic lysis of bones on both sides of the joint, unlike a primary bone tumor, which is restricted to one side of the joint. (Courtesy of J. Berg)*

sonography of the joint space may provide additional information as to the location and extent of the tumor and may guide a biopsy.[55] Some synovial sarcomas of the stifle have recurred at the stump of an amputation; therefore, margins should be evaluated with CT or MRI before surgery.

Of 72 dogs with synovial sarcoma, 20 (23%) had metastases detected at the time of diagnosis and 23 (32%) ultimately developed metastatic tumors. Metastases to the lungs, regional lymph node, and kidney (five dogs) were seen between 6 weeks and 18 months after diagnosis.[49,50]

Histologically, synovial sarcoma is biphasic,[50] meaning that the tumor has varying amounts of epithelioid (synovioblastic) and fibroblastic components. Although one study found that the presence of cytokeratin (an epithelial marker) in tumor cells was a negative prognostic factor,[50] a smaller study found no synovial sarcomas that stained for cytokeratin.[51] To further complicate the picture, two large studies found that only 20% of joint tumors were synovial sarcomas and stained positive for cytokeratin.[52,53] In one study, 57% of dogs with a joint tumor had histiocytic sarcomas based on positive immunostaining for CD18. Synovial sarcomas had a 25% metastatic rate compared with 91% of histiocytic sarcomas. Synovial myxomas did not metastasize.[53]

Part of the staging for a dog with a suspected synovial sarcoma should include immunostaining for cytokeratin and CD18.

PROGNOSTIC FACTORS

A histologic grading system, outlined in Table 62-3, was applied to a study of 36 synovial sarcomas in dogs.[50] Dogs with tumors that had a high mitotic rate, a high degree of nuclear pleomorphism, and a high percentage of necrosis had poor survival, and their tumors were more likely to recur. This same system also showed that dogs with grade 3 tumors had a median survival of 7 months compared with 35.5 months for dogs with grade 1 or 2 tumors. Dogs that had tumors with a high epithelial component as measured by cytokeratin immunohistochemistry had shorter tumor-free remission times than those with tumors that were cytokeratin negative (3.5 months versus >14 months). Cytokeratin staining may be conducted at certain veterinary pathology laboratories.

TREATMENT

Tumors removed by marginal resection recur rapidly (median: 4.5 months); however, amputation improves local tumor control. In one study of 29 dogs that were treated by amputation, the overall median survival time was 30 months. Two dogs had a local stump recurrence, and four developed metastases in a median of 5 months (range: 2–13 months). Of the remainder, more than half were tumor-free 3 years after surgery.[50]

In another study, dogs with synovial tumors of histiocytic origin had a median survival time of 5.3 months; survival times for dogs with undifferentiated sarcomas, synovial sarcomas, and myxomas were 3.5, 31.8, and 30.7 months,

SOFT TISSUE SARCOMAS

Table 62-3 Variables Used to Determine Histologic Grade of Canine Synovial Sarcoma[50]

Score	Giant cells	Demarcation	Mitotic index	Multinucleated cells	Tumor necrosis	Invasiveness
0	None	—	—	None	None	—
1	Few	Well	0–10	Few	1%–14%	Into connective tissue
2	Moderate	Moderate	11–20	Moderate	15%–30%	Into muscle
3	Marked	Poor	21–30	Marked	>30%	Into bone
4	—	—	>30	—	—	—

Grade	Description
1	Cumulative score of ≤4
2	Cumulative score of 5–7
3	Cumulative score of ≥8

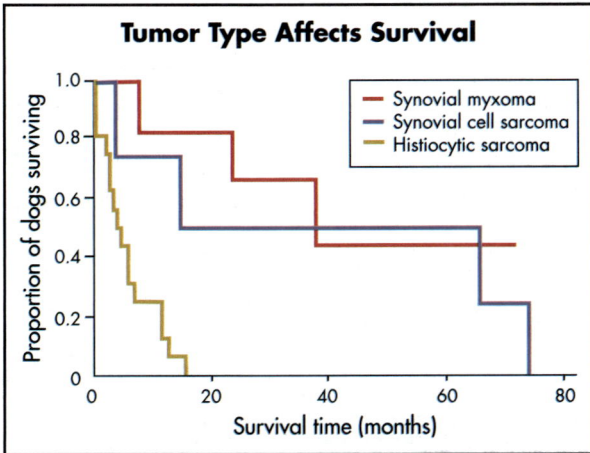

Figure 62-13. Recurrence-free survival curves for synovial tumors that were of histiocytic origin (median: 5.3 months), synovial sarcomas (median: 31.8 months), and myxomas (median: 30.7 months). (From Craig LE, Julian ME, Ferracone JD: The diagnosis and prognosis of synovial tumors in dogs: 35 cases. Vet Pathol 39:66–73, 2002; with permission)

respectively (Figure 62-13).[53] Two dogs with synovial myxomas were treated only with palliative antiinflammatory drugs and were alive more than 2 years after diagnosis,[53] as was another dog treated surgically.[56]

Adjunctive radiation therapy as described for other soft tissue sarcomas would be the most likely therapy to improve local control rates in dogs not suitable for amputation. Only anecdotal information of efficacy exists, with one dog having tumor control for more than 18 months after radiation (four 10-Gy doses) for a tumor that had recurred twice after surgery alone.[57] Another dog had radiation therapy after an incomplete excision and died without recurrence 2 years later.[50]

Chemotherapy using doxorubicin (30 mg/m² IV) has been reported to provide long-term response in dogs with synovial sarcoma.[22,58] In contrast, five dogs that received doxorubicin (one dog); doxorubicin and cyclophosphamide (one dog); cyclophosphamide, vincristine, and prednisone (one dog); cyclophosphamide and prednisolone (one dog); or piroxicam (one dog) showed no measurable tumor responses.[50,52] Other dogs have received doxorubicin, mitoxantrone, or cyclophosphamide as an adjunct to surgery, but the contribution to survival is difficult to assess.[51,53]

REFERENCES

1. Williamson MM, Middleton DJ: Cutaneous soft tissue tumours in dogs: Classification, differentiation, and histogenesis. Vet Dermatol 9:43–48, 1998.
2. Vascellari M, Melchiotti E, Bozza MA, Mutinelli F: Fibrosarcomas at presumed sites of injection in dogs: Characteristics and comparison with non-vaccination site fibrosarcomas and feline post-vaccinal fibrosarcomas. J Vet Med A Physiol Pathol Clin Med 50:286–291, 2003.
3. Rowland PH, Moise NS, Severson D: Myxoma at the site of a subcutaneous pacemaker in a dog. JAAHA 27:649–651, 1991.
4. Kuntz CA, Dernell WS, Powers BE, et al: Prognostic factors for surgical treatment of soft-tissue sarcomas in dogs: 75 cases (1986–1996). JAVMA 211:1147–1151, 1997.
5. Baker-Gabb M, Hunt GB, France MP: Soft tissue sarcomas and mast cell tumours in dogs; clinical behaviour and response to surgery. Aust Vet J 81:732–738, 2003.
6. Bostock DE, Dye MT: Prognosis after surgical excision of canine fibrous connective tissue sarcomas. Vet Pathol 17:581–588, 1980.
7. Dernell WS, Withrow SJ, Straw RC, et al: Intracavitary treatment of soft tissue sarcomas in dogs using cisplatin in a biodegradable polymer. Anticancer Res 17:4499–4505, 1997.
8. Saik JE, Diters RW, Wortman JA: Metastasis of a well-differentiated liposarcoma in a dog and a note on nomenclature of fatty tumours. J Comp Pathol 97:369–373, 1987.
9. Selting KA, Powers BE, Mittleman E, et al: Adjuvant chemotherapy for canine high-grade soft tissue sarcomas. Proc 23rd Annu Conf Vet Cancer Soc:53, 2003.
10. Evans SM: Canine hemangiopericytoma. A retrospective analysis of response to surgery and orthovoltage radiation. Vet Radiol 28:13–16, 1987.
11. Seitz SE, Foley GL, Marretta SM: Evaluation of marking materials for cutaneous surgical margins. Am J Vet Res 56:826–833, 1995.
12. Banks TA, Straw RC, Withrow SJ, et al: Prospective study of canine soft tissue sarcoma treated by wide surgical excision: Quantitative evaluation of surgical margins. Proc 23rd Annu Conf Vet Cancer Soc:21, 2003.
13. Trout NJ, Pavletic MM, Kraus KH: Partial scapulectomy for management of sarcomas in three dogs and two cats. JAVMA 207:585–587, 1995.
14. Connery NA, Bellenger CR: Surgical management of haemangiopericytoma involving the biceps femoris muscle in four dogs. J Small Anim Pract 43:497–500, 2002.

15. Hilmas DE, Gillette EL: Radiotherapy of spontaneous fibrous connective-tissue sarcomas in animals. *J Natl Cancer Inst* 56:365–368, 1976.
16. Brewer WG Jr, Turrel JM: Radiotherapy and hyperthermia in the treatment of fibrosarcomas in the dog. *JAVMA* 181:146–150, 1982.
17. Graves GM, Bjorling DE, Mahaffey E: Canine hemangiopericytoma: 23 cases (1967–1984). *JAVMA* 192:99–101, 1988.
18. McChesney SL, Withrow SJ, Gillette EL, et al: Radiotherapy of soft tissue sarcomas in dogs. *JAVMA* 194:60–63, 1989.
19. McChesney SL, Gillette EL, Dewhirst MW, Withrow SJ: Influence of WR 2721 on radiation response of canine soft tissue sarcomas. *Int J Radiat Oncol Biol Phys* 12:1957–1963, 1986.
20. Simon D, Ruslander DM, Rassnick KM, et al: Combination of orthovoltage radiation therapy and weekly low-dose doxorubicin for incompletely excised soft tissue sarcomas in 39 dogs. *Vet Rec*, in press.
21. McKnight JA, Mauldin GN, McEntee MC, et al: Radiation treatment for incompletely resected soft-tissue sarcomas in dogs. *JAVMA* 217:205–210, 2000.
22. Ogilvie GK, Reynolds HA, Richardson RC, et al: Phase II evaluation of doxorubicin for treatment of various canine neoplasms. *JAVMA* 195:1580–1583, 1989.
23. Schoster JV, Wyman M: Remission of orbital sarcoma in a dog, using doxorubicin therapy. *JAVMA* 172:1101–1103, 1978.
24. Ogilvie GK, Obradovich JE, Elmslie RE, et al: Efficacy of mitoxantrone against various neoplasms in dogs. *JAVMA* 198:1618–1621, 1991.
25. Rassnick KM, Frimberger AE, Wood CA, et al: Evaluation of ifosfamide for treatment of various canine neoplasms. *J Vet Intern Med* 14:271–276, 2000.
26. Payne SE, Rassnick KM, Northrup NC, et al: Treatment of vascular and soft-tissue sarcomas in dogs using an alternating protocol of ifosfamide and doxorubicin. *Vet Comp Oncol* 1:171–179, 2003.
27. Hahn KA, Richardson RC: Use of cisplatin for control of metastatic malignant mesenchymoma and hypertrophic osteopathy in a dog. *JAVMA* 195:351–353, 1989.
28. Orenberg EK, Luck EE, Brown DM, Kitchell BE: Implant delivery system: Intralesional delivery of chemotherapeutic agents for treatment of spontaneous skin tumors in veterinary patients. *Clin Dermatol* 9:561–568, 1992.
29. Theon AP, Madewell BR, Ryu J, Castro J: Concurrent irradiation and intratumoral chemotherapy with cisplatin: A pilot study in dogs with spontaneous tumors. *Int J Radiat Oncol Biol Phys* 29:1027–1034, 1994.
30. London CA, Hannah AL, Zadovoskaya R, et al: Phase I dose-escalating study of SU11654, a small molecule receptor tyrosine kinase inhibitor, in dogs with spontaneous malignancies. *Clin Cancer Res* 9:2755–2768, 2003.
31. McCaw DL, Payne JT, Pope ER, et al: Treatment of canine hemangiopericytomas with photodynamic therapy. *Lasers Surg Med* 29:23–26, 2001.
32. Goldschmidt MH, Shofer FS: Cutaneous fibrosarcoma, in Goldschmidt MH, Shofer FS (eds): *Skin Tumors of the Dog and Cat.* Tarrytown, NY, Pergamon Press, 1992, pp 158–167.
33. Goldschmidt MH, Shofer FS: Canine hemangiopericytoma, in Goldschmidt MH, Shofer FS (eds): *Skin Tumors of the Dog and Cat.* Tarrytown, NY, Pergamon Press, 1992, pp 168–174.
34. Perez J, Bautista MJ, Rollon E, et al: Immunohistochemical characterization of hemangiopericytomas and other spindle cell tumors in the dog. *Vet Pathol* 33:391–397, 1996.
35. Mazzei M, Millanta F, Citi S, et al: Haemangiopericytoma: Histological spectrum, immunohistochemical characterization and prognosis. *Vet Dermatol* 13:15–21, 2002.
36. Goldschmidt MH, Shofer FS: Cutaneous myxoma and myxosarcoma, in Goldschmidt MH, Shofer FS (eds): *Skin Tumors of the Dog and Cat.* Tarrytown, NY, Pergamon Press, 1992, pp 179–183.
37. Goldschmidt MH, Shofer FS: Uncommon skin tumors, in: Goldschmidt MH, Shofer FS (eds): *Skin Tumors of the Dog and Cat.* Tarrytown, NY, Pergamon Press, 1992, pp 291–295.
38. Goldschmidt MH, Shofer FS: Cutaneous tumors of neural differentiation, in: Goldschmidt MH, Shofer FS (eds): *Skin Tumors of the Dog and Cat.* Tarrytown, NY, Pergamon Press, 1992, pp 184–191.
39. Bradley RL, Withrow SJ, Shyder SP: Nerve sheath tumors in the dog. *JAAHA* 18:915–921, 1982.
40. Forterre F, Matiasek K, Schmahl W, Brunnberg L: Periphere nervenerkrankungen: Teil I Monoparese, -plegie bei hund und katze: Retrospective studie über 94 fälle. *Kleintierpraxis* 48:141–150, 2003.
41. Brehm DV, Vite CH, Steinberg HS, et al: A retrospective evaluation of 51 cases of peripheral nerve sheath tumors in the dog. *JAAHA* 31:349–359, 1995.
42. Rudich SR, Feeney DA, Anderson KL, Walter PA: Computed tomography of masses of the brachial plexus and contributing nerve roots in dogs. *Vet Radiol Ultrasound* 45:46–50, 2004.
43. Bagley RS, Wheeler SJ, Klopp L, et al: Clinical features of trigeminal nerve-sheath tumor in 10 dogs. *JAAHA* 34:19–25, 1998.
44. Simpson DJ, Beck JA, Allan GS, Culvenor JA: Diagnosis and excision of a brachial plexus nerve sheath tumour in a dog. *Aust Vet J* 77:222–224, 1999.
45. Liptak JM, Dernell WS, Ehrhart EJ, et al: Retroperitoneal sarcomas in dogs: 14 cases (1992–2002). *JAVMA* 224:1471–1477, 2004.
46. Robinson TM, Dubielzig RR, McAnulty JF: Malignant mesenchymoma associated with an unusual vasoinvasive metastasis in a dog. *JAAHA* 34:295–299, 1998.
47. Munday JS, Prahl A: Retroperitoneal extraskeletal mesenchymal chondrosarcoma in a dog. *J Vet Diagn Invest* 14:498–500, 2002.
48. Rhind SM, Welsh E: Mesenchymal chondrosarcoma in a young German shepherd dog. *J Small Anim Pract* 40:443–445, 1999.
49. McGlennon NJ, Houlton JEF, Gorman NT: Synovial sarcoma in the dog—A review. *J Small Anim Pract* 29:139–152, 1988.
50. Vail DM, Powers BE, Getzy DM, et al: Evaluation of prognostic factors for dogs with synovial sarcoma: 36 cases (1986–1991). *JAVMA* 205:1300–1307, 1994.
51. Fox DB, Cook JL, Kreeger JM, et al: Canine synovial sarcoma: A retrospective assessment of described prognostic criteria in 16 cases (1994–1999). *JAAHA* 38:347–355, 2002.
52. Whitelock RG, Dyce J, Houlton JE, Jefferies AR: A review of 30 tumours affecting joints. *Vet Comp Orthop Traumatol* 10:152, 1997.
53. Craig LE, Julian ME, Ferracone JD: The diagnosis and prognosis of synovial tumors in dogs: 35 cases. *Vet Pathol* 39:66–73, 2002.
54. Madewell BR, Pool R: Neoplasms of joints and related structures. *Vet Clin North Am* 8:511–521, 1978.
55. Kramer M, Stengel H, Gerwing M, et al: Sonography of the canine stifle. *Vet Radiol Ultrasound* 40:282–293, 1999.
56. Berrocal A, Millan Y, Ordas J, de las Mulas JM: A joint myxoma in a dog. *J Comp Pathol* 124:223–226, 2001.
57. Lipowitz AJ, Fetter AW, Walker MA: Synovial sarcoma of the dog. *JAVMA* 174:76–81, 1979.
58. Tilmant LL, Gorman NT, Ackerman N, et al: Chemotherapy of synovial cell sarcoma in a dog. *JAVMA* 188:530–532, 1986.

TUMORS OF THE BODY CAVITIES

Antony S. Moore and Gregory K. Ogilvie

CLINICAL BRIEFING

Minimum database (MDB) includes a CBC, biochemical profile, and urinalysis, as well as thoracic radiography (three views).

Mesothelioma

Clinical presentation	• Effusion of body cavities causing abdominal discomfort, tachypnea, and respiratory distress. • In decreasing order of incidence, affects pleural, peritoneal, or pericardial cavities. • Epithelial-type mesothelioma is most common. • Occurs in older dogs. • Exposure to asbestos and pesticide powders may be associated with development of mesothelioma.
Staging and diagnosis	• MDB and thoracic and abdominal ultrasonography. • Metastasis uncommon.
Prognostic factors	• None identified.
Treatment Initial	• Surgery is unlikely to be curative. • Chemotherapy with intracavitary cisplatin may provide palliation; responses to IV doxorubicin and mitoxantrone have been noted.
Supportive	• Drainage of fluid may be palliative. • Analgesia postoperatively and nutritional support as needed.

Thymoma

Clinical presentation	• Cough; less commonly, dyspnea, regurgitation and lethargy; rarely, polyuria/polydipsia from hypercalcemia. • May have aspiration pneumonia secondary to myasthenia gravis and megaesophagus. • Epithelial malignant component associated with mature lymphocytes and mast cells. • Older dogs and female dogs possibly predisposed. • Usually large, invasive, slowly growing tumors with low metastatic rate. • Paraneoplastic syndromes are common. Myasthenia gravis is most common; polymyositis, hypercalcemia, and second malignancies may occur.
Staging and diagnosis	• MDB and thoracic ultrasonography. • Metastasis uncommon.
Prognostic factors	• Dogs with megaesophagus have very poor prognosis.

SPECIFIC DISEASES

Treatment	
Initial	• Surgery may be curative for small or encapsulated tumors; dogs with megaesophagus need to be monitored for aspiration pneumonia; most thymomas are unresectable.
Adjunctive	• Radiation therapy may be useful in reducing tumor before surgery or to palliate nonresectable thymoma.
	• Chemotherapy uncertain; prednisone and platinum agents may be most active. Lymphocyte-rich thymomas may respond to drugs used to treat lymphoma.
Supportive	• Corticosteroids and possibly anticholinesterase therapy (pyridostigmine) before surgery to reduce myasthenia gravis and resolve megaesophagus. Antibiotics to reduce the risk of aspiration pneumonia.
Histiocytic Diseases	
Common presentation	• Benign cutaneous histiocytoma.
	• Reactive histiocytic diseases: Cutaneous histiocytosis, systemic histiocytosis, splenic histiocytic nodules, and splenic histiocytosis.
	• Malignant histiocytic diseases: Disseminated histiocytic sarcoma (malignant histiocytosis), localized histiocytic sarcoma.
	• These diseases have a spectrum of signs and outcomes.
Staging and diagnosis	• MDB and abdominal ultrasonography.
	• Bone marrow aspiration.
	• Used to separate reactive from malignant forms.
	• Immunohistochemistry to differentiate malignant forms from other neoplasms (CD18 positive).
Prognostic factors	• Thrombocytopenia and hypoalbuminemia are predictors of poor prognosis for malignant forms.
Treatment	
Benign cutaneous histiocytoma	• Surgery curative.
	• Even multiple tumors regress spontaneously.
Reactive histiocytic diseases	• Some regress spontaneously.
	• Immunosuppressive therapy (corticosteroids, cyclosporine, leflunomide).
Malignant histiocytic diseases	• Initial: Surgery for localized disease (usually skin).
	• Adjunctive: Radiation therapy may be palliative. Chemotherapy for localized and disseminated forms. CCNU and other lymphoma drugs may be useful. Immunosuppressive therapy not reported.
	• Supportive: Blood products and plasma transfusions, antibiotics.

Mesothelioma

Normal mesothelial cells line the serosal surfaces of the pleural, pericardial, and peritoneal cavities and the surface of the testes as a single layer. When mesothelial cells are altered by malignancy or inflammation, they take on cytologically similar reactive characteristics, making it difficult to distinguish between neoplastic and activated mesothelial cells.

Neoplastic involvement of the visceral or parietal serosa is almost invariably associated with effusion. Pleural and peritoneal fluids are normally present in minute amounts that are controlled by hydrostatic and colloid osmotic pressures. The small amount of protein normally leaked from capillaries is reabsorbed by lymphatic drainage. Neoplastic involvement of the serosa disrupts capillary integrity, which allows increased protein exudation. Tumor cells may obstruct lymphatic drainage and cause accumulation of fluid. The process may be accelerated by inflammatory reaction to the tumor cells.

Mesothelioma is rare in dogs. Malignant effusion is often a result of other tumors, such as metastatic or primary lung tumors, mammary or prostatic carcinomas, or tumors from other sites. These tumors are rarely large enough to be seen by radiography, ultrasonography, or computed tomography (CT), although effusion may be identified.

INCIDENCE, SIGNALMENT, AND ETIOLOGY

Mesotheliomas are rare in all species. In humans, the development of mesothelioma after exposure to asbestos by inhalation is well documented, although it may take decades to arise. Some dogs with mesothelioma have higher levels of chrysotile asbestos fibers in their lungs than control dogs.[1,2] Affected dogs seem to have greater environmental exposure to asbestos than control dogs.[1] Exposure to pesticides is a cofactor that apparently increases the risk of mesothelioma formation, and dogs in urban environments seem to be at higher risk.[1]

Mesothelioma generally occurs in older dogs; the average age is 8 years,[1–8] although affected dogs range from 11 months to 15 years of age.[2,9–11] The tumor is more common in males than in females. There does not seem to be any strong breed predilection, but one study found that Bouvier des Flandres, Irish setters, and German shepherds are at increased risk.[1]

CLINICAL PRESENTATION AND HISTORY

Clinical signs largely depend on the site of involvement with mesothelioma. Involvement of single body cavities such as the pleural cavity, pericardial sac, or peritoneal cavity is most common. More than one cavity (e.g., pleural and peritoneal cavities,[1,2] pericardial sac and pleural[2] or peritoneal cavities[6]) may be involved. Mesothelioma of the tunica vaginalis has also been documented.[7] Most reported cases involve the thoracic cavity, reflected by the common clinical findings of tachypnea, respiratory distress, decreased exercise tolerance, and cough.[2,4,10] Clinical signs have usually been obvious to the owner for 1 month.[2] The clinical course

> **KEY POINT**
>
> *The clinical history for a dog with mesothelioma may be prolonged.*

of this disease can be prolonged; one dog with mesothelioma remained asymptomatic for pleural masses and effusion for 33 months,[11] another dog had a 2.5-year history of ascites treated by periodic drainage,[8] and a third dog was treated for pericardial effusion for more than 15 months before mesothelioma was diagnosed.[12]

On physical examination and auscultation, dogs with thoracic malignant effusion caused by mesothelioma often have muffled heart sounds and decreased lung sounds with weak peripheral pulses. Dogs with abdominal mesothelioma usually present with abdominal distention because of ascites and nonspecific signs of lethargy and anorexia. Peritoneal effusion is easily recognized on physical examination. Pericardial effusion attributable to mesothelioma cannot be distinguished from idiopathic (nonneoplastic) causes on the basis of clinical signs and physical examination unless a discrete pericardial or intrapericardial mass can be identified.[12]

STAGING AND DIAGNOSIS

In any dog with malignant effusion, blood work, urinalysis, radiography, and ultrasonography provide valuable staging information. On radiography, pleural effusion may be extensive. In cases of pericardial involvement, the cardiac silhouette is enlarged and globoid and the trachea is elevated dorsally. Other radiographic findings, depending on the site of the tumor, include pulmonary edema, mild hepatomegaly, and peritoneal effusion. When present, effusion usually obliterates visualization of lymph nodes and other structures in these cavities.

Ultrasonography is useful in determining the involvement of intrathoracic or intraabdominal viscera, although mesotheliomas rarely penetrate beneath the surface of these organs. It may be difficult to identify a specific cause of the effusion because mesotheliomas may not form discrete mass lesions[13] but instead produce a diffuse thickening of the coelomic surfaces that is not visualized by ultrasonography or CT. In one dog that had a prolonged clinical course, cystic structures that ultimately were shown to be mesothelioma were identified on serosal surfaces of the abdomen by ultrasonography.[8] Pericardial effusion attributable to mesothelioma cannot be reliably distinguished from idiopathic (nonneoplastic) causes on the basis of imaging (radiography or echocardiography).[12]

Thoracoscopy- and laparoscopy-guided biopsies are becoming more common in veterinary practice; these techniques can provide a definitive histopathologic diagnosis with little morbidity to the patient.[14,15] Exploratory surgery is an alternative diagnostic method, but it is rarely therapeutic. The exception is pericardial mesothelioma, in which pericardectomy provides palliative relief. Surgery may also allow removal of grossly visible mass lesions, thereby reducing tumor burden before adjunctive therapy.[16]

Cytologic evaluation of fluid aspirated from the affected body cavity should be undertaken; however, in any benign or malignant transudative process, mesothelial cells undergo extensive hypertrophy and may exfoliate into the fluid. These cells may be binucleate or even multinucleate; therefore, strict criteria of malignancy may be difficult to impose even on biopsy.[12] In one study, exfoliative cytology was suggestive in only one of six dogs with mesothelioma.[5] Mesothelioma

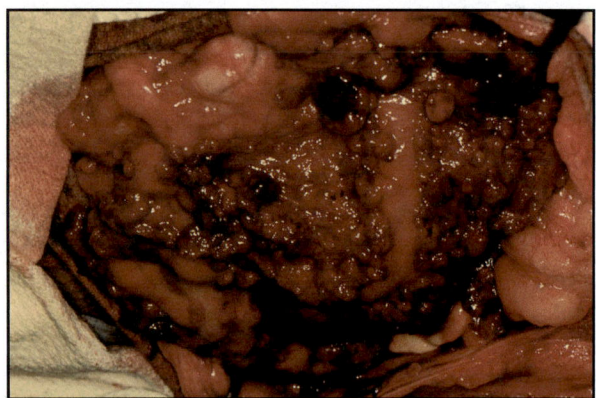

Figure 63-1. *Diagnosis of mesothelioma is rarely made by cytology; however, pleuroscopy or exploratory thoracotomy allows tissue biopsy. A thoracotomy is unlikely to be of therapeutic benefit because of the diffuse nature of this tumor. (Courtesy of John Berg, DVM, Tufts Cummings School of Veterinary Medicine)*

cells may also appear to be carcinoma.[17] It is more likely that a definitive diagnosis will be made by biopsy. Evaluation of the pH of pericardial effusion was not helpful in distinguishing benign causes from mesothelioma in one study.[18]

Epithelial-type mesothelioma is most common in dogs.[3] It may be confused cytologically or histologically with carcinomatosis. Mesotheliomas do not contain the neutral mucosubstances seen in adenocarcinoma cells and do not stain with mucicarmine or periodic acid–Schiff reaction (PAS) stains. Some mesotheliomas stain for the intermediate filament cytokeratin, making it difficult to use this immunostain to differentiate carcinomatosis from mesothelioma.[19] A monoclonal antibody (MAb 3B5) that is sensitive, but not specific, for mesothelioma stained more than 90% of mesotheliomas but fewer than 40% of carcinomas in one evaluation. It also stained more than 80% of hemangiosarcomas.[20] This antibody does not distinguish benign (reactive) mesothelial cells from malignant ones.[19]

Visceral metastasis from mesothelioma is rare in dogs, although evidence of lymphatic invasion by tumor cells[2] or involvement of mediastinal and sternal lymph nodes has been described.[5,12] Widespread metastasis has also been reported.[5,6,9,11]

TREATMENT

Aggressive surgery is rarely feasible or warranted in dogs with mesothelioma because of extensive serosal involvement (Figure 63-1). Palliation of clinical signs caused by effusion can be achieved by repeated thoracocentesis or pericardiocentesis, which can be tolerated by the patient for several months.[3,4] In most animals treated in this way, it eventually becomes necessary to perform centesis every few days,[10] but in one dog, relief of clinical signs of ascites was possible for more than 5.5 years.[8] Obliteration of the pleural space by

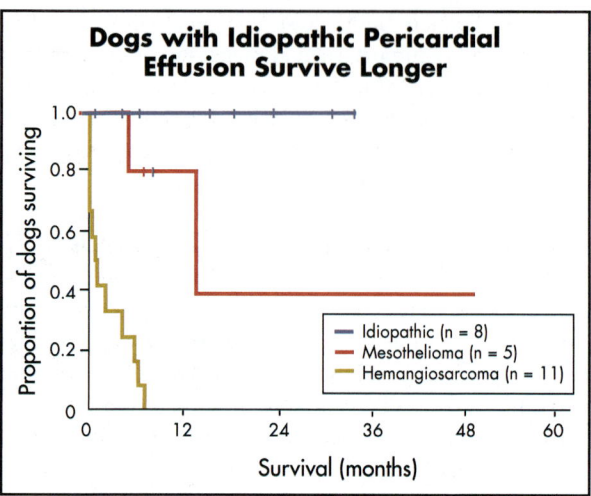

Figure 63-2. *Kaplan-Meier curves for dogs with pericardial effusion caused by mesothelioma, hemangiosarcoma, or idiopathic causes. (From Dunning D, Monnet E, Orton EC, Salman MD: Analysis of prognostic indicators for dogs with pericardial effusion: 46 cases (1985–1996). JAVMA 212:1276–1280, 1998; with permission)*

sclerosis has a palliative benefit in humans, but the role of sclerotherapy in dogs is less clearly defined. Tetracycline or talc has been used with some success in human patients, but in dogs, responses vary, which may be more attributable to technique than to the substance used. In dogs, tetracycline pleurodesis was no better than a placebo in managing experimentally produced pleural effusion.[21] The optimal dose and method have not been established, and this therapy is not recommended for dogs.[22]

Pericardectomy has been used to relieve the clinical signs of pericardial effusion and the potential for cardiac tamponade.[12] Survival of eight dogs with pericardial mesothelioma in one study was 2 months, and dogs that survived beyond 4 months were much more likely to have idiopathic pericardial effusion than mesothelioma.[12] Five of six dogs that were treated by pericardectomy ultimately died because of pleural effusion. In another study, 11 dogs with pericardial mesothelioma had a median survival time of 13.6 months, with 80% of dogs alive 1 year after diagnosis and 40% alive 2 years after diagnosis. Pericardectomy did not affect recurrence of effusion. All dogs with idiopathic effusion were alive 2 years after diagnosis (Figure 63-2).[23] It seems that pericardectomy may provide a diagnosis but not alter the progression of disease in these animals. Thoracoscopy may be a better alternative to obtain a diagnosis because it results in less morbidity than thoracotomy.

Chemotherapy with mitoxantrone resulted in complete remission for 42 days in one dog with mesothelioma,[24] and doxorubicin caused complete remission in one dog for an unstated period.[25] There was no response to cyclophosphamide, vincristine, and prednisone (COP) in another dog.[16] Intracavitary cisplatin chemotherapy (50 mg/m^2 q3wk)

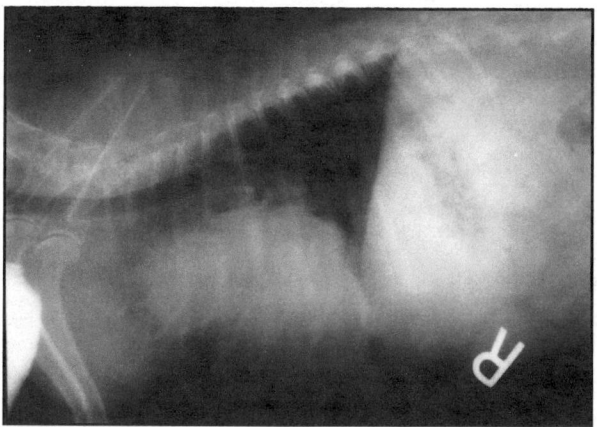

Figure 63-3. *Thymoma in dogs is usually visible radiographically as a poorly defined anterior mediastinal mass that should be differentiated histologically from lymphoma by an abundance of mature lymphocytes and an obvious malignant epithelial component.* (Courtesy of Kenneth M. Rassnick, DVM, Cornell University College of Veterinary Medicine)

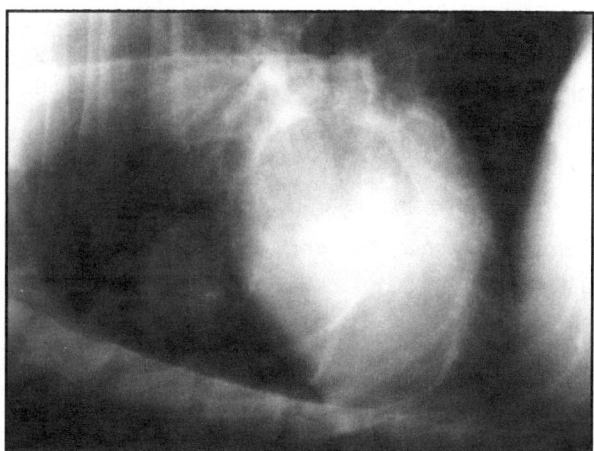

Figure 63-4. *Occasionally, a thymoma may be seen as a small anterior mediastinal mass on thoracic radiographs obtained for an unrelated reason.*

was used to treat three dogs with pleural mesothelioma. Complete control of fluid accumulation was seen in all three dogs for 129 days, 289 days, and 306 days. One dog survived 410 days, and another dog survived more than 306 days; the third dog was lost to follow-up.[16] Intracavitary cisplatin seems to reduce fluid accumulation rapidly if it is going to be effective. If the dog does not respond after one or two treatments, it is unlikely to respond to subsequent treatments.[26] Intracavitary cisplatin is the treatment of choice for mesothelioma in dogs, and concurrent systemic doxorubicin may improve the response rate.[12] One dog with pericardial mesothelioma treated with this protocol was alive and free of disease 27 months after treatment.[27]

Thymoma

INCIDENCE, SIGNALMENT, AND ETIOLOGY

Thymomas originate from the thymic epithelium but often contain a significant proportion of mature lymphocytes. Thymomas invariably occur in the cranial mediastinum,[28] although their exact location may vary. These tumors occur mainly in older dogs with a median age of about 10 years, although dogs as young as 2.5 years of age may be affected. No obvious breed predilection has been reported. Of 61 reported cases, 40 (65%) occurred in female dogs.[28-30] In one study, individual factors associated with prognosis were age, histologic cell type, and the presence or absence of megaesophagus.[28] Old dogs fared better than young dogs, and dogs with lymphocyte-rich thymomas lived longer. On multivariate analysis, however, only the absence of megaesophagus was associated with longer survival. Median survival time was 6 days for 11 dogs with thymoma and megaesophagus and 14.5 months for seven dogs without megaesophagus. The finding of megaesophagus and early postsurgical mortality overwhelm other factors that may become more important when the dog has survived surgery.

CLINICAL PRESENTATION AND HISTORY

Predictably, most of the clinical signs relating to thymoma in dogs involve the respiratory tract; coughing is the most common sign. Dogs with thymoma may also have dyspnea, listlessness, and decreased exercise tolerance. Decreased appetite and weight loss are nonspecific signs associated with thymoma. Some dogs may show dysphagia or regurgitation, presumably from mechanical obstruction by a large compressive mass or from megaesophagus secondary to myasthenia gravis, which is a paraneoplastic syndrome associated with thymoma. Dogs with large compressive tumors may have precaval syndrome and forelimb edema, although this is uncommon and occurred in only seven of 61 (11%) reported cases.[28-31] Precaval syndrome may also occur secondary to invasion of the cranial vena cava.[32] Polydipsia and polyuria occasionally occur secondary to paraneoplastic hypercalcemia.[28] The most common abnormalities detected on physical examination are decreases in heart and ventral lung sounds on auscultation. Small dogs may have an incompressible cranial thorax on palpation.[31]

STAGING AND DIAGNOSIS

The high proportion of paraneoplastic diseases in dogs with thymoma may make it necessary to conduct specialized diagnostic testing, such as electromyography, in addition to routine staging procedures. Thoracic radiographs are very useful in determining whether a dog has an anterior mediastinal mass. Often, the heart is displaced caudodorsally and the trachea is compressed dorsally. In rare cases, however, the thymoma may be in the craniodorsal anterior mediastinum (Figure 63-3).[28] A small thymoma is occasionally discovered on routine radiographs[29] (Figure 63-4). Pleural effusion and megaesophagus may be noted, and changes consistent with pneumonia may be present, possibly after regurgitation and aspiration.[29] Pleural effusion may prevent detection of a thymoma on radiographs.[28]

> **KEY POINT**
> *Pleural effusion may prevent radiographic detection of a thymoma.*

Ultrasonography is the most useful tool for obtaining fine-needle aspirates and needle biopsies while avoiding vessels that may be surrounded or displaced by the thymoma. Ultrasonography and CT or magnetic resonance imaging (MRI) may be useful in determining whether a tumor is encapsulated or invasive; however, for very large tumors, it may be impossible to distinguish between compression and invasion around vital thoracic structures. Whereas thymomas are often described ultrasonographically as being cystic (Figure 63-5), anterior mediastinal lymphomas are usually poorly echogenic. Distant metastases have rarely been described in dogs with thymoma; sites include epicardium, bone, liver, lung, and pleura.[13,29,30]

Fine-needle aspirates may be difficult to evaluate cytologically because of the variable proportion of mature lymphocytes that can be present. As the other most frequent anterior mediastinal tumor in dogs is lymphoma, this presents a diagnostic dilemma. Mast cells are frequently identified in thymomas,[28] and the coincidence of these cells with numerous mature lymphocytes should increase suspicion for thymoma.

> **KEY POINT**
> *Thymomas contain a relatively large number of mature lymphocytes, which may make diagnosis based on cytologic samples difficult.*

Definitive diagnosis requires a biopsy specimen that demonstrates the malignant epithelial portion of thymoma, which may not be evident on aspiration cytology. Thymomas may be subclassified on the basis of their histologic appearance, depending on the proportion and differentiation of the epithelial component; however, this is probably of little prognostic significance.[28]

If radiation therapy is being considered, CT of the thorax may assist in planning, although it may be difficult to distinguish between residual disease and postsurgical reactive tissue if surgery has already been performed.

Thymoma is associated with a high proportion of paraneoplastic syndromes. The best described syndrome is myasthenia gravis. It is thought that thymic myocytes or epithelial cells become immunogenic, leading to the production of autoantibodies against acetylcholine receptors by thymic lymphocytes. The diagnosis of myasthenia gravis was confirmed in 14 of 38 dogs in two reviews of dogs with thymoma.[28,29] All but one of these 14 dogs[28] had evidence of megaesophagus (Figure 63-6). Clinical signs associated with myasthenia gravis, such as exertional muscle weakness and regurgitation, often leading to aspiration pneumonia, were present for 5 days to 3 weeks. One dog, however, had shown signs for more than 3 years.[29] Focal myasthenia may be associated with a thymoma. These dogs have no evidence of appendicular weakness, but they do have focal weakness in the facial, pharyngeal, esophageal, or laryngeal musculature.[33,34] Diagnosis of myasthenia gravis may be confirmed by demonstrating improvement after administration of edrophonium chloride ("Tensilon test") at a dose of 0.11 to 0.22 mg/kg IV; response should be dramatic but transient. Electromyography may demonstrate multifocal fibrillation or other abnormalities but is not widely available. The most specific test is for the presence of serum acetylcholine receptor antibody (AChRAb), which is elevated in most dogs with thymoma and myasthenia gravis.[28,29,31] Normal serum concentrations of AChRAb are less than 0.03 nM. Although myasthenia gravis usually resolves rapidly (within days[33]) of surgery to remove a thymoma, it may persist or develop after surgical removal of the thymoma.[19] The reason for this phenomenon is not clear; however, it is possible that immunologic abnormalities persist even after tumor removal because of the long survival of thymic lymphocytes. Even when AChRAb levels decline to normal, there may be persistent esophageal dysfunction.[35]

Polymyositis has been described in dogs in association with a thymoma[28,29] and resulted in third-degree atrioventricular block in three dogs because of myocardial involvement.[28] This effect may be attributable to antibodies against other skeletal muscle proteins such as titin and ryanodine

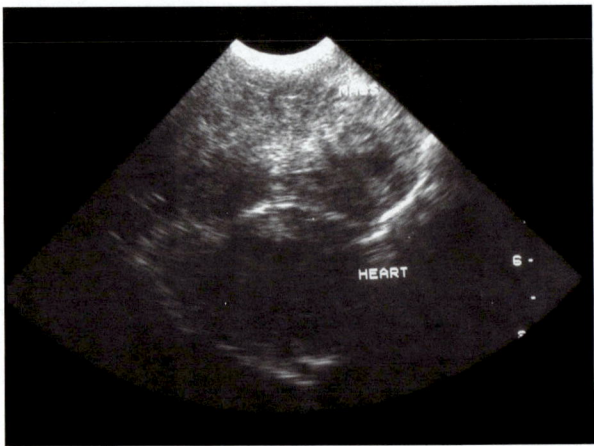

Figure 63-5. *Ultrasonography of the same dog as in Figure 63-3 discloses a multiple cystic mass. (Courtesy of K. M. Rassnick)*

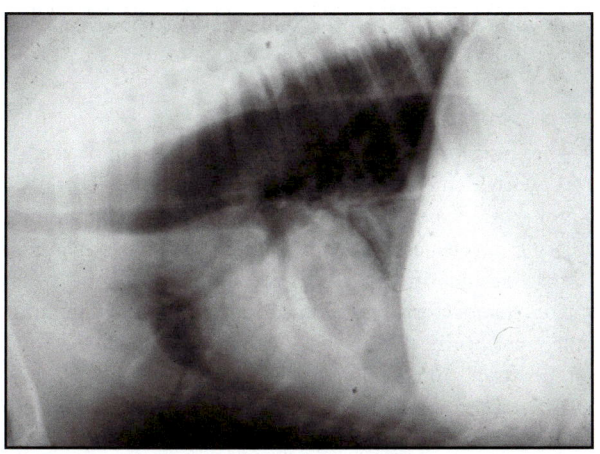

Figure 63-6. Paraneoplastic myasthenia gravis may be associated with megaesophagus and aspiration pneumonia, as in this dog with a thymoma.

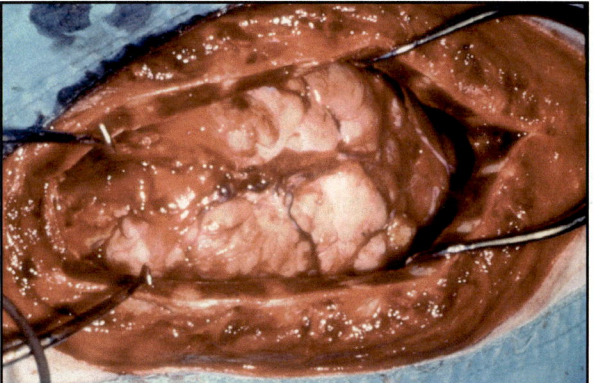

Figure 63-7. Surgery by median sternotomy may give the best exposure to attempt removal of a thymoma, but adhesions and the invasive tendency of this tumor make surgery complicated. A CT scan before surgery may help. (Courtesy of J. Berg)

receptors and may be associated with more severe forms of myasthenia gravis.[36] Hypercalcemia has been described as a paraneoplastic syndrome in dogs with thymoma[28,30] and may resolve after successful treatment.[28] Anterior mediastinal lymphoma is also commonly associated with hypercalcemia, so increased serum calcium cannot be considered as specific for either tumor. Secondary malignancies have been reported to be common in dogs with thymoma and occurred in 15 of 61 dogs.[28–31] These tumors include lymphoma, osteosarcoma, hemangiosarcoma, and various adenocarcinomas and may be the cause of death.[37]

> **KEY POINT**
>
> *Dogs with a confirmed thymoma should be tested for serum AChRAb. Complete staging may help to rule out the presence of other primary malignancies.*

PROGNOSTIC FACTORS

In one study, individual factors associated with prognosis were age, histologic cell type, and the presence or absence of megaesophagus.[28] Older dogs fared better than young dogs, and dogs with lymphocyte-rich thymomas lived longer. On multivariate analysis, however, only the absence of megaesophagus was associated with longer survival. The median survival time was 6 days for 11 dogs with thymoma and megaesophagus and 14.5 months for seven dogs without megaesophagus.

TREATMENT

The best treatment for canine thymoma has yet to be determined. Dogs with myasthenia gravis should be treated with prednisone to reduce AChRAb levels or with anticholinesterase therapy (pyridostigmine; 1.0–1.5 mg/kg PO bid to tid), which may ameliorate clinical signs. Dogs with megaesophagus should be monitored closely for aspiration pneumonia. Before surgery, samples should be obtained by transtracheal aspiration for bacterial culture before beginning antibiotic therapy. The prognosis for dogs with thymoma and megaesophagus is very poor.

Surgery should probably be reserved for dogs without megaesophagus that have well-encapsulated tumors. Radiation therapy and chemotherapy may be useful in reducing the size of the tumor so that surgery may be performed.

The treatment of choice for small thymomas is surgical excision. For these tumors, surgery is potentially curative, but thymoma in dogs is frequently a large and invasive tumor. Even when the tumor is encapsulated, there may be extensive intrathoracic adhesions (Figure 63-7). If surgical margins cannot be assured for larger tumors, incisional biopsy may be preferred to an attempted excision. Other treatment modalities should be considered, particularly if the dog has megaesophagus; careful attention should be given to reducing the risk of developing aspiration pneumonia.

In one study, 13 dogs were treated with surgery alone, and survival times ranged from 1 day to 45 months, with a median survival of 7 days. Three dogs lived more than 1 year.[29] In another study, three dogs without paraneoplastic signs were treated with surgery alone. Two dogs died within 2 days of surgery, and one had local recurrence at 4 months.[29] Two of seven other dogs treated with surgery died perioperatively, and four dogs lived for 6 months, 1 year, 4 years, and 5 years, respectively.[30] Pleural nonchylous effusion may persist after surgery for an encapsulated thymoma. In one dog, placement of a pleuroperitoneal pump reduced the effusion, which ceased 6 weeks later.[38]

Radiation therapy is important in the treatment of thymoma in humans. Its use was described in one dog treated with 54 Gy of orthovoltage radiation in nine weekly fractions.[31] This dog had a 60% reduction in tumor mass and normalization of elevated AChRAb levels for 6 months before signs of myasthenia recurred. The dog was also treated with prednisone (2.2 mg/kg PO every other day). Radiation may reduce tumor size to a point at which surgical excision is feasible, but risks of radiation toxicity to the lungs and myocardium are dose limiting. In a larger report, 13 dogs were treated for thymoma with megavoltage radiation therapy. The radiation protocol varied but mostly consisted of either (1) 3- to 4-Gy fractions given daily or three times a week to 21 to 54 Gy (definitive therapy) or (2) weekly 5-Gy fractions to 15 Gy (palliative therapy) through parallel opposed portals. Three dogs had complete and five had partial (>50%) reduction in tumor size for a median of 3 to 6 months. Two of the dogs with a complete response had a partial surgical excision before definitive radiation therapy. It is unclear whether and which dogs had primarily epithelial or lymphocyte-rich thymomas.[39]

> **KEY POINT**
>
> *Dogs with thymoma and megaesophagus have a very poor prognosis because aspiration pneumonia commonly develops.*

The most active chemotherapeutic agents for treatment of thymoma in human patients are prednisone and cisplatin. In dogs, chemotherapy has been used alone, usually when thymoma is mistakenly diagnosed as lymphoma, and dogs with lymphocyte-rich tumors would be expected to respond. One dog with thymoma did not respond to chemotherapy with COP.[29,30] In contrast, one dog that received this drug protocol after surgery was in complete remission 29 months later, and another dog that received COP for 2 weeks and then prednisone alone maintained stable tumor measurements for 14 months.[28] A dog treated with cisplatin and doxorubicin for osteosarcoma had no change the in size of an incidental thymoma.[28] Doxorubicin and platinum drugs have anecdotally been associated with responses in epithelial thymomas in other dogs. If chemotherapy is to be used with concurrent radiation therapy, and if the heart is in the radiation field, doxorubicin should be used with caution because the cardiomyopathic effects of both are additive, and dogs are more sensitive than humans to doxorubicin-induced cardiomyopathy.

Supportive care may be very important, particularly if myasthenia gravis does not resolve after successful surgery. In these dogs, continued management with prednisone may control the paraneoplastic disease. The addition of anticholinesterase therapy (pyridostigmine; 1.0–1.5 mg/kg PO bid to tid) may result in clinical improvement and may be preferred for long-term management of dogs that do not tolerate corticosteroids.[40] Improved immunosuppression may be obtained by adding azathioprine.[41]

Histiocytic Diseases

The histiocytic disorders are confusing, controversial, and poorly defined in dogs (as in humans). They represent a group of diseases that are seemingly related but appear to fall into several categories, including cutaneous histiocytoma, cutaneous histiocytosis, systemic histiocytosis, splenic histiocytosis or fibrohistiocytic nodules (which can range into histiocytic sarcoma, also called *malignant fibrous histiocytoma*), and malignant histiocytosis (also called *disseminated histiocytic sarcomas*). Some of the confusion stems from the apparent similarity of the cell of origin for disorders that behave differently and the realization that cells that appear similar on light microscopy may have a different origin or function and could be differentiated by histochemistry or immunohistochemistry. For example, it remains controversial whether the tumor described as histiocytic sarcoma or malignant fibrous histiocytoma of the spleen should be considered primarily a soft tissue sarcoma or a histiocytic disease.

In the skin, the disease spectrum is from histiocytoma to cutaneous histiocytosis, malignant histiocytosis, and histiocytic sarcoma. In the spleen, the spectrum is from fibrohistiocytic nodules to histiocytic sarcoma. In the central nervous system (CNS), the spectrum is from granulomatous meningoencephalitis (GME) to malignant histiocytosis. Clinicians are understandably challenged in knowing the best therapeutic approach for any affected individual.

BENIGN CUTANEOUS HISTIOCYTOMA
Incidence, Signalment, and Etiology

Cutaneous histiocytoma is a neoplasm that is unique to the canine skin. It has no similarities to the cutaneous histiocytoma found in humans, nor is it encountered in any other species. It may be misdiagnosed by pathologists who analyze human tissue as histiocytic lymphoma. This tumor should not be confused with malignant fibrous histiocytoma, which is a soft tissue sarcoma, or with systemic histiocytosis. Histiocytomas are far more common in young than in old dogs (mean age: 3.6 years). Most cases occur in dogs younger than 2 years of age, but histiocytoma should not be ruled out just because a dog is older. This skin tumor is more likely to be diagnosed in male dogs. Purebred dogs have a higher incidence than mixed-breed dogs. In one series of 3,497 dogs, breeds that were predisposed (more than three times more likely than the general population) to developing histiocytoma included English bulldogs, Scottish terriers, greyhounds, boxers, Boston terriers, flat-coated retrievers, English cocker spaniels, Parson Russell terriers, American pit bulls, bull terriers, rottweilers, pugs, and shar-peis.[42] Interest-

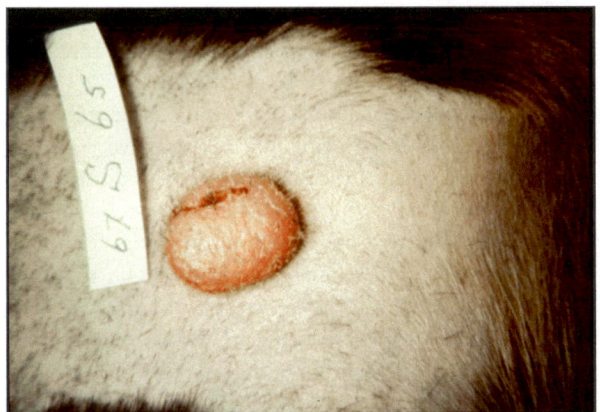

Figure 63-8. *Cutaneous histiocytomas are usually solitary, raised, and hairless. They regress after lymphoid infiltration.*

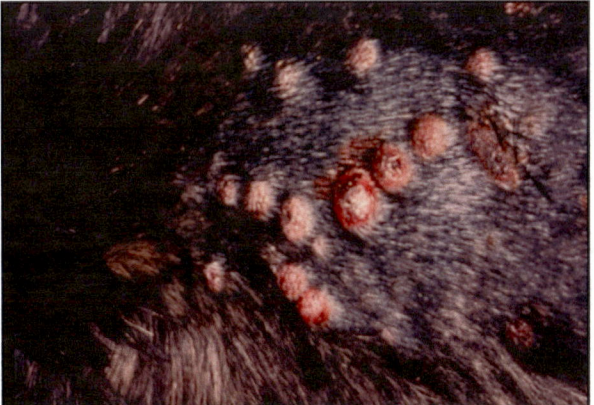

Figure 63-9. *Multiple cutaneous histiocytomas, as seen in this 8-month-old Scottish terrier, usually regress spontaneously.*

ingly, the flat-coated retriever appeared predisposed to developing both cutaneous histiocytomas (215 of 449 [48%] benign lesions) and undifferentiated sarcomas (141 of 411 [34%] malignant tumors), which may represent histiocytic sarcomas.[43,44]

The cause of the tumor is unknown. Intracytoplasmic reticular aggregates, suggestive of viral causation, have been found on electron microscopic examination of tumor cells. No causative agent has been isolated, however, and attempts to transmit the tumor have been unsuccessful.

Clinical Presentation and History

Histiocytomas are rapidly developing, circular, dome-shaped lesions of the skin (Figure 63-8). They are most common on the head (especially the pinnae; 38%), limbs (35%), and thorax (11%). The neck and tail are sometimes involved. The surface of the skin is shiny and alopecic or ulcerated. Although erythematous in appearance, these tumors cause no discomfort to the animal. Tumors range in size from 0.5 to 4.0 cm in diameter; most are 1.0 to 2.0 cm. Multiple histiocytomas represented 0.6% of 3,497 cases.[42] In contrast, multiple histiocytomas were seen in 6% of 206 affected flat-coated retrievers.[43]

> **KEY POINT**
> *Canine cutaneous histiocytoma usually regresses spontaneously after lymphoid infiltration.*

Treatment

Although rapid growth and high mitotic index are highly suggestive of a malignant tumor, these are benign tumors that usually regress spontaneously with lymphoid infiltration composed mainly of CD3-positive lymphocytes (T cells).[45,46] A new histiocytoma arose on other body sites in only 16 of 400 (4%) dogs treated surgically, and only one of 400 tumors recurred at the site of excision.[42]

Multiple histiocytomas have rarely been reported. These tumors also resolve without therapy over 8 to 12 weeks, although their disappearance may not be synchronous[47] (Figure 63-9). Multiple histiocytomas in a flat-coated retriever that metastasized to a lymph node and did not regress may have been systemic histiocytosis.[48]

REACTIVE HISTIOCYTIC DISEASES
Cutaneous Histiocytosis
Incidence, Signalment, and Etiology

Cutaneous histiocytosis is an uncommon disease that occurs in Bernese mountain dogs in what may be an inherited manner. Beagles and golden retrievers (age range: 2–11 years) were more commonly affected than Bernese mountain dogs in another study.[49] The disease principally affects middle-aged male dogs. No etiologic agent has been identified, but cutaneous histiocytosis is considered to be a nonneoplastic disease. The proliferating cell in cutaneous histiocytosis has been suggested to be the epidermal Langerhans cell. Another disease has been described, idiopathic periadnexal multinodular granulomatous dermatitis,[50] which appears in some dogs to form confluence with cutaneous histiocytosis, and the distinction may be an artificial division of a continuum.[51]

Clinical Presentation and History

Dogs with cutaneous histiocytosis have multiple ulcerated, crusted, or alopecic cutaneous masses measuring up to 4 cm in diameter in the skin and subcutaneous tissue. These masses develop predominantly on the head, neck, and extremities (scrotum, feet) and less commonly on the trunk. There are no lesions in other organs. Clinical signs of illness are uncommon, and most dogs present with lesions that have been noticed by the client.[49] The clinical course may be one of waxing and waning lesions, with new lesions appearing at different sites.[52]

Cutaneous and systemic histiocytosis present with identical histologic changes characterized by a nodular to diffuse pleocellular infiltrate dominated by histiocytes, lymphocytes, and neutrophils.

Staging and Diagnosis

In addition to histology, cutaneous histiocytosis is partly a diagnosis of exclusion. Thoracic radiographs should be obtained to check for sternal lymphadenopathy and pulmonary nodules. Abdominal ultrasonography should be conducted to assess the spleen and liver. For completeness, a bone marrow aspirate should be obtained. These tests are to rule out the possibility of systemic histiocytosis and malignant histiocytosis.

In an effort to differentiate histiocytosis from other diseases (e.g., lymphoma), immunohistochemistry may be helpful.[53] In addition to morphologic features, immunostains appear to be the most useful criteria to indicate likely histiocytic origin. Both CD3 (T cell) and CD79a (B cell) are lymphocyte markers, and CD18 is histiocytic. If the lesion is a lymphoma, then one of the T-cell or B-cell markers is usually positive. Histiocytes would be CD18+, CD3-, and CD79a-.

Treatment

Spontaneous regression may occur. The waxing and waning course makes it difficult to assess the efficacy of therapy. In a series of 18 dogs, two dogs had a spontaneous regression and one dog had seasonal relapses. In the same series of dogs, surgical management was successful in another dog. Eight of the remaining dogs had partial regression of skin lesions after either parenteral or intralesional corticosteroid treatment. Leflunomide treatment caused a complete remission in yet another dog. The rest of the dogs were lost to follow-up.[48]

Based on the small numbers reported, it seems that treatment with immunosuppressive medications that are more potent than corticosteroids may be warranted. It has been suggested that the response to immunosuppressive agents is a result of suppression of T cells that are a common infiltrate in the lesions of reactive histiocytosis.[49]

Cyclosporine at a dose of 5 to 10 mg/kg PO divided into two doses per day has been used to treat perianal fistulas in dogs, and this would be the dosage to use in dogs with systemic histiocytosis. The recommended formulation is Neoral (Novartis Pharmaceuticals) rather than Sandimmune (Novartis Pharmaceuticals). Regression might be expected to take 6 to 8 weeks. If long-term therapy is planned, the trough blood levels (just before a dose is due) should be checked periodically, and the level should be higher than 500 ng/ml.[54]

An alternative to cyclosporine, leflunomide, has been used at 4 mg/kg PO once every 24 hours initially, with the dose adjusted to obtain a trough level of 20 µg/ml.[54]

If immunosuppressive therapy is not successful, then more aggressive chemotherapy may be warranted, based on response in the malignant counterparts of this disease. Historically, chemotherapy for malignant histiocytosis and histiocytic sarcoma has not been encouraging. However, combination chemotherapy with an emphasis on alkylating agents has had some success (see Malignant Histiocytic Diseases section, below). L-Asparaginase was successful in causing complete remission in nine of 10 dogs with histiocytic nodular proliferative dermatitis, which may have been this disease; continued therapy was necessary to control lesions.[55]

Systemic Histiocytosis
Incidence, Signalment, and Etiology

This is an uncommon disease that occurs most frequently in Bernese mountain dogs in what may be an inherited manner.[56] Bernese mountain dogs accounted for 11 of 26 dogs in one study; rottweilers and Labrador retrievers were the next most common breeds affected.[49] Systemic histiocytosis principally affects middle-aged male dogs with no gender predilection (age range: 1–9 years).[49] No etiologic agent has been identified, but systemic histiocytosis is considered to be a nonneoplastic disease. The clinical similarities between systemic histiocytosis and malignant histiocytosis make it difficult to distinguish between the two diseases, although involvement of the skin and peripheral lymph nodes is more often described in association with systemic histiocytosis than with malignant histiocytosis.

Clinical Presentation and History

Dogs with systemic histiocytosis have multiple cutaneous masses measuring up to 4 cm in diameter that are ulcerated, crusted, or alopecic in a similar distribution to those in cutaneous histiocytosis, with the exception that their distribution seems to follow vessels.[49] In addition, affected dogs are usually depressed and anorectic and often show other signs because of involvement of organs. These additional lesions develop within predilection sites that include the lymph nodes, sclera, eyelids, nasal cavity, lungs, liver, spleen, and bone marrow. The nasal cavity was the most common systemic site affected, occurring in 14 of 26 dogs, followed by the eyes and adnexae (10 dogs) and lymph nodes (nine dogs). Hypercalcemia was seen in two of 26 dogs.[49]

Staging and Diagnosis

Dogs with cutaneous and systemic histiocytosis present with identical histologic changes characterized by a nodular to diffuse pleocellular infiltrate dominated by histiocytes, lymphocytes, and neutrophils. These cells form perivascular cuffs.[49] Progression to coalescence of nodules and a diffuse, deep panniculitis and dermatitis has been seen. Dogs with systemic histiocytosis may have vascular invasion causing ischemic necrosis.

The lymph nodes should be carefully assessed and the owner questioned about nasal or other signs. Thoracic radiographs should be obtained to check for sternal lymphadenopathy and pulmonary nodules. Abdominal ultrasonography should be conducted to assess the spleen and liver. For completeness, a bone marrow aspirate should be obtained. These tests are done to assess the extent of disease and to rule out the possibility of malignant histiocytosis.

In an effort to differentiate histiocytosis from other diseases (e.g., lymphoma), immunohistochemistry may be helpful. In addition to morphologic features, immunostains appear to be the most useful criteria to indicate likely histiocytic origin. In formalin-fixed biopsies, a limited number of antibodies are available for further characterization of a lesion suspected to be histiocytosis. Both CD3 (T cell) and CD79a (B cell) are lymphocyte markers, and CD18 is histiocytic. If the lesion is a lymphoma, then one of the T- or B-cell markers is usually positive. Histiocytes would be CD18+, CD3-, and CD79a-.

Bone marrow infiltration occurs in systemic and malignant histiocytosis. This makes it difficult for clinicians to decide what disease to treat if the bone marrow contains histiocytes. Distinguishing between the two diseases may be helped by flow cytometry; histiocytic cells in malignant histiocytosis were suggested to be larger than those in benign disease and account for a higher percentage of nucleated cells.[57] Obtaining an appropriate diagnosis of this condition requires the expertise of an excellent pathologist who is very aware of the current literature about histiocytic diseases. This area of the literature is often confusing, and the understanding of these histiocytic diseases has evolved dramatically over the past several years.

Treatment

Unlike cutaneous histiocytosis, spontaneous regression of systemic histiocytosis is rare. In a series of 26 dogs, only one dog had a spontaneous regression. In the same series of dogs, surgical management was successful in two dogs, and eight dogs had regression after medical management consisting of corticosteroid treatment (two dogs), cyclosporine (three dogs), leflunomide (two dogs), or doxorubicin (one dog). Most of these dogs required long-term medication to avoid relapse. The rest either died or were lost to follow-up.

In another report, three of four Bernese mountain dogs treated with corticosteroids had complete responses; two remained disease-free 6 and 12 months after treatment ceased; a third dog relapsed after 4 months but then remained stable on no treatment; and a fourth dog failed to respond to prednisolone and azathioprine. Systemic histiocytosis was diagnosed in these four dogs because of the presence of ocular lesions in addition to skin lesions; no other lesions were found. Again, the distinction between cutaneous histiocytosis and this disease may be difficult to understand clinically.[51]

> **KEY POINT**
>
> *The reactive histiocytic diseases may regress with immunosuppressive treatment. However, the distinction between these and malignant forms is often blurred.*

Although one dog has been reported to respond to chemotherapy with doxorubicin, chemotherapy should probably not be the first choice. Based on the small numbers reported, it seems that an initial therapeutic trial with prednisone or other, more potent immunosuppressive medications may be warranted. It has been suggested that the response to immunosuppressive agents results from suppression of T cells, which are a common infiltrate in the lesions of reactive histiocytosis.[49]

Cyclosporine at a dose of 5 to 10 mg/kg PO divided into two doses per day has been used to treat perianal fistulas in dogs, and this would be the dosage to use in dogs with systemic histiocytosis. The recommended formulation is Neoral rather than Sandimmune. Regression might be expected to take 6 to 8 weeks. If long-term therapy is planned, the trough blood levels (just before a dose is due) should be checked periodically, and the level should be higher than 500 ng/ml.[54]

An alternative to cyclosporine, leflunomide, has been used at 4 mg/kg PO once every 24 hours initially, with the dose adjusted to obtain a trough level of 20 μg/ml.[54]

If immunosuppressive therapy is not successful, then more aggressive chemotherapy may be warranted, based on response in the malignant counterparts of this disease. Historically, chemotherapy for malignant histiocytosis and histiocytic sarcoma has not been encouraging. However, combination chemotherapy with an emphasis on alkylating agents has had some success (see Malignant Histiocytic Diseases section, below).

A human cytotoxic T-cell line (TALL-104) was able to induce remission in four dogs affected with malignant histiocytosis in a preliminary trial of this therapy.[58] Three treated dogs did not have systemic involvement but had only skin and lymph node involvement, which is more suggestive of systemic histiocytosis. Immunotherapy may have a role in the management of both diseases.

SPLENIC HISTIOCYTOSIS OR FIBROHISTIOCYTIC NODULES

A complex of splenic disorders summarized as *splenic histiocytosis* or *fibrohistiocytic nodules* appears to describe a continuum of histiocytic disease from reactive to malignant.[59,60] This may also be true of other histiocytic diseases described as reactive and malignant.

Incidence, Signalment, and Etiology

Although it is often possible to characterize a dog into one of the two groups described by Spangler and Kass,[59,60] many dogs display features of both. Splenic fibrohistiocytic nodules can range into histiocytic sarcoma, also called *malignant fibrous histiocytoma*. It remains controversial whether the tumor described as histiocytic sarcoma or malignant fibrous histiocytoma of the spleen should be considered primarily a soft tissue sarcoma or a histiocytic disease. It is described separately below. Fibrohistiocytic nodules occurred most commonly in older (average age: 11 years) female dogs. The most commonly affected breeds were German shepherds, cocker spaniels, Labrador and golden retrievers, and poodles.[60]

Clinical Presentation and History

Affected dogs may present with nonspecific clinical signs of vomiting, lethargy, fever, and malaise. There were no consistent findings on either complete blood count (CBC) or biochemical profiles for affected dogs.[60]

Staging and Diagnosis

Fibrohistiocytic nodules are characterized by a mixed population of histiocytic and spindle cells in varying proportions intermixed with hematopoietic elements, plasma cells, or lymphocytes.[60] Hematologic and biochemical abnormalities in dogs with fibrohistiocytic nodules are not consistent but include trends toward anemia, neutrophilia with a left shift, and elevated alkaline phosphatase levels.[60] Spangler and Kass[60] argue that these nodules form a continuum between splenic lymphoid nodular hyperplasia (i.e., smaller lesions with >70% lymphocytes with interspersed fibrohistiocytic cells) to malignant splenic stromal neoplasms (i.e., histiocytic sarcoma or malignant fibrous histiocytoma; larger lesions composed of primarily fibrohistiocytic cells with <40% lymphocytes interspersed) and grade the lesions 1 to 3, respectively, with grade 2 falling between the two extremes. Approximately half of the dogs that died had metastases, including to the liver. Some dogs may also have diffuse splenomegaly and other clinical characteristics not addressed in this study.[60]

Prognostic Factors

Spangler and Kass[60] found that the lymphoid:fibrohistiocytic cell ratio in the lesion was the most important prognostic indicator for dogs with this syndrome, with dogs that had less than 40% lymphocytes having a substantially poorer prognosis (1-year survival: 55%) than those with a higher proportion of lymphocytes (1-year survival: 87%). The mitotic index also had some prognostic value, but it was overshadowed by the lymphoid:fibrohistiocytic cell ratio.[60]

Treatment

Splenectomy is the treatment of choice and may be all that is required for the benign forms of the disease (grade 1 lesions based on lymphoid infiltration). For grade 3 lesions (histiocytic sarcoma), systemic therapy is also required (see Malignant Histiocytic Diseases section, below). For grade 2 lesions, the ideal treatment is not certain, but systemic therapy should be considered.

SPLENIC MYELOID METAPLASIA, HISTIOCYTOSIS, AND HYPERSPLENISM
Incidence, Signalment, and Etiology

This syndrome is described as diffuse splenomegaly with distinctive histology that consists of extramedullary hematopoiesis (myeloid metaplasia), histiocytosis, erythrophagocytosis, and thrombosis. This is a disease of older (median age: 8 years) female dogs. The most commonly affected breeds are golden and Labrador retrievers and rottweilers.[59]

Clinical Presentation and History

There is one large report of 65 dogs with this disease.[59] Affected dogs present with clinical signs of vomiting, lethargy, fever, malaise, and cytopenias (usually anemia, thrombocytopenia, or both). All had severe, sustained, progressive splenomegaly. Approximately 35% of the dogs had elevated leukocyte counts, and 30% of the dogs were icteric. Although this disorder primarily affects the splenic parenchyma and is classified as a reactive disease, more than half of the dogs also had histiocytic nodules of varying size in other organs consistent with metastases, so this is not a strictly benign disease.

Prognostic Factors

The only clear prognostic indicator was the presence of giant cells in the lesions, which indicated a uniformly fatal outcome. Although some dogs without giant cells also died, none of the survivors had giant cells.[59]

Treatment

Splenectomy is the treatment of choice and may be all that is required for dogs without other lesions and no giant cells seen on splenic biopsy. The overall 1-year survival for all dogs was 30%, and half of the dogs that died did so in the first month postoperatively; approximately half of these had hepatic metastases. For metastatic lesions, systemic therapy is also required and would be as described for histiocytic sarcomas (see next section).

MALIGNANT HISTIOCYTIC DISEASES
Malignant Histiocytosis
Incidence, Signalment, and Etiology

Also called *disseminated histiocytic sarcoma*, this is an uncommon disease that has been reported most frequently in Bernese mountain dogs, in which it is suspected to be inherited on a polyclonal mode basis.[61-63] It has been reported in this breed in most countries.[64] The same family lines affected by systemic histiocytosis are also affected by malignant histiocytosis.[63] The disease has also been noted in rottweilers, Doberman pinschers, and Labrador, flat-coated, and golden retrievers.[65] These are the same breeds affected with systemic histiocytosis, and the clinical similarities may make it difficult to distinguish between the two diseases. The disease occurs with equal frequency in both genders and is most common in older dogs. Based on immunophenotypic studies, malignant histiocytosis is derived from myeloid dendritic antigen-presenting cells.[66]

Clinical Presentation and History

The tumor frequently involves the lung as solitary or multiple nodular opacities on thoracic radiographs (Figure 63-10). It may occasionally occur as diffuse pulmonary infiltrates with or without hilar lymph node involvement.[65] Although respiratory signs predominate, neurologic signs are common and include posterior paresis, paralysis, or seizures. Bone marrow is frequently involved, with resultant cytopenias and their sequelae. In addition, the lymph nodes, spleen, liver, and, occasionally, other abdominal organs may be involved.[63,66] Involvement of the skin is uncommon.[67]

Staging and Diagnosis

Complete clinical staging includes thoracic radiographs to check for sternal lymphadenopathy and pulmonary nodules as well as routine blood work and urinalysis. Abdominal ultrasonography should be conducted to assess the spleen and liver. Ultrasonography may demonstrate hypoechoic nodules in the spleen, liver, and kidneys as well as mesenteric and medial iliac lymphadenopathy. Dogs with liver involvement may have low serum albumin levels and peripheral edema, which can complicate treatment. These findings are nonspecific, and definitive diagnosis requires cytologic or histologic examination.[68] Abdominal ultrasonography may enable needle (Tru-Cut) biopsies to obtain a definitive diagnosis. Care should be taken when biopsying dogs with bone marrow infiltration and consequent cytopenias because thrombocytopenia may be marked and the patient may be prone to bleeding. For completeness, a bone marrow aspirate should be obtained.

Malignant histiocytosis can affect the CNS,[69,70] where it may be difficult to distinguish clinically or even histologically from focal GME using histiocytic markers.[71,72] In one study, malignant histiocytosis occurred in two forms, as either a diffuse infiltrate throughout the leptomeninges or with nodule formation in the parenchyma. Focal GME was very difficult to distinguish from malignant histiocytosis that had low cellular atypia. An immunomorphologic study of the inflammatory lesions in canine GME showed that they consisted of a heterogeneous population of major histocompatibility complex class II antigen-positive macrophages and predominantly CD3 antigen-positive lymphocytes, which is strikingly similar to the cells found in patients with malignant histiocytosis.[73] Staining for histiocytic markers, lysozyme, α-1 antitrypsin, and lectin RCA-1 was also positive in both malignant histiocytosis and GME.[71] The prognosis for five dogs with malignant histiocytosis of the CNS was poor; their survival times ranged from 4 days to 3 months, with a median of 1 month.[71] Malignant histiocytosis may also affect the pericardium and cardiac muscle.[13]

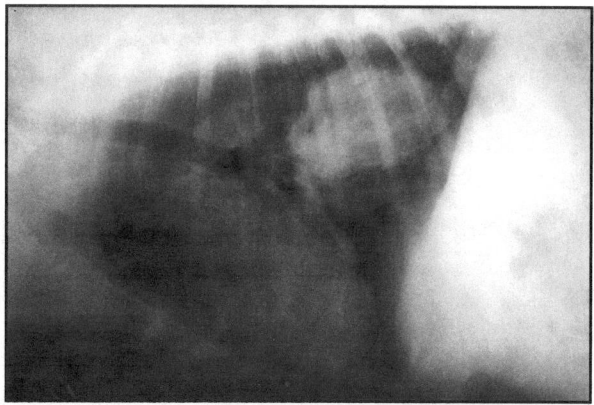

Figure 63-10. *Pulmonary involvement is common in dogs with disseminated histiocytic sarcomas (malignant histiocytosis) and may be a solitary mass that is difficult to distinguish clinically from a primary lung carcinoma. (Courtesy of K. M. Rassnick)*

Bone marrow infiltration occurs in systemic and malignant histiocytosis. There are difficulties in distinguishing between the two diseases on the basis of cytology alone. Variable numbers of large histiocytic cells with some characteristics of malignancy are seen in both disorders.[74] These difficulties in cytopathology make it difficult for clinicians to decide what disease to treat when the bone marrow is involved. Differentiation may be helped by flow cytometry; histiocytic cells in malignant histiocytosis have been suggested to be larger than those in benign disease and account for a higher percentage of nucleated cells.[57] Multinucleated giant cells and phagocytosis of erythrocytes and leukocytes are prominent features in most cytologic preparations from the organs and bone marrow in dogs with malignant histiocytosis. Suppression of normal hematopoiesis may occur, affecting one or all cell lines. In a series of 110 dogs with pancytopenia, malignant histiocytosis was the primary disease process in 5%.[75] Paraneoplastic hypercalcemia has been reported in a dog with malignant histiocytosis.[76]

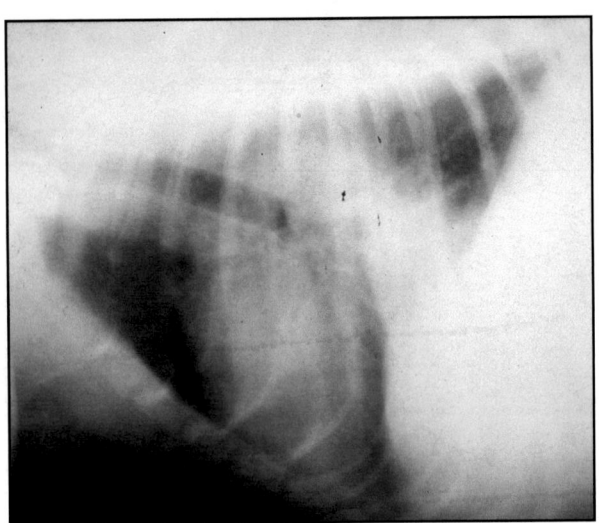

Figure 63-11. *Pulmonary involvement may be diffuse in disseminated histiocytic sarcomas, as in this dog before treatment with CCNU. (Courtesy of K. M. Rassnick)*

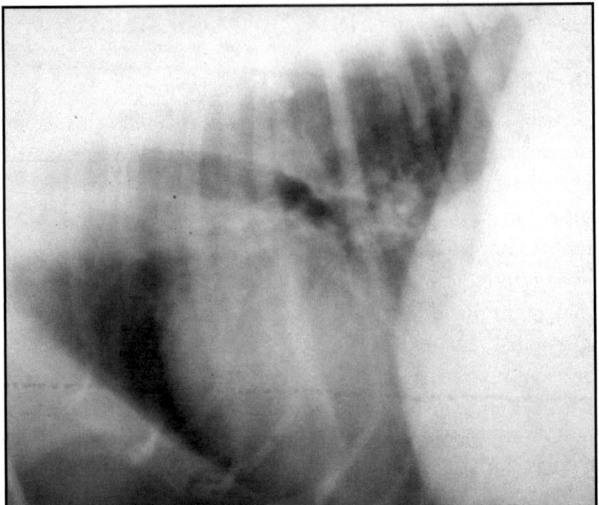

Figure 63-12. *Diffuse lung changes seen in Figure 63-11 have partially resolved after treatment with CCNU. (Courtesy of K. M. Rassnick)*

In an effort to differentiate malignant histiocytosis from other diseases (e.g., histiocytic lymphoma [an obsolete term] and lymphomatoid granulomatosis), immunohistochemistry may be helpful. In addition to morphologic features, immunostains appear to be the most useful criteria to indicate likely histiocytic origin. Whereas both CD3 (T cell) and CD79a (B cell) are lymphocyte markers, CD18 is histiocytic. If the lesion is a lymphoma, then one of the T- or B-cell markers is usually positive. Histiocytes would be CD18+, CD3-, and CD79a. Other stains include lysozyme and lectin RCA-1, both of which stain histiocytes.[56] Lysozyme staining can be used on cytology specimens as well as tissue sections.[77]

Prognostic Factors

A preliminary report of treatment for histiocytic sarcoma using lomustine (CCNU) found thrombocytopenia and hypoalbuminemia to be significant independent predictors of poor prognosis.[78]

Treatment

Systemic treatment is required for dogs with malignant histiocytosis, although it may be difficult to distinguish this disease from systemic histiocytosis, which occurs with a similar breed distribution and similar organs affected.

Some anecdotal reports have shown clinical remission after treatment with COP or doxorubicin-based chemotherapeutic protocols used for the treatment of lymphoma (see Chapter 47), but these remissions are of relatively short duration. One preliminary report discussed an overall 50% response rate in 24 dogs with measurable histiocytic sarcoma (19 with metastases) treated with CCNU, with an overall median survival of 4 months.[78] That report included dogs that responded for as little as 7 days, so the encouraging figures may be misleading. Of an additional 27 dogs treated, we have seen some complete and partial responses, but nowhere near the 50% observed by Drs. Moore and Rassnick (Figures 63-11 and 63-12). A preliminary report of paclitaxel chemotherapy documented partial response in one of two dogs with malignant histiocytosis. The response was for less than 6 months.[79]

Either single-agent CCNU or a combination chemotherapeutic protocol based on CCNU and other agents active against lymphoma may be the treatment of choice for patients with this disease. As a principle of chemotherapy, combination therapy is always expected to provide better outcomes than single-agent treatment. Doxorubicin-containing protocols have been successful in some dogs in Dr. Ogilvie's experience. Some suggest alternating doxorubicin and CCNU at 3-week intervals for the treatment of this disorder.

> **KEY POINT**
>
> *Malignant histiocytosis responds poorly to therapy; chemotherapy is the treatment most likely to be successful.*

A human cytotoxic T-cell line (TALL-104) was able to induce long-term (median: 15 months) remission in all four affected dogs in a preliminary trial of this therapy.[58] However, three dogs did not have systemic involvement but had only skin and lymph node involvement, which is more suggestive of systemic histiocytosis. Immunotherapy may have a role in the management of both diseases. Chemotherapy using doxorubicin and dacarbazine in addition to TALL-104 was used in one dog to achieve a complete remission.[58]

Radiation therapy has been successful in causing remission of GME in dogs and may be palliative for dogs with CNS malignant histiocytosis.

Supportive treatment in the form of blood transfusions, plasma transfusions, and the use of dextrans or hetastarch for hypoproteinemic dogs may be as important as chemotherapy in prolonging survival of severely affected dogs.

Histiocytic Sarcoma

It is unclear whether localized histiocytic sarcomas represent part of the continuum in the spectrum of histiocytic disease or whether they are a variant of soft tissue sarcomas. Our tendency is to treat these tumors as high-grade soft tissue sarcomas. Therefore, further information may be gained from reading Chapter 62.

Incidence, Signalment, and Etiology

Histiocytic sarcoma is also known by other terms (e.g., *malignant fibrous histiocytoma, malignant [grade 3] fibrohistiocytic nodules of the spleen*). In one study of 263 dogs with either malignant histiocytosis or histiocytic sarcoma, 77 cases were considered to be malignant histiocytosis, 110 were histiocytic sarcoma, and the remaining 76 dogs had neoplasms with features of both diseases.[80] This serves to confuse the issue of staging and treatment in affected dogs. Another report characterized tumors as localized histiocytic sarcoma if there was a history of initially single-site involvement and metastasis to the regional lymph node. In that study, 19 of 39 dogs met the criteria, and primary tumors arose mostly in the skin and subcutis but also in the spleen, lung, brain nasal cavity, and bone.[66]

> **KEY POINT**
> *Some dogs have features of disseminated and localized histiocytic sarcomas.*

Histiocytic sarcoma is histologically composed of pleomorphic spindle cells as the major cell population with histiocytic cells (often bizarre) and sometimes multinucleated cells scattered through the tissue.[80] Dogs with malignant histiocytosis had tumors composed of individualized histiocytic cells and multinucleated cells with common phagocytosis. Dogs that had a hybrid neoplasm had tumors in the same or different locations that had features of both neoplasms.[81] As already stated, Bernese mountain dogs and rottweilers are overrepresented in studies of malignant histiocytosis, and they accounted for a high percentage of the dogs with hybrid neoplasms but not histiocytic sarcomas. Golden retrievers were the most commonly affected breed in all three histologic subgroups.[66,80] A cutaneous histiocytic sarcoma was diagnosed in a 4-month-old dog.[81]

Localized histiocytic sarcoma, but not malignant histiocytosis, was diagnosed in flat-coated retrievers in one study.[65] Further investigations showed that undifferentiated sarcomas are a common malignancy in this breed, accounting for 141 of 411 (34%) malignant tumors, and are often confirmed as histiocytic sarcomas.[43,44] Most sarcomas in flat-coated retrievers arose in the deep soft tissues of the limbs, with only 18% arising from internal organs.[43]

A recent study found that most synovial sarcomas were histiocytic sarcomas and that rottweilers accounted for more than 60% of this group. The most commonly affected site was the stifle.[82]

Based on immunophenotypic studies, malignant histiocytosis and histiocytic sarcomas are derived from myeloid dendritic antigen-presenting cells.[65]

Clinical Presentation and History

The clinical signs in a dog with histiocytic sarcoma depend on the primary site of the disease. Dogs with splenic histiocytic sarcoma present with nonspecific signs of lethargy and anorexia and usually have a palpable splenic mass on physical examination.[83] Dogs with synovial histiocytic sarcoma present with a mass or with lameness.[84]

Staging and Diagnosis

The most common primary site of histiocytic sarcomas appears to be the skin and subcutaneous tissue, particularly on the limbs and around joints.[81,82,84] The next most common primary site appears to be the spleen. These tumors have also been described to arise in the tongue, vertebral bone, and nasal cavity.[65] The lungs were affected as metastatic sites in nearly 20% of dogs with histiocytic sarcoma; other, less common sites (10% affected) were the lymph nodes, spleen, liver, and kidney. The same distribution pattern for metastases was seen in dogs with malignant histiocytosis or hybrid neoplasms, but higher percentages of dogs were affected at each site.[80] Involvement of the CNS or bone marrow is rare in dogs with localized histiocytic sarcomas and probably should warrant a diagnosis of malignant histiocytosis.[66]

Of 18 dogs with synovial histiocytic sarcomas based on positive immunostaining of tumor cells for CD18, more than 90% developed metastases, most commonly to the lungs, lymph nodes, and liver.[82]

Complete clinical staging includes thoracic radiography to check for sternal lymphadenopathy and pulmonary nodules as well as routine blood work and urinalysis. Abdominal ultrasonography should be conducted to assess the spleen and liver. Ultrasonography may demonstrate hypoechoic nodules in the spleen, liver, and kidneys as well as mesenteric and medial iliac lymphadenopathy. Dogs with liver involvement may have low serum albumin levels and peripheral edema, which can complicate treatment. These findings are nonspecific, and definitive diagnosis requires cytologic or histologic examination.[67] Abdominal ultrasonography may enable needle (Tru-Cut) biopsies to obtain a definitive diagnosis. Care should be taken when biopsying dogs with bone marrow infiltration and consequent cytopenias because thrombocytopenia may be marked and the patient may be prone to bleeding. For completeness, a bone marrow aspirate should be obtained.

In an effort to differentiate histiocytic sarcoma from other diseases (e.g., other undifferentiated soft tissue sarcomas), immunohistochemistry appears to be the most useful criterion to indicate likely histiocytic origin. Whereas both CD3 (T cell) and CD79a (B cell) are lymphocyte markers, CD18 is histiocytic. If the lesion is a lymphoma, then one of the T- or B-cell markers is usually positive. Histiocytes would be CD18+, CD3-, and CD79a-. Other stains include lysozyme and lectin RCA-1, both of which stain histiocytes.[76]

Prognostic Factors

A preliminary report of treatment for dogs with histiocytic sarcoma using CCNU found thrombocytopenia and hypoalbuminemia to be significant independent predictors of poor prognosis.[78]

A study of splenic fibrohistiocytic nodules found the lymphoid:fibrohistiocytic cell ratio in the lesion to be the most important prognostic indicator for dogs with this syndrome, with dogs that had less than 40% lymphocytes having a substantially poorer prognosis (1-year survival: 55%) than those with a higher proportion of lymphocytes (1-year survival: 87%). The mitotic index also had some prognostic value, but it was overshadowed by the lymphoid:fibrohistiocytic cell ratio.[60]

Treatment

Surgical excision of histiocytic synovial sarcomas is rarely successful, with a median survival time for 15 treated dogs of 4.5 months, which was considerably less than for dogs with synovial tumors of other derivation. The longest survivors were those that were treated by surgery and chemotherapy; three of four dogs lived longer than 12 months. Unfortunately, details of chemotherapy were not reported.[82] Excision of cutaneous histiocytic sarcoma was reported for 13 dogs, five of which had no recurrence, but eight dogs were lost to follow-up.[65]

Histiocytic sarcoma often affects the spleen and may represent the more malignant end of a spectrum of fibrohistiocytic nodules in that organ.[60] Five dogs were treated by splenectomy, but clinical outcome for four of them was not reported. One dog was treated with doxorubicin but developed hepatic metastases 9 months after surgery.[83] Chemotherapy should be considered investigational for patients with this tumor.

Radiation therapy was successful in treating a histiocytic sarcoma of the tongue, although the duration of remission was not reported.[65]

> **KEY POINT**
>
> *Dogs with localized histiocytic sarcomas are best treated by surgery and chemotherapy because the metastatic rate of these tumors is high.*

A preliminary report showed an overall 50% response rate in 24 dogs with measurable histiocytic sarcoma (19 with metastases) treated with CCNU, with an overall median survival of 4 months.[78] That report included dogs that responded for as little as 7 days, so the encouraging figures may be misleading. Of a further 27 dogs treated, Moore and Rassnick have seen some complete and partial remissions but nowhere near the 50% observed in that study. Either single-agent CCNU or a combination chemotherapy protocol based on CCNU and other agents active against lymphoma may be the treatment of choice for this disease. As a principle of chemotherapy, combination therapy is always expected to provide better outcomes than single-agent treatment.

REFERENCES

1. Glickman LT, Domanski LM, MacGuire TG, et al: Mesothelioma in pet dogs associated with exposure of their owners to asbestos. *Environ Res* 32:305–313, 1983.
2. Harbison ML, Godleski JJ: Malignant mesothelioma in urban dogs. *Vet Pathol* 20:531–540, 1983.
3. Trigo FJ, Morrison WB, Breeze RG: An ultrastructural study of canine mesothelioma. *J Comp Pathol* 91:531–537, 1981.
4. Ikede BO, Zubaidy A, Gill CW: Pericardial mesothelioma with cardiac tamponade in a dog. *Vet Pathol* 17:496–501, 1980.
5. Thrall DE, Goldschmidt MH: Mesothelioma in the dog: Six case reports. *J Am Vet Radiol Soc* 19:107–115, 1978.
6. Smith DA, Hill FW: Metastatic malignant mesothelioma in a dog. *J Comp Pathol* 100:97–101, 1989.
7. Cihak RW, Roen DR, Klaassen J: Malignant mesothelioma of the tunica vaginalis in a dog. *J Comp Pathol* 96:459–462, 1986.
8. DiPinto MN, Dunstan RW, Lee C: Cystic, peritoneal mesothelioma in a dog. *JAAHA* 31:385–389, 1995.
9. Kim JH, Choi YK, Yoon HY, et al: Juvenile malignant mesothelioma in a dog. *J Vet Med Sci* 64:269–271, 2002.
10. Breeze RG, Lauder IM: Pleural mesothelioma in a dog. *Vet Rec* 96:243–246, 1975.
11. Morrison WB, Trigo FJ: Clinical characterization of pleural mesothelioma in seven dogs. *Compend Contin Educ Pract Vet* 6:342–348, 1984.
12. Stepien RL, Whitley NT, Dubielzig RR: Idiopathic or mesothelioma-related pericardial effusion: Clinical findings and survival in 17 dogs studied retrospectively. *J Small Anim Pract* 41:342–347, 2000.
13. Girard C, Helie P, Odin M: Intrapericardial neoplasia in dogs. *J Vet Diagn Invest*: 11, 73–78. 1999.
14. Kovak JR, Ludwig LL, Bergman PJ, et al: Use of thoracoscopy to determine the etiology of pleural effusion in dogs and cats: 18 cases (1998–2001). *JAVMA* 221:990–994, 2002.
15. Jackson J, Richter KP, Launer DP: Thoracoscopic partial pericardiectomy in 13 dogs. *J Vet Intern Med* 13:529–533, 1999.
16. Moore AS, Kirk C, Cardona A: Intracavitary cisplatin chemotherapy experience with six dogs. *J Vet Intern Med* 5:227–231, 1991.
17. Geninet C, Bernex F, Rakotovao F et al: Sclerosing peritoneal mesothelioma in a dog: A case report. *J Vet Med A Physiol Pathol Clin Med* 50:402–405, 2003.
18. Fine DM, Tobias AH, Jacob KA: Use of pericardial fluid pH to distinguish between idiopathic and neoplastic effusions. *J Vet Intern Med* 17:525–529, 2003.
19. Peters M, Tenhundfeld J, Stephan I, Hewicker-Trautwein M: Embolized mesothelial cells within mediastinal lymph nodes of three dogs with idiopathic haemorrhagic pericardial effusion. *J Comp Pathol* 128:107–112, 2003.
20. Liu KX, Bird AE, Lenz SD, et al: Antigen expression in normal and neoplastic canine tissues defined by a monoclonal antibody generated against canine mesothelioma cells. *Vet Pathol* 31:663–673, 1994.
21. Gallagher LA, Birchard SJ, Weisbrode SE. Effects of tetracycline hydrochloride on

22. Birchard SJ, Gallagher L: Use of pleurodesis in treating selected pleural diseases. *Compend Contin Educ Pract Vet* 10:826–832, 1988.
23. Dunning D, Monnet E, Orton EC, Salman MD: Analysis of prognostic indicators for dogs with pericardial effusion: 46 cases (1985–1996). *JAVMA* 212:1276–1280, 1998.
24. Ogilvie GK, Obradovich JE, Elmslie RE, et al: Efficacy of mitoxantrone against various neoplasms in dogs. *JAVMA* 198:1618–1621, 1991.
25. Ogilvie GK, Reynolds HA, Richardson RC, et al: Phase II evaluation of doxorubicin for treatment of various canine neoplasms. *JAVMA* 195:1580–1583, 1989.
26. Balli A, Lachat M, Gerber B, et al: [Cardiac tamponade due to pericardial mesothelioma in an 11-year-old dog: diagnosis, medical and interventional treatments]. *Schweiz Arch Tierheilkd* 145:82–87, 2003.
27. Closa JM, Font A, Mascort J: Pericardial mesothelioma in a dog: Long-term survival after pericardiectomy in combination with chemotherapy. *J Small Anim Pract* 40:383–386, 1999.
28. Atwater SW, Powers BE, Park RD, et al: Thymoma in dogs: 23 cases (1980–1991). *JAVMA* 205:1007–1013, 1994.
29. Aronsohn MG, Schunk KL, Carpenter JL, King NW: Clinical and pathologic features of thymoma in 15 dogs. *JAVMA* 184:1355–1362, 1984.
30. Bellah JR, Stiff ME, Russsell RG: Thymoma in the dog: Two case reports and review of 20 additional cases. *JAVMA* 183:306–311, 1983.
31. Hitt ME, Shaw DP, Hogan PM, et al: Radiation treatment for thymoma in a dog. *JAVMA* 190:1187–1190, 1987.
32. Hunt GB, Churcher RK, Church DB, Mahoney P: Excision of a locally invasive thymoma causing cranial vena caval syndrome in a dog. *JAVMA* 210:1628–1630, 1997.
33. Lainesse MF, Taylor SM, Myers SL, et al: Focal myasthenia gravis as a paraneoplastic syndrome of canine thymoma: Improvement following thymectomy. *JAAHA* 32:111–117, 1996.
34. Dewey CW, Bailey CS, Shelton GD, et al: Clinical forms of acquired myasthenia gravis in dogs: 25 cases (1988–1995). *J Vet Intern Med* 11:50–57, 1997.
35. Stenner VJ, Parry BW, Holloway SA: Acquired myasthenia gravis associated with a non-invasive thymic carcinoma in a dog. *Aust Vet J* 81:543–546, 2003.
36. Shelton GD, Skeie GO, Kass PH, Aarli JA: Titin and ryanodine receptor autoantibodies in dogs with thymoma and late-onset myasthenia gravis. *Vet Immunol Immunopathol* 78:97–105, 2001.
37. Klebanow ER: Thymoma and acquired myasthenia gravis in the dog: A case report and review of 13 additional cases. *JAAHA* 28:63–70, 1992.
38. Smeak DD, Birchard SJ, McLoughlin MA, et al: Treatment of chronic pleural effusion with pleuroperitoneal shunts in dogs: 14 cases (1985–1999). *JAVMA* 219:1590–1597, 2001.
39. Smith AN, Wright JC, Brawner WR Jr, et al: Radiation therapy in the treatment of canine and feline thymomas: A retrospective study (1985–1999). *JAAHA* 37:489–496, 2001.
40. Rusbridge C, White RN, Elwood CM, Wheeler SJ: Treatment of acquired myasthenia gravis associated with thymoma in two dogs. *J Small Anim Pract* 37:376–380, 1996.
41. Dewey CW, Coates JR, Ducoté JM, et al: Azathioprine therapy for acquired myasthenia gravis in five dogs. *JAAHA* 35:396–402, 1999.
42. Goldschmidt MH, Shofer FS: Canine cutaneous histiocytoma, in Goldschmidt MH, Shofer FS (eds): *Skin Tumors of the Dog and Cat*, ed 1. Tarrytown NY, Pergamon Press, 1992, pp 222–230.
43. Morris JS, Bostock DE, McInnes EF, et al: Histopathological survey of neoplasms in flat-coated retrievers, 1990 to 1998. *Vet Rec* 147:291–295, 2000.
44. Morris JS, McInnes EF, Bostock DE, et al: Immunohistochemical and histopathologic features of 14 malignant fibrous histiocytomas from flat-coated retrievers. *Vet Pathol* 39:473–479, 2002.
45. Cockerell GL, Slauson DO: Patterns of lymphoid infiltrate in the canine cutaneous histiocytoma. *J Comp Pathol* 89:193–203, 1979.
46. Kipar A, Baumgartner W, Kremmer E, et al: Expression of major histocompatibility complex class II antigen in neoplastic cells of canine cutaneous histiocytoma. *Vet Immunol Immunopathol* 62:1–13, 1998.
47. Bender WM, Muller GH: Multiple, resolving, cutaneous histiocytoma in a dog. *JAVMA* 194:535–537, 1989.
48. Linek M, Mecklenburg L: Multiple kutane histiozytome bei einem flat coated retriever. *Kleintierpraxis* 46:507–511, 2001.
49. Affolter VK, Moore PF: Canine cutaneous and systemic histiocytosis: Reactive histiocytosis of dermal dendritic cells. *Am J Dermatopathol* 22:40–48, 2000.
50. Carpenter JL, Thornton GW, Moore FM, King NW Jr: Idiopathic periadnexal multinodular granulomatous dermatitis in twenty-two dogs. *Vet Pathol* 24:5–10, 1987.
51. Paterson S, Boydell P, Pike R: Systemic histiocytosis in the Bernese mountain dog. *J Small Anim Pract* 36:233–236, 1995.
52. Calderwood-Mays M, Bergeron JA: Cutaneous histiocytosis in dogs. *JAVMA* 188:377–381, 1986.
53. Baines SJ, McCormick D, McInnes E, et al: Cutaneous T cell lymphoma mimicking cutaneous histiocytosis: Differentiation by flow cytometry. *Vet Rec* 147:11–16, 2000.
54. Gregory CR: Immunosuppressive agents, in Bonagura JD (ed): *Kirk's Current Veterinary Therapy, XIII.* Philadelphia, WB Saunders, 2000, pp 509–513.
55. Moriello KA, MacEwen G, Schultz KT: PEG-L-asparaginase in the treatment of canine epitheliotropic lymphoma and histiocytic proliferative dermatitis, in Ihrke, PJ, Mason, IS, White SD (eds): *Advances in Vet Dermatology*, vol 2. Tarrytown, NY, Pergamon Press, 1992.
56. Moore PF: Utilization of cytoplasmic lysozyme immunoreactivity as a histiocytic marker in canine histiocytic disorders. *Vet Pathol* 23:757–762, 1986.
57. Weiss DJ: Flow cytometric evaluation of hemophagocytic disorders in canine. *Vet Clin Pathol* 31:36–41, 2002.
58. Visonneau S, Cesano A, Tran T, et al: Successful treatment of canine malignant histiocytosis with the human major histocompatibility complex nonrestricted cytotoxic T-cell line TALL-104. *Clin Cancer Res* 3:1789–1797, 1997.
59. Spangler WL, Kass PH: Splenic myeloid metaplasia, histiocytosis, and hypersplenism in the dog (65 cases). *Vet Pathol* 36:583–593, 1999.
60. Spangler WL, Kass PH: Pathologic and prognostic characteristics of splenomegaly in dogs due to fibrohistiocytic nodules: 98 cases. *Vet Pathol* 35:488–498, 1998.
61. Ramsey IK, McKay JS, Rudorf H, Dobson JM: Malignant histiocytosis in three Bernese mountain dogs. *Vet Rec* 138:440–444, 1996.
62. Padgett GA, Madewell BR, Keller ET, et al: Inheritance of histiocytosis in Bernese mountain dogs. *J Small Anim Pract* 36:93–98, 1995.
63. Moore PF, Rosin A: Malignant histiocytosis of Bernese mountain dogs. *Vet Pathol* 23:1–10, 1986.
64. Shimizu Y, Nakamura S, Harada T, Takahashi K: Malignant histiocytosis of a Bernese mountain dog. *J Vet Med (Tokyo)* 52:370–374, 1999.
65. Schmidt ML, Rutteman G, Wolvekamp P: Canine malignant histiocytosis (MH): Clinical and radiographic findings. *Tijdschr Diergeneeskd* 117(suppl 1):43–44, 1992.
66. Affolter VK, Moore PF: Localized and disseminated histiocytic sarcoma of dendritic cell origin in dogs. *Vet Pathol* 39:74–83, 2002.
67. Goldschmidt MH, Shofer FS: Uncommon skin tumors, in Goldschmidt MH, Shofer FS (eds): *Skin Tumors of the Dog and Cat*, ed 1. Tarrytown NY, Pergamon Press, 1992, pp 291–295.
68. Ramirez S, Douglass JP, Robertson ID: Ultrasonographic features of canine abdominal malignant histiocytosis. *Vet Radiol Ultrasound* 43:167–170, 2002.
69. Uchida K, Morozumi M, Yamaguchi R, Tateyama S: Diffuse leptomeningeal malignant histiocytosis in the brain and spinal cord of a Tibetan terrier. *Vet Pathol* 38:219–222, 2001.
70. Chandra AM, Ginn PE: Primary malignant histiocytosis of the brain in a dog. *J Comp Pathol* 121:77–82, 1999.
71. Suzuki M, Uchida K, Morozumi M, et al: A comparative pathological study on granulomatous meningoencephalomyelitis and central malignant histiocytosis in dogs. *J Vet Med Sci* 65:1319–1324, 2003.
72. Braund KG: Granulomatous meningoencephalomyelitis. *JAVMA* 186:138–141, 1985.
73. Kipar A, Baumgartner W, Vogl C, et al: Immunohistochemical characterization of inflammatory cells in brains of dogs with granulomatous meningoencephalitis. *Vet Pathol* 35:43–52, 1998.
74. Weiss DJ: Cytologic evaluation of benign and malignant hemophagocytic disorders in canine bone marrow. *Vet Clin Pathol* 30:28–34. 2001.
75. Weiss DJ, Evanson OA, Sykes J: A retrospective study of canine pancytopenia. *Vet Clin Pathol* 28:83–88, 1999.
76. Hugnet C, Hugnet-Bruchon C, Degorie-Rubiales F, Poujadee A: Histiocytose maligne associee a une hypercalcemie paraneoplasique. *Pract Med Chirurgicale* 36:23–27, 2001.
77. Brown DE, Thrall MA, Getzy DM, et al: Cytology of canine malignant histiocytosis. *Vet Clin Pathol* 23:118–123, 1994.
78. Skorupski KA, Clifford CA, Paoloni MC, et al: CCNU for the treatment of dogs with metastatic or disseminated histiocytic sarcoma. *Proc 23rd Annu Conf Vet Cancer Soc*:36, 2003.
79. Poirier VJ, Hershey AE, Burgess KE, et al: Efficacy and toxicity of paclitaxel (Taxol) for the treatment of canine malignant tumors. *J Vet Intern Med* 18:219–222, 2004.
80. Kerlin RL, Hendrick MJ: Malignant fibrous histiocytoma and malignant histiocytosis in the dog: Convergent or divergent phenotypic differentiation? *Vet Pathol* 33:713–716, 1996.
81. Pires MA: Malignant fibrous histiocytoma in a puppy. *Vet Rec* 140:234–235, 1997.
82. Craig LE, Julian ME, Ferracone JD: The diagnosis and prognosis of synovial tumors in dogs: 35 cases. *Vet Pathol* 39:66–73, 2002.
83. Hendrick MJ, Brooks JJ, Bruce EH: Six cases of malignant fibrous histiocytoma of the canine spleen. *Vet Pathol* 29:351–354, 1992.
84. Booth MJ, Bastianello SS, Jiminez M, van Heerden A: Malignant fibrous histiocytoma of the deep peri-articular tissue of the stifle in a dog. *J S Afr Vet Assoc* 69:163–168, 1998.

TUMORS OF THE SKIN AND SURROUNDING STRUCTURES

Antony S. Moore and Gregory K. Ogilvie

CLINICAL BRIEFING

MDB includes a CBC, biochemical profile, and urinalysis, as well as thoracic radiography (three views).

Cutaneous Squamous Cell Carcinoma

Clinical factors
- Ulcerated cutaneous lesions.
- Most often on the trunk (induced by sunlight; actinic)
- Most cutaneous SCCs are well differentiated and rarely metastasize.
- Digital (subungual) lesions are more likely to metastasize.
- Large, black-breed dogs are prone to subungual tumors.
- Light-skinned dogs are prone to actinically induced tumors.

Staging and diagnosis
- MDB.
- Careful examination of regional nodes for subungual.
- CT or MRI if involves nasal planum.

Prognostic factors
- Higher-grade tumors are more likely to be invasive and, therefore, more difficult to excise; they are also more likely to metastasize.

Treatment

Initial
- Early lesions: Surgical excision, retinoids, topical 5-FU or BCNU ointments, and cryotherapy if lesions are <1 cm.
- Invasive lesions: Surgery with or without radiation therapy and intralesional chemotherapy.
- Metastatic lesions: Cisplatin or mitoxantrone chemotherapy.

Supportive
- Analgesia postoperatively.

Cutaneous and Extramedullary Plasmacytomas

Clinical factors
- Solitary cutaneous mass in trunk or limbs.
- May affect oral cavity, ears, and head; less commonly, may occur in multiple sites.
- Older dogs; cutaneous tumors are usually benign.

Staging and diagnosis
- MDB.

Prognostic factors
- Tumors with amyloid may be more likely to recur.

Treatment	
Initial	• Surgery with wide surgical margins is curative in most cases of cutaneous plasmacytomas.
Adjunctive	• Radiation rarely needed but should be sensitive.
	• Chemotherapy with melphalan, prednisone, and doxorubicin have all caused tumor responses.
Supportive	• Analgesia postoperatively.
Cutaneous Lymphoma	
Clinical factors	• Solitary or multiple dermal masses or as a chronic unresolved or progressive case of dermatitis.
	• T-cell variant is usually epitheliotropic and is called *mycosis fungoides*.
Staging and diagnosis	• MDB, abdominal ultrasonography, bone marrow aspiration (as for lymphoma).
	• Often systemic involvement is not seen until later stages.
Prognostic factors	• B-cell lymphoma has a better prognosis than T-cell lymphoma.
Treatment	
Initial	• Surgery with adequate surgical margins for solitary lesions (rare).
	• Radiation also for localized lesions.
Adjunctive	• Early lesions may respond to retinoids or linoleic acid PO.
	• Chemotherapy, usually with alkylating agents. Lomustine, dacarbazine, and L-asparaginase all reported single-agent activity.
	• Radiation may be palliative for painful lesions.
Supportive	• Treat secondary skin infections.
	• Pain relief may be necessary for generalized lesions.
	• Nutritional support, particularly if exudative and debilitating.
Skin Tumors Reviewed in Separate Chapters	
	• Cutaneous melanoma: Chapter 54.
	• Cutaneous hemangioma and hemangiosarcoma: Chapter 56.
	• Cutaneous lymphangioma and lymphangiosarcoma: Chapter 56.
	• Soft tissue sarcomas (fibroma, fibrosarcoma, hemangiopericytoma, neurofibroma, neurofibrosarcoma, schwannoma, rhabdomyoma, rhabdomyosarcoma, leiomyoma, leiomyosarcoma, lipoma, and liposarcoma): Chapter 62.
	• Histiocytoma and histiocytosis: Chapter 63.
	• Mast cell tumors: Chapter 65.

As the major barrier between animals and their environment, the skin is exposed to a high level of environmental carcinogens. This exposure is reflected in the number and variety of primary skin tumors that occur in the skin, subcutis, and adnexae of dogs. The skin is one of the most common sites of tumors in animals. Tumors that occur on the skin are likely to be discovered by the animal's owner. Management of skin tumors (i.e., identifying them and deciding whether to remove them and whether further treatment is necessary after removal) is an important part of small animal practice. Most skin tumors in dogs are benign.

In the largest survey of skin tumors in dogs from the United States, accounting for 29,150 lesions, 35% of tumors were derived from the epithelium; 85% of these were benign, and only 15% were malignant. Mesenchymal tumors accounted for 50% of the tumors, and 57% of these were benign histologically[1] (Table 64-1). Melanomas, which accounted for 4% of skin tumors, are covered separately in

Table 64-1 **Distribution of Skin Tumors in Dogs**[1]

Epithelial Tumors (n = 10,300)	Dogs (%)	Mesenchymal Tumors (n = 14,500)	Dogs (%)
Anal sac carcinoma	2	Cutaneous histiocytoma	24
Apocrine gland adenoma	5	Fibroma	4
Apocrine ductal adenoma	1	Fibrosarcoma	3
Apocrine adenocarcinoma	2	Giant-cell tumor	<1
Basal cell tumor	11	Hemangioma	9
Basal cell carcinoma	<1	Hemangiopericytoma	14
Basosquamous carcinoma	1	Hemangiosarcoma	2
Ceruminous adenoma	1	Lipoma	16
Ceruminous adenocarcinoma	1	Liposarcoma	<1
Hepatoid adenoma	27	Lymphoma	2
Hepatoid adenocarcinoma	1	Lymphangioma	<1
Intracutaneous cornifying epithelioma	5	Mast cell tumor	20
Meibomian adenoma	9	Myxoma and myxosarcoma	1
Meibomian adenocarcinoma	<1	Neural tumors	1
Papilloma	<1	Plasmacytoma	3
Pilomatrixoma	3	Others	<1
Sebaceous adenocarcinoma	2		
Sebaceous adenoma	12		
Squamous cell carcinoma	5		
Trichoepithelioma	12		

Chapter 54. Tumorlike lesions accounted for 11% of skin masses; these include epidermal cysts, follicular cysts, apocrine cysts, sebaceous hyperplasia, adnexal nevi, and skin tags.[1] Some authors have grouped tumors of the basal cells, sebaceous adenomas, and sebaceous epitheliomas as adnexal tumors.[2] This classification accounts for between 20% and 30% of all skin tumors.

Some canine breeds are predisposed to developing particular skin tumors (e.g., boxers and mast cell tumors [MCTs], cocker spaniels and sebaceous tumors). Certain skin characteristics seem to promote other types of tumors (e.g., dogs with poorly pigmented, lightly haired ventral abdominal skin are predisposed to developing squamous cell carcinoma [SCC] and cutaneous hemangiosarcomas).

Skin tumors are often superficial and their margins obvious. Infiltrative masses (e.g., MCTs and soft tissue sarcomas) often have diffuse neoplastic margins that are not easily identified. For skin tumors that attach to underlying tissue or interfere with function, ultrasonography and computed tomography (CT) may be useful adjuncts for staging and delineating tumor borders before surgical excision. In one series of 26 dogs with cutaneous tumors, these two modalities identified 18 dogs that had more advanced disease than was expected on clinical examination, and the surgical plan was subsequently altered.[3] In any case, a preoperative biopsy is recommended if its results might change either the owner's willingness to treat (benign versus malignant) or the type of treatment that would be offered (e.g., sebaceous adenoma versus a grade 3 anaplastic MCT). A needle core biopsy was able to accurately diagnose more than 90% of skin lesions in one study.[4]

An Australian survey from the subtropics found a very similar distribution of tumor types, except that SCCs were the third most common tumor after MCTs and histiocytomas.[5] In another Australian survey from a more temperate climate, SCC was the fourth most common diagnosis.[6]

Epithelial Tumors
CUTANEOUS PAPILLOMAS (WARTS)
Incidence, Signalment, and Etiology

The papillomavirus that induces this benign tumor of stratified squamous epithelium is the same type of virus that has been known to cause cervical cancer and SCCs in many species. Many tumors identified clinically as warts are actually other tumors such as sebaceous adenomas. Papillomas occur with no gender predilection. Middle-aged and older dogs are most often affected (median age: 6 years).[7] Breeds that are predisposed include whippets and Bernese mountain dogs (64 and 32 times more likely than the general population, respectively). Irish setters and beagles are more than three times as likely as other breeds to develop papillomas.[7] Cutaneous squamous papilloma, cutaneous inverted papilloma, and canine pigmented epidermal nevus have all been associated with papillomaviruses, although more than one virus is probably responsible.[8]

Clinical Presentation and History

Papillomas are usually solitary, superficial, pedunculated nodules that are smaller than 1 cm in diameter. They are firm and have a rough, corrugated surface. They are found mainly on the head (including the eyelids), limbs, perineum, and tail. Papillomas are multiple in less than 3% of cases.[7] Numerous small, fungiform projections arise from a broad, flat base. When subjected to trauma, they may bleed and become secondarily infected.

Inverted papillomas appear as 1- to 2-cm circumscribed, flask-like structures below the level of the surrounding skin and look more like an intracutaneous cornifying epithelioma.[9]

Treatment

Some papillomas regress spontaneously over weeks to months. Therefore, therapy includes benign neglect, surgical removal, or cryotherapy. If cryotherapy is used, a 2% lidocaine with bicarbonate (10:1) block is applied subcutaneously and the surface of the tumor is excised for histopathology. The base of the papilloma is then frozen twice with a spray or focal-contact applicator. After surgical excision or cryotherapy, a good prognosis can be given.

Vaccination may reduce the incidence, particularly of the oral variant, but SCCs may develop at the site of papilloma vaccination between 1 and 3 years later.[7,10]

BASAL CELL TUMORS (BASAL CELL EPITHELIOMA)
Incidence, Signalment, and Etiology

Basal cell tumors are usually benign tumors originating from basal cells of the epidermis, hair follicles, sweat glands, or sebaceous glands. Dogs with basal cell tumors are middle-aged to old. Breeds that are more than three times more likely than the general population to develop basal cell tumors include wirehaired pointing griffons, Kerry blue and Wheaton terriers, Welsh springer spaniels, pulis, bichons frisés, spitzes, bearded collies, and cockapoos.[11]

Clinical Presentation and History

These tumors usually appear as well-demarcated, small, firm nodules that sharply elevate the overlying epidermis. They are usually freely movable and rarely multiple. Basal cell tumors are most common on the head and neck (accounting for nearly 80% of cases in one study).[11] On cut surface, they are usually white and may appear lobulated; however, cystic spaces and a darkly pigmented appearance are not uncommon.

Staging and Diagnosis

Basal tumors are considered benign. Occasionally, a truly malignant basal cell tumor may be diagnosed (see below). Thoracic radiographs are still indicated for older animals as part of a minimum database (MDB) and to detect other problems. Cytologic features are nonspecific, although some benign tumors show cytologic criteria of malignancy and could therefore be diagnosed as a more malignant tumor (e.g., melanoma, SCC).[12] Resection is generally all that is needed for diagnosis.

Treatment

Local recurrence has not been described after adequate surgical removal.

MALIGNANT BASAL CELL TUMORS (BASOSQUAMOUS CARCINOMA)
Incidence, Signalment, and Etiology

Malignant basal cell tumors may have areas of squamous differentiation and invade adjacent tissues. Dogs with basosquamous carcinomas are older. Breeds that are more than three times more likely than the general population to develop malignant basal cell tumors include Saint Bernards, Scottish terriers, and Norwegian elkhounds.[11]

Clinical Presentation and History

These tumors usually appear as firm nodules that are fixed because of invasion of the deep dermis and subcutaneous tissues. They are rarely multiple, accounting for less than 2% of cases. Basal cell tumors are most common on the head, neck, back, and limbs.[11] On cut surface, they are usually white and may appear lobulated; however, cystic spaces and a darkly pigmented appearance are not uncommon.

Staging and Diagnosis

If the lesion is a malignant basal cell tumor histologically, the regional lymph nodes should be palpated and fine-

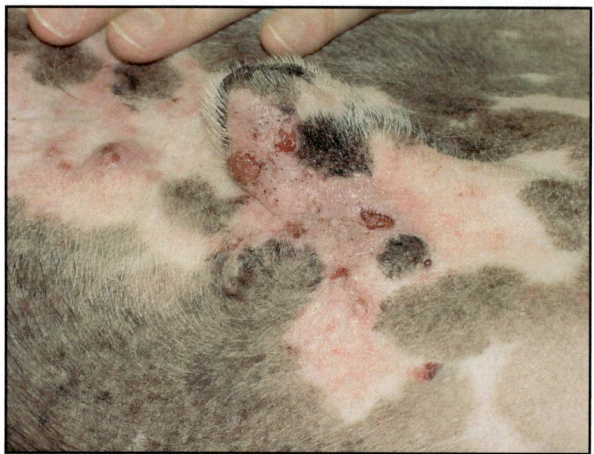

Figure 64-1. *Actinically induced cutaneous SCC on the lightly haired, poorly pigmented abdomen of a dog. Note the erythematous lesions progressing to masses and ulcerated areas. (Courtesy of Nicole Northrup, DVM, University of Georgia College of Veterinary Medicine)*

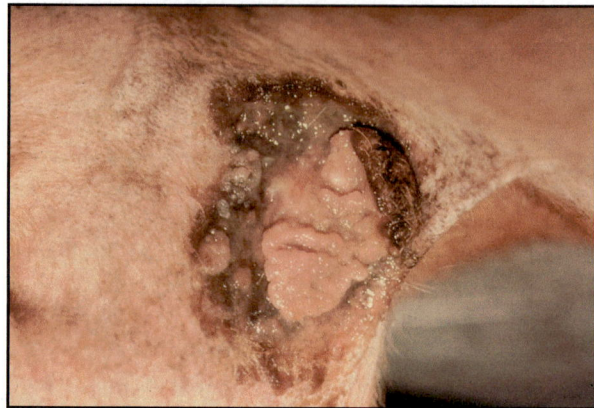

Figure 64-2. *Cutaneous SCC in the axilla of a dog. This lesion has metastasized to the regional lymph node.*

needle aspiration conducted. An MDB that includes thoracic radiographs should be obtained.

Treatment

For incompletely excised or metastatic lesions, the use of radiation therapy and chemotherapy may be appropriate, but this has not been reported in the veterinary literature. The therapeutic approach outlined for SCC is probably appropriate for malignant basal cell tumors as well.

SQUAMOUS CELL CARCINOMAS
Incidence, Signalment, and Etiology

These tumors are firm, nodular masses that may be proliferative or erosive and may extend deep into the dermis. Sites exposed to solar radiation are at greatest risk, especially in dogs with areas of low skin pigmentation. Broad-based erosive SCCs that are presumably actinically (sunlight) induced have been observed on the bellies of lightly pigmented dogs that like to sunbathe.[13] These tumors are found in areas of chronic inflammation that progress to actinic keratoses and, eventually, malignant tumors. Large, black-breed dogs are predisposed to subungual SCCs (see separately below). In one study, bloodhounds and basset hounds were predisposed to developing SCC.[14]

A single case of malignant transformation of follicular cysts to metastasizing SCC over a 2-year period has been reported, but this is extremely rare.[15] A similarly rare transformation of untreated discoid lupus erythematosus to SCC over a 4- to 6-year period was described in two German shepherds.[16]

Clinical Presentation and History

SCCs in dogs most frequently involve the head, limbs, abdomen, and perineum. Tumors are rarely multiple, although dogs with actinically induced SCC may have multiple areas that include not only SCC but also areas of preneoplastic skin changes that appear reddened, edematous, and scaly. Brown, crusty lesions may precede cancer formation.[17] Tumors are often ulcerated and bleed easily, forming crusts and deep erosions; however, they may be proliferative. SCC is usually fixed to the underlying skin because of invasion of the subcutis (Figures 64-1 and 64-2).

Staging and Diagnosis

Most SCCs that arise in the skin are well differentiated and have a good prognosis after adequate surgical removal. Although an SCC will occasionally invade underlying tissue, metastasis is rare. If the lesion is poorly differentiated histologically, however, the regional lymph nodes should be palpated and fine-needle aspiration conducted in addition to an MDB. Highly anaplastic tumors may metastasize to regional lymph nodes and subsequently to the lungs.[17] Therefore, these tumors warrant a guarded prognosis. The staging system for cutaneous SCC is found in Table 64-2.

A histologic grading system may also have some value in predicting behavior and is outlined in Table 64-3.[14] Higher-grade tumors are more likely to be invasive and, therefore, more difficult to excise; they are also more likely to metastasize. Metastasis is usually to the regional lymph nodes and rarely to the lungs.

Some tumors are termed *adenoid squamous cell carcinomas* because they have pseudoglandular structures surrounding acantholytic keratinocytes.[14] One author suggested that invasive SCCs have an affinity for nerve invasion.[14]

Treatment

For solitary SCC, surgical excision is the treatment of choice. Some tumors, particularly actinically induced SCCs, may be multiple. For these tumors, and for tumors that

Table 64-2 World Health Organization Staging Scheme for Cutaneous Tumors

Tumor Size	Criteria
T1	Tumor <2 cm, superficial or exophytic
T2	Tumor 2–5 cm or minimal invasion (regardless of size)
T3	Tumor >5 cm or invasion of subcutis (regardless of size)
T4	Tumor invading muscle, bone, or cartilage

Table 64-3 Histologic Grading of Cutaneous Squamous Cell Carcinoma[14]

Grade	Description
1	SCCs that are well differentiated with abundant cytoplasm, intercellular bridges, and keratin pearls. Minimal nuclear pleomorphism and mitoses. Invasion is accompanied by proliferative fibrous reaction.
2 and 3	SCCs that are moderately differentiated with less abundant cytoplasm. Intercellular bridges and keratin pearls are rare. Moderate nuclear pleomorphism and more numerous mitoses, some bizarre. Invasion is prominent.
4	SCCs that are poorly differentiated with little squamous differentiation, pleomorphic nuclei, with marked mitoses. Invasion is deep and often involves individual cells, with a desmoplastic matrix.

metastasize, other treatment modalities should be considered (Figure 64-3).

Retinoids are synthetic derivatives of vitamin A that may reverse preneoplastic or metaplastic changes in human dermatologic conditions. Etretinate (a synthetic retinoid) at a dosage of 1 mg/kg orally twice daily caused complete resolution of some preneoplastic SCC lesions in dogs.[18] Etretinate is no longer available, but a newer synthetic retinoid, acitretin, may have similar effects at the same dosage. This therapy may be beneficial for dogs with multifocal preneoplastic lesions.

SCCs in dogs express cyclooxygenase-2 (COX-2), and 40% show intense staining on immunohistochemistry.[19] This has led to trials of nonsteroidal drugs that target COX-2. Piroxicam, an NSAID that primarily targets COX-2, was administered orally at 0.3 mg/kg every 24 hours to dogs with oral SCC.[20] Approximately 18% of treated dogs had a measurable response for an average of 6 months. Similar results may be seen in cutaneous lesions. Some oncologists have recommended piroxicam for dogs with multiple SCC lesions that cannot be treated surgically.

Superficial and noninvasive (in situ) lesions may be treated with topical 5-fluorouracil (5-FU) or carmustine (BCNU) ointments.[21] These ointments create an intense inflammatory reaction as part of their antineoplastic effect. Gloves should be worn when applying these ointments. Even if there is no response to 5-FU ointment, the tumor may still respond to intralesional 5-FU (see discussion below).[22] Imiquimod cream is an immunomodulator that has been recently approved for the treatment of superficial skin cancer in human patients. Its exact mechanism of action is unknown. Recommended use in humans is five times per week for 5 to 16 weeks until complete resolution of the tumor is seen. In veterinary patients, we have used it daily for 7 days, then every other day for 14 days, then every third day for 2 additional weeks. The antiviral cream induces a response of the local immune system and thus an intense inflammatory response at the site of treatment in some animals. It is only useful for very superficial (in situ or precancerous) lesions, although, in Dr. Ogilvie's experience, small T1 lesions may respond.

In one study, intralesional chemotherapy using bovine collagen matrix combined with 5-FU or cisplatin resulted in 81% of dogs with SCC having a greater than 50% reduction in tumor size; 55% had complete tumor resolution.[23] Dogs with large tumors or with a large area (mean: 40 cm^2) affected by multiple smaller lesions were treated with three weekly treatments of 5-FU. If there was no response to 5-FU, cisplatin was administered.[22] Five of 13 dogs had a complete response to 5-FU, and the remainder had a greater than 50% reduction in tumor size. Of five dogs that had a partial response to 5-FU and received cisplatin intralesionally, two had a complete response. Duration of tumor control for all 13 dogs was a median of 91 weeks.[22]

Cryotherapy may control small (<1 cm), noninvasive lesions; however, treatment may have to be repeated.

Photodynamic therapy (PDT) is an appropriate treatment for superficial lesions less than 1 cm in depth. In PDT, a drug that can be activated by a certain wavelength of light is given systemically. After a variable period (dependent on the drug), drug levels are higher in the tumor than in the surrounding normal tissue. The tumor and a normal tissue margin are irradiated with a laser of a specific wavelength to activate the drug, and the tumor tissue is damaged by oxygen free radical formation that is absent or minimal in the surrounding normal tissue. The tumor size limitation is attributable to poor light penetration into tissue and blood below a depth of 1 cm. Most photosensitizers are porphyrin derivatives, and most veterinary reports are in cats, but the principles should also apply to SCC in dogs. Responses in oral SCC have been documented in dogs.[24,25] Access to PDT

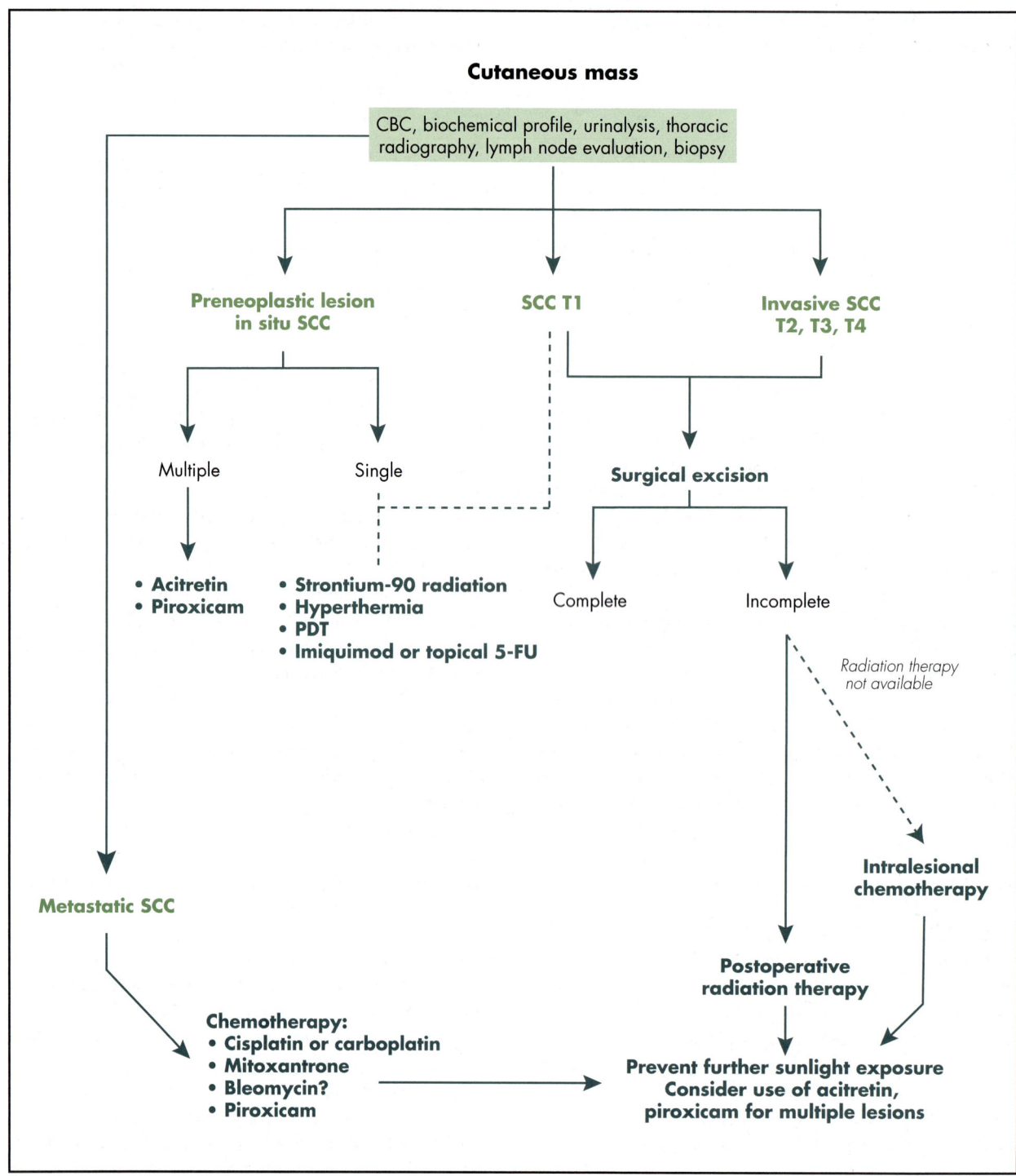

Figure 64-3. *A schematic depicting the treatment of cutaneous SCC in dogs.*

is limited because of the small number of facilities that perform the procedure.

SCC is considered radiation sensitive. For tumors that cannot be excised and have not metastasized, external beam teletherapy should be considered.

Cisplatin has caused objective tumor response in subungual SCCs that have metastasized to the lymph nodes and lung.[26] It is likely that similar responses may be achieved for metastatic SCC from other sites, and platinum derivatives are probably the drugs of choice for dogs with this tumor.

Bleomycin chemotherapy caused a partial response in one dog with actinically induced SCC.[27] The efficacy of this drug in dogs has not been further investigated. Mitoxantrone every 3 weeks caused short-term (42–147 days) responses in four of nine dogs with SCC[28] and may be considered for treatment of dogs with metastatic disease.

SUBUNGUAL SQUAMOUS CELL CARCINOMAS

Incidence, Signalment, and Etiology

Locally destructive SCC of the digit (subungual SCC) is an aggressive tumor. Large, black dogs are predisposed to this particular tumor. In one series, breeds with a risk greater than three times that of the general population were giant schnauzers, Gordon setters, briards, Kerry blue terriers, standard poodles, standard schnauzers, and Afghan hounds.[14] Multiple nail bed SCCs have been seen in related giant schnauzers.[29] Affected dogs are older, with an average age of 10 years in one study.[14]

Clinical Presentation and History

Subungual SCC is usually single but may occur in multiple digits[30] simultaneously or over a period of months and often years.[29,31] These tumors may affect the same foot or, more usually, different feet. Tumors arising from the digit may destroy the nail and, eventually, the phalanx (Figure 64-4). Affected dogs may show nail deformity, paronychia, fissuring, and inflammation. The affected digit is often very painful, particularly if bone invasion is present.

Staging and Diagnosis

These tumors metastasize uncommonly, but the regional lymph nodes and lungs are the most likely sites.[32–34] In one study, seven of 29 dogs (25%) with digital SCC developed metastases either before (three dogs) or after surgery.[35] Multiple digits may be affected simultaneously or over a period of months and often years; these tumors represent de novo tumors rather than metastases from the original SCC.[29,31]

> **KEY POINT**
> *Despite appearing aggressive histologically, subungual SCCs in dogs uncommonly metastasize.*

Radiographs of the affected digit show lysis of P3 in approximately 80% of dogs with subungual SCC. This is in contrast to digital melanomas (another common digital tumor), which rarely cause bony destruction (5% of cases).[32,35] Lysis may cross the joint space to involve P2. Digital SCCs are not pigmented.

Angiogenesis may be pronounced in SCC of the digit, perhaps reflecting the aggressive clinical nature of tumors in this location and suggesting that treatment strategies targeting antiangiogeneis may be effective for tumor control.[36]

Staging should include an MDB (including thoracic radiographs), lymph node palpation, and aspiration cytology (if indicated), as well as high-detail radiographs of the affected foot.

Treatment

Single digital SCC is best treated by high digital amputation. Although they commonly invade the lymphatics of the toe, these tumors often have an indolent course. In two studies totaling 50 dogs with digital SCC, 80% of dogs were alive 1 year after surgery, and just over half the dogs survived 2 years.[32,35] In one of these studies, dogs with tumors that were *not* subungual had poorer survival rates (60% versus 95% and 40% versus 74% at 1 and 2 years after surgery, respectively).[35]

Multiple digits on one foot may be affected, necessitating amputation of the limb. Dogs with multiple lesions or dogs of breeds that are thought to be at risk for developing future subungual SCC may benefit from strategies to prevent future SCC. Unfortunately, no data support this approach in affected dogs. Retinoids are synthetic derivatives of vitamin A that may reverse preneoplastic or metaplastic changes in human dermatologic conditions. Etretinate (a synthetic retinoid) at 1 mg/kg orally twice daily caused complete resolution of some preneoplastic SCC lesions in dogs.[18] Etretinate is no longer available, but a newer synthetic retinoid, acitretin, at the same dosage may have similar effects. This therapy may be beneficial for dogs at high risk for multifocal lesions or dogs that cannot be treated surgically.

SCCs in dogs express COX-2, and 40% show intense staining on immunohistochemistry.[19] This has led to trials of nonsteroidal drugs that target COX-2. Piroxicam, an NSAID that primarily targets COX-2 and is thought to be antiangiogenic, was administered orally at 0.3 mg/kg every 24 hours to dogs with oral SCC.[20] Approximately 18% of treated dogs had a measurable response for an average of 6 months. Similar results may be seen in subungual lesions. Some oncologists have recommended piroxicam for dogs with multiple SCC lesions or to prevent the occurrence of new lesions in dogs that cannot be treated surgically.

Cisplatin has caused objective tumor response in subungual SCCs that metastasized to lymph nodes and lung. In one dog, an escalating dose produced a partial response at 40 mg/m^2 and complete response at 60 mg/m^2.[26] In another dog, partial response occurred at a dose of 60 mg/m^2, but the patient relapsed after the fourth therapy. Three of five dogs treated with cisplatin for SCC of the head and neck had partial responses of 14, 70, and 105 days.[37] The platinum drugs may be the drugs of choice for chemotherapy of metastatic SCC. Cisplatin should not be combined with piroxicam because the potential for nephrotoxicity is enhanced.

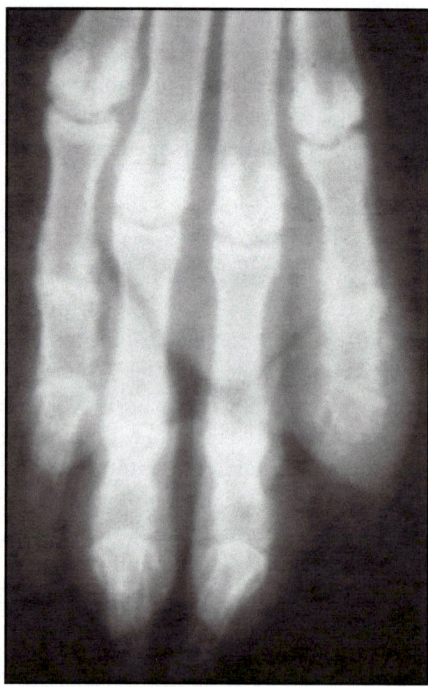

Figure 64-4. *Radiograph showing extensive lysis of the digit in a dog with subungual SCC. (Courtesy of John Berg, DVM, Tufts Cummings School of Veterinary Medicine)*

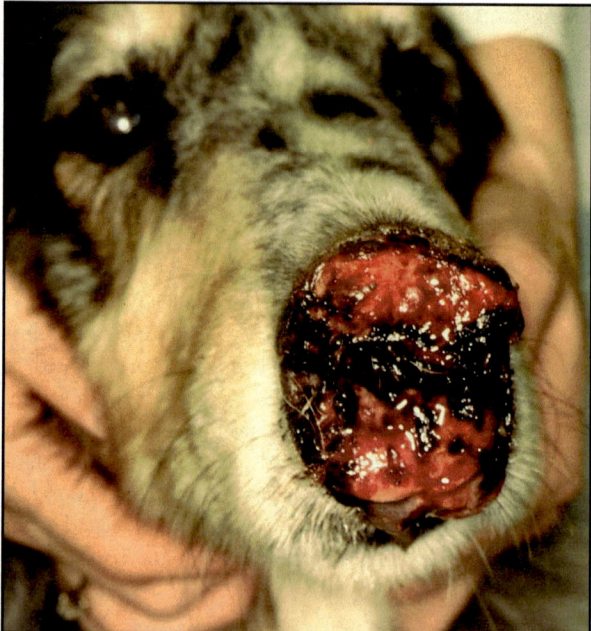

Figure 64-5. *SCC of the nasal planum is a rapidly progressive tumor that is usually advanced at the time of diagnosis, as in this collie. Radical resection is the best treatment.*

NASAL PLANUM SQUAMOUS CELL CARCINOMAS
Incidence, Signalment, and Etiology

In dogs, SCC of the nasal planum is an extremely aggressive and erosive disease, in contrast to SCC of the nasal planum in cats. Affected dogs are older; in two studies totaling 25 dogs, only one dog was younger than 7 years.[38,39] Retrievers (Labrador or golden) accounted for 17 of 25 dogs (70%) in the same two studies, and most other affected dogs were large-breed dogs.[38,39] In three studies, 26 of 31 dogs (>80%) were males, and most were intact.[38–40]

Labrador retrievers have a hereditary nasal planum hyperkeratosis, which may play a role in the precancerous formation of SCC.[41] Transformation over a 4- to 6-year period of untreated discoid lupus erythematosus to an invasive and erosive SCC of the nasal planum was described in two German shepherds.[16]

Clinical Presentation and History

The most common signs that lead an owner to present a dog with nasal planum SCC are epistaxis, sneezing, and ulceration of the planum.[38] The lesion is usually unilateral but can extend to involve both sides of the nasal planum (Figure 64-5). Tumors are usually advanced at presentation; 16 of 25 dogs had a T4 tumor (invasive into underlying muscle, cartilage, or bone), and another six dogs had a T3 tumor (>5 cm in diameter or invading the subcutis; Table 64-2).[38,39]

Staging and Diagnosis

Radiography is rarely helpful in determining the margins of these tumors, which often invade more than 3 cm into and along the nasal cavity, evading clinical detection. CT or magnetic resonance imaging (MRI) is recommended to enhance the accuracy of obtaining surgical margins. These modalities may show bone involvement that is not obvious on radiographs and may even show nasal conchal thickening caused by tumor invasion that cannot be appreciated on physical examination. Without adequately evaluating the tumor margins, excision or radiation therapy is likely to be inadequate.

The small number of dogs treated makes information about staging difficult to interpret, but dogs with smaller tumors should be easier to treat. In one small study, the mitotic rate of the tumor did not seem to influence survival.[39]

It is rare for these tumors to metastasize, and lymph node metastasis at presentation was seen in only one of 25 cases.[38,39] Three other dogs developed lymph node metastasis at the time of tumor recurrence; lymph nodes (mandibular) should be evaluated by cytopathology.

Distant metastases have only been reported in one dog,[42] although few dogs have had long survivals. Thoracic radiographs should be evaluated as part of the staging MDB.

Treatment

Dogs that were not treated had a median survival time of 4 months, and only one of five dogs was alive more than 6 months after diagnosis.[38]

Local excision is only rarely effective.[43] Wide excision (nosectomy) may be curative in some cases when the tumor is localized. Owners should be warned about alterations in the appearance of their dog. The major problem is in assessing margins.[44] For this reason, CT or MRI is recommended. In three studies, 17 dogs were treated surgically. If margins were complete histologically, the prognosis was excellent: only one of 10 had a recurrence, and median control was 24 months, with seven dogs alive without evidence of recurrence more than 1 year after surgery.[39,44,45] In contrast, all seven dogs with an incomplete resection had a recurrence despite the addition of low-dose radiation therapy.[39] Cosmetics can be challenging for owners and caregivers; presurgical consultation is vital to acceptance of the dog's appearance after surgery (see also Chapter 53).

The tumor does not often respond to radiation therapy or chemotherapy.[40] For 14 dogs treated with radiation alone, the median survival time was less than 6 months, with only three dogs alive for more than 1 year.[38–40] One of these three dogs had a T1 tumor and was apparently cured.[39] Radiation was often given to large (T4) tumors and to a low total dose.[39] More aggressive radiation therapy given in smaller fractions to a larger cumulative dose may be more efficacious, as it is in human patients. Radiation therapy given to dogs that had an incomplete surgery did not improve survival either.[39]

Chemotherapy has rarely been used to treat this disease. Three dogs with nasal planum SCCs were treated with interstitial hyperthermia and intralesional cisplatin in bovine collagen matrix. One dog had a complete response for more than 36 weeks; another dog that had a partial response developed distant metastases 9 weeks after treatment.[42] Platinum drugs and possibly piroxicam may be used to treat metastatic disease, as described under SCC above.

Glandular Tumors
SEBACEOUS GLAND TUMORS

These tumors represent 6% to 35% of all skin tumors in dogs. Sebaceous gland tumors are often misdiagnosed as sebaceous cysts. They are similar in appearance to basal cell tumors and trichoepitheliomas. Sebaceous glands are found in many different areas of the body, and the tumors are named accordingly. For example, there are tumors of the meibomian glands and tumors of the perianal (circumanal or hepatoid) glands.

Tumors of the sebaceous glands can be subdivided into three major categories according to the level of maturation of the cells involved: adenomatous hyperplasia of sebaceous glands, sebaceous gland adenomas, and sebaceous gland adenocarcinomas. Adenomatous hyperplasia of sebaceous glands is most common. Adenomas are more common than carcinomas, which are rarely encountered in the skin of dogs. Spaniel breeds are at higher risk of developing all forms of

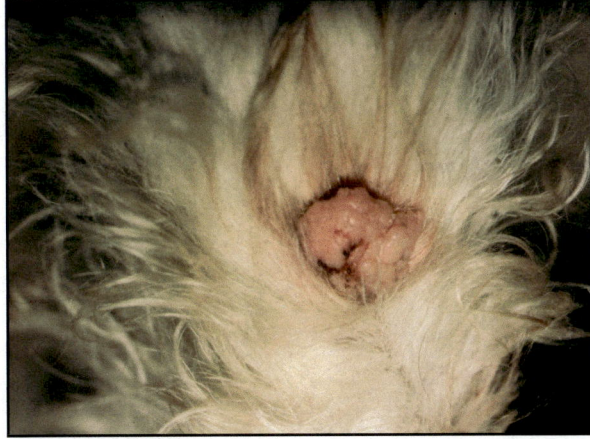

Figure 64-6. *Sebaceous adenomatous hyperplasia, a common disease of terriers.*

sebaceous gland tumors. All three categories of sebaceous tumors affect old dogs and most often occur on the head.

Adenomatous Hyperplasia
Incidence, Signalment, and Etiology

Older dogs, especially males and spayed females, are predisposed, which indicates a possible connection to androgen. The head and limbs are most commonly affected. The most common site is the meibomian glands of the eyelid. Commonly affected breeds are mostly terriers; standard Manchester, Wheaton, Welsh and Kerry blue terriers are at more than three times the risk of developing this condition than the general population. Additional breeds at risk are bichons frisés and miniature poodles.[46]

Clinical Presentation and History

Adenomatous hyperplasia may present as multiple lesions and appears as small (<0.5 cm), superficial, rubbery nodules covered by a thin, shiny, hairless epithelium. The lesions may be multilobulated and are grossly indistinguishable from adenomas (Figure 64-6).

Treatment

Treatment consists of local resection, followed by cryotherapy if excision is incomplete. Dogs are likely to develop new areas of hyperplasia. In one study, dogs with sebaceous gland hyperplasia were treated with isotretinoin or etretinate, and approximately half had successful outcomes.[47] Etretinate is no longer available, but a newer synthetic retinoid, acitretin, may have similar effects at the same dosage.

Sebaceous Adenomas
Incidence, Signalment, and Etiology

Adenomas are seen in dogs of either sex that are older, with an average age of 11 years.[46] Among 1,189 dogs, breeds

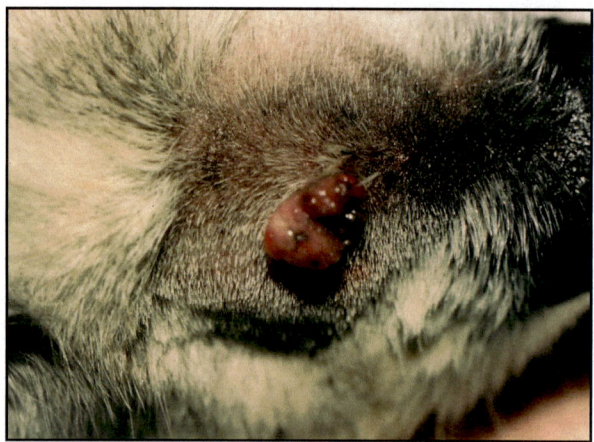

Figure 64-7. Sebaceous adenomas are most common on the head of dogs and are cured by excision.

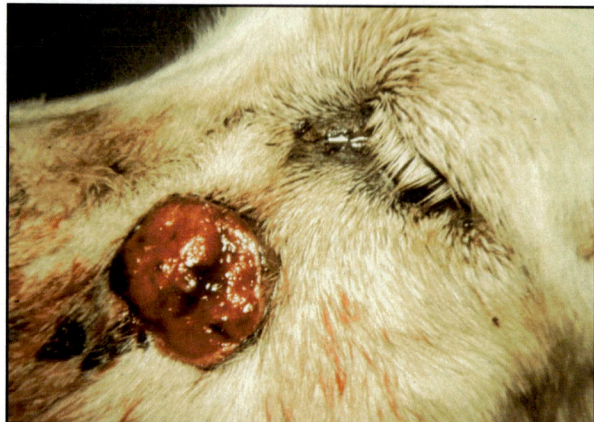

Figure 64-8. Sebaceous adenocarcinomas are most common on the head of dogs, as in this 12-year-old English setter. They are larger and more often ulcerated than their benign counterparts. (Courtesy of Gordon H. Theilen, DVM, University of California, Davis)

that had a risk of developing sebaceous adenomas that was higher than three times that of the general population were coonhounds, English cocker spaniels, and cocker spaniels.[46]

Clinical Presentation and History

Nearly half of recorded sebaceous adenomas occurred on the head, with the limbs the next most commonly affected site.[46] Most commonly, adenomas are solitary, although there may be multiple tumors (4% were multiple in one study) coexisting with other skin tumors. Adenomas are usually small (5 to 10 mm in diameter), raised, multilobulated, domed or pedunculated, well circumscribed, and greasy (Figure 64-7). They may be differentiated from hyperplasia of the sebaceous glands by usually being larger than 5 mm in diameter, mostly solitary, and often ulcerated.[46] Tumors may ooze toothpaste-like material when squeezed. If perianal gland adenomas occur in females, hyperadrenocorticism should be suspected; excessive hormone production is trophic for these adenoma cells.

Treatment

Treatment consists of local resection, followed by cryotherapy if excision is incomplete. Perianal gland adenomas are androgen responsive and usually regress after castration. External-beam radiation at low doses shrinks perianal adenomas; however, this modality is probably best used when the tumor is nonresponsive to hormonal manipulations or if rapid tumor reduction is required.

Sebaceous Adenocarcinomas
Incidence, Signalment, and Etiology

Sebaceous carcinomas accounted for less than 15% of the sebaceous tumors in one study.[46] They occur in older dogs, and intact males appear to be predisposed. The breeds at higher risk of developing sebaceous carcinomas than the rest of the population are cavalier King Charles spaniels (nearly 90 times the risk); cocker spaniels; Scottish, Cairn, and West Highland white terriers; samoyeds; and Siberian huskies.[46]

Clinical Presentation and History

Sebaceous gland carcinomas can be distinguished from benign adenomas by their rapid rate of growth and early ulceration through the skin. They have a predilection for the head, neck, and limbs (Figure 64-8). Malignant tumors are large, usually solitary, poorly circumscribed, ulcerated, and invasive. Whereas sebaceous adenomas are usually slow growing and only rarely recur after surgical removal, sebaceous adenocarcinomas may metastasize to local lymph nodes and to the lungs. Sebaceous carcinomas are rarely multiple; in one study, more than one tumor was seen in approximately 1% of cases.[46]

Treatment

If surgical removal is inadequate, local recurrence may be a problem. In castrated male and in female dogs, most perianal adenocarcinomas metastasize early to the sublumbar lymph nodes (see Chapter 53).

Radiation therapy may cause adenomas to regress, but it has little utility, other than palliation, for adenocarcinomas because of their high metastatic rate. Anecdotal reports show that cisplatin causes regression of metastatic lymph node lesions in dogs.

SWEAT GLAND TUMORS

Sweat gland tumors are less common than sebaceous gland tumors in dogs.[27] The sweat glands of the skin in dogs are mainly apocrine glands; eccrine glands are found only on the footpads. Therefore, most tumors of sweat gland origin are of the apocrine type. Apocrine glands are found in many different parts of the body, and their tumors are named accordingly. In the ear, for example, they are called *ceruminous gland tumors*. In a survey of ear canal tumors, ceruminous adenocarcinoma was the most common malignancy in dogs (see Chapter 50). Other apocrine tumors include mammary gland tumors (see Chapter 59), anal sac tumors, and tumors of the glands at the anal mucocutaneous junction (see Chapter 53).

Apocrine Adenomas
Incidence, Signalment, and Etiology

Apocrine adenomas of the skin affect dogs with an average age of 9.5 years and without gender predilection. Golden retrievers and spaniel breeds were reported to have an increased incidence of these tumors in one study.[48] In another study, Great Pyrenees, chow-chows, and Alaskan malamutes were all at more than three times the risk of the general population.[49] Apocrine adenomas have the same clinical behavior as sebaceous adenomas. Ductal adenomas occurred more frequently in American pit bull terriers, peekapoos, Old English sheepdogs, and English springer spaniels than in the general dog population.[49]

Clinical Presentation and History

Adenomas are small, elevated, well-demarcated nodules. They often have an ulcerated surface as a result of trauma and are generally firm but may have cystic areas. Sweat gland adenomas develop most frequently on the head, neck, and limbs and are multiple in about 1% of cases. Ductal adenomas are more common on the limbs and are evenly distributed between the head, neck, back, thorax, and abdomen.[49]

Adenocarcinomas of the sweat glands were more common than adenomas in one study[48] but not in another.[49]

Staging and Diagnosis

Because of the difficulty in clinically distinguishing between adenomas and adenocarcinomas, veterinarians should consider either presurgical biopsy or a wide surgical excision as an initial therapeutic approach.

Treatment

Surgical removal of sweat gland adenomas is usually curative.

Apocrine Adenocarcinomas
Incidence, Signalment, and Etiology

Apocrine adenocarcinomas of the skin most often affect dogs at an average age of 10.5 years with no gender predilection. Walker coonhounds and Norwegian elkhounds reportedly have an increased incidence of these tumors.[49]

Clinical Presentation and History

Malignant tumors of sweat gland origin are often indistinguishable from adenomas. Some sweat gland tumors, however, present as firm, poorly circumscribed masses diffusely infiltrating the skin, producing an ulcerated, moist, and sometimes hemorrhagic skin surface that is frequently misdiagnosed as acute dermatitis. Adenocarcinomas of the sweat glands were more common than adenomas in one study[48] but not in another.[49] Apocrine gland carcinomas arise on the forelimbs in nearly 30% of cases; the hindlimbs, thorax, and head are the other predilection sites.[49,50] In one study, the ventral abdomen, legs, axilla (Figure 64-9), and inguinal area were predisposed sites,[48] and another study found that tumors in these locations were often inflammatory.[49] These are also predilection sites for inflammatory mammary carcinomas (see Chapter 59).

Staging and Diagnosis

Sweat gland carcinomas may metastasize, primarily via the lymphatics to regional lymph nodes; hematogenous spread to the lungs has been noted. In one study, approximately 20% of carcinomas metastasized,[48] but the rate was considerably lower in other studies.[50] Regardless, an MDB that includes thoracic radiographs should be obtained. Pulmonary metastases from inflammatory apocrine gland carcinomas may have a diffuse interstitial pattern on radiographs.[49] The regional lymph nodes should be palpated, aspirated if enlarged, and removed at surgery for complete staging.[51] Because of the difficulty in clinically distinguishing between adenomas and adenocarcinomas, veterinarians should consider either presurgical biopsy or a wide surgical excision as an initial therapeutic approach. Poorly differentiated tumors are more likely to metastasize,[49] as are tumors that invade the vasculature.[50]

Treatment

Surgical removal of sweat gland adenomas is usually curative, but carcinomas may recur locally after surgical removal. In a study of 25 dogs with apocrine adenocarcinomas treated by surgery alone, only one dog developed metastasis (this dog had evidence of capsular and vascular invasion), seven dogs died from other diseases, and the remaining 70% of patients were alive and free of disease with a median survival of 30 months.[50] For localized tumors (i.e., no lymphatic or vessel invasion and no metastasis), radiation therapy may be palliative, although the few animals treated preclude definitive recommendations.

Chemotherapy for metastatic tumors is anecdotal only, although cisplatin may be a useful agent in dogs. Three of five dogs with circumanal gland malignancies treated with doxorubicin had objective responses (two complete responses, one partial response), although the duration of these responses was not documented.[52] This agent may be active in the treatment of cutaneous apocrine carcinomas. Apocrine gland tumors are similar histologically and clinically to mammary adenocarcinomas, so a therapeutic approach as for mammary tumors may be appropriate (see Chapter 59).

Follicular (Cystic) Tumors

These tumors form cystic structures that may be filled with glandular secretions, keratin, or other epidermal or dermal structures. Most are benign, and their differentiation is mainly of pathologic, rather than clinical, interest. For most of these tumors, rupture, whether by the veterinarian or by the patient, may cause a dramatic inflammatory reaction and require tumor excision.

INTRACUTANEOUS CORNIFYING EPITHELIOMA
Incidence, Signalment, and Etiology

Other terms for this tumor include *squamous papilloma*, *keratoacanthoma*, and *intracutaneous keratinized epithelioma*. This benign neoplasm is of epidermal origin but extends into the dermis and subcutaneous tissues. It is most common in young to middle-aged dogs, with no gender predisposition. Norwegian elkhounds are nearly 30 times more likely to develop this tumor than the general population, and this breed and the Lhasa apso are more likely to develop multiple lesions. Other predisposed breeds are Belgian sheepdogs, bearded collies, bichons frisés, Pekingeses, and soft-coated Wheaton, Kerry blue, and Yorkshire terriers.[53] Most breeds develop solitary tumors; however, Norwegian elkhounds show numerous growths in various stages of development within the skin.

Clinical Presentation and History

This tumor appears as a dermal or subcutaneous nodule measuring 0.5 to 5.0 cm in diameter that may elevate the overlying epidermis and give it a tannish-brown appearance. A pore leading into the mass may be observed. Rupture produces a severe pyogranulomatous dermatitis in reaction to the keratin contents of the cyst. These tumors are most common on the limbs, back, and tail and are multiple in nearly 10% of cases.

Treatment

Surgical resection of solitary tumors is curative; for multiple tumors, surgery is often impractical. The retinoid etretinate (1 mg/kg PO bid) was useful in treating multicentric keratoacanthomas, causing complete remission in all four treated dogs.[54] Etretinate is no longer available, but a newer synthetic retinoid, acitretin, may have similar effects at the same dosage.

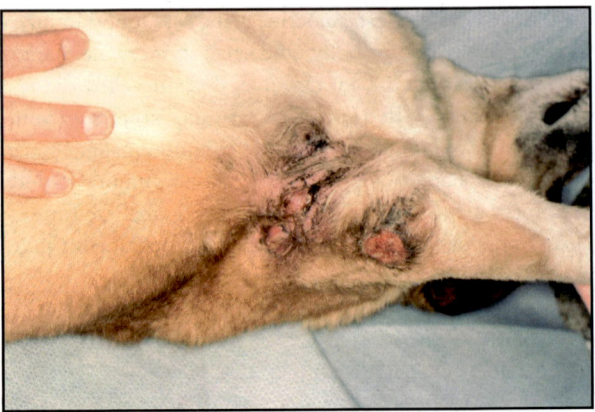

Figure 64-9. *Sweat gland adenocarcinomas are often found in the axillae of dogs. They are often ulcerated and metastasize to regional lymph nodes.*

TRICHOEPITHELIOMA
Incidence, Signalment, and Etiology

Trichoepitheliomas, or *hair matrixomas*, also called are derived from primitive hair-matrix cells that differentiate into either mature or incompletely developed hair follicles. Most trichoepitheliomas occur in female dogs older than 5 years. Basset hounds, English and Walker coonhounds, bullmastiffs, Gordon setters, and soft-coated Wheaton terriers are predisposed to developing these tumors.[55]

Clinical Presentation and History

These tumors often resemble basal cell tumors, but they may be cystic and contain keratin. They are most frequently found on the back, although the limbs, thorax, and neck are commonly affected.[55] The overlying epidermis is atrophic, hairless, and often ulcerated as a result of trauma. These tumors are slow growing, minimally invasive, and usually well encapsulated. Most are solitary, with multiple tumors occurring in less than 6% of cases (usually in basset hounds and English springer spaniels).[55]

Staging and Diagnosis

One author[55] described most (90%) trichoepitheliomas as benign, 9% as infiltrative, and less than 1% as malignant. A benign subtype of these tumors is called *tricholemmoma*. Malignant trichoepitheliomas are very similar in histologic appearance to infiltrative tumors but may show vascular or lymphatic invasion. Metastasis has been described to regional lymph nodes and lungs. An MDB should be obtained for dogs with these tumors.

Treatment

Recurrence after adequate surgical excision is rare. Infiltrative trichoepitheliomas are surrounded by a fibrovascular stroma and, because of their invasive nature, recur in about

10% of cases. Wide excision is recommended.[55] Adjunctive treatment has not been described.

PILOMATRICOMAS
Incidence, Signalment, and Etiology

Pilomatricomas (*pilomatrixomas, necrotizing* and *calcifying epitheliomas*) are tumors that originate from the small, dark-staining cells of the pilar (hair) matrix. Kerry blue terriers are more than 30 times as likely as other breeds to develop these tumors. Other breeds at risk include soft-coated Wheaton terriers, Bouvier des Flandres, bichons frisés, and standard poodles (all >10 times risk), as well as bearded collies, Old English sheepdogs, briards, Irish wolfhounds, standard schnauzers, Airedale terriers, and basset hounds. Older dogs are most commonly affected, with no gender predilection.[56]

Clinical Presentation and History

These are firm, well-defined nodules composed of either multiple cysts filled with tan, pasty material or cysts containing a gritty, granular, mineralized material. Most cases are confined to the hindlimbs, skin of the rump, and shoulder area. The back, neck, and tail are less frequently affected. Multiple tumors are found in 3% of affected dogs. The tumors may be darkly pigmented.

Staging and Diagnosis

These tumors are slow growing and well encapsulated. Histologic evidence of vascular invasion and lymph node involvement are indicators of malignancy. Rarely, malignant pilomatricomas metastasize to local lymph nodes and internal organs, such as the mammary glands, the lymph nodes, bone, the central nervous system (CNS), and the lungs.[56–60] The histologic appearance of malignant tumors may not differ substantially from that of benign tumors.[60,61]

Treatment

Surgical excision should be curative if adequate margins are resected. There are no reports of therapy for metastatic tumors; however, doxorubicin and platinum drugs may be most likely to cause a response.

CYSTS
Incidence, Signalment, and Etiology

Cutaneous cysts may be epidermal, follicular, or apocrine. Clinically, there is little to distinguish them, although affected breeds differ.[62] Epidermal cysts are believed to arise in response to degenerative changes in hair follicles or cystic changes in ducts or cells of sebaceous glands. Follicular cysts may arise after traumatic displacement of epidermal fragments. The lesions are usually acquired and rarely congenital. They may be single or multiple and are most common on the head, neck, and limbs. Cysts are very common in dogs and may occur in any breed. Boxers are predisposed to developing epidermal cysts, bullmastiffs are predisposed to developing follicular cysts, and Old English sheepdogs are predisposed to developing apocrine cysts.[62] Middle-aged to old animals usually are affected.

Clinical Presentation and History

These cysts appear as a single, soft, fluctuant nodule that is freely movable in the dermis and beneath the elevated overlying skin. The cut surface of epidermal and follicular cysts is thin walled and contains tan to yellow pasty material. Apocrine cysts are filled with a clear fluid. Follicular cysts are often inflamed and traumatized. Cysts are multiple in 3% to 5% of affected dogs.

Treatment

As with cystic tumors, when an epidermal or follicular cyst ruptures and the contents of the cyst are released into the dermis, a severe foreign-body reaction occurs. Surgical excision is usually curative for all cysts.

A single case of multiple follicular cysts (i.e., hundreds) that underwent malignant transformation to SCC has been reported, but this is exceedingly rare.[15]

Mesenchymal Tumors
LIPOMAS
Incidence, Signalment, and Etiology

Lipomas are benign tumors of adipose cells and are most common in middle-aged to older dogs. Females are affected twice as frequently as males. The tumor may occur anywhere, although the thorax, abdomen, legs, and axillae are the most frequent sites. Doberman pinschers and Labrador retrievers are at slightly higher than average risk for these tumors, but lipomas occur in most breeds.[63] In humans with lipoma, there is a tendency to develop multiple lesions, and there are often cytogenetic abnormalities. Similar cytogenetic mutations have been seen in dogs with lipomas, and this may raise the suspicion for development of future lipomas in affected dogs.[64] Cutaneous angiolipomas have a similar clinical course to lipomas but contain blood vessels as well as adipocytes.[65]

Clinical Presentation and History

Lipomas are common and are usually solitary, of variable size and shape, slow growing, well circumscribed, and subcutaneous. They usually feel soft, but lipomas that develop between muscle planes may feel firm. These tumors are slow growing and enlarge by expansion rather than by invasion. Approximately 7% of dogs with lipomas have multiple tumors.[63]

Infiltrative lipomas can cause pain and pressure atrophy of muscles; more detail is provided below.

Treatment

Excision of a lipoma is warranted if the lipoma interferes with function and mobility, is rapidly growing, or is bothersome to the owner (Figure 64-10). In most cases, surgery is curative. Intralesional use of calcium chloride was successful in causing regression of tumors in one study, but cutaneous necrosis and discharging wounds were common, limiting the clinical applicability of this treatment.[66] Surgery is preferred.

Lipomas of other sites (intraabdominal and intrathoracic) are also cured by surgery.[67]

> **KEY POINT**
> *Excision of a lipoma is warranted if it interferes with function and mobility, is rapidly growing, or is bothersome to the owner.*

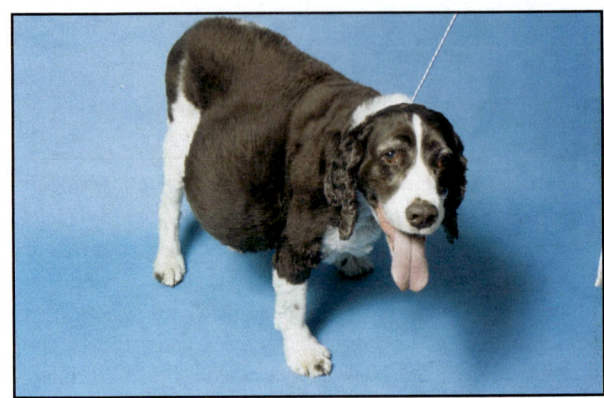

Figure 64-10. Lipoma is a biologically benign tumor, but it may reach a large size and interfere with ambulation. Tumors such as this lipoma in a 13-year-old dog should be removed before they cause problems.

INFILTRATIVE LIPOMAS
Incidence, Signalment, and Etiology

Infiltrative lipomas are tumors of well-differentiated adipose cells that invade surrounding tissues. Similar to lipomas, they are most common in middle-aged to older dogs. Females are affected twice as frequently as males. Standard schnauzers and Labrador retrievers are at slightly higher than average risk for these tumors, which can occur in any breed.[63]

The syndrome of lipomatous infiltration of the mandibular and parotid salivary glands is usually cured by excision.[68]

Clinical Presentation and History

The tumor may occur anywhere, although the limbs are the most common location, followed by the thorax and abdomen. Infiltrative lipomas can cause pain and pressure atrophy of muscles and can interfere with movement. In one study of 16 dogs with infiltrative lipoma, five were Labrador retrievers, and most of the others were large-breed dogs.[69] In most cases, the tumor was present for 1 year or longer before presentation to a veterinarian.

Staging and Diagnosis

These tumors are invasive but do not metastasize. Although one report found an infiltrative lipoma to be a metastatic, well-differentiated liposarcoma, this is rarely a differential problem on histopathology.[70] Staging using an MDB should be conducted, as well as imaging to determine tumor margins, either to predict the surgery needed or to plan the extent of radiation therapy. Both CT and MRI are used for this purpose and are superior to radiography.[71]

Treatment

Although excision of a lipoma is curative, treatment of infiltrative lipoma is more complex. Infiltrative lipomas should be treated with aggressive, initial surgery; even then, recurrence is likely[72] (Figures 64-11 and 64-12). A second surgery is rarely successful.[73] Amputation may be required if the tumor involves a limb, and even then an infiltrative lipoma may track between muscle planes to extend beyond surgical margins. A study of 11 dogs with infiltrative lipomas of the thigh found that the local recurrence rate was 42% after aggressive surgery (including some with amputation), and the median time to recurrence after first surgery was 7 months. Median times to second and third recurrences were 5 months and less than 2 months (i.e., recurrence becomes more rapid). In addition, the authors noted an increased tendency toward invasiveness after each surgery.[74] In another study, 13 dogs had 14 tumors removed surgically, and five tumors (36%) recurred. Median time to recurrence for these five tumors was 8 months (range: 3–16 months). Two-thirds of the dogs were tumor-free 1 year after surgery.[69]

Radiation therapy may be indicated postoperatively for infiltrative lipomas if residual disease is suspected. In a report of radiation therapy for 13 dogs with infiltrative lipomas, cytoreductive surgery was performed before radiation in 10 dogs, although only three dogs had microscopic disease at the time of radiation therapy. Dogs received a total dose of 45.6 Gy to 63 Gy in 2.5- to 4-Gy fractions. Survival time (from the time of completion of radiation therapy) ranged from 6 months to 94 months, with a median of 40 months.[75]

One dog with an infiltrative lipoma had a partial (>50%) reduction after two doses of doxorubicin.[52]

LIPOSARCOMAS
Incidence, Signalment, and Etiology

Liposarcomas are rarer than lipomas. They occur without gender predilection. In a series of 76 cases, both Shetland sheepdogs and beagles appeared to be at higher risk for this tumor.[63]

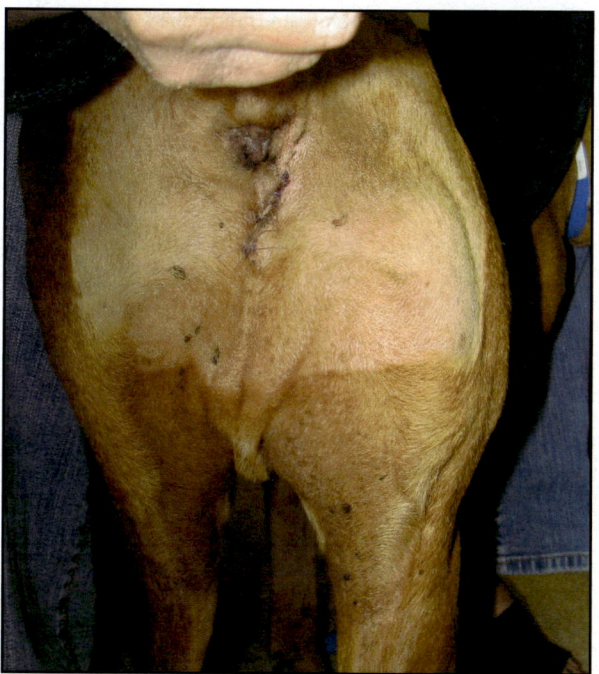

Figure 64-11. *Infiltrative lipoma is not encapsulated and invades surrounding tissue. Therefore, it is treated as a soft tissue sarcoma rather than as a lipoma. (Courtesy of J. Berg)*

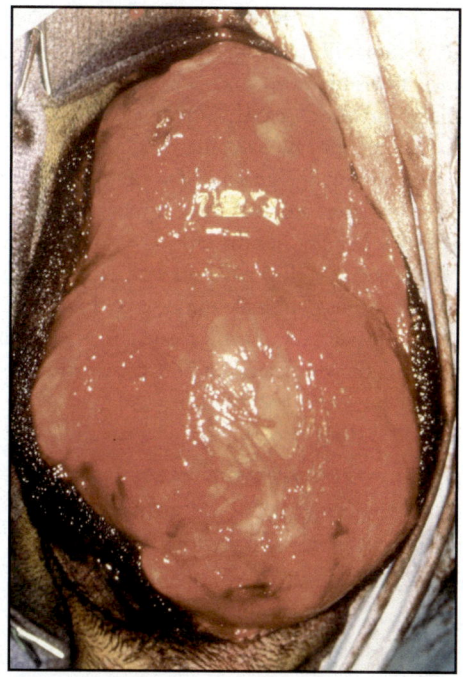

Figure 64-12. *Surgical exposure of an infiltrative lipoma. Apparent encapsulation is illusory, and excision without amputation in this dog will be incomplete. (Courtesy of J. Berg)*

Liposarcoma in response to a foreign body has been reported twice in dogs; glass[76] and a microchip[62] were the offending materials.

Clinical Presentation and History

Liposarcomas are usually solitary; vary in shape, size, and consistency; and are poorly demarcated, subcutaneous, and invasive. The skin is the most common site, and liposarcomas often occur in the same locations as infiltrative lipomas.[77] In one study of 49 dogs with cutaneous liposarcoma, distribution was equally divided between the limbs and the axial areas.[78]

Staging and Diagnosis

Liposarcomas are soft tissue sarcomas; staging for these tumors should include an MDB as well as CT or MRI of the tumor to determine margins for surgery or radiation therapy.

On cytology, liposarcomas are very cellular rather than sparsely cellular like lipomas; they are cytologically more similar to soft tissue sarcomas. Well-differentiated liposarcoma more closely resembles infiltrative lipoma histologically, but this is a rare variant.[63,70] Liposarcomas are, however, rarely metastatic. Individual case reports have documented metastasis to the lungs, lymph nodes, bone, spleen, and liver, leading to early speculation that this is a highly metastatic tumor.[70,79–82] However, in a study of 11 cases of liposarcoma, only one patient developed metastasis to regional lymph nodes and the lung,[77] and of 25 dogs in another study, with known cause of death, only two dogs had developed metastases and seven had developed local tumor recurrence.[78] This behavior is much more similar to other soft tissue sarcomas, and a clinical distinction is probably artificial.

Treatment

Liposarcomas are best treated as soft tissue sarcomas, as detailed in Chapter 62. Excision of the tumor with wide margins may be curative, and the recurrence rate is moderate, as for most soft tissue sarcomas. In one study, the only factor that significantly affected survival in dogs with liposarcomas was whether they had a surgery with wide margins (median survival: 39 months) or a marginal excision (median survival: 21 months); dogs that were not treated lived a median of 6 months.[78] Dogs that had a wide excision were likely to have complete surgical margins based on histopathology. Appendicular or axial location did not affect outcome.

A complete response was seen in a dog after two doses of doxorubicin.[52]

SOFT TISSUE SARCOMAS OF THE SKIN AND SURROUNDING STRUCTURES

Nomenclature for this group of tumors largely depends on microscopic appearance. Because this may change depending on site of biopsy or stage of growth, the same tumor may be given different names at different stages. This is initially frustrating to clinicians; however, very little difference in biologic behavior exists between these tumors. Thus, whether a tumor is labeled fibroma, fibrosarcoma, hemangiopericytoma, neurofibroma, neurofibrosarcoma, schwannoma, rhabdomyoma, rhabdomyosarcoma, leiomyoma, leiomyosarcoma, liposarcoma, or histiocytic sarcoma may not matter as much as the site of tumor, the grade of the tumor, and the thoroughness of excision. Some of these tumors may initially be characterized as benign, but the term *benign tumor* may be a misnomer; it is more clinically correct to consider these as histologic gradations of a single tumor type. Local recurrence is a common problem for any soft tissue sarcoma that has not been excised with wide margins. Soft tissue sarcomas often spread locally but rarely metastasize.

> **KEY POINT**
>
> *Soft tissue mesenchymal tumors are rarely biologically benign; wide and deep surgical margins should be taken regardless of histologic appearance.*

In Chapter 62, the incidence, clinical presentation, and staging for each tumor type are discussed separately. Treatment of all soft tissue sarcomas is identical and is discussed at the end of that chapter.

Round (Discrete) Cell Tumors

Round cell tumors may equally be called *discrete cell tumors*, and cytologically, they appear as clumps or individual cells that have no obvious attachment to other cells. Round cell tumors include mast cell tumors (see Chapter 65), histiocytoma (see Chapter 63), lymphoma, plasmacytoma, and transmissible venereal tumors (see Chapter 58). Melanomas may also look like round cell tumors. Merkel cell tumors (i.e., neuroendocrine tumors that are benign in the skin) are also rarely diagnosed.[83] These tumor types are distinguished by cytology or routine histopathology in most cases, but occasionally special stains may be needed.[84,85]

Plasma Cell Tumors of Extramedullary Sites

Extramedullary is a term given to neoplasms of plasma cells that occur in sites outside the marrow. These tumors rarely produce abnormal paraproteins and are not classified as multiple myeloma. There seems to be a clear difference in the biologic behavior of cutaneous plasmacytomas and plasmacytomas of other extramedullary sites.

Cutaneous and Oral Mucocutaneous Plasmacytoma

INCIDENCE, SIGNALMENT, AND ETIOLOGY

The most common sites of canine extramedullary plasmacytomas are the skin and oral cavity. This is a recently diagnosed tumor, and there are no published reports before 1987. Five reports since that time have documented tumors in 282 dogs,[86–91] with an additional 400 cases described in a monograph.[92]

Canine cutaneous plasmacytomas show no gender predilection. Tumors are usually solitary in middle-aged to older dogs (mean age: 9 years). Cocker spaniels, Airedale terriers, Scottish terriers, and standard poodles are overrepresented.[92] Mixed-breed dogs accounted for more than 25% of 206 dogs with plasma cell tumors of the skin and oral mucosa.[87,88] The mean age of affected dogs is between 9 and 10 years; affected dogs range in age from 2 to 22 years.[92]

CLINICAL PRESENTATION AND HISTORY

Tumors range in diameter from 0.2 to 10.0 cm, but most measure between 1.0 and 2.0 cm. Tumors occur most frequently on the trunk and limbs (48%),[86–90,93] on the head (30%), and in the oral cavity (22%). In one study,[87] 50% of plasmacytomas on the head occurred in the ear canal or on the ear. In another study, nearly 50% of 406 cutaneous plasmacytomas occurred on the head, with 25% on the ears and 16% on the lips.[92] Most cutaneous plasmacytomas are solitary; only 2% to 5% of affected dogs have multiple lesions.

Caregivers often report that tumors grow rapidly; however, few clinical signs are associated with cutaneous or mucosal plasma cell tumors. Most tumors appear as smooth, pink-to-red, raised, circumscribed nodules[86,88] that are occasionally polypoid (particularly in the ear canal) and sometimes ulcerated (especially on the digits).[89] Dogs with aural tumors often have signs of otitis.

STAGING AND DIAGNOSIS

Plasmacytomas of the skin and oral mucosa are rarely associated with systemic disease. In one study, two of 131 dogs had elevated serum protein levels (although protein levels were not measured in most dogs), and serum protein electrophoresis was not conducted for either dog.[87] One of these two dogs also had a rectal tumor and bled excessively after surgery, indicating that this dog may have had multiple myeloma. The dog was euthanatized 2 months later. One dog with nearly 200 cutaneous tumors had evidence of systemic plasma cell tumors and may have had multiple myeloma.[91] In another study, two dogs with a solitary cutaneous plasmacytoma also had multiple myeloma with lytic vertebral lesions.[88] Most cutaneous plasmacytomas are benign. If the clinician wishes to be complete, however, patients should be evaluated with immunoelectrophoresis, radiography, hemogram, biochemistry profile, and urinalysis to rule out the possibility that the cutaneous tumor is a lesion associated with multiple myeloma.

Only one canine cutaneous plasmacytoma is documented to have metastasized to regional lymph nodes.[94]

Special stains for plasma cell tumors include methyl green pyronine; these tumors stain negative with toluidine blue, which is a specific mast cell stain. Although occasional tumors show more cellular atypia and the mitotic index may be high, these tumors are benign, almost without exception.[95] Second cutaneous tumors are considered to be de novo rather than metastases.

Amyloid is present in cutaneous plasmacytoma in approximately 3% of cases. This finding may have some clinical significance because two reports suggest that these tumors are more likely to recur after surgical excision.[90,92]

TREATMENT

Occasional vessel invasion has been reported, but there is no systemic spread. Excision has been curative in nearly all reported dogs, although tumors near the oral cavity may be more difficult to excise.

For dogs with solitary plasmacytomas, surgical excision is nearly always curative unless excision is incomplete on histopathology. In one study, surgical excision completely controlled the tumors in 194 of 213 dogs treated.[86-90] Tumors recurred locally in 11 dogs,[87,89,90] and one dog had both distant and local recurrences.[90] One study found that eight of nine local recurrences were predictable because of incomplete surgical excision; four of these dogs had oral lesions that were difficult to excise completely.[87] Distant recurrences after surgical excision are probably attributable to unrelated or asynchronous primary (de novo) tumors rather than to metastasis.[87]

Based on responses seen in dogs with multiple myeloma, this tumor is probably sensitive to radiation. To date, however, radiation therapy has been reported in only two dogs with plasmacytoma. One dog received radiation treatment with cesium-137 after four surgical excisions failed to control the tumor; the dog was free of disease 3 months later.[30] Another dog with a recurrent oral plasmacytoma was treated with cobalt-60 teletherapy, and there was no recurrence by 6 months after treatment.[96]

Chemotherapy has been reported in only a few dogs with multiple cutaneous or mucosal plasmacytomas, and Susan M. Cotter, DVM, reports that responses are difficult to assess because of occasional, apparently intermittent, spontaneous regressions. Individual reports of tumor response after chemotherapy with doxorubicin[97] and responses to prednisone and melphalan imply that these drugs may be useful for the treatment of nonresectable or widespread disease. Two dogs had tumor regression and were disease-free 16 months after treatment with melphalan and prednisone.[89] Another dog was treated with melphalan and prednisone and had a 7-month remission.[86] On relapse, the dog was treated homeopathically, and the tumors again regressed. Another dog had tumor regression after treatment with cyclophosphamide and prednisone, but new tumors appeared despite continued treatment.[90]

Cutaneous Lymphoma
INCIDENCE, SIGNALMENT, AND ETIOLOGY

This disease may primarily involve the skin or may be part of the manifestations of generalized lymphoma. Further information is found in Chapter 47.

Cutaneous lymphoma is more common in older dogs, with a median age of 9 to 10 years. In a series of 260 dogs, there was no gender predilection, but briards, English cocker spaniels, bulldogs, and Scottish terriers were all at higher risk than the rest of the canine population.[98]

CLINICAL PRESENTATION AND HISTORY

Cutaneous lymphoma can present as solitary or multiple dermal masses of recent onset or as a chronic unresolved or progressive case of dermatitis in which a positive diagnosis is rendered on histopathologic examination of skin biopsy specimens. Pruritus is common. Chronic unresolved dermatitis may eventually produce multiple skin nodules or show the formation of generalized plaques, pustules, or ulcerative skin disease. The dermal nodules vary in size from several millimeters to several centimeters in diameter (Figure 64-13). The covering skin may show partial or complete alopecia. Some of the nodules are covered by a thick, dry crust, which reveals a pink, healing epidermis upon removal. Other areas show epidermal ulceration with a peripheral rim of erythema. Most dogs with mycosis fungoides, a specific form of cutaneous lymphoma in which the malignancy involves T cells, have only plaquelike or nodular lesions and a chronic history of progressive skin disease (see Mycosis Fungoides section, below).

STAGING AND DIAGNOSIS

Definitive diagnosis is made by biopsy. Multiple and serial biopsy specimens should be taken until the diagnosis is confirmed; a single lesion may not contain all the histologic characteristics necessary to confirm the diagnosis. Because of the possibility of systemic disease, a complete blood count (CBC), biochemical profile, urinalysis, radiography, and bone marrow aspiration are appropriate. Immunohistochemistry for T- (CD3) and B-cell (CD79a) markers should be requested on a biopsy. Tumors that are epitheliotropic are usually thought to be T cell, and nonepitheliotropic (nodular) lymphomas are thought to be B cell. However, this generalization is not always true; in one study, three of seven epitheliotropic lymphomas were T cell, and the rest were "null" cell (stained with neither B- or T-cell markers). Also, eight of 10 nonepitheliotropic lymphomas were T cell, and the other two were B cell.[99] There is prognostic advantage to differentiating whether the lymphoma is T cell or B cell, just as for multicentric lymphoma.

638 MANAGING THE CANINE CANCER PATIENT

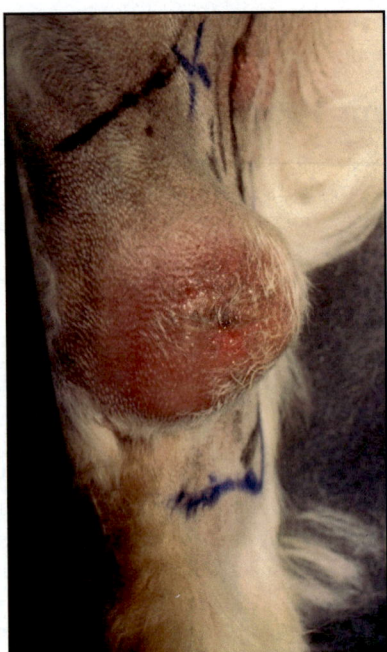

Figure 64-13. *A solitary nodular cutaneous lymphoma may be excised or treated with radiation therapy, as in this dog. Before proceeding with local therapies such as these, staging including an MDB, abdominal ultrasonography, and bone marrow cytology should be conducted because systemic disease is likely.*

Organ involvement is common in the later stages of both B- and T-cell cutaneous lymphoma, occurring in about 70% of affected dogs. Reported sites of involvement include (in descending order) generalized lymphadenopathy, liver, spleen, bone marrow and blood, and intestinal tract.[100]

Paraneoplastic myasthenia gravis has been reported with T-cell, nonepitheliotropic, cutaneous lymphoma.[101]

TREATMENT

Biologic behavior is extremely variable with this type of tumor. Some dogs with a solitary mass show no evidence of recurrence, progression to other skin sites, or internal metastasis after surgical excision.[102] Other dogs develop additional skin nodules and show progression of the disease. In general, it is believed that dogs with B-cell cutaneous lymphoma are more likely to have a complete response to treatment and to have extended survival. Complete response to therapy in these dogs is often long (>1 year). The appropriate therapy for these dogs is combination chemotherapy. Many therapeutic options are available for dogs with mycosis fungoides, but none is very successful in the long term (see below).

Dogs with solitary lesions may be treated with radiation therapy and usually respond rapidly and completely.

Chemotherapy is recommended as an adjunct to surgery or radiation therapy because lymphoma is always considered to be a systemic disease. Combination chemotherapy protocols are most likely to result in clinical response. Response to lymphoma chemotherapy protocols varies, but remissions are usually shorter than those that occur with multicentric lymphoma. Dogs with B-cell cutaneous lymphoma may have a good prognosis with chemotherapy, particularly if the number of lesions is small.

A preliminary study reported complete responses of 2 to 15 months to CCNU (lomustine) chemotherapy in seven dogs with cutaneous lymphoma. T- and B-cell markers were not performed, but five were epitheliotropic and two were not.[103]

MYCOSIS FUNGOIDES
Incidence, Signalment, and Etiology

Mycosis fungoides is a primary cutaneous lymphoma in humans as well as dogs. The neoplastic cell has been immunologically determined to be a helper T cell. The tumor tends to occur in the epidermis, in the superficial dermis, and periadnexally (epitheliotropic). There are characteristic microabscesses (i.e., Pautrier's microabscesses) of tumor cells within the skin. Mycosis fungoides tends to occur in older animals (mean age: 11 years), and no gender predilection is seen. There is a possible overrepresentation of poodles and cocker spaniels.

CLINICAL PRESENTATION AND HISTORY

Mycosis fungoides has a protracted clinical course with three apparent clinical stages:

1. **Premycotic stage (erythroderma stage):** Skin lesions are characterized by eczema, erythema (erythroderma), pigmentation or depigmentation, telangiectasis, atrophy, alopecia, and variable pruritus, which can lead to self-trauma and worsening of lesions. Skin lesions usually start over the trunk or neck and may progress to involve more of the body. Lesions sometimes show a primarily mucocutaneous-junction distribution (Figure 64-14). The oral region is commonly affected in this form, and lesions may be solitary.

2. **Mycotic stage (plaque stage):** Skin lesions are characterized by erythematous, raised, thickened, firm plaques. Lesions may be ulcerated and exudative. These lesions may develop where previous skin lesions existed or in new areas (Figure 64-15).

3. **Tumor stage:** Skin lesions are characterized by distinct, proliferative, protruding nodules, and the skin may be ulcerated (Figure 64-16). Systemic spread to lymph nodes or other organs may occur; this manifestation resembles multicentric lymphoma.

Sézary syndrome is a leukemic variant of mycosis fungoides characterized by circulating, malignant helper T cells

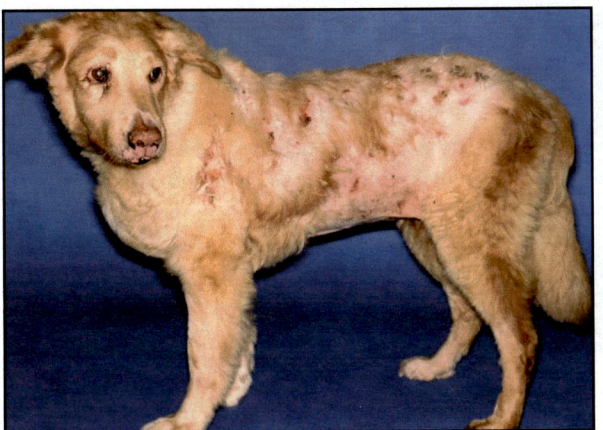

Figure 64-14. *Mycosis fungoides is a specific T-cell variant of lymphoma that occurs within the epidermis. Dry, exfoliative lesions that progress to ulceration, as seen in this 13-year-old golden retriever, are typical. Note involvement of the mucocutaneous junctions around the eyes and nasal planum.*

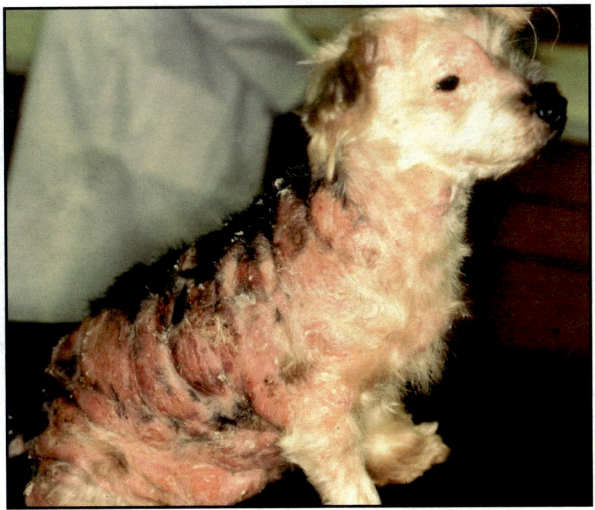

Figure 64-15. *Mycosis fungoides may be generalized, severe, and exacerbated by secondary infection. It causes significant morbidity.*

with similar morphology and antigenic markers as malignant cells in skin lesions. This syndrome can occur during any stage of mycosis fungoides and does not alter the usual progression of the disease or long-term prognosis. Mycosis fungoides complicated with Sézary syndrome is characterized by splenomegaly, lymphadenopathy, and cyclic episodes of generalized erythroderma. The number of peripheral Sézary cells increases immediately before episodes of erythroderma and declines rapidly during the episodes. This suggests migration of these cells from blood to skin and sequestration of Sézary cells in the skin. This syndrome is rarely described in dogs.[104–106]

A solitary variant of mycosis fungoides occurs in the oral mucosa of dogs. This may progress to systemic mycosis fungoides, but it often has an indolent course over many years. One dog with unilateral conjunctival mycosis fungoides has been described.[107]

STAGING AND DIAGNOSIS

Definitive diagnosis is made by biopsy. Multiple and serial biopsy specimens should be taken until the diagnosis is confirmed; a single lesion may not contain all the histologic characteristics necessary to confirm the diagnosis. Earlier lesions in the premycotic and mycotic stages are better samples for histology. Secondary pyodermas are common with mycosis fungoides and may complicate diagnosis and treatment.

Lymph node enlargement may occur at any stage of mycosis fungoides, but in the early stages, it usually represents a reactive response to chronic dermatitis rather than malignant spread of the tumor (i.e., dermatopathic lymphadenopathy). Nevertheless, enlargement is an indication for lymph node biopsy. Similarly, dogs with mycosis fungoides may have splenomegaly or hepatomegaly caused by infiltration at presentation. Because of the possibility of disease elsewhere, a CBC, biochemical profile, urinalysis, radiography, and bone marrow aspiration are appropriate.

Mycosis fungoides usually terminally progresses to involve other organs. The lungs[104] and CNS[108] have been reported to be involved in dogs with mycosis fungoides, as have peripheral lymph nodes and other organs more usually expected to be involved in systemic multicentric lymphoma.[109]

Primary mycosis fungoides of the oral mucosa may be localized to a single lesion or a group of lesions without affecting the skin. This variant still has the potential to spread systemically, although it may be many months before other lymphoma is clinically apparent.

TREATMENT

Many different treatments have been used for mycosis fungoides. None has proven entirely satisfactory, but some success has been achieved with each. If the lesions are limited to the skin, a variety of therapies seem efficacious.

Topical nitrogen mustards, such as mechlorethamine or BCNU, have been the most widely used treatment in humans. These compounds are potent carcinogens, however, which is of more concern to humans in contact with the chemicals than to the animals treated. Reports of the use of these compounds in veterinary medicine are few and usually combine them with other drugs such as prednisone, so the efficacy of these compounds in dogs is difficult to assess.[110]

A treatment widely used in humans with mycosis fungoides is vitamin A analogues (retinoids) such as isotretinoin (Accutane, Roche; 1 to 3 mg/kg PO sid). The mechanism of action of these compounds is by inducing terminal differentiation of tumor cells, and improvement has been reported

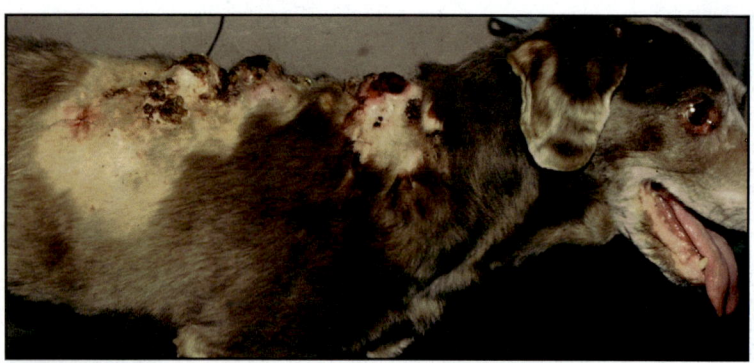

Figure 64-16. *Mycosis fungoides may progress to a nodular form and often to systemic lymphoma, as in this Labrador retriever.*

in dogs. In one study, remission was achieved in six of 14 dogs with cutaneous lymphoma.[54] A newer synthetic retinoid, acitretin, at 1 mg/kg body weight PO once daily has also been reported to cause responses but with less risk of hepatic toxicity than isotretinoin. Most oncologists suggest a 6-week trial before deciding that it is not effective. For dogs that have small numbers of lesions, this may be a valuable therapeutic option.[107] For dogs that are in obvious discomfort and have rapid disease progression, it may be difficult to rely on this treatment alone.

In a similar category is linoleic acid (safflower oil), which has been shown to cause long-term remissions, occasionally over 2 years in duration, in a very small preliminary study. The dose is 3 ml/kg body weight PO on food once daily.[111] No clinical toxicity has been reported. Lesions that responded best were small and localized. This treatment can be used in addition to retinoids. Again, it is best to treat for 6 weeks before deciding this approach is not working and to not delay more aggressive therapies for dogs with more advanced lesions.

If neither option is effective, then prednisolone may cause a tumor response. Prednisolone should not be used long-term if combination chemotherapy is being considered because of the risk of fostering drug resistance.

> **KEY POINT**
>
> *Cutaneous lymphoma and mycosis fungoides may not respond to systemic combination chemotherapy.*

The use of systemic chemotherapy protocols has been suggested for cases in which the disease has disseminated; however, these tumors have proven to be poorly responsive to most commonly used chemotherapeutic agents despite occasional responses.[105,110] The complete response rate (approximately 35%–40%) is probably a little lower than that in dogs with systemic T-cell lymphoma. Just as for dogs with systemic T-cell lymphoma, the addition of alkylating agents (e.g., dacarbazine, CCNU, procarbazine) to the protocol would be beneficial because T-cell patients with lymphoma seem to respond better to this class of agents. Further information is found in Chapter 47. Some oncologists suggest that retinoids should be used concurrently with chemotherapy because they may enhance tumor response.

A preliminary study reported a good response to lomustine (CCNU) chemotherapy in seven dogs with cutaneous lymphoma. T- and B-cell markers were not conducted, but five dogs had epitheliotropic lymphoma and two did not.[103] Complete responses were seen in all dogs for between 2 and 15 months, with epitheliotropic forms responding slightly longer. In two larger studies, 77 dogs with cutaneous epitheliotropic lymphoma were treated with CCNU (70 mg/m^2; range, 50–100 mg/m^2). Twenty dogs (26%) had a complete response; median remission duration was not reached in one report[112] but was 4 months in the other.[113] A partial response was seen in 43 dogs (56%) for a median duration of 3 months.[112,113]

There is a report of long-term response to dacarbazine in a dog with early and localized mycosis fungoides (this dog received only three treatments and had no recurrence at 1 year).[114]

Long-term responses have also been reported to long-term L-asparaginase treatment. In one study, approximately half of the treated dogs had waxing and waning control of plaque-like lesions; dogs with tumor formation did not respond as well.[115]

External-beam radiation therapy may provide long-term remission and occasional cure of lesions that cannot be excised. Although response of localized lesions to radiation therapy may occur at low doses (5 Gy in one report[106]), whole-body radiation above 2 Gy is invariably fatal because of bone marrow aplasia.[106] Electron-beam radiation therapy is theoretically safer because penetration of low-energy electrons spares the underlying tissue, including the bone marrow. Electron-beam therapy has been used extensively in humans with mycosis fungoides with good results. This technology is limited in availability for veterinary medicine. Although details of the protocol were not given, a preliminary report of four canine patients with cutaneous mycosis fungoides treated by electron-beam radiation daily for 20 treatments documented responses in all dogs, with the longest control for more than 20 months.[116]

A technique called *PUVA (psoralen ultraviolet AA)* has been reported as a treatment for mycosis fungoides in humans. A compound, 8-methoxypsoralen, is given orally and is converted to psoralen in the body. Psoralen is activated by ultraviolet (UV) light and binds to the DNA of cells in the epidermis and superficial dermis where UV light has penetrated. Therefore, an antineoplastic effect is localized to the areas exposed to and penetrated by UV light. The use of this method has not yet been reported in veterinary medicine.

One dog was treated with intradermal injections of placental lysate and prednisone orally, and clinical remission of severe skin lesions was achieved for 25 months. No skin lesions were seen at necropsy. In this dog, skin lesions relapsed if either medication was removed from the protocol. All of the above treatments may be effective for the early stages of mycosis fungoides but are less effective once organ involvement is seen.

REFERENCES

1. Goldschmidt MH, Shofer FS: Introduction, in Goldschmidt MH, Shofer FS (eds): *Skin Tumors of the Dog and Cat*, ed 1. Tarrytown, NY, Pergamon Press, 1992, pp 1–10.
2. Pulley LT, Stannard AA: Tumors of the skin and soft tissues, in Moulton JE (ed): *Tumors in Domestic Animals*, ed 3. Berkeley, CA, University of California Press, 1990, pp 23–87.
3. Hahn KA, Lantz GC, Salisbury SK, et al: Comparison of survey radiography with ultrasonography and x-ray computed tomography for clinical staging of subcutaneous neoplasms in dogs. *JAVMA* 196:1795–1798, 1990.
4. Aitken ML, Patnaik AK: Comparison of needle-core (TruCut) biopsy and surgical biopsy for the diagnosis of cutaneous and subcutaneous masses: A prospective study of 51 cases (November 1997–August 1998). *JAAHA* 36:153–157, 2000.
5. Er JC, Sutton RH: A survey of skin neoplasms in dogs from the Brisbane region. *Aust Vet J* 66:225–227, 1989.
6. Rothwell TL, Howlett CR, Middleton DJ, et al: Skin neoplasms of dogs in Sydney. *Aust Vet J* 64:161–164, 1987.
7. Goldschmidt MH, Shofer FS: Cutaneous papillomas, in Goldschmidt MH, Shofer FS (eds): *Skin Tumors of the Dog and Cat*, ed 1. Tarrytown NY, Pergamon Press, 1992, pp 11–15.
8. Nicholls PK, Stanley MA: Canine papillomavirus: A centenary review. *J Comp Pathol* 120:219–233, 1999.
9. Campbell KL, Sundberg JP, Goldschmidt MH, et al: Cutaneous inverted papillomas in dogs. *Vet Pathol* 25:67–71, 1988.
10. Bregman CL, Hirth RS, Sundberg JP, Christensen EF: Cutaneous neoplasms in dogs associated with canine oral papillomavirus vaccine. *Vet Pathol* 24:477–487, 1987.
11. Goldschmidt MH, Shofer FS: Basal cell tumors and basosquamous carcinomas, in Goldschmidt MH, Shofer FS (eds): *Skin Tumors of the Dog and Cat*, ed 1. Tarrytown, NY, Pergamon Press, 1992, pp 16–36.
12. Stockhaus C, Teske E, Rudolph R, Werner HG: Assessment of cytological criteria for diagnosing basal cell tumours in the dog and cat. *J Small Anim Pract* 42:582–586, 2001.
13. Nikula KJ, Benjamin SA, Angleton GM, et al: Ultraviolet radiation, solar dermatosis, and cutaneous neoplasia in beagle dogs. *Radiat Res* 129:11–18, 1992.
14. Goldschmidt MH, Shofer FS: Squamous cell carcinoma, in Goldschmidt MH, Shofer FS (eds): *Skin Tumors of the Dog and Cat*, ed 1. Tarrytown, NY, Pergamon Press, 1992, pp 37–49.
15. Scott DW, Teixeira EAC: Multiple squamous cell carcinomas arising from multiple cutaneous follicular cysts in a dog. *Vet Dermatol* 6:27–31, 1995.
16. Scott DW, Miller WH Jr: Squamous cell carcinoma arising in chronic discoid lupus erythematosus nasal lesions in two German shepherd dogs. *Vet Dermatol* 6:99–104, 1995.
17. Madewell BR, Conroy JD, Hodgkins EM: Sunlight-skin cancer association in the dog: A report of three cases. *J Cutan Pathol* 8:434–443, 1981.
18. Marks SL, Song MD, Stannard AA, Power HT: Clinical evaluation of etretinate for the treatment of canine solar-induced squamous cell carcinoma and preneoplastic lesions. *J Am Acad Dermatol* 27:11–16, 1992.
19. Pestili de Almeida EM, Piché C, Sirois J, Doré M: Expression of cyclo-oxygenase-2 in naturally occurring squamous cell carcinomas in dogs. *J Histochem Cytochem* 49:867–875, 2001.
20. Schmidt BR, Glickman NW, DeNicola DB, et al: Evaluation of piroxicam for the treatment of oral squamous cell carcinoma in dogs. *JAVMA* 218:1783–1786, 2001.
21. Gross TL, Brimacomb BH: Multifocal intraepidermal carcinoma in a dog histologically resembling Bowen's disease. *Am J Dermatopathol* 8:509–515, 1986.
22. Kitchell BE, Orenberg EK, Brown DM, et al: Intralesional sustained-release chemotherapy with therapeutic implants for treatment of canine sun-induced squamous cell carcinoma. *Eur J Cancer* 31(suppl A):2093–2098, 1995.
23. Orenberg EK, Luck EE, Brown DM, Kitchell BE: Implant delivery system: Intralesional delivery of chemotherapeutic agents for treatment of spontaneous skin tumors in veterinary patients. *Clin Dermatol* 9:561–568, 1992.
24. McCaw DL, Pope ER, Payne JT, et al: Treatment of canine oral squamous cell carcinomas with photodynamic therapy. *Br J Cancer* 82:1297–1299, 2000.
25. Frimberger AE, Moore AS, Cincotta L, et al: Photodynamic therapy of naturally occurring tumors in animals using a novel benzophenothiazine photosensitizer. *Clin Cancer Res* 4:2207–2218, 1998.
26. Himsel CA, Richardson RC, Craig JA: Cisplatin chemotherapy for metastatic squamous cell carcinoma in two dogs. *JAVMA* 189:1575–1578, 1986.
27. Buhles WC, Theilen GH: Preliminary evaluation of bleomycin in feline and canine squamous cell carcinoma. *Am J Vet Res* 34:289–291, 1973.
28. Ogilvie GK, Obradovich JE, Elmslie RE, et al: Efficacy of mitoxantrone against various neoplasms in dogs. *JAVMA* 198:1618–1621, 1991.
29. Paradis M, Scott DW, Breton L: Squamous cell carcinoma of the nail bed in three related giant schnauzers. *Vet Rec* 125:322–324, 1989.
30. Madewell BR, Pool RR, Theilen GH, Brewer WG: Multiple subungual squamous cell carcinomas in five dogs. *JAVMA* 180:731–734, 1982.
31. Guerin SR, Jones BR, Alley MR, Broome C: Multiple digital tumours in a rottweiler. *J Small Anim Pract* 39:200–202, 1998.
32. O Brien MG, Berg J, Engler SJ: Treatment by digital amputation of subungual squamous cell carcinoma in dogs: 21 cases (1987–1988). *JAVMA* 201:759–761, 1992.
33. Liu S-K, Hohn RB: Squamous cell carcinoma of the digit of the dog. *JAVMA* 153:411–424, 1968.
34. Brewer WG Jr, Mitley E, Ogilvie GK, et al: Canine digital tumors: Retrospective review of 63 cases (1980–1990): A VCOG cooperative study—Preliminary results. *Vet Cancer Soc News*, 2003.
35. Marino DJ, Matthiesen DT, Stefanacci JD, Moroff SD: Evaluation of dogs with digit masses: 117 cases (1981–1991). *JAVMA* 207:726–728, 1995.
36. Maiolino P, De Vico G, Restucci B: Expression of vascular endothelial growth factor in basal cell tumours and in squamous cell carcinomas of canine skin. *J Comp Pathol* 123:141–145, 2000.
37. Shapiro W, Kitchell BE, Fossum TW, et al: Cisplatin for treatment of transitional cell and squamous cell carcinomas in dogs. *JAVMA* 193:1530–1533, 1988.
38. Rogers KS, Helman RG, Walker MA: Squamous cell carcinoma of the canine nasal planum: Eight cases (1988–1994). *JAAHA* 31:373–378, 1995.
39. Lascelles BDX, Parry AT, Stidworthy MF, et al: Squamous cell carcinoma of the nasal planum in 17 dogs. *Vet Rec* 473–476, 2000.
40. Thrall DE, Adams WM: Radiotherapy of squamous cell carcinomas of the canine nasal plane. *Vet Radiol* 23:193–196, 1982.
41. Peters J, Scott DW, Erb HN, Miller WH: Hereditary nasal parakeratosis in Labrador retrievers: 11 new cases and a retrospective study on the presence of accumulations of serum ("serum lakes") in the epidermis of parakeratotic dermatoses and inflamed nasal plana of dogs. *Vet Dermatol* 14:197–203, 2003.
42. Theon AP, Madewell BR, Moore AS, et al: Localized thermocisplatin therapy: A pilot study in spontaneous canine and feline tumors. *Int J Hypertherm* 7:881–892, 1991.
43. Holt D, Prymak C, Evans S: Excision of tumors in the nasal vestibule of two dogs. *Vet Surg* 19:418–423, 1990.
44. Withrow SJ, Straw RC: Resection of the nasal planum in nine cats and five dogs. *JAAHA* 26:219–222, 1990.
45. Kirpensteijn J, Withrow SJ, Straw RC: Combined resection of the nasal planum and premaxilla in three dogs. *Vet Surg* 23:341–346, 1994.
46. Goldschmidt MH, Shofer FS: Sebaceous tumors, in Goldschmidt MH, Shofer FS (eds): *Skin Tumors of the Dog and Cat*, ed 1. Tarrytown, NY, Pergamon Press, 1992, pp 50–65.
47. White SD, Rosychuk RA, Scott KV, et al: Sebaceous adenitis in dogs and results of treatment with isotretinoin and etretinate: 30 cases (1990–1994). *JAVMA* 207:197–200, 1995.
48. Kalaher KM, Anderson WI, Scott DW: Neoplasms of the apocrine sweat glands in 44 dogs and 10 cats. *Vet Rec* 127:400–403, 1990.
49. Goldschmidt MH, Shofer FS: Apocrine gland tumors, in Goldschmidt MH, Shofer FS (eds): *Skin Tumors of the Dog and Cat*, ed 1. Tarrytown, NY, Pergamon Press, 1992, pp 80–95.
50. Simko E, Wilcock BP, Yager JA: A retrospective study of 44 canine apocrine sweat gland adenocarcinomas. *Can Vet J* 44:38–42, 2003.
51. Kusters AH, Peperkamp KH, Hazewinkel HA: Atrichial sweat gland adenocarcinoma in the dog. *Vet Dermatol* 10:51–54, 1999.

52. Ogilvie GK, Reynolds HA, Richardson RC, et al: Phase II evaluation of doxorubicin for treatment of various canine neoplasms. *JAVMA* 195:1580–1583, 1989.
53. Goldschmidt MH, Shofer FS: Intracutaneous cornifying epithelioma, in Goldschmidt MH, Shofer FS (eds): *Skin Tumors of the Dog and Cat*, ed 1. Tarrytown, NY, Pergamon Press, 1992, pp 109–114.
54. White SD, Rosychuk RA, Scott KV, et al: Use of isotretinoin and etretinate for the treatment of benign cutaneous neoplasia and cutaneous lymphoma in dogs. *JAVMA* 202:387–391, 1993.
55. Goldschmidt MH, Shofer FS: Trichoepithelioma, in Goldschmidt MH, Shofer FS (eds): *Skin Tumors of the Dog and Cat*, ed 1. Tarrytown, NY, Pergamon Press, 1992, pp 115–124.
56. Goldschmidt MH, Shofer FS: Pilomatrixoma, in Goldschmidt MH, Shofer FS (eds): *Skin Tumors of the Dog and Cat*, ed 1. Tarrytown, NY, Pergamon Press, 1992, pp 125–130.
57. Goldschmidt MH, Thrall DE, Jeglum KA, et al: Malignant pilomatricoma in a dog. *J Cutan Pathol* 8:375–381, 1981.
58. Rodriguez F, Herraez P, Rodriguez E, et al: Metastatic pilomatrixoma associated with neurological signs in a dog. *Vet Rec* 137:247–248, 1995.
59. Sells DM, Conroy JD: Malignant epithelial neoplasia with hair follicle differentiation in dogs. Malignant pilomatrixoma. *J Comp Pathol* 86:121–129, 1976.
60. Rodriguez F, Herráez P, Rodriguez E, et al: Metastatic pilomatrixoma associated with neurological signs in a dog. *Vet Rec* 137:247–248, 1995.
61. Lüttgenau H, Flaig K, Kirchhoff A: Malignes pilomatrixom bei einem hund. *Kleintierpraxis* 46:653–660, 2001.
62. Vascellari M, Mutinelli F, Cossettini R, Altinier E: Liposarcoma at the site of an implanted microchip in a dog. *Vet J* 168:188–190, 2004.
63. Goldschmidt MH, Shofer FS: Cutaneous lipoma and liposarcoma, in Goldschmidt MH, Shofer FS (eds): *Skin Tumors of the Dog and Cat*, ed 1. Tarrytown, NY, Pergamon Press, 1992, pp 192–203.
64. Reimann N, Nolte I, Bonk U, et al: Cytogenetic investigation of canine lipomas. *Cancer Genet Cytogenet* 111:172–174, 1999.
65. Liggett AD, Frazier KS, Styer EL: Angiolipomatous tumors in dogs and cats. *Vet Pathol* 39:286–289, 2002.
66. Albers GW, Theilen GH: Calcium chloride for treatment of subcutaneous lipomas in dogs *JAVMA* 186:492–494, 1985.
67. Mayhew PD, Brockman DJ: Body cavity lipomas in six dogs. *J Small Anim Pract* 43:177–181, 2002.
68. Brown PJ, Lucke VM, Sozmen M, et al: Lipomatous infiltration of the canine salivary gland. *J Small Anim Pract* 38:234–236, 1997.
69. Bergman PJ, Withrow SJ, Straw RC, Powers BE: Infiltrative lipoma in dogs: 16 cases (1981–1992). *JAVMA* 205:322–324, 1994.
70. Saik JE, Diters RW, Wortman JA: Metastasis of a well-differentiated liposarcoma in a dog and a note on nomenclature of fatty tumours. *J Comp Pathol* 97:369–373, 1987.
71. McEntee MC, Thrall DE: Computed tomographic imaging of infiltration lipoma in 22 dogs. *Vet Radiol Ultrasound* 42:221–225, 2001.
72. McChesney AE, Stephens LC, Lebel J, et al: Infiltrative lipoma in dogs. *Vet Pathol* 17:316–322, 1980.
73. Kramek BA, Spackman CJA, Hayden DW: Infiltrative lipoma in three dogs. *JAVMA* 186:81–82, 1985.
74. Thomson MJ, Withrow SJ, Dernell WS, Powers BE: Intermuscular lipomas of the thigh region in dogs: 11 cases. *JAAHA* 35:165–167, 1999.
75. McEntee MC, Page RL, Mauldin GN, Thrall DE: Results of irradiation of infiltrative lipoma in 13 dogs. *Vet Radiol Ultrasound* 41:554–556, 2000.
76. McCarthy PE, Hedlund CS, Veazy RS, et al: Liposarcoma associated with a glass foreign body in a dog. *JAVMA* 209:612–614, 1996.
77. Strafuss AC, Bozarth AJ: Liposarcoma in dogs. *JAAHA* 9:183–187, 1973.
78. Baez JL, Hendrick MJ, Shofer FS, et al: Liposarcomas in dogs: 56 cases (1989–2000). *JAVMA* 224:887–891, 2004.
79. Bozarth AJ, Strafuss AC: Metastatic liposarcoma in a dog. *JAVMA* 162:1043–1044, 1973.
80. Zwicker GM: Liposarcoma in a dog. *Pathol Vet* 7:145–147, 1970.
81. Davis PE, Dixon RT, Johnson JA, Paris R: Multiple liposarcoma of bone marrow origin in a Greyhound. *J Small Anim Pract* 15:445–456, 1974.
82. Meierhenry EF: Metastatic liposarcoma with extensive osteolysis in the dog. *JAAHA* 10:478–481, 1974.
83. Konno A, Nagata M, Nanko H: Immunohistochemical diagnosis of a Merkel cell tumor in a dog. *Vet Pathol* 35:538–540, 1998.
84. Duncan JR, Prasse KW: Cytology of canine cutaneous round cell tumors. Mast cell tumor, histiocytoma, lymphosarcoma and transmissible venereal tumor. *Vet Pathol* 16:673–679, 1979.
85. Sandusky GE, Carlton WW, Wightman KA: Diagnostic immunohistochemistry of canine round cell tumors. *Vet Pathol* 24:495–499, 1987.
86. Lucke VM: Primary cutaneous plasmacytomas in the dog and cat. *J Small Anim Pract* 28:49–55, 1987.
87. Clark GN, Berg J, Engler SJ, Bronson RT: Extramedullary plasmacytomas in dogs: Results of surgical excision in 131 cases. *JAAHA* 28:105–111, 1992.
88. Rakich PM, Latimer KS, Weiss R, Steffans WL: Mucocutaneous plasmacytomas in dogs: 75 cases (1980–1987). *JAVMA* 194:803–810, 1989.
89. Baer KE, Patnaik AK, Gilbertson SR, Hurvitz AI: Cutaneous plasmacytomas in dogs: A morphologic and immunohistochemical study. *Vet Pathol* 26:216–221, 1989.
90. Rowland PH, Valentine BA, Stebbons KE, Smith CA: Cutaneous plasmacytomas with amyloid in six dogs. *Vet Pathol* 28:125–130, 1991.
91. Walton GS, Gopinath C: Multiple myeloma in a dog with some unusual features. *J Small Anim Pract* 13:703–708, 1972.
92. Goldschmidt MH, Shofer FS: Cutaneous plasmacytoma, in Goldschmidt MH, Shofer FS (eds): *Skin Tumors of the Dog and Cat*, ed 1. Tarrytown, NY, Pergamon Press, 1992, pp 265–270.
93. Brener W, Colbatzky F, Platz S, Hermanns W: Immunoglobulin-producing tumours in dogs and cats. *J Comp Pathol* 109:203–216, 1993.
94. Trigo FJ, Hargis AM: Canine cutaneous plasmacytoma with regional lymph node metastasis. *Vet Med Small Anim Clin* 78:1749–1751, 1983.
95. Platz SJ, Breuer W, Pfleghaar S, et al: Prognostic value of histopathological grading in canine extramedullary plasmacytomas. *Vet Pathol* 36:23–27, 1999.
96. Morton LD, Barton CL, Ellissalde GS, Wilson SR: Oral extramedullary plasmacytoma in two dogs. *Vet Pathol* 26:637–639, 1986.
97. Brunnert SR, Dee LA, Herron AJ, Altman NH: Gastric extramedullary plasmacytoma in a dog *JAVMA* 200:1501–1502, 1992.
98. Goldschmidt MH, Shofer FS: Cutaneous lymphosarcoma, in Goldschmidt MH, Shofer FS (eds): *Skin Tumors of the Dog and Cat*, ed 1. Tarrytown, NY, Pergamon Press, 1992, pp 252–264.
99. Day MJ: Immunophenotypic characterization of cutaneous lymphoid neoplasia in the dog and cat. *J Comp Pathol* 112:79–96, 1995.
100. Kleiter M, Wagner R, Day MJ: Eine generalisierte demodikose in verbindung mit einem kutanen B-zell lymphosarkom beim adulten hund. *Kleintierpraxis* 43:537–548, 1998.
101. Ridyard AE, Rhind SM, French AT, et al: Myasthenia gravis associated with cutaneous lymphoma in a dog. *J Small Anim Pract* 41:348–351, 2000.
102. O Brown NO, Nesbitt GH, Patnaik AK, MacEwen EG: Cutaneous lymphosarcoma in the dog: A disease with variable clinical and histologic manifestations. *JAAHA* 16:565–572, 1980.
103. Graham JC, Myers RK: Pilot study of the use of lomustine (CCNU) for the treatment of cutaneous lymphoma in dogs. *J Vet Intern Med* 13:257, 1999.
104. Foster AP, Evans E, Kerlin RL, Vail DM: Cutaneous T-cell lymphoma with Sezary syndrome in a dog. *Vet Clin Pathol* 26:188–192, 1997.
105. Thrall MA, Macy DW, Snyder SP, Hall RL: Cutaneous lymphosarcoma and leukemia in a dog resembling Sezary syndrome in man. *Vet Pathol* 21:182–186, 1984.
106. DeBoer DJ, Turrel JM, Moore PF: Mycosis fungoides in a dog: Demonstration of T-cell specificity and response to radiotherapy. *JAAHA* 26:566–572, 1990.
107. Donaldson D, Day MJ: Epitheliotropic lymphoma (mycosis fungoides) presenting as blepharoconjunctivitis in an Irish setter. *J Small Anim Pract* 41:317–320, 2000.
108. Czasch S, Risse K, Baumgartner W: Central nervous system metastasis of a cutaneous epitheliotropic lymphosarcoma in a dog. *J Comp Pathol* 123:59–63, 2000.
109. Brain PH, Howlett CR: Two cases of epidermotropic lymphoma in dogs. *Aust Vet J* 68:247–248, 1991.
110. McKeever PJ, Grindem CB, Stevens JB, Osborne CA: Canine cutaneous lymphoma. *JAVMA* 180:531–536, 1982.
111. Iwamoto KS, Bennett LR, Norman A, et al: Linoleate produces remission in canine mycosis fungoides. *Cancer Lett* 64:17–22, 1992.
112. Williams LE, Rassnick KM, Power H, et al: CCNU (lomustine) for the treatment of canine epitheliotropic lymphoma. *J Vet Intern Med* 2006, in press.
113. Risbon R, Burgess K, Skorupski K, et al: Response of epitheliotropic lymphoma to CCNU. *Proc 24th Annu Conf Vet Cancer Soc*:2004.
114. Lemarié SL, Eddlestone SM: Treatment of cutaneous T-cell lymphoma with dacarbazine in a dog. *Vet Dermatol* 8:41–46, 1997.
115. Moriello KA, MacEwen G, Schultz KT: PEG-L-asparaginase in the treatment of canine epitheliotropic lymphoma and histiocytic proliferative dermatitis, in Ihrke, PJ, Mason, IS, White SD (eds): *Advances in Veterinary Dermatology*, vol 2. Tarrytown, NY, Pergamon Press, 1992.
116. Prescott DM, Gordon J: Total skin electron beam irradiation for generalized cutaneous lymphoma. *Proc 24th Annu Conf Vet Cancer Soc*:2004.

MAST CELL TUMORS

Antony S. Moore and Gregory K. Ogilvie

65

CLINICAL BRIEFING

Minimum database includes a CBC, biochemical profile, and urinalysis, as well as thoracic radiography (three views).

Clinical factors
- Raised or ulcerated intracutaneous mass; may be hairless or hairy; single or multiple.
- Can look and feel like anything.
- Most are grade 2 (moderately differentiated).
- Bulldog-derived breeds (boxers, Boston terriers) and golden retrievers are predisposed, but MCTs can occur in any breed and at any age.

Staging and diagnosis
- Metastasis similar to other hematopoietic tumors: To regional lymph nodes as well as to liver, spleen, and bone marrow.
- Staging includes minimum database and abdominal radiography or ultrasonography as well as bone marrow aspiration.

Prognostic factors
- The most important prognostic factor is histologic grade.
- Tumors on limbs have better prognosis than those on the trunk.
- Slow growth and long duration of presence may be favorable.
- Complete surgical margins are associated with long control.
- Intestinal location is associated with a high metastatic rate and a poor prognosis.

Treatment
Initial and adjunctive
- Grade 1 tumors: Wide surgical excision.
- Grade 2 tumors: Wide surgical excision; adjunctive radiation therapy if incompletely excised (86% achieve 5-year control); chemotherapy only with disseminated or metastatic disease; vinblastine, CCNU, and prednisone appear to be most active agents.
- Grade 3 tumors: Surgery with or without radiation therapy to the regional lymph node may provide local control; chemotherapy using agents listed above; H_1 and H_2 blockers may be palliative.

Supportive
- Analgesia postoperatively and nutritional support as needed. H_1 and H_2 blockers may be palliative.

Normal mast cells are derived from hematopoietic and connective tissue cells. They are present throughout the body in perivascular locations, particularly the skin and subcutaneous tissues, lung parenchyma, digestive tract, and liver, where they play an integral role in allergic reactions and inflammatory processes. Mast cells are seen only occasionally in bone marrow and almost never in the systemic circulation. After immunoglobulin E (IgE) binds to the cell surface, mast cells elicit an immediate hypersensitivity response by releasing vasoactive amines (e.g., histamine and heparin) both locally and into the circulation, causing vasodilation, blood stasis, and edema. Histamine chemotactically attracts eosinophils, which neutralize histamine.

Cutaneous Mast Cell Tumors
INCIDENCE, SIGNALMENT, AND ETIOLOGY

In dogs, mast cell tumors (MCTs) are most commonly found in the cutaneous tissue. Tumors are solitary in most dogs but are multiple in about 6%. Tumors usually occur in older dogs (mean age: 9 years) with no gender predilection. However, MCTs may be seen in dogs as young as 6 months of age. Boxers, Rhodesian ridgebacks, pugs, Boston terriers, pit bull terriers, and weimaraners are at high risk (four to

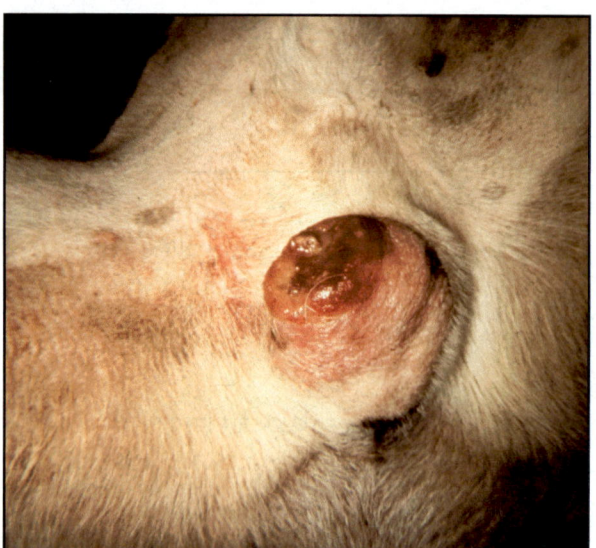

Figure 65-1. *MCTs in the inguinal area were thought to be more aggressive than their counterparts at other cutaneous sites. It now appears that prognostically, tumor grade is more important than site. Shown is a scrotal tumor in a male Boston terrier. (Courtesy of Gordon H. Theilen, DVM, University of California, Davis)*

eight times the risk of the general population) of developing MCTs.[1,2] Boxers, pugs, and weimaraners are more likely to develop multiple MCTs than other breeds.[2] MCTs in the bulldog-derived breeds, such as boxers and pugs, and, possibly, in golden retrievers are usually of a lower (well-differentiated) histologic grade than MCTs in other breeds. Shar-peis, particularly young dogs, are predisposed to developing MCTs, and these tumors are often poorly differentiated and biologically aggressive.[3]

In dogs, MCTs have been experimentally transmitted using cell-free extracts, which suggests a viral origin. However, ultrastructural examination of numerous MCTs of different species has failed to reveal viral particles. Recent studies have found that mutations in the protooncogene *c-kit* may be associated with MCTs in dogs, correlating with a higher histologic grade and opening possibilities for therapeutic strategies.[4-6] Mutations in *c-kit* may also be used to distinguish a very poorly differentiated, nongranulated MCT from lymphoma.[7]

CLINICAL PRESENTATION AND HISTORY

In dogs, it is uncommon to diagnose MCTs without skin involvement. MCTs vary greatly in appearance, and no estimate of their malignancy or prediction of their behavior can be made on clinical appearance alone. Some MCTs may be present for months to years before rapidly disseminating; others act aggressively from the beginning.

Most cutaneous MCTs present as intracutaneous nodules that can be 10 cm or more in diameter. Some cause ulceration of the overlying epidermis; others present as single or multiple elevated, erythematous nodules with alopecia of the overlying skin. MCTs may be edematous on palpation or present as firm, intracutaneous nodules. The tumors usually arise in the dermis and frequently extend into the underlying subcutaneous tissue and musculature. Extension occurs most frequently with rapidly growing tumors (Figures 65-1 and 65-2).

MCTs most commonly occur on the limbs, with the abdominal and thoracic skin as the next most common sites. They are least common in cutaneous sites around the tail and back. Approximately 6% of dogs develop multiple cutaneous MCTs.[2]

> **KEY POINT**
> *Mast cell tumors may "grow" and "shrink" rapidly because of inflammation caused by mast cell degranulation.*

Occasionally, mechanical manipulation during examination of these tumors causes degranulation of mast cells, producing erythema and wheal formations. This phenomenon has been observed in both dogs and cats (Darier's sign) and is considered of diagnostic significance. Owners may report that the tumor enlarges rapidly and then diminishes in size over a period of about 24 hours. Such a history should increase the clinician's suspicion of MCT.

STAGING AND DIAGNOSIS

The clinical appearance of MCTs in dogs may vary widely, but diagnosis is relatively easy using aspiration cytology. Presurgical aspiration of these tumors provides a cytology specimen characterized by round cells that may have well-stained, large cytoplasmic (well-differentiated) granules or may be more anaplastic, with small, poorly staining cytoplasmic granules (see Chapter 19). Other examples of round cell tumors are lymphoma, cutaneous plasmacytoma, histiocytoma, transmissible venereal tumor, and melanoma. Cells from these tumors lack the blue-to-purple cytoplasmic granules of MCTs. Eosinophils are often seen in aspirates of MCTs because of eosinophil chemotaxis to histamine release.

Diagnosis of MCT often can be made by fine-needle aspiration (FNA) cytology, but excisional biopsy is required for accurate histologic grading of the tumor. Histopathologic grading of the tumor has been correlated with both recurrence and survival.

All dogs with MCTs should be staged to determine the extent of their disease. This is especially important for dogs being considered for aggressive surgery such as amputation or radiation therapy. The current staging scheme is shown in Table 65-1.

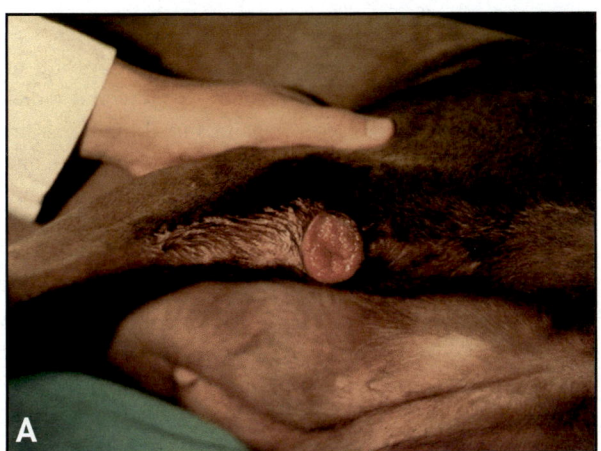 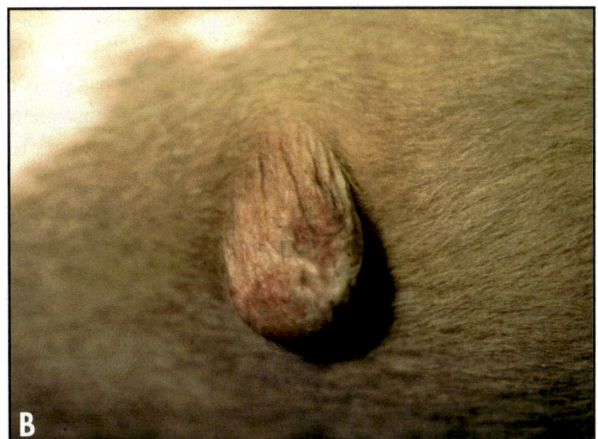

Figure 65-2. MCTs (**A** and **B**) with vastly different appearances found on the same weimaraner. External appearance does not indicate a diagnosis. (Courtesy of Anne G. Evans, DVM, Veterinary Information Network)

To establish the stage of a dog with a cutaneous MCT, information should be obtained from the following:

- **Complete blood count:** The complete blood count (CBC) may reveal anemia or a regenerative or degenerative left shift that could suggest gastrointestinal (GI) bleeding or perforation, respectively. Either may arise from chronic histamine release from the tumor. A CBC is also valuable in assessing animals with MCTs because those with systemic mastocytosis occasionally have peripheral eosinophilia and basophilia in addition to large numbers of circulating mast cells.
- **Lymph node aspirates:** The clinician should conduct FNA of the regional lymph node if the node is enlarged. The presence of clusters of mast cells (and eosinophils) is an indication that the MCT may no longer be confined to the primary site. Mast cells may infiltrate a regional lymph node in a dog with an MCT as an inflammatory response to the tumor; therefore, a suspicious cytology result should be confirmed by biopsy.
- **Radiographs and ultrasonographs:** Splenomegaly or hepatomegaly may indicate systemic spread of MCTs. Enlarged regional nodes (especially sublumbar nodes for

> **KEY POINT**
> *Pulmonary metastasis from canine cutaneous MCTs is extremely rare; therefore, thoracic radiographs are rarely useful for staging.*

perineal tumors) may be identified. FNA may confirm the suspicion of metastasis. Pulmonary metastasis of MCTs is rare. A recent ultrasonography study showed that although both the liver and spleen were subjectively enlarged and showed a diffuse increase in echogenicity as

Table 65-1 **Staging Scheme for MCTs**

Stage	Description
0	One neoplasm incompletely excised (to microscopic disease) without regional lymph node involvement
1	One neoplasm confined to the dermis without regional lymph node involvement
2	One neoplasm confined to the dermis with regional lymph node involvement
3	Multiple dermal neoplasms or large infiltrating neoplasms with or without regional lymph node involvement*
4	Any neoplasm with distant metastasis or systemic involvement

*See the discussion of multiple mast cell tumors on p. 647.

well as hypoechoic nodules when affected with MCT, ultrasonographically unremarkable canine livers and spleens were also found to be infiltrated by mast cells. This implies that ultrasonography is most useful for staging dogs with MCT if it is used in conjunction with histopathology or cytology.[8]

- **Bone marrow aspirates:** The presence of more than 10 mast cells per 1,000 nucleated cells indicates systemic spread of the neoplasm. Because mast cells may be accompanied by eosinophils, the presence of eosinophilia in the marrow should alert the clinician to search carefully for mast cells.[9] In a study involving 16 dogs with systemic mastocytosis, bone marrow aspiration was deemed superior to either buffy-coat or blood smear examination.[10] In a recent report, seven of 157 dogs (4.5%) with cutaneous MCT had either more than 1% mast cells or abnormal mast cells in a bone marrow aspirate.[11]

- **Miscellaneous tests:** In one study, eight of 16 (50%) dogs with systemic disease had signs of systemic illness.[10] Of these eight dogs, five were necropsied and three had gastric ulceration.[10] Histamine release by MCTs and subsequent histamine binding at H_2-receptor sites has been shown to stimulate hydrochloric acid secretion by gastric parietal cells, causing ulceration and GI bleeding.[12] Fecal occult blood tests may be useful in evaluating patients with mast cell disease. In many cases, feces may contain small amounts of blood that are insufficient to produce melena. Evidence of GI bleeding in a patient with an MCT should prompt the clinician to treat with medications that block the effects of mast cell hyperhistaminemia (i.e., H_2 blockers such as cimetidine, ranitidine, famotidine).
- **Buffy-coat smears:** Care must be exercised in interpreting buffy-coat smears because mastocythemia has been reported in a variety of canine acute inflammatory diseases. For this reason, some oncologists now believe that this test has limited applicability to staging of dogs with MCTs. We no longer recommend it as part of staging for MCTs.

> **KEY POINT**
> *Buffy-coat smears are no longer considered to be a valuable staging test for dogs with cutaneous MCTs.*

Systemic mastocytosis refers to disease in which two or more of the following are observed in addition to cutaneous MCTs in an affected dog:

1. Liver or spleen involvement
2. Distant nodal involvement
3. Bone marrow containing more than 10 mast cells per 1,000 nucleated cells
4. Mast cells circulating or on a buffy-coat smear (no longer thought to be specific for MCT; see below)

Alone, these findings are not diagnostic for systemic mastocytosis. In one study, normal dogs had mast cells seen on lymph node cytology in 11 of 46 dogs (25%) with a median of five mast cells per slide; the bone marrow contained a single mast cell in two of 51 normal dogs (5%), and no mast cells were seen in any of 53 buffy-coat smears.[9] In contrast, when dogs with a positive buffy-coat smear were categorized, only 27% of dogs with MCTs had more than 10 mast cells per slide (average number: 71) compared with 76% of dogs with inflammatory disease (average number: 276). More than 95% of the time, a positive buffy-coat smear was not indicative of an MCT; therefore, this test should not be used to screen for occult MCT.[13]

PROGNOSTIC FACTORS

Recent clinical research has led to the identification of prognostic factors for dogs undergoing surgery and radiation therapy, which has led to changes in thinking about other previously well-accepted prognostic factors. In one study, male dogs had a worse prognosis after chemotherapy treatment for MCT,[14] and in another study, dogs older than 8 years were nearly three times more likely to die from their disease after treatment for MCT.[15] Dogs with tumors that grow at a rate greater than 1 cm per week appeared to have a worse prognosis in an early study of dogs treated with surgery alone.[16]

Tumor Grade

Histologic grade has long been believed to be the most important prognostic factor for a dog with a cutaneous MCT. Although grading has been conducted on cytology specimens,[17] histopathology remains the most reliable method to grade a canine MCT. In an early study of 300 dogs from which MCTs were excised with "grossly clear margins," recurrence was seen in 25% of well-differentiated (grade 1) tumors.[18] This percentage increased to 44% for moderately differentiated (grade 2) tumors and to 76% for undifferentiated (anaplastic; grade 3) tumors. Survival was also shown to depend on grade; 6% of dogs with grade 3 tumors, 45% of dogs with grade 2 tumors, and 93% of dogs with grade 1 tumors survived 4 years after surgical excision.[19]

Recent studies using a more aggressive surgical technique and histology to examine margins (rather than the surgeon's clinical impression) have shown that dogs with grade 2 MCTs have a much lower rate of local recurrence and longer survival times. Nonetheless, grading is still an important prognostic factor.[20] In one study, grade 3 tumors were more likely to be incompletely excised and more likely to metastasize.[21] In another study, grade 3 tumors were nearly four times more likely to result in death than tumors of lower grades.[14] In a third study, the disease-free interval was significantly shorter in dogs with grade 3 MCTs.[15] Another British study of 280 dogs with MCTs found that only 18% were grade 3 but that the median survival of this group of dogs was less than 10 months; median survival for dogs with grade 1 or 2 tumors was more than 3.5 years.[22] Tumor regrowth was more likely to occur in dogs that had grade 3 tumors (19%) than dogs with grade 2 (6%) or grade 1 (1%) MCTs.[22]

The Patnaik scheme for grading MCTs is the most common grading system; it is shown in Table 65-2.

Some have suggested that individual pathologists may grade MCTs differently, leading to poor agreement about the grade of any individual canine MCT.[23] Veterinarians are encouraged to read the pathologic description as well as the stated grade and to discuss any uncertain results or apparent inconsistencies with the pathologist before making treatment recommendations.

Surgical Margins

The completeness of excision (i.e., whether the surgical margins are "dirty") is an important prognostic factor and is also important in determining whether further surgery or adjunctive radiation therapy is needed. There is often disparity between the surgeon's assessment of margins and those assessed by histopathology. In one study, 22 of 59 tumors thought to have been excised widely had either questionable (10 tumors) or incomplete (12 tumors) excision based on histologic examination.[21]

Another study defined three levels of surgical excision based on histopathology. The tumors were sectioned in one plane and twice more in a plane perpendicular to the first to give at least four lateral margins and a deep margin. This procedure is probably very important to confidently determine the completeness of surgical excision. Margins were considered complete if there was more than 1 mm of normal tissue around the tumor cells, complete but close if the margin was less than 1 mm, and incomplete if tumor cells were seen at the margin.[24] Other investigators have considered margins to be complete but close if they are between 1 and 10 mm wide.[25]

> **KEY POINT**
>
> *The most important prognostic factor for canine MCTs is histologic grade of the tumor.*

In a study of 214 dogs that had surgical margins examined, there were 23 recurrences at the surgical site.[22] Fourteen of 83 dogs (17%) with incomplete margins had regrowth compared with two of 41 dogs (5%) with marginal (<5 mm) margins and three of 90 dogs (3%) with complete margins.[22] Another study indicated that some dogs with incomplete excisions may not have tumor recurrence after surgery.[26] This may be because it is impossible to distinguish truly infiltrating tumor cells from inflammatory mast cells at the surgical margin except in grade 3 tumors.[22] Another study found that dogs with incomplete excisions were more likely to develop metastatic disease.[21] Because of this finding, and because tumor recurrence is still more common after incomplete excision, clinicians are counseled to obtain clear surgical margins when possible and to not rely on a marginal excision.

Tumor Location

In some studies, dogs with neoplasms of the extremities had longer tumor-free and survival times than dogs with tumors on the trunk,[27] although this is not a consistent finding.[24,26,28]

Although it was often reported that MCTs in the inguinal and perineal regions had a poor prognosis regardless of histologic grade, this has recently been shown to not always be true. Although MCTs in this location have long been thought to be more likely to recur than MCTs in other subcutaneous locations, aggressive local therapy often results in long-term control,[29] and there is no difference in recurrence rate, time to recurrence, or survival time compared with dogs with MCTs at other locations.[15]

MCTs of the muzzle were often found to be grade 3 tumors and to have a higher rate of regional lymph node metastasis in one study (nearly 60% of dogs evaluated; Figure 65-3).[20]

Multiple Tumors

Although the staging scheme detailed in Table 65-1 includes multiple tumors as being a higher clinical stage, the occurrence of multiple tumors has not been shown to be a worse prognostic factor.[24] In a study that compared 145 dogs with a single MCT and 50 dogs with multiple MCTs, there was no significant difference in survival times between these two groups. Survival rates at 1 year were 88% and 86% for these groups. Two years after surgery, 83% of dogs with single tumors and 86% of dogs with multiple tumors were still alive. Whereas eight dogs with stage 2 disease (single MCT with lymph node metastases) had a median survival time of 431 days, dogs with stage 3 disease (multiple tumors) and dogs with stage 1 disease (single tumors) had not reached a median survival time.[30] Similar preliminary findings were

Table 65-2 **Patnaik Grading Scheme for MCTs**

Grade	Description
1	MCT confined to the dermis and interfollicular spaces. Cells are monomorphic with ample cytoplasm with distinct boundaries and medium-sized intracytoplasmic granules. There are no mitoses and minimal edema and necrosis.
2	MCT infiltrating or replacing the lower dermal or subcutaneous tissue. Cells are moderately pleomorphic with scattered spindle and giant cells. Cytoplasm is mostly but not always distinct with fine or occasionally large intracytoplasmic granules. Mitoses rare (0–2 per high-power field). Areas of diffuse edema and necrosis are present.
3	MCT replacing the subcutaneous and deep tissues. Cells are pleomorphic with many binucleate, giant, and multinucleated cells. Cytoplasm is indistinct with fine or absent intracytoplasmic granules. Mitoses are common (3–6 per high-power field). Hemorrhage, edema, and necrosis are common.

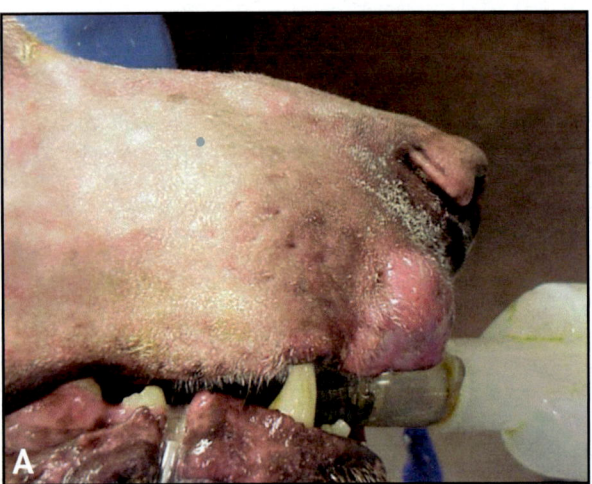 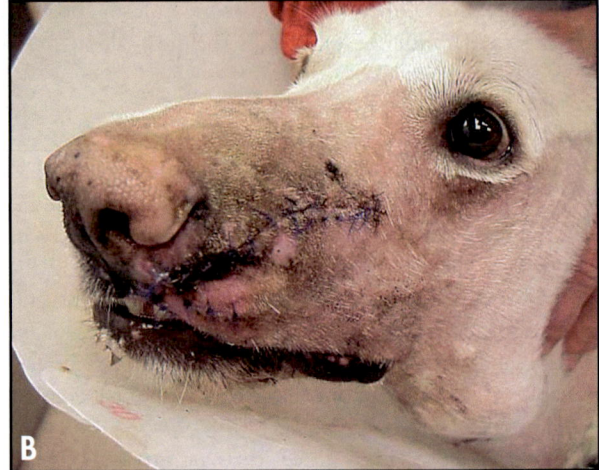

Figure 65-3. *MCTs on the muzzle appear to have a higher metastatic rate than their counterparts at other cutaneous sites. (A) An MCT on the muzzle of a male crossbreed dog after receiving preoperative radiation therapy. Radiation therapy before surgical excision may improve the chance of obtaining complete excision. (B) Same dog as in A after surgery. Note the enlarged mandibular node that contained metastatic disease.*

reported in another study.[31] It appears that the staging scheme described above should be amended to exclude multiple stage 3 tumors (Figure 65-4).

Tumor Stage

It may be that the presence of metastases is a clearer indicator of a poor prognosis than stage, as described above. Three studies have shown that the presence of metastases at the time of diagnosis, rather than clinical stage, was a predictor of poor survival; dogs with lymph node metastases were nearly eight times as likely to die from MCT in one study,[20] and the finding of metastatic disease correlated with a 12- to 30-fold greater chance of dying in another study.[14] In a study that compared populations of dogs with tumors in the perineal location, the finding of nodal metastases (rather than location) meant a more than three times greater chance of dying from the disease.[15] A potential problem with staging is that small numbers of mast cells may be found in the circulation, spleen, liver, and bone marrow, so the significance of such a finding is unclear. In one study, the presence of small numbers of mast cells in theses locations did not seem to influence survival in dogs with grade 2 MCTs.[24] Mast cells may infiltrate a regional lymph node in a dog with an MCT as an inflammatory response to the tumor; therefore, a suspicious cytology result should be confirmed by biopsy.

Measurement of Tumor Proliferation

Argyrophilic nucleolar organizer regions (AgNORs) are present in the nucleus, take up silver stain, and are an indirect measure of cellular proliferation. The average number of AgNORs per cell correlates well with the tumor grade in both histologic and cytologic specimens[32,33] and appears to be an independent predictor of tumor-related death.[32] In one study, AgNOR counts were higher in dogs that developed metastatic disease.[34]

Another method of measuring cellular proliferation, staining for proliferating cell nuclear antigen (PCNA), was also a predictor of metastasis and poor survival in dogs with cutaneous MCTs.[34] The association between PCNA and survival was less clear in another study.[35] The authors of one study proposed using a combination of histopathologic grade, AgNOR staining, and PCNA staining to determine the prognosis. When they used this model, an accurate prognosis still could not be determined for 20% of dogs with MCT, underscoring the heterogeneity of this disease.[34]

A third method of measuring cellular proliferation, staining for Ki67, was found to correlate well with tumor grading.[36] The mean number of Ki67-positive cells was significantly higher in dogs that died from MCT.[35] Furthermore, when dogs with grade 2 MCT were grouped on the basis of Ki67 staining, there was a significant correlation with survival after surgery.[35]

Dogs with MCTs that had a mitotic index greater than 10 figures per 10 high-power (400×) fields were more likely to die from MCT than were dogs with lower scores.[32]

The DNA content of cells in MCTs was reported to be abnormal in about 30% of tumors.[37] There was a tendency for dogs with abnormal DNA content to survive for a shorter time.

Recent studies have found that mutations in the proto-oncogene *c-kit* may be associated with a higher histologic grade.[4-6] Immunohistochemical staining patterns for *c-kit* were found to correlate with recurrence and survival of dogs with MCTs treated by surgery alone.[38]

Levels of proenzyme matrix metalloproteinase 9 (MMP-9) were higher in grade 3 than in grade 2 MCTs.[39] This is not surprising because MMPs are involved in tumor cell invasion into surrounding tissue. Correlation with prognosis has not yet been reported.

Mutations in the tumor-suppressor gene *p53* were found in nearly 50% of cutaneous MCTs in one study and were less common in grade 3 tumors.[40] In another study, cells with mutated *p53* were more common in grade 3 tumors.[41] Although one of these studies showed a correlation with survival time, the association was not greater than the association between grade and survival.[41] The other study showed no association between *p53* and survival.[40]

TREATMENT

Spontaneous regression of multiple cutaneous MCTs in a puppy has been reported,[42] but this is a rare occurrence. Control of canine MCTs involves the use of surgery, chemotherapy, or radiation therapy, either individually or in combination (Figure 65-5).

Surgery

Surgical excision is indicated if the tumor is solitary and evidence of lymph node involvement or systemic spread is lacking. The excision should be wide and deep to a minimum margin of 2 to 3 cm around the perceived borders of the tumor and one fascial plane below. With this aggressive surgical approach, recurrence of grade 1 and grade 2 MCTs is very low. A recent study examined the completeness of surgical excision at margins 1, 2, and 3 cm from the edges of grade 1 and 2 MCTs. All grade 1 tumors were excised 1 cm from the tumor borders, but only 75% of grade 2 tumors were completely excised at the same distance. All grade 2 tumors were excised 2 cm from the tumor borders, leading the authors to speculate that it may be possible to completely excise MCTs with these narrower than usually prescribed margins.[43]

As previously stated, surgical excision should be aggressive. All excised tissue should be examined histologically for completeness of tumor excision, as described above in the prognostic factors section. If the tumor is grade 1 or 2 and excision is complete, no further treatment is necessary. Extension of the tumor beyond the surgical borders or a report of "close" margins (as defined in Surgical Margins section, above) should prompt wider excision, if possible. A second excision should include the previous excision site *plus* lateral margins of 2 to 3 cm and additional deep tissue. If the tumor cannot be completely excised because of tumor location or other factors, or if it is a grade 3 MCT, further therapy is indicated. The animal should be evaluated for radiation therapy, if available. Chemotherapy may be considered if staging discloses metastases or if the MCT is grade 3.

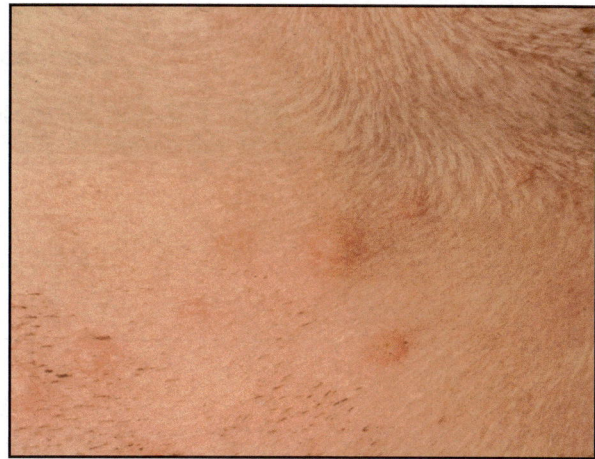

Figure 65-4. *Golden retriever with multiple cutaneous MCTs. Multiple tumors do not always indicate metastatic disease; de novo tumors often arise.*

Grade 1 Tumors

Dogs with grade 1 MCTs have a high likelihood of complete tumor control after complete surgical excision. A recent study showed that all grade 1 MCTs were completely excised with a 1-cm clinical margin. However, because tumor grading is performed histologically, not on cytology, all MCTs for which a grade is as yet uncertain should be excised for biopsy with wide (2- to 3-cm) margins.

Grade 2 Tumors

Three recent studies have challenged early assumptions[16,19] that dogs with grade 2 MCTs have a high likelihood of local recurrence even after apparently complete excision. These studies showed that with a more aggressive surgical technique and histology to examine margins (rather than the surgeon's clinical impression), dogs with grade 2 MCTs have a much lower rate of local recurrence and longer survival times than previously reported. Specifically, between 5% and 10% of dogs had a local recurrence of MCT a median of 7 months after surgery (range: 2–24 months).[24,26,28] More than 30% of these dogs had an MCT on the limb, for which some limbs were amputated. On the other hand, many of these dogs developed another MCT at a distant cutaneous site. These were considered to be de novo tumors (rather than cutaneous metastases, which have not been reported) and were diagnosed from 2 months to 4 years later, with a median time to diagnosis of about 1 year. Metastasis was rare, occurring in fewer than 3% of dogs.[24,28]

Grade 3 Tumors

One study found that grade 3 tumors were more likely to be incompletely excised and more likely to metastasize than grade 1 or 2 MCTs.[21] Radiation therapy is probably war-

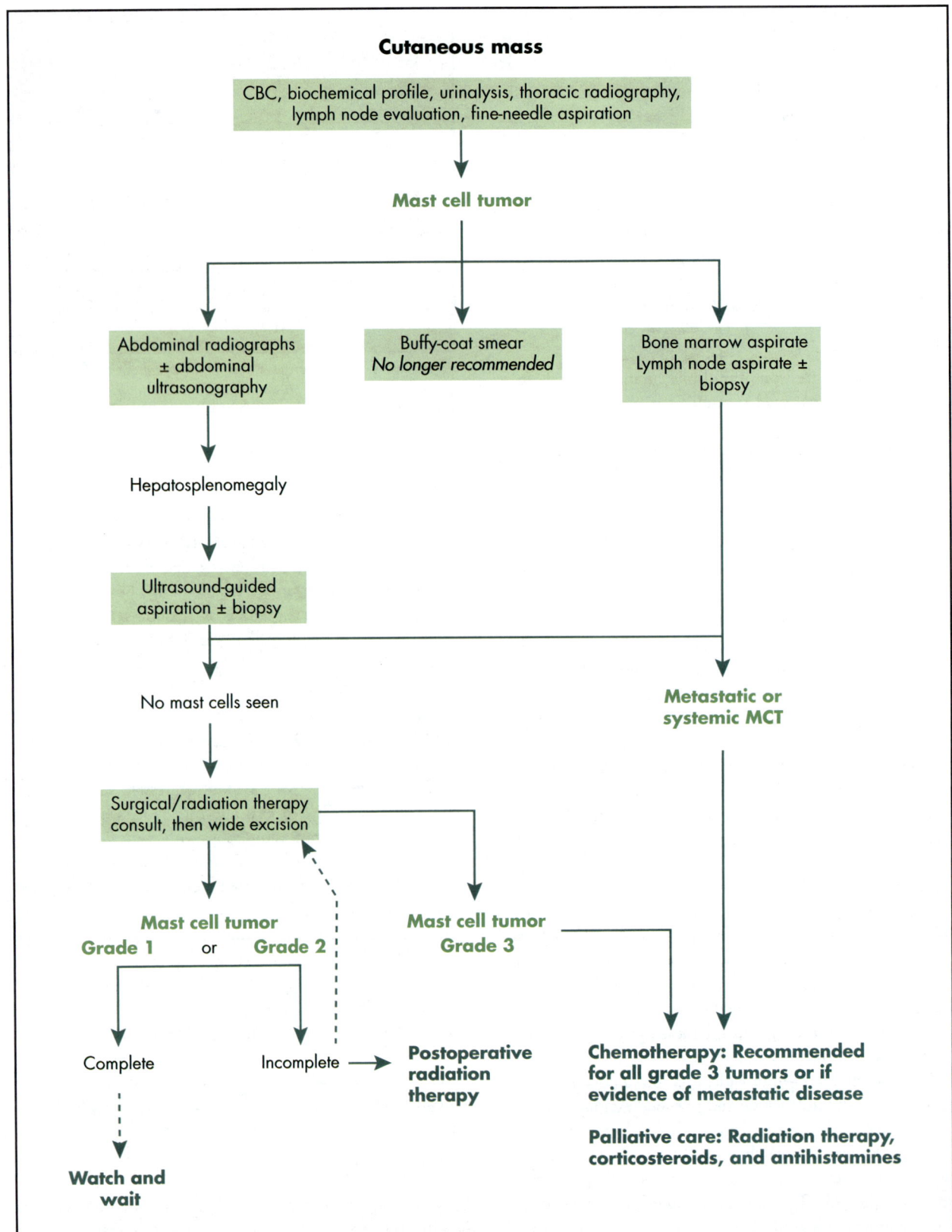

Figure 65-5. *A schematic flowchart for the treatment of MCTs in dogs.*

ranted (see below), and chemotherapy should be considered for grade 3 MCTs.

Radiation Therapy

MCTs are sensitive to the effects of radiation therapy, even at moderate doses. In one study, 44% of 23 dogs had satisfactory responses to radiation therapy, with tumor control of greater than 12 months and an average longevity of 24 months.[44]

Another study using external-beam radiation to treat 95 MCTs on 85 dogs found mean and median tumor-free times of 63 and 17 months, respectively; 79% of dogs were tumor-free at 1 year and 77% were tumor-free at 2 years.[27] In this study, survival was shorter in dogs that had higher tumor grades, and recurrence and survival were affected by tumor location. Dogs with neoplasms on the limbs had longer tumor-free times and survived longer than dogs with tumors on the trunk. Dogs with grade 2 tumors survived longer than dogs with grade 3 MCTs.

The long control and survival times in this study[27] are influenced by the inclusion of dogs that had no measurable evidence of disease after surgical removal of MCTs but had incomplete excision on histologic examination of excised tissues (stage 0). This group of dogs has significantly longer tumor control and survival than other dogs. A similar result was obtained in a more recent study, in which dogs with measurable MCT disease had local disease control for a median of 12 months compared with 54 months for dogs with microscopic disease.[45] Thus, postsurgical radiation therapy for incompletely excised tumors seems beneficial. MCTs of the extremities often present the greatest challenge for complete surgical excision. For well- or moderately differentiated tumors in these locations, combined modalities of less aggressive surgical "debulking" followed by radiation therapy may be a more acceptable treatment, both functionally and cosmetically.

Acute and self-limiting radiation reactions occur at a higher incidence and with greater severity in dogs with MCTs, possibly because of mast cell degranulation and release of proteolytic enzymes and vasoactive amines. Reactions can be of great significance in the distal extremities,

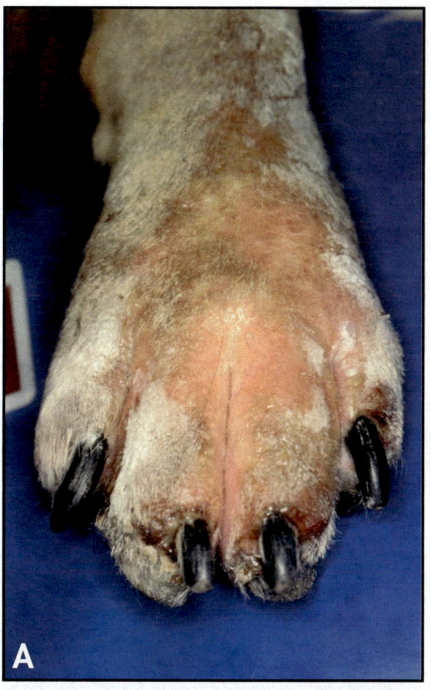 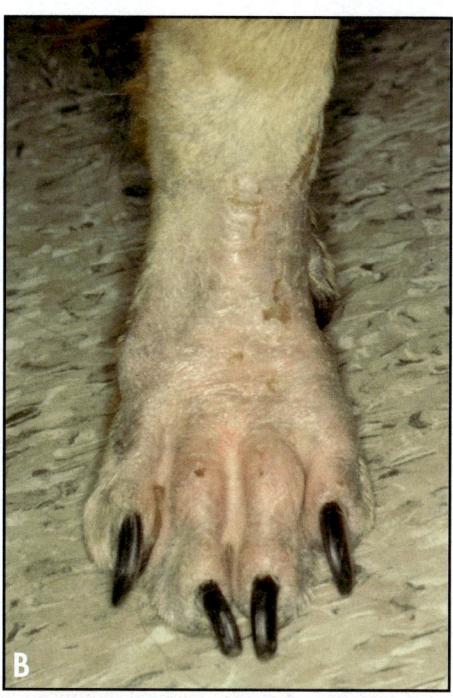

Figure 65-6. *(A)* An MCT on the foot of a male Bernese mountain dog immediately after radiation therapy showing moist desquamation typical of the treatment. *(B)* Same dog as in *A* 2 weeks later. Hair loss is obvious, but healing of the reaction is complete.

where the skin is thin, and great care to prevent self-injury should be taken with dogs undergoing this therapy.[27] The acute effects of radiation therapy usually subside within 2 weeks of completing therapy (Figure 65-6).

Grade 2 Tumors

In one study, 32 dogs with intermediate-grade (grade 2) MCTs that were incompletely excised received adjunctive cobalt-60 radiation therapy to a cumulative dose of 54 Gy.[46] Tumor-free survival rates were 96% at 1 year and 88% at 2 through 5 years. Similar results were achieved using orthovoltage or linear accelerator radiation to doses of 48 Gy.[47] Therefore, adjunctive radiation seems to be the treatment of choice for incompletely excised grade 2 MCTs. Nearly 70% of the MCTs in these two studies were on the limbs, and these tumors present the greatest challenge to achieving complete surgical margins. Tumor control was not as good in a small series of dogs treated with surgery and iridium-192 (^{192}Ir) interstitial brachytherapy in which nearly half (five of 11) of the dogs had a recurrence, although that recurrence was more than 3 years after treatment in three dogs.[48] The benefit of brachytherapy is that fewer anesthetics are required, making brachytherapy possibly useful in dogs if the risk for complications during anesthesia precludes the multiple anesthetics required for fractionated teletherapy.

Some investigators have recommended prophylactic irradiation of the regional lymph node in dogs with grade 2 MCTs that have mast cells observed on cytologic examination of a lymph node needle aspirate.[49] A positive cytology result should prompt surgical biopsy for confirmation because mast cells may infiltrate a regional lymph node as an inflammatory response to an MCT. Eleven dogs with cutaneous MCTs were treated with surgery and ^{192}Ir interstitial brachytherapy. Minimum tumor doses ranged from 47.2 to 63.3 Gy. Treated tumors were classified as grade 2 (n = 7) or 3 (n = 4). Five dogs had recurrences with a median progression-free interval of 1,391 days, and six dogs had no recurrence at a median follow-up time of 942 days. Acute adverse effects were well tolerated, and late effects were mild. One dog developed a second tumor of a different cell type in the radiation treatment field.[48]

Grade 3 Tumors

Radiation therapy (52.2 Gy in 2.9-Gy fractions given three times a week) was used to treat 31 dogs with grade 3 MCTs that had only residual microscopic disease after surgery. In all cases, the regional lymph node was also irradiated. Local control of the MCTs was excellent, with a median remission time of 28 months. More than half (16 of 31) of the dogs eventually developed lymph node metastases, underscoring the need for systemic therapy in dogs with this disease.[50]

Palliative Radiation Therapy

Radiation therapy may alleviate signs of extensive or systemic disease. When the tumor is poorly differentiated or metastasis is already confirmed, the use of high-dose intermittent radiation treatments may improve the quality of life by stopping bleeding or reducing the size of a bulky or irritating tumor. In these cases, a fully fractionated course would be costly and reduce the amount of time spent by owners with the dog. A coarsely fractionated series of three 8-Gy treatments on a schedule of days 0, 7, and 21 provides relief from signs, although it does not increase life span. Systemic therapy can also be considered.

A recent study investigated the efficacy of coarsely fractionated radiation therapy (4 weekly 8-Gy fractions) in treating 35 dogs with nonresectable MCTs of all grades on the head or limb; 17 dogs had cytologic evidence of lymph node metastasis.[51] All dogs received concurrent 40 mg/m² prednisolone daily for 10 to 14 days before radiation therapy and half that dose for 2 months afterward. A complete response was seen in 12 dogs and a partial response in 19. With long-term follow-up, 11 dogs experienced local recurrence. The median tumor control was 34 months, with 1- and 2-year control rates of 60% and 52%, respectively. Tumor grade did not predict the prognosis for this group of dogs, but dogs with tumors located on the head were more likely to have recurrences or metastases. Severe late effects were not seen in this group of dogs

Other Local Therapies

Injection of deionized water into the site of incomplete surgical resection was initially reported to reduce local recurrence of MCTs compared with marginal surgery alone. For moderately differentiated MCTs examined in one study, seven of 27 tumors recurred locally after injection.[52] In a larger study, 30% of grade 2 and 60% of grade 3 tumors recurred after four injections.[53] The duration of remission was not provided. Injections were painful if large volumes were used, and some dogs required heavy sedation or anesthesia. In contrast, a study that evaluated the time to recurrence found that dogs treated with surgery and deionized water were more likely to have tumor recurrence and had a more rapid recurrence than dogs treated with surgery alone.[54] The injection of deionized water is discouraged because it may delay or preclude more appropriate therapy.

Anecdotally, intralesional injections of triamcinolone at a dose rate of 1 mg/cm diameter of tumor every 2 weeks gives good palliative local tumor control.

Systemic Therapy

Metastatic disease was found to occur more frequently in dogs with grade 3 MCT and in dogs with incomplete surgical excision of cutaneous tumors.[21] When MCTs have metastasized or spread systemically, localized therapies, such as surgery or radiation, are appropriate only as palliation for discomfort or mechanical obstruction. For these dogs, systemic therapy is required.

Corticosteroids are primarily palliative, but some long-term responses do occur. Oral prednisone (2 mg/kg/day for 2 weeks, then 1 mg/kg/day for 2 weeks, then 1 mg/kg every other day) is given as long as the tumor does not progress. Anecdotally, dogs that are tumor-free after 6 months have a lower incidence of recurrence[16]; therefore, therapy is usually discontinued at this time.

The exact mechanism by which **glucocorticoids** exert their cytotoxic effects on MCTs is unknown, although the process may parallel their effects on lymphocytes. Glucocorticoid receptor sites were found in the cytoplasm of canine mast cells; these sites may be involved with the susceptibility of MCTs to glucocorticoids.[55] The type of glucocorticoid administered is immaterial, but intralesional application of corticosteroids may be more effective than systemic therapy. Fewer cushingoid side effects have been seen with short-acting glucocorticoids such as prednisone. Remission times are usually 10 to 20 weeks. The only controlled study using prednisone to treat dogs with measurable MCT found that five of 21 dogs (24%) showed an objective response (one complete and four partial).[56] Of the five dogs that responded, two had solitary tumors, two had multiple tumors, and one had regional lymph node metastasis.

Although receptors for progesterone and estrogen have been described in the tumor cells of dogs with canine MCTs, the role of **sex steroids** in the treatment of canine MCTs has yet to be investigated.

Interestingly, the **multidrug resistance proteins** p-glycoprotein and multidrug resistance–associated protein were found in up to 25% of canine cutaneous MCTs. These proteins are important in the resistance of tumor cells to corticosteroids and to chemotherapeutics such as doxorubicin and vincristine. Both proteins were absent in grade 3 tumors, which is encouraging because these are the tumors that most often require chemotherapy.[57]

Chemotherapy in dogs with grade 3 MCTs has been investigated in retrospective studies, small case series, and anecdotal reports. Some articles have combined reported results of adjunctive chemotherapy for dogs with grades 2 and 3 MCTs, so it is difficult to interpret the data clearly for dogs with grade 3 disease only. However, several agents with some objective efficacy against MCT in dogs have been identified, including vinblastine and CCNU (lomustine). The overall response rate for protocols containing these drugs seems to be between 40% and 50%, although some of the responses are short lived.

Vinblastine (2 mg/m^2 IV weekly) and prednisone were used to treat MCTs in one study. The overall response rate in 15 dogs with measurable disease was 47% (seven of 15); there were five complete responses and two partial responses. The median response duration was 5 months (range: 1 to >22 months). Dogs with lower-grade tumors seemed to respond better.[58] A protocol that used the same two drugs was given to 15 dogs with inadequately excised MCTs. Only one dog (7%) had a local recurrence, although this dog and two others developed new cutaneous MCTs. Although toxicity was considered mild, one dog died from sepsis during treatment.[25] Another 25 dogs that received vinblastine and prednisone after incomplete grade 2 MCT excision had a median survival time of 24 months.[59] Vinblastine is myelosuppressive, and a weekly CBC should be conducted before administering the drug at this intertreatment interval. It is difficult to evaluate the efficacy of adjuvant chemotherapy because some dogs with incompletely excised MCTs may not have a recurrence.

In a different study, vinblastine 2 to 3 mg/m^2 IV every 3 weeks and cyclophosphamide 250 to 300 mg/m^2 PO over 4 days (days 8 to 11) every 3 weeks were combined with prednisone 1 mg/kg PO daily. All treated patients had lymph node metastases. The overall response rate in 14 evaluable dogs with measurable disease was 73% (11 of 15). All were partial responses, and the median survival time for these 11 dogs was 6 months (4 to 10 months).[60]

> **KEY POINT**
>
> ***Vinblastine* (not vincristine) *and lomustine (CCNU) are the most active chemotherapy agents for systemic treatment of canine MCTs.***

CCNU (lomustine) is an alkylating agent used to treat hematopoietic tumors in humans. It was given to 19 dogs at 90 mg/m^2 PO every 4 weeks. One dog had a complete response for 15 months, and seven dogs had a partial response for an average of 3 months (1 to 9 months).[61] This drug can be safely combined with prednisone. If using CCNU, CBC (especially platelet count) and liver enzymes should be assessed before each administration and CCNU discontinued if thrombocytopenia or increased liver enzymes are seen.

Vincristine was found to be an inactive agent for the treatment of MCT.[62] In that study, only two dogs (7%) had partial remissions, and nine dogs (32%) had their treatments discontinued because of severe GI toxicity. Vincristine is not recommended as a first-line chemotherapy agent for the treatment of dogs with MCT.

L-Asparaginase has been recommended as an active agent in treating dogs with MCTs. In one study, three of six dogs with cutaneous MCTs showed an objective response (whether complete or partial was not specified) for the short interval of 1 to 2 months.[63] One of two other dogs treated with L-asparaginase showed an objective response to therapy for 6 months.[64]

Doxorubicin and prednisolone were given to nine dogs with measurable disease. There was no response in any of seven dogs with MCT that had recurred after combination chemotherapy, and there was a single partial response in a dog that had not been treated.[14] Doxorubicin is not recommended for treatment of this disease.

Anecdotally, other chemotherapeutic agents, such as chlorambucil, have been used to treat MCTs. Kenneth M. Rassnick, DVM, reports that hydroxyurea failed to cause a response in 21 dogs with MCTs.

Other combination therapy has been reported. A protocol using vincristine, cyclophosphamide, prednisolone, and hydroxyurea was used to treat 15 dogs with cutaneous MCT. The overall response rate was 60% (nine dogs), with three complete responses (all alive between 29 and 30 months after treatment) and six 6 partial responses (median: 3 months).

Two preliminary reports have discussed a protocol that alternates vinblastine (2 mg/m^2 IV) and CCNU (60–70 mg/m^2 PO) every 2 weeks for eight total treatments. The overall response rate in 29 dogs with measurable disease was 72% (21 of 29), with 14 complete responses and seven partial responses.[65,66] In one report, the remission duration was short, but in the larger report, the median remission duration was 10 months.[66]

The chemotherapy recommendation (in addition to surgery) for dogs with grade 3 MCT, positive staging for metastasis, or systemic spread is a protocol of vinblastine and prednisolone. A more aggressive protocol alternating between vinblastine and CCNU has also been recommended, but only preliminary data exist to evaluate its efficacy.

Immunotherapy

Recurrence was seen in 70% of MCTs after injection of the nonspecific immunomodulator *Corynebacterium parvum* into the site of incomplete surgical excision.[67] This rate is consistent with that reported for dogs treated by surgery alone. Also, a dog with multiple cutaneous MCT had long-term control and regression of cutaneous masses during intralesional treatment with the nonspecific immunomodulator *Propionibacterium acnes* (immunoregulin).[68] Therefore, there is insufficient information to recommend immunotherapy for MCTs at this time.

Novel Therapies

Mutations in the protooncogene *c-kit* were shown to lead to constitutive phosphorylation of the gene product, and these mutations are believed to be important in the development and progression of canine MCT.[69] There is no evidence that such mutations are breed associated. Abnormalities in *c-kit* are more common in grade 2 and 3 tumors than in grade 1 MCTs, implying a role in the biologic behavior of MCT in dogs.[5,6,70] Mutations in one study were seen in more than one-third of dogs with grade 2 or 3 MCTs.[6]

The therapeutic implication of such a finding is that kinase inhibitors may be useful. Imatinib mesylate has been reported to cause clinical remissions in human patients with similar *c-kit* mutations.[6] Imatinib mesylate has anecdotally caused serious morbidity and mortality when used in dogs, limiting its clinical usefulness for veterinary medicine. However, clinical trials using drugs with a similar mode of action are under way in canine patients, with preliminary encouraging results with one such drug (SU11654).[71]

Palliation of Paraneoplastic Signs

Ancillary drug therapy is important with canine MCTs. Animals with mastocytosis or bulky mast cell disease should receive H_2 antagonists because rapid degranulation of neoplastic mast cells may occur after surgery or chemotherapy. Elevated systemic histamine levels may also be seen with recurrent disease.[72] The objective of the therapy is to prevent GI ulceration associated with elevated levels of histamine and to treat ulcers already present. This is most likely to occur in dogs with larger, bulky disease, recurrence of cutaneous disease, or systemic spread of MCTs.[12] Cimetidine reduces gastric acid production by competitive inhibition of the action of histamine on H_2 receptors of the gastric parietal cells. Ranitidine and famotidine, H_2 antagonists that require less frequent administration, may be used for a similar effect. Omeprazole, which inhibits gastric acid production by the gastric parietal cells through proton pump inhibition, may also be used. Dogs with evidence of GI ulceration and bleeding may benefit from sucralfate therapy at a dose of 0.5 to 1.0 g PO tid. Sucralfate reacts with stomach acid to form a highly con-

> **KEY POINT**
>
> *Famotidine reduces gastric acid production and ulceration that results from degranulation of bulky or disseminated mast cell tumors.*

densed, viscous, adherent, pastelike substance that binds to the surface of gastric and duodenal ulcers. The barrier formed protects the ulcer from potential ulcerogenic properties of pepsin, acid, and bile and allows it to heal. Such H_1 antagonists as diphenhydramine should be considered for use along with cimetidine before and after surgical removal of canine MCTs to help prevent the negative effects of local histamine release on fibroplasia and wound healing. A second-generation H_1 antagonist, loratadine, has been shown to be very effective at inhibiting histamine release by blocking degranulation from normal canine mast cells and, therefore, may be a good choice for palliation of dogs with MCTs.[73]

Intestinal Mast Cell Tumors

INCIDENCE, SIGNALMENT, AND ETIOLOGY

MCTs are rarely found at noncutaneous sites. MCTs of the GI tract have been described in two reports from Japan.[74,75] Tumors usually occur in older dogs (mean age: 10 years) with no gender predilection. Miniature breeds, particularly Maltese terriers, are at high risk for developing GI MCTs.

CLINICAL PRESENTATION AND HISTORY

Tumors mostly affected the duodenum (33%), small intestine (28%), and stomach (20%) with fewer MCTs found in the large intestine (10%). Multiple tumors were seen in fewer than 10% of affected dogs.[74] Mucosal ulceration was common, and the most common presenting signs were vomiting, diarrhea, and melena in almost all cases. GI perforation was seen in some dogs.[75]

STAGING AND DIAGNOSIS

Tumor cells invaded from the mucosa to the serosa, sometimes replacing all layers of the intestinal wall. Mucosal ulceration was common. Histologically, multinucleated giant cells were seen in more than 30% of the tumors, indicating poor differentiation. Cells were granular after staining with toluidine blue (a specific stain for mast cell granules), but the number of granules was small.

Anemia was common in one study, as was hypoproteinemia,[75] and circulating mast cells were noted on some hemograms.

On histopathology, there was lymphatic or blood vessel invasion seen in 30% and 13% of affected dogs, respectively. Lymph node metastasis at the time of diagnosis was seen in 11 of 14 dogs in which the lymph nodes were examined, and systemic metastasis to the lungs, heart, kidney, liver, adrenal gland, and other sites in the intestine was seen in some dogs.[74] Staging should include thoracic radiography, abdominal ultrasonography, and biopsy of suspicious lesions. Regional lymph nodes should be identified and biopsied in dogs in which intestinal MCT is suspected.

TREATMENT

One study reported no obvious effect of glucocorticoid or chemotherapy treatment in any dog, but details were not provided.[75] In the other report, it was unclear how many dogs were treated with curative intent with surgery, but the median survival time was less than 1 month from diagnosis, and only two dogs lived longer than 6 months. This is obviously an aggressive disease with a high propensity to metastasize. Chemotherapy (as described in the Systemic Therapy section, above) is recommended adjunctively until further data become available.

REFERENCES

1. Macy DW: Canine and feline mast cell tumors: Biologic behavior, diagnosis, and therapy. *Semin Vet Med Surg (Small Anim)* 1:72–83, 1986.
2. Goldschmidt MH, Shofer FS: Mast cell tumors, in Goldschmidt MH, Shofer FS (eds): *Skin Tumors of the Dog and Cat*, ed 1. Tarrytown, NY, Pergamon Press, 1992, 1992, pp 231–251.
3. Miller DM: The occurrence of mast cell tumors in young shar-peis. *J Vet Diagn Invest* 7:360–363, 1995.
4. London CA, Kisseberth WC, Galli SJ, G, et al: Expression of stem cell factor receptor (*c-kit*) by the malignant mast cells from spontaneous canine mast cell tumours. *J Comp Pathol* 115:399–414, 1996.
5. Zemke D, Yamini B, Yuzbasiyan-Gurkan V: Mutations in the juxtamembrane domain of *c-KIT* are associated with higher grade mast cell tumors in dogs. *Vet Pathol* 39:529–535, 2002.
6. Downing S, Chien MB, Kass PH, et al: Prevalence and importance of internal tandem duplications in exons 11 and 12 of *c-kit* in mast cell tumors of dogs. *Am J Vet Res* 63:1718–1723, 2002.
7. Zemke D, Yamini B, Yuzbasiyan-Gurkan V: Characterization of an undifferentiated malignancy as a mast cell tumor using mutation analysis in the proto-oncogene *c-KIT*. *J Vet Diagn Invest* 13:341–345, 2001.
8. Sato AF, Solano M: Ultrasonographic findings in abdominal mast cell disease: A retrospective study of 19 patients. *Vet Radiol Ultrasound* 45:51–57, 2004.
9. Bookbinder PF, Butt MT, Harvey HJ: Determination of the number of mast cells in lymph node, bone marrow, and buffy coat cytologic specimens from dogs. *JAVMA* 200:1648–1650, 1992.
10. O'Keefe DA, Couto CG, Burke-Schwartz C, Jacobs RM: Systemic mastocytosis in 16 dogs. *J Vet Intern Med* 1:75–80, 1987.
11. Endicott MM, Charney SC, McKnight JA, Bergman PJ: Incidence of bone marrow infiltration and hematologic abnormalities in canine cutaneous mast cell tumors: 157 cases (1999–2002). *Proc 23rd Annu Conf Vet Cancer Soc*:22, 2003.
12. Howard EB, Sawa TR, Nielsen SW, Kenyon AJ: Mastocytoma and gastroduodenal ulceration. Gastric and duodenal ulcers in dogs with mastocytoma. *Pathol Vet* 6:146–158, 1969.
13. McManus PM: Frequency and severity of mastocytemia in dogs with and without mast cell tumors: 120 cases (1995–1997). *JAVMA* 215:355–357, 1999.
14. Gerritsen RJ, Teske E, Kraus JS, Rutteman GR: Multi-agent chemotherapy for mast cell tumours in the dog. *Vet Quart* 20:28–31, 1998.
15. Sfiligoi G, Rassnick KM, Scarlett JM, et al: Outcome of dogs with mast cell tumors in the inguinal or perineal region versus other cutaneous locations: 124 cases (1990–2001). *JAVMA* 226:1368–1374, 2005.
16. Bostock DE: The prognosis following surgical removal of mastocytomas in dogs. *J Small Anim Pract* 14:27–41, 1973.
17. Strefezzi RF, Xavier JG, Catao-Dias JL: Morphometry of canine cutaneous mast cell tumors. *Vet Pathol* 40:268–275, 2003.
18. Hottendorf, GH, Nielsen SW: Pathologic study of 300 extirpated canine mastocytomas. *Zbl Vet Med* A14:272–281, 1967.
19. Patnaik AK, Ehler WJ, MacEwen EG: Canine mast cell tumor: Morphologic grading and survival time in 83 dogs. *Vet Pathol* 21:469–474, 1984.
20. Gieger TL, Theon AP, Werner JA, et al: Biologic behavior and prognostic factors for mast cell tumors of the canine muzzle: 24 cases (1990–2001). *J Vet Intern Med* 17:687–692, 2003.
21. Baker-Gabb M, Hunt GB, France MP: Soft tissue sarcomas and mast cell tumours in dogs; clinical behaviour and response to surgery. *Aust Vet J* 81:732–738, 2003.
22. Murphy S, Sparkes AH, Smith KC, et al: Relationships between the histological grade of cutaneous mast cell tumours in dogs, their survival and the efficacy of surgical resection. *Vet Rec* 154:743–746, 2004.
23. Northrup NC, Howerth EW, Harmon BG, et al: Variation among pathologists in histopathologic grading of canine cutaneous mast cell tumors. *Proc 23rd Annu Conf Vet Cancer Soc*:73, 2003.
24. Séguin B, Leibman NF, Bregazzi VS, et al: Clinical outcome of dogs with grade-II mast cell tumors treated with surgery alone: 55 cases (1996–1999). *JAVMA* 218:1120–1123, 2001.
25. Davies DR, Wyatt KM, Jardine JE, et al: Vinblastine and prednisolone as adjunctive therapy for canine cutaneous mast cell tumors. *JAAHA* 40:124–130, 2004.
26. Michels GM, Knapp DW, DeNicola DB, et al: Prognosis following surgical excision of canine cutaneous mast cell tumors with histopathologically tumor-free versus nontumor-free margins: A retrospective study of 31 cases. *JAAHA* 38:458–466, 2002.
27. Turrel JM, Kitchell BE, Miller LM, Theon A: Prognostic factors for radiation treatment of mast cell tumor in 85 dogs. *JAVMA* 193:936–940, 1988.
28. Weisse C, Shofer FS, Sorenmo K: Recurrence rates and sites for grade II canine cutaneous mast cell tumors following complete surgical excision. *JAAHA* 38:71–73, 2002.
29. Cahalane AK, Payne S, Barber LG, et al: Prognostic factors for survival of dogs with inguinal and perineal mast cell tumors treated with surgery with or without adjunctive treatment. 68 cases. *JAVMA* 225:401–408, 2004.
30. Murphy S, Sparkes AH, Blunden AS, et al: Canine cutaneous mast cell tumours: Do dogs with multiple tumours have a poorer prognosis? *Vet Rec* 2006, in press.
31. Mullins M, Dernell W, Ehrhart E, et al: Multiple cutaneous canine mast cell tumors: A retrospective analysis. *Proc 24th Annu Conf Vet Cancer Soc*:13, 2004.
32. Bostock DE, Crocker J, Harris K, Smith P: Nucleolar organiser regions as indicators of post-surgical prognosis in canine spontaneous mast cell tumours. *Br J Cancer* 59:915–918, 1989.
33. Kravis LD, Vail DM, Kisseberth WC, et al: Frequency of argyrophilic nucleolar organizer regions in fine-needle aspirates and biopsy specimens from mast cell tumors in dogs. *JAVMA* 209:1418–1420, 1996.
34. Simoes JPC, Schoning P, Butine M: Prognosis of canine mast cell tumors: A comparison of three methods. *Vet Pathol* 31:637–647, 1994.
35. Abadie JJ, Amardeilh MA, Delverdier ME: Immunohistochemical detection of proliferating cell nuclear antigen and Ki-67 in mast cell tumors from dogs. *JAVMA* 15:1629–1634, 1999.
36. Sakai H, Noda A, Shirai N, et al: Proliferative activity of canine mast cell tumours evaluated by bromodeoxyuridine incorporation and Ki-67 expression. *J Comp Pathol* 127:233–238, 2002.
37. Ayl RD, Couto CG, Hammer AS, et al: Correlation of DNA ploidy to tumor histologic grade, clinical variables, and survival in dogs with mast cell tumors. *Vet Pathol* 29:386–390, 1992.
38. Kiupel M, Webster JD, Kaneene JB, et al: The use of KIT and tryptase expression patterns as prognostic tools for canine cutaneous mast cell tumors. *Vet Pathol* 41:371–377, 2004.
39. Leibman NF, Lana SE, Hansen RA, et al: Identification of matrix metalloproteinases in canine cutaneous mast cell tumors. *J Vet Intern Med* 14:583–586, 2000.

40. Ginn PE, Fox LE, Brower JC, et al: Immunohistochemical detection of p53 tumor-suppressor protein is a poor indicator of prognosis for canine cutaneous mast cell tumors. *Vet Pathol* 37:33–39, 2000.
41. Jaffe MH, Hosgood G: Immunohistochemical and clinical evaluation of p53 in canine cutaneous mast cell tumors. *Vet Pathol* 37:40–46, 2000.
42. Davis BJ, Page R, Sannes PL, Meuten DJ: Cutaneous mastocytosis in a dog. *Vet Pathol* 29:363–365, 1992.
43. Simpson AM, Ludwig LL, Newman SJ, et al: Evaluation of surgical margins required for complete excision of cutaneous mast cell tumors in dogs. *JAVMA* 224:236–240, 2004.
44. Slusher R, Roengik WJ, Wilson GP: Effect of x-irradiation on mastocytoma in dogs. *JAVMA* 151:1049–1054, 1967.
45. LaDue T, Price S, Dodge R, et al: Radiation therapy for incompletely resected canine mast cell tumors. *Vet Radiol Ultrasound* 39:57–62, 1998.
46. Al Sarraf R, Mauldin GN, Patnaik AK, Meleo KA: A prospective study of radiation therapy for the treatment of grade 2 mast cell tumors in 32 dogs. *J Vet Intern Med* 10:376–378, 1996.
47. Frimberger AE, Moore AS, LaRue SM, et al: Radiotherapy of incompletely resected, moderately differentiated mast cell tumors in the dog: 37 cases (1989–1993). *JAAHA* 33:320–324, 1997.
48. Northrup NC, Roberts RE, Harrell TW, et al: Iridium-192 interstitial brachytherapy as adjunctive treatment for canine cutaneous mast cell tumors. *JAAHA* 40:309–315, 2004.
49. Chaffin K, Thrall DE: Results of radiation therapy in 19 dogs with cutaneous mast cell tumor and regional lymph node metastasis. *Vet Radiol Ultrasound* 43:392–395, 2002.
50. Hahn KA, King GK, Carreras JK: Efficacy of radiation therapy for incompletely resected grade-III mast cell tumors in dogs: 31 cases (1987–1998). *JAVMA* 224:79–82, 2004.
51. Dobson J, Cohen S, Gould S: Treatment of canine mast cell tumours with prednisolone and radiotherapy. *Vet Compar Oncol* 2:132–141, 2004.
52. Grier RL, DiGuardo G, Schaffer CB, et al: Mast cell tumor destruction by deionized water. *Am J Vet Res* 51:1116–1120, 1990.
53. Grier RL, DiGuardo G, Myers R, Merkley DF: Mast cell tumour destruction in dogs by hypotonic solution. *J Small Anim Pract* 36:385–388, 1995.
54. Jaffe MH, Hosgood G, Kerwin SC, et al: Deionised water as an adjunct to surgery for the treatment of canine cutaneous mast cell tumours. *J Small Anim Pract* 41:7–11, 2000.
55. Takahashi T, Kadosawa T, Nagase M, et al: Inhibitory effects of glucocorticoids on proliferation of canine mast cell tumor. *J Vet Med Sci* 59:995–1001, 1997.
56. McCaw DL, Miller MA, Ogilvie GK, et al: Response of canine mast cell tumors to treatment with oral prednisone. *J Vet Intern Med* 8:406–408, 1994.
57. Miyoshi N, Tojo E, Oishi A, et al: Immunohistochemical detection of P-glycoprotein (PGP) and multidrug resistance-associated protein (MRP) in canine cutaneous mast cell tumors. *J Vet Med Sci* 64:531–533, 2002.
58. Thamm DH, Mauldin EA, Vail DM: Prednisone and vinblastine chemotherapy for canine mast cell tumor: 41 cases (1992–1997). *J Vet Intern Med* 13:491–497, 1999.
59. Santoro SK, Chun R, Garret, LD: Vinblastine and prednisone for the treatment of grade 2 mast cell tumors in dogs. *Proc 24th Annu Conf Vet Cancer Soc*:10, 2004.
60. Elmslie RE: Combination chemotherapy with and without surgery for dogs with high grade mast cell tumors with regional lymph node metastases. *Vet Cancer Soc Newsletter* 20:6–7, 1997.
61. Rassnick KM, Moore AS, Williams LE, et al: Treatment of canine mast cell tumors with CCNU (lomustine). *J Vet Intern Med* 13:601–605, 1999.
62. McCaw DL, Miller MA, Bergman PJ, et al: Vincristine therapy for mast cell tumors in dogs. *J Vet Intern Med* 11:375–378, 1997.
63. Hardy WD Jr, Old LJ: L-Asparaginase in the treatment of neoplastic diseases of the dog, cat and cow. *Cancer Res* 33:131–139, 1970.
64. Legrand J-J, Carlier B, Parodi A-L: Apport de la cytologie au diagnostic, au pronostic et au suivi thérapeuticque du mastocytome chez le chien. *Bull Acad Vet* 60:269–278, 1987.
65. Hershey AE, Jones PD, Klein MK: Evaluation of combination vinblastine, lomustine and prednisone for the treatment of canine mast cell tumors. *Proc 23rd Annu Conf Vet Cancer Soc*:71, 2003.
66. Bennett P, Langova V: Response of mast cell tumours to combination therapy with lomustine and vinblastine. *Proc 24th Annu Conf Vet Cancer Soc*:76, 2004.
67. Owen LN, Lewis JC, Morgan DR, Gorman NT: The effects of *Corynebacterium parvum* in dogs and a study of its distribution following intravenous injection. *Eur J Cancer* 16:999–1005, 1980.
68. Tinsley PE Jr, Taylor DO: Immunotherapy for multicentric malignant mastocytoma in a dog. *Mod Vet Pract*:225–228, 1987.
69. London CA, Galli SJ, Yuuki T, et al: Spontaneous canine mast cell tumors express tandem duplications in the proto-oncogene *c-kit*. *Exp Hematol* 27:689–697, 1999.
70. Reguera MJ, Ferrer L, Rabanal RM: Evaluation of an intron deletion in the c-kit gene of canine mast cell tumors. *Am J Vet Res* 63:1257–1261, 2002.
71. Pryer NK, Lee LB, Zadovaskaya R, et al: Proof of target for SU11654: kit inhibition in canine mast cell tumors. *Proc 23rd Annu Conf Vet Cancer Soc*:72, 2004.
72. Ishiguro T, Kadosawa T, Takagi S, et al: Relationship of disease progression and plasma histamine concentration in 11 dogs with mast cell tumors. *J Vet Intern Med* 17:194–198, 2003.
73. Garcìa G, DeMora F, Ferrer L, Puigdemont A: Effect of H1 antihistamines on histamine release from dispersed canine cutaneous mast cells. *Am J Vet Res* 58:293–297, 1997.
74. Ozaki K, Yamagami T, Nomura K, Narama I: Mast cell tumors of the gastrointestinal tract in 39 dogs. *Vet Pathol* 39:557–564, 2002.
75. Takahashi T, Kakosawa T, Nagase M, et al: Visceral mast cell tumors in dogs: 10 cases (1982–1997). *JAVMA* 216:222–226, 2000.

SECTION 6

ABRIDGED FORMULARY AND GUIDE TO ABBREVIATIONS

Abridged Formulary 659

Abbreviations 669

ABRIDGED FORMULARY FOR THE CANINE CANCER PATIENT*

ACEPROMAZINE

Use:	Preanesthetic, sedative
How supplied:	Injectable: 10 mg/ml in 50 ml vials
	Oral: 10 and 25 mg tablets
Dose:	0.062–0.25 mg/kg (0.03–0.11 mg/lb) parenteral
	Maximum IV dose: 3 mg/dog
	1.1–2.2 mg/kg (0.5–1.0 mg/lb) oral

ACTINOMYCIN D

Use:	Antineoplastic agent
How supplied:	Injectable: 0.5 mg vials
Dose:	0.5–0.9 mg/m^2 IV slow infusion (over 20 min) q1–3wk

AMOXICILLIN

Use:	Broad-spectrum antibiotic
How supplied:	Injectable: 250 mg/ml in 25 g vials
	Oral: 50, 100, 200, and 400 mg tablets
	50 mg/ml suspension in 15 ml bottles
Dose:	11–22 mg/kg (5–10 mg/lb) bid to tid PO

AMOXICILLIN–CLAVULANIC ACID

Use:	Broad-spectrum antibiotic (effective against many penicillinase-producing pathogens)
How supplied:	Oral: Fixed combination with four parts amoxicillin and one part clavulanic acid as the potassium salt
	62.5, 125, 250, and 375 mg tablets of drug combination
	62.5 mg/ml suspension in 15 ml bottles
Dose:	13.75 mg/kg (6.25 mg/lb) of combination bid

AMPICILLIN SODIUM

Use:	Broad-spectrum antibiotic
How supplied:	Injectable: 1 g vials
Dose:	22 mg/kg (10 mg/lb) IM or IV tid

L-ASPARAGINASE

Use:	Antineoplastic agent
How supplied:	Injectable: 10,000 U/vials
Dose:	10,000–20,000 U/m^2 or 400 U/kg weekly IM
Note:	Watch for anaphylaxis!

AZATHIOPRINE

Use:	Immunosuppressive, antimetabolite
How supplied:	Oral: 50 mg tablets
Dose:	2.2 mg/kg/day for 4 days, then 1 mg/kg PO every other day

BLEOMYCIN

Use:	Antineoplastic agent
How supplied:	Injectable: 15 U vials (1 U = 1 mg)
Dose:	0.3–0.5 U/kg IM or SC weekly to total cumulative dose of 125–200 U/m^2; IV push over at least 10 min

BUPIVACAINE

Use:	Long-duration local anesthetic
How supplied:	Injectable: 0.75% in 30 ml single-dose vials
Dose:	7 mg/kg (maximum) per site

BUPRENORPHINE

Use:	Opioid partial agonist
How supplied:	Injectable: 0.3 mg/ml in 1 ml ampules
Dose:	0.007–0.02 mg/kg IM or SC

*Note: This section contains information on the most important and most commonly discussed drugs in this book. Highly experimental agents and those with limited availability are not included here.

BUTORPHANOL

Use:	Central-acting analgesic; narcotic agonist/antagonist
How supplied:	Injectable: 10 mg/ml in 50 ml vials
	Oral: 5 mg tablets
Dose:	0.1 mg/kg (0.045 mg/lb) IV
	0.1–0.4 mg/kg (0.045–0.18 mg/lb) SC or IM q6–12h
	0.55 mg/kg (0.25 mg/lb) PO q6–12h
Note:	Do not give butorphanol within 12 hours of any preoperatively or intraoperatively administered narcotic.
	Controlled substance

CALCIUM GLUCONATE (BOROGLUCONATE)

Use:	Hypocalcemia
How supplied:	Injectable: 10% solution in 10 ml ampules
	23% solution in 500 ml vials
	26% solution with magnesium, phosphorus, and dextrose in 500 ml vials
Dose:	10–30 ml 10%

CARBOPLATIN

Use:	Antineoplastic agent
How supplied:	Injectable: 50, 150, and 450 mg vials
Dose:	250–300 mg/m^2, depending on size of patient

CARPROFEN

Use:	Analgesic, antiinflammatory
How supplied:	Oral: 25, 75, and 100 mg tablets
Dose:	2.2 mg/kg (1 mg/lb) bid

CCNU

See Lomustine

CEFADROXIL

Use:	First-generation cephalosporin antibiotic
How supplied:	Oral: 50, 100 mg tablets
Dose:	11–22 mg/kg (5–10 mg/lb) PO bid

CEFAZOLIN

Use:	First-generation cephalosporin antibiotic
How supplied:	Injectable: 1 g vials
Dose:	22 mg/kg (10 mg/lb) IV, IM, or SC q8h
	For surgical prophylaxis, give within 30 min of surgery and repeat every 2.5 h.

CEFOXITIN

Use:	Second-generation cephalosporin antibiotic
How supplied:	Injectable: 1 g vials
Dose:	22 mg/kg (10 mg/lb) tid

CEPHALEXIN

Use:	First-generation cephalosporin antibiotic
How supplied:	Oral: 25 mg/ml suspension in 100 ml bottles
	250 and 500 mg capsules
Dose:	11–22 mg/kg (5–10 mg/lb) tid

CHLORAMBUCIL

Use:	Antineoplastic agent
How supplied:	Oral: 2 mg coated tablets
Dose:	0.2 mg/kg or 6 mg/m^2 daily or every other day

CHLORPHENIRAMINE

Use:	Antihistamine
How supplied:	Oral: 4 mg tablets
Dose:	4–8 mg bid to tid

CHLORPROMAZINE

Use:	Tranquilizer, antiemetic
How supplied:	Injectable: 25 mg/ml in 2 ml ampules
Dose:	0.11 mg/kg (0.05 mg/lb) (antiemetic)
	1–2 mg/kg (0.5–0.9 mg/lb) (tranquilization) IM or IV q8h

CIMETIDINE

Use:	H$_2$-receptor antagonist
How supplied:	Injectable: 150 mg/ml in 8 ml vials
	Oral: 300 mg tablets
Dose:	4 mg/kg (1.8 mg/lb) PO or IV q6h or 5.5 mg/kg (2.5 mg/lb) IV tid

CISAPRIDE

Use:	Cholinergic enhancer, GI-emptying adjunct
How supplied:	Oral: 10 mg tablets
Dose:	0.1–0.5 mg/kg PO up to tid given 30 min before meals

CISPLATIN

Use:	Antineoplastic agent
How supplied:	Injectable: 1 mg/ml in 50 ml vials
Dose:	Follow oncology protocol (50–70 mg/m^2 IV with diuresis)

CLINDAMYCIN

Use:	Antibiotic
How supplied:	Oral: 25, 75, and 150 mg capsules
	25 mg/ml solution in 20 ml bottles
Dose:	5.5–11.0 mg/kg (2.5–5.0 mg/lb) bid

CODEINE/ACETAMINOPHEN

Use:	Analgesic
How supplied:	Oral: tablets containing codeine 60 mg/acetaminophen 300 mg
Dose:	0.5–2 mg/kg (of codeine) q6–8h
Note:	Controlled substance—schedule III

CYCLOPHOSPHAMIDE

Use:	Antineoplastic
How supplied:	Oral: 25 and 50 mg tablets
	Injectable: 200 mg and 500 mg vials (reconstituted with 20 ml of D5W to make 10 mg/ml)
Dose:	50 mg/m^2 once daily 3–4 days per week or every 3 weeks, or 250 mg/m^2 PO or 200 mg/m^2 IV once every 3 weeks; give with furosemide to reduce the risk of cystitis

CYPROHEPTADINE

Use:	Appetite stimulant
How supplied:	Oral: 4 mg (scored) tablets
Dose:	0.5 mg/kg PO tid

CYTARABINE

Use:	Antineoplastic agent
How supplied:	Injectable: 100 mg vials (reconstituted to 20 mg/ml)
Dose:	Low dose: 10 mg/m^2 SC or IM sid or q12h
	High dose: 60 mg/m^2 SC, IM, or IV sid for 4 days q3wk
	For granulomatous meningoencephalomyelitis: 200 mg/m^2 as a constant rate infusion over 48 hours or 50 mg/m^2 bid SC for 2 consecutive days
	Repeat dosage schedule every 3 weeks.

DACARBAZINE

Use:	Antineoplastic agent
How supplied:	Injectable: 100 and 200 mg vials
Dose:	800 mg/m^2 every 3–4 weeks or 20 mg/m^2 daily for 5 consecutive days every 3 weeks
Note:	Give dolasetron as a prophylactic antiemetic.

DACTINOMYCIN

See Actinomycin D

DESMOPRESSIN (DDAVP)

Use:	ADH derivative, increases factor VIII activity
How supplied:	Injectable: 0.01% solution
Dose:	1 µg/kg (0.45 µg/lb) SC 20–30 min before collecting blood or performing surgery

DEXTRAZOXANE

Use:	Cardioprotectant
How supplied:	Injectable: 500 mg vials with diluent
Dose:	30 mg for every 1 mg of doxorubicin

DIAZEPAM

Use:	Tranquilizer, anticonvulsant
How supplied:	Injectable: 5 mg/ml in 2 ml or 10 ml vials
Dose:	1 mg/kg (0.5 mg/lb) IM
	0.2 mg/kg/hr constant-rate infusion (starting dose)
	1 mg/kg IV to effect (increase in 5 mg increments)
	1–2 mg/kg per rectum to effect up to maximum dose of 40 mg

DIPHENHYDRAMINE

Use:	Antihistamine
How supplied:	Injectable: 50 mg/ml in 1 ml vials
	Topical: 2% conditioner in 8 oz bottles
Dose:	2–4 mg/kg, IV or IM q6–8h

DOLASETRON MESYLATE

Use:	Antiemetic
How supplied:	Injectable: 12.5 mg ampules
Dose:	0.6–1 mg/kg PO or IV slowly

DOXORUBICIN

Use:	Antineoplastic agent
How supplied:	Injectable: 2 mg/ml in 100 ml vials
Dose:	30 mg/m^2 IV (1 mg/kg for dogs <10 kg) repeated every 21 days to an accumulated dosage of 180 mg/m^2
Note:	Give **slowly**.

DOXYCYCLINE

Use:	Long-acting broad-spectrum tetracycline
How supplied:	Oral: 10 mg/ml suspension in 16 oz bottles; 100 mg tablets
Dose:	5 mg/kg (2.3 mg/lb) PO daily to bid

ENROFLOXACIN

Use:	Broad-spectrum antibacterial (fluoroquinolone)
How supplied:	Injectable: 22.7 mg/ml in 20 ml bottles
	Oral: 22.7 and 68 mg tablets
Dose:	5 mg/kg (1.13 mg/lb) PO or IM daily
	Dose may be increased up to 20 mg/kg daily.
	Daily dose may be divided and given bid.

EPOETIN ALFA

Use:	Stimulation of RBC production
How supplied:	Injectable: 4000 U/ml in 1 ml vials
Dose:	100 U/kg SC three times weekly initially
	May be decreased to twice weekly or increased in 50 U/kg increments depending on response.

ETOMIDATE

Use:	Anesthetic, hypnotic
How supplied:	Injectable: 2 mg/ml in 20 ml vials
Dose:	1 mg/kg IV

FAMOTIDINE

Use:	H_2-receptor antagonist
How supplied:	Injectable: 10 mg/ml in 20 ml vials
	Oral: 10 mg tablets
Dose:	0.5–1 mg/kg PO, SC, or IV daily or bid

FATTY ACIDS

Use:	Fatty acid supplement
How supplied:	Oral: Capsules in small, medium, and large dog sizes
	Liquid: 60 ml bottles
Dose:	100–200 mg/kg

FENTANYL

Use:	Narcotic analgesic
How supplied:	Injectable: 0.05 mg/ml in 5 ml ampules and in 20 ml and 50 ml vials
	Transdermal: 2.5 mg, 5.0 mg, 7.5 mg, and 10 mg patches
Dose:	4 µg/kg (1.9 µg/lb) IV
	2–4 µg/kg/h constant-rate infusion
	4–10 µg/kg (1.8–4.5 µg/lb) SC or IM
	Total dose not to exceed 500 µg (0.5 mg) per dog
	2.5 mg transdermal patch for 10–25 lb dog, 5 mg transdermal patch for dogs that weigh 26–50 lb, and 10 mg transdermal patch for dogs that weigh more than 75 lb
Note:	Controlled substance—schedule II

5-FLUOROURACIL

Use:	Antineoplastic agent
How supplied:	Injectable: 500 mg in 5 g ampules or vials
	Topical: 1% or 2% ointment or solution
Dose:	5–10 mg/kg weekly IV

GEMCITABINE

Use:	Antineoplastic agent
How supplied:	Injectable: 200 mg and 1 g vials
Dose:	250–300 mg/m^2 IV weekly for 4 weeks with a 1 week rest before reinitiating therapy
	Toxicity and probably efficacy depend on the rate at which the drug is infused. Preliminary studies suggest that the drug should be infused over a 30- to 90-min period.

GENTAMICIN

Use:	Aminoglycoside antibiotic
How supplied:	Injectable: 100 mg/ml in 100 ml vials
Dose:	6.6 mg/kg IM, IV, or SC as a single daily dose or may be **divided** bid or tid
Note:	If given IV, administer slowly.

GLYCOPYRROLATE

Use:	Anticholinergic agent
How supplied:	Injectable: 0.2 mg/ml in 20 ml vials
Dose:	11 µg/kg (5 µg/lb) IM, IV, or SC

HALOTHANE

Use:	Inhalant anesthetic
How supplied:	Liquid: 250 ml bottles
Dose:	3% (induction); 0.5%–1.5% (maintenance)

HEPARIN SODIUM

Use:	Anticoagulant in vivo and in vitro
How supplied:	Injectable: 1,000 U/ml in 10 ml vials
Dose:	2 U/ml intraocular irrigation
	1–2 U/ml for heparinized saline
	300 U/kg IV bolus, 600 U/kg/day constant-rate infusion

HETASTARCH

Use:	Plasma volume expansion
How supplied:	Injectable: 6% in normal saline in 500 ml vials

HYDROCODONE–HOMATROPINE

Use:	Antitussive
How supplied:	Oral: Hydrocodone 5 mg/homatropine 1.5 mg tablets
Dose:	0.22 mg/kg (of hydrocodone) bid to tid
Note:	Controlled substance—schedule III
	Calculate dose considering 5 mg/tablet.

HYDROXYUREA

Use:	Antineoplastic agent
How supplied:	Oral: 500 mg capsules
Dose:	80 mg/kg PO q3d (reformulate)

IFOSFAMIDE

Use:	Antineoplastic agent
How supplied:	Injectable: 1 g vials
Dose:	350 (dogs <10 kg) to 375 mg/m^2 every 3 weeks
Note:	Must give with IV saline diuresis and mesna (included in package)

ISOTRETINOIN

Use:	Antineoplastic agent for mycosis fungoides
How supplied:	10, 20, and 40 mg capsules
Dose:	1–3 mg/kg/day

KETAMINE

Use:	Neuroleptoanalgesia
How supplied:	Injectable: 100 mg/ml in 10 ml vials
Dose:	10–21 mg/kg (4.5–9.5 mg/lb) IM
	2.2–4.4 mg/kg (1–2 mg/lb) IV

KETOPROFEN

Use:	Antiinflammatory agent
How supplied:	Injectable: 100 mg/ml in 100 ml vials
Dose:	1 mg/kg single dose postsurgical

LIDOCAINE

Use:	Local and topical anesthetic, antiarrhythmic
How supplied:	Injectable: 2% solution in 100 ml vials
	Oral topical: 2% (viscous) in 100 ml bottles

Dose:	2–5 mg/kg IV bolus administered over 2–3 min
	50–120 µg/kg/min constant-rate infusion
Note:	Use caution. Start CRI at 60 µg/kg/min and increase by 10 µg increments q2h if no or minimal response is noted.

LOMUSTINE (CCNU)

Use:	Antineoplastic agent
How supplied:	Oral: 10, 40, and 100 mg capsules
Dose:	Initial: 60–90 mg/m² PO q4–6wk

MECHLORETHAMINE HCL

Use:	Antineoplastic agent
How supplied:	Injectable: 10 mg powder
Dose:	3 mg/m² IV as part of MOPP protocol

MEDETOMIDINE

Use:	Small animal sedative, analgesic
How supplied:	Injectable: 1 mg/ml in 10 ml vials
Dose:	0.75 mg/m² IV or 1 mg/m² IM

MEGESTROL

Use:	Appetite stimulant
How supplied:	Oral: 5 mg tablets
Dose:	0.5 mg/kg daily for 3 days, then every 2–3 days thereafter to enhance appetite

MELPHALAN

Use:	Antineoplastic agent
How supplied:	Oral: 2 mg tablets
Dose:	0.1 mg/kg daily for 10 days, then reduce to every other day

MESNA

Use:	Uroprotectant for cyclophosphamide and ifosfamide to prevent hemorrhagic cystitis
How supplied:	Injectable: 100 mg/ml solution
Dose:	60% of the daily ifosfamide mg dosage IV

METHOTREXATE

Use:	Antineoplastic agent
How supplied:	Oral: 2.5 mg tablets
	Injectable: 5 mg, 20 mg, 50 mg, 100 mg, 200 mg, 250 mg, and 1 g vials
Dose:	2.5 mg/m² PO, IV, IM, or SC sid

METOCLOPRAMIDE

Use:	Antiemetic, GI disorders
How supplied:	Injectable: 5 mg/ml in 20 ml vials
	Oral: 10 mg tablets
	1 mg/ml solution
Dose:	1–2 mg/kg/day constant rate infusion IV
	0.2–0.4 mg/kg (0.1–0.2 mg/lb) tid, 1/2 hr before meals PO

METRONIDAZOLE

Use:	Amoebiasis, giardiasis, trichomoniasis, balantidiasis, anaerobic infections
How supplied:	Oral: 250 mg tablets
	25 mg/ml suspension (compounded)
Dose:	32 mg/kg (15 mg/lb) bid for 8 days for giardiasis
	10–15 mg/kg q8h × 5 days for *Clostridium perfringens* infection
	Caution! Avoid overdosing, especially in larger dogs. Deaths have been reported at the 32 mg/kg dose in larger dogs.

MISOPROSTOL

Use:	Prevention of NSAID-induced gastric ulcers
How supplied:	100 µg (scored) tablets
Dose:	2–4 µg/kg PO tid to qid

MITOXANTRONE

Use:	Antineoplastic agent
How supplied:	Injectable: 2 mg/ml concentrate to be diluted for IV administration
Dose:	5.5 mg/m² IV every 3 weeks

MORPHINE

Use:	Analgesic
How supplied:	Injectable: 1 mg/ml in 10 ml single-dose ampules (for epidural use only)
	15 mg/ml in 1 ml and 20 ml vials
Dose:	Epidural: 0.1 mg/kg (dogs use preservative-free formulation)
	0.5–2 mg/kg (0.25–1 mg/lb) IM or SC
	0.05–0.1 mg/kg (0.025–0.045 mg/lb) for pulmonary edema
	1.1–2.2 mg/kg SC as an emetic in dogs

NALBUPHINE

Use:	Narcotic agonist-antagonist
How supplied:	20 mg/ml in 10 ml multiple-dose vials
Dose:	Premedication: 0.5–1 mg/kg SC or IM

NALOXONE

Use:	Narcotic antagonist
How supplied:	Injectable: 400 µg/ml in 1 ml and 10 ml vials
Dose:	15 µg/kg (6.8 µg/lb)
	Usually 400 µg IM, IV, or SC

OMEPRAZOLE

Use:	Antisecretory compound
How supplied:	20 mg sustained-release capsules
Dose:	0.7 mg/kg once daily (approximately one capsule per dog)

ONDANSETRON

Use:	Prevention of nausea and vomiting associated with chemotherapy, surgery, and other therapies
How supplied:	Injectable: 4 mg/ml in 2 ml vials
	Oral: 4 mg tablets
Dose:	0.1 mg/kg PO or IV 15 min before and 4 hr after chemotherapy
Note:	Give slowly IV (over 2–5 min) or dilute

OXACILLIN SODIUM

Use:	Treatment of penicillinase-producing *Staphylococcus* spp.
How supplied:	Oral: 250 mg capsules
Dose:	12–24 mg/kg (5.5–11 mg/lb) PO tid

OXYMORPHONE

Use:	Narcotic analgesic
How supplied:	Injectable: 1.5 mg/ml in 1 ml ampules or 10 ml vials
Dose:	0.11–0.22 mg/kg (0.05–0.1 mg/lb), IM, IV, or SC (maximum dose: 4.5 mg/dog)

PACLITAXEL

Use:	Antineoplastic agent
How supplied:	50 mg/5 ml in 5 ml vials
Dose:	130 mg/m^2 IV q3wk slow infusion *after* dexamethasone, diphenhydramine, and cimetidine therapy
Note:	Dilute with 0.9% NaCl to a concentration of 0.6–0.7 mg/ml

PAMIDRONATE

Use:	Treatment of hypercalcemia
How supplied:	30 and 90 mg vials
Dose:	1–2 mg/kg IV over 2 hours 3 hours after and 1 hour before a saline diuresis at 18.3 ml/kg/h

PENTOBARBITAL, SODIUM

Use:	Sedative, anticonvulsant, IV anesthetic, euthanasia
How supplied:	Injectable: 50 mg/ml in 50 ml vials
	400 mg/ml in 250 ml vials (euthanasia solution)
Dose	Approximately 25–30 mg/kg IV for anesthesia 3–15 mg/kg given slowly IV until effect for anticonvulsant
	88 mg/kg (40 mg/lb) IV for euthanasia

PHENOBARBITAL

Use:	Sedative, anticonvulsant
How supplied:	Injectable: 130 mg/ml (sodium salt) in 1 ml vials
	Oral: 15, 30, 60, 100 mg tablets
Dose:	2 mg/kg bid PO to start; base increases in dose on serum levels
Note:	Controlled substance—schedule IV
	One-time loading dose: 6–20 mg/kg IV
	Diazepam (IV or rectally) may be given concurrently because IV phenobarbital requires 20–30 min to exert an anticonvulsant effect.

PIROXICAM

Use:	Analgesic, antiinflammatory
How supplied:	10 mg capsules (2.5 mg and 5 mg capsules commonly compounded)
Dose:	0.3 mg/kg daily for 3–5 days, then q24h thereafter
Note:	Use cautiously! GI ulceration is common. May compound nephrotoxicity of chemotherapeutics.

POTASSIUM BROMIDE

Use:	Anticonvulsant
How supplied:	Oral: 250 mg/ml
Dose:	10–30 mg/kg (4.5–13.6 mg/lb) PO bid
Note:	Steady state is reached more rapidly if an oral loading dose (400–600 mg/kg) of sodium bromide is given in divided multiple doses over a 48-hour period.

PREDNISOLONE

Use:	Corticosteroid therapy
How supplied:	Injectable: 50 mg/ml acetate suspension in 30 ml vials
	Oral: 5 mg tablets
Dose:	0.5–2.2 mg/kg (0.23–1 mg/lb) IM or PO

PREDNISOLONE SODIUM PHOSPHATE

Use:	Corticosteroid therapy
How supplied:	Injectable: 20 mg/ml (14.8 mg of prednisolone base per ml) in 50 ml vials
Dose:	0.5–2.2 mg/kg (0.23–1 mg/lb) IV

PREDNISONE

Use:	Corticosteroid therapy
How supplied:	Oral: 5 and 20 mg tablets
	1 mg/ml solution
Dose:	0.5–2.2 mg/kg (0.23–1 mg/lb) PO

PROCARBAZINE

Use:	Antineoplastic agent
How supplied:	May need to be compounded
Dose:	50 mg/m^2 daily for 14 days as part of MOPP protocol

PROPOFOL

Use:	Anesthesia
How supplied:	Injectable: 10 mg/ml in 20 ml ampules
Dose:	4–6 mg/kg IV, titrated to effect

PROPRANOLOL

Use:	β-Blocker
How supplied:	Injectable: 1 mg/ml in 1 ml ampules
Dose:	0.04–0.06 mg/kg (0.02–0.03 mg/lb) IV, slowly

RANITIDINE

Use:	H_2-receptor antagonist
How supplied:	Injectable: 25 mg/ml in 6 ml vials
	Oral: 15 mg/ml syrup
	150 and 300 mg tablets
Dose:	2 mg/kg PO, IV, or SC bid to tid

STREPTOZOCIN (STREPTOZOTICIN)

Use:	Antineoplastic agent for insulinoma
How supplied:	Injectable: 1 mg/ml in 1 ml ampules
Dose:	500 mg/kg IV every 2–3 weeks. IV 0.9% saline at 18.3 ml/kg/hr for 7 hours. The dose of streptozocin is included in the infusion during hours 3 and 4. Butorphanol 0.4 mg/kg IM is given at the end of the streptozocin portion of the infusion as an antiemetic, although ondansetron or dolasetron may be more effective.

SUCRALFATE

Use:	Duodenal ulcer treatment
How supplied:	Oral: 100 mg/ml solution, 1 g tablets
Dose:	0.5–1 g tid 1 hour before feeding (12.5 mg/lb) PO or IV daily

SULFASALAZINE

Use:	Sulfonamide
How supplied:	Oral: 500 mg tablets
Dose:	12.5 mg/kg (5.7 mg/lb) qid for 2 weeks With improvement, may reduce dose to 6.25 mg/kg (2.85 mg/lb) qid for 2 weeks.

THIOPENTAL SODIUM

Use:	Ultra–short-acting barbiturate
How supplied:	Injectable: 5 g vial for preparation of 2.5% and 10% solution
Dose:	To effect (about 18 mg/kg)

TRIMETHOPRIM–SULFAMETHOXAZOLE

Use:	Antibacterial
How supplied:	Combination product containing one part trimethoprim to five parts sulfamethoxazole
	Oral: 120 mg coated tablets
	480 and 960 mg tablets
	48 mg/ml suspension
Dose:	15 mg/kg (7 mg/lb) PO bid for routine infections. May double dose for unique or difficult infections.
Note:	The dose listed above is for the combination of the two ingredients. This dose (i.e., 15 mg/kg) is based on the combined weight of the two ingredients.

TYLOSIN

Use:	Macrolide antibiotic
How supplied:	Oral powder: 25 g (base)/318.6 g bottles
Dose:	11 mg/kg (5 mg/lb) PO tid (approximately 0.25 tsp powder per 20 lb body weight)

URSODIOL

Use:	Dissolution of radiolucent gallstones; cholesterol-lowering agent
How supplied:	Oral: 300 mg capsules (60 mg commonly compounded)
Dose:	15 mg/kg/day

VINBLASTINE

Use:	Antineoplastic agent
How supplied:	Injectable: 1 mg/ml in 10 ml vials
Dose:	2 mg/m^2 weekly

VINCRISTINE

Use:	Antineoplastic agent
How supplied:	Injectable: 1 mg/ml in 2 ml vials
Dose:	0.5–0.75 mg/m^2 weekly

VINORELBINE

Use:	Antineoplastic agent
How supplied:	Injectable: 10 mg/ml vials
Dose:	15–18 mg/m^2 weekly to every 2 weeks

XYLAZINE

Use:	Sedative, analgesic, emetic in cats
How supplied:	Injectable: 20 mg/ml in 20 ml vials
	100 mg/ml in 50 ml vials
Dose:	1 mg/kg (0.45 mg/lb) IM or IV

YOHIMBINE

Use:	α_2 antagonist
How supplied:	Injectable: 5 mg/ml in 20 ml vials
Dose:	0.1–0.5 mg/kg IV

GUIDE TO ABBREVIATIONS

2,4 D	2,4 dichlorophenoxyacetic acid	cm	centimeter(s)
5-FU	5-fluorouracil	CML	chronic myeloid leukemia
5-HT-3	5-hydroxytryptamine	CNS	central nervous system
6-MP	6-mercaptopurine	Co	cobalt
AChRAb	acetylcholine-receptor antibody	CO_2	carbon dioxide
ACT	activated clotting (coagulation) time	COAP	cyclophosphamide (Cytoxan), vincristine (Oncovin), ara-C (cytosine arabinoside), prednisone
ACTH	adrenocorticotropic hormone (corticotropin)		
ADH	antidiuretic hormone	COP	cyclophosphamide (Cytoxan), vincristine (Oncovin), prednisone
AgNOR	argyrophilic nucleolar organizer region		
AIGR	amended insulin:glucose ratio	COPA	cyclophosphamide (Cytoxan), vincristine (Oncovin), prednisone, doxorubicin, (Adriamycin)
ALL	acute lymphoblastic leukemia		
ALP	alkaline phosphatase		
ALT	alanine aminotransferase	CPR	cardiopulmonary resuscitation
AML	acute myeloid leukemia	CR	complete response (remission)
AMM	anterior mediastinal mass	Cs	cesium
ANLL	acute nonlymphoid leukemia	CSF	cerebrospinal fluid
APTT	activated partial thromboplastin time	CT	computed (computerized) tomography
ara-C	cytosine arabinoside	CTZ	chemoreceptor trigger zone
AST	aspartate aminotransferase	DIC	disseminated intravascular coagulation
AT	adrenal tumor	dl	deciliter(s)
AT-III	antithrombin III	DM	diabetes mellitus
ATLS	acute tumor lysis syndrome	DNA	deoxyribonucleic acid
ATP	adenosine triphosphate	DPG	diphosphoglycerate
AV	atrioventricular	DTIC	dacarbazine
BAG	bone marrow suppression, alopecia, gastrointestinal toxicity	ECG	electrocardiogram
		EDTA	ethylenediamine tetraacetic acid
BCG	bacillus Calmette-Guerin	e.g.	for example
BCNU	carmustine	FDA	U.S. Food and Drug Administration
BER	basal energy requirement	FDP	fibrin degradation product
bid	twice a day	Fr	French
bpm	beats per minute	g	gram(s)
BRM	biologic response modifier	ga	gauge
BSA	body surface area	G-CSF	granulocyte colony-stimulating factor
BUN	blood urea nitrogen	GH	growth hormone
°C	degrees Celsius	GI	gastrointestinal
CBC	complete blood count	GM-CSF	granulocyte-macrophage colony-stimulating factor
CCNU	lomustine		
CLL	chronic lymphocytic leukemia	Gy	gray (radiation dose)
		H	hydrogen

ABRIDGED FORMULARY

HDDS	high-dose dexamethasone suppression	MDB	minimum database: includes CBC, biochemical profile, urinalysis, and thoracic radiography (three views)
HDL-CH	high-density lipoprotein cholesterol		
Hg	mercury		
HIV-1	human immunodeficiency virus-1	MDR	multiple drug resistance
hr	hour	MDS	myelodysplasia
I	iodine	M:E	myeloid:erythroid ratio
i.e.	that is	mEq	milliequivalent
IER	illness energy requirement	MeV	million electron volts
IgA	immunoglobulin A	MF	mycosis fungoides
IgE	immunoglobulin E	mg	milligram(s)
IgG	immunoglobulin G	min	minute(s)
IgM	immunoglobulin M	ml	milliliter(s)
IL-1	interleukin-1	MLO	multilobular osteochondrosarcoma
IL-2	interleukin-2	mm	millimeter(s)
IL-3	interleukin-3	MMP	matrix metalloproteinase
IM	intramuscular	MOPP	mechlorethamine, vincristine (Oncovin), procarbazine, prednisone
INF	interferon		
IP	intraperitoneal	MRC	Medical Research Council
IU	international unit(s)	MRI	magnetic resonance imaging
IV	intravenous	n	number
K	potassium	N	lymph node metastasis (TNM classification)
kcal	kilocalorie		
KCl	potassium chloride	Na	sodium
kg	kilogram(s)	NaCl	sodium chloride
L	liter(s)	NaPO$_4$	sodium phosphate
lb	pound(s)	Nd:YAG	neodymium:yttrium–aluminum–garnet
LDDS	low-dose dexamethasone suppression		
L-MTP-PE	liposome-encapsulated muramyl tripeptide-phosphatidylethanolamine	Ng	nanogram(s)
		nM	nanomole(s)
		No.	number
LRS	lactated Ringer's solution	NSAID	nonsteroidal antiinflammatory drug
µg	microgram(s)	OAF	osteoclast-activating factor
µl	microliter(s)	o,p'-DDD	mitotane
µm	micrometer(s)	OSHA	Occupational Safety and Health Administration
µU	micro unit(s)		
M	distant metastasis (TNM classification)	OSPT	one-step prothrombin time
m^2	square meters	OSPTT	one-step partial thromboplastin time
m^3	cubic meters	P	phosphorus
MBq	megabecquerel	PAS	periodic acid–Schiff reaction
mCi	millicurie	PCNA	proliferating cell nuclear antigen
MCT	mast cell tumor	PCV	packed cell volume
MCV	mean corpuscular volume	PD	progressive disease
		PDH	pituitary-dependent hyperadrenocorticism
		PEG	polyethylene glycol
		PET	positron emission tomography

pH	negative logarithm of hydrogen ion activity	sid	once a day
PO	oral	SPECT	single-photon emission computed tomography
PR	partial response (remission)	Sr	strontium
PRN	according to circumstances; as needed	SUN	serum urea nitrogen
PT	prothrombin time	T	tumor size (TNM classification)
PTH-rP	parathyroid hormone-related peptide	T3	triiodothyronine
PTU	propylthiouracil	T4	thyroxine
PUVA	psoralen ultraviolet-A	TCC	transitional cell carcinoma
PVC	polyvinyl chloride	tid	three times a day
q	every	TNF	tumor necrosis factor
qid	four times a day	TNM	tumor size, lymph node metastasis, distant metastasis (tumor staging)
RBC	red blood cell	TRH	thyrotropin-releasing hormone
rcG-CSF	recombinant canine granulocyte colony-stimulating factor	TSH	thyroid-stimulating hormone (thyrotropin)
rhG-CSF	recombinant human granulocyte colony-stimulating factor	TVT	transmissible venereal tumor
RNA	ribonucleic acid	U	unit(s)
SC	subcutaneous	WBC	white blood cell
SCC	squamous cell carcinoma	WHO	World Health Organization
SD	stable disease	wt	weight
SIADH	syndrome of inappropriate secretion of antidiuretic hormone		

SECTION 7

CLIENT INFORMATION SERIES

Introduction 675

What Is Cancer? 676

Caring for Your Dog with Cancer: The First Steps 678

Nutritional Support of Your Dog with Cancer 680

How Will I Know If My Dog Is in Pain? 682

Caring for Your Dog with Radiation Therapy 684

Caring for Your Dog with Surgery 686

Caring for Your Dog with Chemotherapy 688

Caring for Your Dog with Carboplatin Chemotherapy 692

Caring for Your Dog with Doxorubicin Chemotherapy 694

Caring for Your Dog with Cryosurgery 696

Medication Information Sheet 697

When It's Time to Say Good-Bye: Euthanasia and Your Dog . . . 698

Demystifying Cancer Care: A Glossary for Caregivers 701

Introduction

This section contains information geared toward the owners of dogs with cancer. The handouts are designed to be photocopied and distributed to caregivers to help educate families and individuals who have a dog with cancer about what to expect during the treatment of their pet. Because client caregivers are important members of the veterinary health care team, it is critical that they understand what is being done for their dog and have the necessary knowledge to make informed decisions regarding the care and treatment of their beloved pet. They also need to know what to expect and need to be prepared to deal with reactions to, and complications of, diagnostic and therapeutic procedures. The more clients know and understand about cancer and its treatment, the better able they are to focus on what is best for their dog.

Permission is hereby granted to photocopy these forms and distribute them to your clients for instructional purposes only. The forms are also available on the Internet at www.CompassionateCancerCare.com/handouts.

What Is Cancer?

Cancer is an unrestrained growth of cells that occurs despite the body's anticancer defense mechanisms or immune system. Cancer begins with a single cell that fails to respond to orderly growth. This cell divides, and the cancer grows undetected for months to years. Cancer is caused by many things, including genetic abnormalities that may result from exposure to tobacco smoke, certain nutrients, radiation, drugs, toxins, viruses, inflammation, pollution, chemicals, or any other substance that can damage the foundation of life, DNA.

Most cancers in veterinary medicine can be prevented by limiting exposure to tobacco smoke, pollutants, chemicals, and, possibly, viruses. Early spaying and neutering, preventing obesity throughout life, and providing food that is likely to prevent cancer are additional ways to prevent the disease. The single most important thing that can be done to enhance the cure rate of cancer is early detection and diagnosis. Therefore, presenting your pet to your veterinary health care team is absolutely essential so that cancer can be detected early, before it is likely to spread throughout the body.

The word *cancer* is as dark and empty as the disease it defines. A cancer diagnosis often brings feelings of overwhelming fear, loss of control, and, most devastating of all, loss of hope. This can happen regardless of whether the patient is a friend, family member, or precious pet. When we face the diagnosis of cancer in a beloved pet, it is even more difficult because we must make important and life-changing decisions for our animal friend, who relies totally on our judgment for its well-being. Pets share not only our homes, our lives, and our experiences but also our hearts. We have experienced their love as unconditional, and we seek through our own decision-making process to provide them with the highest quality and dignity of life that we know they deserve. Seeking the most appropriate care for these wonderful friends is the very least we can do as a response to their love and affection. Our goal becomes to share as many moments as possible within this wonderful relationship.

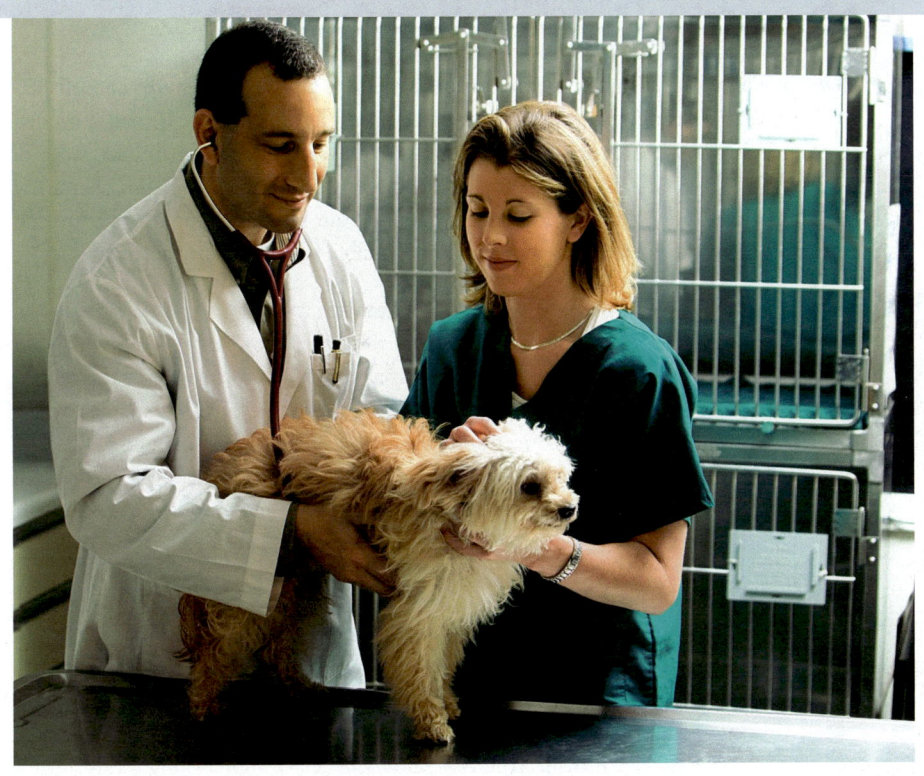

Knowledge is power, and we gain power over cancer by understanding what it is, where it is, and how fast it is growing.

Knowledge is power, and we gain power over cancer by understanding what it is, where it is, and how fast it is growing. If your pet has a growth or tumor, your veterinary health care team will first work to determine whether the tumor is benign or malignant. Benign growths do not often aggressively spread throughout the body, but leaving them untreated can result in the death of the pet. Therefore, complete surgical excision of a benign tumor is necessary.

If the tumor or growth is malignant, your veterinary health care team will first determine its particular type and usual behavior. There are many different types of malignant tumors, all of which behave differently. Understanding the grade, type, and stage of the cancer is very important to begin to develop strategies to defeat it. The *grade* of the cancer is determined after the tumor is surgically removed to determine how fast it grows and how often it spreads throughout the body. The *stage* of the tumor or cancer is determined by common diagnostic tests to determine how big the tumor is and where it is in the body. The *histopathologic* or *cytologic* diagnosis is the determination of the name and type of the cancer. There are *round cell tumors, carcinomas,* and *sarcomas,* and within each category, there are different types of tumors. For example, mammary adenocarcinoma, salivary gland adenocarcinoma, and thyroid carcinoma are a few of the dozens of different types of carcinomas. Determining the stage, grade, and histopathologic or cytologic diagnosis empowers your veterinary health care team with knowledge of the prognosis and the best way to defeat the cancer locally and, if needed, throughout the body.

The word *cancer* is feared throughout the world, yet cancer is the most curable of all chronic diseases, and it is controllable in many patients that are not cured. Having accurate information about this disease empowers you, the caregiver, and the veterinary health care team with important knowledge about the options for care.

Caring for Your Dog with Cancer: The First Steps

Cancer. The word is frightening in part because there are so many myths and misperceptions about cancer. However, almost all dogs with cancer can be helped. Empowering yourself with appropriate information allows you to begin finding ways of joining with your veterinary health care team to help your best friend. Your dog shares not only your home, your life, and your experiences but also your heart. Seeking the most appropriate care will allow you to spend as much time as possible with your special friend.

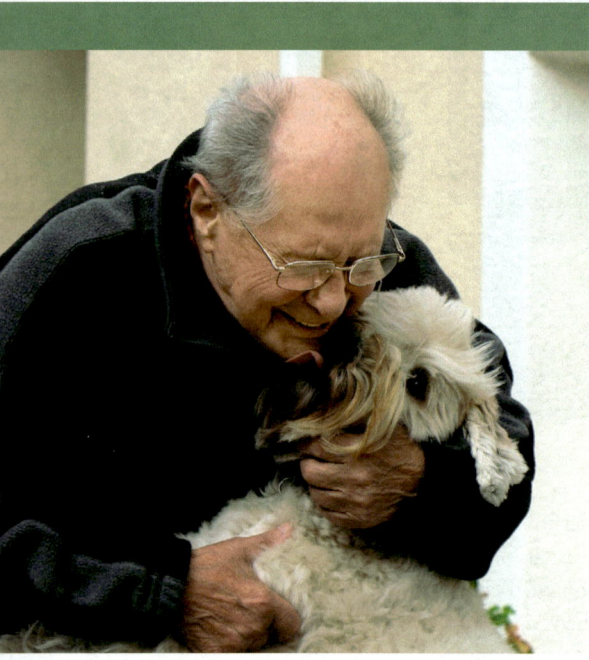

Empower Yourself with Information

You can defeat the darkness of cancer with knowledge. Work with your veterinary health care team to learn as much as possible about the disease and its treatment. Be proactive. Ask questions and obtain resources to tear away the many misconceptions about cancer and cancer therapies. Tackling the emotional aspects of cancer can enhance your ability to think clearly, make decisions, and begin to find the hope and opportunities that lie before you as you deal with your dog's cancer.

Pick a Good Team

As your dog's primary caregiver, you are in the best position to know and meet your dog's needs and desires. Your greatest task is to find a veterinary health care team that is experienced in cancer care and committed to working with you as a member of that team. Once the right team is forged, everyone can provide true *compassionate care*. Compassionate care means that your dog is as free as possible from the adverse effects that may be associated with cancer and cancer care. This includes freedom from pain, nausea, and starvation. Ask your veterinary health care team about what supportive care measures can be undertaken to enhance the quality of your dog's life.

Empowerment Tips

- **Take notes.** Record all discussions about your dog's disease or recommended treatments with the veterinary health care team. Repeat the information back to them to ensure that you understand completely.

- **Seek support.** Bring a friend or spouse with you when you talk to the veterinary health care team.

- **Include the whole family.** All discussions should involve everyone who is intimately associated with your dog, including your children. Allow everyone, including your children, to ask questions and to voice their opinions.

- **Ask for printed materials or information.** Obtain resources to help you understand your dog's disease and the treatment options. The Internet can be a powerful resource of both truth and misinformation. Work with your health care team to understand the validity of all information you obtain.

- **Understand that there are no correct decisions, only decisions that are right for you.** Do not worry what other people will think about your decisions. You know your dog better than anyone else in the world. *Once you are empowered with the information you need, listen to your heart, and you will make the right decisions.*

Questions You May Want to Ask Your Veterinary Health Care Team

About your dog's cancer and treatment:
- What is the name of my dog's tumor?
- Is the tumor benign or malignant (cancerous)?
- How often does this type of tumor metastasize (spread to other parts of the body)?
- If left untreated, what will the cancer do to my dog?
- What diagnostic tests do we need to perform to determine the location and extent of the cancer (i.e., the stage of the disease)?
- What are all the treatment options, and what are the costs, side effects, time involved, and effectiveness of each treatment?

About your dog's pain management:
- Is my dog in any discomfort?
- How do you treat cancer pain?
- Is pain management important at this practice?
- What happens if my dog's pain is not relieved with the usual treatment?
- Is severe pain considered an emergency at this practice?
- Who do I call after hours?
- Will I receive directions in writing?
- Who can help when you are away?
- What happens if my dog's pain does not go away?
- Who will show me how to give pain medication to my dog?

About your dog's nutrition:
- Is there anything special my dog should eat?
- How much should my dog eat?
- When should appetite stimulants be used?
- What is "assisted tube feeding?"
- How important is it to keep my dog from losing weight?
- How can we prevent my dog from losing its appetite?

About ensuring your dog does not have an upset stomach:
- How can I tell if my dog has an upset stomach?
- How can we prevent nausea and vomiting?
- When should I call for help if my dog seems nauseated or is vomiting?
- Who should I call?
- What can be done if my dog seems nauseated or is vomiting?
- What can we do to enhance appetite and ensure good nutrition?

Date and time of my next appointment: _____

Time required for the next appointment: _____

Purpose of my next appointment: _____

Once you are empowered with the information you need, listen to your heart, and you will make the right decisions.

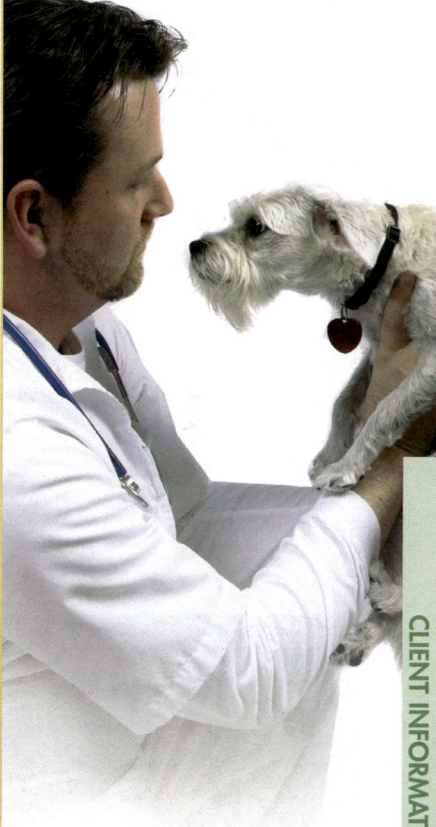

Nutritional Support of Your Dog with Cancer

Good nutrition goes hand in hand with quality of life. Indeed, good nutritional support has been shown in people and in animals to improve not only quality but also length of life by enhancing the beneficial effects of surgery, chemotherapy, and radiation therapy while reducing the side effects of these therapies. You can play a key role in enhancing your pet's quality of life by providing good nutritional support.

The first question many people ask is, "What do I feed my dog with cancer?" The answer is quite simple: Anything your dog will eat! If your dog will eat, then you and your veterinarian should develop a dietary plan to specifically benefit him or her. Although the ideal cancer diet for dogs is not known, there are some simple concepts that can be followed:

- Provide a diet with good aroma and taste.
- Minimize simple carbohydrates (starches and sugars).
- Provide a diet that has high-quality protein sources (meat, fish).
- When possible, consider enhancing the levels of n-3 fatty acids, such as algae-based or fish-based docosahexaenoic acid (DHA).

A big challenge for pets with cancer is the prevention and treatment of a finicky appetite. You can take several steps to encourage your dog to eat, including:

- **Provide a variety of fresh, tasty, and good-smelling foods.** Warming the food to just below body temperature can enhance the appeal of many foods.
- **Work with your veterinary health care team to prevent and treat any discomfort.** Your dog will have a better appetite when it is comfortable.
- **Work with your veterinary health care team to prevent and treat nausea.**
- **Work with your veterinary health care team to prevent and treat dehydration.** A dehydrated pet often has a poor appetite.

If the above suggestions do not work, consider the addition of appetite stimulants as prescribed by your veterinarian.

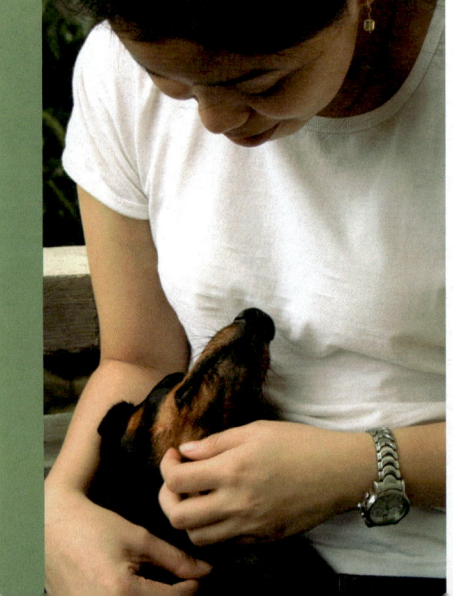

Do not change your dog's diet at the same time as chemotherapy or other drugs are administered if these drugs have the chance of causing nausea. This results in "food aversion," in which your pet may associate the uncomfortable feeling with the food rather than the true culprit, chemotherapy or other drugs or procedures.

When your dog cannot or will not eat, assisted tube feeding is a great option to enhance your dog's quality and length of life. This method also ensures that you can give medicines, fluids, and nutrition without worrying about your pet's desire to eat. Assisted tube feeding is the placement of a small tube into the dog's throat (esophagostomy tube), stomach (gastrostomy tube), or intestine (jejunostomy tube) to allow the nonpainful administration of food, water, and medicine. The key is to begin assisted tube feeding before significant weight loss is observed. Assisted tube feeding should be considered as a great way of preventing any decline in your pet's health and should be used early in the course of your pet's disease. You must be an advocate for your pet. Don't hesitate to contact your veterinary health care team to discuss the importance of nutritional care of your pet.

The Internet and other sources of information are brimming with promises of the health benefits of a wide variety of dietary supplements. Most are unfounded and unproven, but your veterinary health care team welcomes discussion of any treatments that may help your pet. *Discuss any and all treatments and supplements with your veterinarian before you administer them to your dog.*

There is a commercially available diet for dogs with cancer, called Hill's Prescription Diet n/d. Alternatively, a homemade diet can be made.

Next appointment: _____

Don't hesitate to contact your veterinary health care team to discuss the importance of nutritional care of your pet.

Homemade Canine Cancer Food

This is a balanced homemade formula for dogs with cancer. The following recipe will make 3 days' worth of food for a 25- to 30-pound dog.

Ingredients	Amount
Lean ground beef, fat drained	454 grams (1 pound)
Rice, cooked	227 grams (1⅓ cups)
Liver, beef	138 grams (⅓ pound)
Vegetable oil	63 grams (4½ Tbs)
Fish oil	9 grams (nine 1,000-mg fish oil capsules)*
Calcium carbonate	3.3 grams**
Dicalcium phosphate***	2.9 grams (¾ tsp)
Salt substitute (potassium chloride)	1.9 grams (⅓ tsp)

Directions
Cook the rice with salt substitute added to the water. Cook the ground beef and drain the fat. Cook the liver and dice or finely chop it into small pieces. Pulverize the calcium carbonate and vitamin/mineral tablets. Mix the vegetable oil, fish oil (break open the capsules), and supplements with the rice. Add the cooked ground beef and liver. Mix well, cover, and refrigerate. Feed approximately one-third of this mixture each day to a 25- to 30-pound dog. Palatability will be increased if the daily portion is heated to approximately body temperature. (Caution: when using a microwave, be careful of "hot spots," which can burn the mouth.)

Nutrient Profile (% dry matter basis)

Protein	35.3	Sodium	0.36
Fat	41.6	Potassium	0.68
Carbohydrate	17.8	Magnesium	0.05
Calcium	0.65	Energy	1,989 kcal/kg as fed
Phosphorus	0.54		

*Note: Fish oil or, preferably, algae-based DHA should be added.
**Calcium carbonate is available as oyster shell calcium tablets or Tums tablets (0.5 g regular Tums, 0.75 g Tums Extra, or 1.0 g Tums Ultra).
***Bone meal can be used in place of dicalcium phosphate.

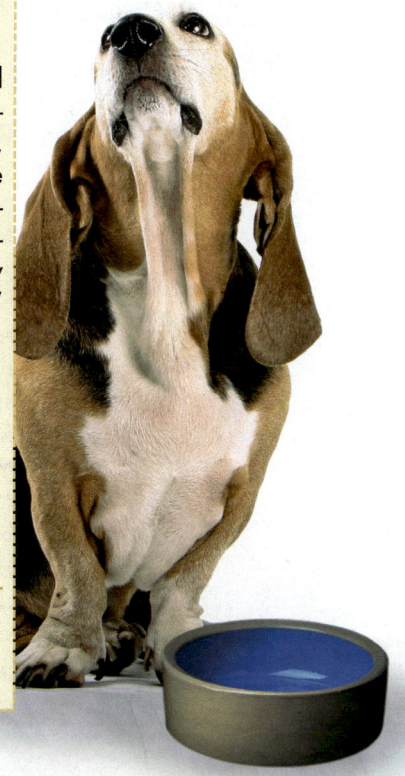

How Will I Know If My Dog Is in Pain?

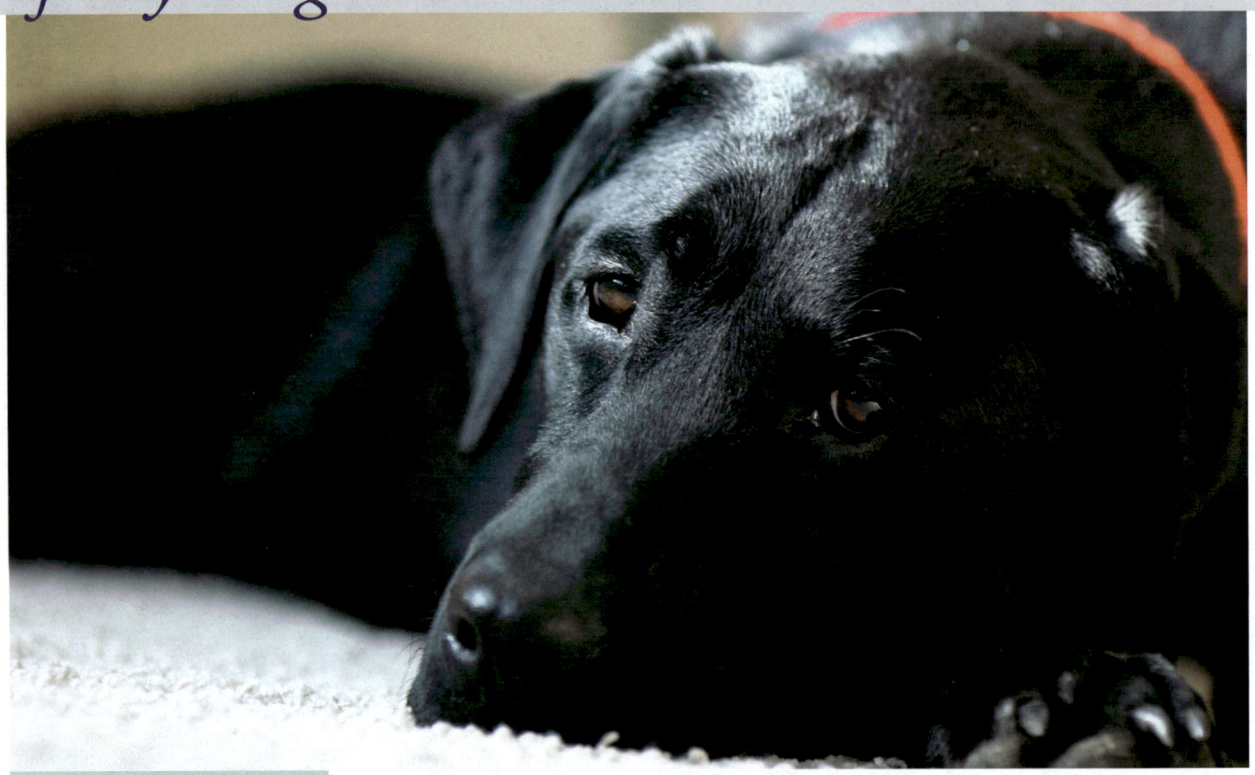

The best practitioners anticipate and intervene early rather than waiting for clinical signs associated with discomfort.

Compassionate care is the watchword of your veterinary health care team, and pain control is the cornerstone of the caring process. Pain management can be difficult because pets may be secretive, making it hard to identify pain early, when it is easiest to treat. The key to compassionate pain control is to intervene early with analgesics before pain receptors ever identify discomfort.

Recognizing Pain

Some dogs rarely exhibit signs of pain until discomfort is quite advanced. Indeed, the clinician's only indicator of pain and discomfort may be increased blood pressure. Experienced veterinary team members and caregivers watch for subtle changes in activity level, appetite, and movements. Vocalization is another sign, although it is not a specific indicator of pain, especially when discomfort is significant. Some pets become more reclusive, but others, especially younger dogs, pace and may thrash around. Increased breathing rate, increased heart rate, and dilated pupils can be used to assess pain in dogs even when they are not fully conscious.

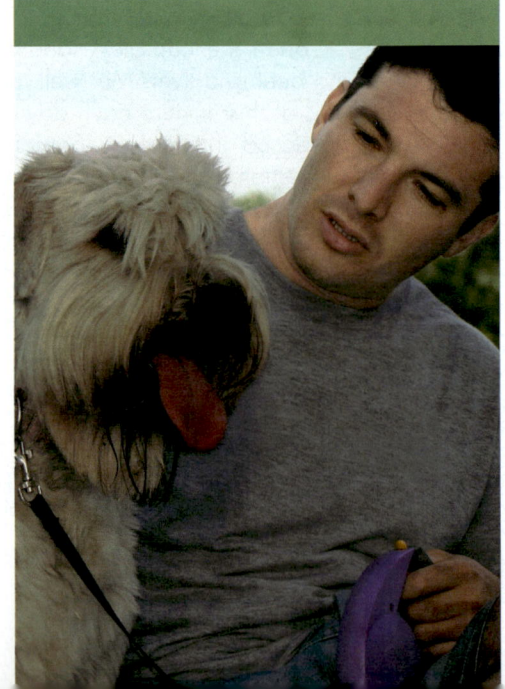

Questions You May Want to Ask Your Veterinary Health Care Team
- Is my dog in pain?
- How can I recognize pain and discomfort?
- What medicines are safe and effective for controlling pain in my dog?

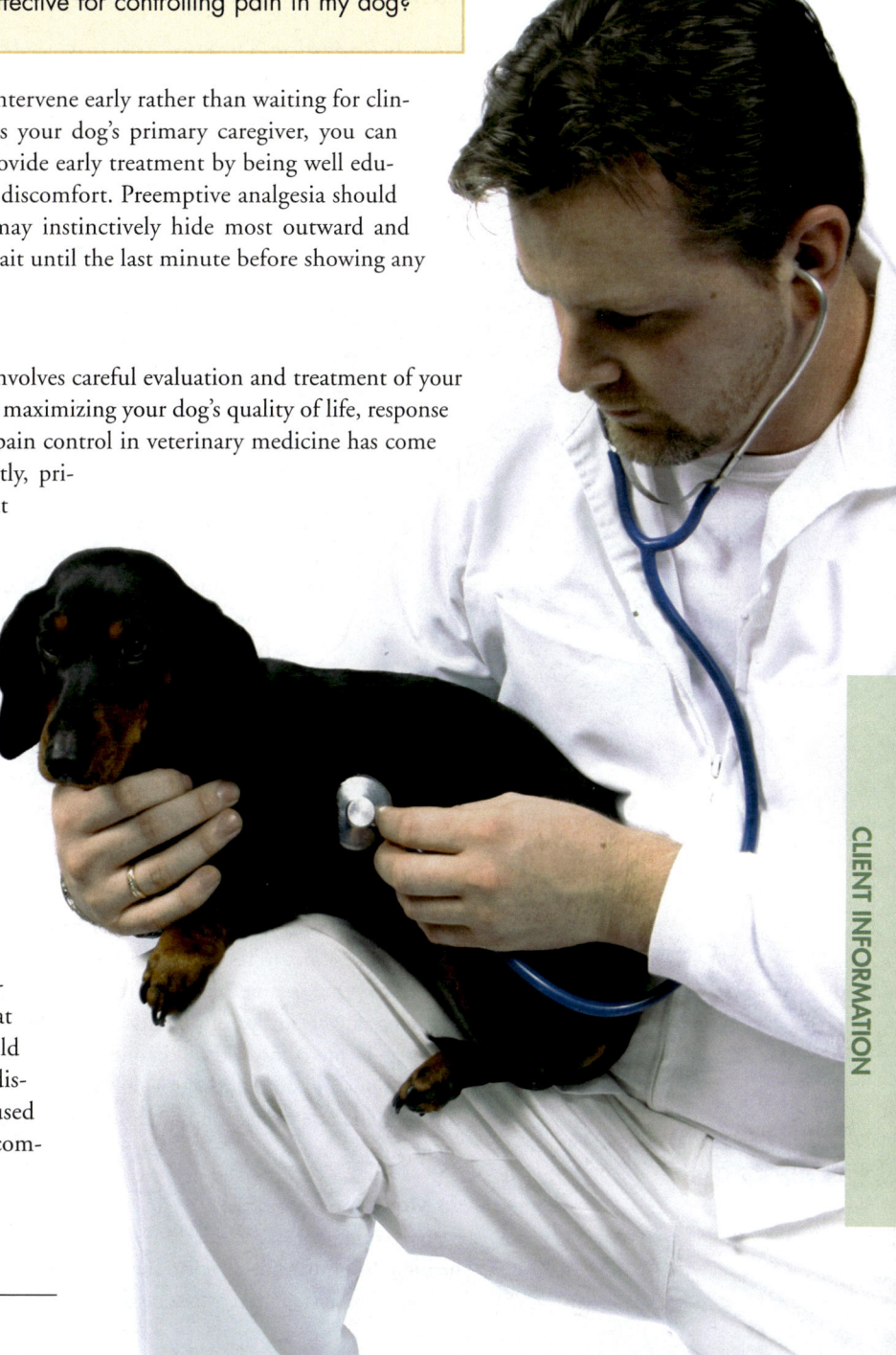

The best practitioners anticipate and intervene early rather than waiting for clinical signs associated with discomfort. As your dog's primary caregiver, you can help your veterinary health care team provide early treatment by being well educated about procedures that could cause discomfort. Preemptive analgesia should be practiced whenever possible. Dogs may instinctively hide most outward and measurable manifestations of pain and wait until the last minute before showing any signs of pain.

Managing Pain

Comprehensive management of pain involves careful evaluation and treatment of your dog. Adequate pain control is essential to maximizing your dog's quality of life, response to therapy, and survival time. However, pain control in veterinary medicine has come to the forefront of attention only recently, primarily because of lack of knowledge about pain medications, pain assessment, and appropriate therapies in dogs. In many cases, analgesics have been withheld because of fear of adverse side effects and because little research has demonstrated the beneficial effects of pain relief in dogs. Client demand has been an important force in bringing pain control to the forefront of compassionate care.

The management of pain begins with high-quality, compassionate care by every member of the veterinary health care team. Careful nursing with gentle handling and provision of a comfortable, relaxing environment is of great benefit to the dog. Local anesthesia should be used whenever possible to alleviate discomfort. Systemic analgesia should be used whenever there is a possibility that discomfort is not alleviated by local analgesia.

Next appointment:
_____

Caring for Your Dog with Radiation Therapy

Many people have preconceived notions about what radiation therapy does and what its effects are. Radiation therapy is often shrouded in negative misconceptions, and the term "radiation" alone may conjure up horrible images. However, radiation's healing power has been used to help dogs with cancer for decades. To ensure that your dog receives the best care possible, we want to enhance your understanding of radiation therapy.

How Is Radiation Therapy Administered?

Whenever radiation therapy is planned for a dog with cancer, maintaining quality of life and freedom from discomfort are the highest goals. In order to minimize the adverse effects and to enhance control of the cancer, small doses are administered over several weeks. During each treatment, your dog will be placed under a light level of anesthesia, and a machine will be used to safely and precisely direct the healing radiation therapy beams over a period of several minutes. The radiation therapist will determine the appropriate dosage and number of treatments to ensure the best possible outcome. When radiation is used with the intent of eliminating or controlling cancer for a long period of time, nine to 40 treatments are administered over 3 to 6 weeks. These treatments take only a few minutes to administer, and they are not painful.

Are There Any Side Effects?

In the course of radiation treatment, some surrounding normal tissue will be affected. Radiation-induced effects to normal tissues usually do not begin until the end of the therapy period, and they continue for weeks after the treatment has ended. These are called the **acute side effects**, and they usually resolve within weeks after radiation has been completed. Other adverse effects associated with radiation therapy may occur months or years after radiation is complete. These are called **delayed adverse effects**. The adverse effects associated with radiation therapy are much less in dogs than in most other species, including people. Indeed, most adverse effects are mild and self-limiting. Your veterinary health care team will work with you to ensure that your dog is as comfortable as possible during this 2- to 4-week period when adverse effects are noted. The side effects that *may* be seen are checked below:

❑ **Skin**

Radiation reactions that may appear toward the end of therapy include hair loss and a sunburn-like effect to the skin, which may become itchy, dry, or moist. Most dogs keep the area clean. Oral or injectable medication to reduce itching or discomfort may be helpful. Applying oily creams or ointments usually slows down healing in dogs. Most dogs develop a change in the color of the skin and hair in the area being treated, and occasionally, their hair falls out and does not regrow in that area. Other changes to the skin that are much less common include formation of a nonhealing wound or of thickened scar tissue in the treatment area.

❑ **Mouth**

If your dog is being treated for a tumor in or around the mouth, injury to this area can include a sunburn-like effect to the tongue and the tissues lining the mouth. This can result in loss of appetite, altered tongue function, and tenderness to the lining of the mouth. In these cases, one of the best things that can be done to ensure your dog has a good quality of life is to consider assisted tube feeding. A small tube is placed into the dog's throat (esophagostomy tube), stomach (gastrostomy tube), or intestine (jejunostomy tube), bypassing the mouth area, to allow the nonpainful administration of food, water, and medicine. The key is to begin this assisted tube feeding before any weight loss is observed. During radiation therapy, you may want to gently rinse your dog's mouth out with a solution of salt and water (1 teaspoon salt in 1 quart of water). Some recommend adding Maalox (Novartis Consumer Health) to this saltwater solution to coat the mouth. Some dogs appreciate cool tea solutions to reduce the discomfort of the oral cavity and freshen the breath. Your veterinarian may recommend some additional therapies if your dog stops producing enough saliva.

Radiation's painless healing power has been used to help dogs with cancer for decades.

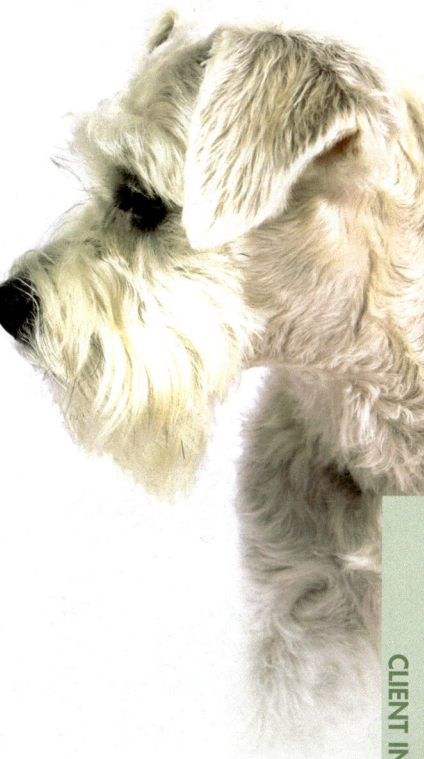

❏ Large Intestine and Rectum

Occasionally, the large intestine (colon) and rectum (area just inside the anal opening underneath the tail) are affected when tumors in this area of the body are being treated. Most dogs have only mild, transient side effects that can include diarrhea that may contain blood and some discomfort passing stool. A special diet, stool softeners, and, in some cases, steroid enemas may be beneficial in some dogs. Whenever the anus and the area around it are injured by radiation therapy, the area should be gently cleansed using soap and water and then dried thoroughly.

❏ Eye

The eye is often in the treatment field when tumors of the skin, sinuses, or nasal cavity are treated. Although most dogs do not show any acute effects associated with damage to the eye, delayed effects can include cataract formation months to years after therapy is finished, damage to the retina (the back of the eye), decreased tear production, and irritation to the tissues around the eye. Occasionally, an ulcer of the cornea (the outer layer of the eye) may be noted. In some cases, medicines may be needed to treat these conditions.

Next appointment: _____

Questions You May Want to Ask Your Veterinary Health Care Team

- What is the probability of controlling my dog's tumor with radiation therapy?
- What, if anything, is known about how long this tumor will be controlled for the average dog with this type of tumor?
- What additional therapies, such as chemotherapy, are recommended to enhance the control of the cancer?
- What are the possible acute adverse effects associated with my dog's radiation plan?
- What are the possible delayed adverse effects associated with my dog's radiation plan?
- I understand that the radiation treatments themselves do not hurt; however, what can be done to prevent or reduce the adverse effects associated with radiation therapy?

Caring for Your Dog with Surgery

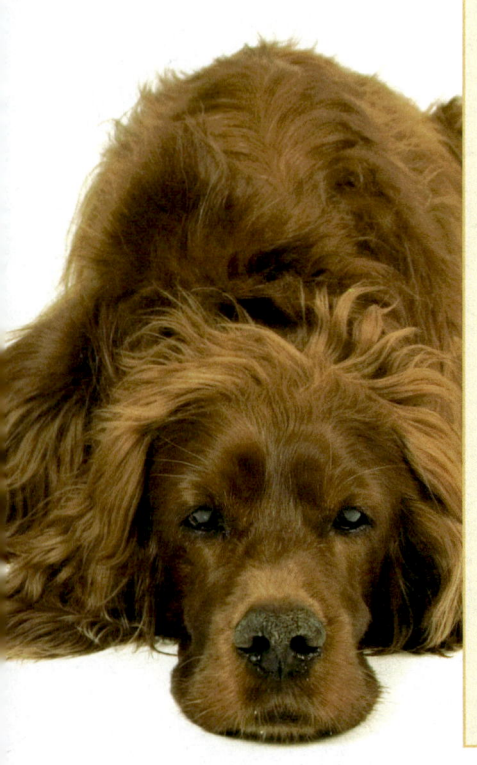

Surgery is the oldest form of cancer therapy in human and canine medicine and has been responsible for the cure of more patients than any other treatment. It can also make other treatments work better. Indeed, surgery plays an important role in the prevention, diagnosis, definitive treatment, and rehabilitation of canine cancer patients.

Although surgery is a critical step in the treatment of most canine malignancies and will help your dog, surgical procedures can be frightening. To make sure that you understand the risks and benefits of surgery, have a frank and open discussion with the entire veterinary

Caring for Surgical Wounds

Surgery can result in some adverse effects, most of which are resolvable. You should examine the incision every day for excess swelling or discharge. Keep the incision clean, but be aware that it is tender to the touch. If you have questions, contact your veterinary health care team. The following are some specific effects that you might observe and the actions you should take to care for them.

You See:	You Should:
Mild "oozing" of blood or body fluids at the surgery site	Keep the area clean by gently washing with mild soap and water.
Visible, continued bleeding at the surgery site	Contact your veterinary health care team immediately.
Redness, swelling, or crusting of the stitches	Keep the area clean by gently washing with mild soap and water and contact your veterinarian. Monitor your dog's body temperature and make sure it does not go above 102°F.
Infection of the surgery sites—may be noticeable as depression, loss of appetite, swelling, discharge, and fever (rectal temperature >102°F)	Contact your veterinary health care team immediately.
Stitches (sutures) that have come untied or that your dog has licked or scratched out	Contact your veterinary health care team and consider a "shirt" or an Elizabethan collar.
Discomfort	Contact your veterinary health care team to ensure your dog has appropriate pain control therapy.
Poor healing	Contact your veterinarian if the wound does not heal within the amount of time discussed.

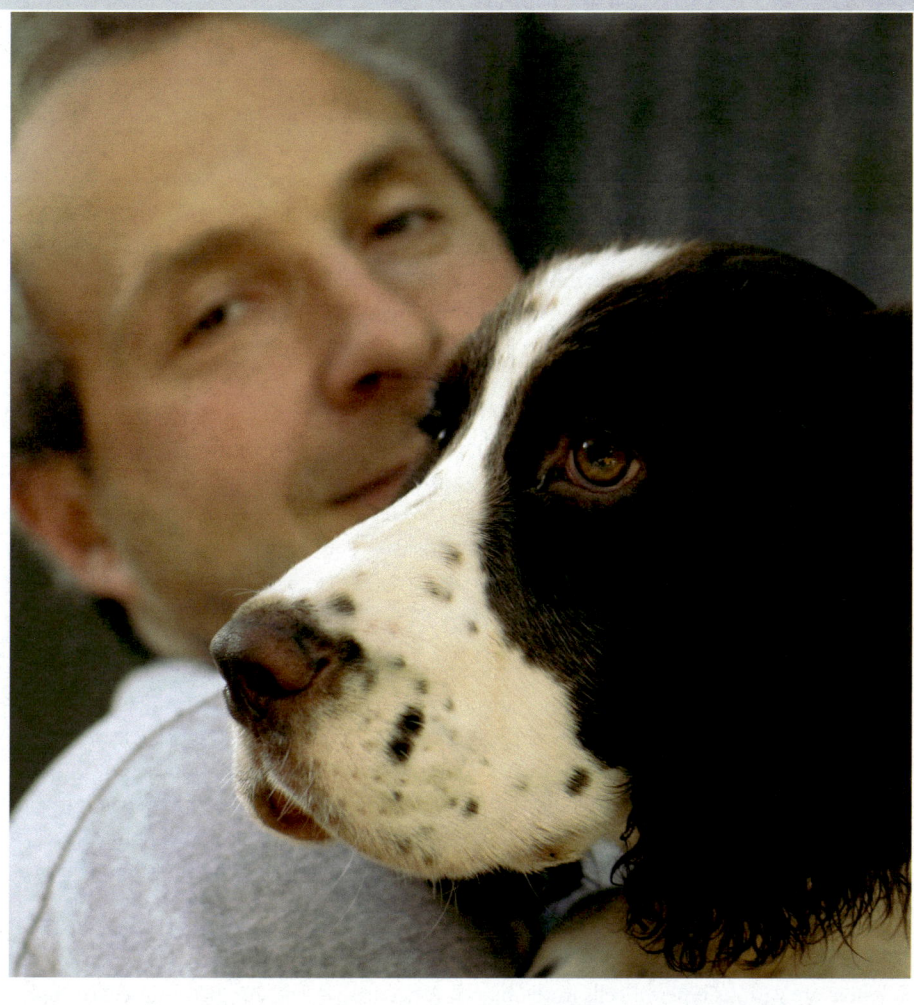

Surgery has been responsible for the cure of more patients with cancer than any other treatment.

health care team about the procedure recommended for your dog. This discussion may help dispel unfounded myths. For example, you may be afraid that the surgery may be disfiguring or that the procedure will result in a decreased quality of life. Your veterinary health care team can help you understand why this is not true.

Before your dog has surgery, consult your veterinary health care team to determine what can be done to ensure that your dog is appropriately prepared. In general:

- No food should be given after 10 p.m. the night before surgery.
- Consult with your veterinary health care team to determine whether water and medication should be given up to the time of surgery.
- Please leave your telephone contact number(s) in case your veterinary health care team needs to contact you before surgery.

Next appointment: _____

Suture removal: _____

Caring for Your Dog with Chemotherapy

Chemotherapy is a word that creates an instant emotional response in almost everyone. Chances are that you or someone you know has experienced chemotherapy for the treatment of cancer. The reality of chemotherapy for dogs is generally different from that for human cancer patients. Most people are pleasantly surprised at how well their dogs seem to feel while undergoing chemotherapy.

Most of the drugs are administered by the veterinary health care team by injection (vincristine, doxorubicin, cyclophosphamide, L-asparaginase) or by mouth (prednisone and sometimes cyclophosphamide). If therapy is to be administered by injection, the patient lies quietly on a padded table during administration and rarely needs any form of sedation.

Practically all anticancer drugs have side effects. However, their potential effect against cancer generally outweighs the risk of these effects. Although serious adverse effects can occur with any chemotherapy, there is less than a 5% chance that your pet will be hospitalized with side effects and less than a 1% chance of fatality. The possible side effects of chemotherapy are listed below. Please consult your pet's doctor with any questions you may have about chemotherapy.

Hair Loss (Alopecia)

When a person loses hair as a result of chemotherapy, it can be devastating. However, dogs rarely lose their hair, and if they do, they are not bothered by it as much as people are. In most dogs, hair does not grow continually throughout their lives like it does in people; therefore, hair loss in dogs is not common unless your dog is a breed that has constantly growing hair, such as poodles, Old English sheepdogs, schnauzers, and Scottish terriers. In general, if your dog needs to visit a groomer periodically to be clipped, then it may experience some degree of hair loss as a result of chemotherapy. All dogs may, however, lose all or most of their whiskers. Please ask your pet's doctor about the possibility of hair loss in your dog.

Reduction in the Number of White Blood Cells (Neutropenia)

There are various types of cells in the blood. A decrease in the number of infection-fighting white blood cells is known as *neutropenia*. Many chemotherapeutic agents impair the

---

Combination Chemotherapy Protocol for Lymphoma

A "protocol" is a chemotherapy treatment regimen used to fight lymphoma. Most of the drugs in the regimen are administered by the veterinary health care team by injection (vincristine, doxorubicin, cyclophosphamide, L-asparaginase) or by mouth (prednisone and sometimes cyclophosphamide). If therapy is to be administered by injection, the patient lies quietly on a padded table during administration and rarely needs any form of sedation.

The combination chemotherapy protocol involves the use of several different drugs over 18 to 25 weeks. Although it is one of the most aggressive and time-consuming protocols available, it is also one of the most successful. In fact, this kind of use of multiple drugs has been shown to be very effective in inducing remissions in lymphoma. Treatments take place once weekly for the first 9 weeks and then every other week for the remaining 16 weeks.

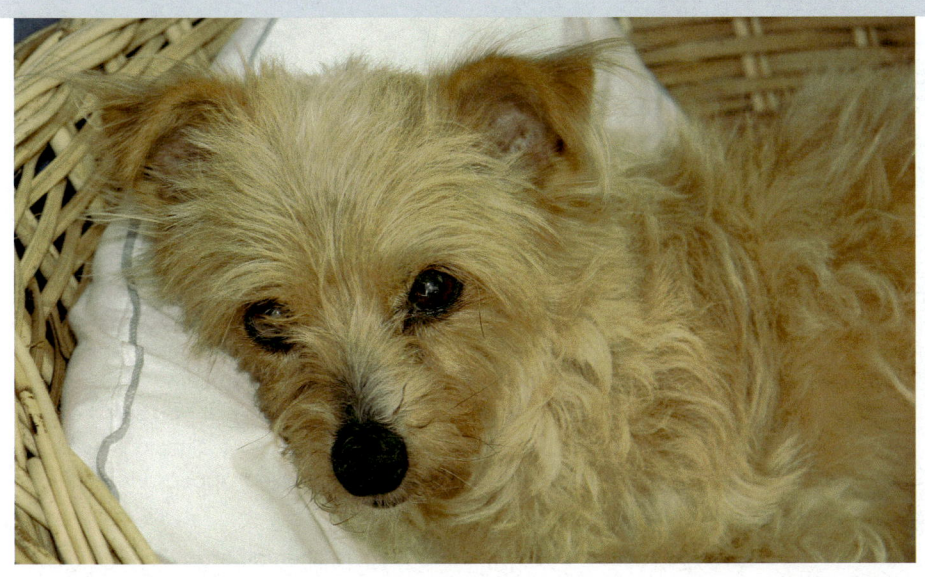

Most people are pleasantly surprised at how well their dogs seem to feel while undergoing chemotherapy.

bone marrow's ability to produce cells. As a result, neutropenia may occur 7 to 10 days after chemotherapy. Neutropenia alone is not a danger to your pet. However, your pet's ability to fight off infection is impaired by neutropenia. Before each drug treatment, your dog will be given a complete physical examination, and a blood test called a *complete blood count (CBC)* will be performed. If your pet has a significant reduction in the number of white blood cells, your veterinarian may wish to perform periodic blood tests, prescribe antibiotics to protect your pet from infection, or both.

Stomach or Intestinal (Gastrointestinal) Discomfort

Some dogs experience some form of stomach or intestinal discomfort 2 to 7 days after a chemotherapy treatment. Your veterinarian will prescribe medication to try to prevent or treat the discomfort. Below are listed some steps you can take at home.

Upset Stomach (Nausea)
- If your pet begins to show any signs of upset stomach (drooling, "smacking" the lips) or loss of appetite, administer the medicine your doctor prescribed for nausea.
- Offer ice cubes every few hours.
- After 12 hours, feed your pet small, frequent meals instead of one large meal.
- Call your veterinary health care team if you have concerns or if the condition persists for more than 24 hours.

Vomiting
- Do not give your dog any food or water for 12 hours.
- After 12 hours, offer your dog ice cubes, then water, then small, bland meals.
- Call your veterinary health care team if you have concerns or if the condition persists for more than 24 hours.

Loss of Appetite
- If your dog begins to show any signs of upset stomach or loss of appetite, administer the medicine your doctor prescribed for nausea.

Caring for Your Dog with Chemotherapy (cont.)

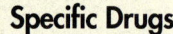

Specific Drugs

The following is a brief synopsis of each drug and the uncommon adverse effects that can occur with each one.

Prednisone: Prednisone is an oral medication you will be required to give your pet at home. It is a steroid that can cause side effects such as increased water intake and urine output, increased appetite, and panting. With long-term use and high doses, this drug can result in ulceration of the stomach or intestinal tract and can cause blood in vomit or bowel movements. If you see these signs, discontinue all medications and call your clinician. Additional long-term side effects include a potbellied appearance, thinning of hair, and pigmentation of the skin.

Cyclophosphamide: Cyclophosphamide is chemotherapy agent that can be administered into the vein or given orally at home. As a true chemotherapy agent, this drug must be handled appropriately. Wear latex gloves provided by the pharmacy when handling this medication. A unique side effect seen with cyclophosphamide is bloody urine. This may be a result of irritation of the bladder caused by the metabolites of cyclophosphamide. If this occurs, do not administer any more cyclophosphamide, and call your clinician immediately.

Vincristine: Vincristine is a clear liquid that is administered directly into a vein. The intravenous administration of vincristine usually takes only a few minutes. In some patients, a side effect called peripheral neuropathy may result from the repeated use of vincristine. Peripheral neuropathy is a neurological abnormality that causes weakness in the limbs. If you witness any irregularity in your pet's gait or excessive licking or chewing of the toes, notify the clinician or nurse at your next visit. Your pet will be thoroughly examined for neurological deficits, and the health care team will determine if this drug should be continued.

Doxorubicin: Doxorubicin is an orange-red liquid that is diluted and painlessly administered directly into a vein. The administration of doxorubicin usually takes about 15 to 20 minutes. The patient lies quietly on a padded table and rarely needs any form of sedation. Although this drug is quite effective, it has been shown to cause cardiomyopathy (heart disease) in patients that have received high or repeating doses. However, the dose of doxorubicin prescribed for your pet is below the dose that usually causes heart disease. About 5% of patients develop heart disease as a result of doxorubicin chemotherapy. In combination chemotherapy, your pet will be administered this drug only four times. Therefore, the risk of heart damage is minimal. However, this is a side effect you should be aware of, and if there is any indication your pet is not a candidate for this drug, your clinician will notify you immediately and further discuss this with you.

- Offer your pet four to six small bland meals a day. Examples include cooked rice, chicken, and turkey.
- Add warm broth, animal fats, and favorite foods to increase flavor and appeal.

Diarrhea
- If your pet begins to show signs of diarrhea, administer the medicine your veterinarian prescribed for diarrhea.
- Keep water available at all times.
- If your pet is also not eating, offer chicken or beef broth.
- Call your veterinarian if you have concerns or if the condition persists for more than 24 hours.

The potential benefits of anticancer drugs generally outweigh the risk of adverse side effects.

Tissue Damage

If the chemotherapy is accidentally given outside the vein, severe tissue reactions can result. Therefore, drugs such as doxorubicin, vincristine, and vinblastine are handled with the utmost care and are only administered by highly trained professionals. If irritation of the injection site develops in the form of pain or redness, apply ice packs for 15 minutes every 3 hours. Call your veterinary health care team if you have concerns or if the condition persists for more than 24 hours.

Allergic Reactions

Allergic reactions to chemotherapeutic agents are very rare and generally not a problem you will have to treat at home. If your pet has an allergic reaction to any drug, the reaction would develop upon administration, and your veterinarian and the hospital staff are trained to treat patients for allergic reactions.

Heart Damage

Heart damage almost never occurs in dogs that receive anticancer agents. However, in some rare cases, doxorubicin can irreversibly damage the heart muscle. The dose of doxorubicin prescribed for your pet is below the dose that usually causes heart disease. This is an exceedingly rare adverse effect in dogs. Some specialists argue that it is not a concern. Your veterinarian will discontinue the use of doxorubicin if heart disease is detected at any time.

Important During Every Visit

It is important to make an appointment for each chemotherapy administration. At each visit, the veterinary health care team will admit your dog. You will be asked how your pet has been doing since the last visit. This is a good time to express concerns you have about your pet's condition and let your veterinary health care team know if you need refills of any medications. Your dog will receive a complete physical examination by a doctor, and blood may be drawn for a CBC. Once the blood values have been reviewed and are determined to be within normal limits, your pet will receive a treatment. This entire process may take 2 to 3 hours. You may wait in the lobby during this time, or you may leave and return later in the day.

Next appointment: _____

Caring for Your Dog with Carboplatin Chemotherapy

The word *chemotherapy* often conjures up negative images and emotions. For some people, the word can be even more frightening than the cancer it is used to treat. Fortunately, most dogs do very well with chemotherapy. Your veterinary health care team is dedicated to working with you to enhance the quality and length of your dog's life.

Carboplatin is a specific chemotherapeutic drug that interferes with the growth of cancer cells. The purpose of this information sheet is to give you an idea of the potential risks associated with carboplatin chemotherapy. Like all anticancer drugs, carboplatin has the potential to produce

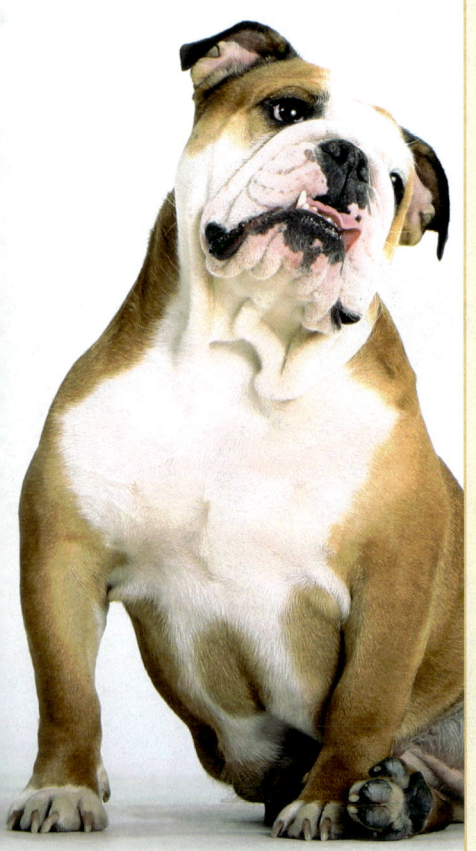

Treatment of Side Effects

Loss of Appetite
- Provide a variety of fresh, tasty foods that smell great to dogs. Warming the food to just below body temperature can enhance the appeal of many foods. Dogs are intermittent eaters, so food should be available throughout the day.
- Work with your veterinary health care team to prevent and treat any discomfort. A dog that is in pain will often not show interest in eating.
- Work with your veterinary health care team to prevent and treat nausea.
- Work with your veterinary health care team to prevent and treat dehydration. A dehydrated dog will often have a poor appetite. Your veterinarian may teach you how to administer fluids under the skin to prevent or to treat dehydration.
- If the above suggestions do not work, consider the addition of appetite stimulants as prescribed by your veterinary health care team.

Nausea or Vomiting
- Temporarily withhold food. Offer ice cubes every few hours.
- Feed smaller, more frequent meals versus one large meal.
- Offer small, bland meals such as chicken or veal baby food. Gradually reintroduce your dog's normal diet after the nausea or vomiting resolves.
- Call your veterinary health care team if the condition persists longer than 24 hours.

Not Drinking
- Offer chicken or beef broth.
- Call your veterinary health care team if the condition persists longer than 24 hours.

Diarrhea
- Feed bland food such as chicken or veal baby food, boiled chicken, or lamb mixed with cooked rice. Gradually reintroduce your dog's normal diet after the diarrhea resolves.
- Call your veterinary health care team if the condition persists.

Increased Thirst or Urination
- Call your veterinary health care team if this persists for more than 4 to 5 days.

adverse side effects. However, in most cases, its potential benefits against the cancer outweigh its possible side effects. While rare, serious adverse effects—including death—can occur with any drug therapy, including carboplatin. Most dogs do very well with carboplatin chemotherapy.

Testing and administration of carboplatin will take several hours. Your dog will be hospitalized on an outpatient basis during this time. This is because carboplatin administration must be preceded by blood tests to minimize the likelihood of adverse effects, and this drug must be given into a vein. Your dog will not experience any pain or discomfort during this procedure. Treatments are usually given 4 weeks apart.

> *Carboplatin is a specific chemotherapeutic drug that interferes with the growth of cancer cells. Most dogs do very well with carboplatin chemotherapy.*

Potential Side Effects

Upset stomach, diarrhea, or loss of appetite. These types of adverse effects are temporary and often self-limiting. Medications may need to be prescribed to prevent or control upset stomach.

Low blood cell counts. This type of adverse effect is also temporary and often self-limiting. A lowered white blood cell count is actually expected and is not commonly associated with clinical problems such as infection. A complete blood cell count (CBC) will be run before each drug administration. The dose of carboplatin may be lowered or administration delayed if the CBC is abnormal.

Whisker or hair loss. This is not a common problem after carboplatin administration; however, shaved areas will be slow to regrow.

Kidney damage. This is also not a common problem after carboplatin administration. Kidney function will be assessed before each carboplatin administration by performing blood work and urine tests. If any abnormalities are detected, your veterinary health care team can usually prevent further kidney damage by "flushing" your dog's kidneys with plenty of fluids before administering carboplatin.

Deafness. This adverse effect has never been reported to occur in dogs, but it is a rare problem in human patients and is difficult to evaluate in dogs.

Preparation

1. Withhold food the morning of the visit.
2. Call 1 week in advance to schedule an appointment.

It is recommended that you wait 2 months after your dog receives chemotherapy to resume vaccinations.

If you have any problems or questions, please call your veterinary health care team at:
_____

Next appointment: _____

Caring for Your Dog with Doxorubicin Chemotherapy

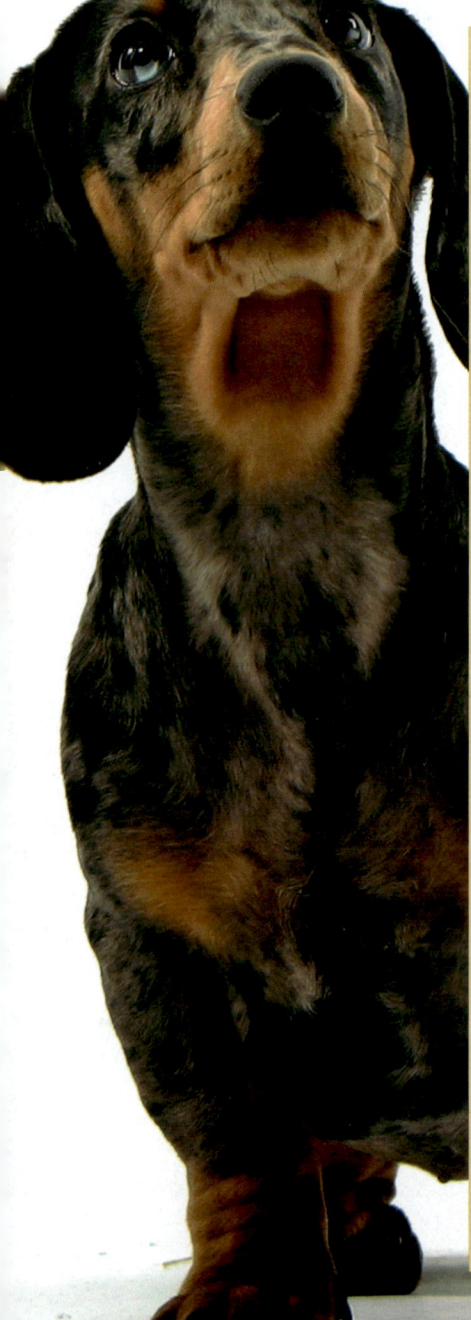

The word *chemotherapy* often conjures up negative images and emotions. For some people, the word can be even more frightening than the cancer it is used to treat. Fortunately, most dogs do very well with chemotherapy. Your veterinary health care team is dedicated to working with you to enhance the quality and length of your dog's life.

Doxorubicin is a specific chemotherapeutic drug that interferes with the growth of cancer cells. The purpose of this information sheet is to give you an idea of the risks associated with doxorubicin chemotherapy. Like all anticancer drugs, doxorubicin has the potential to pro-

Treatment of Side Effects

Loss of Appetite
- Provide a variety of fresh, tasty foods that smell great to dogs. Warming the food to just below body temperature can enhance the appeal of many foods. Dogs are intermittent eaters, so food should be available throughout the day.
- Work with your veterinary health care team to prevent and treat any discomfort. A dog that is in pain will often not show interest in eating.
- Work with your veterinary health care team to prevent and treat nausea.
- Work with your veterinary health care team to prevent and treat dehydration. A dehydrated dog will often have a poor appetite. Your veterinarian may teach you how to administer fluids under the skin to prevent or to treat dehydration.
- If the above suggestions do not work, consider the addition of appetite stimulants as prescribed by your veterinary health care team.

Nausea or Vomiting
- Temporarily withhold food. Offer ice cubes every few hours.
- Feed smaller, more frequent meals versus one large meal.
- Offer small, bland meals such as chicken or veal baby food. Gradually reintroduce your dog's normal diet after the nausea or vomiting resolves.
- Call your veterinary health care team if the condition persists longer than 24 hours.

Not Drinking Fluids
- Offer chicken or beef broth.
- Call your veterinary health care team if the condition persists longer than 24 hours.

Diarrhea
- Feed bland food such as chicken or veal baby food, boiled chicken or lamb mixed with cooked rice. Gradually reintroduce your dog's normal diet after the diarrhea resolves.
- Call your veterinary health care team if the condition persists.

Increased Thirst or Urination
- Call your veterinary health care team if this persists for more than 4 to 5 days.

duce adverse side effects. However, in most cases, its potential benefits against the cancer outweigh its possible side effects. While rare, serious adverse effects—including death—can occur with any drug therapy, including doxorubicin. Most dogs do very well with doxorubicin chemotherapy.

Testing and administration of doxorubicin will take several hours. Your dog will be hospitalized on an outpatient basis during this time. This is because doxorubicin administration must be preceded by blood tests to minimize the likelihood of adverse effects, and this drug must be given into a vein. Your dog will not experience any pain or discomfort during this procedure. Treatments are usually given 3 weeks apart.

Potential Side Effects

Upset stomach, diarrhea, or loss of appetite. These types of adverse effects are temporary and often self-limiting. Medications may need to be prescribed to prevent or control upset stomach.

Low blood cell counts. This type of adverse effect is also transient and often self-limiting. A lowered white blood cell count is actually expected and is not commonly associated with clinical problems such as infection. A complete blood cell count (CBC) will be run before each drug administration. The dose of doxorubicin may be lowered or administration delayed if the CBC is abnormal.

Tissue damage. Doxorubicin does not cause any tissue damage if it is administered inside the vein; however, if the drug accidentally gets outside the vein, it can cause significant, potentially permanent damage to the tissue near the area where it was injected. An intravenous catheter is used for each administration.

Whisker or hair loss. This is not a common problem after doxorubicin administration, however, shaved areas will be slow to regrow.

Kidney damage. This is also not a common problem after doxorubicin administration. Kidney function will be assessed before each doxorubicin administration by performing blood work and urine tests. If any abnormalities are detected, your veterinary health care team can usually prevent further kidney damage by "flushing" your dog's kidneys with plenty of fluids before administering doxorubicin.

Heart damage. This adverse effect has not been reported to happen very commonly in pet dogs treated with doxorubicin; however, it has been seen in about 5% of dogs. Your veterinary health care team will evaluate your dog's heart before therapy to make sure this problem is an unlikely complication of therapy.

Next appointment: _____

> *Doxorubicin is a specific chemotherapeutic drug that interferes with the growth of cancer cells. Most dogs do very well with doxorubicin chemotherapy.*

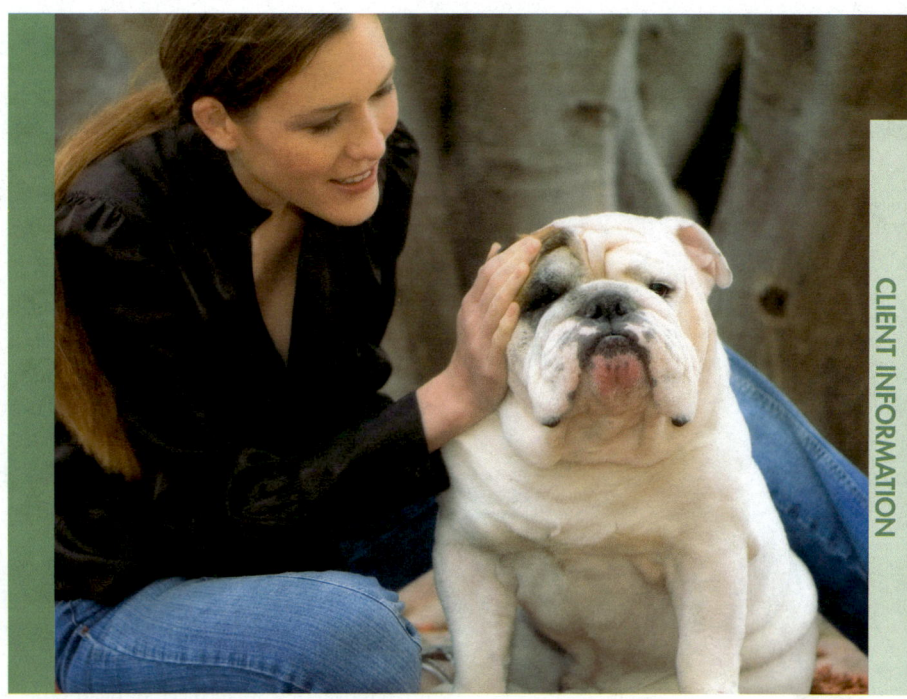

Caring for Your Dog with Cryosurgery

Cryosurgery is a standard treatment for a variety of localized, small malignancies in canine medicine.

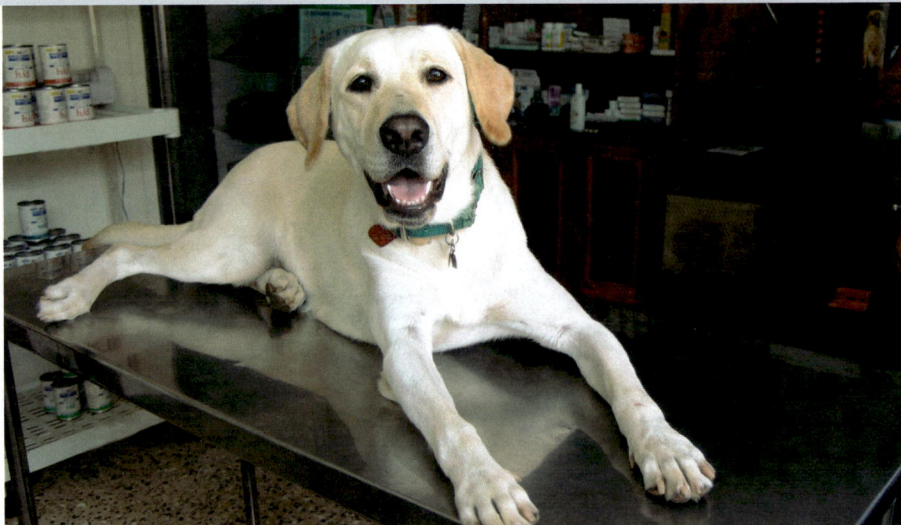

Cryosurgery is the use of very cold temperatures to kill tumor cells and their blood supply. Initially, cryosurgery was used to treat a wide variety of types and sizes of malignant and nonmalignant tumors. Currently, it is used most effectively to treat selected, very small tumors. Because cryosurgery is fast, cost-effective, and can be comfortably performed with medicines to prevent and to treat discomfort, it remains a standard treatment for a variety of localized, small malignancies in canine medicine.

Expected Effects of Cryosurgery

0–24 Hours
- Slight oozing of blood or serum from the cut surface of the tumor
- Swelling (only of concern if severe)
- Occasional irritation or mild pain that can be prevented or treated with relatively mild analgesics

1–14 Days after Treatment
- The tissue should form a slightly moist to dry scab that requires no special care and does not need to be removed.
- The scab will fall off on its own, revealing a pink to red area of healing tissue.
- The red area should soon be covered by normal skin or a flat pink layer of thin skin.
- Some areas may remain hairless or have some white hair regrowth.

During the procedure, the area is injected with a local anesthetic (numbed), a biopsy sample is taken, and the remaining tissue is frozen to -4°F. The area is frozen two or three times in one treatment period. Several changes are to be expected in the area that was treated.

For benign cancers, a routine recheck is not necessary. Some cancers in the mouth may require removal of a small piece of dead bone if it has not healed by 2 months.

Next appointment: _____

Medication Information Sheet

MEDICATION DISPENSED:

- ☐ Analgesic
- ☐ Antibiotic
- ☐ Prevention/treatment of nausea
- ☐ Prevention/treatment of diarrhea
- ☐ Other: _____

DOSAGE (GIVE THE MEDICATION):

- ☐ Once a day
- ☐ Twice a day
- ☐ Three times a day
- ☐ Other: _____
- ☐ By mouth ☐ In the food ☐ Other: _____

DIET:

_____
_____
_____

EXERCISE:

- ☐ None
- ☐ Unlimited
- ☐ Other: _____

OTHER INSTRUCTIONS:

_____
_____
_____
_____
_____

*If you have any problems or questions, please call us at:*_____

CLIENT INFORMATION

When It's Time to Say Good-Bye: Euthanasia and Your Dog

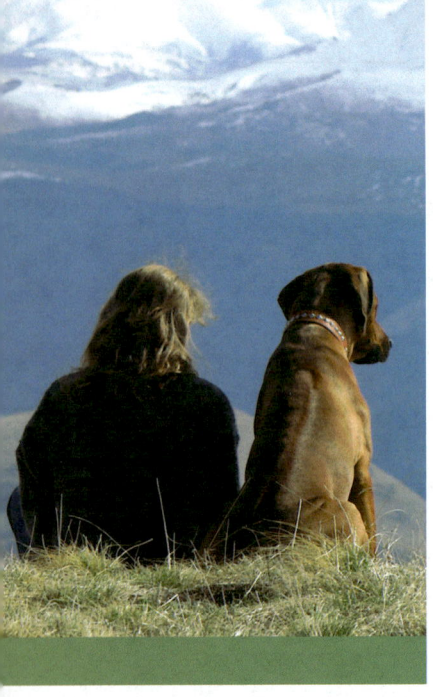

The decision to euthanize a beloved dog is not an easy one. At this very emotional time, concerns about the quality and dignity of your dog's life become increasingly important. For this reason, you must work as a team with your veterinarian and his or her staff. It is vitally important that your concerns and wishes are honored and that you are given complete and accurate information to make all of the decisions that lie ahead. The entire veterinary health care team can assist you by providing information as well as a listening and understanding ear. It is important to realize that your options may also include at-home hospice care, during which your dog's pain and suffering can be sufficiently alleviated until natural death occurs.

What Is Euthanasia?

Euthanasia is the medical procedure of alleviating pain and suffering by administering intravenous drugs that stop the heart permanently to allow for a painless death. Every veterinary health care team performs euthanasia a bit differently, yet these different processes have many similarities. It is very important for you to realize that you are the ultimate decision maker. You have control of the decision-making process as well as the ability to guide and select options for this final step in the care of your beloved dog.

When Will I Know It's Time?

The actual "time" that euthanasia is performed is a very personal decision. There is no one

What to Expect

Many people decide they want to be present at the time of euthanasia, but others do not. Regardless of which path is chosen, the family needs to have an understanding of what will transpire. Every hospital performs euthanasia differently. The following is just one example of how the process may unfold:

- A quiet time and place will be selected so that the veterinary health care team, you, and your family and friends can be involved. You should be comfortable stating how you would like this process to proceed.
- A member of the veterinary health care team will describe the euthanasia process while other members of the team place a catheter in the vein. Euthanasia is the process of injecting an anesthetic agent into a catheter placed in the vein until unconsciousness occurs and the heart stops forever. Although this may sound very frightening, it is almost always accomplished in a tender, gentle manner with no pain, suffering, or struggle.
- You may wish to spend some time alone with your special friend before and after euthanasia.
- Euthanasia can be performed with many drugs. These medicines cause a smooth transition to a state of total relaxation, sleep, and then death within seconds to minutes. As your dog comes to this loss of consciousness, he or she may take a breath or make a slight movement.
- After your dog has passed away, it is normal for the bladder and bowels to release and for the eyes to stay open.

correct decision. There is, however, a decision that will be right for you. There are many issues to take into account during this time. Some are your dog's quality of life, the cost of continued care, the time you must invest to care for your dog during this illness, and the kind of life you want your dog to live. Quality of life is a subjective assessment, but it can be judged in part by accounting for things such as appetite, activity and energy level, grooming habits, and attention to daily rituals, such as sleeping in favorite places. It is often very helpful for you to keep some sort of record of your dog's home "lifestyle." You may want to ask yourself questions such as:

- Do the good days and times outnumber the bad?
- Is my dog able to do the things that in the past have made him or her happy?
- How does my dog's day differ now compared with days before he or she was sick?

The decision to euthanize can profoundly affect your memories and actions for months to years. During this time of assessment, decision making, and action, it is important to realize that your dog's veterinary health care team can be a vital support system for you and any involved family and friends.

The first step of becoming comfortable with euthanasia is to realize that you can personalize this time to meet the needs of you, your family, and, most importantly, your precious dog. This is best done through advance planning whenever possible. Before the time of euthanasia, you may want to consider the following:

- If it is comfortable for you and your dog, you may wish to spend some time doing some of those special activities or rituals that have held meaning for you during the lifetime of your dog. This may be something as simple as allowing your dog to bask in the sun in a favorite place or sit on your lap as you read the paper.
- It is important that children not be "sheltered" from this important decision-making process and time. Many studies have shown that excluding children or making up stories (e.g., "Fluffy ran away") is destructive in the long run. It is also important for parents to appreciate the ability to comprehend the concepts of death and euthanasia at different ages.
- You may wish to take pictures, clip hair, or make paw imprints (on paper or in clay) as a lasting memorial.
- You may find it easier to discuss body care (cremation, burial, disposal, and so on) before euthanasia.

Grief is a normal manifestation of loss regardless of whether the beloved friend is a person or a dog. There are many ways for you to work through the grief process. You should be aware that the loss of an animal, like the loss of a family member or friend, could cause physical and emotional changes that can last for weeks or months. You may wish to contact a pet loss support group, pet loss hotline, or local specialist who is knowledgeable about loss and receptive to helping people who have lost a beloved dog. Ask your veterinarian for a referral.

> *You are the ultimate decision maker. You have control of the decision-making process as well as the ability to guide and select options for this final step in the care of your beloved dog.*

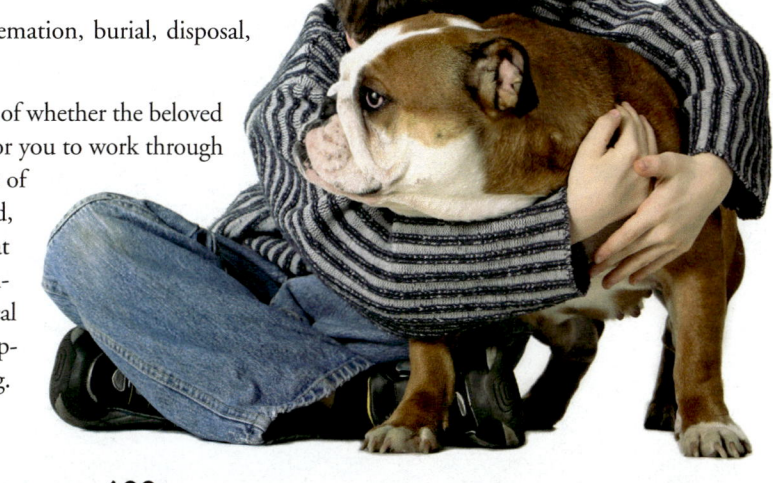

Demystifying Cancer Care: A Glossary for Caregivers

Cancer and cancer therapy are frightening partly because the language used can be confusing. The following abridged glossary may help you understand some of the key words that might be used by the team caring for your dog with cancer.

A

Acute: A sudden onset of symptoms or disease

Adenocarcinoma: A malignant tumor arising from glandular tissue

Adenoma: A benign tumor made up of glandular tissue

Adrenal glands: Two small organs near the kidneys that release hormones

Alopecia: The loss of hair, which may include all body hair besides scalp hair

Analgesic: Any drug that relieves pain

Anemia: A condition in which a decreased number of red blood cells may cause symptoms such as tiredness, shortness of breath, and weakness

Anorexia: The loss of appetite

Antibody: A substance formed by the body to help defend it against infection

Antiemetic: A drug that prevents or controls nausea and vomiting

Antigen: Any substance that causes the body to produce natural antibodies

Antineoplastic agent: A drug that prevents, kills, or blocks the growth and spread of cancer cells

Arrhythmia: An irregular heartbeat

Aspiration: The process of removing fluid or tissue from a specific area

Autoimmunity: A condition in which the body's immune system mistakenly fights and rejects the body's own tissues

Axilla: The area under the front leg; the "armpit"

B

Barium enema: The milky solution (barium sulfate) given by an enema to allow x-ray examination of the lower intestinal tract

Barium swallow: The milky solution (barium sulfate) given orally to allow x-ray examination of the upper intestinal tract

Benign: A swelling or growth that is not cancerous and does not spread from one part of the body to another

Biopsy: The surgical removal of tissue for microscopic examination for diagnosis

Blood cells: Minute structures made in the bone marrow; they consist of red blood cells, white blood cells, and platelets

Blood count: The number of red blood cells, white blood cells, and platelets in a sample of blood

Bone marrow: The spongy material found inside the bones; most blood cells are made in the bone marrow

Bone marrow biopsy and aspiration: The procedure by which a needle is inserted into a bone to withdraw a sample of the bone marrow

Bone marrow suppression: A decrease in the production or number of blood cells

Bone scan: A picture of the bones using a radioactive dye that shows any injury, disease, or healing; this is a valuable test to determine if cancer has spread to the bone

Bronchoscopy: The insertion of a flexible, lighted tube through the mouth and into the lungs to examine the lungs and airways

C

Cancer: A group of diseases in which malignant cells grow out of control and spread to other parts of the body

Cancer in situ: The stage in which the cancer is still confined to the tissue in which it started

Carcinogen: A substance that causes cancer (e.g., nicotine in cigarettes is a carcinogen that has been shown to increase the risk of cancer in dogs, cats, and people)

Carcinoma: A kind of cancer that starts in the skin or the lining of organs

- **Adenocarcinoma:** A malignant tumor arising from glandular tissue
- **Basal cell carcinoma:** The most common type of skin cancer
- **Bronchogenic carcinoma:** Cancer originating in the lungs or airways
- **Squamous cell carcinoma:** Cancer arising from the skin or the surfaces of other structures, such as the mouth or lungs

CLIENT INFORMATION

Cardiomegaly: An enlargement of the heart

Cellulitis: The inflammation of an area of the skin (epithelial layer)

Central venous catheter: A special intravenous tube that is surgically inserted into a large vein near the heart and exits from the chest or abdomen; it allows medications, fluids, or blood products to be given and blood samples to be taken

Chemotherapy: The treatment of cancer with drugs

- **Adjuvant chemotherapy:** Chemotherapy given to kill any remaining cancer cells, usually after all detectable tumor is removed by surgery or radiotherapy
- **Combination chemotherapy:** The use of more than one drug during cancer treatment

Chronic: Persisting over a long period of time

Colonoscopy: A procedure for looking at the colon or large bowel through a lighted, flexible tube

Congestive heart failure: A buildup of fluid in the lungs, extremities (especially the legs), or both; this occurs because the heart cannot pump the blood adequately

CSF (colony-stimulating factor): An injectable substance used to stimulate the bone marrow to produce more cells

CT/CAT scan: A test that uses computers and x-rays to create images of various parts of the body

Cyst: An accumulation of fluid or semisolid material within a sac

Cystitis: An inflammation of the bladder

D

Drug resistance: The result of cancer cells' ability to resist the effects of a specific drug

Dysphagia: Difficulty swallowing

Dyspnea: Difficult or painful breathing; shortness of breath

Dysuria: Difficult or painful urination

E

Edema: The accumulation of fluid in part of the body

Effusion: A collection of fluid in a body cavity, usually between two adjoining tissues (e.g., a pleural effusion is the collection of fluid between two layers of the pleura, the lung's covering)

Electrocardiogram (EKG or ECG): A test that records the electrical activity of the heart

Endoscopy: A procedure looking at the inside of body cavities, such as the esophagus or stomach

Erythema: Redness of the skin

Erythrocyte: The red blood cell that carries oxygen to body cells and carbon dioxide away from body cells

Esophagitis: Inflammation of the esophagus

Esophagostomy tube (e-tube): A tube that is placed surgically into the esophagus that can be used to administer food, fluids, and medicine; it can stay in place for hours or years before being removed

Excision: Surgical removal

Extravasation: The leaking of intravenous fluids or medications into tissue surrounding the infusion site; may cause tissue damage

F

Fine-needle aspiration: A procedure in which a needle is inserted under local anesthesia to obtain a sample for the evaluation of suspicious tissue

Frozen section: A technique in which tissue is removed and then quick frozen and examined under a microscope by a pathologist

G

Grade: For a tumor, the categorization of the aggressiveness of the cancer based on its microscopic characteristics

Granulocyte: A type of white blood cell that kills bacteria

H

Hematocrit (Hct): The percentage of red blood cells in the blood; a low hematocrit indicates anemia

Hematologist: A veterinarian who specializes in the problems of blood and bone marrow

Hematology: The science that studies the blood

Hematuria: Blood in the urine

Hormone: A substance that regulates growth, metabolism, and reproduction and is secreted by various organs in the body

Hospice: A concept of supportive care to meet the special needs of the dog and family during the terminal stages of illness; the care may be delivered in the home or hospital by a specially trained team of professionals

I

Immunity (immune system): The body's ability to fight infections and disease

Immunosuppression: Weakening of the immune system that causes a lowered ability to fight infections and disease

Immunotherapy: The artificial stimulation of the body's immune system to treat or fight disease

Infiltration: The leaking of fluid or medicines into tissues, which can cause swelling

Infusion: The delivery of fluids or medications into the bloodstream over a period of time

Injection: Pushing a medication into the body with the use of a syringe and needle

- **Intramuscular (IM):** Into the muscle
- **Intravenous (IV):** Into the vein
- **Subcutaneous:** Into the fatty tissue under the skin

L

Lesion: A lump or abscess that may be caused by injury or disease, such as cancer

Leukemia: Cancer of the blood; white blood cells may be produced in excessive amounts and are unable to work properly

Leukocyte: *See* White blood cells

Leukopenia: A low number of white blood cells

Lumpectomy: The simple and conservative removal of a mass

Lymphangiogram: A test to look at the lymph nodes

Lymphatic system: A network including lymph nodes, lymph, and lymph vessels that serves as a filtering system for the blood

Lymph nodes: Hundred of small oval bodies that contain lymph and that act as the first line of defense against infections and cancer

Lymphocytes: White blood cells that kill viruses and defend against the invasion of foreign material

Lymphoma, lymphosarcoma: A cancer of the lymphatic system. Veterinarians determine the different lymphomas by the type of cell that makes up the tumor. Treatments depend on the type of cell that is seen as well as the location of the lymphoma.

M

Malignant tumor: A tumor made up of cancer cells of the type that would spread to other parts of the body. This type of tumor needs treatment.

Mast cell tumor: A tumor of the skin that may involve the liver, spleen, lymph nodes, and bone marrow

Mastectomy: Surgical removal of the breast

- **Lumpectomy:** Removal of the lump and a small amount of surrounding breast tissue
- **Simple mastectomy (modified mastectomy):** Removal of the entire breast
- **Radical mastectomy:** Removal of the entire breast along with underlying muscle and possibly lymph nodes

Melanoma: A cancer of the pigment-forming cells of the skin or the retina of the eye

Metastasize: To spread from the first cancer site, such as bone cancer spreading to the lung

MRI (magnetic resonance imaging): A sophisticated test that provides in-depth images of organs and structures in the body

Mucosa (mucous membrane): The lining of the mouth and gastrointestinal tract

Myelogram: An x-ray procedure during which a dye is injected into the spinal column to show any pathology of the spinal cord

Myeloma: A malignant tumor of the bone marrow associated with the production of abnormal proteins

Myelosuppression: A decrease in the production of red blood cells, platelets, and some white blood cells by the bone marrow

N

Neoplasm: A new growth of tissue or cells; a tumor that is generally malignant

Neutropenia: A decreased number of neutrophils, a type of white blood cell

O

Oncologist: A veterinarian who specializes in oncology

Oncology: The study and treatment of cancer

P

Palliative treatment: Treatment aimed at the relief of pain and symptoms of disease but not intended to cure the disease

Pathologic fracture: A break in a bone usually caused by cancer or some disease condition

Pathologist: A veterinarian who specializes in pathology

Pathology: The study of disease by the examination of tissues and body fluids under a microscope

Petechiae: Tiny areas of bleeding under the skin, usually caused by a low platelet count

Phlebitis: A painful inflammation of a vein

Photosensitivity: Extreme sensitivity to the sun, leaving the patient prone to sunburns. Some cancer drugs and radiation have this side effect.

Placebo: An inert substance often used in clinical trials for comparison

Platelet (Plt): Cells in the blood that are responsible for clotting

Platelet count: The number of platelets in a blood sample

Polyp: A benign or malignant growth of tissue protruding into a body cavity, such as the nose or rectum

Primary tumor: The original cancer site (e.g., breast cancer that has spread to the bone is still called breast cancer)

Prognosis: The outcome of a disease; the life expectancy

Prosthesis: Artificial replacement of a missing body part

Protocol: A cancer treatment plan

R

Radiation therapy: X-ray treatment that damages or kills cancer cells

Radiologist: A veterinarian who specializes in the use of x-rays to diagnose and treat disease

Recurrence: The reappearance of cancer after a period of remission

Red blood cells (erythrocytes): Cells in the blood that bring oxygen to tissues and take carbon dioxide from them

Red blood count (RBC): The number of red blood cells seen in a blood sample

Regression: The shrinkage of cancer growth

Relapse: The reappearance of cancer

Remission: Complete or partial disappearance of the signs and symptoms of disease

Risk factor: Anything that increases an animal's chance of developing cancer

S

Sarcoma: A malignant tumor of muscles or connective tissue such as bone and cartilage

- **Chondrosarcoma:** A malignant tumor of cartilage that usually occurs near the ends of the long bones
- **Osteosarcoma:** A tumor of the bone; usually occurs in large-breed dogs

Side effects: Secondary effects of cancer treatment

Staging: Determination of extent of the cancer in the body

Steroid: A type of hormone

Stomatitis: Temporary inflammation and soreness of the mouth

Systemic disease: A disease that affects the whole body instead of a specific organ

T

Thoracentesis (pleural tap): A procedure to remove fluids from the area between the two layers (pleura) covering the lung

Thrombocytopenia: An abnormally low number of platelets (thrombocytes); if the platelets are too few, bleeding could occur

Tracheostomy: A surgical opening through the trachea in the neck to provide an artificial airway

Tumor: An abnormal overgrowth of cells; tumors can be either benign or malignant

U

Ultrasound examination: The use of high-frequency sound waves for the purpose of diagnosis

V

Venipuncture: Puncturing the vein to obtain blood samples, to start an intravenous drip, or to give a medication

Vesicant: An intravenous medication that, if leaked into tissues, could cause pain, swelling, tissue damage, and destruction

Virus: A tiny infectious agent that is smaller than a bacterium

W

White blood cells (WBCs; leukocytes): General term for a variety of cells responsible for fighting invading germs, infections, and allergy-causing agents; specific white blood cells include granulocytes and lymphocytes

White blood count (WBC): The actual number of white blood cells seen in a blood sample

X

X-ray: High-energy electromagnetic radiation used to diagnose and treat disease; diagnostic test using high energy to visualize internal body organs (*see* Radiation therapy)

SECTION 8

INDEX

INDEX

A

ABCDEs, of pain management, 214
Abdomen
 chemotherapeutic agent administration into, 124
 malignant effusion in, 605–607
 paracentesis of, 98
Acanthomatous epulides, 428–430, 429f, 430t
Acemannan, 169
Acepromazine
 for biopsy
  bone marrow, 78
  liver, 94
  lymph node, 67
  respiratory tract, 71
  skin, 63, 64
  urinary tract, 83, 85
 for procedural pain, 223, 224
Acetaminophen, dosage for, 218t
Acitretin, for mycosis fungoides, 640
ACOPA-2 protocol, for lymphoma, 346
ACTH (adrenocorticotropic hormone)
 ectopic production of, 325
 from pituitary tumors, 385–387, 497, 498f, 499–500
Actinomycin D, extravasation of, 296–297, 296t
Acupuncture, 181, 182t, 219
Acute lymphoblastic leukemia (ALL), 366–367, 366f
Acute myeloid (nonlymphoid) leukemia (AML), 364–366, 364t
Acute tumor lysis syndrome, 306–308, 307f, 307t
Acutely responding tissues, 154
Acute-phase proteins, in diagnosis, 42
Adamantinoma (acanthomatous epulides), 428–430, 429f, 430t
Adenocarcinoma(s)
 anal sac, 450–454, 451f–453f
 ceruminous gland, 402–403
 colorectal, 446–449, 447f, 447t, 449f
 definition of, 37
 gastric, 442–444, 443f
 large intestinal, 446–449, 447f, 447t, 449f
 mammary, 103f, 107, 542, 542t, 544
 nasal, 406–411
 ovarian, 523–524
 perianal gland, 449–450, 450f
 pituitary, 385–388, 386f, 387f
 renal, 550–551, 551f
 sebaceous, 629–630, 630f
 small intestinal, 444–446
Adenoid squamous cell carcinoma, 624
Adenoma(s)
 adrenal, 500–505
 apocrine, 631
 cytology of, 107–108
 definition of, 37
 pancreatic, 476–477
 parathyroid, 515–517, 516f
 perianal, 104f, 107, 449–450, 450f
 pituitary, 385–388, 386f, 387f
 sebaceous, 104f, 107, 629–630, 629f, 630f
 thyroid, 510–514, 517t, 519t
Adenomatous hyperplasia, sebaceous glands, 629, 629f
Adjuvant chemotherapy, 128
Adrenal gland tumors
 adenomas and adenocarcinomas as, 49, 500–503, 501f, 502f, 515, 517t, 519t
 pheochromocytoma as, 503–505, 504t, 505f, 517–518, 518t, 519t
Adrenalectomy, for hyperadrenocorticism, 499
Adrenocorticotropic hormone
 ectopic production of, 325
 from pituitary tumors, 385–387, 497, 498f, 499–500
Aerobic glycolysis (Warburg effect), 231–232, 231f, 232f
Alanine aminotransferase, in diagnosis, 41t
Albumin, in diagnosis, 41t
Alendronate
 for osteosarcoma, 577
 for pain management, 219
Alkaline phosphatase, in diagnosis, 41t, 570, 570t
Alkylating agents, 126, 135–138
ALL (acute lymphoblastic leukemia), 366–367, 366f
Allergic reactions, in chemotherapy, 133, 298–300, 299f
Allogeneic bone marrow (stem cell) transplantation, 191–192
Alloxan, for insulinoma, 508
Aloe vera, 185t
Alopecia, in chemotherapy, 131
α_2-agonists, 217, 217t
α-fetoprotein, in liver tumors, 472
Alternative medicine, see Complementary and alternative medicine
Amantadine, dosage for, 218t
Ameloblastoma (acanthomatous epulides), 428–430, 429f, 430t
Amended insulin:glucose ratio, in insulinoma, 506
Amifostine, 144, 302
Amine precursor uptake and decarboxylation (APUD) system, tumors of, 272–273, 505–510, 506f–508f
Amino acids, dietary, 233
9-Aminocamptothecin, 144, 343t
Aminoglycosides, for sepsis, 289t, 290
Amitriptyline, dosage for, 218t
AML (acute myeloid/nonlymphoid leukemia), 364–366, 364t
Ampicillin, for sepsis, 289t
Amputation
 for cutaneous squamous cell carcinoma, 627

Note: Page numbers followed by *f* indicate an illustration; those followed by *t*, a table.

for fibrosarcoma, 584–585
for osteosarcoma, 571, 573f
for soft tissue sarcomas, 593–594, 594f
Anal sac, adenocarcinoma of, 450–454, 451f–453f
Analgesia
  acupuncture for, 181, 182t, 219
  administration routes for, 221
  antidepressants with, 219
  nerve blocks for, 220–221, 220f, 221f
  preventive, 222–224, 223f
  selection of, 216–219, 217t–218t, 219f
  tranquilizers with, 219
Anaphylaxis, in chemotherapy, 298–300, 299f
Anaplasia, definition of, 37
Anemia, 16, 280–282, 281t
  in chemotherapy, 131
  in lymphoma, 333–334
  refractory (myelodysplasia), 362–363, 363t
  transfusion for, 248–249
Anesthesia
  for biopsy, 59–60
    bone marrow, 79
    liver, 93, 95
    lymph node, 67, 68f, 69
    oral cavity, 88
    respiratory tract, 71
    skin, 61–64, 62f
  local, 218t
  for nerve blocks, 220–221, 220f, 221f
Angioendotheliomatosis, malignant, 355
Angiogenesis inhibitors, *see* Antiangiogenesis therapy
Angiography, 45t, 46
Angiotrophic lymphoma, 355
Anion gap, in diagnosis, 41t
Anorexia
  in chemotherapy, 121, 131
  in lymphoma, 337, 337f
Antebrachial joint, osteosarcoma distal to, 577
Anterior vena cava syndrome, in lung tumors, 413
Antiangiogenesis therapy, 170–172, 209–210
  for lymphoma, 352, 354
  for osteosarcoma, 576
  for splenic hemangiosarcoma, 485
Antibiotics
  for chemotherapy, 126, 138–140
  for sepsis, 289–290, 289t
Anticancer drugs, *see* Chemotherapeutic agents
Anticholinesterase therapy, for thymoma, 609, 610
Antidepressants, for pain, 219
Antidiuretic hormone, inappropriate secretion of, 274–275, 275t
Antiemetics, in chemotherapy, 131, 227–229, 227f, 228t
Antigens, for cancer vaccines, 207–208
Antihistamines, for vomiting, 229
Antimetabolites, 126, 140–141
Antineoplastic drugs, *see* Chemotherapeutic agents
Antineoplastons, 185
Aortic body tumors, 420–423, 421f, 422f

Apocrine glands, tumors of, 631–632, 632f
APUD (amine precursor uptake and decarboxylation) system, tumors of, 272–273, 505–510, 506f–508f
Argentaffin cells, in carcinoid tumors, 473
Arginine supplements, 233
Argyrophilic nuclear organizer region numbers
  in lymphoma, 339
  in mast cell tumors, 648
Arrhythmias, treatment-related, 262–265
Ashwagandha, 185t
L-Asparaginase, 142, 237
  for leukemia, 367
  for lymphoma, 342–343, 343t, 345–348
  for mast cell tumors, 653
  toxicity of, 132, 343
    allergic reactions in, 298–300, 299f
    central nervous system, 315
Aspiration cytology
  bone marrow, 78–81, 79f–81f
  respiratory tract, 72–74, 73f
Astragalus, 185t
Astrocytomas, brain, 379–385, 380t, 382f, 383t
Atenolol, for heart failure, 263, 265
Atrium, right, hemangiosarcoma of, 485–487, 486f, 487f
Atropine
  for biopsy
    bone marrow, 78
    liver, 94
    lymph node, 67
    respiratory tract, 71
    skin, 63, 64
    urinary tract, 83, 85
  for procedural pain, 223, 224
Auricle, hemangiosarcoma of, 485–487, 486f, 487f
Autologous bone marrow (stem cell) transplantation, 191
Axial skeleton, osteosarcoma of, *see* Osteosarcoma, of axial skeleton
Azathioprine, for hemolytic anemia, 281

B

Bacillus Calmette-Guérin, 168, 575
Bacteria, as biologic response modifiers, 168
Basal cell epithelioma, 623
Basophils, increased, 278t
Basosquamous carcinoma, 623–624
B-cell lymphoma, prognostic factors in, 335–336, 335f, 336t, 637–638
BCNU, *see* Carmustine (BCNU)
Bence Jones proteins, 40, 372–374
Bereavement, support for, 27–28
Bicarbonate, for sepsis, 290
Bile acids, in diagnosis, 41t
Biliary carcinoma, 473, 473f
Bilirubin, in diagnosis, 41t
Biofield therapy, 183
Biologic response modifiers, 167–173
  agents for, 167, 168
  antiangiogenesis agents as, *see* Antiangiogenesis therapy

nonspecific immunomodulators as, 167–170
specific monoclonal antibodies as, 172
Biologic safety cabinet, for chemotherapeutic agent handling, 112–114, 112*f*
Biopsy, *see also specific malignancies and locations*
  anesthesia for, 59–60
  bladder, 82–84, 83*f*, 84*f*
  bone marrow, 78–81, 79*f*–81*f*
  catheter, 82–85, 83*f*
  colon, 90–92, 90*f*, 91*f*
  complications of, 59
  contraindications to, 59
  CT-guided, 47
  cystoscopic, 83–84, 84*f*
  duodenum, 88–89, 89*f*, 90*f*
  esophagus, 88–89, 90*f*
  excisional, 63–64, 63*f*, 66–67, 67*f*
  fine-needle aspiration, 96–99, 98*f*
  gastrointestinal tract, 87–92
    lower, 90–92, 90*f*, 91*f*
    oral cavity, 87–88
    upper, 88–89, 89*f*, 90*f*
  guidelines for, 57–59, 57*f*–59*f*
  importance of, 56
  incisional, 62–63, 63*f*, 591–592
  liver, 92–95, 93*f*, 95*f*
  lung, 70–75, 71*f*–74*f*
  lymph node, 66–69, 67*f*, 68*f*
  mediastinum, 74–75, 74*f*
  needle core
    lymph node, 67–69, 68*f*
    prostate, 84–85
    skin, 64–65, 64*f*, 65*f*, 591–592
  oral cavity, 87–88
  pericardium, 74–75, 74*f*
  pleura, 74–75, 74*f*
  prostate, 84–86, 85*f*, 530
  punch, skin, 61–62, 62*f*, 63*f*, 591–592
  rectum, 90–92
  respiratory tract, 70–77
    bronchoscopy in, 70–72, 71*f*–72*f*
    nasal cavity, 75–77, 76*f*, 77*f*
    thoracic cavity, 70–75, 71*f*–74*f*
  scraping for, 99
  sedation for, 59–60
  skin, 61–65
  specimens for, 57–59, 57*f*–59*f*
  in staging, 60
  stomach, 88–89, 89*f*, 90*f*
  surgeon consultation on, 58
  surgical, principles of, 176
  thoracoscopic, 74–75, 74*f*
  tissue impressions and, 99
  types of, 56–57
  ultrasound-guided, 49
  urogenital tract, 82–86, 83*f*–85*f*

Bisphosphonates, 172
  for hypercalcemia, 270, 270*t*
  for pain management, 219
Bladder
  biopsy of, 82–84, 83*f*, 84*f*
  chemotherapeutic agent effects on, 134, 134*f*
  radiation therapy effects on, 159
Bladder tumor(s), 554–562
  carcinoma as, 164
  clinical presentation of, 555, 556*f*
  diagnosis of, 555–557, 556*f*, 557*f*
  etiology of, 554–555
  incidence of, 554–555
  prognostic factors in, 557–558, 557*t*
  rhabdomyosarcoma as, 562
  staging of, 555–557, 556*f*, 557*f*
  treatment of, 558–562, 558*f*, 559*f*, 561*f*
  types of, 55*t*
  ultrasonography in, 50*f*
Bladder tumor antigen test kit (V-BTA), 42–43
Bleomycin, 138
  for cutaneous squamous cell carcinoma, 626
  for testicular tumors, 528
  toxicity of, 132*t*
Blood
  disorders of, *see* Hematologic disorders
  typing of, 246–247, 248*t*
Blood transfusions, 246–250, 247*f*, 248*f*, 248*t*
Blood urea nitrogen, in diagnosis, 41*t*
Blood vessel tumors, *see* Hemangiomas; Hemangiosarcomas
Body surface area, chemotherapy dosing based on, 120, 121*t*
Bone
  hemangiosarcoma of, 490–491
  hypertrophy of, 324–325, 325*f*, 413, 413*f*
  lymphoma of, 355
  metastasis to, 46–47, 46*f*, 53*f*
  multiple myeloma of, 372–376
  radiation therapy effects on, 158, 159*f*
  resorption of, hypercalcemia of malignancy in, 266–270, 268*f*, 269*f*, 270*t*
  tumors of, *see also* Osteosarcoma
    nonosteosarcoma, 584–587, 585*f*–587*f*
Bone graft, for limb-sparing surgery, 571–572, 572*f*
Bone marrow
  aspiration of, in mast cell tumors, 645
  biopsy of, 78–81, 79*f*–81*f*, 334
  chemotherapeutic agent effects on, 131
  malignant histiocytosis of, 615
  neoplasia of, *see also* Leukemia(s)
    multiple myeloma as, 102*f*, 372–376, 373*f*–375*f*
    myelodysplasia as, 362–364, 362*f*, 363*t*
    polycythemia as, 277, 278*t*, 279*t*, 370–372
    thrombocytopenia as, 370
  radiation therapy effects on, 158
  transplantation of, *see* Hematopoietic stem cell transplantation
Bone scintigraphy, 51–52
BOPP protocol, for lymphoma, 354

Botanical preparations, 184, 185t–186t, 186–187
Bowman-Birk inhibitor, 237
Brachytherapy, 150, 151f, 651
Brain
    biopsy of, 381
    herniation of, 315
    radiation therapy effects on, 159
    seizures involving, 315–317, 316t
Brain tumors, 379–388
    cavernous hemangioma as, 491
    choroid plexus, 385
    clinical presentation of, 380
    computed tomography in, 47, 47f
    diagnosis of, 380–381, 381f, 382f, 383t
    incidence of, 379–380, 380t
    lymphoma as, 354–355
    metastatic, 315
    MRI in, 50, 51f
    pituitary, 385–388, 386f, 387f
    prognostic factors in, 381–382
    radiation therapy for, 164
    staging of, 380–381, 381f, 382f, 383t
    treatment of, 382–385, 384f
    types of, 379–380, 380t
Brain-heart syndrome, 315
Bronchogenic carcinoma, 104f
Bronchoscopy, in biopsy, 70–72, 71f–72f
Bupivacaine
    dosage for, 218t
    for nerve blocks, 220–221
Buprenorphine, dosage for, 217t
Burial, 26
Burnout, vs. compassion fatigue, 29–30
Busulfan, 135
    for leukemia, 365, 369–370
    toxicity of, 132t
Butorphanol, 218
    dosage for, 217t
    for vomiting, 228, 229
Butterfly catheter, for drug administration, 123
Bystander effect, in gene therapy, 206

C

Cachexia, cancer, 231–237, 231f–232f, 320–322, 322f
Calcifying epithelial odontogenic tumors, 430
Calcitonin, for hypercalcemia, 270, 270t
Calcium
    abnormal levels of, see Hypercalcemia; Hypocalcemia
    in diagnosis, 41t, 42
    supplementation with, 239
Calcium gluconate
    for hypocalcemia, 271, 513
    for seizures, 316t
Cancer cachexia
    clinical presentation of, 321, 322f
    diagnosis of, 321
    mechanisms of, 320–321
    nutrition for, 231–237, 231f–232f
    treatment of, 322
Cancer pain
    factors influencing, 215–216
    management of, see Pain management
    mechanisms of, 214
    prevention of, 222–224, 223f
    recognition of, 214–215
    severity of, 215t, 216t, 222–224, 223f
Cancer prevention by delay, 128–129, 234–235
Cancer vaccines, see Vaccines, cancer
Canine lymphoma/monoclonal antibody 231, 172
Canine lymphomatoid granulomatosis, 417
Canine metabolic epidermal necrosis, 510
Cannabinoids, for vomiting, 229
Capecitabine, 140
Carbohydrates, in cancer, 231–233, 231f, 232f, 239
Carboplatin, 144–145
    for bladder tumors, 560–561
    for mammary tumors, 544
    for oral melanoma, 462
    for osteosarcoma, 573–575, 574t
Carcinogens, environmental, 8
Carcinoid tumors
    large intestinal, 448
    liver, 473
    small intestinal, 445
Carcinoma(s), see also Adenocarcinoma(s)
    adrenal, 500–505, 501f
    basosquamous, 623–624
    biliary, 473, 473f
    bladder, 164
    bronchogenic, 104f
    ceruminous gland, 162, 402, 402f, 403f
    choroid plexus, 385
    cytology of, 107–108
    definition of, 37
    hepatocellular, 472–473, 474f
    inflammatory mammary, 545–547, 546f
    intestinal, 103f
    laryngeal, 411–412
    nasal, 48f, 51f, 406–411
    pancreatic, 476–477
    parathyroid, 515–517
    prostatic, 529–532, 530f–532f
    renal, 550–551
    salivary gland, 440–441, 441f, 441t
    squamous cell, see Squamous cell carcinoma
    thyroid, 49f, 510–515, 511f–513f
    transitional cell, renal, 554–560
    uterine, 525
Cardiac tumors, see Heart, tumors of
Cardiomyopathy, treatment-related, 261–265, 262t, 264t
Care, compassionate, see Compassionate care
Carmustine (BCNU)
    for brain tumors, 385

for lymphoma, 345, 354
toxicity of, 132t
Carotid body tumors, 53f, 423, 423f
Carprofen
  for biopsy
    bone marrow, 78
    liver, 94
    lymph node, 67
    oral cavity, 88
    respiratory tract, 71
    skin, 62, 64
    urinary tract, 85
  dosage for, 217t
  for procedural pain, 223, 224
Cartilage products, 185
Catecholamines, secretion of, from pheochromocytoma, 503–504
Catheter(s)
  biopsy with
    bladder, 82–83, 83f
    prostate, 84–85
  chemotherapeutic agent extravasation from, 295–297, 296t, 297f
  for drug administration, 122–123
  for enteral nutrition, 239–243, 238f, 240f–243f
  for parenteral nutrition, 244
  sepsis due to, 285, 286f
Cavernous hemangioma, brain, 491
CAVM, *see* Complementary and alternative medicine
CCNU, *see* Lomustine (CCNU)
Cecum, tumors of, 444–446, 445f, 446f
Cefazolin, for sepsis, 289t
Cefoxitin, for sepsis, 289t
Cell cycle, radiation therapy and, 149
Central nervous system, *see also* Brain; Spinal cord
  paraneoplastic syndromes of, 314–319, 316t, 319t
  radiation therapy effects on, 317–318
  tumors of, *see also* Brain tumors
    hemangiosarcoma as, 490
    lymphoma as, 354–355
    malignant histiocytosis as, 615
Cephalosporins, for sepsis, 289t, 290
Ceruminous gland tumors, 162, 402–403, 403f
Chelation therapy, 184
Chemo pins, in drug preparation, 115–116
Chemodectoma, 420–423, 421f–423f
Chemoimmunotherapy, for lymphoma, 351–352
Chemoprotection, gene therapy for, 207
Chemoreceptor trigger zone, 226, 227f
Chemotherapeutic agents, *see also specific drugs*
  administration of
    intracavitary, 124
    intralesional, 123–124
    intramuscular, 123–124
    intravenous, 122–123
    oral, 124
    timing of, 130
  alkylating, 126, 135–138
  antibiotics as, 126, 138–140

  antimetabolites as, 126, 140–141
  combinations of, 129–130
    with NSAIDs, 169–170
    for osteosarcoma, 574–575, 575f
  cytokines as, 141–142
  disposal of, 114, 114f, 119
  dosing of, 120–122, 121t, 122t, 130
  emetic potential of, 226
  enzymes as, 127, 142–143, 237
  exposure to, 112
  handling of, 112–113, 112f
  hematopoietic growth factors with, 141–142, 251–255, 253f
  hormones as, 127, 143
  indications for, 126–127
  Material Safety Data Sheets for, 113
  matrix metalloproteinases and, 171–172, 210
  plant alkaloids as, 127, 143–144
  polyunsaturated fatty acids with, 235
  preparation of, 113–119
    guidelines for, 113–114
    intralesional agents, 117–118
    intravenous agents, 115–117, 118f
    oral agents, 117
    PhaSeal system for, 115, 116f, 117f
    precautions with, 118–119
    safety in, 112–115, 112f, 114f, 118–119
    standard method for, 115–118
  radiation therapy interactions with, 149, 594–595
  resistance to, 130, 339, 341–342
  sepsis due to, *see* Sepsis
  spills of, 119
  therapy with, *see* Chemotherapy
  topoisomerase-I inhibitors as, 144
  toxicity of, 111–112, 126–127, 130–135, 132t–133t
    acute tumor lysis syndrome in, 306–308, 307f, 307t
    allergic reactions in, 133, 298–300, 299f
    alopecia in, 131
    bone marrow, 131
    cardiac, 133–134, 261–265, 262t, 264t
    central nervous system, 314–319, 316t, 319t
    cystitis in, 134, 134f
    dermatologic, 135
    gastrointestinal, 131, *see also* Nausea and vomiting
    hematologic, 280–281, *see also* Sepsis
    in lymphoma, 340
    neurologic, 134
    pulmonary, 135
    renal, 134, 301–305, 302t–304t
  vesicant, 295
Chemotherapy, *see also specific malignancies*, chemotherapy for
  agents for, *see* Chemotherapeutic agents
  cancer vaccines with, *see* Vaccines, cancer
  consolidation, 128, 129
  hematopoietic stem cell rescue in, 190–191
  immunocytokines with, 209
  for lymphoma, *see* Lymphoma, chemotherapy for
  myths about, 128

nausea in, *See* Nausea and vomiting
principles of, 128–129
protective gene therapy with, 207
quality of life issues in, 18–22
team approach to, 119
vaccination during, 341
vomiting in, *See* Nausea and vomiting
Chiropractic science, 181–182
Chlorambucil, 135
    for chronic lymphocytic leukemia, 368–369
    for lymphoma, 342
    toxicity of, 132*t*
Chlorpromazine, for vomiting, 228, 229
Chondroitin, dosage for, 218*t*
Chondrosarcoma
    bone, 585–586, 585*f*–587*f*
    nasal, 406–411, 407*f*
CHOP protocol, for chronic lymphocytic leukemia, 369
Choroid plexus tumors, 385
Chromosomal abnormalities, in lymphoma, 339
Chronic myeloid leukemia (CML), 369–370
Ciliary body tumors, 397–398
Cimetidine, 169
    for anaphylaxis, 300
    for kidney failure, 304*t*
    for oral melanoma, 462
Cisplatin, 145
    for bladder tumors, 560
    for cutaneous squamous cell carcinoma, 625–627
    for lymphoma, 354
    for mammary tumors, 544
    for mesothelioma, 606–607
    for oral fibrosarcoma, 439
    for oral melanoma, 462
    for oral squamous cell carcinoma, 435
    for osteosarcoma, 572–575, 573*f*, 573*t*, 574*t*, 575*f*
    for soft tissue sarcomas, 596, 596*f*
    for testicular tumors, 528
    for thymoma, 610
    for thyroid tumors, 515
    for tonsillar squamous cell carcinoma, 436–437
    toxicity of, 132*t*, 301–303, 315
Citrate toxicity, in transfusion, 250
Clear cell melanoma, 464
Clinical cancer chemoprevention, 129
Clinical chemistries, 40, 41*t*–42*t*, 42–43
Clodronate, for hypercalcemia, 270, 270*t*
CML (chronic myeloid leukemia), 369–370
COAP protocol, for lymphoma, 345–346
Coarse fractionation, in radiation therapy, 160, 162–164, 163*f*
Colon
    biopsy of, 90–92, 90*f*, 91*f*
    radiation therapy effects on, 158
    tumors of, 165, 446–449, 447*f*, 447*t*, 449*f*
Colonoscopy, 90–92, 90*f*, 91*f*, 447
Compassionate care
    cure in, 23, 24*f*

delivery of, steps for, 13–14
fatigue in, 29–31
goals of, 23–24, 24*f*
information for, 4–5
myths interfering with, 4, 11–12
pain management in, *see* Pain management
philosophy of, 11–14
preventive, 6–10, 7*f*, 9*t*
quality of life issues in, 18–22
team for, 12–13
Complementary and alternative medicine, 179–189
    acupuncture in, 181, 182*t*
    advantages of, 180
    biofield therapy in, 183
    biologic treatments in, 184
    chiropractic science in, 181–182
    ethics and, 180–181
    herbal and botanical preparations in, 184, 185*t*–186*t*, 186–187
    homeopathy in, 183–184, 184*t*
    limitations of, 180
    massage therapy in, 182–183
    nutritional therapy in, 187
    pharmacologic, 184
    for quality of life enhancement, 180
    usage statistics on, 179–180
Complete blood count, in lymphoma, 333–334, 338
Compound melanoma, 464
Compton absorption, in radiation therapy, 150
Computed tomography, 45*t*, 46–48, 47*f*, 48*f*
    in adrenal tumors, 501, 501*f*
    in aortic body tumors, 421
    in brain tumors, 380–381, 381*f*–382*f*
    in lung tumors, 414
    in nasal tumors, 407, 407*f*, 408, 408*f*
    in neurofibrosarcoma, 598, 598*f*
    in oral fibrosarcoma, 437
    in pituitary tumors, 386–387, 386*f*
    in spinal tumors, 389–390
    in staging, 16–17, 16*f*
Conformal radiation therapy, 151
Congestive heart failure, treatment-related, 261–265, 262*t*, 264*t*
Connective tissue tumors, cytology of, 103, 105*f*–106*f*, 108
Consolidation, in chemotherapy, 128, 129, 348–349, 349*t*
Contrast agents
    for computed tomography, 46
    for MRI, 50
COP protocol, for lymphoma, 345–346, 346*t*
COPA protocol, for lymphoma, 346
Corticosteroids, *see also specific agents*
    for hypercalcemia, 270*t*
    for insulinoma, 508
    for lymphoma, 339–340, 339*f*
    for mast cell tumors, 652–653
    for nasal tumors, 411
    for radiation-induced skin lesions, 157
    for sepsis, 290
    for vomiting, 228, 229

Cortisol, excess of, *see* Hyperadrenocorticism
Corynebacterium parvum
    for mast cell tumors, 654
    for oral melanoma, 462–463
Cremation, 26
Critical incidents, triggering compassion fatigue, 29
Cryoprecipitate, 248
Cryotherapy, 199–201, 200*f*
    for eye tumors, 398
    for large intestinal tumors, 448
    for warts, 623
Cryptorchidism, tumors in, 527
CT, *see* Computed tomography
Culture, in sepsis, 287, 287*f*
Cushing's syndrome, ectopic, 325
Cyclophosphamide, 135–136
    for bladder rhabdomyosarcoma, 562
    for canine lymphomatoid granulomatosis, 417
    for epulides, 430
    for leukemia
        acute lymphoblastic, 367
        acute myeloid, 365
        chronic lymphocytic, 369
        chronic myeloid, 370
    for lymphoma, 342, 343*t*, 345–348, 346*t*
    for mammary tumors, 544–545
    for multiple myeloma, 375
    for prostate tumors, 532
    for splenic hemangiosarcoma, 484
    toxicity of, 132*t*, 134, 134*f*
Cyclosporine
    for cutaneous histiocytosis, 612
    for systemic histiocytosis, 613
    for thrombocytopenia, 283
Cyst(s), cutaneous, 633
Cystadenocarcinoma complex, renal, 551–553, 552*f*
Cystectomy, for bladder tumors, 558–559
Cysteine supplements, 233
Cystic (follicular) tumors, cutaneous, 632–633
Cystitis, in chemotherapy, 134, 134*f*
Cystoscopic biopsy, 83–84, 84*f*
Cystostomy, for bladder tumors, 559, 559*f*
Cytarabine (cytosine arabinoside), 140
    for acute myeloid leukemia, 365
    liposomal, 141
    for lymphoma, 343*t*, 344–346, 354
    for myelodysplasia, 363
    for spinal tumors, 391
    toxicity of, 132*t*, 315
Cytokeratins, 97
Cytokines
    for chemotherapy, 141–142, 170, 206–207
    hematopoietic, 254
Cytology, 96–108
    abdominal paracentesis in, 98
    advantages of, 96
    in connective tissue tumors, 108
    in epithelial cell tumors, 107–108
    fine-needle aspiration in, 96–99, 98*f*
    interpretation of, 99–104, 100*f*–105*f*
    in lymphoma, 331–332
    in mast cell tumors, 645
    in mesothelioma, 605–606
    in respiratory tract tumors, 72–74, 73*f*
    in round cell tumors, 105–107
    thoracentesis in, 98–99
Cytopenia, in myelodysplasia, 362–363, 363*t*
Cytosine arabinoside, *see* Cytarabine (cytosine arabinoside)
Cytotoxic drugs, *see* Chemotherapeutic agents

D

Dacarbazine, 136
    for lymphoma, 353
    for oral melanoma, 462
    toxicity of, 132*t*
Dactinomycin, 138
    for lymphoma, 344–345, 353–354
    toxicity of, 132*t*
Darier's sign, in mast cell tumors, 644
Daunorubicin
    for acute myeloid leukemia, 365
    extravasation of, 296–297, 296*t*
    toxicity of, 132*t*
DEAs (dog erythrocyte antigens), 246–247, 248*t*
Death, *See* Euthanasia
Debulking surgery, 177
Definitive fractionation, in radiation therapy, 160, 162–164
Definitive therapy
    radiation, vs. palliative, 151
    surgical, 176–177
Dehydration
    in kidney failure, 305
    in vomiting, 227–228, 228*t*
Deionized water injections, for mast cell tumors, 652
Demeclocycline, for syndrome of inappropriate secretion of antidiuretic hormone, 275
Dendritic cell vaccines, 208
Deprenyl, for ectopic Cushing's syndrome, 500
Deracoxib
    dosage for, 217*t*
    for procedural pain, 224
Dermatofibrosarcoma, 596–597
Dermatofibrosis, in renal cystadenocarcinoma complex, 551–553, 552*f*
Desmin, 97
Dexamethasone
    for adrenalectomy, 501–502
    for anaphylaxis, 299, 300
    for brain herniation, 315
    for hypercalcemia, 270*t*
    for sepsis, 290
    for vomiting, 228, 229
Dexamethasone suppression test, 497, 500

Dexrazoxane, 145
    for cardiac toxicity prevention, 263
    for extravasation, 296t
Diarrhea
    in chemotherapy, 131
    prevention of, 19
Diazepam
    for appetite stimulation, 238
    for seizures, 316t, 317
Diazoxide
    for hypoglycemia, 273
    for insulinoma, 508
Diff-Quik stain, 99
Digestive system, see Gastrointestinal tract; Liver; Pancreas
Digoxin, for heart failure, 263–265
Dihydrotachysterol, for hypocalcemia, 513
Diltiazem, for heart failure, 263, 265
Dimenhydrinate, for vomiting, 228, 229
Dimethylsulfoxide, for extravasation, 296t, 297
Diphenhydramine
    for anaphylaxis, 299, 300
    for vomiting, 228, 229
Disseminated intravascular coagulation, 309–313
    anemia in, 280
    diagnosis of, 310–311, 310t, 311f, 312f
    predisposing factors in, 309–310
    transfusion for, 249
    treatment of, 311–313
Diuretics, for kidney failure, 302–305, 303t
DNA vaccination, 207, 207f, 463
Dobutamine, for heart failure, 264, 264t
Docetaxel, 145, 545
Docosahexaenoic acid
    anticancer effects of, 171–172, 234–235
    for tumor sensitization, in radiation therapy, 159, 235
Dog erythrocyte antigens, 246–247, 248t
Dolasetron, for vomiting, 228–229
Domperidone, for vomiting, 228
Dopamine, for kidney failure, 304t
DOPP protocol, for lymphoma, 354
Doppler studies, 50
Doramectin, for *Spirocerca lupi* infestations, 441
Dosing
    of analgesics, 217t–218t
    of chemotherapeutic agents, 120–122, 121t, 122t, 130, see also individual drugs
Doxorubicin, 138–139
    administration rate for, 122–123
    for anal sac adenocarcinoma, 453
    for bladder rhabdomyosarcoma, 562
    for cardiac hemangiosarcoma, 487
    for cutaneous hemangiosarcoma, 489–490
    dose calculation for, 120
    for epulides, 430
    extravasation of, 296–297, 296t
    for leukemia, 365
    liposomal, 139
    for lymphoma, 342–344, 343t, 344t, 346–348, 353
    for malignant histiocytosis, 616
    for mammary tumors, 545
    for mast cell tumors, 653–654
    for oral fibrosarcoma, 439
    for oral melanoma, 462
    for osteosarcoma, 573–575, 574t, 575f
    for prostate tumors, 532
    for soft tissue sarcomas, 594–596
    for splenic hemangiosarcoma, 484–485
    for synovial cell sarcoma, 601
    for thyroid tumors, 514–515
    for tonsillar squamous cell carcinoma, 436–437
    toxicity of, 132t, 133–134
        allergic reactions in, 298–300
        cardiac, 261–265, 262t, 264t
        renal, 403
    for vaginal tumors, 525
Dry mouth, in radiation therapy, 157–158, 158f
Duodenum, biopsy of, 88–89, 89f, 90f
Dysplasia, definition of, 37

E

Ear, tumors of, 400t, 401–403, 401t, 402f, 403f
Eastern Cooperative Oncology Group Evaluation, Modified, 20t
Echocardiography
    in aortic body tumors, 421, 421f
    in cardiac hemangiosarcoma, 486
Edrophonium chloride test, in thymoma, 608
Eicosapentaenoic acid
    anticancer effects of, 171–172, 234–235
    for tumor sensitization, in radiation therapy, 159, 235
Electron microscopy, 38
Electron-beam therapy, 150
Embryonal nephroma (nephroblastoma), 553–554, 553f, 553t
Emergencies, oncologic
    anaphylaxis as, 298–300, 299f
    central nervous system, 314–319, 316t, 319t
    disseminated intravascular coagulation, 249, 280, 309–313, 311f, 312f
    extravasation as, 135, 295–297, 296t, 297f
    hypercalcemia as, 266–270, 268f, 269f, 270t
    hypocalcemia as, 271
    hypoglycemia as, 272–273
    overview of, 260
    sepsis as, 284–290, 285t, 286f–288f, 289t
    sodium abnormalities as, 274–275, 275t
    surgery for, 177–178
    tumor lysis syndrome, 306–308, 307f, 307t
Emesis, see Nausea and vomiting
Enalapril, for heart failure, 264t
Endocrine tumors
    adrenal, 49, 500–505, 501f, 502f, 504t, 505f
    multiple endocrine neoplasia, 517–518, 517t–519t
    pancreatic, 505–510, 506f–508f
    parathyroid, 515–517, 516f, 517t
    pheochromocytoma as, 503–505, 504t, 505f, 517–518, 518t, 519t

pituitary, 385–388, 386f, 387f, 497–500, 498f
thyroid, 510–515, 511f–513f
Endoscopy
  gastrointestinal
    in gastric cancer, 443
    in large intestinal tumors, 447
    lower tract, 90–92, 90f, 91f
    in small intestinal tumors, 445
    upper, 88–89, 89f, 90f
  respiratory tract, 72, 74–75, 74f
Enemas, for colonoscopy, 91–92
Energy requirements, for enteral feeding, 248
Enrofloxacin, for sepsis, 289t
Enteral nutrition, 238–243, 322
  calculating contents and volumes for, 238–239
  routes of, 239–243, 240f–243f
Enterochromaffin cells, in carcinoid tumors, 473
Enucleation, for eye tumors, 398
Enzymes
  anticancer effects of, 347
  for chemotherapy, 127, 142–143, 237
Eosinophils, abnormal levels of, 278t
Epidural analgesia, 221
Epinephrine, for anaphylaxis, 299
Epirubicin
  extravasation of, 296–297, 296t
  for lymphoma, 343t, 344
  for uterine carcinoma, 525
Epithelial cell tumors
  cutaneous, 622t, 623–629, 624f, 625t, 626f, 628f
  cytology of, 101, 103f–105f, 107–108
  mesothelioma as, 606
Epithelioma(s)
  basal cell, 623
  cytology of, 107–108
Epulides, 161, 428–430, 429f, 430t
Erythrocytosis, 277, 278t–279t, 279, 370–372
Erythropoietin, 141–142, 251–252
  for anemia, 281
  elevated, in erythrocytosis, 277, 278t–279t, 279
  for myelodysplasia, 363
Esophagostomy tubes, 239
Esophagus
  biopsy of, 88–89, 90f
  thymoma manifestations in, 607–609, 609f
  tumors of, 441–442
Estrogen levels, in ovarian tumors, 523–524
Ethics, of complementary and alternative medicine, 180–181
Ethylenediaminetetraacetic acid chelation therapy, 184
Etidronate, for hypercalcemia, 270, 270t, 454
Etodolac
  for biopsy
    bone marrow, 78
    lymph node, 67
    oral cavity, 88
    respiratory tract, 71
    skin, 62, 64

dosage for, 217t
for procedural pain, 223, 224
Etoposide, 143
  extravasation of, 296–297, 296t
  for lymphoma, 353
  toxicity of, 132t, 298–300, 299f
Etretinate
  for cutaneous squamous cell carcinoma, 625
  for intracutaneous cornifying epithelioma, 632
Euthanasia, 24, 25–28
  bereavement support in, 28
  follow-up communication after, 27
  owner reactions to, 27
  preparation for, 25–26
  procedure for, 26–27, 26f
  smooth process for, 27–28
  timing of, 25
Excisional biopsy
  lymph node, 66–67, 67f
  skin, 63–64, 63f
External-beam radiation therapy (teletherapy), 149–150, 150f
Extravasation, of chemotherapeutic agents, 135, 295–297, 296t, 297f
Eye
  biopsy of, 399–400
  radiation therapy effects on, 158, 159f, 411
  tumors of, 397–398
    hemangiosarcoma as, 490
    melanoma as, 465–468, 468f
    metastatic, 397–398
Eyelid tumors, 201, 201f, 397–398

F

Factor VIII, in immunohistochemistry, 97
Famotidine, for gastrinoma, 509
Fat(s), dietary, 233–235, 239
Fatigue, compassion, 29–31
Fatty acids, dietary, 234–235, *see also* Polyunsaturated fatty acids
  for tumor sensitization, 159, 171–172
Feeding, enteral, 239–243, 238f, 240f–243f, 322
Female reproductive system tumors, *see under* Reproductive system tumors
Fentanyl, 218, 219f
  for biopsy
    bone marrow, 78
    lymph node, 67
    oral cavity, 88
    respiratory tract, 71
    skin, 64
  dosage for, 217t
  for procedural pain, 223, 224
Fever, 250, 324
Fibrohistiocytic nodules, splenic, 613–614
Fibromas, 596
Fibromatous epulides, 428–430, 429f, 430t
Fibrosarcomas, 596
  bone, 584–585

oral, 105*f*, 161, 437–439, 437*f*, 439*t*
retrobulbar, 398
Filgrastim, 152
Fine-needle aspiration biopsy, 96–99, 98*f*
Fixatives, for biopsy specimens, 58, 58*f*
Flow cytometry, 38–39, 336
Fluid therapy
for acute tumor lysis syndrome, 307*t*, 308
for anaphylaxis, 299
for disseminated intravascular coagulation, 312
for erythrocytosis, 279
for hypercalcemia, 268–269, 270*t*
for kidney failure, 302–305, 303*t*
for sepsis, 288, 289*t*
for vomiting, 227–228, 228*t*
Fluoroscopy, in transthoracic aspiration, 72–73
5-Fluorouracil, 140
for cutaneous squamous cell carcinoma, 625
for mammary tumors, 544–545
toxicity of, 132*t*
Follicular tumors, cutaneous, 632–633
Fractionation, in radiation therapy, 160–165
Fractures, osteosarcoma formation at, 567–568, 568*f*
Freezing, *see* Cryotherapy
Fresh frozen plasma, 248
Furosemide
for heart failure, 264, 264*t*
for hypercalcemia, 269, 270*t*
for kidney failure, 304*t*
for lymphoma, 348

G

Gallbladder carcinoma, 473, 474
Gallium nitrate, 145, 270
γ-Glutamyltransferase, in diagnosis, 41*t*
Ganglioneuroblastoma (peripheral neuroblastoma), 393
Ganglioneuroma (peripheral neuroblastoma), 393
Garlic, 185*t*, 187
Gastrinoma, 509
Gastrointestinal trac*t*
biopsy of, 87–92
lower, 90–92, 90*f*, 91*f*
oral cavity, 87–88
upper, 88–89, 89*f*, 90*f*
chemotherapeutic agent effects on, 131
tumors of, 425–456
anal sac adenocarcinoma as, 450–454, 451*f*–453*f*
cecal, 444–446, 445*f*, 446*f*
esophageal, 441–442
large intestinal, 446–449, 447*f*, 447*t*, 449*f*
lymphoma as, 354
mast cell, 654–655
oral, *see* Oral cavity tumors
perianal gland, 449–450, 450*f*
salivary gland, 440–441, 441*f*, 441*t*
small intestinal, 444–446, 445*f*, 446*f*
stomach, 442–444, 443*f*
ultrasonography of, 92
Gastrostomy tubes, 239–243, 241*f*, 242*f*
Gemcitabine, 140–141
Gene therapy, 205–207, 205*f*, 207*f*, 463
Genetic factors, in cancer, 8
Gentamicin, for sepsis, 289*t*
Germ cell tumors, testicular, 527–528
Ginger, 185*t*
Ginseng, 185*t*, 186*t*
Glandular tumors, cutaneous, 629–632, 629*f*, 630*f*, 632*f*
Glaucoma, in melanoma, 466
Glial fibrillary acidic protein, 97
Glioblastoma multiforme, 380
Gliomas, brain, 379–385, 380*t*, 382*f*, 383*t*
Gliomatosis cerebri, 380
Globulin, in diagnosis, 41*t*
Glossectomy, for carcinoma, 439–440
Glucagon
for hypoglycemia, 273
for insulinoma, 509
Glucagonoma, 509–510
Glucocorticoids, *see* Corticosteroids
Glucosamine, dosage for, 218*t*
Glucose
altered homeostasis of, 272–273
blood, in diagnosis, 41*t*
for sepsis, 290
Glutamine supplements, 233
Glycolysis, aerobic (Warburg effect), 231–232, 231*f*, 232*f*
Grading, pathology in, 37
Graft, for hematopoietic stem cell transplantation, 192–193
Graft-versus-host disease, 193–194
Graft-versus-tumor effect, 193–194
Granular cell tumors, of tongue, 440
Granulocyte colony-stimulating factor, 142, 252–253, 253*f*, 289*t*, 290
Granulocyte-macrophage colony-stimulating factor, 253–254
Granulomatosis, lymphomatoid, 417
Granulomatous inflammation, 99
Granulosa cell tumors, 523–524, 523*f*
Green tea, 185*t*, 187
Gross tumor volume, in radiation therapy, 152, 152*f*

H

Hair loss, in chemotherapy, 131
Hair matrixoma (trichoepithelioma), 632–633
Half-body irradiation, 165, 349
Haloperidol, for vomiting, 228, 229
Hazardous Drug Safety and Health Plan, 113
Healing touch, 183
Health and wellness program, 8–9, 9*t*
Heart
chemotherapeutic agent effects on, 133–134, 261–265, 262*t*, 264*t*
radiation therapy effects on, 159, 261–265, 262*t*, 264*t*
tumors of
aortic body, 420–423, 421*f*, 422*f*

carotid body, 423, 423f
chemodectoma as, 420–423, 421f–423f
hemangiosarcoma as, 485–487, 486f, 487f
lymphoma as, 355
sarcomas as, 423–424
ultrasonography in, 50f
Hemangiomas
cavernous, brain, 491
cutaneous, 487–488, 488f
L-MTP-PE for, 168–169
Hemangiopericytomas, 106f, 594f, 596–597
Hemangiosarcomas
anemia in, 280
bone, 490–491
cardiac, 485–487, 486f, 487f
cutaneous, 488–490
liver, 490, 490f
muscle, 490
nervous system, 490
ocular, 490
retroperitoneal, 491, 599
splenic, 474–476, 481–485, 482f–484f, 482t, 484t
urogenital, 490
Hematocrit, 278t
Hematologic disorders
anemia as, see Anemia
disseminated intravascular coagulation as, 249, 280, 309–313, 311f, 312f
erythrocytosis as, 277, 278t–279t, 279
laboratory findings in, 278t
leukocytosis as, 283–284
neutropenia as, 284–290, 285t, 286f–288f, 289t
thrombocytopenia as, 249, 282–283, 283f, 370
Hematoma, vs. hemangiosarcoma, 481
Hematopoietic growth factors
with chemotherapy, 141–142, 251–255, 253f
for sepsis, 290
Hematopoietic stem cell transplantation, 190–196
autologous vs. allogeneic, 191–192
cell population for, 193
complications of, 193–194
donor selection for, 191–192
graft source for, 192–193
indications for, 190–191
for lymphoma, 349–350
nonmyeloablative, 194
process for, 191
recommendations for, 194
syngeneic, 192
Hemoglobin, 278t
Hemolysis, in transfusion, 249–250
Hemolytic anemia, 248, 280–282, 281t
Hemorrhage
anemia in, 280–282, 281t
transfusion for, 248
Heparin, for disseminated intravascular coagulation, 312–313
Hepatectomy, for liver tumors, 473–474, 474f

Hepatocellular carcinoma, 472–473, 474f
Hepatoid (perianal) gland tumors, 104f, 107, 449–450, 450f
Herbal preparations, 184, 185t–186t, 186–187
Herniation, brain, 315
Histiocytic diseases, 610–618, see also Histiocytomas
benign cutaneous, 610–611, 611f
cutaneous histiocytosis as, 611–612
histiocytic sarcoma as, 617–618
malignant, 615–618, 615f, 616f
reactive, 611–613
splenic, 613–614
systemic histiocytosis as, 612–613
terminology of, 610
Histiocytic sarcoma, 617–618
Histiocytomas
benign cutaneous, 610–611, 611f
cytology in, 101f, 106
Histiocytosis
cutaneous, 611–612
malignant, 615–617, 615f, 616f
Homeopathic medicine, 183–184, 184t
Hormonal therapy, 127, 143
for brain tumors, 384
for prostate tumors, 532
Hormone receptors, in mammary tumors, 540, 546
Horner's syndrome, 318–319
Hospice care, 24
Human–animal bond, 6–7
Hyaluronidase, for extravasation, 296t
Hydralazine, for heart failure, 264t
Hydrocortisone
for adrenalectomy, 501
for brain herniation, 315
for extravasation, 296t
for sepsis, 290
Hydromorphone
dosage for, 217t
for procedural pain, 224
Hydroxyurea, 136
for erythrocytosis, 371
for leukemia, 369–370
for polycythemia, 279
for thrombocytopenia, 370
toxicity of, 132t
Hyperadrenocorticism
in adrenocortical tumors, 500–503, 501f, 502f
as paraneoplastic syndrome, 325
in pheochromocytoma, 503–505, 504t, 505f, 517–518, 518t, 519t
pituitary-dependent, 385–388, 386f, 387f, 497, 498f, 499–500
Hypercalcemia
in anal sac adenocarcinoma, 451, 453f, 454
in multiple myeloma, 372, 374
in parathyroid tumors, 515–517, 516f, 517t
Hypercalcemia of malignancy, 266–270, 268f, 269f, 270t, 334, 338
Hyperfractionation, in radiation therapy, 160, 162
Hypergammaglobulinemia, 292–294
Hyperkalemia, in acute tumor lysis syndrome, 306–308

Hyperparathyroidism, in parathyroid tumors, 515–517, 516f, 517t
Hyperplasia
    cytology in, 100, 101
    definition of, 37
Hypersensitivity reactions, in chemotherapy, 298–300, 299f
Hypersplenism, 614
Hyperthermia, 197–199, 198f, 199f
    for mammary tumors, 545
    for oral fibrosarcoma, with radiation therapy, 439
Hypertrophic osteopathy, 324–325, 325f, 413, 413f
Hyperviscosity syndrome (hypergammaglobulinemia), 292–294, 372–373, 373f
Hypervolemia, in hyponatremia, 275t
Hypoalbuminemia, in lymphoma, 340
Hypocalcemia, 271
    in acute tumor lysis syndrome, 306–308
    after thyroidectomy, 513
    treatment of, 513
Hypofractionation, in radiation therapy, 160–165
Hypoglycemia, in insulinoma, 272–273, 505–509
Hyponatremia, in syndrome of inappropriate secretion of antidiuretic hormone, 274–275, 275t
Hypophosphatemia, in acute tumor lysis syndrome, 306–308
Hypophysectomy, for pituitary tumors, 499
Hypoproteinemia, plasma transfusion for, 249
Hypothyroidism, after thyroidectomy, 513
Hypovolemia, in hyponatremia, 275t
Hypoxia, erythrocytosis in, 279, 279t

I

Idarubicin, 139, 296–297, 296t
Ifosamide, 136
    for bladder tumors, 561, 562
    for lymphoma, 353
    for soft tissue sarcomas, 595
    for splenic hemangiosarcoma, 485
    toxicity of, 315
Imaging, see also specific modes
    functional, 54
    types of, 44–45, 45t
Imatinib mesylate, for mast cell tumors, 654
Imiquimod cream, for cutaneous squamous cell carcinoma, 625
Immunoaugmentive therapy, 184
Immunocytokines, 209
Immunodeficiency, sepsis in, 285
Immunohistochemistry, 38
    in brain tumors, 381
    concepts of, 97
    in liver tumors, 472
    in melanoma, 464
Immunomodulation, 206–207, 207f
Immunotherapy
    for brain tumors, 385
    for mast cell tumors, 654
    for oral melanoma, 462–463
    for osteosarcoma, 575–576

Impressions, tissue, for cytology, 99
In situ tumors, definition of, 37
Incisional biopsy, skin, 62–63, 63f, 591–592
Inclusions, cytology of, 107–108
Induction, of chemotherapy, 129
Indwelling catheter, for drug administration, 123
Infections, in chemotherapy, 131, 284–290, 285t, 286f–288f, 289t
Infiltrative lipoma, 634, 635f
Inflammation
    cytology in, 100–101, 100f
    pain in, 214
    types of, 99
Inflammatory mammary carcinoma, 545–547, 546f
Infraorbital nerve block, 220, 221f
Infusion port, subcutaneous, for drug administration, 123
Insulin, excess of, in cancer, 231–232, 231f
Insulin:glucose ratio, in insulinoma, 506
Insulinomas, 272–273, 505–509, 506f–508f
Intensification, in chemotherapy, 128
Intercostal nerve block, 220, 220f
Interferon-α, 142, 170, 211
Interferon-γ, 206
Interleukin-2, 142, 170, 206–207, 211, 576
Interleukin-3, 254
Intermediate filaments, 97
Interstitial brachytherapy, 150, 151f
Interstitial cell tumors, testicular, 527–528, 527f
Intestine, see also Colon; Small intestine
carcinoma of, cytology of, 103f
Intracavitary administration, of chemotherapeutic agents, 124
Intracutaneous cornifying epithelioma, 107–108, 632
Intradural–extramedullary tumor of young dogs (nephroblastoma), 391–392
Intralesional administration, of chemotherapeutic agents
    preparation of, 117–118
    technique for, 123–124
Intramuscular administration
    of analgesics, 221
    of chemotherapeutic agents, 123–124
Intravascular lymphoma, 355
Intravenous administration
    of analgesics, 221
    of chemotherapeutic agents, 115–117, 118f, 122–123
Islet cell tumors
    gastrinoma as, 509
    glucagonoma as, 509–510
    insulinoma as, 272–273, 505–509, 506f–508f
    in multiple endocrine neoplasia, 517, 517t, 518t
    PPoma as, 510
Isotretinoin, 145–146

J

Jamshidi needle, for bone marrow biopsy, 79, 80, 81f
Jejunostomy tubes, 243, 243f
Junctional activity, in melanoma, 463
Juzen-taiho-to, 186t

K

Karnofsky's Performance Criteria, 19
Keratoacanthoma (intracutaneous cornifying epithelioma), 632
Ketamine, 218–219
    dosage for, 218*t*
    for oral cavity biopsy, 88
    for procedural pain, 224
Ketoconazole
    for adrenal tumors, 503
    for adrenalectomy, 501–502
    for ectopic Cushing's syndrome, 325, 499
Ketoprofen
    for biopsy
        bone marrow, 78
        liver, 94
        lymph node, 67
        oral cavity, 88
        respiratory tract, 71
        skin, 62–64
        urinary tract, 83, 85
    dosage for, 217*t*
    for procedural pain, 223
Keyhole liver biopsy, 94
Ki67 antigen
    in lymphoma, 339
    in mammary tumors, 542
    in mast cell tumors, 648
    in melanoma, 464, 466*f*
Kidney
    chemotherapeutic agent effects on, 134
    dysfunction/failure of, 301–305
        diagnosis of, 302
        drugs causing, 301, 302*t*
        erythrocytosis in, 279, 279*t*
        hypercalcemia in, 266–270, 268*f*, 269*f*, 270*t*
        predisposing factors in, 301–302
        prevention of, 302–303
        treatment of, 303–305, 303*t*, 304*t*
    metastasis to, 49*f*
    tumors of, 550–551, 551*f*
    hemangiosarcoma as, 490
    multifocal cystadenocarcinoma complex as, 551–553, 552*f*
    nephroblastoma as, 553–554, 553*f*, 553*t*

L

Lactate, excess of, in cancer, 231–232, 232*f*
Laparoscopic liver biopsy, 94–95, 95*f*
Large intestine, *see* Colon
Laryngectomy, for laryngeal tumors, 412
Larynx, tumors of, 411–412
Laser surgery
    for mammary tumors, 545
    for ocular melanoma, 467–468
Leflunomide
    for cutaneous histiocytosis, 612
    for systemic histiocytosis, 613
Leiomyoma, 597
    gastric, 442–444
    uterine, 524–525, 525*f*
    vaginal, 524–555, 524*f*
Leiomyosarcoma, 444–446, 445*f*, 597
Leukemia(s)
    acute lymphoblastic (ALL), 366–367, 366*f*
    acute myeloid (nonlymphoid), 364–366, 364*t*
    chronic lymphocytic (CLL), 367–369, 368*f*
    chronic myeloid (CML), 369–370
    hematopoietic stem cell transplantation for, 190–196
    treatment of, acute tumor lysis syndrome in, 306–308, 307*f*, 307*t*
Leukocytosis, 283–284
Levamisole, 169
Leydig cell tumors, testicular, 527–528, 527*f*
Lidocaine
    for biopsy
        bone marrow, 79
        liver, 93, 95
        lymph node, 68*f*, 69
        nasal cavity, 75–76
        skin, 61, 62*f*, 65
    dosage for, 218*t*
    for heart failure, 263, 265
    for nerve blocks, 220–221
    for thoracentesis, 99
Ligustrum, 185*t*
Limbs, osteosarcoma of, *see* Osteosarcoma, of appendicular skeleton
Limb-sparing surgery, for osteosarcoma, 571–572, 572*f*
Linoleic acid, for mycosis fungoides, 640
Lipase, in diagnosis, 42*t*
Lipids, *see* Fat(s); Fatty acids
Lipomas, 108, 633–634, 634*f*, 635*f*
Liposarcomas, 634–635
Liposomal cytosine arabinoside, 141
Liposomal doxorubicin, 139
Liver
    biopsy of, 92–95
        keyhole, 94
        laparoscopic, 94–95, 95*f*
        transabdominal percutaneous, 93–94, 93*f*
    tumors of, 471–474, 472*f*–474*f*, 490, 490*f*
L-MTP-PE (liposome-encapsulated muramyl tripeptide-phosphatidylethanolamine), 168–169, 210–211
    for oral melanoma, 463
    for osteosarcoma, 576
    for splenic hemangiosarcoma, 485
Lobaplatin, for osteosarcoma, 573–574, 574*t*
Lobectomy, for lung tumors, 415–416, 416*f*
Lomustine (CCNU), 136–137
    for brain tumors, 385
    for histiocytic sarcoma, 618
    for lymphoma, 348, 353
    for malignant histiocytosis, 616, 616*f*
    for mast cell tumors, 653
    for mycosis fungoides, 640

toxicity of, 132t
Luer-Lok syringe, 115–117, 117f, 118f
Lumpectomy, for mammary tumors, 544
Lung
  biopsy of
    bronchoscopic, 70–72, 71f–72f
    thoracoscopic, 74–75, 74f
    transthoracic aspiration, 72–74, 73f, 414
  chemotherapeutic agent effects on, 135
  malignant histiocytosis of, 615–617, 615f, 616f
  radiation therapy effects on, 158–159, 160f
  tumors of, 333, 333f, 413–417, 413f, 414f, 415t, 416f–417f
Lymph nodes
  biopsy of, 66–69, 67f, 68f
  examination of, 15
  normal cytology of, 100f
Lymphadenopathy
  in lung tumors, 415, 416f
  lymph node biopsy in, 66–69, 67f, 68f
  in lymphoma, 330–331, 331f
  in tonsillar squamous cell carcinoma, 436, 437f
Lymphangiomas, 491–492
Lymphangiosarcomas, 491–492, 491f
Lymphoblastic leukemia, acute (ALL), 366–367, 366f
Lymphocytes, 278t
Lymphocytic leukemia, chronic (CLL), 367–369, 368f
Lymphoma, 329–358
  aerobic glycolysis in, 231–232, 231f, 232f
  angiotrophic, 355
  B-cell, 335–336, 335f, 336t
  body weight and, 338
  cardiac, 355
  chemotherapy for, 342–356
    alkylating agent consolidation in, 348–349, 349t
    combination, 345–351, 346t, 349t, 351f, 353–354
    current recommendations for, 350–351, 351f
    discontinuous, 347–348
    extranodal, 354–356
    increased dose intensity, 349–350
    nutritional therapy with, 351, 352t
    radiation therapy with, 349
    rescue, 352–354
    single-agent, 342–345, 343t, 352–353
    supportive therapy with, 351, 352t
  chromosomal abnormalities in, 339
  clinical presentation of, 330–331, 331f, 637, 638f
  complete blood count in, 333–334, 338
  cutaneous, 637–641, 638f–640f
  cytology in, 100f, 331–332, 106
  diagnosis of, 331–335, 331, 332f, 333f, 637–638
  etiology of, 330, 637
  gastrointestinal, 354
  gender differences in, 340
  hematopoietic stem cell transplantation for, 190–196
  histologic type of, 338
  history of, 330–331
  hypercalcemia in, 338
  hypoalbuminemia in, 340
  imaging in, 332–333, 333f
  immunohistochemistry in, 332
  incidence of, 330, 637
  intravascular, 355
  low-grade, 339
  lymph node biopsy in, 66–69, 67f, 68f
  vs. lymphosarcoma, 330
  monoclonal antibodies for, 208–209
  multidrug-resistant
    prognostic factors in, 339
    treatment of, 341–342
  musculoskeletal, 355
  mycosis fungoides as, 638–641, 639f, 640f
  nasal, 355
  nervous system, 354–355
  nutritional therapy for, 351, 352t
  paraneoplastic syndromes in, 334–335
  pericardial, 355
  physical examination in, 332
  prognostic factors in, 335–340, 335f–337f, 336t, 337t, 339f
  retrobulbar, 398
  signalment of, 330
  splenic, 50f, 340
  stage of, vs. prognosis, 337–338, 337f
  staging of, 331–335, 332f, 333f, 637–638
  substage of, 336–337, 336f, 337f, 337t
  T-cell, 335–336, 335f, 336t
  treatment of, 340–356
    acute tumor lysis syndrome in, 306–308, 307f, 307t
    chemoimmunotherapy in, 351–352
    chemotherapy in, see Lymphoma, chemotherapy for
    client discussion on, 340–341
    combination, 342, 342t
    corticosteroids in, 339–340, 339f
    cutaneous, 638
    discontinuous, 347–348
    extranodal, 354–356
    multidrug-resistant, 341–342
    remission in, 341
    response to, 338
    toxicity of, 340
  tumor proliferation measurement in, 339
  urinary tract, 355
  urine tests in, 333–334
Lymphopenia, in lymphoma, 334
Lysis, of tumors, 306–308, 307f, 307t

M

Macroadenomas, pituitary, 385–388, 386f, 387f, 497, 498f, 499–500
Macroglobulinemia, vs. multiple myeloma, 375–376
Magnetic resonance imaging, 45t, 50, 51f, 52f
  in adrenal tumors, 501
  in brain tumors, 381, 382f
  in liver tumors, 471
  in pituitary tumors, 386–387, 386f

in spinal tumors, 389–390, 390f
in splenic tumors, 475
in staging, 16–17
Magnetic resonance spectroscopy, 50
Maintenance therapy, with chemotherapeutic agents, 128, 129
Maitake mushroom, 185t
Male reproductive system tumors, *see under* Reproductive system tumors
Malignant effusion, in mesothelioma, 604–607, 606f
Malignant histiocytosis, 615–617, 615f, 616f
Mammary tumors, 537–548
    clinical presentation of, 538–539, 539f
    cytology of, 103f, 107
    diagnosis of, 539–540, 539f, 540t
    etiology of, 538, 538t
    incidence of, 538
    inflammatory mammary carcinoma as, 545–547, 546f
    in males, 543
    prevention of, 543–544
    prognostic factors in, 540–543, 540t, 541f, 542t, 543f
    staging of, 539–540, 539f, 540t
    treatment of, 164–165, 543–545, 544t
Mammectomy, for mammary tumors, 544
Mammography, 45–46
Mandible, osteosarcoma of, 579, 579t
Mandibular nerve block, 220–221, 221f
Mandibulectomy
    for fibrosarcoma, 438
    for melanoma, 461
    for oral tumors, 430–431, 431f–433f
    for osteosarcoma, 579
    for squamous cell carcinoma, 434–435
Mannitol
    for brain herniation, 315
    for kidney failure, 304t
Markers, *See* Tumor markers
Massage therapy, 182–183
Mast cell tumors
    cutaneous, 643–654
        clinical presentation of, 644, 644f, 645f
        diagnosis of, 644–646, 645t
        etiology of, 643–644
        incidence of, 643–644
        prognostic factors in, 646–649, 647t, 648f, 649f
        staging of, 644–646, 645t
        treatment of, 649–654, 650f, 651f
    cytology of, 102f, 107
    intestinal, 654–655
    lymph node biopsy in, 66–69, 67f, 68f
    radiation therapy for, 163–164
    retrobulbar, 398
Mastectomy, for mammary tumors, 544
Mastocytosis, systemic, 645
Material Safety Data Sheets, for chemotherapeutic agents, 113
Matrix metalloproteinases and inhibitors, 171–172, 210, 576
Matrixoma, hair (trichoepithelioma), 632–633
Maxilla, osteosarcoma of, 581

Maxillectomy
    for fibrosarcoma, 438
    for melanoma, 461
    for oral tumors, 430–431, 433f
    for squamous cell carcinoma, 434–435, 436f
Mechlorethamine, 137
    extravasation of, 296–297, 296t
    for lymphoma, 348, 353–354
    toxicity of, 132t
Medetomidine, dosage for, 217t
Mediastinum
    biopsy of, 74–75, 74f
    lymphoma of, 333, 333f
Megaesophagus, in thymoma, 607–609, 609f
Megavoltage teletherapy, 150
Megestrol acetate, 146, 238, 238f
Melan A, 97, 459, 464
Melanoma, 457–469
    benign, 463, 464f
    cytology of, 103f, 107
    ocular, 397
    oral, 458–463
        clinical presentation of, 458, 459f
        diagnosis of, 458–460, 460f, 460t
        incidence of, 458
        prognostic factors in, 450, 461f, 461t
        radiation therapy for, 161
        staging of, 458–460, 460f, 460t
        treatment of, 460–463, 462t
Meloxicam
    for biopsy
        bone marrow, 78
        lymph node, 67
        oral cavity, 88
        respiratory tract, 71
        skin, 62, 64
    dosage for, 217t
    for procedural pain, 223, 224
Melphalan, 137
    for hypergammaglobulinemia, 294
    for leukemia, 369
    for multiple myeloma, 375, 376
    for oral melanoma, 462
    toxicity of, 133t
Memory of water theory, in homeopathic medicine, 183
Meningiomas
    brain, 164, 379–384, 380t, 381f, 383t, 384f
    retrobulbar, 398–400
    spinal, 388–391
Meperidine, dosage for, 217t
Mepivacaine, dosage for, 218t
Mercaptopurine, 141
    for lymphoma, 345
    toxicity of, 133t
Mesenchymal skin tumors, 622t, 633–636, 635f
Mesenchymomas
    liver, 473

splenic, 475, 475t
Mesna, 146
Mesothelioma, 604–607, 606f
Metabolism, cancer cachexia and, 231–237, 231f–232f, 320–322, 322f
Metalloproteinases and inhibitors, 171–172, 210, 352
Metaplasia, definition of, 37
Metastasis
　from adrenal gland, 501, 504
　from anal sac tumors, 451, 452f
　from apocrine adenocarcinoma, 631, 632f
　from bladder, 556–557, 557f
　to bone, 46–47, 46f, 53f
　from bone hemangiosarcoma, 491
　from brain, 381
　to brain, 315
　from cardiac hemangiosarcoma, 486–487
　from colorectal cancer, 447–448
　from cutaneous hemangiosarcoma, 488–489
　from cutaneous melanoma, 464–465
　from gastrinoma, 509
　from glucagonoma, 510
　from insulinoma, 505–507, 507f
　from kidney, 550–551
　to kidney, 49f
　from liver tumors, 472–473
　from lung, 414–415, 416f
　from lymphangiosarcoma, 492
　from mammary tumors, 539–542, 539f, 541f, 542t
　from mast cell tumors, 647, 648f, 649
　from multilobular osteochondrosarcoma, 582
　from nephroblastoma, 553–554
　from ocular melanoma, 466–467
　from oral fibrosarcoma, 438
　from oral melanoma, 458–463
　from osteosarcoma, 569, 576
　from ovary, 523–524
　from pheochromocytoma, 504
　from prostate, 530, 531, 531f
　from small intestine, 445–446
　from soft tissue sarcoma, 592, 593, 594f
　from splenic hemangiosarcoma, 481–484
　from stomach, 443–444
　surgery for, 177
　from synovial cell sarcoma, 600
　from testicular tumors, 528
　from thyroid, 511, 513–514
　from tonsils, 436
　from transmissible venereal tumor, 533–535, 534f
Methadone, dosage for, 217t
Methimazole, for thyroid tumors, 515
Methotrexate, 141
　for lymphoma, 343t, 345
　for osteosarcoma, 572
　toxicity of, 133t, 315, 403
Methylprednisolone, for sepsis, 290
Metoclopramide, for vomiting, 131, 227, 228
Metronidazole, for sepsis, 289t

Mexiletine, for heart failure, 263
Microadenomas, pituitary, 497, 498f, 499–500
Microscopy, electron, 38
Milk thistle, 186t
Milrinone, for heart failure, 264t
Minerals, requirements for, 236–237, 239
Minocycline, 172, 485
Mithramycin, see Plicamycin
Mitotane, 146
　for adrenal tumors, 502–503
　for ectopic Cushing's syndrome, 325, 499
　toxicity of, 133t
Mitoxantrone, 139
　for bladder tumors, 561, 561f
　for cutaneous squamous cell carcinoma, 626
　for lymphoma, 343t, 344, 352–353
　for mesothelioma, 606
　for oral squamous cell carcinoma, 435
　for prostate tumors, 532
　for soft tissue sarcomas, 595
　toxicity of, 133t
Molecularly targeted therapy, 209–211
Monoclonal antibodies
　anticancer effects of, 172, 208–209
　for lymphoma, 352
Monoclonal gammopathy
　hypergammaglobulinemia in, 292–294
　in multiple myeloma, 372–373, 374f
Monocytes, 278t
MOPP protocol, for lymphoma, 353–354
Morphine, 217
　for biopsy
　　bone marrow, 78
　　liver, 94
　　lymph node, 67
　　oral cavity, 88
　　respiratory tract, 71
　　skin, 64
　　urinary tract, 85
　dosage for, 217t
　for heart failure, 264t
　for procedural pain, 223, 224
Mouth, see Oral cavity
MRI, see Magnetic resonance imaging
M-syndrome (hypergammaglobulinemia), 292–294
Mucocutaneous plasmacytoma, 636–637
Mucositis, in radiation therapy, 157–158, 158f, 411
Multilobular osteochondrosarcoma, 581–582, 582f, 583t, 584f
Multiple endocrine neoplasia, 517–518, 517t–519t
Multiple myeloma, 372–376
　clinical presentation of, 372–373, 373f
　cytology of, 102f
　diagnosis of, 373–374, 374f
　hypergammaglobulinemia in, 292–294
　prognostic factors in, 374, 375f
　spinal, 388
　treatment of, 375–376

Multiple-drug resistance, to chemotherapeutic agents, 130, 339, 341–342
Muramyl tripeptide-phosphatidylethanolamine, *see* L-MTP-PE (liposome-encapsulated muramyl tripeptide-phosphatidylethanolamine)
Musal, 237
Muscle, hemangiosarcoma of, 490
Mustargen, *see* Mechlorethamine
Myasthenia gravis, in thymoma, 608–610
Mycosis fungoides, 638–641, 639*f*, 640*f*
Myelodysplasia, 362–364, 362*f*, 363*t*
Myeloid leukemia
    acute (AML), 364–366, 364*t*
    chronic (CML), 369–370
Myeloma, multiple, *see* Multiple myeloma
Myelosuppressive potential, of chemotherapeutic agents, 121, 131, 285, 285*t*
Myxoma, 597
Myxosarcoma, 597

N

Nails
    melanoma under, 463, 465*f*
    squamous cell carcinoma under, 627, 628*f*
Nalbuphine
    for biopsy
        liver, 94
        lymph node, 67
        respiratory tract, 71
        skin, 64
        urinary tract, 85
    dosage for, 217*t*
    for procedural pain, 223
Nasal cavity, biopsy of, 75–77, 76*f*, 77*f*
Nasal planum, squamous cell carcinoma of, 628–629, 628*f*
Nasal tumors, 406–411
    angiomatous proliferation as, 491
    clinical presentation of, 406–407
    computed tomography in, 48*f*
    diagnosis of, 407–408, 407*f*
    etiology of, 406
    incidence of, 406
    lymphoma as, 356
    magnetic resonance imaging in, 51*f*
    osteosarcoma as, 581
    prognostic factors in, 408–409, 408*f*
    radiation therapy for, 162
    staging of, 407–408
    treatment of, 409–411, 409*f*, 410*f*
Nausea and vomiting, 225–229
    in chemotherapy, 131
    mechanism of, 226, 227*f*
    prevention of, 19
    treatment of
        agents for, 228–229
        guidelines for, 226, 227*f*
        homeopathic remedies for, 184*t*
        life-threatening, 227–228
        self-limiting, 227, 228*t*
Needle aspiration biopsy, 96–99, 98*f*
Needle core biopsy
    lymph node, 67–69, 68*f*
    prostate, 84–85
    skin, 64–65, 64*f*, 65*f*, 591–592
Needle-off method, for fine-needle aspiration biopsy, 97, 98*f*
Needle-on method, for fine-needle aspiration biopsy, 97, 98*f*
Neoadjuvant chemotherapy, 128
Neoplasia
    cytology in, 100, 101
    definition of, 37
Nephrectomy, for renal tumors, 551, 551*f*
Nephroblastoma, 391–392, 553–554, 553*f*, 553*t*
Nephrotoxicity, of chemotherapeutic agents, 134, 301–305, 302*t*–304*t*
Nerve blocks, 220–221, 220*f*, 221*f*, 223, 224
Nerve sheath tumors, *see* Neurofibrosarcomas (nerve sheath tumors)
Nervous system, *see also* Brain; Central nervous system; Spinal cord
    chemotherapeutic agent effects on, 134
    lymphoma of, 354–355
Neuritic pain, 214
Neuroblastomas, peripheral, 393
Neurofibrosarcomas (nerve sheath tumors)
    cutaneous, 597
    nerve root, 597–599, 598*f*, 599*f*
    peripheral nerve, 393
    spinal, 388–389, 390*f*, 391
Neurokinin-1 receptor antagonists, for vomiting, 229
Neuropathic pain, 214
Neuropathy, paraneoplastic, 318–319, 319*t*
Neurotoxicity, of chemotherapeutic agents, 134
Neutropenia, 278*t*
    differential diagnosis of, 286*f*
    sepsis related to, *see* Sepsis
Neutrophilia, 16, 278*t*
Nitroglycerin, for heart failure, 264, 264*t*
Nitroprusside
    for heart failure, 264, 264*t*
    for pheochromocytoma, 504
Nonregenerative anemia, transfusion for, 248–249
Nonsteroidal antiinflammatory drugs, 216–217, 217*t*
    anticancer effects of, 169–170
    for biopsy
        bone marrow, 78
        liver, 94
        lymph node, 67
        respiratory tract, 71
        skin, 62, 64
        urinary tract, 85
    for pain prevention, 222
Nose, *see* Nasal cavity; Nasal tumors
NSAIDs, *See* Nonsteroidal antiinflammatory drugs
Nuclear medicine, 51–52, 53*f*, 54*f*
Nutrition, 187, 230–245
    appetite stimulation in, 238, 238*f*, 239
    for cancer prevention, 7–8, 7*f*, 237

carbohydrates in, 231–233, 231f, 232f, 239
enteral, 238–243, 238f, 240f–243f, 322
enzymes in, 237
homemade food for, 239
lipids in, 233–235, 322
for lymphoma, 351
mammary tumors and, 541
minerals in, 236–237, 239
for nausea and vomiting, 227
parenteral, 244, 444
promotion of, 19
proteins in, 233, 239
for small intestinal tumors, 446
vitamins in, 236
water needs in, 235–236

O

Obesity, avoidance of, 237
Occupational Safety and Health Administration, chemotherapeutic agent guidelines of, 112
Octreotide, for insulinoma, 508
Oligodendrogliomas, brain, 379–385, 380t, 382f, 383t
Omeprazole, for gastrinoma, 509
Oncocytomas, laryngeal, 411–412
Oncofetal antigens, 40, 42
Ondansetron, for vomiting, 228–229
Opioid(s), 217–218, 219f, 217t, 228, 229
Opioid agonist-antagonists, 217t, 218
Oral administration
    of analgesics, 221
    of chemotherapeutic agents
        preparation of, 117
        technique for, 124
Oral cavity
    biopsy of, 87–88
    radiation therapy effects on, 157–158, 158f
Oral cavity tumors, 428–440
    cryotherapy for, 201
    epulides as, 428–430, 429f, 430t
    fibrosarcoma as, 105f, 437–439, 437f, 438f, 439t
    lingual, 439–440, 440f
    melanoma as, see Melanoma, oral
    plasma cell, 636–637
    radiation therapy for, 161
    squamous cell carcinoma as, 432–435, 434f, 434t, 435t, 436f
    surgery for, 430–431, 431f–433f
    tonsillar, 435–437, 437f
Orbit
    osteosarcoma of, 581
    tumors of, 398–400, 399f
Orchiectomy, for cancer prevention, 8
Orthovoltage teletherapy, 149–150
Ossifying epulides, 428–430, 430t
Osteochondromas, tracheal, 412
Osteochondrosarcomas, multilobular, 581–582, 582f, 583t, 584f
Osteogenesis, in limb-sparing surgery, 572

Osteopathy, hypertrophic, 324–325, 325f, 413, 413f
Osteosarcoma
    of appendicular skeleton, 567–568, 567–577
        clinical presentation of, 568, 568f–569f
        diagnosis of, 568–570, 569f
        distribution of, 568, 568f
        etiology of, 567–568
        incidence of, 567–568
        nonweightbearing, 577, 578f
        prognostic factors in, 570–571, 570t
        staging of, 568–570, 569f
        treatment of, 571–577, 572f–573f, 573t, 574t, 575f, 577f, 578f
    of axial skeleton, 578–584
    cytology of, 106f, 108
    extraskeletal, 583–584
    histopathology of, 570
    L-MTP-PE for, 168
    mandibular, 579, 579t
    maxillary, 581
    multilobular, 581–582, 582f, 583t, 584f
    nasal, 581
    orbital, 581
    patellar, 577
    pelvic, 581
    radiation therapy for, 165
    retrobulbar, 398
    rib, 580, 580f
    spinal, 388, 389f, 390, 580–581
    splenic, 474–475, 475t
    surface, 582–583
    zygomatic arch, 581
Ovarian tumors, 523–524, 523f
Ovariohysterectomy
    for cancer prevention, 8
    mammary tumor prognosis and, 543, 543f
    for mammary tumors, 544
Over-the-needle catheter, for drug administration, 123
Oxaliplatin, 146
Oxygen, radiation therapy response and, 149
Oxyglobin blood substitute, 248
Oxymorphone, 217–218
    for biopsy
        skin, 63
        urinary tract, 83
    dosage for, 217t
    for procedural pain, 223

P

p53 tumor suppressor gene mutations
    in mast cell tumors, 649
    in osteosarcoma, 568
Paclitaxel, 146–147
    allergic reactions to, 298–300, 299f
    for mammary tumors, 545
Pain management, 213–224, see also Analgesia; Anesthesia
    ABCDEs of, 214

acupuncture for, 181, 182*t*, 219
acute vs. chronic, 222–223
analgesics for, *see* Analgesia; *specific drugs*
antidepressants for, 219
approach to, 215–216, 215*t*–216*t*
chronic vs. acute, 222–223
concepts of, 215–216, 215*t*–216*t*
nerve blocks for, 220–221, 220*f*, 221*f*
pain mechanisms and, 214
pain recognition for, 214–215
vs. pain severity, 222–224, 223*f*
preventive care in, 222–224, 223*f*
for procedural discomfort, 216*t*, 222–223, 223*f*
for quality of life improvements, 18–19
radiation therapy for, 219
tranquilizers for, 219
Palliative care, 23–24
for anal sac adenocarcinoma, 453–454
for bladder tumors, 559, 559*f*
for brain tumors, 382
for inflammatory mammary carcinoma, 547
for liver tumors, 474
for mast cell tumors, 652, 654
for mesothelioma, 606–607, 606*f*
for nasal tumors, 410
for osteosarcoma, 576–577, 577*f*
radiation therapy in, 151, 165
for renal cystadenocarcinoma complex, 552–553
surgery in, 178
Pamidronate, 147
dosage for, 218*t*
for hypercalcemia, 270, 270*t*, 454
for osteosarcoma, 577
for pain management, 219
Pancreas, tumors of
endocrine, 272–273, 505–510, 506*f*–508*f*
exocrine, 476–477
insulinoma as, 272–273, 505–509, 506*f*–508*f*
Pancreatectomy, partial, for insulinoma, 506–507, 507*f*
Pancreatic polypeptide tumor (PPoma), 510
Pancytopenia, in myelodysplasia, 362–363, 363*t*
Papillary squamous cell carcinoma, 435
Papillomas
choroid plexus, 385
cutaneous, 623
definition of, 37
Paracentesis, abdominal, 98
Paranasal sinus tumors, *see* Nasal tumors
Paraneoplastic syndromes
anemia as, 280–282, 281*t*
cancer cachexia as, 231–237, 231*f*–232*f*, 320–322, 322*f*
central nervous system, 314–319, 316*t*, 319*t*
corticosteroid alterations as, 325
Cushing's syndrome as, 325
erythrocytosis as, 277, 278*t*–279*t*, 279
fever as, 324
hypercalcemia as, 266–270, 268*f*, 269*f*, 270*t*

hypergammaglobulinemia as, 292–294
hypertrophic osteopathy as, 324–325, 325*f*, 413, 413*f*
hypocalcemia as, 271
hypoglycemia as, 272–273
leukocytosis as, 283–284
in lung tumors, 413–414, 413*f*
in mast cell tumors, 654
neutropenia as, 284–290, 285*t*, 286*f*–288*f*, 289*t*
overview of, 259–260
peripheral neuropathy as, 318–319, 319*t*
in renal tumors, 551
sepsis as, 284–290, 285*t*, 286*f*–288*f*, 289*t*
sodium abnormalities as, 274–275, 275*t*
thrombocytopenia as, 282–283, 283*f*
in thymoma, 607–608
Parathyroid glands
hyperplasia of, in multiple endocrine neoplasia, 517, 517*t*, 518*t*
tumors of, 515–517, 516*f*, 517*t*
Parathyroid hormone, 42
Parenteral nutrition, 244, 444
Patella, osteosarcoma of, 577
Pathology, 35–39, *see also* Biopsy
cancer terminology, 37–38
in grading, 37
information obtained from, 36–37
specimens for, 57–59, 57*f*–59*f*
in staging, 16, 37
in therapy response evaluation, 37–38
tools for, 38–39
in tumor margin evaluation, 37
Patnaik scheme, for mast cell tumor grading, 646, 647*t*
Pegaspargase, 142–143
Pelvic osteosarcoma, 581
Penicillin(s), for sepsis, 289*t*, 290
Penile tumors, 528–529
Pentazocine, dosage for, 217*t*
Pentobarbital, for euthanasia, 26
Peptic ulcer
in gastrinoma, 509
in mastocytosis, 654
Perianal gland tumors, 104*f*, 107, 449–450, 450*f*
Pericardectomy
for aortic body tumors, 422, 422*f*
for mesothelioma, 606, 606*f*
Pericardium
biopsy of, 74–75, 74*f*
lymphoma of, 355
mesothelioma of, 604–607
Periodontal ligament, tumors of (epulides), 429–430
Peripheral blood stem cells, transplantation of, 192–193
Peripheral neuropathy, 318–319
Personal protective equipment, for chemotherapeutic agent handling, 113–115
Pesticides, bladder tumors due to, 554–555
PET (positron emission tomography), 44–45, 45*t*, 53–54
Pezzer-tip gastrostomy tube, 242*f*
Pharynx, radiation therapy effects on, 157–158, 158*f*

PhaSeal system, 114, 116f, 117f
Phenobarbital
    for brain tumors, 382
    for seizures, 316t, 317
Phenothiazines, for vomiting, 229
Phenoxybenzamine, for pheochromocytoma, 504
Phentolamine, for pheochromocytoma, 504
Pheochromocytoma, 503–505, 504t, 505f
Phlebotomy, for erythrocytosis, 279, 371
Phosphorus, in diagnosis, 42t
Photodynamic therapy, 201–202, 201f
    for bladder tumors, 561–562
    for cutaneous squamous cell carcinoma, 625–626
    for esophageal tumors, 442
    for nasal tumors, 411
    for prostate tumors, 532
    for soft tissue sarcomas, 596
Pills, for chemotherapy
    administration of, 124
    preparation of, 117
Pilomatricoma, 633
Pimozide, for vomiting, 228, 229
Piroxicam, 147
    anticancer effects of, 169–170
    for biopsy
        bone marrow, 78
        lymph node, 67
        oral cavity, 88
        respiratory tract, 71
        skin, 62, 64
    for bladder tumors, 560–561
    for cutaneous squamous cell carcinoma, 625, 627
    dosage for, 217t
    for large intestinal tumors, 448
    for lymphoma, 352
    for nasal tumors, 411
    for oral squamous cell carcinoma, 435
    for procedural pain, 223, 224
    for prostate tumors, 532
    for tonsillar squamous cell carcinoma, 437
Pituitary tumors, 385–388, 386f, 387f, 517t, 519t
PIXY321 fusion protein, 254
Plant alkaloids, 127, 143–144
Plasma, transfusion of, 248–249
Plasma cell tumors
    bone, 586–587
    cytology of, 102f, 106–107
    extramedullary, 636–637
Plasmacytomas, 636–637
Plasmacytosis, in multiple myeloma, 372, 374
Plasmapheresis, for hypergammaglobulinemia, 294
Platelet(s)
    decreased, *see* Thrombocytopenia
    increased, 278t
    transfusion of, 283
Pleomorphism, definition of, 37
Pleura
    biopsy of, 74–75, 74f
    mesothelioma of, 604–607, 606f
Pleural effusion, in lung tumors, 414
Pleurodesis, for mesothelioma, 606
Plicamycin, 139–140, 270, 270t
Pneumonitis, radiation, 158–159, 160f
Polycythemia, 279, 279t, 370–372
Polymerase chain reaction, 39, 43
Polyps
    colorectal, 446–448
    ureteral, 554
Polyunsaturated fatty acids
    anticancer effects of, 171–172, 234–235, 322
    for lymphoma, 351
    for tumor sensitization, in radiation therapy, 159, 235
Positron emission tomography, 44–45, 45t, 53–54
Potassium
    in diagnosis, 42t
    for hypercalcemia, 268, 270t
    for vomiting, 227, 228t
PPoma (pancreatic polypeptide tumor), 510
Prednisolone, for leukemia, chronic myeloid, 369
Prednisone, 143
    for adrenalectomy, 501–502
    for brain tumors, 382
    for canine lymphomatoid granulomatosis, 417
    for hemolytic anemia, 281
    for hypercalcemia, 269, 270t
    for hypergammaglobulinemia, 294
    for hypertrophic osteopathy, 324
    for hypoglycemia, 273
    for insulinoma, 508
    for leukemia
        acute lymphoblastic, 367
        acute myeloid, 365
        chronic lymphocytic, 368–369
    for lymphoma, 342, 343t, 345–348, 346t, 353–354
    for mast cell tumors, 652
    for multiple myeloma, 375
    for myelodysplasia, 363
    for sepsis, 290
    for spinal cord compression, 318
    for spinal tumors, 391
    for thrombocytopenia, 283
    for thymoma, 609
Preleukemia (myelodysplasia), 362–364, 362f, 363t
Preventive care, 6–10
    chemotherapy in, 129
    epidemiology and, 7–8
    health and wellness program for, 8–9, 9t
    human–animal bond in, 6–7
    kidney protection in, 302–303, 302t
    for mammary tumors, 543–544
    pain management in, 222–223, 223f
    for sepsis avoidance, 286
    surgery in, 175
Primidone, for seizures, 316t

Procainamide, for heart failure, 263, 265
Procarbazine, 137, 348, 353–354
Prochlorperazine, for vomiting, 228, 229
Propofol
    for appetite stimulation, 238
    for biopsy
        bone marrow, 78
        liver, 94
        lymph node, 67
        oral cavity, 88
        respiratory tract, 71
        skin, 63, 64
        urinary tract, 83, 85
    for procedural pain, 223, 224
Propranolol
    for heart failure, 263, 265
    for hypoglycemia, 273
Prostate
    biopsy of, 84–86, 85f, 530
    tumors of, 529–532, 530f–532f
        hemangiosarcoma as, 490
        radiation therapy for, 165
Prostatectomy, for prostate tumors, 531–532, 532f
Protein, dietary, 233, 239
Proton-beam therapy, 150
Psoralen ultraviolet therapy, for mycosis fungoides, 640–641
Pubic osteotomy, for urethral tumors, 558
Punch biopsy, skin, 61–62, 62f, 63f, 591–592
Pyridostigmine, for thymoma, 609, 610

Q

Quality of life, 18–22
    commandments for, 18–19
    complementary and alternative medicine for, 180
    in hospice care, 24
    quantitating, 19, 20t, 21, 21f
Quinidine, for heart failure, 263

R

Radial carpal bone, osteosarcoma of, 577, 578f
Radiation therapy, 148–166
    adverse effects of, 153–159, 155f
        acute tumor lysis syndrome, 306–308, 307f, 307t
        bone, 158, 159f
        bone marrow, 158
        central nervous system, 317–318
        colon, 158
        eye, 158, 159f
        heart, 261–265, 262t, 264t
        kidney failure, 301
        lung, 158–159, 160f
        oral cavity, 157–158, 158f
        pharynx, 157–158, 158f
        rectum, 158
        skin, 156–157, 156f, 157f, 409, 410f
    for anal sac adenocarcinoma, 453
    for bladder tumors, 164, 559–560, 562
    for bone lesions, in multiple myeloma, 376
    for brain tumors, 164, 383–384, 384f
    for ceruminous gland tumors, 162, 403
    chemotherapy interactions with, 149, 594–595
    clinical uses of, 160–165
    conformal, 151
    for cutaneous melanoma, 465, 467f
    electron-beam, 150
    for epulides, 430
    external-beam (teletherapy), 149–150, 150f
    fatty acids and, 159, 235
    half-body, 165
    hematopoietic stem cell rescue in, 190–191
    implanted (brachytherapy), 150, 151f, 651
    for infiltrative lipomas, 634
    for large intestinal tumors, 448
    for lymphoma, 349
    for mammary tumors, 164–165, 545
    for mast cell tumors, 163–164, 651–652, 651f
    for melanoma, 461–462, 462t, 465, 467f
    for mycosis fungoides, 640
    for nasal tumors, 162, 409–411, 410f, 629
    for neurofibrosarcoma, 598–599
    for oral tumors, 161
        fibrosarcoma, 438–439, 439t
        melanoma, 461–462, 462t
        squamous cell carcinoma, 434–435
    for osteosarcoma, 165, 576–577, 577f
    for pain management, 219
    palliative, 165
        vs. definitive, 151
    for pituitary tumors, 387–388, 500
    planning for, computed tomography in, 48
    postoperative, 153, 154f
    preoperative, 153, 154f
    properties of, 148–149
    for prostate tumors, 532
    protocols for, 160–161
    proton-beam, 150
    for salivary gland tumors, 441
    second malignancies after, 155, 155f
    for soft tissue sarcomas, 162–163, 163f, 594–595, 595f
    for spinal cord compression, 318
    for spinal tumors, 390–391
    for squamous cell carcinoma, 161–162
    systemic, 151
    for thymoma, 164, 609–610
    for thyroid tumors, 164, 514
    timing of, 153, 154f
    for tonsillar squamous cell carcinoma, 436–437
    for transmissible venereal tumor, 534
    treatment planning in, 152–153, 152f, 153f
    types of, 149–151, 150f, 151f
    uses of, 148–149
    whole-body, 165

Radiofrequency treatment, 198–199, 199f
Radiography, 45–46, 45t, 46f
  in adrenal tumors, 500–501
  in aortic body tumors, 421, 421f
  in bladder tumors, 566, 566f
  in cardiac hemangiosarcoma, 486, 486f
  in large intestinal tumors, 447
  in liver tumors, 471, 472f
  in lung tumors, 414, 414f
  in lymphoma, 332–333, 333f
  in mast cell tumors, 645
  in nasal tumors, 407, 407f
  in osteosarcoma, 568, 569f
  in prostate tumors, 530, 530f
  in small intestinal tumors, 445
  in splenic tumors, 475
  in staging, 16–17
  in thymoma, 607, 607f
Radioimmunotherapy, 151
Radioiodine therapy, for thyroid tumors, 514
Radionuclide studies, 51–52, 53f, 54f
  in lymphoma, 333
  in thyroid tumors, 511–512, 512f
Radionuclide therapy, 151
Radioresistance, of tumors, 154
Radiosensitivity, of tumors, 154
Radiosurgery, 151, 164
Rappaport system, for lymphoma histology, 338
Reactive histiocytic diseases, 611–613
Recombinant proteins, 211
Reconstruction, surgery for, 178
Rectum
  biopsy of, 90–92
  radiation therapy effects on, 158
  tumors of, 165, 446–449, 447f, 447t, 449f
Red blood cells
  decreased, see Anemia
  increased (erythrocytosis), 277, 278t–279t, 279
Refractory anemia (myelodysplasia), 362–363, 363t
Rehabilitation, surgery for, 178
Reiki healing touch, 183
Reishi mushroom, 186t
Remifentanil, dosage for, 217t
Remission, in chemotherapy, 128, 341
Renal cystadenocarcinoma complex, 551–553, 552f
Reproductive system tumors, 522–536
  female
    ovarian, 523–524, 523f
    transmissible venereal, 533–535, 534f
    uterine, 525
    vaginal, 524–526, 524f, 525f
  male
    penile, 528–529
    prostatic, 529–532, 530f–532f
    testicular, 527–528, 527f
    transmissible venereal, 533–535, 534f
Rescue chemotherapy, 129, 352–354
Residual disease, surgery for, 177
Resistance, to chemotherapeutic agents, 130, 339, 341–342
Respiratory tract
  biopsy of, 70–77
    nasal cavity, 75–77, 76f, 77f
    thoracic cavity, 70–75, 71f–74f
  thymoma manifestations in, 607–610, 607f–609f
Respiratory tract tumors, 405–419
  laryngeal, 411–412
  lung, 413–416, 413f, 414f, 415t, 416f–417f
  nasal, see Nasal tumors
  tracheal, 412
Retinoids (vitamin A), 236
  for cutaneous squamous cell carcinoma, 625
  for mycosis fungoides, 639–640
Retrobulbar tumors, 398–400, 399f
Retroperitoneal sarcomas, 491, 599
Rhabdomyomas, laryngeal, 411–412
Rhabdomyosarcomas, bladder, 562
Rhinoscopy, in nasal tumors, 407–408
Rhinotomy, in nasal tumors, 408
Rib
  chondrosarcoma of, 586, 586f
  osteosarcoma of, 580, 580f
Ring enhancement, in brain tumors, 380, 382f
Romifidine, dosage for, 217t
Ropivacaine, dosage for, 218t
Round cell tumors, see also specific type
  cutaneous, 636
  cytology of, 101, 101f–103f, 105–107

S

S-100 protein, 97
Safety, in handling chemotherapeutic agents, 112–115, 112f, 114f, 118–119
Salivary glands, tumors of, 440–441, 441f, 441t
Samarium-153-ethylene diamine tetramethylene phosphonate, for osteosarcoma, 577
Sarcomas
  blood vessel, see Hemangiosarcomas
  bone, see Osteosarcoma
  cardiac, 423–424
  definition of, 37
  fibrous, see Fibrosarcomas
  histiocytic, 617–618
  leiomyosarcoma as, 444–446, 445f, 597
  lymphangiosarcoma as, 491–492, 491f
  myxosarcoma as, 597
  nerve sheath, see Neurofibrosarcomas (nerve sheath tumors)
  retroperitoneal, 599
  soft tissue, see Soft tissue sarcomas; specific types
  spindle cell, 596–597
  splenic, 474–476, 475t, 476f
  synovial cell, 599–602, 600f, 601f, 601t
Schisandra, 186t
Scintigraphy, see Radionuclide studies

Scirrhous response, definition of, 37
Scraping, tissue, for cytology, 99
Sebaceous glands, tumors of, 104*f*, 107, 629–630, 629*f*, 630*f*
Sedation, for biopsy, 59–60
Seizures, 315–317, 316*t*, 380
Selenium, requirements for, 237
Seminomas, testicular, 527–528
Sepsis, 284–290
    diagnosis of, 286–288, 286*f*, 288*f*
    predisposing factors for, 285–286, 285*t*, 286*f*
    treatment of, 288–290, 288*f*, 289*t*
Serotonin antagonists, for vomiting, 228–229
Sertoli cell tumors, testicular, 527–528
Sertoli-Leydig tumors, ovarian, 523–524, 523*f*
Sex, lymphoma prognosis and, 340
Sézary syndrome, 638–639
SHEN therapy, 183
Shiitake mushroom, 186*t*
Shock
    in anaphylaxis, 298–300
    septic, *see* Sepsis
Single-photon emission computed tomography, 44–45, 45*t*, 53
Sinus tumors, *see* Nasal tumors
Skin
    biopsy of, 61–65
        excisional, 63–64, 63*f*
        incisional, 62–63, 63*f*, 591–592
        needle core, 64–65, 64*f*, 65*f*, 591–592
        punch, 61–62, 62*f*, 63*f*, 591–592
    chemotherapeutic agent effects on, 135
    fibrosis of, in renal cystadenocarcinoma complex, 551–553, 552*f*
    necrosis of, in glucagonoma, 510
    radiation therapy effects on, 156–157, 156*f*, 157*f*
    tumors of, *see* Skin tumors
Skin tumors, 620–642
    basal cell, 623–624
    benign histiocytoma as, 610–611, 611*f*
    cryotherapy for, 201
    cysts as, 633
    epidemiology of, 621–622, 622*t*
    epithelial, 622*t*, 623–629, 624*f*, 625*t*, 626*f*, 628*f*
    follicular, 632–633
    glandular, 629–632, 629*f*, 630*f*, 632*f*
    hemangioma as, 487–488, 488*f*
    hemangiosarcoma as, 488–490
    histiocytic sarcoma as, 617–618
    histiocytosis as, 611–612
    intracutaneous cornifying epithelioma as, 632
    lipoma as, 108, 633–634, 634*f*, 635*f*
    liposarcoma as, 634–635
    lymphangioma and lymphangiosarcoma as, 491–492, 491*f*
    lymphoma as, 637–641, 638*f*–640*f*
    mast cell, *see* Mast cell tumors, cutaneous
    melanoma as, 463–465, 464*f*–466*f*
    mesenchymal, 622*t*, 633–636, 635*f*
    mycosis fungoides as, 638–641, 639*f*, 640*f*
    papillomas as, 623
    pilomatricoma as, 633
    plasma cell, 636–637
    round cell, 636
    sarcomas as, *see* Soft tissue sarcomas
    sebaceous gland, 629–630, 629*f*, 630*f*
    squamous cell carcinoma as, 624–627, 624*f*, 625*t*, 626*f*, 628*f*
    sweat gland, 630–632, 632*f*
    trichoepithelioma as, 632–633
    types of, 621–622, 622*t*
Skull, osteosarcoma of, 581–582, 582*f*, 583*t*, 584*f*
Slides, specimen placement on, for cytology, 97, 99
Small intestine
    biopsy of, 88–89, 89*f*, 90*f*
    tumors of, 444–446, 445*f*, 446*f*, 654–655
Sodium, abnormalities of, 274–275, 275*t*
Sodium chloride, hypertonic, for syndrome of inappropriate secretion of antidiuretic hormone, 275
Soft tissue sarcomas, 590–602, 635–636
    clinical presentation of, 591, 591*f*
    cytology of, 108
    diagnosis of, 591–592, 592*t*–593*t*
    etiology of, 591
    incidence of, 591
    prognostic factors in, 592–593, 592*f*, 593*t*, 594*f*
    radiation therapy for, 162–163, 163*f*
    staging of, 591–592, 592*t*–593*t*
    treatment of, 593–596, 594*f*–596*f*
    types of, 590–591
Solar elastosis, 488–489
Somatic pain, 214
Sotalol, for heart failure, 263, 265
Specimens, for pathology, 57–59, 57*f*–59*f*
SPECT (single-photon emission computed tomography), 44–45, 45*t*, 53
Spinal cord, compression of, 317–318
Spinal tumors, 388–392
    classification of, 388
    clinical presentation of, 389
    diagnosis of, 389–390, 389*f*, 390*f*
    etiology of, 388–389
    extradural, 388–390, 389*f*, 391*f*
    incidence of, 388–389
    intradural–extramedullary, 388–391, 390*f*
    intramedullary, 388–389, 391
    lymphoma as, 354–355
    nephroblastoma as, 391–392
    osteosarcoma as, 580–581
    staging of, 389–390, 389*f*, 390*f*
    treatment of, 390–391, 391*f*
Spindle cell sarcoma, 596–597
Spirocerca lupi, esophageal tumors related to, 441
Spleen, tumors of, *see* Splenic tumors
Splenectomy
    for fibrohistiocytic nodules, 614
    for myeloid metaplasia, histiocytosis, and hypersplenism syndrome, 614
    sepsis after, 285

for splenic hemangiosarcoma, 483–484, 484f
for splenic tumors, 475–476
Splenic tumors, 474–476, 475t, 476f
    fibrohistiocytic nodules, 613–614
    hemangiosarcoma as, 481–485, 482f–484f, 482t, 484t
    histiocytic sarcoma as, 617–618
    histiocytosis as, 613–614
    lymphoma as, 50f, 340
    myeloid metaplasia, histiocytosis, and hypersplenism syndrome, 614
    osteosarcoma as, 583–584
Squamous cell carcinoma
    adenoid, 624
    cutaneous, 624–627, 624f, 625t, 626f, 628f
    cytology of, 107
    laryngeal, 411–412
    lingual, 439–440, 440f
    oral, 161, 432–435, 434f–436f, 434t, 435t
    papillary, 435
    subungual, 627, 628f
    tonsillar, 161–162, 435–437, 437f
Squamous papilloma (intracutaneous cornifying epithelioma), 632
Squash-prep, for fine-needle aspiration biopsy, 97
Staging, 15–17, 16f, see also specific malignancies
    biopsy in, 60
    clinical chemistries in, 40–43
    pathology in, 37
    surgery in, 175–176
Stains, for pathology, 38, 99
Staphylococcus aureus enterotoxin A, in gene therapy, 206–207, 463
Status epilepticus, 316t
Stem cell factor, 254
Stem cell transplantation, 190–196
Stomach
    biopsy of, 88–89, 89f, 90f
    enteral nutrition through, 239–243, 238f, 240f–243f, 322
    mast cell tumors of, 654–655
    tumors of, 442–444, 443f
Streptozocin, 137–138
    for hypoglycemia, 273
    for insulinoma, 508
    toxicity of, 403
SU11654
    for mammary tumors, 545
    for soft tissue sarcomas, 596
Subarachnoid analgesia, 221
Subcutaneous administration, of analgesics, 221
Subcutaneous infusion port, for drug administration, 123
Subungual squamous cell carcinoma, 627, 628f
Sucralfate, for mast cell tumors, 654
Suction capsule biopsy instruments, for bladder biopsy, 83
Sufentanyl, dosage for, 217t
Suicide genes, in gene therapy, 206
Superficial necrolytic dermatitis, in glucagonoma, 510
Support resources, for bereavement, 27
Supportive care, 24
Surface osteosarcoma, 582–583

Surgery, 174–178
    for adrenal tumors, 501–502, 502f
    for anal sac adenocarcinoma, 452–453
    for aortic body tumors, 422, 422f
    for apocrine adenocarcinoma, 631
    for bladder tumors, 558–559, 558f, 559f
    for bone hemangiosarcoma, 490–491
    for brain tumors, 382–384
    for cardiac hemangiosarcoma, 487, 487f
    for carotid body tumors, 423, 423f
    for cutaneous hemangiosarcoma, 489
    for cutaneous melanoma, 464–465, 464f, 465f
    for cutaneous squamous cell carcinoma, 624–625, 626f, 627
    definitive, 176–177
    for ear tumors, 401–403
    for emergencies, 177–178
    for epulides, 429–430
    for esophageal tumors, 442
    for eye tumors, 398
    for fibrohistiocytic nodules, 614
    for fibrosarcoma, 584–585
    for gastric carcinoma, 444
    for gastrinoma, 509
    for glucagonoma, 510
    for infiltrative lipomas, 634, 635f
    for insulinoma, 273, 506–507, 507f, 508f
    for large intestinal tumors, 448–449
    for laryngeal tumors, 412
    for liver tumors, 473–474, 474f
    for lung tumors, 415–416, 416f
    for lymphangioma and lymphangiosarcoma, 492
    for mammary tumors, 544, 544t
    for mast cell tumors, 649, 651
    for metastasis, 177
    for myeloid metaplasia, histiocytosis, and hypersplenism syndrome, 614
    for nasal tumors, 409, 409f
    for nephroblastoma, 553–554
    for neurofibrosarcoma, 598
    for ocular melanoma, 467
    for oral fibrosarcoma, 438
    for oral melanoma, 460–461
    for oral squamous cell carcinoma, 434–435, 436f
    for osteosarcoma, 571–572, 572f, 574t, 579–584
    for ovarian tumors, 524
    for palliation, 178
    for pancreatic tumors, 477
    for parathyroid tumors, 516–517, 516f
    for penile tumors, 529
    for pheochromocytoma, 504, 505f
    for pituitary tumors, 387, 499
    for plasma cell tumors, 637
    for prevention, 175
    for prostate tumors, 531–532, 532f
    for reconstruction and rehabilitation, 178
    for renal tumors, 551, 551f
    for residual disease, 177

for retrobulbar tumors, 400
for salivary gland tumors, 440–441
for small intestinal tumors, 446
for soft tissue sarcoma, 593–594, 594f
special knowledge for, 175
for spinal tumors, 390–391, 391f
for splenic hemangiosarcoma, 483–484, 484f
for splenic tumors, 475–476
for staging, 175–176
for synovial cell sarcoma, 600–601, 601f
for testicular tumors, 528
for thymoma, 609, 609f
for thyroid tumors, 513–514, 513f
for tracheal tumors, 412
training for, 175
for treatment, 176–178
Sweat glands, tumors of, 630–632, 632f
Syndrome of inappropriate secretion of antidiuretic hormone, 274–275, 275t
Syngeneic bone marrow (stem cell) transplantation, 191–192
Synovial cell sarcoma, 599–601, 600f, 601f, 601t
Systemic histiocytosis, 612–613

T

T lymphocytes, cytotoxic, 172
TALL-104 cells, 172
    for malignant histiocytosis, 616
    for mammary tumors, 545
    for systemic histiocytosis, 613
Tamoxifen, for mammary tumors, 545
Tarsocrural joint, osteosarcoma distal to, 577
T-cell lymphoma, prognostic factors in, 335–336, 335f, 336t, 637–638
Tea, 185t, 187
Technetium compounds, in scintigraphy, 51–52
    in lymphoma, 333
    in thyroid tumors, 511–512, 512f
Teletherapy, 149–150, 150f
Ten significant tonic decoction, 186t
Tensilon test, in thymoma, 608
Testicular tumors, 527–528, 527f
Tetracyclines, 172
Thalidomide, 147, 172, 210, 315
Therapeutic touch, 183
6-Thioguanine, for leukemia, 365
Thiopental
    for biopsy
        bone marrow, 78
        liver, 94
        lymph node, 67
        oral cavity, 88
        respiratory tract, 71
        skin, 63, 64
        urinary tract, 83, 85
    for euthanasia, 26
    for procedural pain, 223, 224
Thiotepa, 133t, 138

Thoracentesis, 72–74, 73f, 98–99
Thoracic cavity
    biopsy of
        bronchoscopy in, 70–72, 71f–72f
        thoracoscopic, 74–75, 74f
        transthoracic aspiration in, 72–74, 73f, 414
    chemotherapeutic agent administration into, 124
    mesothelioma of, 604–607, 606f
Thrombocytopenia, 249, 282–283, 283f, 370
    in lymphoma, 334
    transfusion for, 249
Thrombocytosis (essential thrombocytopenia), 370
Thymidine kinase, in diagnosis, 43
Thymoma, 164, 607–610, 607f–609f
Thyroid hormones, in diagnosis, 42, 42t
Thyroid tumors, 510–515
    clinical presentation of, 511, 511f
    computed tomography in, 49f
    diagnosis of, 511–512, 512f
    ectopic, 512
    etiology of, 510–511
    incidence of, 510–511
    in multiple endocrine neoplasia, 517, 517t–519t
    prognostic factors in, 512–513, 512f
    radiation therapy for, 164
    scintigraphy in, 52, 53f
    staging of, 511–512, 512f
    treatment of, 513–515, 513f
Thyroidectomy, for thyroid tumors, 513–514, 513f
Thyroxine, for hypothyroidism, 513
Tissue impressions, for cytology, 99
TNM system, for staging, 15
α-Tocopherol (vitamin E), 236
Tolfenamic acid, dosage for, 217t
Tongue, tumors of, 439–440, 440f
Tonsil, squamous cell carcinoma of, 161–162, 435–437, 437f
Topoisomerase-I inhibitors, 144
Toxicity
    of chemotherapy, see Chemotherapeutic agents, toxicity of
    of radiation therapy, see Radiation therapy, adverse effects of
Trachea, tumors of, 412
Tramadol, dosage for, 218t
Tranquilizers, for pain, 219
Transabdominal percutaneous liver biopsy, 93–94, 93f
Transdermal administration, of analgesics, 221
Transfusions, 246–250
    for anemia, 281, 281t
    calculating amount, 249
    complications of, 249–250
    components for, 247–248, 247f, 248f
    for disseminated intravascular coagulation, 312
    indications for, 248–249
    for leukemia, 367
    for myelodysplasia, 363–364
    neutrophil-rich, for sepsis, 290
    serology of, 246–247, 248t
    for thrombocytopenia, 283

Transitional cell carcinoma
    bladder, 164
    renal, 554–560
Transmissible venereal tumors, cytology of, 106
Transmucosal administration, of analgesics, 221
Transplantation, bone marrow (hematopoietic stem cell), *see* Hematopoietic stem cell transplantation
Transrectal needle core biopsy, prostate, 85–86, 85*f*
Transthoracic aspiration cytology, 72–74, 73*f*, 414
Transurethral resection, for urethral tumors, 559
Triamcinolone, for mast cell tumors, 652
Trichoepithelioma, 632–633
Triethylene thiophosphoramide (thiotepa), 133*t*, 138
Trigeminal nerve paralysis, 318–319
Trilostane, for ectopic Cushing's syndrome, 499–500
Trimethobenzamide, for vomiting, 228, 229
Trimethoprim–sulfamethoxazole, for sepsis, 289*t*, 290
Troponins, in cardiac hemangiosarcoma, 486
Tubes
    esophagostomy, 239
    gastrostomy, 239–243, 241*f*, 242*f*
    jejunostomy, 243, 243*f*
Tufts University, VELCAP-SC protocol of, 348–350, 351*f*, 352*t*
Tumor(s), definition of, 37
Tumor margins
    pathologic evaluation of, 37
    samples for, 59, 59*f*
Tumor markers, 40–43
    clinical applications of, 43
    for melanoma, 459
    types of, 40, 41*t*–42*t*, 42–43
Tumor necrosis factor, anticancer effects of, 170
Tumor volume, in radiation therapy, 152, 152*f*
TVT cells, 101*f*
Typing, blood, 246–247, 248*t*
Tyrosine kinase inhibitors, 209

U

Ulna, osteosarcoma of, 577
Ultrasonography, 45*t*, 48–50, 49*f*, 50*f*
    in adrenal tumors, 500–501, 501*f*, 503
    in bladder tumors, 566
    in gastric cancer, 443, 443*f*
    in intestinal tumors, 92
    in large intestinal tumors, 447, 447*f*
    in liver tumors, 471, 472*f*
    in lymphoma, 333, 333*f*
    in mast cell tumors, 645
    in mesothelioma, 605
    in pancreatic tumors, 477
    in parathyroid tumors, 515, 517, 517*t*
    in pheochromocytoma, 503
    in prostate tumors, 531, 531*f*
    for renal tumors, 550
    in retrobulbar tumors, 399–400
    in small intestinal tumors, 445, 445*f*
    in splenic tumors, 475, 482, 483*f*
    in staging, 16–17
    thymoma manifestations in, 608, 608*f*
    in thyroid tumors, 511
    in transthoracic aspiration, 72
Ureteral tumors, 554
Urethral tumors
    clinical presentation of, 555*t*
    diagnosis of, 555–557, 556*f*, 557*f*
    incidence of, 554
    staging of, 555–557, 556*f*, 557*f*
    treatment of, 558–562
    types of, 555*t*
Urinary tract tumors, 549–564
    bladder, *see* Bladder tumor(s)
    lymphoma as, 355
    renal, 550–554, 551*f*–553*f*, 553*t*
    ureteral, 554
Urine tests
    in lymphoma, 333–334
    tumor markers in, 40, 41*t*–42*t*, 42–43
Urogenital tract, *see also* Reproductive system tumors; Urinary tract tumors
    biopsy of, 82–86, 83*f*–85*f*
    hemangiosarcoma of, 490
Uterine tumors, 525

V

Vaccines
    cancer, 207–208
        for lymphoma, 352
        for melanoma, 352
        for infectious diseases, during chemotherapy, 341
Vaginal tumors, 524–526, 524*f*, 525*f*
Vascular endothelial growth factor, in splenic hemangiosarcoma, 483
V-BTA (bladder tumor antigen test kit), 42–43
Vectors, for gene therapy, 205–206, 205*f*
VELCAP-L protocol, for lymphoma, 346–347
VELCAP-S protocol, for lymphoma, 346–347, 350, 351*f*, 352*t*
VELCAP-SC protocol, for lymphoma, 348–350, 351*f*, 352*t*
Vesicants, 295
Vestibular tumors, 524–526, 524*f*, 525*f*
Vimentin, 97
Vinblastine, 143
    extravasation of, 296–297, 296*t*
    for leukemia, 365
    for lymphoma, 343*t*, 345, 353
    for mast cell tumors, 653
    toxicity of, 133*t*
    for transmissible venereal tumor, 535
Vincristine, 143–144
    for canine lymphomatoid granulomatosis, 417
    extravasation of, 296–297, 296*t*
    for leukemia, 367–369
    for lymphoma, 342–343, 343*t*, 345–348, 346*t*, 353–354
    for mast cell tumors, 653

for multiple myeloma, 375
for thrombocytopenia, 283
toxicity of, 133*t*
for transmissible venereal tumor, 534–535, 534*f*
Vinorelbine, 144
Viruses, as gene therapy vectors, 205–206
Visceral pain, 214
Vitamin(s), 236
Vitamin D, for hypocalcemia, 271
Vomiting, *see* Nausea and vomiting
VP16, *see* Etoposide
Vulvovaginectomy, for vaginal tumors, 525

W

Warburg effect, 231–232, 231*f*, 232*f*
Warts, 623
Water
requirements for, 235–236
restriction of, in syndrome of inappropriate secretion of antidiuretic hormone, 275
Weight, chemotherapy dosing based on, 120, 121*t*
White blood cell count, increased, *see* Leukocytosis
Whole-body hyperthermia, 198–199, 198*f*
Whole-body irradiation, 165
Wisconsin protocol, for lymphoma, 348, 350, 351*f*, 352*t*
Wobenzym, 237
World Health Organization
lymphoma clinical stages of, 331, 331*t*, 332*f*
melanoma stages of, 459–460, 460*t*
WR-2721, *see* Amifostine

X

Xerostomia, in radiation therapy, 157–158, 158*f*
Xylazine
dosage for, 217*t*
for procedural pain, 223

Y

Yohimbine, for vomiting, 228

Z

Zoledronic acid, 147
Zollinger-Ellison syndrome, 509
Zygomatic arch, osteosarcoma of, 581